Textbook of Acute Trauma Care

Peter Lax
Editor

Textbook of Acute Trauma Care

Springer

Editor
Peter Lax
Tactical Medical Wing
Royal Air Force
Brize Norton
Oxfordshire
UK

ISBN 978-3-030-83627-6 ISBN 978-3-030-83628-3 (eBook)
https://doi.org/10.1007/978-3-030-83628-3

This Springer imprint is published by the registered company Springer Nature Switzerland AG
The registered company address is: Gewerbestrasse 11, 6330 Cham, Switzerland

To my wife Emma, without whom this book would have not been possible.
And to Jim, William, Olivia, and Archie, without whom this book would have been finished eighteen months earlier...
...I love you all

Foreword

Injured patients' survival depends on expert, time-critical, complex, and specialised care. Patients are looked after by teams of teams, who must work in synchrony, smoothly handing over care to the next phases of care. Expert teams are made of expert individuals, and experts fundamentally need a deep understanding of the disease they are managing. Their knowledge must extend to not only their own specific area of care, but to know holistically what a patient needs now, and how their specific actions will integrate with those of others to deliver the best possible outcomes. Hence this textbook.

Trauma care is often taught as a set of protocols—semi-rigid approaches to be followed in the same way, patient after patient. But the essence of trauma care is to tailor diagnosis and treatment to the condition of the patient. The team must adjust their approach, adjust their techniques, and adjust their whole tempo in response to the patient—how quickly they are bleeding, how bad their brain injury is, how old they are, and how cold they have become. Understanding why and how management has to be bespoke for each patient requires an understanding of the pathophysiology associated with different injuries, and how these are modulated by our interventions. In other words, there is a science to trauma care.

As a trauma care provider, there is something in this book for you, regardless of your profession or specialty. Written by contemporary multi-professional trauma care specialists, this book gives the reader a wide but deep knowledge of the human response to injury. "Textbooks are dead" is a common refrain. Blogs, FOAMed, webinars, YouTube videos, and even twitter all offer versatile, rapid, and free access to learning resources. Writing and editing a textbook is a major undertaking, and one that mostly carries less kudos than getting a research paper published. But despite all this, textbooks are still surviving and thriving. A book can pull all the strings of a subject together to give a deeper, holistic view of a subject. It is often only by covering the breadth of a subject that one can gain an understanding of its whole and hence of its parts. So I'd congratulate the editor and all the contributors of this textbook in having the enthusiasm, drive, and endeavour to see this project through to completion, and of course I'd congratulate you on your wisdom to purchase it.

Trauma is not going away. Our world is getting hotter, more crowded, and more unequal. Conflict from social pressures and lack of resources is growing on micro and macro scales. The stresses of modern living are fuelling a rise in mental health problems and attempted suicide. An expanding, more active elderly population are sustaining injuries complicated by their pre-existing conditions. While most of the world's diseases are reducing in incidence and severity, accidental and non-accidental injuries are increasing in incidence and severity. But we have never had a better understanding of injury that we do now, and we have never had better knowledge and tools to save and rebuild peoples' lives.

Now is a good time to be reading a new textbook of trauma care.

Karim Brohi
Queen Mary University of London, London, UK
Barts Health NHS Trust, London, UK

The original version of this book was revised. The correction to this book can be found at https://doi.org/10.1007/978-3-030-83628-3_45

Acknowledgements

No work like this could be achieved without a vast amount of help from a multitude of people, and indeed I have been supported by quite a few!

To my family—you are the reason why I can keep doing this. Thank you for your unwavering support throughout my training, Consultancy, and ongoing work—I really could not have done this without your patience, understanding, and forbearance through late nights, early mornings, and deadlines. Mostly, thank you for keeping me supplied with therapeutic caffeine and gin when needed!

To doctors Sikorski, Galvagno, Conti, Koerner, Bucci, Grissom, Stephens, Samet, Hyder, Fouche-Weber, Scalea, Habashi, and O'Connor, all the CRNAs, anaesthetics, and ICU staff at Shock Trauma—you are the reason why I know how to do this. The teaching and exposure I had in your programme has been a massive influence in how I've practised as a Consultant and has had an impact on patient care many years after I graduated the Shock Trauma Fellowship.

To Elaine Giles and Mike Thomas—thank you for three years of real-time technical support! From figuring out the finer parts of Scrivener and the Affinity programmes, help with design elements during the creation of this textbook, and my work during COVID, this book could not have been produced without your help, support, and teaching. You've directly contributed to saving patients in all the work you've helped me with.

To Jocko Willink—thanks for the discipline to write 1,000 words a day, good or bad! It really helped when I was struggling and made the whole thing more manageable.

This textbook represents the total of my trauma teaching and experience over the last 15 years on a variety of courses and rotations. The principles outlined in this textbook have been drawn with experience from not only "traditional" courses such as ATLS, but also involvement with more modern courses such as ATACC, ETC, work in the R Adams Cowley Shock Trauma Centre, the RAF Critical Care Air Support Team (CCAST), and as a PHEM doctor for the Air Ambulance Service (TAAS) in the UK.

I am indebted to the supervisors that I have had since I started in trauma care as a slightly over-keen medical student. I hope that this textbook will be used by doctors, nurses, paramedics, and other healthcare providers internationally to support their decision-making and improve patient care. I am active on social media, and you can find me on Twitter (@DrPeteLax).

I welcome any questions, suggestions for improvements, or clarifications that you have regarding the textbook. The authors have produced some great chapters and all credit goes to them, but as the editor any omissions or errors are exclusively my fault. If you have spotted any mistakes or wish to suggest any amendments or have any other general comments, then please let me know. Of note, this textbook has taken many years to write. With Brexit, a pandemic and the extended time taken to go from authorship to publication, some recommendations and policies that may have been superseded in this time. Readers are advised to check their local policies for accepted practices in their instututions rather than relying on one source.

This textbook represents the most up-to-date evidence available at the time of publishing, but if you are aware of a new paper that may change recommendations or current practice, then please let me know so I can update the textbook in line with this in the event of a second edition!

PL, Tactical Medical Wing, 2021

Contents

Part IX Post-Incident Care

Contributors

Matthew Beardmore Department of Anaesthesia, Royal Cornwall Hospitals NHS Trust, Cornwall, Truro, UK

Devon Air Ambulance Trust, Exeter, Devon, UK

M. D. Dominic Bell Department of Anaesthesia and Critical Care Medicine, Leeds General Infirmary, Leeds, UK

Robin D. Berry Department of Anaesthesia and Critical Care Medicine, Derriford Hospital, Plymouth, UK

Tactical Medical Wing, Royal Air Force, Brize Norton, Oxfordshire, UK

Steven Bland Queen Alexandra Hospital, Portsmouth Hospitals NHS Trust, Portsmouth, UK

Royal Navy, Portsmouth, UK

Peter G. Brindley Department of Critical Care Medicine, Department of Anesthesiology and Pain, Medicine, University of Alberta, Edmonton, Canada

Dosseter Ethics Centre, University of Alberta, Edmonton, Canada

Samantha K. Brooks Health Protection Research Unit, King's College London, London, UK

Holly A. Chambers Department of Anaesthesia and Critical Care Medicine, Derriford Hospital, Plymouth, UK

Tactical Medical Wing, Royal Air Force, Brize Norton, Oxfordshire, UK

Hannah M. Clancy Royal Army Medical Corps, Leuchars, UK

Steve Dick East Midlands Ambulance Service NHS Trust, Nottingham, UK

The Air Ambulance Service (TAAS), Rugby, Warwickshire, UK

Ryan Fransman Surgical Department, The Johns Hopkins Hospital, Baltimore, MD, USA

Richard J. Gould Department of Anaesthesia and Critical Care Medicine, Leeds General Infirmary, Leeds, UK

Neil Greenberg Health Protection Research Unit, King's College London, London, UK

Robert Greig Emergency Medicine, Jersey, Channel Islands, UK

Thomas Irving Liverpool University Hospitals NHS Foundation Trust, Liverpool, UK

Jonathan Jones Emergency Medicine Department, Leeds General Infirmary, Leeds, UK

Nikolaos K. Kanakaris Department of Orthopaedic Surgery, Leeds General Infirmary, Leeds, UK

Timothy Knight Royal Orthopaedic Hospital, Birmingham, UK

Birmingham Children's Hospital, Birmingham, UK

Peter Lax Tactical Medical Wing, Royal Air Force, Brize Norton, Oxfordshire, UK

The Air Ambulance Service (TAAS), Rugby, Warwickshire, UK

Caroline Leech Emergency Department, University Hospitals Coventry and Warwickshire NHS Trust, Coventry, UK

The Air Ambulance Service (TAAS), Rugby, Warwickshire, UK

Kathryn Lowery Department of Orthopaedic Surgery, Leeds General Infirmary, Leeds, UK

Jenny Mealey The Air Ambulance Service (TAAS), Rugby, Warwickshire, UK

Rashmi Menon Department of Anaesthesia and Critical Care Medicine, Leeds General Infirmary, Leeds, UK

Chris Miller Radiology Department, Leeds General Infirmary, Leeds, UK

Alan Mistlin Royal Army Medical Corps, Defence Medical Rehabilitation Centre Stanford Hall, Loughborough, UK

Shaun C. Moeller Department of Anesthesiology and Critical Care Medicine, The Johns Hopkins Hospital, Baltimore, MD, USA

Joe Moore Sloane Helicopters, Sywell, Northampton, UK

The Air Ambulance Service (TAAS), Rugby, Warwickshire, UK

Jill Neale Regional Rehabilitation Unit, RAF Cranwell, Sleaford, Leicester, UK

University Hospitals of Leicester NHS Trust, Leicester, UK

Matthew O'Meara EMRTS Wales, Llanelli, UK

Deprtment of Anaesthesia and Critical Care Medicine, University Hospital of North Staffordshire, Stoke, UK

Oliver O'Sullivan Royal Army Medical Corps, Defence Medical Rehabilitation Centre Stanford Hall, Loughborough, UK

Jowan Penn-Barwell Royal Navy, Portsmouth, UK

Department of Orthopaedic Surgery, John Radcliffe Hospital, Oxford, UK

Graham M. Percival Emergency Medical Retrieval Service, Paisley, Scotland

Tactical Medical Wing, Royal Air Force, Brize Norton, Oxfordshire, UK

Alexander G. Porthouse Royal Army Medical Corps, Catterick Garrison, UK

Rebecca Powell Leeds Children's Hospital, Leeds, UK

Chris Press Department of Anaesthesia and Critical Care Medicine, Sheffield Teaching Hospitals, Sheffield, UK

The Air Ambulance Service (TAAS), Rugby, Warwickshire, UK

Alex Psirides Intensive Care Unit, Wellington Regional Hospital, Wellington, New Zealand

Wellington Aeromedical Retrieval Service, Wellington, New Zealand

University of Otago, Wellington, New Zealand

Haripriya Ramotar Department of Clinical Radiology, Whittington Health, London, UK

Darren Reid Royal Centre for Defence Medicine, Birmingham, UK

The Air Ambulance Service (TAAS), Rugby, Warwickshire, UK

Jonathan Ritson Addenbrooke's Hospital, Cambridge University Hospitals NHS Foundation Trust, Cambridge, UK

Royal Navy, Portsmouth, UK

Alice Roberts Department of Anaesthesia and Critical Care Medicine, Sheffield Teaching Hospitals, Sheffield, UK

Edward Rothera Department of Anaesthesia and Critical Care Medicine, Leeds General Infirmary, Leeds, UK

Leeds Children's Hospital, Leeds, UK

Neil Roy Department of Anaesthesia and Critical Care Medicine, Leeds General Infirmary, Leeds, UK

Paul Savage OBE Health Sciences Department, Bournemouth University, Bournemouth, UK

UK Search and Rescue Medical Group, London, UK

Robert A. Sikorski Deparment of Anesthesiology and Critical Care Medicine, The Johns Hopkins Hospital, Baltimore, MD, USA

Tejinder S. Swaran Singh Department of Anesthesiology, University of Iowa Healthcare, Iowa City, IA, USA

Priyank Sinha Department of Neurosurgery, Leeds General Infirmary, Leeds, UK

James Sira Department of Anaesthesia and Critical Care Medicine, Leeds General Infirmary, Leeds, UK

Jocelyn M. Slemko Department of Critical Care Medicine, University of Alberta, Edmonton, Canada

Brendan D. R. Sloan Department of Anaesthesia and Critical Care Medicine, The Yorkshire Regional Burns Centre, Pinderfields Hospital, Wakefield, UK

Justin Squires The Air Ambulance Service (TAAS), Rugby, Warwickshire, UK

Emergency Medicine Department, Sheffield Teaching Hospitals, Sheffield, UK

Tim J. Stansfield The Leeds Vascular Institute, Leeds Teaching Hospitals NHS Trust, Leeds, UK

Royal Army Medical Corps, London, UK

Clare Thompson West Yorkshire Deanery, Yorkshire, UK

Leeds Children's Hospital, Leeds, UK

Andrew Thurgood Mercia Accident Rescue Service, Hereford, UK

Constantinos Tingerides Radiology Department, Leeds General Infirmary, Leeds, UK

Sam Todd Emergency Medicine Department, Addenbrookes Hospital, Cambridge, UK

Tactical Medical Wing, Royal Air Force, Brize Norton, Oxfordshire, UK

Jake Turner Department of Anaesthesia, Nottingham University Teaching Hospitals NHS Trust, Nottinghamshire, UK

The Air Ambulance Service (TAAS), Rugby, Warwickshire, UK

Midland's Air Ambulance (MAA), West Midlands Ambulance Service, West Midlands, UK

Jonathan Veitch Department of Anaesthesia, Nottingham University Teaching Hospitals NHS Trus, Nottingham, UK

212 Field Hospital (Reserves), Sheffield, UK

Alexander M. Wood Orthopaedic Department, John Radcliffe Hospital, Oxford, UK

Thomas G. D. Woolley Royal Army Medical Corps, Department of Anaesthesia, Nottingham University Teaching Hospitals NHS Trust, Nottingham, UK

The Air Ambulance Service (TAAS), Rugby, Warwickshire, UK

Bhavana Yalamuru Department of Anesthesiology and Perioperative Medicine, University of Massachusetts Memorial Medical Group, Worcester, MA, USA

Alia Yaqub Emergency Medicine Department, Leeds General Infirmary, Leeds, UK

Part I

Trauma Systems and Teams

1 Human Factors in Trauma Care

Why the Human Factor Is Always a Factor

Peter G. Brindley and Jocelyn M. Slemko

- Definition and importance of human factors in trauma resuscitation
- Causes of Error: flow disruption and active or latent failures
- Individual Human Factors: adverse physiologic states, managing stress and cognitive bias
- Task Based Factors: mastery and the use of checklists
- Human Factors and Teams: pre-briefing and debriefing, communication, and leadership/followership
- Environmental Factors: physical layout, resource utilization, and the Zero Point Survey
- Organizational and System Factors

The authors composed, revised and approved this manuscript. The work is original. There are no conflicts or relevant disclosures.

P. G. Brindley (✉)
Department of Critical Care Medicine, Department of Anesthesiology and Pain, Medicine, University of Alberta, Edmonton, Canada

Dosseter Ethics Centre, University of Alberta, Edmonton, Canada
e-mail: brindley@ualberta.ca

J. M. Slemko
Department of Critical Care Medicine, University of Alberta, Edmonton, Canada
e-mail: jmslemko@ualberta.ca

Who is in charge of the clattering train?
The axels creak, and the couplings strain.
For the pace is hot, and the points are near,
And sleep hath deadened the driver's ear;
And signals flash through the night in vain.
Death is in charge of the clattering train!
–Edwin James Milliken, 1890

Introduction

When humans, and their systems, are pushed beyond their limits then disasters follow: it is just a matter of time. Milliken's poem was relevant over a century ago when a train crashed due to poor working conditions and distracted drivers. Half-a-century on it was just as relevant when Winston Churchill repurposed it for his history of World War II, *The Gathering Storm.* Fast forward another 50 years and it offers a useful starting point for discussing human performance in modern trauma medicine. It will likely continue to be all too familiar until we humbly accept that 'the human factor is always a factor", and adopt a culture of constant reflection and improvement. Having hopefully captured your precious cognitive band-width, we now offer practical insights that can save patients' lives and keep medical teams strong.

Hyperbole aside, it is not difficult to liken the modern trauma bay to a clattering Victorian train: with people in peril and workers straining to halt death. Despite all of medicine's giddy technical advances, it can still be unclear who is in charge.

P. Lax (ed.), *Textbook of Acute Trauma Care*, https://doi.org/10.1007/978-3-030-83628-3_1

There is still every likelihood that resuscitators are sleep-deprived, that judgements are distracted, and that performance is stymied by maddening bureaucracy and dysfunction. "Red flags" go unnoticed, technology can falsely reassure, and chaos can predominate. That is, unless we commit to understanding the good, bad and ugly of human performance. This is because, following major trauma, a patient's aortic dissection, cerebral oedema, and unstable pelvis are certainly a threat to their life, but so are our prehistoric human responses and sclerotic systems [1].

Accordingly, this chapter focuses on non-technical skills, otherwise known as Human Factors (HF). These are often taught under the rubric of Crisis Resource Management (CRM) which contains six subsections: situation awareness, decision-making, communication, task-resource management, leadership and followership, and teamwork [2]. Our goal is to offer insights at the level of the individual, team, task, and environment. Importantly, non-technical competence should not be assumed, or intuited, any more than technical competence. For example, we do not assume you can insert a central venous line without instruction and practise; the same applies to working in complex resuscitation teams. Fortunately, HF knowledge, and CRM skills, can be learnt, mastered and maintained. Like many things in Medicine, improvement starts by giving a damn, and refusing to accept the status quo.

What Are Human Factors and Why Should We Care?

HFs can be broadly defined as the interplay between individuals, teams, tasks and the environment. They are largely synonymous with CRM in that the focus is not on the technical aspects of medical care (i.e. medications and procedures) but rather the ergonomics of how humans identify threats, make decisions, and coordinate activity. HF and CRM are scientific disciplines. However, HF solutions may be little more than codified common sense, or lessons redeployed from everyday life. As such, HF may be the best way to understand why errors occur in complex human systems, and the best way to mitigate their harm. An understanding of HFs also explains why we need regular simulation, and structured debriefs. Once you grasp the importance of HF you are also likely to see medicine not only a science and art, but also a branch of engineering and psychology [3].

Deliberate study of HF and CRM began approximately half-a-century ago. Commercial aviation industry led the way, and because 70% of adverse events were attributable [4]. The percentage of attributable errors is similar in medicine, but we continue to be laggards. Both medicine and transportation should strive to manage people safely and predictably. There is, however, a danger of oversimplifying the comparisons with aviation. After all, resuscitation rarely allows us to delay "take off" until everyone is rested and familiar, or "return to base" if things go awry. As such, low performing trauma teams should look to learn from high performing trauma teams not just Top Gun pilots. You may prefer to compare trauma medicine to symphony orchestras or sports team: it does not matter. What matters is that medical practitioners are open to any translatable insight no matter their source. Aviation represents the best starting point because it has been formally studied, and because, like doctors, pilots face individual stress, unfamiliar players, dizzying technology, and pervasive bureaucracy. Aviation also offers an important reminder that medical patients and practitioners are at the mercy of the very system designed to keep them safe.

Importantly, better resuscitation is not about just replacing humans with computers and checklists, or assuming that humans are an unmitigated liability. Instead HF and CRM are about understanding the strengths and limitations of each component in a system (self, team, environment, patient, technology) and designing better work environments (i.e. more resilient team structures, more sensible work-rosters, and more appropriate fail-safes). It means leveraging ergonomics and psychology and engineering to help humans be more thoughtful, efficient, vigilant, safe and caring. It is about making Safety (with a big S) everybody's business and a system wide imperative; every bit as important as throughput [5]. It means minimizing errors while also accepting that they will inevitably occur in complex systems. It means looking beyond the traditional approach of "name-blame-shame". Clearly, we have work to do.

Factual knowledge still matters and so does manual dexterity. Moreover, healthcare professionals and administrators must still accept appropriate individual-responsibility. However, HF emphasizes the need to also look at the wider system, context and culture. It moves us beyond simplistic questions such as "why did you do that?" and onto "why at the time did that occur and seem appropriate?". It means working on our verbal dexterity and team dexterity. HFs aims to help the individual patient in the here and now, but also to build a medical culture that is mature and just. It is why medical practitioners should see themselves as "culture change agents" not just "all-knowing" clinicians who do discrete shifts. If we fail to learn these lessons then we will continue to make repetitive mistakes in high stake situations, and patients will needlessly suffer [6].

An understanding of HFs also offers a road map for the future; even a healthcare revolution. This is because it helps us understand that complexity outstrips any individual, and that resuscitation is now a team pursuit [7]. It explains why experts (especially experts) ask for help, incorporate double checks, and insist on closed loop communication. It means building a system where simulations are not a luxury, nor a soul-crushing embarrassment. HFs is about making team members feel safe, and communicating that we are all lifelong learners and change agents. HFs are also not about buzzwords, or endless meetings, but rather building a system where the best practitioners want to work, where the best administrators want to help, and where you would want your mother cared for.

Causes of Error

General Principles

As stated by Alexander Pope, in the 1700s- and repeated by the Institute for Health Improvement in 1999- "to err is human". In other words, humans are not perfect, life is not perfect, and therefore trauma care is not perfect. Therefore, mistakes (typically understood as decisions that turn out to be wrong) and errors (typically defined as actions that go against accepted rules or norms) will occur. Our job is to minimize their likelihood, severity and consequence. Medical errors- also understood as predictable human errors that occur in a medical setting- are more likely when situations are convoluted and people are unfamiliar, distracted or biased. The consequences increase when patients are frail (i.e. they lack physiologic reserve) and when systems are stressed or dogmatic (i.e. they lack administrative reserve). Consequential mistakes and errors are more likely when teams consist of individuals from different backgrounds and experience levels, especially when if humans fail to check inherent biases, egos, or put others ahead of their needs.

Trauma is inherently risky. It comes with diagnostic uncertainty, high stakes, time pressure, unsociable hours and even uncooperative patients. Regardless, the majority of trauma-associated errors are not from insufficient technical proficiency, but rather non-technical issues. These include CRM deficits such as ineffective situational awareness (i.e. a lack of a shared mental model; team members not being on the same page), poor decision making (i.e. cognitive overload and insufficient cognitive offloading), inappropriate communication (which can be subdivided into verbal, non-verbal and paraverbal communication), poor task resource management (i.e. insufficient prioritization, allocation, delegation, mobilization), insufficient leadership (i.e. poor role clarity and diffusion of responsibility), insufficient followership (i.e. failing to ascertain how we can be most helpful) and insufficient teamwork (after all, "a team of experts is not an expert team") [2, 8].

The "swiss cheese model of error"—usually credited to James Reason- explains why, when mistakes and errors occur, we often "get away with it" [9]. This is because, for an error to become a bad outcome, several "holes" need to line up in time and place. In other words, not all errors lead to bad outcomes, but bad outcomes are usually multifactorial. Similarly, it explains why higher functioning (i.e. more resilient) systems have numerous safeguards and fail-safes. It is why a single shortcoming (i.e. sleep-deprived team members), or even two shortcomings (sleep-deprived team members plus faulty equipment) need not result in disaster. Importantly, the swiss chess model also emphasizes why we should not to equate being "lucky" with being "good".

These ideas also explain why safety reviews are not witch hunts but rather core business. We should be reviewing cases that go badly (so called "safety-one"- see below) but also the greater number that go well (so called "safety-two"- see below). In other words, a robust system learns from failure but understands the mechanics of success. As outlined, when root causes are explored, it is common to identify numerous issues [10]. Accordingly, substantial improvements are often the cumulation of multiple marginal gains [11]. System weaknesses (and successes) can be understood by looking at how, when, where and why errors (and successes) occur, and minimizing (though not ignoring) the "who" [12]. It means that errors (and successes) are rarely unpredictable or random. Every system really does produce the results it is "designed" to.

Flow Disruptions

Flow disruptions are deviations from the predictable chain of events. These threaten safety because they create confusion, complexity and inefficiency [12]. Within trauma care, flow disruptions are most likely to be aberrations in coordination, communication, or equipment. Importantly, these are more likely to occur in 'ectopic' areas (i.e. radiology departments or operating rooms (OR), rather than comparatively controlled environments (i.e. Intensive Care Units (ICUs) or Emergency Rooms (ERs) [12]. Catchpole et al. showed that implementing HF interventions that focused on reducing flow disruptions- for example, having the Radiology Department pre-alerted to traumas or having a structured OR handover- was associated with shorter hospital stay. In other words, standardization can help, and simulations should occur throughout the hospital. The importance of flow disruptions highlights the importance of addressing the patient's entire journey, including potentially perilous handovers from one team or location to the next. After all, relay races are usually won or lost on the baton pass.

Active and Latent Failures

As the term suggests, active failures are committed by those in closer patient contact. They are also more likely to have an immediate and obviously detrimental effect [1]. This, in turn, means that active failures are often easier to identify and more likely to be addressed [13]. An example is when an intubator inserts an endotracheal tube into the oesophagus. In short, everyone from the intubator to the most junior nurse likely knows an error occurred. In contrast, latent failures occur more at a system level, and, therefore, may be harder to identify and attribute. It may also take longer for latent failures to be linked to bad outcomes. Latent failures typically, lay in waiting and require the right trigger [1]. An example is having the difficult airway cart far from patients, not clearly marked, or inconsistently stocked. This could result in staff being unable to find the right equipment, which in turn means they attempt intubation despite suboptimal conditions. As such, the endotracheal tube still ends up in the oesophagus and the patient suffers the same consequence. By addressing both active and latent failures a system increases its resilience, closes more "holes in the swiss cheese", and become more proactive. There is also an increased sense of shared responsibility and, hopefully, less finger-pointing [13].

Key Points

- Trauma resuscitation can be error prone due to its chaotic environment, diagnostic challenges, and high stakes nature.
- Flow disruptions introduce multiple threats to patient safety and team resilience.
- Active failures have an immediate adverse effect, while latent failures are more difficult to identify and are deeply rooted within a system. Both need to be addressed.

Individual Factors

Example

Imagine it is your first week on the trauma service: whether as a nurse, registrar, or student. You are 15 hours into a busy shift, having hardly eaten or used the bathroom, and the trauma team has just been called overhead. You have only participated in one other trauma resuscitation, you believe it went badly, and you felt you were "in over your head". You are petrified that you are going to make another mistake. You have little obvious backup, and you are working under a senior doctor who is known to be patronising and influential. You enter the room and see that CPR is in progress and you are handed a laryngoscope. You hear that the patient has multiple life-threatening injuries that will require simultaneous emergent intervention—some of which you have never done before. Perhaps we can start with a simple but fundamental question: How do you feel? ◄

Stress and Adverse Physiologic States

An old medical maxim asserts that before checking the patient's pulse you should check your own. In other words, stress affects our performance and needs to be managed. A small "dose" of stress is helpful, as it usually focuses attention. Manageable stress also propels humans beyond denial and deliberation into deliberate action. Most people need "physiologic arousal" in order to engage, but, excessive stress impairs performance. This is because excess physiologic arousal impairs higher-level thought and action. Excessive stress causes "attentional narrowing", meaning it impairs our ability to step back, and appraise the larger situation. Rather than apply innovative thinking we are more likely to fall back on what we did before. In extreme cases we simply freeze.

Excessive stress impairs global situational awareness and creates tunnel vision. This means we can miss important peripheral clues. Stress can also create "tunnel action", and perseverance. In other words, overstressed people persist in the same action and same thoughts, whether right or wrong. It means we tend to do the same old things, even if unwarranted, and because they offer us comfort, control and familiarity. A mea culpa example is when we simply wish to intubate, insert central lines, or fire up the echo machine…regardless of whether the patient will benefit or not [14].

The "goldilocks" of stress ("not too much, not too little") is illustrated by the Yerkes-Dodson curve [15]. While perhaps an oversimplification, it is the "sweet spot" where we avoid under arousal (associated with disengagement) and also avoid hyperarousal (which threatens task execution, especially requiring fine motor skills or nuanced judgement) [7]. Importantly, stress is subjective- what some people find exhilarating others find terrifying. Stress also depends on prior experience and personality traits such as risk-tolerance and rule-adherence [7]. It can be improved by stress inoculation training. This is where deliberate, graduated repeated and realistic exposure is used to inoculate the resuscitator to stress. Incorporation of stress inoculation is also one way to prevent simulations from becoming predictable and unrealistic. In short, it is a simple, cheap and profound way in which to improve performance. As such, we highly recommend you give it a go [14].

Stress also matters because perception becomes reality. If an individual (or team or organization) assesses that their resources are insufficient then they are more likely to perform poorly. This could include not thinking that they are capable, not believing they have the appropriate help or equipment, or not accepting that they work in a culture that "has their back". Obviously, these beliefs may be valid. The issue is that feeling stressed makes it difficult to execute higher level task because you are burdened by excessive tachycardia, elevated catecholamine levels, and general sympathetic overactivity [16]. It stands to reason that it is more difficult to resuscitate trauma patients with sweaty, shaky hands, and a nagging (and often self-fulfilling) sense of dread.

Myriad physiologic states can worsen human performance. In addition to excessive subjective stress, providers can be ill, intoxicated, or taking medications [13]. Fatigue is also a substantial risk factor, akin to intoxication [17]. We may be able to function in the moment when sleep deprived, because adrenaline kicks in, but this cannot be maintained for ever. Not surprisingly, long cumulative hours and shift work have both been shown to compromise higher cognitive skills and bespoke decision making in the short term. Sleep deprivation also impairs mental and cardiovascular health in the longer term [18]. The fact that our profession continues to blithely ignore the importance of sleep shows we have a long way to go in understanding even the basics of HFs.

The acronym "IM SAFE"—which stands for illness, medication, stress, alcohol, and fatigue-offers a useful acronym for self-reflection and self-improvement. It was developed by the aviation industry and is readily translatable to trauma team members [19]. We recommend a self-check before starting a shift, during the hospital commute, or when taking the elevator down to the trauma bay. After all, to do well you must be well.

Managing Stress and Increasing Cognitive Readiness

If you work in trauma then you will be exposed to stress: no ifs, ands or buts. We may not be able to wholly eliminate high-stakes decision-making, diagnostic uncertainty, or unsociable hours. We can, however, increase cognitive readiness and decrease sympathetic nervous system overload [20]. Three effective strategies are breathing techniques, self-affirmation, and mental rehearsal [20]. All are easy to learn and cost-free. Perhaps the only obstacle is giving yourself permission in the midst of chaos. Even just feeling your feet on the ground and your chest rising and falling can help you feel "centered" and more in control.

Controlled breathing simply involves four steps: slow deep inspiration, then breath holding, then slow full expiration, then breath holding. Each is done for four seconds, hence this is also known as square breathing. These can be done prior to, during, or after stressful events [5]. It will be familiar to anyone who has tried meditation. Fortunately, it should be familiar to anyone who has breathed in and out during regular life: in other words, every one of us can do this.

The second stratagem is self-affirmation or positive self-talk. Reminding yourself that "I've done loads of chest tubes" can decrease doubt and help you to cognitively reframe [7]. Thirdly, athletes mentally or pre-imagine their moves prior to big events, and we should too. Mental rehearsal, aka mental imagery, aka cognitive imagining is associated with higher confidence, greater sense of control, and better performance [16]. In other words, the human brain is a great simulator, so use it. Mental practice may not always make perfect but it does mitigate panic. Mentally preparing for success can make it more likely to happen. We believe you would have to be out of your mind not to use this!

Cognitive Bias

Beliefs and behaviours are influenced by prior experiences; for good and bad. Especially in stressful situations, we tend fall back on what we have seen before and done before. This is summarized as the Gestalt effect or pattern recognition. These can be immensely beneficially because is reduces delays (so-called 'analysis paralysis') and means not ever solution has to be built from the bottom up. The danger is that even when not fatigued we tend to favour inappropriately simple answers to complex problems [21].

In other words, we may see patterns where we should not, and we need self-discipline not to be lazy.

Other common biases include premature closure (downplaying contradictory evidence), availability heuristics (favouring those ideas at the forefront of the mind), anchoring heuristics (staying with initial assumptions), and fixation errors (ignoring evidence that points us in another direction) [21]. Once again, these HF principles emphasize that errors are often driven by unconscious or semi-conscious processes. They are rarely deliberate of insufficient factual knowledge or lack of moral fibre.

In this digital age, it is worth emphasizing that humans are capable of genius, abstraction, nuance, deep thought and emotional connection. Accordingly, it is not time for a wholesale replacement of humans in healthcare. However, all humans- including your authors- can be unpredictable, irrational, distractible, and fatigable. This is why metacognition- namely taking time to think about thinking- is important. Each of us needs to put in the work to make the unconscious conscious: otherwise we will be lousy teachers. We also need to accept our fallibility, but then use that to spur ourselves towards constant iterative improvement. We need to recognize those triggers that make us more prone to error. Now that we are primed as individuals, it is time to shift to the task at hand.

Key Points

- Stress, and other adverse physiologic states, can substantially impact human performance
- Breathing techniques, self-talk and mental rehearsal can optimize stress levels (not too little stress, not too much)
- Awareness of one's own cognitive biases is imperative to minimize error

Task Factors

Good trauma resuscitation means being able to complete myriad tasks swiftly and safely. Importantly, there is a difference between taskwork (those actions required to complete a task: in other words, "the what") and teamwork (the extra work that enables members to function collaboratively: in other words, "the how") [7]. Failure to appreciate the difference is another reason why we over rely (and over blame) individuals. It is also why we refuse to attribute success and failure to teams and systems.

The next lesson is that by 'overlearning' we can save more lives. In other words, we should practise well beyond the point of mastery. Honing our reflexes, such that some responses are subconscious, frees up cognitive bandwidth for other tasks (i.e. it improves task work), and communicates a sense of calm to the team (i.e. it improves team work). This should mitigate chaos and increase the sense of control, both internal (in the individual's brain) and external (i.e. to all team members). The only caution is that automaticity should not mean inflexibility or laziness [7]. We do simple things in the same predictable ways in order to free up time and bandwidth so we can tackle the more complicated. This segues into the good, bad and the decerebrate of checklists.

Checklists

Relying solely on our memory can be dangerous, especially during stress. As a result, there is a strong argument for cognitive aids. These aide memoires typically come in the form of checklists (a series of key items), and mnemonics (a memorable word, phrase or letters that also summarizes key items). These can be used both during crisis care, and routine endeavours. The most important thing is to test whether they make us smarter or dumber. Understand that checklists can save lives, but do not assume we need a checklist for everything. Moreover, do not assume that once a checklist is created then the work is done. It needs to be stress-tested and stress-finessed.

An example of an evidence-based checklist is the Surgical Time Out, developed by the World Health Organization (WHO). This has been associated with improve mortality, especially in the developing world. It has since been widely adopted [22]. Checklists are intended to increase team communication, improve delegation, and flatten the social hierachy [22]. Importantly, however, checklists are only a tool, and like any tool will only be as good as the people that use them. After all, a hammer can be used to build things or smash things.

Checklists should be "dosed". In other words, just like our other therapies they should be administered at the right time by the right people and in the right situation. Importantly, they appear to be best when limited to seven or fewer items (just like phone numbers), and when they demand answers (what will you do when…) [23]. In other words, a 20-item checklist is not fit for task, and nor is the human tendency to mindlessly tick boxes. Cognitive aids should justify the extra time that they consume. They should be incorporated into simulations, posted in highly visible common areas and be co-created by both senior and junior team members [22].

After the Surgical Time Out, The WHO developed a Trauma Care checklist, in order to complete the primary and secondary survey plus other key steps [24]. In the same vein, Fitzgerald et al. (2019), developed a Trauma Team Time Out. This is intended for the first thirty minutes of trauma resuscitation. Once again, the goal is not to replace humans, nor is it to replace human judgement. Instead cognitive aids should ensure that we do not miss critical steps. They should free the brain up for higher level thought, and unite the team [25].

Team Factors

Trauma teams need to assemble quickly and be ready for coordinated action. Teamwork is more than just the sum of its parts; it is a larger integration of mental, manual, and social expertise [26]. As mentioned, a team of experts is not automatically an expert team [27]. In addition to the individual task skills discussed above, the success of the trauma resuscitation relies equally on the interpersonal functioning of the trauma team [26]. Not surprisingly, Cohen et al. (2018) found that success and failure are substantially influenced by the team's communication, coordination, and planning [13].

Justice Potter Stewart famously opined that while he couldn't define pornography he knew it when he saw it. The same could be said of the less salacious topic of teamwork. We all know a high functioning team when we see one: to reference our opening poem it resembles a well-oiled machine devoid of creak and strain. Regardless, effective teams have well-defined structures (i.e. the team knows how to give and take instructions, and knows how to confirm instructions were heard and completed). Nowadays, it involves "more we and less me". Empathic teams also perform hot debriefs (immediately after in order to address emotions) and cold debriefs (after a short lag to address what could be done better). All of this cross monitoring promotes better team resilience in the longer run [8]. Importantly, however, there are ways to improve performance before the patient even arrives. Welcome to the prebrief…

Don't Just Debrief, Prebrief

It has been argued that failing to prepare is like preparing to fail. Regardless, generations of healthcare professionals have been taught that all resuscitation begins with the primary survey or ABCs: airway, breathing and circulation. This is not always true. The primary survey is still fundamental, but, as will also be discussed under the section entitled the "Zero Point Survey" [14], we need not wait until the patient arrives. Instead, preassemble your team, identify the overall leader, and identify each sub-team (i.e. airway team, transfusion team etc.). Ensure that roles are delegated (thereby minimizing 'diffusion of responsibility'). Use this time to explicitly tell team members that you value their presence and authorize everyone to speak up if they have significant concerns. Once you have done this you can add the polite coda that interruptions should be brief and only if necessary for the patient's well-being.

The pre-brief is the first opportunity to build the team, to apportion tasks, and to develop a shared mental model. Ideally, everyone should have the opportunity to verbalize what they know, what they are concerned about, and their proposed solution (aka Plan A) [7]. This team huddle allows the team to own the plan. It bolsters both teamwork and taskwork and gives everyone a structure to rally around if chaos builds. Done right it creates a team that provides updates and cross monitors. Done right and a group of relative strangers can become nimble enough to manage complex trauma, overcome human biases, and put aside interpersonal concerns.

Team Structure: Leadership and Followership

Attend enough lectures and somebody will eventually highlight the importance of culture. The problem is they rarely go on to define what 'culture' actually means. A deep dive is beyond the remit of this chapter but the Dutch Psychologist, Geert Hofstede offers a good place to start [28]. In brief, his group outlined six indices of culture. These are: Power Distance Index (i.e. how the powerful and less powerful accept their status); Individualism (i.e. loyalty vs everyone for themselves); Masculinity vs Femininity (i.e. money-focus; self-centeredness); Uncertainty Avoidance (i.e. comfort with uncertainty; reliance on rules vs style); Long Term Orientation (i.e. persistence, and the importance of shame), and Indulgence vs Restraint (i.e. individual freedom vs societal norms).

In broad strokes, building a better medical culture means hard work over years rather than the typical trauma timescale. It means ensuring that empathy is cultivated and shared, and that workplace toxicity or complacency is not tolerated. It means accepting that hierarchy must exist but balancing that against creating the creation of a safe and respectful work environment. This is because we need to structure but also to leverage everybody's knowledge and skills [26]. It means making team members feel safe. This is done by committing to team members' longer-term career development rather than casting people aside after one mistake. It means understanding that those actively talking (i.e. resuscitating by voice) are as important as those actively listening [26]. It means understanding that while team leaders may be largely responsible for setting the dynamic, we all own culture.

Better leadership improves team performance, satisfaction and efficiency [8]. However, just like culture, leadership can be hard to define. An effective leader knows when to be hands-on (explicit leadership) and when to step back and delegate (implicit leadership) [26]. Leadership is hard and cannot always be intuited. Leaders have to simultaneously earn the team's trust, present an acceptable shared mental model, centralize information flow, coordinate tasks and overcome emotions (their own and other's) [29]. They manage and monitor the overall situation, and they accept disproportionate responsibility (i.e. including when it is not even their fault). Leaders step up and get their hands dirty when required. Leaders also teach, mentor, and set a standard for the whole team [8]. This is why hierarchy matters- you earn the right to lead; it isn't just awarded on day one.

Importantly, followership skills are no less important than leadership skills, even if this is not reflected in the literature. To date, there are 60 publications on leadership for every one publication on followership [30]. Moreover, there is likely still a stigma associated with self-identifying as a follower (i.e. a relative subordinate), even though 85% of healthcare workers are better understood to be followers. Healthcare simply could not function without skilled followers, and once again these skills can and should be taught [2]. Effective followers are able to step up when required and not taking it personally when they need to step back. In short, followership is an advanced impressive skill and should be valued as such.

Followers are able to self-manage and use their emotional intelligence to size up what they can and should contribute in any moment [26]. Clearly, the binary ideas of leader versus follower is outdated. Instead, members of the trauma team move in and out of leadership and followership roles. Therefore, it is better to simply talk about high functioning team members, who, in turn, are those with the dexterity to adapt to *what* (rather than *who*) is right. As outlined, effective leaders and followers also cross monitor. This means that while we manage ourselves, we also remain vigilant to the needs of others. Part of being a good trauma team member is having that 'sixth sense', where you size up a situation and step up or step back in whatever way best serves the patient and team.

Complex resuscitations often require sub teams. In HF terms, this minimizes task overload and ensures cognitive offload. While each team member maintains a global perspective, sub teams divide up the work and can thereby narrow their focus [7]. Examples include an airway team, or vascular access team. This breaks the resuscitation into more manageable chunks, and enables the leader to maintain a more supervisory role, or 'thousand-foot view' [7]. This mirrors the two attention types seen in nature types. System-1 is a focused spotlight gaze. This is exemplified in nature by the predator who focuses on only what truly matters, namely catching prey. System-2 means scanning from stimulus to stimulus. In nature, this is the potential prey who must avoid fixating on one spot and instead moves their attention constantly [8].

Shared Mental Models

Situational awareness consists of three parts: how we absorb cues, synthesize these into meaning, and predict what will happen next [8]. If all three steps occur then teams are better able to perform 'adaptive coordination'. In aviation terms this means we "fly ahead of the plane". In trauma terms it means not letting the patient go anywhere that your brain has not already been, and modifying errant behaviours well before disaster strikes [2, 7]. For the team to able to adapt, members need to be on the same page especially as things evolve. In other words, they need a robust but adaptable shared mental model. This is usually managed by the team leader, and strengthened and/or modified by team members sharing information. Trauma team leaders promote adaptive coordination by seeking input from others and then providing regular updates [7].

A mental model, or psychological map, includes an understanding of the task, context and resources [5, 21]. While we should avoid excessive noise, the process of "thinking out loud" keeps team members on the same page as the trauma progresses. This should optimize stress, enhance situational awareness, and communicate the team's priorities and each individual's role [31]. Hierarchy is important in managing the shared mental model. If excessive it discourages subordinates from speaking up. If inadequate it can lead to diffusion of responsibility. Experienced trauma teams often use a low authority gradient (also known as horizontal authority). This is where team members speak up and the leader says less [29]. In contrast, less experienced teams often need more explicit coordination and a more vertical authority gradient, akin to command and control [2].

Communication

Just as manual dexterity is needed to insert a chest tube, verbal dexterity is essential in complex trauma care [26]. Too often words that are meant are not said, words that are said are not heard, words that are heard are not understood, and words that are understood are not done. As such, it takes time, humility and commitment to become an expert communicator. Moreover, it takes skill to hear and to shut up [32]. Silence is not always golden, but nor is cacophony [29]. Three pillars of effective communication are closing the loop, verbalizing thoughts and plans, and maintaining a "sterile" resuscitation bay.

Language should be concise and precise. It should also be commonly understood, so avoid jargon, or words known only to your specialty. We also need to avoid vague statements, aka mitigating phrases. There really is no room for maybes or perhaps-es; instead be concise and direct. Moreover, every request should be amplified by somebody confirming that it was heard and confirming again when it is done (this is known as closed loop communication). Mitigating language is so dangerous that it the number one reason that commercial planes crash. It is often because we are afraid to offend, lack confidence, or are embarrassed [29]. However, one need not be rude to be clear. An example of communication that is closed loop and mitigation-free could be as simple as:

Example

Trauma team leader: Anaesthesia, please intubate the patient, and confirm when successful (NOT "Would someone be able to intubate the patient").

Anaesthesia resident: I am going to intubate the patient now.

Anaesthesia resident: The patient has been intubated successfully. ◄

As seen above, the three steps of closed loop communication include directing a request to a specific individual, verbal acknowledgment of that request, and confirmation that the request has been successfully completed [7]. Graded assertiveness is also important when overcoming authority. A useful approach is using the Concerned-Uncomfortable-Safety rule [7]. Using the above example, this is how to CUS:

Example

Trauma team leader: Anaesthesia, please intubate the patient, and confirm when successful.

Anaesthesia resident: I am concerned that this will be a difficult airway due to facial trauma.

(Then, if response received is not adequate)

Anaesthesia resident: I am uncomfortable intubating this patient without assistance and advanced equipment. ◄

If neither of these red flags are acknowledged, a safety threat can be declared. Because both members of the team understand the CUS model, it should simultaneously decrease reluctance and offense. Another method to advocate and raise concerns is to use a five-step approach. Developed by the aviation industry, it involves: i) an attention getter, ii) statement of concern, iii) statement of the problem as you see it, iv) a solution, and v) a request for agreement [29]. This would look like:

Example

Excuse me Dr. Smith. I am concerned that this airway is difficult. I do not believe I have the equipment to manage it successfully. I think we should obtain the difficult airway cart and get anaesthesia backup. Do you agree? ◄

As outlined above, it helps to verbalizing thoughts and plans (i.e. the leader asks 'what am I missing" during a floundering cardiac arrest), and to double check that potentially dangerous actions are indicated (i.e. a nurse announces they are giving a medication). This not only promotes sharing, but allows for confirmation, and reassessments [29]. In emergency situations, this type of communication needs to be dispassionate and direct. The most important messages/questions should come first ("Nurse, does she have a pulse?") followed by why the message is critical ("The end tidal CO_2 is dropping he may be about to arrest") [31].

Effective communication is less likely when messages are excessively complex or if there is distraction from noise, emotion, and time pressure [32]. These increase the likelihood of misinterpretation and results in "channel overload". This is why we should strive for a "sterile" resuscitation environment. Team members must speak up when required, while recognizing that critical moments (like intubation) should be silent. During these moments, the leader is given extra temporary power such that everyone else's comments are held, and those being silenced cannot take offense [29].

The word communication means sharing meaning and make understanding common. Accordingly, it is the most important HF and the best way to identify a high functioning team. Importantly, communication is more than just delivered words. Delivery can be divided into verbal (what is said), paraverbal (how it is said) and nonverbal (eye contact, facial expression, hand gestures). Just as expert teams know when to share key pieces of information[31] they are skilled (whether consciously or unconsciously) in each type of communication. They also ensure that it is consonant, not dissonant. This means that words (verbal) match tone (paraverbal) and both match facial expression (non verbal). This is because words are actually the least important of the three communication subtypes. Saying "I don't need help" but in a tone that suggestions otherwise simply increases confusion and danger. Just ask for help if you want it.

As outlined, equally important to what is being said is how it is delivered. Four main tones have been outlined: aggressive, submissive, cooperative, and assertive [10, 33]. The problem with excessively aggressive or submissive language is that it shifts the focus from what the patient needs to the status and ego of various team members. Modern clinicians are increasingly expected to use more cooperative/assertive styles, and further fine tune based on the situation's urgency and the team's maturity.

In short, communication (or lack thereof) is the important nontechnical skill in medicine, and the largest hole in the swiss cheese of medical error. It is insufficiently taught [34], and too often left to chance. We need to get better. This means we need to commend good communicator and condemn bad communicators. We cannot say it any clearer than that.

Handovers and Debriefs

If communication matters then it follows that the handover from one team to another can be equally perilous. This is why we need to practice and perfect handovers, every bit as much as handwashing. As patients make their way from pre-hospital, to the emergency room, to the operating room and beyond—each creates an opportunity for error, akin to that children's game of broken telephone. SBAR (Situation, Background, Assessment, and Recommendation) is a widely recognized, effective strategy. It was developed by the military and ensures that handover is delivered succinctly and comprehensively. Importantly, its structure is widely known. For example, this means those of the receiving end will recognize when the last component (i.e. the all-important recommendation) is missing. Having the deliver and receiver familiar with the same communication tool can be the difference between aggression- "so what the **** do you want me to do?" versus polite redirection "so, are you calling for advice or transfer?" [29].

Another handover tool is the 'ATMIST' mnemonic, which was designed for trauma and showed its usefulness in Camp Bastion, Afghanistan [35]. Sequentially, it includes i) age of patient, ii) time of incident, iii) mechanism of injury, iv) injuries (head to toe), v) vital signs, and vi) treatments given so far. It is similar to the more familiar AMPLE mnemonic which incorporates i) allergies, ii) medications iii) past medical history iv) last meal v) events surrounding the trauma. Whichever handover system is chosen, it should be concise and logical with a sequential structure. Once again it should be familiar to both deliver and receiver. We need to be on eth same wavelength.

Debriefings allow teams to explore and highlight what went well and what did not. They are an opportunity to learn, and to identify when a formal quality or review is required [25]. They are also a time to let off steam, share emotions, bond, and work through ethical or moral concerns [35]. Debriefing should be routine rather than exceptional, should be non-threatening, and should take place soon after the linked event. They used to occur in the pub. If this is no longer deemed appropriate then we need to find other ways.

Key Points

- Successful team perform pre-briefs, and develop and cultivate shared mental models.
- A strong leader is able to anticipate team members needs and make team members feel safe.
- Followership skills are no less important than leadership skills but have been underemphasized to date.
- Effective communication involves closing the loop, verbalizing thought processes, and maintaining a "sterile resuscitation bay".

- Handovers should be practiced and perfected, and critical events should be followed by deliberate debriefs.

Environmental Factors

The Zero Point Survey

The Zero Point survey, shown in Fig. 1.1, uses the mnemonic STEP UP to prepare Self, Team, Environment and Patient [20]. It is also a practical way to improve ergonomics (i.e. the interaction between the work environment and the worker). The first three steps precede the patient's arrival, and precedes the primary survey. Personal readiness includes seemingly mundane iterative improvements, such as using the toilet or obtaining a snack before a long resuscitation. After the team has been prepared the focus turns to optimizing the resuscitation environment. This means appraising whether space and equipment restrictions will compromise patient management. If so then we need to move things before the patient arrives. Examples include creating space around the patient, ensuring adequate lighting, and implementing crowd control [20]. It might mean moving things out of the way (so that patients can be rushed to the Operating Room (OR), or closer (so that the Difficult Airway Kit is at hand).

Physical Layout

As outlined, there is more to safe resuscitation than just clever people and shiny equipment. Halls should be wide enough, obstacles removed, kit nearby and elevators free and functioning. We should ensure that phones (and any other communication devices) are strategically placed and actually work (for example, land lines may be needed in lead lined areas such as Radiology Departments or ERs). It means knowing that security personnel are available. The trauma bay itself should have adequate lighting, visible monitors, supplies, and enough room for the team to function. On the other hand, it should not to so large that team members cannot see or hear one another.

Inadequate space, misplaced equipment and haphazard wires and tubing can all be latent threats [7, 13]. Key anatomic areas, such as the patient's head and thorax should also be kept clear. The location of equipment and how it is labelled should be known by all in order to minimize delays. Team members should familiarize

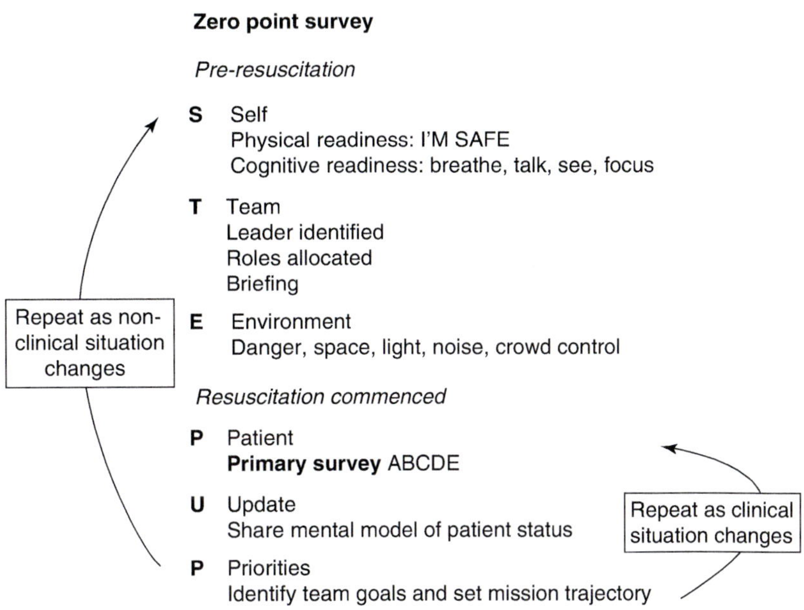

Fig. 1.1 The STEP-UP approach to the Zero-Point Survey, preceding and commencing with patient arrival [20]

themselves with the physical environment and location of equipment prior to patient arrival. More recently, courtesy of COVID-19, it has become necessary to delegate somebody not only to crowd control, but to supervising during donning and doffing of personal protective equipment: the so-called "dofficer" [7].

Resource Utilization

In practical terms, resource utilization is about how we help or hinder ourselves and how well we prioritize tasks. Importantly, "more" does not always mean "more". For example, eight people might be optimal number of staff members around a patient's bed (the so-called Dunbar's number- named after the psychologist Robin Dunbar). In contrast, larger teams can create distraction, excessive noise and the bystander effect (i.e. humans are less likely to help when others are present). This means that it can be appropriate during resuscitation to remove unnecessary personnel. However, it is usually best to have them close (i.e. just outside of the room) in case you need a "go-for" (to grab supplies), a procedural expert (in case that airway is difficult) and a cognitive resource (in case the trauma becomes more complex than expected).

Key Points

- Using the Zero Point Survey can improve the likelihood of success even before the patient arrives.
- Attending to the physical layout of the trauma bay can further optimize individual and team performance.
- Resource utilization matters: It's important to find the optimal balance between too much and too little help.

Organizational and System Factors

To ensure that there is a consistent, iterative, proactive approach to safety, there must also be support from the overarching system. The system or organization should also understand HF, and for the simple reason that healthcare is still run by humans and for humans. The organizational climate encompasses its vision, policies and culture [13]. All three should be informed by regular feedback and from all levels: frontlines and backrooms. A useful example is the Massive Transfusion Protocol used in trauma resuscitation [36]. Mangers who are visible and approachable are equally important [36]. Trauma team members are unlikely to respect desk jockeys.

Safety-I and Safety-II

Patient Safety is often fallaciously understood as just the absence of failure. Similarly, an "error-is-everywhere" mindset has led to idea that all we need is minimal variation and maximal compliance. This has also meant that Safety (with a big S) has been largely defined by administrators, regulators, and external mandates [37, 38] It has led to a "find and fix" strategy and relies on adverse events to guide safety, without acknowledging the irony of this approach [38]. This approach- now known as Safety-1—largely assumes that systems are bimodal (i.e. things go right or wrong) and decompostable (i.e. complexity can be broken down into individual repairable parts). Safety-1 is more likely to see humans as a liability, because we introduce variability into a system that would work perfectly if we just followed the protocol [38]. This "scooby-doo principle"- namely, "it would be fine if it wasn't for those meddling kids"- is short sighted.

Unfortunately, Safety-I can be highly attractive to some administrators and programmers, especially those far from frontline care. Complex healthcare is often so nuanced, and its components are so intertwined, that they cannot be broken down or summarized on a one-page linear algorithm. This means that we may be better looking at complexity theory (as attributed to Gloubermann and Zimmermann) or chaos theory (often attributed to Lorenz). Regardless, when things are unpredictability it is hard to dictate a single way, or precisely define 'ideal behaviour'– except in the most basic cases. This means that Patient Safety means we also need to understand how humans get things right most of the time. This in turn means empowering humans and respecting gestalt and experience. This study of 'how most things go right' is known as Safety-II, and is a profound advance in terms of highlighting the importance of humans (and their HFs), and exposing the shortcomings of computers.

Safety-II is the study of success rather than failure. It relies on the adaptation, improvisation, tenacity, and everyday problem-solving skills of practical people. Accordingly, "expertise" is recognized and rewarded. It means respecting intuition, and accepting that some are better able to deal with unpredictability and chaos. Safety-II aims to learn how teams adapt, and sees humans as an essential resource because of their flexibility, practicality and experience [38]. In means the excessive standardization can be a liability (not a state of administrative nirvana) if it prevent necessary adaptability and creativity. Safety-II, does not forgive error, or human laziness, or human inexperience. It also does not give humans maverick license to do as they please. Instead, Safety-II matures our understanding of what humans bring to healthcare. It helps explain adverse events as transient phenomena at a specific time and place. It reinforces the idea that improvements come from numerous iterative everyday adjustments [38].

Going forward, our understanding of HF will need to combine the two paradigms: with Safety-I predominating for simple matters, and Safety-II predominating for the more complex. Importantly, this updated understanding also adds extra nuance to why so many report burnout and frustration [37]. Without oversimplifying complex HFs like wellbeing and resilience, most healthcare workers will be familiar with feeling despondent because a Safety-1solution (i.e. another unnecessary delay) was implemented without their input, when a Safety-2 solution would have been better (i.e. a senior clinician could have been empowered). If we continue with a Safety-I focus there is every likelihood that front-liners will be disproportionally blamed and disempowered, and forced to endure wrong solutions, rather than just creating workarounds.

Examples of Safety-I versus Safety-II thinking abound. For example, doctors are (rightly) accused of illegible handwriting, and this is needs to stop. However, it likely results from doctors having to write too many orders: after all we weren't selected for bad handwriting; it developed because on the job. A Safety-1 solution would be to force doctors to type all orders, but with the result that we become even less efficient and even more distracted. A Safety-II solutions include allowing more verbal orders, have scribes assigned to busy doctors, or more default orders. Safety-I means we often face numerous security-stops when one, but done properly, would allow doctors to care for patient: Safety-II. The erstwhile focus on Safety-I can mean we overly rely on one laboratory findings (i.e. the SOFA score) rather than a face-to-face assessment of the patient (i.e. how quickly we should get off the sofa) i.e. Safety-II.

Systems that obsess over Safety-I and ignore Safety-II may lead exhausted and frustrated healthcare workers to quit clinical work [37]. After all, anyone who understands even basic HF appreciates humans can only take so much moral distress. We want humans to do the right thing because of the system not despite it. A greater use of Safety-II thinking might help dedicated humans feel valued and able to craft systems that are not only safer but more human-focused. Keeping experienced people engaged means we keep their wisdom in the system, rather than just their wrath. System-II could also mean a more nuanced understanding of the emotional and cognitive demands of working in healthcare, and the (in)human experience of being a patient. After all, none of us wants to be treated like a mere cog in a clattering train.

Summary

The more chaotic and unpredictable the situation, the more that HFs become the difference between success and failure, in both the short and long term. The individual must be equipped to overcome stress and their own biases. Communication, a shared mental model, and mutual respect must underpin every leader, and, just as importantly, every follower. The working environment should be ergonomically designed and the team should be poised for action that is safe, logical and practised. The system in which this occurs should also be supportive and adaptive and should see its humans as resources not liabilities. When these things occur, Death is no longer in charge of the clattering train, and resuscitation is a life-affirming, life-saving and rather wonderous thing.

Questions

1. Stress is an important individual human factor that can be optimized to an appropriate level. Which of the following is NOT an appropriate way to manage stress?
   (a) Self affirmation through positive self talk
   (b) The four steps of controlled breathing
   (c) Self medication with anxiolytics
   (d) Mentally rehearsing the task ahead
2. Which is true regarding effective team structure for a resuscitation?
   (a) Effective leaders are always hands-on and never delegate
   (b) Hierarchy must never exist
   (c) Those actively talking are more important than those listening
   (d) Effective followers know when to speak up and when to step back
3. Highly functioning teams use all of the following communication methods EXCEPT for:
   (a) The use of mitigating language
   (b) "Closing the loop"
   (c) Maintaining a "sterile communication environment"
   (d) Verbalizing thoughts and plans
4. When does the Zero Point Survey ideally start to take place?
   (a) When care is being handed over to another service
   (b) When first alerted that a patient is en route
   (c) Immediately prior to the primary trauma survey
   (d) When debriefing team members after the resuscitation
5. What is the difference between the Safety- I and Safety-II paradigms?
   (a) Safety-I focusses on patient related factors, and Safety-II on system related factors
   (b) Safety-II looks at events taking place after initial resuscitation
   (c) Safety-I focuses on what went wrong, while Safety-II explores what went right
   (d) Safety-II has replaced Safety-I entirely in analysing adverse event

Answers

1. c
2. d
3. a
4. b
5. c

References

1. Nickson C. Human factors. Life in the Fast Lane. 2019 Jun. Available from: https://litfl.com/human-factors/
2. Brindley PG, Cardinal P. Optimizing crisis resource management to improve patient safety and team performance – a handbook for acute care health professionals. 1st ed. Ottawa: Royal College of Physicians and Surgeons of Canada; 2017.
3. Brindley PG. Improving teamwork in anaesthesia and critical care: many lessons still to learn. Br J Anaesth. 2014;112(3):399–401.
4. Helmreich RL. On error management: Lessons from aviation. Br Med J. 2000;320(7237):781–5.
5. Russ AL, Fairbanks RJ, Karsh BT, Militello LG, Saleem JJ, Wears RL. The science of human factors: separating fact from fiction. BMJ Qual Saf. 2013;22(10):802–8.
6. Brindley PG. Patient safety and acute care medicine: lessons for the future, insights from the past. Crit Care. 2010;14(2):1–5.
7. Hicks C, Petrosoniak A. The human factor: optimizing trauma team performance in dynamic clinical environments. Emerg Med Clin North Am. 2018;36(1):1–17.
8. Gillman LM, Widder S, Blaivas M, Karakitsos D. Trauma team dynamics. 1st ed. Cham: Springer; 2016.
9. Reason J. Human error: models and management. Br Med J. 2000;320:768–70.
10. Brindley PG. Communication in crisis: the importance of verbal dexterity. In: Intensive Care Medicine Annual Update. New York: Springer; 2010. p. 581–90.

11. Clear J. Atomic habits. New York: Penguin Random House; 2018.
12. Catchpole K, Ley E, Wiegmann D, Blaha J, Shouhed D, Gangi A, et al. A human factors subsystems approach to trauma care. JAMA Surg. 2014;149(9):962–8.
13. Cohen TN, Cabrera JS, Litzinger TL, Captain KA, Fabian MA, Miles SG, et al. Proactive safety management in trauma care: applying the human factors analysis and classification system. J Healthc Qual. 2018;40(2):89–96.
14. Lauria M, Weingart S, Swaminathan A, Hicks C. Learning to take the heat: The problem with stress. 2020 Aug. Available from https://www.emra.org/emresident/article/stress-management/
15. Arul G, Pugh H, Nott D. Keep calm, pack and pause. Bull R Coll Surg Engl. 2019;101(3):92–5.
16. Kent J, Thornton M, Fong A, Hall E, Fitzgibbons S, Sava J. Acute provider stress in high stakes medical care: implications for trauma surgeons. J Trauma Acute Care Surg. 2020;88(3):440–5.
17. Walker M. Why we sleep. New York: Scribner; 2017.
18. Groombridge CJ, Kim Y, Maini A, Smit DV, Fitzgerald MC. Stress and decision-making in resuscitation: a systematic review. Resuscitation. 2019;144(September):115–22. https://doi.org/10.1016/j.resuscitation.2019.09.023.
19. Norris EM, Lockey AS. Human factors in resuscitation teaching. Resuscitation. 2012;83(4):423–7. https://doi.org/10.1016/j.resuscitation.2011.11.001.
20. Reid C, Brindley P, Hicks C, Carley S, Richmond C, Lauria M, et al. Zero point survey: a multidisciplinary idea to STEP UP resuscitation effectiveness. Clin Exp Emerg Med. 2018;5(3):139–43.
21. Brindley PG. Preventing medical "crashes": psychology matters. J Crit Care. 2010;25(2):356–7. https://doi.org/10.1016/j.jcrc.2010.02.017.
22. Marshall SD, Touzell A. Human factors and the safety of surgical and anaesthetic care. Anaesthesia. 2020;75(S1):e34–8.
23. Brindley PG, Beed M, Law JA, Hung O, Levitan R, Murphy MF, et al. Airway management outside the operating room: how to better prepare. Can J Anesth. 2017;64(5):530–9.
24. Nolan B, Zakirova R, Bridge J, Nathens AB. Barriers to implementing the world health organization's trauma care checklist: a Canadian single-center experience. J Trauma Acute Care Surg. 2014;77(5):679–83.
25. Fitzgerald M, Reilly S, Smit DV, Kim Y, Mathew J, Boo E, et al. The World Health Organization trauma checklist versus trauma team time-out: a perspective. Emerg Med Australas. 2019;31(5):882–5.
26. Gillman LM, Brindley PG, Blaivas M, Widder S, Karakitsos D. Trauma team dynamics. J Crit Care. 2016;32:218–21.
27. Brindley PG. Peak performance under pressure: lessons from a helicopter rescue doctor. Anesth Analg. 2020;131(1):e11–2.
28. Hofstede G. Attitudes, values and organizational culture: disentangling the concepts. Organ Stud. 1998;19(3):477–92.
29. Brindley PG, Reynolds SF. Improving verbal communication in critical care medicine. J Crit Care. 2011;26(2):155–9. https://doi.org/10.1016/j.jcrc.2011.03.004.
30. Leung C, Lucas A, Brindley P, Anderson S, Park J, Vergis A, et al. Followership: a review of the literature in healthcare and beyond. J Crit Care. 2018;46:99–104. https://doi.org/10.1016/j.jcrc.2018.05.001.
31. Mike Lauria. COMM CHECK: more on resuscitation communication. EMCrit Blog. 2020 Jul. Available from https://emcrit.org/emcrit/comm-check-more-on-resuscitation-communication/
32. Brindley PG. Symposium: new challenges to clinical communication in serious illness commentary: communication: the most important "procedure" in healthcare and bioethics. Camb Q Healthc Ethics. 2019;28(3):415–21.
33. Cyna AM, Andrew MI, Tan SGM, Smith AF. Handbook of communication in anaesthesia & critical care: a practical guide to exploring the art. Oxford: Oxford University Press; 2010. p. 288. Available from http://books.google.com/books?id=6Ipf3pdp46QC&pgis=1
34. Brindley PG, Smith KE, Cardinal P, LeBlanc F. Improving medical communication: skills for a complex (and multilingual) clinical world. Can Respir J. 2014;21(2):89–91.
35. Arul GS, Pugh HEJ, Mercer SJ, Midwinter MJ. Human factors in decision making in major trauma in Camp Bastion, Afghanistan. Ann R Coll Surg Engl. 2015;97(4):262–8.
36. Enticott JC, Jeffcott S, Ibrahim JE, Wood EM, Cole-Sinclair M, Fitzgerald M, et al. A review on decision support for massive transfusion: understanding human factors to support the implementation of complex interventions in trauma. Transfusion. 2012;52(12):2692–705.
37. Smaggus A. Safety-I, safety-II and burnout: how complexity science can help clinician wellness. BMJ Qual Saf. 2019;28(8):667–71.
38. Hollnagel E, Wears R, Braithwaite J. From safety-I to safety-II: a white paper. London: The Resilient Health Care Net; 2015.

2 Dealing with Death in Trauma

Alex Psirides

- Epidemiology and timing of traumatic causes of death. Comparison to other hospital deaths
- Theory of death trajectory, how it differs by disease, how trauma deaths are different
- 'Bad' vs 'good' deaths—societal & cultural expectations vs medical reality
- Dealing with death: the family. How television & film inform expectations. Practical advice on breaking the worst news
- Dealing with death: the clinical team. How to debrief the team after a traumatic death
- Dealing with death: the expert. How senior staff can help their colleagues, and themselves

The real problem of humanity is the following: we have Palaeolithic emotions, medieval institutions and God-like technology.

Edward O.Wilson, debate at the Harvard Museum of Natural History, Cambridge, USA. September 2009.

Introduction

Despite significant advances in care with the development of trauma systems, networks, and designated centres within modern healthcare systems, death from a traumatic event remains common. In the UK, the 2007 National Confidential Enquiry into Perioperative Deaths (NCEPOD) report describes trauma as the fourth leading cause of death in the Western world and the leading cause of death in the first four decades of life [1]. For each traumatic death, there is an estimate of 36 life-years lost. In the US, half of all deaths occur within minutes of injury either at the scene or en route to hospital, with significant variation in mortality reported, from 35% in high-income to 63% in low-income settings [2]. A 2010 report from the National Audit Office on major trauma care in England reported 20,000 major trauma events per year resulting in 5400 deaths [3]. Although previous epidemiological studies have described trimodal death distribution (immediate death on scene, early death due to haemorrhage, and late death from organ failure), data from the largest European trauma database has challenged this [4]. The UK Trauma Audit and Research

The author composed, revised and approved this manuscript. The work is original. There are no conflicts or relevant disclosures.

A. Psirides (✉)
Intensive Care Unit, Wellington Regional Hospital, Wellington, New Zealand

Wellington Aeromedical Retrieval Service, Wellington, New Zealand

University of Otago, Wellington, New Zealand
e-mail: alex.psirides@ccdhb.org.nz

P. Lax (ed.), *Textbook of Acute Trauma Care*, https://doi.org/10.1007/978-3-030-83628-3_2

Network (TARN) report into 3632 deaths between 1997 and 2001 showed the majority of trauma deaths occurred soon after hospital admission without further peaks in mortality. This was roughly divided into quarters—the first 25% die within the first two-and-a-half hours after trauma, the second within the first twenty-four hours, and the third within the first week, with the remaining quarter of those who die doing so after this period.

Compared to many deaths encountered within hospital, trauma deaths are usually sudden and therefore unexpected, involve younger patients and, even as trauma systems have evolved to significantly improve care, are often unavoidable. The effect of these factors on both the family members these deaths leave behind, and the clinical staff who have cared for the deceased and may be present at death will be discussed in this chapter.

Death Trajectories

To place death from trauma in context, it is necessary to consider how it differs in comparison to other fatal disease processes. Not only is this relevant to clinicians' experience of the deaths that they encounter during paramedic, nursing and medical training, but also gives context to family and societal expectations when dealing with trauma(tic) death. One method of describing (and graphically representing) these differences is to consider theoretical trajectories of dying—what happens to patients' physical and social function over time in the last year or so preceding their death.

The concept of death trajectories was first suggested in 1968 [5]. Three different models were proposed—sudden 'surprise' death, 'expected' death (short-term and lingering), and 'entry-reentry' deaths where people slowly deteriorate with intervening intermittent hospital admissions. Several studies have since expanded upon this theoretical model using analysis of large administrative and clinical datasets [6, 7]. An analysis of a US Medicare database from 1993–1998 in older claimants who died suggested 92% of decedents were able to be categorised into one of four underlying conditions which determined their trajectories at the end of their life. These were sudden death (7%), cancer (22%) and organ system failure (16%) with the remainder due to frailty.

Figure 2.1 shows differences between theoretical death trajectories superimposed on a single chart, representing functional changes over time. Although these are represented as distinct categories, different trajectories may overlap in single patients (frail patients who die from a traumatic event for example). The progressive decline in function may be influenced to differing degrees

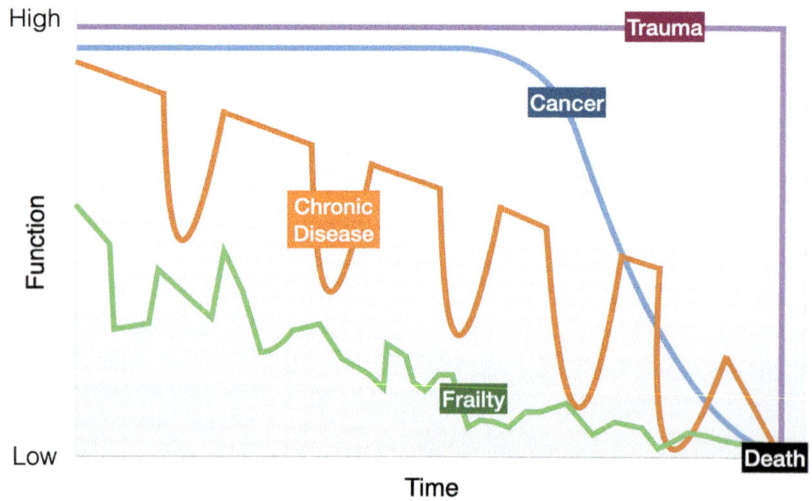

Fig. 2.1 Theoretical comparative death trajectories

by medical intervention. A functional decline from chronic disease—heart failure or chronic obstructive pulmonary disease for example—may result in reversible acute on chronic deterioration where hospitalisation provides short-term improvement. Often such patients do not return to pre-admission baseline. Such acute decrements are expected to become more frequent and move further from a pre-morbid state as the disease progresses towards death. The frailty trajectory has been described as 'prolonged dwindling' where functional decline continues irrespective of medical intervention. Such patients are unlikely to benefit from hospitalisation, where exposure to this environment may even accelerate deconditioning and do more harm than good. Patients on an incurable cancer trajectory, where the underlying disease progression can be delayed but not halted, are more likely to be able to benefit from the expertise of palliative medicine clinicians in managing their symptoms. They also, along with those with chronic disease, may have time to make autonomous decisions regarding the when, where, and how they die. For those in the final category, who die from sudden traumatic events, these opportunities are almost never available. Although death is seldom desired, it is presumed that most people, when it comes, would wish for their ultimate demise to be 'good'.

The Bad Death

As clinicians we are frequently exposed to death and the process that precedes it. What constitutes a 'bad' or 'good' death is considerably subjective. The death we may want for ourselves, our family members or our patients may not be the death they would want for themselves. Although death is inevitable, the low prevalence of advanced care planning suggests that many people are unlikely to have discussed with their families (or their doctors) how they may die. In modern healthcare systems where life expectancy continues to rise, societal expectations of a long and healthy life often preclude consideration of the alternative. This is particularly relevant for deaths related to trauma. The acute nature of the event both selects for a younger population in whom death was previously a far-away ill-considered possibility, and may remove or reduce the ability to have any influence on the process. Many deaths from trauma are likely to happen despite ongoing maximal treatment, not from limitations placed due to futility as may occur with chronic disease states. Indeed, any traumatic event that impairs consciousness or decision making removes the individual from determining what happens to them. Their dying process may then rely instead on the consensus of proxy decision makers made up of clinicians, family members, or even legal authorities.

To determine what is a 'bad' death, one should first consider the alternative. Societal expectations of death are varied and often determined by cultural or religious beliefs. For some, a 'good' death would involve the autonomy to determine where, how or even when they die. A 2016 literature review exploring themes around a good death described thirty-six studies involving interviews with clinicians, family members, and patients [8]. Eleven core themes of a good death were identified. These included being pain-free, dying with dignity, having family members present, and having control over the dying process. Deaths from sudden trauma are unlikely to meet any of these. It is more likely that sudden trauma will lead to a 'bad' death due to a variety of factors. These include:

Key Points

- **Location:** death is more likely to occur either pre-hospital (roadside or in an ambulance or helicopter), in the resuscitation bay of an emergency department (ED), or in an operating theatre or intensive care unit (ICU), rather than at home or another preferred location
- **Timing:** death may occur during or immediately after a treatment or procedure that was unlikely to change outcome, with little control over this from either the patient or clinical staff. There is often no opportunity for family and friends to 'say goodbye' or resolve any outstanding conflicts

- **Personnel:** the patient is more likely to have paramedics, nurses or doctors present, not family or friends
- **Quiet and calm:** the death is more likely to occur in a noisy environment accompanied by monitors and alarms
- **Dignity:** the aggressive nature of trauma resuscitation with exposure, cannulation and intubation does not lend itself to a dignified death
- **Cultural or spiritual needs:** although these may be able to be met after death (subject to local Coronial requirements), these are often unknown, or if known are difficult to address during resuscitative efforts

Accepting that a cost of doing everything to save a life may result in a bad death, the effects of either participating in this process (as clinicians) or being absent as a result of it (family members and friends) will be considered from different viewpoints.

Dealing with Death: The Family

The responsibilities of a clinician caring for a patient who dies from trauma do not end with the patient's death. Although resuscitative efforts may be guided by protocols, what comes after—breaking the worst news—is harder to prescribe. Although some deaths may be discussed and expected (a patient with unsurvivable brain injury in an intensive care unit for example), many trauma deaths occur outside hospitals, in resuscitation rooms, radiology suites or operating theatres. Rapid attendance of family members or friends allows little preparation for what may happen and what could be signposted in advance. The onus usually falls upon the most senior clinician present, sometimes fresh from the resuscitation, to deliver the news that a loved one has died.

Before considering what and how this process should occur, some context around societal expectation (which affects both families and clinicians, although to differing degrees) is relevant. Unless family members have either previous experience of acute traumatic death or have clinicians amongst their group, it is likely their expectations are informed by the outcomes they have been exposed to through television, film and print media. Although this assertion may seem strange on first consideration, it has been subjected to several studies examining outcomes of fictional patients in television dramas [9–12]. An analysis of 88 episodes from 4 different television medical dramas (2 each from England and the US) showed 76 cardiorespiratory arrests and 70 resuscitation attempts. Overall there was an immediate success rate of 46%, with the most common cause of arrest being secondary to trauma. Survival (or not) to discharge was usually not shown. In the real world, survival from traumatic cardiac arrest varies but rates have been reported between 0%–3.5% [13].

For patients who may survive the initial resuscitation but have incurred brain injury resulting in a reduced level of consciousness, television portrayal is even more likely to lead to false hope amongst family members [14]. A study of 64 characters who exhibited unconsciousness exceeding 24 hours duration in 9 US television dramas showed that 89% of patients made a full recovery. Of those who recovered, 86% did so fully on the day of waking. For those with traumatic cause of their coma, 89% were depicted as making a full recovery (compared to 7% in reality).

The gap between expectation and reality should be borne in mind when meeting with family members, particularly if there is uncertainty around outcome. For breaking bad news around a sudden traumatic death however, the outcome is already known. The focus should therefore be on process. Although the complete scope of communication strategies for breaking bad news is beyond this chapter, there are some factors specific to sudden traumatic death that should be considered.

Professor Peter Brindley has described the family meeting as 'the most dangerous procedure in the hospital' [15]. He goes on to discuss that communication skills are rarely innate, do not necessarily improve through years of unstructured experience and that communication training is associated with increased (clinician) confidence, improved patient satisfaction, less anxiety and lower post-traumatic stress. The potential for poor communication to cause lasting harm should not be underestimated. In mitigation, the following points are presented for consideration as a suggested process for breaking the news of sudden death to family or friends:

Key Points

- If possible, find a small quiet private space with seating, away from busy clinical areas. Unless absolutely unavoidable, this is not a conversation for a corridor or resuscitation room
- If clothing or shoes are soiled with blood, change them before going into the room
- Do not keep family members waiting any longer than absolutely necessary
- The meeting should be led by the most senior staff member available and not delegated. Ideally, they would have been involved in the resuscitation process so are able to answer questions from their own experience. Other clinical staff should attend to support the lead and family members or for education purposes, but not in such large numbers that they overwhelm. If other staff are attending, a prebrief from the lead may be helpful, particularly if silence is to be used as a communication tool
- Begin by quickly asking who is in the room and whether anyone else is arriving imminently. Introduce all staff members briefly
- Ask the family what they know about what has happened. Incorporate this into a single-sentence summary of known events. Pause
- Tell the family that, despite the best efforts of the team, their loved one has died. Use the patient's name when you do so. Precede this with an empathic expression of sorrow that you are comfortable using. Do not use euphemisms. Use the words '*died*' or '*dead*'
- **Stop talking and wait**. It is likely that very little said beyond this point will be remembered. Sit with the family, saying nothing. This process has been described by the eminent Australian social worker Dr. Liz Crowe as 'sitting in the rubble' [16].
- Continue to wait until the family are able to ask questions; let them break the silence. Answer questions honestly and simply. If a question cannot be answered at that time, tell the family that an answer will be found (if possible) and take responsibility for providing it yourself or delegating it to someone appropriate
- Communication should be empathic, not sympathetic. It is unlikely clinicians know what family members are experiencing so expressions that suggest so should be avoided
- Once questions have been answered, explaining practicalities about what happens next may be useful if deemed appropriate. If the family wish to be with their relative, ensure that the area where the body is located is accessible and they are presented in as dignified a way as possible before taking them into the room. Any major injuries should be covered if possible. This will likely be the last memory of their loved one
- Make sure a support person remains with them or is easily accessible until they leave the hospital

Death notification in the pre-hospital domain may be more burdensome for clinicians without the resources available in a hospital to assist. Family members may already be on scene (travelling in a vehicle with the deceased for example) and may also be injured themselves. To help with this, death education curricula and tools have been developed [17, 18] and their effects studied [19], suggesting an improvement in paramedics' ability to perform these tasks. Prior to a death notification course, 84% described their training was inadequate to communicate death or help a family with their grief; this rose to 92% self-reporting that they felt better prepared after training.

The poet and civil rights activist, Maya Angelou said "*.. people will forget what you said, people will forget what you did, but people will never forget how you made them feel.*"

Although this is one of the worst days of their lives, small changes in the way death notification is conveyed may make a lasting difference. This applies both to the family and the clinicians involved in the process.

Dealing with Death: The Clinical Team

Trauma deaths are unlike other deaths in hospital. They are less frequent, may progress rapidly, are likely to involve larger numbers of clinicians with differing experience, and, as described by trauma epidemiology, are likely to involve younger patients with few if any co-morbidities. Although traumatic deaths may be increasing, clinical exposure to in-hospital trauma deaths may be decreasing. One US study indicated that all-case deaths in emergency departments halved between 1997 and 2011 [20]. Another US study over a similar time period indicated a change in place of death from acute hospital wards to home or community settings but also reported a rise of deaths within the ICU [21]. If frequency of exposure to death and dying in certain environments is reduced, then the impact upon clinicians when they do experience or witness it may be greater.

Death in ICU is relatively common. ICU mortality varies but is reported as between 10–40% for acute admissions [22, 23] Whereas the majority of death in ICU is hastened by treatment limitation or withdrawal on the grounds of futility, trauma deaths in the prehospital setting, ED or operating theatre are more likely to occur despite ongoing resuscitation. The subtle difference of death being 'allowed' to happen due to an irreversible underlying process, compared to death occurring despite 'heroic' efforts of clinicians working together to avoid that very outcome is important. The outcome is the same; the process is very different. The effects of this distinction upon those involved should not be underestimated when participating in or leading the teams involved.

The trauma team model—where clinicians from different specialties including but not limited to emergency medicine, surgery, anaesthesia, intensive care, or paediatrics—brings together individuals with different skills at different levels of training. The team must function as a single unit with a unified goal under direction. Although the team model lends itself to some diffusion of responsibility, for adverse outcomes or where resuscitation is unsuccessful, more junior team members may feel they contributed to the patient's death, or that they could have done more. Clinical bystanders with less direct responsibility—nursing, medical and paramedical students for example—may be witnessing these events for the first time and require specific support in dealing with their distress, guilt and grief [24]. This may go unnoticed by those immersed in the resuscitation. Even a well-run trauma call proceeding in a quiet, bloody frenzy is not a 'normal' environment for many of the participants to work.

For some individuals or specialties, death may be anathema. One anaesthetic trainee rotating through the author's ICU fed back at the end of their six-month run that "I had no idea there would be so much death". To a specialist who has only worked in the ICU environment for many years, this was an interesting insight into desensitisation when death is frequent and normalised. Compared to ICU, a death in an operating theatre usually results in the team—theatre nurses, surgeon and anaesthetist—being stood down and debriefed. In ICU, the paperwork ritual is completed, the body removed, and the room cleaned ready for the next admission. The differences in mindsets of trauma team members should be considered when managing their experiences after a traumatic death.

Giving team members the opportunity to reflect on their shared experience after traumatic events may be beneficial. The process—debriefing—may be staged with a 'hot' debrief immediately after the event (if competing clinical demands allow) and then a delayed 'cold' debrief where the immediate emotional reaction may have reduced, to improve reflection on team performance. Several debriefing mechanisms have been described [25] with practical guidance available on how to conduct this in the emergency department [26]. Although there is no definitive evidence that debriefing decreases post-traumatic stress, some studies have suggested the process may help to reduce it [27–29].

The full gamut of debriefing is outside the scope of this chapter. However, as a brief summary, the following process for a 'hot' debrief (immediately after the patient's death) could be considered:

Key Points

- After the patient has died, pause. Some centres have described requesting 30–60 seconds of silence to consider what has just happened. This is respectful of the life of the person who has just died as well as the efforts of those who tried to prevent it. Request that team members do not immediately disperse unless they have urgent clinical tasks elsewhere. If the family have arrived or are present then communication with them must be prioritised
- Tie up any loose ends, delegating tasks where possible to those who were not directly involved in the event. Offer the chance to debrief to those who wish to attend, telling them it is not mandatory but may be helpful. The debrief should ideally be led by someone who has been trained to do so, or is comfortable doing so. This does not have to be the trauma team leader, and may not even be someone who was directly involved in the event
- Assemble the team in a quiet area and establish ground rules. What is discussed is confidential, participation is voluntary, anyone may leave at any time and the debrief is informal and supportive, not accusatory or to apportion blame. Explain that the debrief is to get a sense of what just happened from everyone's perspective rather and to prevent individual team members blaming themselves for the outcome
- Check in with those present. Ask directly "is everyone OK?". If not, address why first
- Begin by asking the group to run through the facts, to construct a shared mental model of what just happened
- Once the facts are agreed and established, the emotional responses can be discussed. Ask what people were thinking at various points during the resuscitation and how they felt, how they performed the tasks they were allocated and any difficulties they may have had with them
- Discussion around process should be encouraged rather than discussion around outcome. This can be best considered with 3 simple questions: What went well? What didn't go well? What would we do differently? The last question could be framed as an opportunity to learn from the event
- Close off the debrief with a summary of what has been discussed and the points, if any, to be addressed for improvement in process. If there is feeling that further debrief may be required then offer an opportunity for this to occur. The debrief leader should check in again that everyone involved are able to return to their clinical work and provide support for those who aren't.

Dealing with Death: The Expert

Finally, the effects of traumatic death upon more senior staff should be considered. There are undoubtedly expectations within organisations, specialities and even different cultures as to which qualities strong leaders should model. For some leaders, the outward expression of emotion may be considered a sign of weakness and seen as poor leadership. For some teams, evidence of their leader's humanity may be seen as a positive trait. In politics at least, perceptions around what strong leadership looks like are being challenged [30].

Some insights into the effects of death of patients upon specialists involved in their care are provided by studies in two contrasting specialties—oncology and trauma surgery. The first, a 2012 study of 20 oncologists in 3 Canadian hospitals with a range of 18 months to 30 years clinical experience described their experiences of patient death as 'desiring detachment' but 'struggling with grief' [31]. Grief was considered unprofessional, shameful, and a weakness to be hidden from others. Over half reported feelings of self-doubt and powerlessness. For most, talking to the study authors was the first time they had ever spoken about it. More importantly from the patients' perspective, half had reported their grief had affected treatment decisions with subsequent patients. This included more aggressive chemotherapy, enrolment in experimental studies, or further surgery when palliative care may have been preferable. Their reported experience suggests that not only do doctors grieve, but also that it affects the treatment that may be offered to the next patient.

Secondly, a 2014 study in US trauma surgeons surveyed respondents for symptoms of post-traumatic stress disorder (PTSD) asking about frequencies of a variety of symptoms [32]. These included questions such as 'do you have repeat disturbing memories, thoughts or images?', 'do you avoid thinking or talking about stressful experiences?', 'do you feel distant or cut off from other people?', and 'do you feel emotionally numb?'. The authors reported that 40% of respondents described PTSD symptoms with 15% meeting formal diagnostic criteria. Risk factors for PTSD were male gender and higher frequency of on-call duties; a fifth of respondents were from a military background. The effects of occupational exposure to traumatic events reported in this study and others have led to the development of specific resources to help those affected [33]. One example—Trauma Risk Management (TRiM)—offers a peer-delivered support system to help support individuals after traumatic events within organisations, especially those working in disaster-exposed occupations where injury or death of a colleague may occur [34]. A more detailed approach to preventing and treating trauma-related mental health problems is described in the trauma-related mental health problems chapter of this textbook.

The effect of death upon surgeons has been poorly described. A 2019 systematic review on the impact of patient death found only five studies [35]. The authors concluded that surgeons carry a strong psychological burden when facing death and are more at risk than the general population from developing problems with long-lasting psychological impact. The risk of getting too close to dying patients means loss of objectivity; staying further away prevents a therapeutic relationship. Both may contribute to a progression towards burnout.

Generic advice on how one should deal with the death of a patient is difficult to provide. Each individual will develop coping mechanisms that suit their personality or management style. There are some support mechanisms described by the growing 'wellness' movement that may have some utility. These include the seeking out of peers who understand the environment in which you work and will be able to provide empathic support without judgement. Mentors may be helpful in debriefing one-on-one in either a formal or informal setting. Other factors that have been associated with improved coping mechanisms for abnormal events include autonomy in a positive work environment in which you feel your contribution is valued. Interests and activities away from work that improve work-life imbalances in favour of the latter are recommended. Self-perception around the irreplaceable importance of one's work are likely to be both wrong and harmful in the long term. The faulty vending machine sign stating 'the light inside has broken but I still work' is an unintentional warning for clinicians who fail to recognise they have a problem [36].

The early twentieth century French vascular surgeon René Leriche wrote 'Every surgeon carries about him a little cemetery, in which from time to time he goes to pray, a cemetery of bitterness and regret, of which he seeks the reason for certain of his failures'. Visiting such a place occasionally is likely to keep a clinician grounded and pragmatic; spending too much time there may be harmful. Developing life-long strategies to manage the inevitable conflict between Palaeolithic emotions and god-like technology is recommended for every clinician who deals with death, traumatic or not. This includes managing its effects on the families they also care for, members of the team they are responsible for, and checking in on colleagues who may have differing or absent coping mechanisms.

Summary

Death from a sudden traumatic event differs in a number of ways from the non-traumatic deaths with which clinicians and patients' families are likely more familiar. Not only are they likely to occur despite aggressive treatment rather than as a result of withdrawal of it, but are more likely to involve a younger population, including children. Trauma deaths also differ in trajectory from that of other diseases. Both acuity and aggressive treatment prevent the 'good' death that many would want for themselves or their loved ones. Breaking sudden death news to family members is particularly difficult for many clinicians but empathy and a structured approach may help both parties. The effects of participating in or bearing witness to efforts to stop death from trauma should be considered on all team members, both junior and senior. Structured debriefing may help manage normal emotional responses to awful events and reduce self-blame. Repeated exposure to trauma(tic) events that end in fatality will have effects upon all staff involved to differing degrees. Individual clinicians working in such areas should develop conscious coping strategies to reduce post-traumatic stress disorder or burnout.

Questions

1. Compared to death from other causes, deaths from trauma:
   (a) Are more likely to happen in the elderly
   (b) Occur, in the majority, several weeks after hospital admission
   (c) Are almost always preventable, if the patient reaches hospital alive
   (d) Are often sudden and unexpected
2. Death trajectories:
   (a) Are theoretical models with some support from analysis of administrative and clinical databases
   (b) Hypothesise that, for chronic disease, after hospital admission the patient will always return to baseline
   (c) Suggest that frailty will always benefit from medical intervention
   (d) For trauma, have a long lead time where discussions with patients and their families allow autonomous decision making
3. Recommended methods for informing families of the sudden death of a patient include:
   (a) Use of euphemisms such as 'gone to another place' to soften the blow
   (b) Using sympathy ("I understand what you're going through right now"), not empathy
   (c) Providing as much information as possible regarding the events that led to the death and a detailed explanation of the efforts of the resuscitation team that were, unfortunately, unsuccessful
   (d) Clearly stating the patient has died after which the clinician should stop talking and wait.
4. Debriefing trauma teams after a patient's death:
   (a) Is a waste of time. Everyone is busy
   (b) Should be led by the most junior team member to provide insight into their perspective
   (c) Should begin by establishing a shared understanding of factual events before discussing emotional responses
   (d) Is mandatory for all those involved
5. Senior clinicians:
   (a) Are never affected by the death of their patients and do not experience grief
   (b) In a study of US trauma surgeons, described PTSD symptoms in 40% of respondents
   (c) With regard to surgeons, have been extensively studied to investigate the impact of patient death upon them
   (d) If affected by the death of a patients, should not seek help from others as this is a sign of weakness

Answers

1. d
2. a
3. d
4. c
5. b

References

1. National Confidential Enquiry into Peri-Operative Deaths. Trauma: Who cares? https://www.ncepod.org.uk/2007report2/Downloads/SIP_summary.pdf. Accessed 14 Aug 2020.
2. Jucá Moscardi M, Meizoso J, Rattan R. Trauma Epidemiology. In: Nasr A, Saavedra Tomasich F, Collaço I, Abreu P, Namias N, Marttos A, editors. The trauma golden hour. Cham: Springer; 2020. https://doi.org/10.1007/978-3-030-26443-7_2.
3. National Audio Office. Major trauma care in England. https://www.nao.org.uk/wp-content/uploads/2010/02/0910213.pdf. Accessed 14 Aug 2020.
4. Leckie T, Roberts R, Lecky F. Timing of trauma deaths within UK hospitals. Trauma Audit and Research Network. https://www.tarn.ac.uk/content/downloads/68/leckie1.pdf. Accessed 14 Aug 2020.
5. Glaser B, Strauss AL. Time for dying. Chicago, Ill: Aldine Publishing Co; 1968.
6. Lunney JR, Lynn J, Foley DJ, Lipson S, Guralnik JM. Patterns of functional decline at the end of life. JAMA. 2003 May 14;289(18):2387–92.
7. Lunney JR, Lynn J, Hogan C. Profiles of older medicare decedents. J Am Geriatr Soc. 2002 Jun;50(6):1108–12.
8. Meier EA, Gallegos JV, Thomas LP, Depp CA, Irwin SA, Jeste DV. Defining a good death (successful dying): literature review and a call for research and public dialogue. Am J Geriatr Psychiatry. 2016 Apr;24(4):261–71.
9. Primack BA, Roberts T, Fine MJ, Dillman Carpentier FR, Rice KR, Barnato AE. ER vs. ED: a comparison of televised and real-life emergency medicine. J Emerg Med. 2012 Dec;43(6):1160–6.
10. Harris D, Willoughby H. Resuscitation on television: realistic or ridiculous? A quantitative observational analysis of the portrayal of cardiopulmonary resuscitation in television medical drama. Resuscitation. 2009 Nov;80(11):1275–9.
11. Portanova J, Irvine K, Yi JY, Enguidanos S. It isn't like this on TV: revisiting CPR survival rates depicted on popular TV shows. Resuscitation. 2015 Nov;96:148–50.
12. Berger E. From Dr. Kildare to Grey's anatomy: TV physicians change real patient expectations. Ann Emerg Med. 2010 Sep;56(3):A21–3.
13. Georgescu V, Tudorache O, Nicolau M, Strambu V. Study regarding the survival of patients suffering a traumatic cardiac arrest. J Med Life. 2015;8(Spec Issue):103–9.
14. Casarett D, Fishman JM, MacMoran HJ, Pickard A, Asch DA. Epidemiology and prognosis of coma in daytime television dramas. BMJ. 2005 Dec 24;331(7531):1537–9.
15. Brindley P. The Most dangerous procedure in the hospital? ICU Manag Pract. 2015;15:2. https://healthmanagement.org/c/icu/issuearticle/communicating-about-difficult-medical-decisions. Accessed 14 Aug 2020
16. Morgan M. Matt Morgan: when nothing is the right thing to say. BMJ. 2020 Feb 18;368:m574.
17. Smith TL, Walz BJ, Smith RL. A death education curriculum for emergency physicians, paramedics, and other emergency personnel. Prehosp Emerg Care. 1999 Jan-Mar;3(1):37–41.
18. Hobgood C, Mathew D, Woodyard DJ, Shofer FS, Brice JH. Death in the field: teaching paramedics to deliver effective death notifications using the educational intervention "GRIEV_ING". Prehosp Emerg Care. 2013 Oct-Dec;17(4):501–10.
19. Smith-Cumberland TL, Feldman RH. EMTs' attitudes' toward death before and after a death education program. Prehosp Emerg Care. 2006 Jan-Mar;10(1):89–95.
20. Kanzaria HK, Probst MA, Hsia RY. Emergency department death rates dropped by nearly 50 percent, 1997-2011. Health Aff (Millwood). 2016;35(7):1303–8.
21. Teno JM, Gozalo P, Trivedi AN, Bunker J, Lima J, Ogarek J, et al. Site of death, place of care, and health care transitions among US Medicare beneficiaries, 2000-2015. JAMA. 2018;320(3):264–71.
22. Khan I, Ridley S. Intensive care: who benefits? JICS. 2014;15(4):297–303.
23. Capuzzo M, Volta C, Tassinati T, Moreno R, Valentin A, Guidet B, et al. Hospital mortality of adults admitted to intensive care units in hospitals with and without intermediate care units: a multicentre European cohort study. Crit Care. 2014 Oct 9;18(5):551.
24. Batley NJ, Bakhti R, Chami A, Jabbour E, Bachir R, El Khuri C, et al. The effect of patient death on medical students in the emergency department. BMC Med Educ. 2017 Jul 10;17(1):110.
25. Hale SJ, Parker MJ, Cupido C, Kam AJ. Applications of Postresuscitation debriefing frameworks in emergency settings: a systematic review. AEM Educ Train. 2020 Jul;4(3):223–30.
26. Kessler DO, Cheng A, Mullan PC. Debriefing in the emergency department after clinical events: a practical guide. Ann Emerg Med. 2015 Jun;65(6):690–8.
27. Morrison LE, Joy JP. Secondary traumatic stress in the emergency department. J Adv Nurs. 2016 Nov;72(11):2894–906.
28. Schmidt M, Haglund K. Debrief in emergency departments to improve compassion fatigue and promote resiliency. J Trauma Nurs. 2017 Sep/Oct;24(5):317–22.
29. Spencer SA, Nolan JP, Osborn M, Georgiou A. The presence of psychological trauma symptoms in resuscitation providers and an exploration of debriefing practices. Resuscitation. 2019;142:175–81.
30. https://www.theguardian.com/world/2020/may/31/jacinda-ardern-political-leaders-can-be-both-empathetic-and-strong. Accessed 14 Aug 2020.
31. Granek L, Tozer R, Mazzotta P, Ramjaun A, Krzyzanowska M. Nature and impact of grief over patient loss on oncologists' personal and professional lives. Arch Intern Med. 2012 Jun 25;172(12):964–6.

32. Joseph B, Pandit V, Hadeed G, Kulvatunyou N, Zangbar B, Tang A, et al. Unveiling posttraumatic stress disorder in trauma surgeons: a national survey. J Trauma Acute Care Surg. 2014;77(1):148–54. discussion 154
33. Brooks SK, Rubin GJ, Greenberg N. Traumatic stress within disaster-exposed occupations: overview of the literature and suggestions for the management of traumatic stress in the workplace. Br Med Bull. 2019;129(1):25–34.
34. https://strongmindresilience.co.uk/courses/trim-trauma-risk-management-an-overview/. Accessed 14 Aug 2020.
35. Joliat GR, Demartines N, Uldry E. Systematic review of the impact of patient death on surgeons. Br J Surg. 2019;106(11):1429–32.
36. Ladher N. Shining a light on burnout. BMJ. 2017;358:j3609.

Legal and Ethical Issues in Trauma Care

3

M. D. Dominic Bell

The diversity of the non-clinical aspects of trauma care, coupled with constantly evolving directives by the regulatory bodies or the law, render it impossible to set out enduring 'rules of engagement' for every possible scenario. The chapter is therefore largely formatted as a series of vignettes which illustrate problematical areas, highlight the key challenges and offer directions to optimise public trust, ensure effective collaboration with other agencies, and limit future professional jeopardy.

Contextual Disclaimer

This chapter does not attempt to describe the relationship between healthcare providers and judicial or regulatory agencies beyond the UK. Even within the UK, Scotland has an independent parliament, legal system and inquest process, and whilst English law covers the generic aspects of Welsh life, independent Welsh law governs local aspects. The contents of the chapter, and particularly the individual scenarios, are illustrative of English law but are hopefully formulated to stimulate the reader to consider how the interface would change in a different country or judicial system.

Introduction

It is the primary responsibility of every healthcare practitioner dealing with anything other than minor trauma to initially focus on the nature and systemic impact of the injury. Standardised approaches or algorithms for the different categories and severity of trauma have been set out within the specialised chapters of this book, but ultimately several generic questions should be asked in one format or another from the point of hospital admission:

- what do we know as to the mechanism of injury from the history
- what can we see in terms of injury and systemic impact
- what can't we see and thereby warrants further investigation
- what is the physiological/resilience context in terms of age and comorbidity
- what are the priorities for intervention
- what ancillary treatments do we need to administer, such as antibiotics, antifibrinolytics or blood products
- which other medical/surgical disciplines do we need to engage et cetera.

M. D. Dominic Bell (✉)
Department of Anaesthesia and Critical Care Medicine, Leeds General Infirmary, Leeds, UK
e-mail: dominic.bell@nhs.net

P. Lax (ed.), *Textbook of Acute Trauma Care*, https://doi.org/10.1007/978-3-030-83628-3_3

Learning objective 1: would it be evident from retrospective review of the medical records that either you or the trauma team had systematically considered, acted upon and documented the above elements of care?

Liaison with individuals beyond the healthcare team is understandably and defensibly not a priority at this stage when dealing with life- or limb-threatening pathology. Communication outside the healthcare team may be focussed on updating the next-of-kin initially (rather than statutory bodies) if the scenario makes this relevant. Even if the police are in attendance due to injuries attributable to or in association with some criminal act, at best they can anticipate a summary position on anticipated clinical course and opinion on survivability within the first 24-h. This may be in contrast to their desire to have access to structured information which allows optimal planning for an investigative process running in parallel with healthcare delivery. In a changing world however, it is not just the police that may be in attendance, but other agencies including counter-terrorism officers, as we enter an era of increasing idealogically driven mass casualty events. Even without such overt criminality, certain scenarios such as industrial accidents automatically trigger the engagement of statutory bodies including the HSE (Health and Safety Executive). This in turn requires access to healthcare information and justifies early consideration of investigations not immediately relevant to the above healthcare priorities. These may include toxicological screens for potential contributory factors to injury including alcohol, recreational drugs or prescription medication.

This naturally raises the questions of who, when and where, representatives of external agencies can access the patient or clinical records. Other questions surround the ability of healthcare practitioners to undertake investigations or access information on their behalf. Are clinicians at risk of breaching employment or regulatory expectations in relation to patient confidentiality, data protection or information governance?

Consider the seemingly least contentious scenario of injuries sustained following a fall from a ladder on a domestic DIY project. There may be nothing meriting investigation by external agencies, and therefore nothing to consider beyond the immediate treatment and obligation to update the next-of-kin. In the event of death, however, there will be an obligatory referral to the coroner. It can reasonably be expected that a practitioner will be capable of not only providing a factual narrative, but will be able to explain the pathophysiological process from the point of injury that culminated in death. This may lead to offering a medical cause of death for the coroner in lieu of post-mortem examination. The escalating move by coroners away from a forensic post-mortem is not based on cost reduction or sensitivity to increasing public opposition to an invasive procedure, although these factors do have to be considered [1–3]. Post-mortem examinations may be unnecessary if there is a clear narrative from an appropriate practitioner on the clinical consequences of injury and the pathway followed by the patient. The precise description of injury from a contemporaneous high-resolution trauma CT, coupled with functional investigations such as echocardiography during life should underpin these comments; indeed, post-mortem CT is now replacing formal autopsy in several cases [4, 5]. If there is sufficient evidence as to a cause of death, further physical examination of the body may not be required or desirable.

Provision of such a narrative demands being able to interrogate the medical records for all the answers to the above generic questions. This will be supplemented by an evaluation as to why all surgical and medical support measures were ineffective in this particular situation, with an accompanying explicit and defensible declaration that no window of opportunity was lost. This responsibility on a medical practitioner is grounded in several ethical, regulatory and legal principles. Ethically, the principles of transparency and accountability are obvious. From a regulatory perspective, the General Medical Council make it an explicit duty of a doctor to assist in such investigations when in the public interest or when compelled by court order [6]. Legally, the coroner has a responsibility laid out in The Coroners and Justice Act (2009) [7]. This includes issuing a Regulation 28 Report to an individual, organisation, local authority or government department or their agencies, if the coroner believes that action needs to be taken to prevent future similar deaths in such circumstances [8]. Scrutiny of both process and outcomes from major trauma via engagement in national audit such as TARN (Trauma Audit and Research Network) to identify variant patterns and underpin research activity are well accepted by clinicians. However, those processes will also be under scrutiny by the coroner in the event of death and within civil litigation in the event of an unfavourable outcome. This demonstrates that even the seemingly non-contentious case of the accidental injury in the home can become problematical. Personal and organisational defensibility in the event of any adverse outcome or complaint is therefore reliant on a high standard of documentation, demonstrating that the above introductory generic questions were asked from the outset and re-asked every time the patient deviated from a favourable trajectory towards recovery.

The relationship between clinicians and the coroner's office has traditionally been challenging from both perspectives, due to a seemingly conditioned response of defensiveness to a request for a medical report in relation to treatment and care. This usually translates into the most limited factual statement, invariably sanitised by the risk management department, and forwarded after a long interval from the initial request and date of treatment. Problems such as lack of availability of the clinical records are not infrequently put forward in mitigation. This inevitably leads to frustration on the part of the coroner and their officers, who will be dealing with an increasingly resentful bereaved family. This then leads in turn into an approach on the part of the clinician which may perpetuate defensiveness and less than helpful reports or statements in future.

It is important for clinicians to remember that the primary role of the coroner is to derive a medical cause of death and a conclusion, (previously called the verdict) that best summarises the context of the trauma. This conclusion may be as simple as RTC, accidental death or suicide, but a key goal of the coroner is to reach this point of closure within a short timeframe for all parties. The coroner is specifically prevented from attributing a death to negligence, or finding an individual or organisation culpable from a civil or criminal perspective. Section 10 of the Coroners and Justice Act 2009 [7] section 2 specifically states that "A determination under subsection [1] (a) may not be framed in such a way as to appear to determine any question of criminal liability on the part of a named person or civil liability". Given the explicit responsibility of any doctor to assist with statutory investigations as a condition of registration with the regulatory body, there is an implicit responsibility to understand the broader professional obligations associated with treating trauma. This includes addressing any request by the coroner to provide a report responsively, remembering that helping the next-of-kin understand why someone died is a responsibility that comes with the privileges of being a doctor and has became a statutory obligation, under 'duty of candour'. Many of the patients that die after admission to hospital (as opposed to those that die at the scene of injury) will have been subject to various surgical and medical interventions. This may prove challenging for a pathologist in attempting to differentiate primary injury from those interventions (e.g. stab wound vs surgical incision for thoracostomy). All competent pathologists will reach a conclusion as to the medical cause of death based on an interpretation of the available clinical information as well as the macroscopic/microscopic findings (and possibly toxicology). It is understandable that those conclusions would be erroneously skewed if the clinical information were inaccessible, incomplete or inaccurate, as highlighted within one of the following scenarios. It is the author's practice as an intensivist to submit the pro forma (attached as appendix) if a challenging case is to undergo a forensic post-mortem examination, and when acting as coroner, to request that this is completed by a responsible clinician prior to post-mortem examination for a relatively complex case. It can be seen therefore, that even this seemingly simple trauma case requires early consideration of the predictable expectations associated with an adverse outcome, serving as a reminder of the importance of standards of documentation.

At the opposite end of the spectrum, with an intense presence and scrutiny from the outset, are those scenarios where the external agencies are themselves under scrutiny. If a patient presents with serious injuries in association with either attempted arrest or actual restraint, regardless of whether those injuries were sustained in activity prior to police engagement, there will be obligatory referral to the IOPC (Independent Office for Police Conduct) [9]. This arouses understandable interest in delineating injuries attributable to factors other than police intervention, the predictable consequences of such injuries, and the presence or otherwise of alcohol, medication or recreational drugs. Suicide attempts whilst in the custody of either police or prison services, also trigger scrutiny by external agencies. This is due to the State's obligation under Article 2 (the right to life) of the European Convention of Human Rights [10], to actively prevent suicide and self-harm in custody, to protect prisoners from serious assault, and to investigate any such incidents. It follows from this that there will be intense scrutiny of medical process to determine whether there was any shortfall in care that could be considered causal for or contributory to any adverse outcome. This may also lead to requests to take images and collect specimens including blood, urine and hair for toxicology analysis. HSE inspectors, as alluded to above, have considerable powers under Section 20 of the Health And Safety at Work etc. Act of 1974, and could reasonably under those powers request information and samples if considered relevant to their investigations [11].

Within the wide spectrum between these potential scenarios, perhaps the most common situation testing the duty of disclosure, regardless of whether the patient has the capacity to consent, is knife or gunshot injury. The commonest situation testing provision of samples for drugs and alcohol arises in relation to an RTC where the patient lacks capacity, and the one scenario where a detailed forensic examination is requested by the police would be following serious sexual assault, again where the patient lacks capacity. The other scenarios which straddle the spectrum are those in which there is a safeguarding issue which can range from children to vulnerable adults within care homes or those with mental health or learning difficulties housed within a community setting. The principles of safeguarding children have been standardised within the European Union for over a decade under the umbrella concept of Keeping Children Safe. There exists explicit responsibilities on individuals and organisations under this guidance, which for healthcare practitioners translates into mandatory training and an obligatory component of history taking and examination of any child presenting with any degree of injury. Similarly, the Care Act of 2014 establishes the principles that underpin the safeguarding of adults, with a corresponding obligation on practitioners to consider such a potential background explanation and escalate concerns through very specific pathways [12]. Although these scenarios clearly represent an interface between trauma and statutory authorities, it should not be considered necessary to duplicate within this chapter the obligations that rest upon practitioners in relation to safeguarding, given the accessibility of guidance within other forums.

One of the key purposes of this chapter is to expand on the primary duty of disclosure in certain other circumstances and clarify what can reasonably be anticipated in terms of requests by external agencies in the above settings, acknowledging that every potential trauma scenario cannot be included. The following vignettes should be considered illustrative therefore rather than comprehensive, but aim to highlight key principles and the multiple grey areas where decision-making and action is required without delay, but where questions may be later raised as to professional conduct.

Scenario 1: Injuries Sustained in an RTC and Police Requests for Specimens

Learning objective 2: to have an understanding of what the police can reasonably request when accompanying a trauma patient suspected of criminal activity, the role of the forensic physician, and the limits of medical responsibility.

A young male is brought in by ambulance with multiple injuries sustained in an RTC as driver, and he will require surgical intervention. The police who have accompanied him suspect he may have been under the influence of drugs or alcohol, and have asked him to provide a specimen of blood or urine which he has refused. He has however had blood taken at the point of cannula insertion for a number of investigations and cross-matching of blood products. He is likely to shortly lose capacity due to induction of anaesthesia. The police officers inform you that in the RTC, a pedestrian sustained serious injuries and has been airlifted to the regional Major Trauma Centre. What factors are relevant and what options are open to both the treating clinician and the attendant police officers?

Principles and Opinion

The Police Reform Act of 2002 allows the police within England, Wales and Scotland to obtain blood specimens from people who have been involved in road traffic accidents who are unable to give consent [13]. The assessment of the patient's capacity to undergo or refuse such testing is the responsibility of the attending police officer and the instructed forensic physician (historically referred to as a police surgeon), not the clinician responsible for care. The clinician treating the patient cannot be requested to either make the capacity assessment or to undertake the sampling procedure. If the patient is considered to have capacity to refuse such testing, this cannot be undertaken by the use of force or restraint, and it is the refusal to provide a specimen that becomes the criminal offence [14]. If a specimen is taken from a patient lacking capacity, this cannot be tested without the future consent of the patient, but any such refusal as above then becomes the criminal offence.

Regardless of whether the patient has or lacks capacity, it is the responsibility of the police in these circumstances to confirm with the responsible clinician that either the assessment of capacity or the sampling procedure will not interfere with the process of care. Such confirmation by the treating doctor does not give credence to any subsequent allegation on the part of the patient of aiding and abetting an assault by the forensic physician in undertaking blood sampling without consent, since this procedure is lawful in these circumstances under the legislation. There will inevitably be a number of grey areas within such a scenario which cannot be prescriptively defined within either legislation or professional guidance. In the initial stages of clinical management, any competent police officer is likely to take the view that either the treating doctor or the patient will be likely to refuse such sampling, regardless of the logistical difficulties in achieving the attendance of a forensic physician. There will be an understandable preference for the police to avoid a patient refusal, given the future potential for questioning the validity of capacity for such a refusal in the circumstances of significant injury requiring imminent surgical intervention. This potentially could lead to the patient avoiding conviction on the charge of failing to provide a specimen. The justification for waiting until the patient is anaesthetised, clearly lacking capacity at this stage, and therefore testable under the law, whilst understandable, can reasonably be interpreted as contrary to the spirit of the law, and would therefore require further caveats to be justifiable. If the patient required a short procedure under general anaesthesia (e.g. joint relocation), with an expectation of an early return to full capacity, it would be appropriate for the forensic physician to take the view that the request should be placed before the patient in the post-operative period. If however, it is likely that the patient will require prolonged surgical intervention such that a return of full capacity could not be predicted within any reasonable timeframe, then it would appear reasonable to undertake sampling at an early stage if this did not interfere with the process of clinical care. This is to ensure that the likely administration of significant volumes of blood products and intravenous fluids does not compromise any rational interpretation of later blood results,

Another grey area relates to the actual technique of sampling, since although there are specific procedures that have to be followed including division of the specimen into two samples, there is no absolute specificity that a sample cannot be drawn from an indwelling cannula despite the potential for dilution or contamination of such a specimen. It is however the author's opinion and practice that it is reasonable for a forensic physician, having been fully informed and compliant with infection control procedures, to take a sample from a three-way tap attached to an arterial or central venous cannula. Blood must first be withdrawn in such a volume (e.g. 10 ml) that a subsequent result is predictably representative of plasma levels at that time of sampling, in line with routine clinical practice. It is the author's opinion that such an approach is defensible in terms of patient well-being, reducing the risks of needle-stick injury, and in terms of reliability of the specimen.

Although the vignette hinted at the possibility of utilising specimens already taken for clinical purposes, this would not be considered compliant with long established principles in relation to evidential standards under PACE (Police and Criminal Evidence Act 1984) [15]. If, however, there was any suggestion of neurological dysfunction in the form of confusion, agitation or drowsiness, and the medical team was attempting to distinguish alcohol/drug intoxication from CNS pathology, it would be reasonable to send specimens for toxicology. A request could be made that the laboratory retain the sample, or formally transfer it over as evidence, for any future re-examination, which would allow the police and CPS to consider how the clinical specimen and results could be utilised in any future prosecution.

The vignette also suggests that the doctor should support concepts of justice in view of the serious injuries suffered by an innocent third party, but while such a position is understandable, the consequences as opposed to the actions and potentially criminal behaviour of the driver, do not modify the above principles and professional expectations.

Scenario 2: Medical Deterioration after a Police Arrest

Learning objective 3: to understand the circumstances in which disclosure of clinical information is justified.

A break-in is reported to the police, culminating in the suspect falling approximately 20 feet from a second-floor balcony as officers approached the building and he attempted escape. Although seemingly injured, the suspect forcibly resists arrest, necessitating restraint, and during the process of applying handcuffs he becomes less responsive. Paramedic assistance is requested and he is transferred as an emergency, unresponsive with a systolic blood pressure of 90 mmHg and requiring assisted ventilation with 100% oxygen to maintain an oxygen saturation greater than 90%. The police (with one handcuff still applied) accompany his admission to the emergency department, and are requesting toxicology investigations, an update on the results of the radiological investigations, and a review by a forensic physician.

Principles and Opinion

Despite the current clinical circumstances, the police have made an arrest, the patient correspondingly remains under arrest, and the police officers have an additional responsibility to ensure that the individual does not pose a risk of injury to any third party. Although the clinical picture suggests significant surgical or medical pathology, police and prison services will be both educated in and familiar with prisoners capable of manipulating healthcare practitioners and the hospital environment. There is a requirement on practitioners therefore to confirm and communicate that the clinical picture is not only genuinely indicative of significant pathology, but also does not indicate temporary systemic dysfunction due to a recoverable problem such as a seizure or drug intoxication due to the suspect having swallowed 'evidence'. If it becomes clear after investigation that the patient has sustained significant injury such as intracranial haemorrhage or ruptured spleen that will require general anaesthesia or surgical intervention, this information should be communicated to the responsible officers at the earliest opportunity. This will allow planning for the arrest process that is in harmony with healthcare provision, especially if the patient requires admission to intensive care or a hospital ward.

Disclosure of clinical information is therefore warranted. Disclosure would also be warranted for lesser degrees of injury or medical problems if a patient was to be transferred back into custody. This ensures that healthcare practitioners within the police or prison service are adequately informed as to the nature of the problem. The information is also required to enable the police officers to pass on accurate information to the IOPC to assist in planning of their investigation.

It is unlikely that such clinical information will be challenged by any forensic physician instructed by the police, and nor is it likely that specimens will be requested for toxicology analysis, since the offence lies in the 'breaking and entering' rather than in any associated state of intoxication. However, it is inevitable that questions will be raised as to whether any injuries and the cause of the collapse can be attributed to the primary fall or the secondary period of agitation and restraint. This scenario will therefore require at some stage that a practitioner provide opinion to help not only make this distinction, but also to distinguish between pre-admission findings and post-admission features of surgical intervention. This in turn requires a high standard of documentation, based on a practitioner's understanding and anticipation of such a future request.

It is also likely that the police will ask for an early forensic examination with photography to assist with the IOPC investigation. If the patient has capacity once stabilised, they are free to consent to or decline such an assessment. However, there is no authority for police personnel to undertake such investigations if the patient is sedated or lacks capacity for any other reason, even if the police have sought and gained proxy consent from the next-of-kin.

The police do however have powers of search (including the oral cavity) following an arrest, or indeed pre-arrest if they have reasonable grounds to suspect that a crime has been committed for which arrest would be appropriate. This would make it reasonable to search the patient, their clothing and belongings, for illicit drugs, weapons or stolen property, and to retain such items including clothing, for forensic analysis.

Given the clinical requirement for a full and thorough patient examination in these circumstances, it would be reasonable to engage the police during removal of clothing and other belongings. This is not only in the interests of justice, but also because the police will be vigilant by training when searching an individual for items which generate a risk to the searcher such as contaminated needles.

Confirmation of the individual's identity is important from a clinical perspective in retrieving any relevant past records. The police are empowered under Section 61 of PACE (Police and Criminal Evidence Act 1984) and Code D to undertake mobile biometric testing with fingerprint scanners of an individual where either an offence has been committed or suspected, and either no name is provided or the name provided is suspected to be false [15]. Such a process of identification can not only be advantageous clinically to the patient but can also assist in identifying and mobilising next-of-kin.

It can be concluded therefore that the clinical safety and well-being of the patient must always be a primary consideration for the clinician, but provision of information and a collaborative approach with arresting officers can not only assist that process by early identification but can also protect the safety and well-being of healthcare providers.

Scenario 3: Trauma in Association with Mental Health Disorder Complicated by Non-compliance, Needle-Stick Injury and Data Protection Issues

Learning objective 4: to understand the principles of capacity, justification for medical interventions including sedation against a patient's wishes, and information governance and management of a needle-stick injury where the patient lacks capacity.

An individual with a suspected mental health disorder walks into the road and is hit by a car. They are aggressive and refusing hospital assessment, culminating in being brought into the emergency department having been restrained by the police within an ambulance. They continue to refuse medical attention and respond aggressively to restraint. It is debated and considered by police, paramedics and clinical staff that they represent a danger to themself and others, and the ED doctor asks the police to maintain restraint whilst an intramuscular injection of sedative is attempted. During a violent response to this attempted intervention, a paramedic and police officer suffer needle-stick injuries. The medication is eventually administered and with anaesthetic assistance the patient is sedated and ventilated for the trauma CT scan. The mobile fingerprint scanner does not provide the identity of anyone on the database, but during the police search a phone is found. The ED doctor activates this using the patient's thumbprint, and having looked at various text messages and rung certain numbers, is able to identify the patient. A review of medical records indicates previous interaction with mental health services and a hospital admission with a drug overdose. In the context of the needle-stick injury, the police and paramedics are asking if the records indicate either HIV or hepatitis status.

Principles and Opinion

Every practitioner will be familiar with the interplay between mental health disorders and trauma. There exists a spectrum between a violent suicide attempt such as the jump from a high bridge or before an oncoming train, to the patient unaware of the significance of accidental injury and requirement for medical intervention. The interface between treating clinicians, mental health practitioners and the police, and responsibilities under the Mental Health Act (1983) [16] (MHA), Mental Capacity Act (2005) [17] (MCA), and common law in these nuanced circumstances, remain a challenge. If the police were concerned in this scenario about damage to property or injury to a third-party, the individual could be arrested to 'preserve the peace'. If in the more likely interpretation of this scenario, the police were primarily concerned with the well-being of the individual, they could be detained under Section 136 MHA for a 24-h period. There is an associated requirement for ambulance attendance, with an expectation that a paramedic would make the judgement call as to whether the individual should be taken to an emergency department or to an alternative place of safety for assessment and management of the mental health disorder.

This particular individual having been brought to ED, the injuries and necessity for investigation and treatment steer management away from MHA in the first instance and towards MCA. There is an expectation that an assessment of capacity will be attempted before progression towards sedation under restraint. This would be considered justifiable (and thereby defensible) under the principles of best interests, necessity, immediacy, and the 'least restrictive option' as defined under the MCA.

The attendant police officers could reasonably decline to assist in the proposed sedative strategy, since this falls outwith areas of training, expertise and responsibility. There is also an expectation that any healthcare facility undertaking such an exercise will ensure the availability of appropriately trained staff. This raises the possibility of the hospital carrying legal liability for any injuries sustained by police officers during such an intervention, and places certain moral and ethical obligations on the institution following the needle-stick injuries.

The position at law under the MCA however, is that no intervention can be undertaken on a patient lacking capacity that is not in their best interests. This principle seemingly would preclude blood sampling for HIV and hepatitis status for the benefit of a third party. This principle is consistently and explicitly overridden when undertaking these investigations prior to consideration of patients for organ donation, with endorsement of such practice by the Department of Health [18]. It appears illogical to differentiate between this form of benefit by reduction of risk to a predictably anonymous third-party and not to undertake such testing to allow a healthcare professional to make an early and informed choice regarding post exposure prophylaxis (PEP). Treatment with PEP has its own significant risks, regardless of the destructive impact of worry, particularly when the individual concerned is exposing themselves to risk whilst acting in the patient's best interests. This introduces concepts of 'reciprocity' within the relationship between healthcare practitioner and patient. There may be a reasonable expectation that patients would consent if capacitous to withdrawal of a blood sample from an indwelling cannula for the purpose of testing, given the significance of the result for the practitioner. It has been the author's practice over the timeframe of this impasse to request proxy consent from the next-of-kin, utilising the concept of 'substituted judgement' [19]. This is where the next of kin offers an opinion that this is what the patient would have consented to if they were able to process this request, or to proceed to testing if it is not likely that next-of-kin will be identifiable within a short timeframe. Given that for maximum efficacy, PEP should be started as soon as possible (and certainly within 12 h) this is a time-sensitive issue. It has also been the author's practice to lobby for explicit endorsement of this approach from professional, regulatory and government bodies. Despite the introduction of presumed consent for organ retrieval in law within the UK over this timeframe, there has been consistent disengagement at an appropriately senior level. This is despite the tangible risk of compromised care to patients if practitioners understandably distanced themselves from hazardous procedures if they will not be able to make informed choices, if needle-stick injury or other contamination occurs. This scenario therefore demands moral courage on the part of senior doctors to check existing results or undertake testing. This will optimise not only staff welfare, but actually promote optimal care for patients and not deny their broader best interests by allowing testing for the health and well-being of staff who have put themselves at risk in order to provide clinical care. If, furthermore, optimal patient care depends on optimal multi-agency co-operation and collaboration, this principle should naturally be extended to the police officers who have sought to ensure the well-being of the patient from the outset. It can be noted in relation to this particular issue that in some jurisdictions around the world, individuals can be ordered to undergo HIV testing if they spit at or bite an arresting officer, with criminal charges against anyone refusing to undergo testing [20–22].

The broader issue in this particular case of ensuring the engagement of psychiatric services will be a familiar problem for most practitioners. Liaison psychiatry services will predictably declare the patient unfit for psychiatric assessment until the immediate requirement for medical and surgical investigation and treatment has been met. This usually leads to a delay in instituting an emergency section order, and a suggestion of re-referral once capacity has returned and a psychiatric assessment can be undertaken. This inevitably leaves the responsible healthcare team attempting to treat the patient within the principles of both the MCA and MHA. One difficulty that this leads to is the decision-making around sedative and antipsychotic therapy during attempts at weaning following operative intervention or periods of intensive care. There are a multitude of strategies that will be familiar to intensive care practitioners to wean a patient from conventional sedation, including dexmedetomidine and clonidine infusions. It has been the author's practice to introduce a second-generation antipsychotic agent such as risperidone early in the admission process for not only this category of patient, but in those where aggressive non-compliance is evident at an early stage. This may also be due to diffuse axonal injury or hypoxic brain injury in young male patients, particularly those with a background of recreational drug usage.

The broader interface with psychiatry services is beyond the remit of this chapter but it is anticipated that practitioners will be able to access local policies on this subject.

The ancillary issue within this scenario of unlocking the patient's phone with their own thumbprint is likely to meet with a range of opinion. This is based not only on an understanding of the Caldicott principles [23, 24] within UK law or those of the Data Protection Act (1998) [25], but on uncertainty as to how compliance with information governance will be interpreted by either employing organisation or the regulatory body if a complaint is raised in this regard. On the facts of this case, the approach adopted would be justified if the phone was interrogated solely for the purpose of identifying and communicating with the next-of-kin. The intention was to both identify the patient and ensure early engagement of partner or family, but this is again a scenario requiring moral courage on the part of a senior practitioner.

Scenario 4: Gunshot or Knife Injury

Learning objective 5: understanding the circumstances that dictate a duty of disclosure.

An individual is dropped off outside the ED by 'friends' who then drive away. Reception staff ask for clinical assistance and it becomes apparent that the patient has been stabbed in the chest and abdomen. They volunteer a name and age but not address, next-of-kin, or any information in relation to the assailant. They state they will refuse all care and leave the hospital if the police are called.

Principles and Opinion

This recurring scenario highlights the enduring conflict between duties of confidentiality to the individual patient and of disclosure in the public interest. There has been a long-standing duty of disclosure in relation to communicable disease, but the importance of confidentiality in promoting attendance for and compliance with medical treatment was highlighted by the emerging AIDS epidemic in the 1980s. In the scenario described, in the absence of any reports or features of self-harm, it is apparent that a crime has been committed and it is the responsibility of the police to assess the risk of another attack to the presenting patient, healthcare staff or other members of the general public.

The General Medical Council as regulatory body correspondingly issued guidance on this matter in October 2009 setting out the responsibility on doctors to inform the police whenever they treat a suspected victim of serious knife or gun crime [26]. This particular duty of disclosure remains somewhat ambiguous however, given that there is no specified responsibility to provide identifiable patient details or to allow the police access to the victim. The duty of disclosure only arises in the context of 'serious' crime, without specifying the threshold between serious and non-serious. Such ambiguity therefore requires an exercise in professional judgement by a senior clinician who would be able to shoulder allegations of either an inappropriate breach in confidentiality or the contrary failure to inform police of a serious crime and thereby fulfil responsibilities to protect either the patient or any other party from future injury.

One key question to be asked is how the various regulatory and disciplinary bodies, or civil courts, would interpret the subsequent death of this patient from a further attack after discharge from hospital if the police had not been informed. Increasingly, there is also personal and institutional anxiety regarding how such an outcome might be reported in the lay media.

The situation becomes even more challenging in the context of injuries sustained in potential preparation for terrorist activity. The government-led multi-agency 'Prevent' programme aims to identify radicalisation or potential transition towards terrorist activity, and this exercise has become a component of mandatory training for healthcare practitioners [27]. Disclosure is clearly justified in the public interest in order to prevent a serious threat to public health and national security, but concerns have been raised from within the medical profession that there is an intrinsic risk of racial profiling with all the attendant adverse consequences. Doctors are placed in a difficult position therefore if a patient presents with serious burns injuries in association with potential features of blast, which are reportedly due to a domestic kitchen fire. The focus question as above is to look at the potential adverse consequences for innocent third parties and indeed the treating doctor if either the patient or their associates go on to carry out a terrorist atrocity. Once again, this is clearly the responsibility of a senior decision-maker.

Reporting Domestic Violence

A more common scenario exemplifying conflict in relation to disclosure relates to a suspicion of domestic violence. Doctors have a duty to be alert to signs of domestic abuse under the concept of safeguarding patients from future harm, but also have a responsibility to respect confidentiality, acknowledging that in the context of being offered an accidental explanation for injuries, it is not the primary role of the doctor to act as investigator, judge and jury. Decisions about disclosure should be made in partnership with the patient, but a patient who has capacity can refuse to allow disclosure [6].

Once again the focus question is how re-presentation of the patient with life-threatening or life-changing injuries would be interpreted by various external parties if consideration had not been given at the point of earlier attendance to escalation of concerns and at least some primary attempts at safeguarding, such as requesting GP opinion and review.

Given the inevitable absence of specific direction for every potential scenario, this problem should be addressed by a senior decision-maker and in collaboration with the patient and senior colleagues.

Scenario 5: Serious Sexual Assault and Request for Forensic Examination

Learning objective 6: understanding the circumstances in which the police might request a full forensic examination.

A young woman is found on public land in a semi-conscious state with evidence of multiple areas of external bruising including to the face and head, with rape/sexual assault suspected due to clothing having been removed and evidence of focal injury in the genital area. The police attended at the scene and accompanied the patient to the emergency department. They have requested the attendance of a forensic physician to examine the patient and take specimens. The patient is sedated and intubated prior to a trauma CT scan which reveals the presence of extensive intracranial haemorrhage requiring surgical evacuation.

Principles and Opinion

The police have a responsibility to investigate this crime and given the distinct possibility that the patient will not be able to contribute to the prosecution process given the nature of the head injury, there is critical dependence on forensic evidence in identifying the perpetrator. The immediate clinical priority is however evacuation of the large subdural haematoma and to address any other life or limb-threatening injuries. Gathering pictorial evidence of external injuries prior to wound toilet/suture, historically defaulted to a departmental digital camera or a phone camera, but this practice is contrary to contemporary expectations of data protection and information governance [28, 29]. If however a SOCO (scenes of crime officer) was present and photography during clinical assessment did not interfere with or delay treatment, it would be reasonable to accommodate this request. If the hospital had the support of a medical photography department, this would represent a reasonable alternative from perspective of image quality, acceptability for prosecution purposes and concepts of data protection/information governance. It would not however be reasonable to delay craniotomy for a full forensic examination, but this could be accommodated following definitive surgical intervention. Examination should be performed prior to other interventions such as intimate examination or scrubbing wounds to the hands, thereby avoiding contamination of essential evidence prior to trained forensic examination. If infection control procedures can be complied with, there is no barrier to this process being undertaken in the operating theatre setting given the space, light and equipment such as stirrups to optimise the examination process. It is more conventional however to undertake this examination in the critical care setting once the patient has been stabilised, and staff will be familiar with the logistical difficulties of accommodating specialised light sources et cetera for this process. It is also predictable that the police will request early access to the clinical records to include all findings and observations, and this usually follows provision by the police of a signed consent form by the next-of-kin. Disclosure in these circumstances would be in line with the expectations of the regulatory body on a doctor to assist with investigations directed towards crime solving and justice. The ramifications of such a scenario are escalated if the patient is either in state detention within a mental health facility, or is identifiable as a vulnerable adult by virtue of learning disabilities, with obligatory engagement of additional agencies.

No single source of advice can provide a blueprint for every potential scenario, and these examples necessitate engagement of risk management departments within hospitals.

Scenario 6: Trauma Compounded by Iatrogenic Insult

Learning objective 7: understanding the duty of candour after iatrogenic injury and the potential for professional jeopardy when submitting verbal or written evidence.

A young patient is brought to the emergency department with GCS 3/15 having been assaulted with a blow to the head and a secondary brain injury at the point of impact with the pavement. He was intubated and ventilated and the CT scan demonstrates extradural, subdural and parenchymal haemorrhage. At craniotomy the underlying brain was severely swollen and following evacuation of the haemorrhage the bone flap was not replaced. High ICP was recorded following this procedure and the pupils became fixed and dilated on day three. A forensic post-mortem examination concluded that the cause of death was severe traumatic brain injury. As the intensive care consultant, you are asked to provide a statement for the police. During review of the electronic records, you identify a blood gas result from the emergency department which records a pH of 7, a pO_2 of 6 and a pCO_2 of 24 kPa, raising questions of suboptimal care of a head injured patient. A blood gas undertaken two hours later in the operating theatre was essentially normal apart from a residual acidosis. There is no record of either this result or of any untoward incident within either the paper or electronic records, but your enquiries identify a problem with the setup of the ventilator circuit in the emergency department. How do you proceed?

Principles and Opinion

The practitioner tasked with responding to the police request is placed in a difficult position, since there are significant implications of this discovery within the healthcare setting for individuals, departments and the wider organisation. Having identified an issue that meets the criteria for serious incident reporting under the NHS systems of STEIS (Strategic Executive

Information System) [30] and the NRLS (National Reporting & Learning System) [31], the practitioner is obliged to trigger an incident report within his own institution. A 'duty of candour' exists in relation to the police investigation, due to the inescapable fact that the patient was exposed to significant and sustained recognised secondary cerebral insults. It could be argued that these were contributory to the findings of the grossly swollen brain at surgery and progression to brainstem death. It could correspondingly be argued by any competent criminal defence team provided with such evidence that a 'novus actus interveniens' (a new intervening act) had broken the chain of causation: "my client accepts he inflicted injury, but it was the negligence of the healthcare team that resulted in the death". It would then be left to the prosecution to argue that the deceased was only exposed to negligence within the healthcare system due to the malevolent act of the assailant, and/or that the deceased would ultimately have died as a consequence of the primary injuries albeit at potentially a later stage, and that the accused should still be found guilty of manslaughter. Given the significance of these events in the context of a criminal prosecution, if the intensivist was to deliberately withhold this information in a report statement providing an overview of care, they would be vulnerable to censure from the regulatory body. However, prosecution for perjury would be unlikely given that an omission is not synonymous with giving false information. The 'duty of candour' as set out within the conditions of registration by the GMC as regulatory body also extends to disclosure to the next-of-kin, regardless of the potential for this to trigger litigation [32]. Ultimately however, the success of civil proceedings would depend on the ability to prove causation i.e. that the breach of duty caused a loss that would not otherwise have occurred. The implications of either a causal or contributory role in the patient's death are therefore highly significant on multiple fronts. This raises questions as to whether the intensivist as a witness of fact rather than an independent expert witness should be offering an opinion on this aspect. This situation is completely different to that described within the introduction, emphasising a responsibility to assist either the coroner or a pathologist in interpreting clinical information and offering an opinion on the cause of death. It is predictable therefore that if advice is sought from either the hospital risk management team or a defence organisation, this will be to provide no commentary on the potential contributory role to the patient's death, and to restrict the content of the report to the factual elements of condition and treatment following admission to the intensive care unit. In the event of such advice, it would then become the responsibility of the hospital risk management and legal teams to inform coroner, police and next-of-kin. The police will predictably seek witness statements from the practitioners involved during that initial period. It is likely that the statements will follow an interview by police under caution, emphasising the importance of accuracy and consistency in evidence. Practitioners continue to be charged with perjury, following the naïve assumption that the police or coroner will not be able to understand complex medical detail. In this scenario, it is likely that the responding anaesthetist and emergency department teams will be interviewed over events. A more senior individual within that department will also be interviewed with regards to responsibility for the specification, preparation and testing of ventilatory equipment and breathing circuits. Whilst all these individuals will be covered by the 'crown indemnity scheme', whereby the NHS insures its employees for work carried out on its behalf, this scenario highlights the conflict between support for the individual employee and protection of institutional reputation. No institution would wish to face criticism for corporate negligence in the event of being found responsible for inadequate governance standards in relation to the purchase, sterilisation, maintenance or preparation of equipment that was ultimately not fit for its intended purpose. It would be unedifying but foreseeable if the stance of the hospital was one of accepting that the event demonstrated shortfalls, but that ultimately it was the responsibility of any competent anaesthetist to ensure that a ventilator and breathing circuit was functioning correctly before use. This is particularly true given the availability of both monitors and alarms for these parameters, and nationally agreed minimum monitoring standards. This potential for sacrificing the protection of an employee to maintain institutional reputation emphasises the importance of individual professional indemnity to supplement the NHS scheme, a concept which receives further emphasis when considering other potential ramifications of this scenario. It could be considered reasonably foreseeable that if the individual practitioner is to be 'isolated' from the broader organisation and held solely responsible, that their defence could include criticism of other individuals and departments. This could be for failing to provide adequate levels of supervision, (thereby bringing the on-call consultant into the frame), or failing to provide adequate critical incident training including simulation, thereby bringing everyone from educational supervisors to training programme directors under scrutiny. The importance and value of independent professional indemnity becomes immediately apparent if practitioners are facing criticism from the primary anaesthetist's defence team, at a time when the institution has no wish to embrace corporate responsibility. These issues will predictably not be active during the prosecution of the original assailant, but would surface in any subsequent inquest or GMC investigation. In relation to a potential inquest, once criminal proceedings are initiated against a person who may have caused the death, the investigation/inquest process will be suspended until the criminal case is concluded. This is because an inquest conclusion/verdict has to be compatible with the findings of the 'higher' criminal court. If the accused is convicted of either murder or manslaughter, the coroner will usually close their inquest with a summary conclusion of 'unlawful killing', there being no need for a hearing since the evidence has already been explored in open court. In the scenario described, it is likely however that the coroner will conduct an inquest hearing, given the public interest issues associated with healthcare failings, which would not necessarily be evaluated to any reasonable degree within the setting of the criminal court, and which may activate responsibilities under Regulation 28. It is foreseeable that the defence team acting for the now professionally isolated primary anaesthetist will call the individuals with the various roles as set out above to at least establish various mitigating factors in anticipation of the predictable secondary GMC hearing. It is equally foreseeable that a coroner would hold such an inquest with a jury and allow them, notwithstanding a conviction for manslaughter in the criminal courts, to reach a verdict/conclusion that "hospital failings significantly contributed to the death", with obvious professional repercussions for a number of individuals. The scope of this chapter does not include detailed analysis of GMC disciplinary process, but readers should be aware of how certain high-profile cases have been managed over the last decade. There have been notable differences in process and outcomes depending on the profile of support for the practitioner from the broader professional body[1] [33, 34]. Although mitigating circumstances can be accommodated, ultimately the GMC expects and considers honesty, candour, insight and definitive remedial action when reaching a conclusion on sanctions. This further emphasises the importance of a consistent narrative from the point of initial questioning by senior clinicians or Trust executives, through to police, coroner and regulatory body.

[1] *R v Bawa-Garba* [2016] EWCA Crim 1841 (https://www.bailii.org/ew/cases/EWCA/Crim/2016/1841.html); *R v Sellu* [2016] EWCA Crim 1716 (https://www.bailii.org/ew/cases/EWCA/Crim/2016/1716.html)

Scenario 7: Family Opposing Limitation of Treatment after Severe Traumatic Injury

Learning objective 8: to understand the relative authority of healthcare team versus patient's family when a favourable outcome is not anticipated, and the options and pitfalls when addressing conflict.

A young male overturned a quad bike at high speed and was trapped beneath it. At the time of paramedic attendance, he was unresponsive with an oxygen saturation of 70% and a systolic blood pressure of 70 mmHg. He was intubated at the scene and the trauma CT revealed chest wall injuries, pulmonary contusions and ruptured spleen and liver lacerations. His intra-abdominal injuries were managed conservatively after interventional radiology could not define an active bleeding point. The CT head demonstrated minor traumatic subarachnoid haemorrhage and the early features of hypoxic ischaemic injury. After 48 hours of sedation, his cardio-respiratory parameters were sufficiently stable to permit a clinical neurological assessment, which demonstrated high tone and spontaneous extensor posturing. A repeat CT scan demonstrated progression of the HIE (hypoxic ischaemic encephalopathy) and an EEG on day five was reported as 'alpha coma'. This result is where the alpha activity normally seen in wakefulness is coupled with clinical unresponsiveness/coma, a characteristic feature of brain injury of this nature. The family were unwilling to consider any withdrawal of support and after long debate a tracheostomy was undertaken to facilitate weaning from ventilatory support. An attempt was made to agree ceilings of treatment and DNAR in the event of any future deterioration, but the family were opposed to any such limitation. How do you progress this issue?

Principles and Opinion

The era of medical paternalism is long since dead, replaced not only by patient autonomy, but an accompanying cycle of public suspicion and challenge to medical decision-making. This is not just attributable to the explosion of readily available information on medical matters, or the ease of access to supportive legal advice underpinned by the Human Rights Act 1998 [10], but is also fuelled by the series of healthcare scandals that have undermined public trust. These scandals include paediatric cardiac surgery [35, 36], retained organs [37, 38], empirical DNAR decisions [39, 40] and broader institutional failings such as the Mid-Staffordshire problems [41], with an on-going pattern indicating that these are issues that cannot be dismissed as historical. It may be understandable to any competent healthcare professional that this particular patient will not re-gain a meaningful quality-of-life in the event of survival, and the proposition of a limitation of life-sustaining medical treatment (LSMT) may be a logical next step. However, it is equally understandable that the next-of-kin may not wish to see their hope extinguished. They may also be suspicious that the medical opinion is wrong, premature or based on discrimination due to disability. In more extreme cases there may be a suspicion that this is motivated by resource implications or even a wish to move towards organ donation, particularly given the current context where 'presumed consent' has now been enshrined in law. The simple position at law is that no doctor can be compelled to provide treatment that they do not believe to be in the patient's best interests. However, the nuances of what constitutes a patient's 'best interests' generate an opportunity for challenge if family understanding or trust is limited from the outset. Not many intensive care practitioners would be prepared to declare with confidence that the outcome would inevitably be one of the vegetative state at that stage. It is predictable that a second opinion from neurology or neuro-rehabilitation (who naturally deal with extreme neurological disability) would declare that the outcome can only be specified after the passage of time. Hence, it becomes the pragmatic solution to undertake a tracheostomy, wean from ventilatory support, and transfer the patient under the care of rehabilitation. There is the hope from a critical care perspective that colleagues in rehabilitation would not endorse reintroduction of LSMT or resuscitation in the event of new complications. The challenge arises if the family's position has become polarised by their perspective on the preferred medical position of withdrawing LSMT at the earlier point in time, and are not prepared to countenance any future restriction in medical treatment. This recurring scenario has many facets other than simple occupation of a critical care bed. It is inevitable that a disagreement of this nature will be picked up by other families, leading to an amplified level of suspicion, compromising optimal communication and decision-making within the broader critical care unit. Whilst natural that clinicians of any grade would not wish to be the subject of complaint by continuing to push for ceilings of treatment, this can lead to an adverse impact on other members of the multidisciplinary team. This may disproportionately affect nursing staff and therapists if they are being expected to provide cares that ultimately have no prospect of a satisfactory outcome. An impasse of this nature can have the additional adverse impact from a societal ethics perspective of compromised access to critical care for those patients capable of benefiting; this scenario is at variance with the expectation that resources are rationally utilised. The principles of promoting a patient's 'best interests' in circumstances where there is a loss of capacity are set out within the Mental Capacity Act 2005 [17], and these include both offering and seeking a genuinely independent second opinion in challenging situations. This may ultimately lead to the Court of Protection when these issues cannot be resolved even with techniques such as independent mediation. In these particular circumstances, the majority of the five statutory principles relating to mental capacity are not applicable. This is because it would be agreed by all parties that there can be no presumption of capacity, that the patient cannot be supported to the point of making a capacitous decision, and this is not a scenario therefore where a patient should be allowed to make an 'unwise decision'. The Court will therefore be focused on best interests (which are broad under the Act), but would not be independently responsible for defining the future process of care. This is the responsibility of the healthcare facility making the application, with the Court's role being to reach a conclusion as to whether the application proposal is in line with the patient's broader best interests and therefore lawful. It should be apparent to anyone that if an impasse is maintained by a breakdown of trust, this is unlikely to be restored by the decision of a court, where there will inevitably be a suspicion that there will be deference to medical opinion. Furthermore, if the court sanctions a withdrawal of LSMT, how will this practically take place and be compatible with principles of a good death, if the family remain strongly opposed? Similarly, how would the practicalities of not optimising a progressively deteriorating patient at ward level be managed with an antagonistic family, if the court has declared that the treating team does not have to consider readmission to ICU, escalation of support, or resuscitation manoeuvres? It is difficult to ignore a rising pattern of broader public engagement and activism in these cases fuelled by social media[2] [42], and the demonstrations outside hospitals and explicit hostility towards healthcare practitioners likely represent a future recurring theme. It is understandable and inevitable therefore that there is limited inclination within health care teams to take a firm approach with families resistant to any form of limitation. A significant number of patients are therefore stepped down to long-term care facilities, with the hope that over time the next-of-kin may accept that the patient will not make a meaningful recovery. They may correspondingly accept either palliative management of new complications, or in the case of PVS, withdrawal of artificial nutrition and hydration after the diagnosis has been consolidated by the passage of time. As an aside, one extraneous factor that has currently shifted the pendulum back

[2] https://www.bbc.co.uk/news/health-40554462

towards a more paternalistic approach to healthcare decision-making has been the COVID pandemic. Ceilings of treatment and resuscitation status have been expected to have been defined within the community to avoid hospitalisation, or within a short time after admission for those who have been hospitalised. Given the limitations of attendance of the next-of-kin in these circumstances, it is inevitable that complaints will arise at some future point. The question will be asked whether 'exceptional circumstances' which dictate a requirement to use scarce resources most efficiently, justify processes such as reverse triage or sweeping restrictions such as not countenancing hospital admissions from care homes. There is clearly a requirement for moral courage on the part of healthcare practitioners in such challenging times, but it remains to be seen how complaints will be addressed in the aftermath of these events. This is a subject for a monograph in its own right, but for now, interested readers can consider whether Dr. Pou in the extraordinary circumstances generated by Hurricane Katrina in New Orleans was treated fairly and justly by not only the regulatory agencies but also by the degree of support within the medical profession after exercising 'moral courage' [43].

Scenario 8: Patient with High Spinal-Cord Injury Requesting Withdrawal of Support

Learning objective 9: to understand medical responsibilities when a patient with capacity is requesting discontinuation of life-sustaining medical treatment.

A 34-year-old sustains a high level cervical spine injury during a scrum at a women's rugby match, but with near immediate pitch side resuscitation avoids any hypoxic ischaemic injury. The MRI confirms cord injury extending to C1 and following posterior spinal fixation, a tracheostomy is undertaken with the expectation of long-term dependency on ventilatory support. From the moment of weaning from sedation, it is clear that the patient has recall of the primary injury and expresses a wish for ventilation to be stopped and to be allowed to die. Her partner of 18 months, although upset, explains that the patient had previously discussed the possibility of a severe sports-related injury. The patient had a fixed view that she had no wish for a life with restrictions inherent in the longer term after spinal injuries in a state of limitation and dependency. The patient expected her partner to support any measures to stop such a situation arising or continuing. The patient's parents took the view that she was simply upset and needed time to come to terms with these events and start the process of adjustment, and that they were in a position to provide care for her at home over the longer term. A psychiatry assessment was requested following the patient's refusal to have any discussion with the liaison practitioner from the regional spinal injuries unit. The psychiatrist concluded that the patient did not have capacity because she was not prepared to consider that many individuals made reasonable adjustment and lived a fulfilling life after embarking on a spinal rehabilitation programme. The psychiatrist also recommended that antidepressant therapy be started, but when this was explained to the patient, she refused with forceful expression that she did not consider herself depressed, but was angry that she was continuing to be treated against her will. How can this scenario be progressed?

Principles and Opinion

This scenario will predictably trigger a spectrum of opinion within and between the different healthcare professionals responsible for critical care provision. Medical staff will have less practical interaction with the patient than nursing staff and physiotherapists, who will therefore be exposed to the patient's opposition and anger on a more continuous basis. The basic premise at law is that the consent of a capacitous patient is essential to prevent treatment of any description constituting an assault. A patient's decision that is at variance with medical recommendations cannot be considered indicative of a lack of capacity, and psychiatric opinion that the patient is clinically depressed similarly cannot be utilised to underpin a conclusion that such depression compromises any claim to capacity. Certain intensive care practitioners will state that this is just another scenario requiring moral courage, and at the opposite end of the spectrum there will be those who are reluctant to embrace concepts of futility. Other practitioners may state that they would wish to do the right thing by the patient, but that they have no intention of having their motives and practice challenged at inquest, or by the regulatory body in the event of a complaint by the parents or indeed a member of the healthcare team opposed to such a course of action. It could also be argued that to comply with the patient's wishes would be assisting a suicide, which remains unlawful under the Suicide Act 1961 [44]. This is an additional factor suggesting that no single individual should take responsibility for whichever course of action the overall team takes, the decision should not be hasty, and ideally any decision should be endorsed by the local clinical ethics committee. Ultimately however, the above principles endorsing compliance with the wishes of a competent patient are applicable, regardless of the outcome of death. The position at law and these expectations were clarified by the courts almost 20 years ago in the case of Ms. B, when it was determined that this particular patient had capacity which was not compromised by a refusal to engage with spinal rehabilitation [45]. The court not only endorsed the right to have ventilator support withdrawn within a compassionate palliative approach, but also awarded nominal damages in respect of the continuation with ventilator support against her consistently expressed wishes. Whilst it is likely that many critical care practitioners may not encounter such a scenario during a professional lifetime, it should be noted that the key principles are played out on a more regular basis in respect of patients with motor neurone disease wishing to cease ventilatory support provided either non-invasively or via a tracheostomy. It was clear that this particular situation was not being addressed consistently and confidently, due in no small part to the backdrop of on-going contentious debate on assisted dying [46–49]. After multidisciplinary deliberations, draft guidance was placed before the medical professional bodies, the GMC as regulator and defence organisations and coroner's representatives within the UK. A consensus was achieved that neither the removal of ventilatory support at the patient's request, nor the use of pre-emptive analgesia and sedation made this anything other than a natural causes death from the underlying disease. There is no moral, ethical or legal distinction between the decision-making in both scenarios, despite motor neurone disease falling within the category of a life terminating condition. The fact that certain patients may live for an indefinite period after spinal injury and may appreciate being alive despite extreme disability does not alter the fundamental principle of respect for patient autonomy. The principle whereby it is also lawful to administer pre-emptive medication such as morphine and midazolam parenterally, is based on the fundamental responsibility of a doctor to relieve pain and suffering when there is no effective or acceptable solution to maintaining life. Clearly, if ventilatory support was withheld or withdrawn in the absence of such therapeutic measures, discomfort or distress would be triggered i.e. the medical approach would fall short of the anticipated compassionate care standards. This does raise an interesting aspect however as to which analgesic and sedative regimes would be considered acceptable either within the profession or on scrutiny by external agencies. Whilst certain practitioners have suggested the use of target controlled opioid and propofol infusions within the critical care setting, as would be utilised within anaesthesia (although at higher levels in anticipation of actual surgical intervention), it has been the author's recommendation in these circumstances that morphine and midazolam are utilised, given that these are conventionally used in a palliative setting. Logically however, there is no moral, ethical or legal distinction between differing regimes if the intention is simply to take the patient beyond any potential respiratory discomfort and associated distress prior to extubation, decannulation, or removal of ventilatory support. It can be argued that practitioners have more of a problem with a capacitous patient explicitly wishing to have care withdrawn against a backdrop of relative physiological stability, than with a patient whose wishes are not known but who predictably will never regain capacity.

Overview/Conclusions/Overall Learning Objective

A textbook chapter cannot cover the potential nuances of every trauma scenario or provide foreseeably definitive advice on how ethical challenges and the interface with external bodies and agencies should be anticipated and managed. It is more reasonable therefore to challenge the knowledge base and professional judgement of the reader. This chapter aims to emphasise the key points of considering the contextual implications of trauma, being aware of responsibilities to the broader public and principles of justice, the uneasy dynamic between duty of disclosure and principle of confidentiality, compliance with information governance and data protection, expectations of contributing to statutory investigations, and inevitable scrutiny of not only clinical care, but decision-making on these vexed topics and the standard of documentation in relation to these issues. The issues themselves are inescapable with the likelihood that precise guidance will be either absent or ambiguous, which demand in turn that practitioners demonstrate moral courage in making these judgement calls and have access to the support of colleagues with specific expertise and authority in these areas. The clinical management of trauma can often follow specific algorithms, but the professional expectations generated by the context of the trauma creates less tangible challenges.

Appendix: Post Mortem Narrative Tool

CLINICAL SUMMARY PRIOR TO POST-MORTEM:

Name:
DoB:
Unit No:

Date of Hospital Admission:	**Date of ICU Admission:**
Date of Death:	**Place of Death:**
Parent Specialty:	**Named Consultant:**

Key Injuries or pathologies on admission to intensive care:
1
2
3
4

Past Medical History
1.
2.
3.
4.

Surgical interventions after admission to intensive care:
1
2
3
4

ICU interventions:
Advanced monitoring:
Organ support:
Key drug treatments:
Procedures: (drains, tracheostomy)
Other:

Significant Events on Intensive Care
1.
2.
3.
4.

Relevant Investigation Results:
Microbiology
Biochemistry
Haematology
Radiology

Death occurred;
1. Despite ongoing provision of full support
2. After limitation or withdrawal of active support
(please delete appropriately)

If after limitation or withdrawal of active support this was due to:
1. Physiological futility (unable to achieve survival despite full support)
2. Qualitative futility (unable to achieve the broader goals of intensive care)
3. Both physiological and qualitative futility.

(please delete appropriately)

Medical devices removed after death: none/the following:

Provisional intensive care opinion as to Cause of Death;
1a
1b
1c
11

If cause of death not apparent, pathologies/ diagnoses felt likely to be contributing to death or to need evaluation at post-mortem;	
1	
2	
3	
4	
Completed by:	Status: Consultant/ SpR Critical Care
If completed by SpR, details of ICU consultant with whom discussed;	
Name:	
Mobile:	
e-mail:	
Date:	Signature:

References

1. Jones D. The relationship between homicide rates and forensic post mortem examinations in England and Wales. J Homicide Major Incid Investig. 2014 Nov;9(2):58–72.
2. Pounder D, Jones M, Peschel H. How can we reduce the number of coroner autopsies? Lessons from Scotland and the Dundee initiative. J R Soc Med. 2011 Jan 1;104(1):19–24.
3. Turnbull A, Osborn M, Nicholas N. Hospital autopsy: endangered or extinct? J Clin Pathol. 2015 Aug 1;68(8):601–4.
4. Rutty GN, Morgan B, Robinson C, Raj V, Pakkal M, Amoroso J, et al. Diagnostic accuracy of post-mortem CT with targeted coronary angiography versus autopsy for coroner-requested post-mortem investigations: a prospective, masked, comparison study. Lancet. 2017 Jul 8;390(10090):145–54.
5. Thali MJ, Jackowski C, Oesterhelweg L, Ross SG, Dirnhofer R. VIRTOPSY – the Swiss virtual autopsy approach. Legal Med. 2007 Mar 1;9(2):100–4.
6. General Medical Council. Confidentiality: good practice in handling patient information [Internet]. General Medical Council; 2017 [cited 2020 Oct 2]. Available from https://www.gmc-uk.org/ethical-guidance/ethical-guidance-for-doctors/confidentiality
7. Coroners and Justice Act 2009 [Internet]. [cited 2020 Oct 5]. Available from https://www.legislation.gov.uk/ukpga/2009/25/contents
8. Bass S, Cowman S. Anaesthetist's guide to the Coroner's court in England and Wales. BJA Educ. 2016 Apr 1;16(4):130–3.
9. Independent Office for Police Conduct. Focus – referrals. Focus. 2016;9:12.
10. Human Rights Act 1998 [Internet]. legislation.gov.uk. Statute Law Database; [cited 2020 Oct 5]. Available from: https://www.legislation.gov.uk/ukpga/1998/42/contents
11. Health and Safety at Work etc. Act 1974 [Internet]. legislation.gov.uk. Statute Law Database; [cited 2020 Oct 5]. Available from https://www.legislation.gov.uk/ukpga/1974/37/contents
12. Care Act 2014 [Internet]. legislation.gov.uk. Statute Law Database; [cited 2020 Oct 5]. Available from https://www.legislation.gov.uk/ukpga/2014/23/contents
13. Police Reform Act 2002 [Internet]. legislation.gov.uk. Statute Law Database; [cited 2020 Oct 5]. Available from https://www.legislation.gov.uk/ukpga/2002/30/contents
14. Road Traffic Act 1988 [Internet]. legislation.gov.uk. Statute Law Database; [cited 2020 Oct 5]. Available from https://www.legislation.gov.uk/ukpga/1988/52/contents
15. Police and Criminal Evidence Act 1984 [Internet]. legislation.gov.uk. Statute Law Database; [cited 2020 Oct 5]. Available from https://www.legislation.gov.uk/ukpga/1984/60/contents
16. Mental Health Act 1983 [Internet]. legislation.gov.uk. Statute Law Database; [cited 2020 Oct 5]. Available from https://www.legislation.gov.uk/ukpga/1983/20/contents
17. Mental Capacity Act 2005 [Internet]. legislation.gov.uk. Statute Law Database; [cited 2020 Oct 5]. Available from https://www.legislation.gov.uk/ukpga/2005/9/contents
18. Brown A, Czachorowski M, Davidson J, Delpech V, Glass R, Guerra L, et al. HIV testing in England: 2017 report. 2017;57.
19. Torke AM, Alexander GC, Lantos J. Substituted judgment: the limitations of autonomy in surrogate decision making. J Gen Intern Med. 2008 Sep;23(9):1514–7.
20. Cowan E, Macklin R. Unconsented HIV testing in cases of occupational exposure: ethics, law, and policy. Acad Emerg Med Off J Soc Acad Emerg Med. 2012 Oct;19(10):1181–7.
21. Bayer R, Edington C. HIV testing, human rights, and global AIDS policy: exceptionalism and its discontents. J Health Polit Policy Law. 2009 Jun;34(3):301–23.
22. Harsono D, Galletly CL, O'Keefe E, Lazzarini Z. Criminalization of HIV exposure: a review of empirical studies in the United States. AIDS Behav. 2017 Jan;21(1):27–50.
23. The Caldicott Committee. Report on the Review of Patient-Identifiable Information [Internet]. Department of Health; 1997 Dec [cited 2020 Oct 5] p. 137. Available from http://webarchive.nationalarchives.gov.uk/20130124064947/http://www.dh.gov.uk/prod_consum_dh/groups/dh_digitalassets/@dh/@en/documents/digitalasset/dh_4068404.pdf
24. Crook MA. The Caldicott report and patient confidentiality. J Clin Pathol. 2003 Jun;56(6):426–8.
25. Data Protection Act 1998 [Internet]. Statute Law Database; [cited 2020 Oct 5]. Available from https://www.legislation.gov.uk/ukpga/1998/29/contents

26. General Medical Council. Confidentiality: reporting gunshot and knife wounds [Internet]. 2018 [cited 2020 Oct 5]. Available from https://www.gmc-uk.org/ethical-guidance/ethical-guidance-for-doctors/confidentiality%2D%2D-reporting-gunshot-and-knife-wounds
27. UK Home Office. Prevent duty guidance [Internet]. GOV.UK. 2019 [cited 2020 Oct 5]. Available from https://www.gov.uk/government/publications/prevent-duty-guidance
28. Nabulyato W, Jeyaseelan L, Malagelada F, Heaton S. Legal, ethical and practical considerations of smartphone use in orthopaedics. Bull R Coll Surg Engl. 2016 Jun;98(6):252–7.
29. British Association of Dermatologists. UK Guidance on the use of mobile photographic devices in dematology [Internet]. 2017 [cited 2020 Oct 5]. Available from http://northeast.devonformularyguidance.nhs.uk/documents/Referral-documents/Dermatology/Mobile-photographic-device-national-guidance-2017.pdf
30. Reporting a Serious Incident to the Strategic Executive Information System (StEIS) | NHS Improvement [Internet]. 2018 [cited 2020 Oct 5]. Available from https://improvement.nhs.uk/resources/steis/
31. Learning from patient safety incidents | NHS Improvement [Internet]. 2018 [cited 2020 Oct 5]. Available from https://improvement.nhs.uk/resources/learning-from-patient-safety-incidents/
32. General Medical Council. Openness and honesty when things go wrong: the professional duty of candour. Arch Dis Child. 2015;101(5):243.
33. Sellu V. The Crown [2016] EWCA Crim 1716. 2016. https://www.bailii.org/ew/cases/EWCA/Crim/2016/1716.html
34. Bawa-Garba V. R. [2016] EWCA Crim 1841. 2016. http://www.bailii.org/cgi-bin/format.cgi?doc=/ew/cases/EWCA/Crim/2016/1841.html&query=(bawa)+AND+(garba)
35. Dyer C. Bristol inquiry. BMJ. 2001 Jul 28;323(7306):181.
36. Savulescu J. Beyond Bristol: taking responsibility. J Med Ethics. 2002 Oct 1;28(5):281–2.
37. Burton JL. The Alder hey affair. Arch Dis Child. 2002 Jan 1;86(1):4–7.
38. Bauchner H, Vinci R. What have we learnt from the Alder hey affair? BMJ. 2001 Feb 10;322(7282):309–10.
39. Hall CC, Lugton J, Spiller JA, Carduff E. CPR decision-making conversations in the UK: an integrative review. BMJ Support Palliat Care. 2019 Mar;9(1):1–11.
40. Callus T. 'One day I will find the right words, and they will be simple'—rethinking DNACPR at a national level. J Public Health. 2018 Jun 1;40(2):404–8.
41. Report of the Mid Staffordshire NHS Foundation Trust Public Inquiry [Internet]. GOV.UK. [cited 2020 Oct 20]. Available from https://www.gov.uk/government/publications/report-of-the-mid-staffordshire-nhs-foundation-trust-public-inquiry
42. https://www.independent.co.uk/news/health/charlieg-ard-high-court-judge-great-ormond-street-visitors-hospital-ill-baby-london-a7852846.html
43. Okie SD. Pou and the hurricane — implications for patient care during disasters. N Engl J Med. 2008 Jan 3;358(1):1–5.
44. Participation E. Suicide Act 1961 [Internet]. Statute Law Database; [cited 2020 Oct 20]. Available from https://www.legislation.gov.uk/ukpga/Eliz2/9-10/60/contents
45. Sensky T. Withdrawal of life sustaining treatment. BMJ. 2002 Jul 27;325(7357):175–6.
46. Papadopoulou N. Losing our grip on death: what now for assisted dying in the UK? J Med Law Ethics. 2017 Mar 1;5(1):57–79.
47. Reichstein A. A dignified death for all: how a relational conceptualisation of dignity strengthens the case for Legalising assisted dying in England and Wales. Hum Rights Law Rev. 2019 Dec 31;19(4):733–51.
48. Gerson SM, Bingley A, Preston N, Grinyer A. When is hastened death considered suicide? A systematically conducted literature review about palliative care professionals' experiences where assisted dying is legal. BMC Palliat Care. 2019 Aug 31;18(1):75.
49. Davis J. Most UK doctors support assisted dying, a new poll shows: the BMA's opposition does not represent members. BMJ. 2018 Feb;7:k301.

The Evolution of Trauma Systems

4

Jonathan Jones

Learning Objectives

- To describe the drivers behind the development of the English major trauma networks
- To explain the concept of the major trauma networks
- To examine the evidence supporting their apparent improvements in mortality outcomes
- To recognise current and future challenges to UK trauma systems

- A review of the history of major trauma networks
- Drivers for change in the UK
- The introduction of English Major Trauma Networks
- Major Trauma Networks appear to improve mortality
- Other benefits of an organised trauma system
- Future challenges to the UK trauma system.

J. Jones (✉)
Emergency Medicine Department, Leeds General Infirmary, Leeds, UK
e-mail: jonathanjones1@nhs.net

Introduction

In April 2010 the NHS in London restructured the provision of care for severely injured patients. On scene triage determined whether or not the individual would be taken to the nearest Emergency Department (ED) or instead, transported a potentially greater distance to one of four Major Trauma Centres (MTC). From April 2012 to April 2013 this system was rolled out across England. Twenty-seven MTCs were established, each embedded within a Network of smaller Trauma Units in (mostly) District General Hospitals. At the time of writing North Wales utilises the English Midlands Major Trauma Network (MTN), whilst South Wales and Scotland are in the process of developing their own Trauma Networks.

Each Major Trauma Network (MTN) is responsible for the entire patient pathway from injury to rehabilitation. Each MTC is expected to provide the full range of specialist services necessary for the care of complex major trauma patients, delivered by those whose training and experience has given them particular expertise.

The model feels right. The logic seems self-evident. But it took nearly 50 years from the first supportive Parliamentary report for it to be established in England and the evidence of improved outcomes was, in 2012, by no means conclusive.

P. Lax (ed.), *Textbook of Acute Trauma Care*, https://doi.org/10.1007/978-3-030-83628-3_4

How Did We Get to our Current System and Does it Work?

In 1935 the BMA Committee on Fractures, mourning the loss of expertise developed in the First World War, argued for the introduction of specialised Fracture Units, capable of supporting smaller rural hospitals. They enviously described Böhler's Vienna unit, funded by insurance companies, where the savings generated by "shortness of invalidity and completeness of recovery" far outweighed the costs of the institution. An Interdepartmental Committee established by the Home Secretary in 1936 supported this model in their final report, published a month before the outbreak of World War Two, but explicitly stated that "proposals for the institution of 'general' [as opposed to fracture] traumatic services are not called for, and would under conditions in this country be impracticable".

In 1941 Birmingham was experiencing a 40% increase in industrial injuries as a result of the influx of unskilled labour to its factories in addition to casualties from German air raids. Fortuitously the opening of a new teaching hospital had left the old undergraduate teaching hospital vacant. Sir William Gissane led the development of a new unit modelled on those recommended by the Interdepartmental Committee. The Birmingham Accident Hospital opened its doors on the 1st April and it was intended that "by rebuilding and reorganization" it would "eventually treat the majority of serious injuries in and around Birmingham". The BAH incorporated Medical Research Council teams investigating wound healing, burn care and the nature of road injuries to guide injury reduction schemes. Rehabilitation was prescribed from the "very early stages of in-patient treatment" and continued "during out-patient after-care". The hospital developed 'accident surgeons' who were "preferably young men physically capable of meeting the peculiar tempo of their responsibilities at any hour" with "sound general surgical training and special experience in orthopaedic and plastic surgery" supported by "equally well trained anaesthetists [gender not specified]".

Meanwhile, in the rest of the country, little changed. In the early 1960s Sir Henry Osmond Clarke's BMA accident services review committee recommended a tripartite system of a number of casualty services, and fewer 'accident units' focused around a central major injury unit serving one to two million people. The Platt Report (1962) (generally credited as leading to the development of Accident & Emergency Medicine) recommended that injured patients should be taken to the most *appropriate* hospital to manage their injuries, not the nearest.

Across the Atlantic, islands of excellence in major trauma care were developing but a 1966 National Academy of Sciences report highlighted the lack of a system encompassing the entirety of care from first response to research and rehabilitation. The Vietnam war led, as conflict usually does, to significant learning in trauma systems (specifically the importance of rapid transport to definitive care). The well reported personal tragedy of James Styner in 1976 led to the introduction of ATLS the following year. In 1979 analysis of patients in Orange County, California declared 2/3 of non-CNS related deaths at a non trauma centre to be potentially survivable (based on autopsy findings). Steadily trauma centres spread across the continent. In Orange County itself a regionalised system was introduced in June 1980. By 1983 a re-evaluation of outcome [1] using the autopsy approach claimed significant reductions in the frequency of preventable death.

But in the UK, again, little had changed. In 1987 the Confidential Enquiry into Perioperative Deaths [2] (notable for its striking title font) reviewed ten deaths following major trauma. In 50% the reviewers felt that the patient "would probably have survived in an American or Continental Trauma centre".The Royal College of Surgeons Report of the Working Party on the Management of Patients with Major Injuries (1988) concluded that one third of all deaths occurring after major injury were preventable with appropriately delivered care. The recommendations were predictable: rapid transfer, integrated services between hospitals, investment in rehab and research. A retrospective review [3] of just under 1000 cases of major injury (ISS > 15) in Yorkshire from October 1988 to September 1989 found that only 58% of patients reaching hospital alive survived to discharge.

In 1992 MTOS, the Major Trauma Outcome Study, reviewed the care of nearly 15,000 patients from 33 hospitals through a structured audit. Calculated predicted mortality was compared to reality. Outcomes for blunt trauma were found to be considerably worse than in the US. Outcomes for penetrating trauma (4.1% of the total—a figure largely unchanged to this day) were comparable to the US. Explanations offered focussed around poor initial assessment by too junior clinicians. The visible nature of penetrating trauma was felt to account for the comparatively better care. The closure of the Birmingham Accident Hospital in 1993 seemingly simply as a byproduct of a financially necessitated reorganisation of local services seems, with hindsight, a retrograde step.

Things did improve over the next few years. By 1997 a review of the UK Trauma Audit and Research Network (MTOS evolved) dataset indicated that your chances of surviving major injury had improved (mortality odds ratio 0.72 [0.55–0.92]). An increase in the proportion of such patients first seen by a senior doctor from 32% to 60% may have been a contributing factor.

In 1997 some doubt was cast on the validity of the MTC concept. The Department of Health's Trauma Centre Evaluation Study provided funding to North Staffordshire Royal Infirmary [4] allowing 24 h consultant cover for trauma patients, together with additional A&E and ICU nursing staff and ATLS trauma team training. A review of outcome (comparing Stoke to Preston and Hull), found no significant change in mortality. The lack of evidence of benefit was blamed on the short time elapsed between intervention and analysis and the lack of true regionalisation: there was no evidence of diversion of trauma patients to the MTC.

But in 2002 further review of the TARN data set suggested that the improvement in outcome noted in 1997 had actually stalled in 1994 with no change by 2000 [5]. The reviewers concluded that a plateauing in consultant involvement may have been to blame. In 2005 another TARN report identified a 26% increase in mortality for patients with severe head injuries who were not managed in a specialist neuroscience unit [6].

Meanwhile, on the other side of the world, work was ongoing to develop an integrated major trauma system in Victoria State, Australia. A number of studies had identified that up to 1/3 of road traffic fatalities were preventable and noted recurring deficiencies in trauma management and system response: inadequate prehospital and ED skills, prolonged scene times, reception by junior ED staff, under-resourced hospitals and delays in interhospital transfer. A ministerial taskforce was established in 1997 and recommended the development of strategies to deliver the right patient to the right hospital by the fastest and safest means with concentration of expertise in a few specialist institutions [6].

In Canada work that had commenced in 1993 on the regionalisation of trauma services was demonstrating significant reductions in mortality [7]. In the US further evidence emerged from 14 states suggesting mortality was reduced when patients were managed at a dedicated major trauma centre [8] (one year mortality of 10.4 v 13.8%). A 2006 systematic review and meta-analysis of US trauma systems incorporating work from 1992 to 2004 concluded that the presence of a trauma system was associated with a 15% reduction in mortality [9].

Back in the UK three further reports were critical in finally precipitating wholescale change in the UK system.

In 2007 NCEPOD (the National Confidential Enquiry on Patient Outcome and Death) published the results of an expert casenote review of the care of 795 major trauma patients. The title: "Trauma: Who cares?" provides an insight into the findings. Almost 60% of patients were considered to have "received a standard of care that was less than good practice" as a result of deficiencies in "both organisational and clinical aspects of care". The key recommendations for improvement were:

Key Points

- The development of integrated regional trauma services with trauma centres
- Improved pre-hospital airway management
- 24/7 consultant led trauma teams
- Rapid access to top to toe CT scanning
- Specialist neuroscience critical care for all patients with severe head injury

- Links to specialised paediatric services
- Standardised transfer processes

The same year the review of healthcare in London "A Framework for Action" (commonly known as the Darzi report) recommended the introduction of a major trauma system for the capital. The report used TARN outcome data to highlight better than expected outcomes for patients managed at the Royal London Hospital (the organisation closest to fulfilling the criteria for an MTC) and evidence from Quebec [10] reporting better outcomes for patients taken directly to an MTC as distinct to those transferred from another hospital. That same year Healthcare for London established a programme to deliver these recommendations resulting in a decision to commission four trauma networks for the region.

Outside the traditional health economy global events continued to push forward the management of trauma. From 2005 until 2014 the British Military hospital at Camp Bastion in Helmand Province, Afghanistan acted as a central focus for the development of combat casualty care. Whilst this is outside the scope of this chapter it is important to recognise the impact of the continual drip feed of this experience back into the NHS. Returning clinicians highlighted the extent to which the care provided to civilian casualties lagged behind that delivered in an austere combat environment.

Darzi's next report (High Quality Care for all [11]) extended to England as a whole and again restated the need for regional trauma networks. With clinical and political viewpoints finally aligned in 2009 Professor Keith Willett, who had helped establish 24 h consultant resident trauma care at the John Radcliffe Hospital in Oxford, was appointed National Clinical Director for Trauma Care.

Willett's work was given more impetus by further evidence of deficiencies emerging in a 2010 National Audit Office [12] report. London's trauma system went live in April 2010. By April 2013 the rest of England had followed. A national major trauma system following the recommendations of the national Clinical Reference Group was in place. After decades of inaction in a remarkably short time 27 designated Major Trauma Centres supporting 19 major trauma networks had been established. But has this work led to improvements in outcome?

How Do the English Trauma Networks Function?

Each Trauma Network consists of a number of Trauma Units (TUs), based around a Major Trauma Centre. In 11 cities the MTC is a single hospital serving both adults and paediatrics. In other networks the MTC is in reality more than one hospital either because of the presence of a separate Children's MTC or because all the necessary specialties are not present under one roof.

At the scene of injury the ambulance service will apply a major trauma triage tool. These currently vary from region to region, though work is ongoing at developing a single tool with better utility. The tools use a combination of anatomical, physiological and mechanistic factors to determine whether or not the injured patient should be taken to an MTC. If the MTC can be reached within 60 min then they will be conveyed directly there. There is wide variation in the level of care that can be provided at the scene or en route depending on the extent of local pre hospital emergency medicine care.

Each MTC serves a population of between 1.5 to 3 million and will manage between about 800 to 1800 patients a year with injuries significant enough to merit inclusion on the TARN database.

Patients who present to a TU either as a result of under-triage or self presentation (as is the case for ¼ of significantly injured children [13]) will be assessed by a trauma team at the TU and if necessary rapidly transferred to the MTC.

Each Network is responsible for ensuring that patient care within their region reaches nationally mandated standards. This is done through the provision of clinical guidelines and transfer pathways within a clear governance structure (example www.wymtn.com).

In August 2018 a wide range of UK news outlets [14–16] reported that the introduction of major trauma networks had saved more than 1600 lives over the preceding 6 years. The reports, no doubt stimulated by an NHS England press release [17], were based on a publication [18] in EClinicalmedicine, an online open access journal produced by the Lancet. The authors were from TARN, together with Keith Willett (now National Clinical Director for Acute Care) and Prof Chris Moran, his successor as NCD for Major Trauma.

The authors reviewed TARN submissions from April 2008 to March 2017 for 35 hospitals who had been reliable and consistent providers of data during that time period 15 of which had been designated as MTCs. They focused on the more severely injured patients—those with an Injury Severity Score of 9 or more, arguing that mortality benefits were unlikely in those with relatively minor injury.

What Is the Injury Severity Score?

The ISS was introduced in 1974 [19]. It utilises the Abbreviated Injury Score (AIS) developed by the American Association for the Advancement of Automotive Medicine [20]. The AIS, which has been revised on numerous occasions, assigns a score of 1 to 6 to any injury (with six being reserved for unsurvivable ones such as hemicorporectomy). The body is divided into six regions (Head & Neck, Chest, Abdomen & Pelvis, Extremities, External, Face). The scores for the three most significant injuries (no more than one from each region) are squared and combined to produce the ISS.

So for example: a man is involved in an RTC and sustains a cerebral contusion (AIS 3), a moderate subdural haematoma (AIS 4) (both in the HEAD body region), a major haemothorax (AIS 4), a partial transection of the aortic arch (AIS 4) (both in the CHEST body region), a badly ruptured spleen (AIS 4), a minor liver lacertion (AIS 2), a pelvic ring fracture (AIS 2) (all in the ABDO / PELVIS body region) and a closed tibial fracture (EXTREMITY body region) (AIS 2).

His three most significant injuries for ISS scoring purposes are the subdural haematoma (4), the aortic arch injury (4) and the ruptured spleen (4). His other injuries don't factor in either because there is a more severe injury in that body region or because (like the fractured femur) it isn't severe enough to make the top three injured body regions (which in this case are the head, chest and abdomen/pelvis).

So his ISS is $4^2 + 4^2 + 4^2 = 48$ (note that if you've been unfortunate enough to sustain an injury with an AIS of 6 your ISS is automatically 75).

A widely used definition of major trauma is an ISS of 16 or more. The problem is that this would include (for example) a spontaneous subdural in an 82 year old on warfarin who is fully conscious whilst failing to include bilateral closed femoral fractures. Perhaps a better definition of major trauma is any potentially 'life changing' injury.

Other issues with ISS include the ability to achieve the same score with a constellation of very different injuries (eg fractured femur, minor splenic laceration and a minor pneumothorax = ISS 9 whilst penetrating cardiac injury = ISS 9 but I know which I'd rather have) and the fact that if there are multiple injuries in the same body region (eg as in the abdomen / pelvis body region of the worked example above) only one counts towards your score.

It's also worth noting that the ISS is an ordered categorical variable and in no way normally distributed (though many authors wrongly use mean ISS in their studies). Some ISS values are not possible (eg 7) and there are big peaks at values 1, 4 and 9 (patients with a single body region injured with an AIS of 1, 2 or 3 [21].

110,863 patients were included. The annual number of patients increased from around 5300 (2008/09) to a little over 19,000 in 2016/17. There were some interesting changes in demographics with significant increases in age, co-morbidity and female gender. The mechanism of injury changed too—the much reported epidemic in knife crime is not manifest with the three fold increase in reported penetrating trauma (n = 900 or 4.7% of the total) dwarfed by the five fold increase in injuries resulting from falls from standing and a height of less than 2 m (n = 9064 or 47.2% of the total). Crude mortality however remained remarkably constant across the time period studied (8%).

So how did NHS England conclude that 1600 lives were saved? The answer lies in the analysis of observed mortality vs predicted mortality. TARN methodology involves the calculation of probability of survival for each patient using ISS, GCS, gender, age and (since 2014) co-morbidity. Cumulative observed vs predicted outcome is then summarised to produce the W statistic. The authors analysed the W statistic for the duration of the study and noted an essentially flat line until the introduction of trauma networks followed by a steady improvement in the years from 2012 to 2017. The conclusion was of an odds ratio for survival of 1.19 (95% CI 1.03 to 1.36) comparing 2008/09 and 2016/17. Presumably it was this figure that allowed NHS England to estimate the magnitude of effect.

This is the first time that the effect of a system wide change in major trauma care delivery has been studied on this scale. Unfortunately the analysis is not without some limitations. Perhaps most importantly the study population changed during the period reviewed. A significant financial inducement (the best practice tariff) was introduced. Either £1400 or £2800 (depending on ISS) could be claimed for MTC patients (as long as their data was submitted to TARN). Suddenly large numbers of low energy 'major trauma' patients were being found on Care of the Elderly wards. This has almost certainly been a factor in the shifting demographics and injury mechanisms noted above—the population is ageing, but not so fast to account for the much greater proportion of older patients within the database. A changing study population over the period studied is a potentially significant flaw in the methodology.

In addition, wider use of CT scanning with the introduction of polytrauma CTs during the study period will have led to ISS inflation [22]—more injuries are picked up but these injuries, whilst inflating the ISS, will not actually have a significant impact on mortality—thus outcomes appear to improve through the improved diagnosis of effectively 'incidental' injuries. An example would be a few rib fractures in someone with a distal tibial fracture. They are unlikely to affect mortality but do affect the apparent severity of injury—the patient would have survived either with or without a major trauma centre but their survival looks more impressive after a polytrauma CT scan.

There are other problems with the comparative outcome methodology used by TARN. TARN exclude patients from their database who have died and who have had a postmortem until postmortem results are available. PM results can be notoriously difficult to obtain (depending on the approachability and cooperativeness of the local coroner) and so a potential bias is introduced.

Interesting results also surface that don't seem to fit with observed practice. The Royal London Hospital is considered by many to be an exemplar Major Trauma Centre and is at the forefront of trauma care in the UK. Yet it consistently 'underperforms' on this model [23]. This may be because of the type of trauma demographic—they have a much higher proportion of penetrating trauma than the national average. In addition they may be victims of their own success with the most advanced pre-hospital system in the country potentially delivering patients to the MTC who elsewhere would have died at the scene (TARN does not currently cover pre-hospital systems).

Nonetheless the data demonstrating improved outcomes is very encouraging and on a par with the US results from 2006. Subjectively there are few working in major trauma in the UK who would dispute that the care provided to victims of significant injury has not improved markedly in the last 20 years.

Widening the focus from the UK (and predating the Eclinicalmedicine English review), a 2018 [24] systematic review identified 41 studies examining the impact of trauma system structure on injury outcome and subjected 19 of these to meta-analysis. Accepting the 2006 evidence that *a* trauma system was better than *no* trauma system the review focused on what features of a trauma system led to better results. Low quality evidence was identified supporting inclusive trauma system design aimed at delivering the right patient to the right place (the MTC) first time. Interestingly, the authors suggest that full trauma system maturity takes 10 years—a feature commented upon in the 2018 English study as suggesting that the full mortality benefits of the NHS restructuring may yet not be manifest.

Of course mortality alone is a poor demonstration of the effectiveness of a healthcare system. What other indicators of improved outcome are there? Sadly few that have been explored. TARN has commenced work on Patient Related Outcome Measures (PROMS) but no data has yet been published. In Victoria State (Australia) an initial trend of improvement in quality of life measures following the introduction of the major trauma system [25] has not been sustained and in recent years has regressed [26]. Some evidence exists suggesting that children cared for at MTCs are less likely to have a splenectomy than if managed at a TU [27].

Other benefits of organised networks have become apparent. Dissemination of good practice and new evidence is far faster—the adoption of the use of tranexamic acid being a clear example. Collaborative research involving the majority of MTCs across the country is in place. Examples include the UK-REBOA [28] and CRYOSTAT-2 [29] studies. Some networks are leading the way in work on injury prevention. Redthread work on reducing knife injuries in London through targeted work with young victims [30] and have now developed a Midlands pilot.

What Challenges Remain?

Ironically the apparent success of the development of the English major trauma system is probably its greatest challenge. UK healthcare funding is essentially a zero sum game and trauma has had its time in the political spotlight. It is well recognised that a great deal more remains to be done. Rehabilitation, particularly specialist rehabilitation, has been neglected from the outset. Increasing numbers of survivors, with potentially more significant injuries, place an ever greater burden on a sparse resource. The increasing age and frailty of the population means the trauma population is changing and has greater co-morbidity. Work remains in identifying 'stealth' trauma [31] in both the very young and very old whose injuries are often under-appreciated leading to delays in diagnosis. De-skilling has become apparent at Trauma Units leading to an increased burden on MTCs of patients who may not be those who most benefit from their care, potentially at the expense of those who do. True trauma surgeons are few and far between and the rigours of an intense job do not lead to easy recruitment. Far more work is required to ensure that outcomes beyond mortality are improving and to identify how best to maximise these improvements.

Summary

Objective evidence from a range of countries supports the assertion that major trauma centres, functioning within a developed trauma system, reduce mortality and morbidity from major trauma. Some evidence from Australia argues for broader socio-economic benefits. Less tangible advantages exist in the ability to rapidly disseminate good practice and gain new insights from an increasingly responsive research network. The introduction of the English major trauma system, after many years of prevarication, can be broadly considered a success. The risk now is that complacency leads to stagnation.

Questions

1. The first Major Trauma Centre in the UK was in:
   (a) London
   (b) Edinburgh
   (c) Leeds
   (d) Birmingham
   (e) Manchester

2. Analysis of trauma centre vs non trauma centre care in Orange County, California in the 1970s established that:
   (a) 2/3 of non head injury deaths occurring at the non major trauma centres were preventable
   (b) 40% of head injury deaths occurring at the non major trauma centres were preventable
   (c) Major Trauma Centre time-critical surgery occurred an average of 2 h later than at the non major trauma centre
   (d) Major Trauma Centre care was not associated with improvements in mortality
   (e) Major Trauma Centre care led to worse neurological outcomes
3. In 2018 how many lives did NHS England conclude had been saved by the introduction of major trauma networks?
   (a) 0
   (b) 340
   (c) 900
   (d) 1250
   (e) 1600
4. When considering the Injury Severity score:
   (a) The maximum possible ISS is 80
   (b) An ISS of 75 represents an unsurvivable ISS
   (c) An ISS of 7 is the commonest score
   (d) An ISS of 25 or more is often considered indicative of 'major trauma'
   (e) The ISS is calculated from the four most significant injuries the patient has sustained
5. Since the introduction of the English Major Trauma Networks:
   (a) There has been a large rise in the proportion of people suffering penetrating traumatic injuries.
   (b) There has been a large increase in the average age of trauma patients.
   (c) Overall trauma numbers have decreased 15%
   (d) Low energy mechanism of trauma have been found to account for very few injuries
   (e) Penetrating trauma has been found to be the cause in 26% of cases.

Answers

1. (d) The Birmingham Accident Hospital (1941) was the first recognisable MTC in the UK.
2. (a) Major Trauma Centre care appeared to greatly improve the chance of survival in those who had suffered major injuries to the body (as opposed to the head).
3. (e), although their interpretation of the data is of course open to question.
4. (b). The maximum ISS is 75 and this represents an unsurvivable injury. An ISS is calculated from the most significant injuries in the most significantly injured three body regions. A score of 16 or more is considered to represent major trauma. A score of 7 is not possible.
5. (b) Better data collection and a changing demographic has identified large numbers of injuries resulting from low energy trauma in older patients.

References

1. West JG. Impact of regionalization: the Orange County experience. Arch Surg. 1983 Jun 1;118(6):740.
2. Buck N, Lunn JN, Devlin HB. The report of a confidential enquiry into perioperative deaths. London: Nuffield Provincial Hospitals Trust; 1989.
3. Airey CM, Franks AJ. Major trauma workload within an English health region. Injury. 1995 Jan;26(1):25–31.
4. Nicholl J, Turner J. Effectiveness of a regional trauma system in reducing mortality from major trauma: before and after study. BMJ. 1997 Nov 22;315(7119):1349–54.
5. Lecky FE. Lack of change in trauma care in England and Wales since 1994. Emerg Med J. 2002 Nov 1;19(6):520–3.
6. Patel HC, Bouamra O, Woodford M, King AT, Yates DW, Lecky FE, et al. Trends in head injury outcome from 1989 to 2003 and the effect of neurosurgical care: an observational study. Lancet. 2005 Nov 29;366(9496):1538–44.
7. Sampalis JS, Denis R, Lavoie A, Frechette P, Boukas S, Nikolis A, et al. Trauma care regionalization: a process-outcome evaluation. J Trauma. 1999 Apr;46(4):565–81.
8. MacKenzie EJ, Jurkovich GJ, Frey KP, Scharfstein DO. A National Evaluation of the effect of trauma-center care on mortality. N Engl J Med. 2006;13:150.
9. Celso B, Tepas J, Langland-Orban B, Pracht E, Papa L, Lottenberg L, et al. A systematic review

and meta-analysis comparing outcome of severely injured patients treated in trauma centers following the establishment of trauma systems. J Trauma. 2006;60(2):371–8. discussion 378
10. Moore L, Lavoie A, Sirois M-J, Amini R, Belcaïd A, Sampalis JS. Evaluating trauma center process performance in an integrated trauma system with registry data. J Emerg Trauma Shock. 2013 Jan 4;6(2):95.
11. Great Britain, Department of Health. NHS next stage review final report by Lord Darzi. London: Stationery Office Books.: [distributor] Stationery Office Books; 2008.
12. Great Britain, National Audit Office, Great Britain, Parliament, House of Commons. Major trauma care in England: report. London: Stationery Office; 2010.
13. The Trauma Audit and Research Network. 2 Years of Severe Injury in Children [Internet]. The University of Manchester: Manchester Academic Health Science Centre (MAHSC); 2015 [cited 2020 May 21] p. 24. Available from: https://www.tarn.ac.uk/Content/ChildrensReport2/files/assets/basic-html/page-1.html#
14. Correspondent KL Health. NHS saves 1,600 lives by sending ambulances on longer journeys. [cited 2020 May 21]; Available from https://www.thetimes.co.uk/article/nhs-saves-1-600-lives-by-sending-ambulances-on-longer-journeys-fczsmsjdn
15. Sky News. More lives saved because of major trauma centres [Internet]. Sky News. [cited 2020 May 21]. Available from https://news.sky.com/story/more-lives-saved-because-of-major-trauma-centres-11477258
16. Triggle N. 'I broke every bone in my face – and survived'. BBC News [Internet]. 2018 Aug 20 [cited 2020 May 21]; Available from https://www.bbc.com/news/health-45184373
17. NHS England » More than 1,600 extra trauma victims alive today says major new study [Internet]. [cited 2020 May 21]. Available from https://www.england.nhs.uk/2018/08/more-than-1600-extra-trauma-victims-alive-today-says-major-new-study/
18. Moran CG, Lecky F, Bouamra O, Lawrence T, Edwards A, Woodford M, et al. Changing the system – major trauma patients and their outcomes in the NHS (England) 2008–17. E Clinical Medicine. 2018 Aug 1;2:13–21.
19. Baker SP, O'neill B, Haddon WJ, Long WB. The injury severity score: a method for describing patients with multiple injuries and evaluating emergency care. J Trauma Acute Care Surg. 1974 Mar;14(3):187–96.
20. Abbreviated Injury Scale (AIS) [Internet]. Association for the Advancement of Automotive Medicine. [cited 2020 May 21]. Available from https://www.aaam.org/abbreviated-injury-scale-ais/
21. Stevenson M, Segui-Gomez M, Lescohier I, Scala CD, McDonald-Smith G. An overview of the injury severity score and the new injury severity score. Inj Prev. 2001 Mar 1;7(1):10–3.
22. Gupta M, Gertz M, Schriger DL. Injury severity score inflation resulting from Pan-computed tomography in patients with blunt trauma. Ann Emerg Med. 2016 Jan;67(1):71–75.e3.
23. TARN – Main Hospital Details Royal London Hospital [Internet]. 2019 [cited 2020 May 21]. Available from https://www.tarn.ac.uk/Content.aspx?ca15&c=2897&hid=8003&pcid=3056
24. Moore L, Champion H, Tardif P-A, Kuimi B-L, O'Reilly G, Leppaniemi A, et al. Impact of trauma system structure on injury outcomes: a systematic review and Meta-analysis. World J Surg. 2018;42(5):1327–39.
25. Gabbe BJ, Simpson PM, Sutherland AM, Wolfe R, Fitzgerald MC, Judson R, et al. Improved functional outcomes for major trauma patients in a regionalized, inclusive trauma system. Ann Surg. 2012 Jun;255(6):1009–15.
26. Department of Health and Human Services. Victorian State Trauma Registry annual report 2016-17 [Internet]. 2018. Available from: https://www2.health.vic.gov.au/about/publications/annualreports/victorian-state-trauma-registry-annual-report-2016-17
27. Warwick AM, Jenks T, Fisher R, Garrett-Cox R, Lecky F, Yates D. Disparities in the management of paediatric splenic injury. Br J Surg. 2019;106(3):263–6.
28. UK-REBOA [Internet]. [cited 2020 May 21]. Available from https://w3.abdn.ac.uk/hsru/REBOA/Public/Public/index.cshtml
29. CRYOSTAT-2 Trial [Internet]. CRYOSTAT-2. [cited 2020 May 21]. Available from https://cryostat2.co.uk/
30. Redthread [Internet]. Redthread. [cited 2020 May 21]. Available from https://www.redthread.org.uk/
31. Davies F, Coats TJ. 'Stealth trauma' in the young and the old: the next challenge for major trauma networks? Emerg Med J. 2020 Feb 1;37(2):56–7.

Part II

The Fundamental Approach to Trauma Patients

5 Point of Injury to Rehabilitation

Peter Lax

- Overall assessment and pre-arrival actions
- Importance of massive haemorrhage control
- Airway signs and basic manoeuvres
- Respiratory assessment
- Cardiovascular assessment and signs
- Clinical neurological assessment
- Exposure and burns assessment

Introduction

The approach to trauma patients has several variables that will shift depending on where they are encountered. Amongst these are the skill level of staff and available resources, location (austere pre-hospital taskings versus a patient arriving packaged in a fully equipped Major Trauma Centre) and the leadership and interpersonal dynamics of the team. All of these factors may influence care and patient outcomes. As discussed in the first section of this textbook, leadership and followership are essential attributes of well-functioning teams of any size. Shared mental modelling helps achieve those goals, but a large part of establishing that model is a common baseline understanding of how to assess and treat patients.

When to Start the Assessment?

The assessment of trauma patients usually begins even before the first responder or team see the patient by consideration of the mechanism of injury. Consider two patients described by a person making an emergency phone call; The first has been hit by a car at five miles per hour and is complaining of leg pain. The second has been hit by a truck at 35 miles per hour and is only grunting or snoring. While there has been no medical input into either of these patients, a mental model of how unwell they are and the potential diagnostic tests or interventions they may require, is already starting to build. These initial pictures from a scene by non-medical staff can dictate the level of response that is sent to the patient and the time in which it arrives. The AMPDS criteria [1] are used by UK medical dispatchers to triage both response times and level of care needed. These depend on responses to questions over the phone and is the first triage and assessment mechanism that is used on patients.

The contents of a pre-alert phone call from the scene should also begin to form a mental model of the patient coming in to the hospital. Indeed, trauma triage tools are routinely employed to

P. Lax (✉)
Tactical Medical Wing, Royal Air Force, Brize Norton, Oxfordshire, UK

The Air Ambulance Service (TAAS), Rugby, Warwickshire, UK
e-mail: p.lax@NHS.net

P. Lax (ed.), *Textbook of Acute Trauma Care*, https://doi.org/10.1007/978-3-030-83628-3_5

ensure that the sickest patients are sent directly to Major Trauma Centres rather than peripheral units. Conversely, these tools can also be used to ensure that any patient that is sent to a peripheral unit should be within their capabilities and is unlikely to require a secondary transfer.

The Mechanism of Injury chapter gives further insight into patterns of injury or specific concerns that may be associated with different types of trauma. While these may be immediately apparent to pre-hospital clinicians who meet the patient on scene, they are not always immediately evident to hospital staff. Receiving a patient that is neatly packaged in a well-lit trauma bay without any context can occasionally give a false sense of security. There are two points to note at this stage—for hospital clinicians, a picture paints a thousand words. Photos of a scene can help hospital clinicians immeasurably in gaining an understanding of the forces involved in patients' injuries. It may also help them to understand why everything has not been done to perfection. If only one cannula has been inserted or a blood sugar measurement omitted, it is not uncommon to hear some hospital staff complain. However, when shown a picture of the severely deformed vehicle, upside down, in the rain, at night, in the middle of nowhere from which the patient was extricated, there is suddenly more understanding (and appreciation) of the skill and hard work necessary to get the patient from scene to hospital, resuscitated and packaged well.

The second point is that once the pre-hospital team leaves, so too does any information from the scene that has not been written down or handed over to the hospital team. Make sure that all the relevant information follows the patient! Significant injuries that are seen or suspected should always verbally be handed over to the team leader and documented by the departing staff. Not everything that is said is always heard or understood, and a written record of the scene, injuries and treatment can be of great use when assessing patients later on in intensive care or the ward.

It should be noted that trauma does not always exist in isolation; patients can have traumatic injuries as a result of a medical insult. In the context of a road traffic collision, for example, information from the scene can have a direct influence on management in the hospital. A patient who has crashed their car on a straight road in clear conditions may have had a medical event before their traumatic one, and this may influence subsequent management. A patient who has had an arrhythmia and then suffers a cardiac arrest with minimal traumatic injuries is NOT a candidate for a resuscitative thoracotomy, and this should be borne in mind.

The Reprioritisation of Haemorrhage Control

Historically (and in other non-trauma resuscitation courses), students are taught the ABC approach to patient management—airway, followed by breathing and then assessment of the circulation. Safar first established this in his 1961 publication on ventilation and closed-chest compression [2], an early predecessor to the current Advanced Life Support course. In current trauma practice, this approach is suboptimal because of two factors; firstly, it negates the clinical concept and importance of massive haemorrhage taking priority. Data from military experience has shown that most battle casualty deaths occur within 10 minutes of injury, and the majority of deaths are from exsanguination [3]. Of these deaths, while truncal haemorrhage is the leading cause, the same paper demonstrated that 18% of the deaths that were attributable to bleeding were from limb or neck wounds that were potentially compressible. The paper argues that these deaths were potentially preventable with the correct training. In a traditional ABC approach, these wounds would not have been addressed as a priority, and not at all until airway and breathing had been assessed and treated as needed. The short period from injury to death in these papers emphasises that speed in circulation preservation is necessary. To further highlight this approach, an article by Eastridge in 2012 [4] and a further review in 2019 [5] have concluded that in those who died in combat, 90% of potentially survivable injuries were due to haemorrhage. With more training, reprioritisation of massive haemorrhage control and use of tourniquets in self- and buddy-aid, there was an 85% drop in deaths attributable to limb haemorrhage. A further paper by Kragh et al. [6] showed that early and aggressive tourniquet usage in severe limb trauma before the development of shock was associated with a significant survival improvement (90% vs 10%). These findings, while based on military data and experience, are echoed in civilian practice. A 2007 Canadian paper by Tien et al. [7] concluded that 16% of trauma deaths were potentially preventable with earlier and more aggressive haemorrhage control. A 2005 paper from the USA by Dorlac et al. [8] suggested over 50% of patients who exsanguinated and died from isolated extremity injuries could potentially have been successfully treated with tourniquet application early on in their care. These data have renewed the emphasis on massive haemorrhage control, placing it above airway as the initial priority in trauma care.

The second difference is that the way trauma patients are assessed and treated has evolved, and reflects what has already been discussed in the Trauma Systems and Teams section of this textbook. The Advanced Trauma Life Support course was revolutionary when it was first developed in the late 1970s and has undoubtedly saved many lives by standardising the approach to trauma since its inception. However, the model of trauma care that it was initially aimed at was for a single practitioner with an assistant working in a remote hospital with minimal resources and access to specialist expertise. Out of necessity, it stressed a methodical ABCDE approach with the idea to treat the pathology that kills first before moving onto other systems. Modern trauma care is different in that our understanding of treatment and pathology has evolved over 40 years, and that (except for small pre-hospital teams) most in-hospital trauma teams are large enough to diagnose and treat multiple systems concurrently. While ATLS teaches an individual to assess and treat a patient sequentially, a more modern approach favours a team working in parallel (rather than sequence) to diagnose pathology in multiple systems concurrently, led by a "hands-off" team leader. This has also been termed "horizontal" resuscitation as opposed to the previous "vertical" approach [9]. Earlier, more aggressive investigation and treatment of haemorrhage has led to improved outcomes after reprioritising circulation preservation with tourniquets and other methods as described above. A further adaptation that has been used in horizontal resuscitation is the concept of "3D" resuscitation [9], where the trauma team leader may identify a small group of patients based on pre-hospital information who may benefit from transfer direct to the operating theatre from the ambulance. This approach was employed in Camp Bastion during the Afghanistan conflict where it was termed "Right Turn Resus" as the doors to the operating theatres were originally on the right as the patient was wheeled into the Resus department. The trauma team could assemble in the operating theatre and perform ED resuscitative measures at the same time as surgical control of bleeding and damage control. Patients who benefit from this approach are the most severely injured (e.g. explosive injuries with limb loss and/or multiple torso injuries and cardiovascular collapse) [9, 10].

A Universal Treatment Algorithm

For these reasons (and others outlined in the Massive Haemorrhage Chapter), an MABCDE approach is advocated:

- **Major haemorrhage control**
- **Airway with c-spine consideration when needed**
- **Breathing**
- **Circulation**
- **Disability**
- **Exposure/ Environment/ Everything else.**

This has also been referred to as a MARCH approach (Massive haemorrhage, Airway, Respiration, Circulation, Head injury/ Hypothermia). However, in all honesty, it does not matter which mnemonic is used—the result is the same. This textbook employs the MABCD approach as it is usually the most familiar, or at least provides the least deviation from a well-known and taught system from other areas of medicine while emphasising the importance of aggressive circulation preservation. Each section of the mnemonic has a dedicated chapter later in the textbook. However, the critical thing to bear in mind is that for a primary survey, clinicians should only be looking to detect and treat immediately life-threatening injuries and not perform an exhaustive examination. The availability and speed of modern imaging in hospital usually means that patients can rapidly have appropriate radiological examinations (usually contrast-enhanced CT) within 30 min of arriving in hospital. The MABCD approach emphasises treating conditions which will either kill the patient before they can be detected by imaging, or identify patients who should go straight to the operating theatre and bypass CT altogether if they are too unstable. However, it is essential to point out that the most unstable patients may have the most to gain from whole-body CT imaging [11]. Even in haemodynamically unstable patients, modern CT scanners are so quick that a CT scan may avoid operative management in nearly 50% of patients who previously would have gone straight to theatre [12]. More details are available in the Radiology in Trauma section.

Overarching Principles of MABCD

Each step of the MABCD approach in the initial assessment emphasises a swift damage control approach:

- Preserve circulation
- Ensure adequate oxygenation
- Promote normalising physiology
- Avoid secondary injury

As patients progress further through the chain of resuscitation, the options available to clinicians increase. However, the overarching aim during initial resuscitation remains unchanged—to identify and treat time critical pathology before moving on. While this may occur concurrently in well-resourced teams as described above, the same MABCD sequence and principles apply to both large teams and solo responders. Specific interventions may be beyond the scope of practice of an individual, or impractical due to their location. If severe pathology is suspected, it is incumbent on the clinician to highlight their concerns when handing over the patient to the next level of care to ensure that they are addressed and not forgotten. Time is one of the most precious and scarce commodities trauma patients have, and it should not be wasted. If intervention is needed that is not available, then an expedited transfer should be considered as much a resuscitative measure as an operation. Spending time either on scene or in a resuscitation bay in an attempt to "fully" resuscitate patients before moving them to the operating theatre or CT scanner is wasteful of both time and resources. It may result in worsening hypothermia, acidosis and coagulopathy as described in the Damage Control chapter.

It may be that patients suffer a significant degree of trauma and go into cardiac arrest as a result of this. If there are absent signs of life on any of the ABC assessments, it may be appropriate to perform a resuscitative thoracotomy. This is only appropriate in the presence of specific pathologies, and when the absence of vital signs is thought to be due to a low-flow state. Again, it is worth emphasising the importance of context as a trauma thoracotomy will not fix a medical problem!

Massive External Haemorrhage

Massive external haemorrhage refers to imminently life-threatening bleeding, e.g. a femoral or brachial artery transection that can approach 1000 ml/min blood loss. True massive external haemorrhage rarely presents untreated to hospital. Due to response and transport times, patients who have these injuries and are not rapidly treated will exsanguinate and die before arrival. In pre-hospital medicine, these injuries are critical to identify and promptly treat. As previously described, there has been a significant decrease in preventable mortality as a direct result of education in the military. There are now civilian programmes such as "Stop the Bleed" [13–15] which are teaching the use of tourniquets and other circulation preservation techniques to the public. The general DIT escalation approach (Direct pressure, Indirect Pressure, Tourniquet) is covered in the massive haemorrhage chapter, and it should take less than one minute to establish control.

The total circulating volume of an adult is approximately 70 ml/kg, or around 5000 ml—as much of this volume as possible should be preserved rather than being replaced (see damage control chapter for more information). In children, circulating volume is around 80 ml/kg, but the absolute volume is lower than in adults, so effective haemorrhage control is even more critical. Younger children are not able to adapt their cardiovascular physiology as well as adults and consequently tolerate hypovolaemia poorly, with sudden and catastrophic deterioration when they can no longer compensate. Looking for signs of bleeding and aggressive treatment is necessary. Any blood-soaked clothing or obvious spurting bleeding should be considered due to treatable massive external haemorrhage until proven otherwise in both adults and children.

Tourniquets have enjoyed a resurgence in popularity in the last 15 years, and multiple models are now available for purchase. There are even more options which may be available in-hospital such as pneumatic devices which are in everyday use for elective orthopaedic surgery. These devices increase pressure over a larger area, so may be tolerated better by patients and decrease the risk of nerve or tissue damage in comparison to windlass devices. Another advantage of using any form of tourniquet is freeing up other practitioners. Massive haemorrhage control may only be achievable by constant external pressure over a wound which takes one clinician out of the team. If the injury is amenable to compression with a tourniquet of some description, then the clinician can be freed up to continue with assessment and treatment once the tourniquet is in place and tightened/inflated.

Airway

Trauma patients who can talk are much easier to assess. The fact they can speak at all tells the clinician that the airway reflexes are almost certainly intact, their airway is *currently* patent, they can breathe sufficiently to talk and have a sufficient blood pressure to perfuse their brain. It is also a particularly useful assessment method if the patient is concealed, entrapped or not immediately visible when the clinician arrives on the scene.

If the airway is not clear, it will need addressing as the next priority after massive external haemorrhage has been controlled. There may be a primary airway issue if there is facial or neck trauma. Alternately, airway compromise may be secondary to a decreased level of consciousness following a head injury, administration of drugs, or metabolic disorder such as hypoglycaemia or hypercarbia. Considerations relevant to airway management are discussed more fully in the airway chapter, but all clinicians should have mental schemata in mind to escalate from basic manoeuvres with simple adjuncts to more advanced options. Even if unable to perform some of the more advanced techniques themselves, clinicians should be able to recognise and communicate concerns about a threatened or failing airway. This enables preparations to be made by the next level of care and save valuable time.

Airway obstruction can be partial or complete. Depending on the cause, partial airway obstruction may present as a hoarse voice (in the case of inflammation due to infection or inhalation burns), snoring, gurgling noises or coughing or gagging. If a sound is heard, then some degree of air is moving past the vocal cords, but a noisy airway is a warning of potential imminent obstruction. Airways can become obstructed by a range of substances such as blood, vomitus, teeth, foreign bodies or food or other debris and symptoms and signs seen should be related to the underlying mechanism of injury. Treatment is directed towards the underlying cause and can range from repositioning the patient and suction to intubation or a surgical airway as needed in evolving airway swelling such as in burns or chemical inhalation.

In complete airway obstruction, there is no noise at all; this is an immediately life-threatening emergency. Again, this can be a primary or secondary airway issue, but without manoeuvres or procedures to open the airway unconsciousness and death will swiftly follow. The patient may demonstrate "see-saw" breathing [16], where the diaphragm contracts against a closed airway and distends the abdomen but causes the chest to be drawn inwards during attempted inspiration. During expiration, the opposite occurs, and the abdominal muscles contract inwards in an attempt to increase intrathoracic pressure and expel air. The closed upper airway leads to slight distension of the chest at this point as a result, and a rocking motion is seen across the diaphragm. Again, the treatment can escalate from simple manoeuvres to surgical airway along the airway ladder, depending on the underlying cause.

Reassessment of patients regularly is essential to quantify both responses to treatment and evolution of pathology. Patients who have been given certain medications with analgesic or sedative properties are at risk of losing control of their airway, as are patients with decreased cerebral perfusion due to ongoing hypovolaemia or evolving intracranial pathology.

Breathing

All trauma patients in the initial period should be given high flow oxygen as a safety measure until a rapid primary survey has been concluded and ongoing oxygen requirement has been assessed. This is consistent with the British Thoracic Society guidelines on emergency administration of oxygen [17] and includes patients with a history of lung disease. There is frequent concern about a minority subset of patients who have chronic type two respiratory failure and may not tolerate high flow oxygen without becoming hypercapnoeic. These patients are a tiny minority of patients who suffer from trauma. Frequent reassessment of the patient (which is the hallmark of an excellent primary survey) will alert the clinician to a susceptible patient who may be deteriorating as a result of oxygen administration. Far more harm is likely to come in trauma from restricting access to oxygen for those who require it than giving it for short periods to patients who may not. In patients who are known to have type two respiratory failure and are chronically hypoxic, once the initial survey is complete the oxygen concentration can be decreased to achieve their usual target saturation (usually an SpO_2 of 88–92%). It must be again stressed that this target is for a tiny minority of patients with severe chronic lung disease who have been injured — the vast majority of patients should be given supplementary oxygen to achieve saturations of 94–98%. A full discussion of oxygen-induced hypercarbia is beyond the scope of this textbook, but an excellent article by Abdo and Heunks [18] explains the physiology behind oxygen-induced hypercapnoea and the often quoted myth of "hypoxic drive" for those who are interested.

Monitoring of patients on oxygen is essential, and this is achieved using multiple data points. Firstly by looking at the oxygen mask. This should mist every time the patient exhales due to water vapor in the patients' upper airway. In some models, a brightly coloured polystyrene ball will lift with expiratory effort as a visual aid to count respiratory rate. In some cases, end-tidal waveform capnography can be used to monitor respiratory rate. It must be noted, however, that outside of ventilated patients the absolute $EtCO_2$ value is inaccurate. The respiratory rate can still be used, but due to mixing with entrained air or oxygen, the displayed value of the peak $EtCO_2$ will under-read. In addition to $EtCO_2$ monitoring, the most useful monitor that should be applied at the earliest opportunity is the pulse oximeter. Not only will it give information about oxygen saturation (SpO_2), most models will display a pulse rate and a rhythm plethysmograph, which can indicate an irregular pulse. In addition to this, the oximeter can be a crude surrogate marker of perfusion. A trace will only be picked up in reasonably perfused fingers, and in significantly hypovolaemic states it may not pick up at all. The other clinical pitfalls to avoid are poor or absent traces in patients who are cold or have fake/

painted nails, and unreliable SpO_2 readings in patients with certain abnormal forms of haemoglobin after toxin inhalation (e.g. carboxyhaemoglobin or methaemoglobin). Depending on patient location and available equipment, blood gas analysis may also be possible. This is a useful point of care test that can rapidly give information on oxygenation and ventilation parameters as well as acid-base balance, base deficit, levels of electrolytes, haemoglobin and lactate.

During the primary survey, the initial focus is on detecting and treating life-threatening pathology, which can be found on clinical examination or with the use of near-patient testing modalities such as ultrasonography or plain film x-rays. Due to the initial supine positioning of patients in the trauma bay, it can be challenging to assess for posterior wounds unless the patient is rolled onto their side. Similarly, in patients transported with their arms by their sides, it is not uncommon to miss axillary wounds—these must actively be sought out as part of the primary survey. The neck and abdomen border the thoracic cavity, so injuries in these areas should raise suspicion of intra-thoracic damage too.

There are many mnemonics to use for clinical examination, and FLAPSS (Feel, Look, Auscultate, Percuss, Search Sides and back) is a useful one. A caveat is that in noisy environments (in hospital as well as pre-hospital), the usefulness of auscultation can be limited [19]. An assessment following this methodology should pick up at least some of the signs of chest pathology, which is fully covered in the breathing chapter. Evaluation of the chest should also include the neck, and the mnemonic TWELVE (Tracheal position, Wounds, Emphysema, Laryngeal crepitus, Venous distension and Everything else) can be used.

After any significant intervention, re-examination and reassessment should be performed. Specifically, post-intubation checks should assess for the evolution of pneumothoraces and correct tube placement. As previously mentioned, auscultation can be limited in utility and there may be a role for ultrasonography in detecting significant pathology. For example, lung sliding can be used to assess for pneumothorax—if both lungs are seen to move under the pleura, then this is reassuring that there is no pneumothorax. The sensitivity of ultrasound is much higher than plain film x-ray for anterior pneumothoraces [20] and can be combined into other ultrasonographic assessments for trauma (e.g. e-FAST or RUSH protocols), which may also reveal haemothorax. A pitfall for the unwary is malposition of an endotracheal tube. If the tube is advanced too far, it will usually pass into the right main bronchus and not ventilate the left lung at all. This will also cause an absence of lung sliding (although lung pulsation will still be seen), absent breath sounds on the left and hypoxia, which could equally be suggestive of a pneumothorax. Before intervening, check that the tube is not too far in!

Other respiratory pathology may be apparent following intubation, such as decreased lung compliance (needing higher pressures to inflate the lung than would typically be necessary), increased A:a gradient (hypoxia despite additional oxygen supply) and difficulties in gas exchange.

Circulation

Circulatory assessment is the fourth stage in the primary survey, though some clues may already have been apparent about circulatory status from the initial steps. If a patient is talking coherently, then their circulation is adequate to perfuse their brain. This is to say that perfusion is *sufficient* rather than *normal*. Initial circulatory assessment includes the presence or absence of peripheral pulses (radial, femoral and carotid), a heart rate and capillary refill time.

Further assessments such as blood pressure and heart rate can come when monitoring is applied, but in the initial stage, these first measures can give a gross estimate of current circulatory status within seconds. Historically it was taught that a radial pulse equated to a systolic blood pressure of 80 mmHg, a femoral 70 mmHg and a carotid 60 mmHg. While these specific figures have been debunked [21], the order in which the pulses disappear is generally sound [22]. Patients who have a decreasing level of consciousness should be assessed for bleeding as a cause. This includes patients who appear to be confused, agitated or intoxicated—the underlying cause may be that they are not perfusing their brain due to hypovolaemia.

Patients who are suspected of having ongoing bleeding should be rapidly assessed and appropriately imaged to shorten the time to a definitive haemostatic procedure, either radiologically or surgically. Until diagnostic imaging is obtained, patients with a significant mechanism of injury and clinical signs compatible with ongoing bleeding should be considered to be actively bleeding still. Administration of tranexamic acid, appropriate use of blood products and other resuscitative measures are discussed in the circulatory chapter. Sites of blood loss are generally remembered by the saying "Blood on the floor and four more" This refers to external bleeding and internal bleeding into either the chest, abdominal or pelvic cavities and long bone fractures. Acutely, circulation preservation should be the aim. Treatments such as pelvic binders and long bone traction and splintage should be considered resuscitative measures for circulation, as much as for orthopaedic or analgesic reasons.

Hypoperfusion of tissues will also cause disturbances in acid-base balance as described in the circulation chapter. Hypoperfusion causes the production of lactate, resulting in an increasingly negative base excess and fall in pH. If severe (pH < 7.2) this may adversely affect clotting and other enzymatic dependent systems. Young patients will generally compensate for blood loss for an extended period in terms of maintaining their blood pressure, so hypovolaemia is a relatively late sign of bleeding. One American retrospective study of 115,000 trauma patients showed that by the time patients became hypotensive due to blood loss, their base deficit was already −20 and their overall mortality approached 65% [23]. Potential other causes of hypotension are tension pneumothorax or neurogenic shock; however, all hypotension in trauma should be considered to be due to hypovolaemia until proven otherwise. Similarly, a normal haemoglobin level does not rule out bleeding, as the concentration of the remaining blood will initially remain the same. A low haemoglobin level (<11 g/dl) should definitely raise the concern of acute blood loss and prompt a damage control approach.

Cold patients may have a prolonged capillary refill time (CRT) peripherally, so CRT should always be tested on either the sternum or forehead to ensure validity. As well as increasing CRT, cold patients may be developing a coagulopathy. This is partially because of the reduced effectiveness of enzymes involved in blood clot formation at lower temperatures, but also due to the degree of blood loss that must occur to induce hypothermia. Coagulopathy can occur independently of hypothermia, and as many as 30% of major trauma patients may have developed a coagulopathy by the time they arrive at the emergency department. This traumatic coagulopathy is independently associated with a poorer outcome [24–27]. If present on admission, hypothermia is also associated with a nearly threefold increased mortality in some studies [28–31] and should be aggressively treated by heating the patient, the treatment environment and any IV fluids, including blood products.

If a patient arrests as a result of trauma, then the correct management is to follow a traumatic cardiac arrest protocol, which is different from the usual ALS guidelines. This is discussed further in the traumatic cardiac arrest chapter, and interventions may include resuscitative thoracotomy if indicated in selected patients. This group is mainly those patients who have a witnessed arrest due to chest trauma and relatively short down time with a potentially amenable underlying cause. If a patient suffers a cardiac arrest as a result of a medical reason, resuscitative thoracotomy is not indicated. Medical and traumatic cardiac arrests are very different clinical entities and should be treated as such.

Disability and Head Injuries

Assessment of neurological status is the next step in trauma management, beginning with the level of consciousness. Formally, the Glasgow Coma Scale (GCS) is the accepted and validated method of assessing the level of consciousness in head-injured patients [32, 33]. GCS is a score from 3–15 depending on the level of consciousness, and there is a stepwise progression in mortality as the score falls (I.e. the patient becomes more unconscious) [34]. GCS is a useful score and is understood when making referrals, but can occasionally be challenging to remember how to calculate. A simpler alternative is AVPU. This stands for Alert, responds to Voice, responds to Pain stimuli or Unresponsive. In some areas, Confusion has been added as a variable between "alert" and "responds to voice" as another method of describing the level of consciousness (ACVPU). Trends over time are useful as patients with head injuries who are becoming more drowsy or unconscious should be treated as time-critical patients, mandating urgent imaging. Decreased level of consciousness can be due to medical as well as traumatic causes (e.g. hypoglycaemia, seizures etc.), and a medical cause of unconsciousness may have caused a traumatic injury, e.g. hypoglycaemia causing a patient to crash their car.

Neurological defects that are present at the point of presentation are significant to note, as patients who are becoming progressively more unresponsive may require anaesthesia for airway protection. The opportunity to examine for gross lateralising signs that may indicate a stroke, spinal cord injury or other neurological concerns may be lost once the patient is intubated. In the case of head-injured patients, waking them up to examine them may not be an appropriate course of action. Any coughing against an endotracheal tube may increase intracranial pressure and worsen secondary brain injury, so perform a baseline gross neurological exam before anaesthetising patients whenever possible.

Pupillary reflexes should routinely be examined as part of a neurological assessment, and any differences between sides should prompt urgent evaluation and treatment. If a patients' pupils are unreactive in head injury, then this is an emergency. However, the outcome may not be as nihilistic as previously believed depending on the presenting pathology. In a meta-analysis by Scotter et al., over 50% of patients who presented with fixed dilated pupils as a result of extradural haematoma made a good recovery back to independent living [35]. Traditionally, these patients would have been considered to have unsurvivable injuries.

Exposure

The final stage in the primary survey is exposure. This involves removing clothing and examining the patient for any other injuries that have not yet been found or addressed in the MABCD stages. These injuries may include fractures, burns or other significant soft tissue injuries such as degloving. When exposing patients, a balance must be struck between preserving dignity and body heat versus missing a relevant injury. At this point, the patient should be rolled and an assessment made of their back for injuries which may not have been found. It is also essential to consider other areas which have not been visualised and may have significant injuries such as axillae, groins, perineum and buttocks. Stab wounds in these areas can often be missed in unconscious patients, and the Exposure stage of the primary survey should be a trigger to examine them actively. In come centres where access to CT scanning is virtually immediate, patients may be taken to CT first and then exposure completed as part of the secondary survey. In the pre-hospital environment, full exposure may not be appropriate or possible for the reasons outlined above, even more so if patients are entrapped or immobile for another reason. Indeed, attempting to expose an entrapped patient may decrease the speed of extrication and lower temperature, both of which may increase mortality. Selective exposure should be undertaken if needed and if it may change patient management, especially if there is suspicion of penetrating wounds or significant bleeding. Any suspected but unconfirmed injuries which require further investigation in hospital should be handed over as a routine.

An in-hospital pitfall to avoid is an over-reliance on CT scanning to elucidate all injuries. A CT scan is not a substitute for a full clinical examination and secondary survey! This may have to wait if the patient is intubated or unable to speak, but a formal secondary survey should be undertaken as soon as practicable. CT scans typically will image from the vertex of the skull to mid femurs unless a specific request for additional sites is added. Most trauma centres have moved towards using a biphasic contrast scan (occasionally referred to as the Bastion Protocol [36]) as compared to previous methods for contrast CT scanning in trauma. This protocol can acquire excellent images in a shorter time with less radiation dose [37]. While CT scans can provide detailed images of solid viscera, bleeding sites and bony injuries, they may not image tendinous lesions or some other soft tissues well. To ensure no "minor" injuries are missed and good functional outcomes achieved, a targeted clinical examination should be performed as part of the secondary survey. CT scans can be used as a prompt to examine specific areas (in addition to prompts from the mechanism of injury), but should not be relied on to find every injury that needs treating.

Burns patients should also be exposed fully but should be kept as warm as possible to avoid hypothermia. Some regional burns units are co-located at Major Trauma Centres, but this is not always the case. Patients may need to have their initial trauma dealt with at the MTC and be transferred later to a specialist centre, so basic burns care and communication with specialist burns teams should be available at every MTC. The current UK criteria for referral to or discussion with regional burns centres are [38]:

Paediatrics

- **≥ 30% total body surface area (TBSA) burn of any degree**
- **≥ 15% TBSA if under one-year-old**
- **≥ 20% TBSA full-thickness burns**
- **Burns to face, feet, hands or genitalia**
- **Any chemical, electrical or serious friction burn**
- **Any cold injury**
- **Any burn not healing two weeks post-injury**
- **Any patient requiring ventilation for ≥ 24 h due to their burn injury**
- **Any child who is physiologically unstable as a result of burns or in whom a non-accidental injury is suspected**
- **Any burn in a neonate**

Adults

- **≥ 40% TBSA or ≥ 25% with inhalational injury**
- **≥ 25% TBSA if over 65 years old**
- **Burns to face, feet, hands or genitalia**
- **Any chemical, electrical or serious friction burn**
- **Any cold injury**
- **Any burn not healing two weeks post-injury**
- **All patients with major trauma and burn injury after treatment within a Major Trauma Centre.**

Onward Care

After initial resuscitation and treatment, patients should be admitted to a critical care area or a ward appropriate to deal with their injuries depending on their requirements. All patients with an Injury Severity Score (ISS) > 8 should have a rehabilitation assessment and prescription within 72 h of their injury by a rehabilitation medicine consultant. This timeframe can be extended to up to 96 h if the patient is unable to be assessed for clinical reasons before this point. This rehabilitation assessment should cover not only physical functional aspects of recovery but also cognitive/psychological, social and educational aspects of rehabilitation. This should lead to the formation of a specific rehabilitation prescription which can vary from observation only in the case of more minor injuries, through to formal rehabilitation programs in dedicated specialist national centres (e.g. spinal injury units).

Conclusion

The MABCD system of assessment identifies and treats pathology in a logical manner which can be applied in a variety of clinical settings from pre-hospital to in-hospital environments. It ensures that significant pathology is treated in the order that it may kill patients, and provides a standard system that is understood and applied by all members of the trauma team at each stage of progression of the case. In the event of deterioration, reassessment using the same system provides a solid base for identifying progression or evolution of pathology, or identification of clinical signs that may not have been present during the initial assessment. Even in advanced care, the MABCD methodology still forms the basis of the evaluation, and while the tools available to assess each system may be more complex, the underlying principles are the same.

Questions

1. The correct sequence of clinical assessment of trauma patients is:
   (a) ABCDE
   (b) MABCD
   (c) CABDE
   (d) DABC
2. Noisy breathing/gurgling is a sign of complete airway obstruction
   (a) True
   (b) False
3. An SpO2 reading of over 95% on a standard oximeter always indicates normal tissue oxygenation in burns patients
   (a) True
   (b) False
4. Trauma patients who become cold or present with hypothermia have worse outcomes than those who retain a normal temperature
   (a) True
   (b) False
5. Whole body CT of trauma patients will pick up all injuries
   (a) True
   (b) False

Answers

1. b
2. b—complete airway obstruction is silent due to lack of air movement
3. b—inhalation of carbon monoxide or cyanide compounds from burning plastics can falsely elevate SpO2 by creation of carboxyhaemoglobin or cyano-compounds
4. a
5. b

References

1. Clawson JJ, Dernocoeur KB, Murray C. Principles of emergency medical dispatch. Salt Lake City: International Academy of EMD; 2014.
2. Safar P, Brown TC, Holtey WJ, Wilder RJ. Ventilation and circulation with closed-chest cardiac massage in man. JAMA. 1961 May 20;176:574–6.
3. Katzenell U, Ash N, Tapia AL, Campino GA, Glassberg E. Analysis of the causes of death of casualties in field military setting. Mil Med. 2012 Sep;177(9):1065–8.
4. Eastridge BJ, Mabry RL, Seguin P, Cantrell J, Tops T, Uribe P, et al. Death on the battlefield (2001–2011): implications for the future of combat casualty care. J Trauma Acute Care Surg. 2012 Dec;73:S431–7.
5. Eastridge BJ, Holcomb JB, Shackelford S. Outcomes of traumatic hemorrhagic shock and the epidemiology of preventable death from injury. Transfusion (Paris). 2019;59(S2):1423–8.
6. Kragh JF, Walters TJ, Baer DG, Fox CJ, Wade CE, Salinas J, et al. Survival with emergency tourniquet use to stop bleeding in major limb trauma. Ann Surg 2009 Jan;249(1):1–7.
7. Tien HC, Spencer F, Tremblay LN, Rizoli SB, Brenneman FD. Preventable deaths from hemorrhage at a level I Canadian trauma center. J Trauma. 2007 Jan;62(1):142–6.
8. Dorlac WC, DeBakey ME, Holcomb JB, Fagan SP, Kwong KL, Dorlac GR, et al. Mortality from isolated civilian penetrating extremity injury. J Trauma. 2005 Jul;59(1):217–22.
9. Rasmussen TE, Tai NRM, Rich NM, editors. Rich's vascular trauma. 3rd ed. Philadelphia, PA: Elsevier; 2016. 350 p.
10. Russell RJ, Hodgetts TJ, McLeod J, Starkey K, Mahoney P, Harrison K, et al. The role of trauma scoring in developing trauma clinical governance in the Defence medical services. Philos Trans R Soc B Biol Sci. 2011 Jan 27;366(1562):171–91.
11. Huber-Wagner S, Biberthaler P, Häberle S, Wierer M, Dobritz M, Rummeny E, et al. Whole-body CT in Haemodynamically unstable severely injured patients – a retrospective, multicentre study. PLoS One. 2013 [cited 2019 Aug 26];8(7). e68880. Available from https://www.ncbi.nlm.nih.gov/pmc/articles/PMC3722202/
12. Ordoñez CA, Herrera-Escobar JP, Parra MW, Rodriguez-Ossa PA, Mejia DA, Sanchez AI, et al. Computed tomography in hemodynamically unstable

severely injured blunt and penetrating trauma patients. J Trauma Acute Care Surg. 2016 Apr;80(4):597–603.
13. Stop The Bleed [Internet]. Stop The Bleeding Coalition. [cited 2019 Aug 26]. Available from https://stopthebleedingcoalition.org/
14. Zhao KL, Herrenkohl M, Paulsen M, Bulger EM, Vavilala MS, Moore M, et al. Learners' perspectives on stop the bleed: a course to improve survival during mass casualty events. Trauma Surg Acute Care Open. 2019 Jul 1;4(1):e000331.
15. Zwislewski A, Nanassy AD, Meyer LK, Scantling D, Jankowski MA, Blinstrub G, et al. Practice makes perfect: the impact of stop the bleed training on hemorrhage control knowledge, wound packing, and tourniquet application in the workplace. Injury. 2019 Apr;50(4):864–8.
16. Saraya T, Shimoda M, Hirata A, Takizawa H. Paradoxical respiration: 'seesaw' motion with massive pulmonary consolidation. Case Rep. 2016 Jan 19;2016:bcr2015213449.
17. O'Driscoll BR, Howard LS, Earis J, Mak V. British Thoracic Society guideline for oxygen use in adults in healthcare and emergency settings. BMJ Open Respir Res. 2017 May 1;4(1):e000170.
18. Abdo WF, Heunks LM. Oxygen-induced hypercapnia in COPD: myths and facts. Crit Care. 2012;16(5):323.
19. Noble VE, Lamhaut L, Capp R, Bosson N, Liteplo A, Marx J-S, et al. Evaluation of a thoracic ultrasound training module for the detection of pneumothorax and pulmonary edema by prehospital physician care providers. BMC Med Educ. 2009 Jan 12;9:3.
20. Petrosoniak A, Hicks C. Resuscitation Resequenced: a rational approach to patients with trauma in shock. Emerg Med Clin North Am. 2018 Feb;36(1):41–60.
21. Deakin CD, Low JL. Accuracy of the advanced trauma life support guidelines for predicting systolic blood pressure using carotid, femoral, and radial pulses: observational study. BMJ. 2000 Sep 16;321(7262):673–4.
22. Poulton TJ. ATLS paradigm fails. Ann Emerg Med. 1988 Jan;17(1):107.
23. Parks JK, Elliott AC, Gentilello LM, Shafi S. Systemic hypotension is a late marker of shock after trauma: a validation study of advanced trauma life support principles in a large national sample. Am J Surg. 2006 Dec;192(6):727–31.
24. Maegele M, Lefering R, Yucel N, Tjardes T, Rixen D, Paffrath T, et al. Early coagulopathy in multiple injury: an analysis from the German Trauma Registry on 8724 patients. Injury. 2007 Mar;38(3):298–304.
25. Brohi K. Diagnosis and management of coagulopathy after major trauma. Br J Surg. 2009 Sep;96(9):963–4.
26. MacLeod JBA, Lynn M, McKenney MG, Cohn SM, Murtha M. Early coagulopathy predicts mortality in trauma. J Trauma. 2003 Jul;55(1):39–44.
27. Kushimoto S, Kudo D, Kawazoe Y. Acute traumatic coagulopathy and trauma-induced coagulopathy: an overview. J Intensive Care. 2017 Dec;5(1):6.
28. Balvers K, Van der Horst M, Graumans M, Boer C, Binnekade J, Goslings JC, et al. Hypothermia as a predictor for mortality in trauma patients at admittance to the intensive care unit. J Emerg Trauma Shock. 2016;9(3):97.
29. Wang HE, Callaway CW, Peitzman AB, Tisherman SA. Admission hypothermia and outcome after major trauma. Crit Care Med. 2005 Jun;33(6):1296–301.
30. Shafi S, Elliott AC, Gentilello L. Is hypothermia simply a marker of shock and injury severity or an independent risk factor for mortality in trauma patients? Analysis of a large National Trauma Registry. J Trauma Inj Infect Crit Care. 2005 Nov;59(5):1081–5.
31. Waibel BH, Schlitzkus LL, Newell MA, Durham CA, Sagraves SG, Rotondo MF. Impact of hypothermia (below 36°C) in the rural trauma patient. J Am Coll Surg. 2009 Nov 1;209(5):580–8.
32. Teasdale G, Jennett B. Assessment of coma and impaired consciousness. A practical scale. Lancet Lond Engl. 1974 Jul 13;2(7872):81–4.
33. Jain S, Teasdale GM, Iverson LM. Glasgow coma scale. In: StatPearls [Internet]. Treasure Island: StatPearls Publishing; 2019 [cited 2019 Aug 30]. Available from http://www.ncbi.nlm.nih.gov/books/NBK513298/
34. Gennarelli TA, Champion HR, Copes WS, Sacco WJ. Comparison of mortality, morbidity and severity of 59,713 head injured patients with 114,447 patients with extracranial injuries. J Trauma Inj Infect Crit Care. 1994 Dec;37(6):962–8.
35. Scotter JM, Hendrickson SA, Marcus HJ, Wilson MH. Prognosis of patients with bilateral fixed dilated pupils secondary to traumatic extradural or subdural haematoma who undergo surgery: a systematic review and meta-analysis. Emerg Med J EMJ. 2015;32(8):654–9.
36. Carter NJ, Kirkwood GW, Miles R, Gay DAT. The inception of the Bastion protocol for trauma CT scanning. J R Nav Med Serv. 2018;104(3):183–6.
37. Hakim W, Kamanahalli R, Dick E, Bharwani N, Fetherston S, Kashef E. Trauma whole-body MDCT: an assessment of image quality in conventional dual-phase and modified biphasic injection. Br J Radiol [Internet]. 2016. [cited 2019 Aug 30];89(1063) 20160160. Available from https://www.ncbi.nlm.nih.gov/pmc/articles/PMC5257328/
38. National Network for Burn Care (NNBC). National Burn Care Referral Guidance-2012.pdf [Internet]. 2012 [cited 2019 Aug 30]. Available from https://www.britishburnassociation.org/wp-content/uploads/2018/02/National-Burn-Care-Referral-Guidance-2012.pdf

6 Massive Haemorrhage Control

Alia Yaqub and Peter Lax

- Understand the different types of major haemorrhage
- Know how to manage the different types of haemorrhage
- Understand when advanced techniques, such as REBOA and thoracotomy, might be used

Case Discussion: Massive Haemorrhage in Civilian Settings

A known Intravenous Drug User has self-inflicted wounds to his left antecubital fossa and has bled significantly. Paramedics on scene have applied two tourniquets in an attempt to control the bleeding. They report the patient is pale, confused and sweaty. They will be in the Emergency Department (ED) in 5 minutes.

What should you do?

What are the steps in pre-hospital haemorrhage control?

What should the goals be in resuscitation?

When should pre-hospital or ED thoracotomy be considered?

When might resuscitative endovascular balloon occlusion of the aorta (REBOA) be considered?

Returning to the original case, the patient will arrive shortly. Anticipate needing to give warmed blood quickly. This may require activation of the local massive transfusion pathway. Blood should be given to maintain a central pulse. Pre-hospital haemorrhage control should have included a failure of direct pressure, and a failure to stop the bleeding with a single tourniquet should lead to the application of a second. The aim of resuscitation should be definitive bleeding control. This is likely to be achieved operatively, but for now, the patient may need significant analgesia in order to tolerate the tourniquet. There is no role for thoracotomy or REBOA in this case.

A. Yaqub (✉)
Emergency Medicine Department, Leeds General Infirmary, Leeds, UK
e-mail: aliayaqub@nhs.net

P. Lax
Tactical Medical Wing, Royal Air Force, Brize Norton, Oxfordshire, UK

The Air Ambulance Service (TAAS), Rugby, Warwickshire, UK

P. Lax (ed.), *Textbook of Acute Trauma Care*, https://doi.org/10.1007/978-3-030-83628-3_6

Introduction

Advances in trauma care are often fuelled by conflict, and current understanding and treatment protocols for massive haemorrhage control are no different in this respect. As medicine advances and our understanding of pathophysiological mechanisms expands, treatments for trauma improve, resulting in increased survival. Several case review series have looked at death rates and mechanism of death on the Battlefield from World War 2, through the American experience in Vietnam and, more latterly, to operations in Iraq and Afghanistan. Overall mortality has decreased, from 30% in World War Two to 24% in Vietnam and under 10% in recent conflicts [1] (though the absolute accuracy of these figures has been somewhat disputed due to the methodology used) [2]. While medical advances have played a significant part in reducing in-hospital deaths, the reintroduction of simple and long-known techniques have seen a substantial decrease in the number of soldiers who have died of treatable haemorrhage. In Vietnam, half of the potentially treatable deaths were from limb wounds that were amenable to tourniquet use [3], but this rate fell to 13.5% in Iraq from 2001–2011 [4]. This is due primarily to the training of personnel in the use of massive haemorrhage control techniques, including the use of tourniquets, with subsequent feedback and reinforcement during the military operational medical pathway [4–7]. While deaths in warzones will show a more substantial component of blast and ballistic injuries, the basic principles of massive haemorrhage control and their importance remain the same in civilian practice. With terrorist incidents such as the bombings in Madrid in 2004 [8], Boston Marathon in 2013 [9, 10] and more recent major incidents in Paris [11, 12], military evidence is all the more relevant to civilian trauma care.

Studies and reports on massive haemorrhage in civilian settings [13] have shown a concerning picture. In one review, trauma haemorrhage was identified as the cause of 30–40% of all trauma deaths and 51% of early trauma deaths. A study from Texas into mortality from isolated extremity injury showed approximately half of these patients could have been saved by tourniquet use earlier in their care [14]. A Canadian retrospective review identified that 16% of trauma deaths might have been preventable if sources of bleeding were more aggressively sought and treated [15].

In common with military experience, massive haemorrhage represents the leading cause of potentially treatable trauma deaths in the civilian population. For treatment to be life-saving, it must be instigated as quickly as possible, often by people with minimal or basic medical training. There is also evidence linking duration and depth of hypovolaemic shock with worsening outcome [16–20]. Treating massive haemorrhage earlier may save lives; both at the immediate point of treatment and later by minimising the systemic effects of hypotensive shock, such as coagulopathy and multiorgan failure. The American College of Surgeons Stop the Bleed campaign [21] started in 2015. It highlights how a significant proportion of preventable deaths are from haemorrhage [22] and recognises that professional help will not arrive immediately. The campaign, therefore, aims to train bystanders to manage severe bleeding as quickly as possible using simple techniques. A study performed in 2018/19 into the efficacy of the Stop the Bleed teaching showed that this campaign, with a combination of lectures and hands-on skill workshops, improved knowledge and management in life-threatening bleeding scenarios [23].

This is not a phenomenon seen exclusively in the USA; in the UK, the 1999 Stephen Lawrence inquiry [24] appears to support this need for bystander education. It found the teenager (who was stabbed and bled to death at a bus stop) was dead before the ambulance crew arrived, but that there were bystanders present who could have intervened.

Haemorrhage control efforts can be broadly divided into two categories; temporary and definitive. Most of the methods covered in this chapter fall into the former group, and may buy the patient enough time to reach the latter. The use of pressure and tourniquets will be covered, as well as more advanced measures. As will be discussed, much of our current civilian practice comes from military evidence.

What Is Massive Haemorrhage?

Confusingly, there is not a single universally accepted definition of massive haemorrhage in the literature. Definitions are hugely variable and range from absolute numbers such as 50% blood loss within three hours [25], six units of RBC's in 12 h, 50 units of blood components in 24 h [26], loss of more than one circulating volume within 24 h [27] or a sustained rate of >150 ml/min [25]. There is at least recognition in some publications that these definitions are problematic [26, 28]. In most cases, the criteria are both retrospective and heavily weighted towards hospital practice and the varyingly accurate assumption that blood and blood products will readily be at hand for transfusion. The reality from the previously mentioned data is that patients with massive haemorrhage will, in many cases, not survive the transfer to hospital from the scene of injury unless the source of their massive haemorrhage is at least temporarily addressed at the point of injury. Of the more practical definitions, an ongoing rate of blood loss of equal to or greater than 150 ml/min, or bleeding that leads to a heart rate of more than 110 beats/min or systolic blood pressure of less than 90 mmHg [28] are more useful. Massive haemorrhage may be difficult to define precisely, but to borrow a legal phrase, "I know it when I see it" [29].

Sources of Massive Haemorrhage

External Bleeding

The Advanced Trauma Life Support adage of "blood on the floor and four more" holds true [30]. Large amounts of external bleeding should be very obvious, and ongoing bleeding should be addressed as a priority. Patients may also lose massive amounts of blood into their pelvis or from long bone fractures (humerus and femur), and both long bone and pelvic fractures can be splinted to reduce both pain and bleeding. Bleeding into the chest and abdomen is much more challenging to treat in the pre-hospital setting; management is explored further under the non-compressible haemorrhage section (below) and the damage control surgery and interventional radiology sections of this textbook.

Skin/Scalp Bleeding

Staples, sutures and/or adrenaline dressings (and occasionally devices such as the iTClamp [31, 32]) may be needed to stem bleeding from the scalp, as bandages may provide insufficient pressure when applied circumferentially around the head. The iTClamp is a device that opposes wound edges to encourage clots to form and arrest bleeding (see Videos 6.1–6.3). It has been used by military [33] and civilian [34] personnel in the USA in isolation or combination with other haemorrhage control methods. In common with other mass haemorrhage control strategies, its application can be rapidly learnt and then applied by those with minimal medical training. The iTClamp is now part of the Committee on Tactical Combat Casualty Care's recommendations for Tactical Field Care in combination with haemostatic dressings, as it can apply direct pressure without a practitioner remaining hands-on with the patient [35]. While the device looks painful to use, the patient (by definition) will have a significant wound to require it to be applied in the first place and so require good analgesia *a priori*. Surprisingly, when an assessment of pain was made during application on 26 volunteers, the average pain score on application on a 1–10 scale was self-reported as a mean of 2.0 ± 1.1. On removal, pain scores were 1.9 ± 1.5. The maximum scores on application and removal were 5.0 and 7.0 respectively, with a minimum score of 0 for both [36]. It is also safe in terms of tissue damage. One study demonstrates minimal tissue damage (needle holes only in 59/60 cadaveric and swine applications [37]). The iTClamp also outperforms the Combat Application Tourniquet (CAT) in terms of preservation of marksmanship skills in healthy volunteers on a target range [38]. This may be of relevance if used in tactical environments.

Video 6.1: iTClamp Application to live animal model **[External video link: https://www.youtube.com/watch?v=OGJyzxyLCMs]**

Video 6.2: iTClamp application to the scalp **[External video link: https://www.youtube.com/watch?v=EOvtQsDcEWo]**

Video 6.3: iTClamp self-application by healthy volunteers **[External video link: https://www.youtube.com/watch?v=18U1Jh7idHU]**

Other haemorrhage control methods from large skin edges include adrenaline-soaked dressings and application of sutures or staples for wound opposition. Adrenaline dressings manage bleeding by causing local vasospasm, and staples or sutures allow rapid skin opposition in bleeding wounds. Paramedics may carry staples; sutures are more often instituted by a doctor in the UK.

Facial Trauma

Harris et al. from London HEMS described a technique to manage massive maxillofacial bleeding in 2010 [39]. Several other pre-hospital care providers have since adopted this technique. It involves using a well-fitting cervical collar to splint the face, applying bite blocks between the maxilla and mandibular molars, as well as a nasal epistat in each nostril (Fig. 6.1). Given the significant association between significant maxillofacial injury and head injury, these patients are often intubated. The endotracheal tube also provides a degree of splinting [40]. This method and the anatomical sources of maxillofacial bleeding are more fully explored in the airway chapter of this textbook.

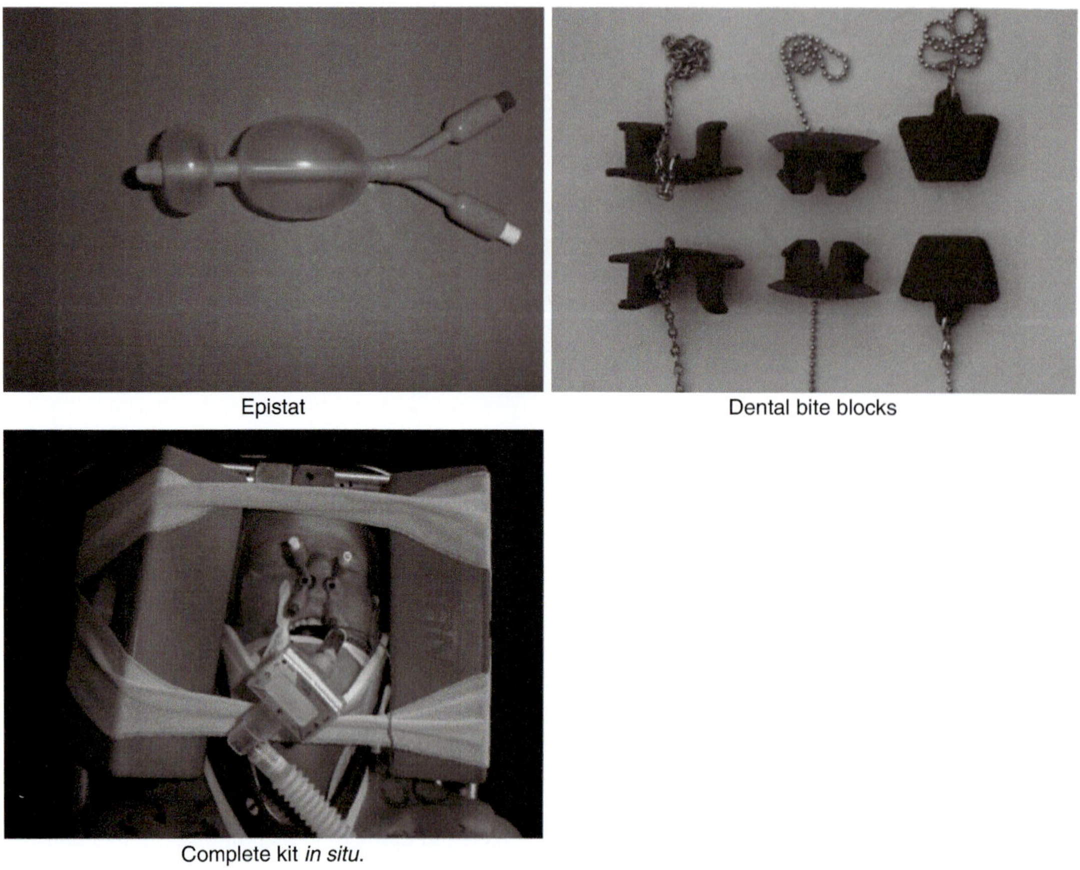

Fig. 6.1 Kit for controlling massive maxillofacial haemorrhage (from Harris et al. [39])

Pelvic Trauma

Bleeding from pelvic injuries can be catastrophic, either from bone edges, associated vascular damage or visceral injuries. Specifics of pelvic injuries are dealt with in the pelvic chapter, but in terms of massive haemorrhage control, the application of a pelvic binder is a haemorrhage control intervention. Their application is now a standard procedure for ambulance crew [41]. The Faculty of Pre-Hospital care made a consensus statement in 2012 reviewing the available evidence and supported their use and that of scoops rather than repeated log rolls [42]. Pelvic binders have been used in an effort to control pelvic haemorrhage for decades [40]. The reduction in pelvic volume is thought to create tamponade and reduce venous bleeding, while reduction and stabilisation of the fracture site is believed to minimise bone edge bleeding and protect against disruption of any initial clot formation [43]. A study examining the effects of pelvic binders published in 2017 showed they significantly reduced mortality and blood transfusion [44]. If a pelvic binder is not available, a simple sheet may be used to reduce the volume of the intra-pelvic cavity and subsequent bleeding into it [45].

Patient handling is now geared to reduce rotational movement with the aim of preserving clot. A patient with significant pelvic fractures found in a semi-prone position was previously log-rolled; such a patient would undergo 510 degrees of rotation rather than 170 degrees which can be achieved with a scoop stretcher [40].

Treatment of Massive Haemorrhage

Massive haemorrhage largely falls into two categories in trauma—compressible and non-compressible. There is also an element of environmental interplay in pre-hospital care. What might be an anatomically compressible injury (e.g. a cut brachial artery) may be temporarily uncompressible based on the patient's location (e.g. arm caught in heavy machinery up to the axilla). Safety of personnel is the prime consideration (see scene safety chapter), so ensure that any dangers are addressed before starting treatment—e.g. machines that are still running may injure those who attempt a rescue. Some treatments are appropriate for haemorrhage in both pre- and in-hospital settings, such as tranexamic acid administration (TXA). The CRASH-2 trial [46] showed a 9% relative risk reduction in mortality in bleeding trauma patients, with the most benefit seen if TXA was given within the first hour of injury, but benefit still seen if administered within three hours of injury. This drug is now a standard medication given by paramedics and other pre-hospital clinicians in the UK [41]. Hypothermia is well-recognised to impair clotting and worsen bleeding, so patients should be kept as warm as possible. This may involve measures such as the removal of wet clothes and the use of blankets, as well as fluid/blood warmers. More detail is available in the circulation and haemostasis in trauma chapters.

Compressible Haemorrhage

The prime example of compressible haemorrhage is an injury to a limb. The more distal the injury, the easier it is to deal with, especially if there is an arterial component. As wounds become more proximal, they become increasingly difficult to either compress or use a tourniquet. Injuries in the neck, axilla or groin are referred to as junctional haemorrhage. They are particularly problematic as they contain large vascular structures which may be quite deep, difficult to control, and are not readily amenable to tourniquet use.

DDIT Escalation of Treatment

- **Direct pressure**
  - Expose the bleeding site and apply direct pressure
- **Direct pressure (again)**
  - If bleeding is not immediately brought under control, quickly reassess that the pressure is applied to the correct site and re-apply. Avoid the temptation of repeated looks or swathes of dressings; remember

all bleeding is blood that is no longer carrying oxygen to vital organs. Once blood has left the body, it cannot be reinfused (at least in the pre-hospital environment).

- **Indirect pressure**
  - If direct pressure has failed to stop the bleeding, apply indirect pressure in addition to direct pressure. This is done over an artery proximal to the bleeding site and compresses the vessel against a bone. Either direct pressure in isolation or in combination with indirect pressure controls the bleeding in most cases.
- **Tourniquet**
  - If the bleeding is still not controlled, apply a tourniquet. The application time should be documented on the tourniquet and form part of the handover to the receiving team.

The escalation from direct pressure through the rest of the treatment pathway as needed must be rapid. If there is a high-volume ongoing blood loss, there is precious little time to arrest it. The progression through the process of assess—intervene—re-check—escalate has to be fast to preserve as much circulating volume as possible. Even if blood is immediately available for transfusion, transfused red blood cells do not function as well as the patient's own blood immediately after admission. How long blood products have been stored may also influence how well they work [47–49]. The best blood to be circulating in a patient's body is their own, so preserving as much of it as possible instead of replacing it should be the aim. Occasionally, an obvious catastrophic bleed will require tourniquet application from the outset (e.g. amputation, major artery transection). In these cases, it is appropriate to use a tourniquet as a first-line haemorrhage control method, as escalation and reassessment steps are unlikely to be effective without tourniquet use. During the time it would take to escalate as described above, the patient is still losing valuable blood. Once the patient is in a more controlled environment, it may be appropriate to de-escalate from tourniquet use when facilities are available to allow appropriate haemorrhage control (e.g. in an operating theatre or emergency department).

Direct pressure onto a bleeding site is a well-accepted first aid measure for most cuts, whether they fall into the definition of massive haemorrhage or not, as is the elevation of the bleeding site above the level of the heart. Direct and continuous pressure with a gauze pad or bandage may be sufficient in itself to stem bleeding, but it may take time to work. One problem often seen is repeated removal of dressings to check if bleeding has stopped. If clots start to form around the wound/dressing interface and then the dressing is removed, the bleeding will restart. For this reason, when a wound is first seen it can be helpful for hospital staff if a picture is taken before dressing if this will not delay treatment. Once a wound has been covered (if superficial) or packed (if deep) to stop bleeding, the dressings should not be taken down or swapped until the patient is in hospital, ideally in an operating theatre if the wounds are severe. If there is bleeding through the dressing, another dressing should be placed on top and the initial dressing left in place to avoid disrupting any clot. Pressure should be focused (where possible) on the specific point of the wound that is bleeding.

Indirect Pressure

If direct pressure is insufficient, indirect pressure over a major pulse point (brachial or femoral artery) in addition to pressure over the wound may help to reduce bleeding. This is resource-intensive, as pressure now needs to be kept on two areas constantly. Simultaneously, other therapeutic interventions that are necessary are undertaken, and this may be impossible for a lone clinician. Indirect pressure may buy time to apply a haemostatic dressing or tourniquet if one is not immediately available. However, it is primarily a short-term temporising measure that is not practical for more extended periods.

Pressure on the aorta is the most extreme example of indirect pressure. There has been some simulation evidence suggesting that indirect pressure can be transmitted effectively to the aorta by two-handed or knee compression of the abdomen [50]. This method cannot currently be advocated for clinical use due to lack of evidence. However, it is a similar thought process for some devices such as the Abdominal Aortic and Junctional Tourniquet (AAJT) [51]. While initial data on healthy individuals for this device were compelling, further studies have failed to live up to the initial promise. The AAJT is less effective than other junctional devices and takes longer to apply [52, 53].

Tourniquets

The final step in the DDIT pathway for managing compressible haemorrhage is the application of tourniquets. Tourniquets work by stopping the arterial blood flow to an injured limb, thereby minimising further blood loss. They have been used since the Middle Ages, with military use first documented in 1674 [54]. They have, at times, fallen out of favour [55] but are currently recognised to be life-saving for bleeding that is uncontrolled by direct pressure. Tourniquets form the last stage in major limb haemorrhage guidance for UK paramedics [41], and the National Institute for Clinical Excellence supports their use [56]. The Faculty of Pre-hospital Care advises that tourniquets are applied as rapidly as possible, directly against the skin, as distal as possible above the wound and tightly enough to arrest haemorrhage [57]. Combat Action Tourniquets (CAT) are the most widely used model [58] and are designed to allow application with one hand—this allows for self-application if necessary (Fig. 6.2). Although each brand has its own instructions, the broad principle is that they are strapped around the limb and pressure increased with a windlass, compressing a single artery against a single bone until bleeding is stemmed.

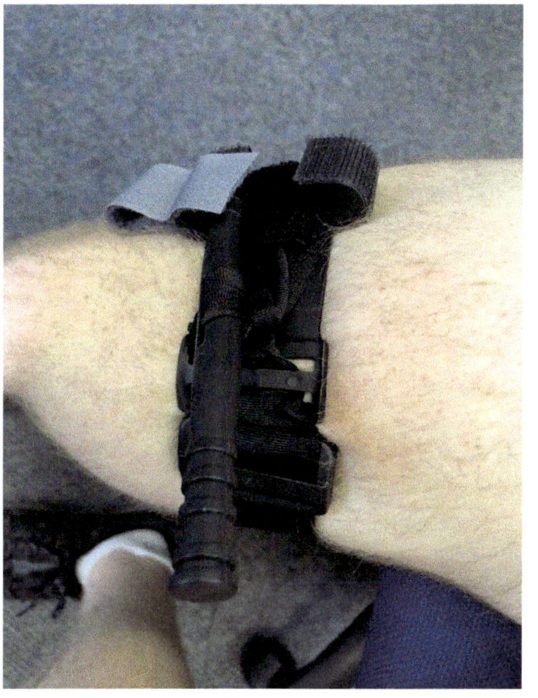

Fig. 6.2 Combat Application Tourniquet with windlass tightened

Many devices, including the CAT, come with a place to write on the time of application. Whether or not this is the case, it is vital to document the application time and hand this over to the receiving team. Additional measures (such as a large "T" and the time of application written on the patients' forehead or another visible area) act as a reminder that a tourniquet has been applied. This is especially important in intubated or unconscious patients who may not complain of the pain due to the tourniquet and suffer ischaemic complications as a result. When properly applied to conscious patients, the resulting ischaemia causes pain in addition to the injury itself; the analgesia requirement is likely to be significant, requiring morphine, ketamine or some other potent analgesic. Tourniquets may be applied in the ED if bleeding cannot be managed in any other way, though pneumatic devices are preferred if available.

There is an ongoing debate about the role of tourniquets in the management of crush injury. Theoretically, there is some benefit in their use after crush to prevent reperfusion injury by stemming blood flow to the affected site and controlling the release of blood from ischaemic tissues back into the central circulation. Due to ongoing ischaemia, rhabdomyolysis and muscle damage, this returning blood may be cold, high in potassium and acidic. This may cause hypotension and arrhythmias, as seen in vascular surgery when clamps are taken off and limbs reperfuse [59, 60]. This concern has been raised with a similar phenomenon reported in knee replacement surgery [61]. In practical terms, pneumatic devices are more effective than windlass devices such as the CAT as they arrest blood flow at lower pressures [62] and cause less tissue damage, hence why they are preferred in hospital practice.

The evidence for the use of any tourniquets in traumatic crush injury is often low quality and contradictory. However, what relevant published literature there is agrees that fluid resuscitation and the avoidance of potassium-containing solutions are important in these patients [63–65]. In these cases, the potential for sudden cardiovascular deterioration should be anticipated when a casualty is released from a crush scenario. Although theoretically attractive, further study is needed before clear recommendations can be made for the routine use of tourniquets in traumatic crush injury. If there is an overt vascular injury that would necessitate tourniquet use in other circumstances, one should still be used. Research is still ongoing on how to best mitigate the ischaemic consequences of tourniquet use [66], but tourniquets are life-saving devices and should be used when necessary.

A key point on tourniquet use is that although these devices are easy to use, training is essential and should be as immersive as possible. Putting a device on a fake limb without any movement or resistance is a straightforward task; however, this does not adequately replicate how the task is achieved *in vivo*. Putting a tourniquet on an aggressive/combative/confused patient in the pre-hospital environment is very different from doing it in a warm, well-lit classroom. Practitioners should "train how they fight" and aim to stretch themselves while training with these devices and ensure familiarity with the particular model that their employer uses. This should increase efficacy and proficiency when they are needed for real.

Other concerns revolve around the length of time they can be applied. The general consensus is that after two hours there is a risk of permanent nerve damage and muscle or skin necrosis, and after six hours this extends to complete muscle damage that is likely to require amputation [67]. This data is primarily based on pneumatic tourniquet use in elective operating theatres. Patients who are hypovolaemic due to trauma, and have a non-pneumatic tourniquet applied, are at higher risk of complications. A battlefield study by Lakstein et al. [68] showed that the mean ischaemic time for tourniquet application without complications was 78 min. However, due to the heterogeneity of injuries it was difficult to demonstrate a minimum time before complications started. There is also uncertainty regarding whether the nature of tourniquet injuries is from direct pressure/compression or ischaemic damage of the nerve. Periodic loosening of tourniquets has been suggested to mitigate this damage; however, this will likely cause incremental bleeding and is therefore not generally advised in the first hour [69]. Once a tourniquet has been applied, the patient should be treated as a time-critical casualty and taken to hospital for immediate evaluation and treatment. Where the pre-hospital phase is prolonged (> 1–2 h), and after application of a direct pressure bandage to the bleeding wound, cautious tourniquet release (but leaving the tourniquet in place) is recommended.

The pain associated with correct tourniquet application has been previously mentioned, but another consideration may be the effects of pain or further resuscitation on the patient's blood pressure. Tourniquets, when applied correctly, should obliterate a distal pulse. However, patients who have bled profusely may have lost distal pulses due to hypovolaemia before the tourniquet is applied. When an extremely painful stimulus such as application of a tourniquet or further resuscitation is given, if the tourniquet is not on tight enough and the blood pressure rises, bleeding may resume. If the tourniquet is maximally tightened and bleeding is still occurring, a second tourniquet may be applied to the same limb more proximally. This is more often required where there is more muscle to compress, typically in the upper leg.

Haemostatic Dressings

In cases of severe haemorrhage, direct pressure can be combined with the use of haemostatic dressings such as Celox, Quik-Clot or Hem-Con. These dressings are impregnated bandages, pads or pellets (depending on the product used) that will increase clotting at the site of injury. In early zeolite-based dressings, such as first- and second-generation Quick-Clot products, this was achieved by absorbing water and concentrating the patients clotting factors at the wound site in an exothermic reaction. However, these were discontinued following reports of wound burns and tissue damage due to the heat created by the exothermic reaction [70–72].

Each product works using different mechanisms. These include direct activation of intrinsic clotting pathways (e.g. kaolin-based third-generation Quik-Clot) or attracting red blood cells into a bandage and creating an adherent seal over the wound (chitosan-based dressings such as HemCon/ChitoFlex/ChitoGauze/Celox). More recent iterations of haemostatic dressings (e.g. the modified rapid deployment haemostat) work on multiple complex mechanisms involving platelet activation, coagulation cascade activation, local vasoconstriction and agglutination of red blood cells, all mediated by fully acetylated poly-N-acetyl-glucosamine [73]. While there are numerous animal studies of these agents, there is little human trial data on differences in effectiveness *between* various products. One concern that is often brought up in chitosan-based dressings is the risk of allergic reaction in patients who are sensitive to shellfish (chitosan is a shellfish polysaccharide derivative). These dressings have specifically been tested on shellfish-sensitive patients and found to be safe [74, 75]. Most of these studies show that haemostatic dressings are effective in clinical use. Due to the widespread use by various military forces of Celox, HemCon and Quikclot, it is unlikely that other products in this class will be able to break into the market [76]. Other novel sealants may be useful in different circumstances (e.g. FloSeal (gelatin granules and human thrombin) or fibrin sealants in surgery).

Future advances in the use of expanding haemostatic foams are focusing on minimising infection whilst optimising compression by using foam impregnated with iodine [77].

Junctional Haemorrhage

These are areas of bleeding such as the neck, axilla or groin where the torso joins the extremities, and tourniquets cannot be easily applied. A ten-year retrospective US battlefield study showed that 17.5% of potentially preventable deaths were due to junctional haemorrhage [4]. Treating and preventing injuries in these areas is problematic for many reasons. There are a large number of vascular structures, but these are in areas where both tourniquets and direct pressure are difficult to apply and maintain, especially in military or other tactical settings.

From a military protection and prevention viewpoint, these areas are also challenging. Increasing the amount of protective body armour around the groin, axilla, or neck reduces the range of movement and can significantly limit mobility. Increasing protection but reducing speed and agility may result in an easier target for the enemy and unwittingly increase the risk of death or injury [78, 79].

The principles of direct pressure with haemostatic dressings are the same for treating junctional haemorrhage. These may be harder to perform successfully, but there are few options for managing bleeding in this area in the pre-hospital environment. Once in hospital, rapid transfer to theatre and control of proximal vessels in the chest or abdomen may be required.

Specific devices for junctional compression are in development and early deployment, such as the Combat Ready Clamp (CRoC), the SAM Junctional Tourniquet (SAM-JT), Junctional Emergency Tool and the previously mentioned AJTT [80]. While there is not a large amount of empirical trial data for the use of these devices, cadaveric studies and isolated case reports show they do have some merit. It is also worth looking at qualitative data from users. If the device is impractical to use *in vivo*, it is largely irrelevant how well it performs in perfect conditions in the manufacturers' lab. When end-users have trialled various devices, the CRoC and SAM-JT were preferred over the JETT and AJTT by US Army medics during training [81]. Feedback from actual battlefield use is equally poor for the AJTT, with units reporting it was "easily broken" and the CRoC was "bulky, heavy and takes too much time to apply" [80]. The AAJT is also contraindicated in penetrating abdominal trauma, so it does not appear to be a device that would be as useful as its manufacturers may hope in the population for which it was designed.

Some devices use haemostatic agents in an applicator for deep narrow track junctional wounds where compression may be difficult or impossible (such as the XStat [82, 83]). The XStat has been trialled favourably against Combat Gauze in animal models of haemorrhage [84], has a good safety profile during *in vivo* use in hospital [85] and has been incorporated into the Tactical Combat Casualty Care guidelines [86]. It is a syringe-like device that contains multiple compressed chitosan-covered cellulose sponges that can be injected into sites of junctional haemorrhage and secured with ordinary bandages [45]. The previously mentioned iTClamp has been successfully evaluated in animal models for use in conjunction with haemostatic agents for junctional haemorrhage [87] and has made its way into ToCCC guidelines [33, 35].

A few pre-hospital teams can also offer resuscitative balloon occlusion of the aorta (REBOA) in select cases. REBOA may be used to stop life-threatening junctional, pelvic or abdominal bleeding where other measures have failed. More and more teams can offer this within the hospital, and there may be a role for this in far-forward military surgical units as a damage control measure in the field, during transfer to higher levels of care or as part of initial damage control resuscitation [88–91]. The femoral artery is cannulated via a Seldinger technique, a balloon passed and subsequently inflated to occlude the aorta to arrest catastrophic bleeding (e.g. into a fractured pelvis) until a more definitive solution is offered. More on REBOA can be found in the dedicated chapter.

Non-compressible Haemorrhage: Torso

Other than rapid transfer to a hospital with as delicate handling as possible, there is little that can be done pre-hospital in this group. The mainstay of treatment is transfer to a surgical facility, where surgery or interventional radiology can be performed, depending on injuries and local set up.

Persistent major haemorrhage in the chest may require a thoracotomy to stop the bleeding and is discussed in the traumatic cardiac arrest chapter. Surgical intervention for abdominal bleeding is not an option in the pre-hospital phase. This is for several reasons, but principally because of the complex surgical manoeuvres to access major vascular structures in the abdomen and the high number of structures that could be injured a priori or iatrogenically. This means that haemorrhage control by laparotomy is a technique that cannot be readily taught to non-surgeons. To facilitate operative management of abdominal haemorrhage, rapid transfer to an operating theatre is necessary. Many pre-surgical adjuncts have been suggested for the management of patients with non-compressible torso haemorrhage (NCTH) in an attempt to reduce the high morbidity and mortality in this group [92]. An American study suggested that the mortality of these patients can be up to 44% [93].

Trials are ongoing, with treatments such as expanding polyurethane foam being suggested for use in intra-abdominal non-compressible haemorrhage before surgery [94, 95]. Such foam expands and becomes solid, occluding bleeding points but risking localised pressure necrosis and subsequent surgical complications such as adhesions. These potential complications may, however, be an acceptable alternative to exsanguination.

Other treatments which have been investigated include:

- Gas insufflation to tamponade bleeding vessels (shown to be effective in animal models [45]).
- Lyophilised and freeze-dried blood products such as thrombosomes. There was some initially good animal safety data and encouraging phase 1 trial data for thrombocytopaenic patients [96–98]. This would have massive logistical advantages over using conventional platelets as they are stable at room temperature for 24–36 months and can be stockpiled and rehydrated quickly. However, further studies are needed (Phase 2 trials of thrombosomes are ongoing). With the extremely limited data currently available, the use of lyophilised platelets in lab-based animal trauma models have shown either decreased [99] or no [100] haemostatic ability.
- Nanoscale injectable therapies—polymers that encourage activated platelets to aggregate and decrease blood loss. Preliminary animal data is mostly positive, but they have a narrow therapeutic window. There exists some concern over the potential for pulmonary infarcts when post-mortem studies of test rats were performed [101–103].
- Other injectable therapies (such as polySTAT [104, 105]) improve fibrin clot cross-linking in rat models. While this decreases blood loss, due to the polymer's size, it is excreted slowly, with up to 7% of the polymer retained in the kidneys a week after administration [106].
- Occlusion of the descending aorta (REBOA) may also be used as a last-ditch attempt to stem bleeding that would otherwise prove fatal, but this comes with high morbidity and mortality as the balloon would have to be inflated in zone 1 or 2 [45] (see REBOA Chapter for further information).

Fluid Management

The circulation and trauma-induced coagulopathy chapters give a more thorough discussion on the theoretical basis, evidence and management of fluids in trauma. Below is a brief summary of current UK guidance. Pre-hospital teams are advised by the National Institute of Clinical Excellence to resuscitate patients in aliquots of 250 ml to a radial pulse in patients bleeding from blunt injuries and to achieve a central pulse in those with penetrating wounds [107].

International guidance advises aiming for a systolic blood pressure of 80–89 mmHg in patients without concomitant head injury [108].

Some pre-hospital services can give blood; since 2012 this has been possible in UK civilian services [40] though the vast majority of services carry crystalloid as a first-line fluid. Either may be used to achieve the outcome measures suggested by NICE. Those able to are advised to obtain intravenous access regardless of whether or not fluid is to be administered pre-hospital, [41] as it may be harder to achieve later. Pre-hospital blood transfusion improves patient physiology at the time of arrival to ED [109]. It makes clear physiological sense to replace what is lost with the same substance, rather than a crystalloid with neither oxygen-carrying capability nor coagulation factors, where this option is available. The currently running RePHILL trial in the UK is looking to provide evidence for the efficacy of pre-hospital blood in trauma patients [110], though realistically even an equivocal outcome is unlikely to decrease the trend of pre-hospital transfusion, as it is becoming an accepted (and anticipated) standard of care.

Criteria for a pre-hospital thoracotomy are essentially the same as an ED thoracotomy provided the appropriate skill-mix is present on scene; if there is a penetrating injury that may be causing cardiac tamponade and the patient has been in cardiac arrest for less than ten minutes [111–114] it may be appropriate. This approach can occasionally also be used to manage life-threatening pulmonary haemorrhage, though with fewer survivors. Further information can be found in the chapter on traumatic cardiac arrest. The Resus Council advise that a thoracotomy be considered in any penetrating trauma arrest with wounds from the nipple to the epigastrium [115]. There is no such guidance for arrests in blunt trauma. The Faculty of Pre-Hospital Care [116] state that any such intervention must be performed within ten minutes of the loss of cardiac output. This is a very narrow timeframe for such measures and makes intervention within the required time difficult without appropriate skills on scene (as opposed to transferring to a hospital within the timelines). Survival rates beyond this time are virtually zero. Specifically, it should be pointed out that a resuscitative thoracotomy is for the treatment of penetrating thoracic trauma, or injuries that may involve the thorax (e.g. epigastric stab wound that traverses the diaphragm). It is not a treatment for hypovolaemia caused by non-thoracic injuries which are otherwise amenable to direct control (e.g. limb haemorrhage). While compression of the descending aorta may arrest blood supply to a bleeding pelvis or leg, tourniquets or other strategies outlined above will do the same. The cornerstone of treatment in these peri-arrest patients is aggressive filling with blood products along with source control, initially with a tourniquet then definitively in an operating theatre. A recent systematic review has suggested a role for this intervention in some instances of isolated, non-compressible abdominal trauma with signs of life (pulse or recent arrest in a PEA rhythm) [117]. However, it excluded pre-hospital thoracotomies and reported a significant increase in morbidity and mortality in polytrauma patients compared to isolated injuries. These data need to be interpreted cautiously as interventions such as REBOA, interventional radiology and improvements in haemostatic resuscitation may mean that while thoracotomy for abdominal trauma was previously seen as a last-ditch effort, the adoption of newer, less invasive treatments may improve survival in this group without the need for thoracotomy. There are individual and organisational learning curves in adopting any new treatment, so the indications for resuscitative thoracotomy may become fewer still as these treatments mature.

Conclusion

Massive haemorrhage can be fatal. The treatment may be simple; direct pressure is often sufficient, but occasionally a more sophisticated approach is required. Any pre-hospital or ED technique may only be temporising. Still, it may allow the patient to survive until a more definitive procedure is possible and should not delay transfer to definitive care. Competence in massive haemorrhage control is an essential skill for all staff involved in providing trauma care, whether in hospital or pre-hospital. While pre-hospital clinicians are more likely to encounter patients with injuries requiring these interventions, patients may self-present with catastrophic injuries at emergency departments or clinics. The majority of skills are easily teachable for the most part and require little in the way of medical knowledge. This is best demonstrated by the proliferation and success of programmes such as the "Stop the bleed" campaign [21] and Public Access and Tourniquet Training Study [118] in the USA, and may potentially save many lives. These courses are both effective and well regarded by attendees [119] but do require top-up training to maintain competence. The dramatic drop in patients who died of treatable injuries in military theatres of operations is also another testament to the importance, practicality and ease of learning of how to implement these vital skills in trauma care [120] outside of the direct supervision of medical personnel. The number of devices and treatments available and in development for the treatment of massive haemorrhage is increasing. Hopefully, it will decrease the number of preventable deaths from junctional and non-compressible haemorrhage further still.

While several dramatic interventions come under the umbrella of massive haemorrhage control, there are diminishing returns in success rates for increasingly invasive procedures. There is a great deal of debate and many publications, courses and simulations dedicated to these interventions in this population. However, increased attention to improving the application of more rudimentary haemorrhage control methods may obviate the need for some of them. By acting early enough and aggressively enough with haemorrhage control and minimising scene times, patients may never require interventions such as REBOA or a resuscitative thoracotomy. Some injuries and circumstances may require these interventions promptly; however, they are the minority of cases rather than the majority and should only be undertaken when there is a realistic prospect of patient benefit [121].

Questions and Answers

What are the two major types of haemorrhage?

Answer: compressible and non-compressible

What bleeding might be halted by tourniquet application?

Answer: limb/extremity bleeding

What is the initial treatment of any bleeding?

Answer: direct pressure

What is the maximum timescale in which thoracotomy could be considered?

Answer: within 10 minutes of arrest

What location of bleeding might REBOA manage?

Answer: junctional, pelvic or abdominal

References

1. Gawande A. Casualties of war — military care for the wounded from Iraq and Afghanistan. N Engl J Med. 2004 Dec 9;351(24):2471–5.
2. Holcomb JB, Stansbury LG, Champion HR, Wade C, Bellamy RF. Understanding combat casualty care statistics. J Trauma. 2006 Feb;60(2):397–401.
3. Bellamy R. Combat trauma overview. In: Bellamy R, Zajtchuk R, editors. Anesthesia and perioperative care of the combat casualty. Borden Institute; 1995. [cited 2020 May 8]. p. 1–42. [Internet] Available from https://www.cs.amedd.army.mil/borden/bookDetail.aspx?ID=3ebfb1fd-2292-4555-9883-80f69fb70df4&pageTitle=Anesthesia%20and%20Perioperative%20Care%20of%20the%20Combat%20Casualty
4. Eastridge BJ, Mabry RL, Seguin P, Cantrell J, Tops T, Uribe P, et al. Death on the battlefield (2001–2011): implications for the future of combat casualty care. J Trauma Acute Care Surg. 2012 Dec;73:S431–7.
5. Hodgetts TJ, Mahoney PF, Russell MQ, Byers M. ABC to <C> ABC: redefining the military trauma paradigm. Emerg Med J. 2006 Oct;23(10):745–6.
6. Cordts PR, Brosch LA, Holcomb JB. Now and then: combat casualty care policies for operation Iraqi freedom and operation enduring freedom compared with those of Vietnam. J Trauma. 2008;64(2 Suppl):S14–20. discussion S20
7. Kotwal RS, Montgomery HR, Kotwal BM, Champion HR, Butler FK, Mabry RL, et al. Eliminating preventable death on the battlefield. Arch Surg. 2011 Dec 1;146(12):1350–8.
8. de Ceballos JPG, Turégano-Fuentes F, Perez-Diaz D, Sanz-Sanchez M, Martin-Llorente C, Guerrero-Sanz J. 11 March 2004: the terrorist bomb explosions in Madrid, Spain – an analysis of the logistics, injuries sustained and clinical management of casualties treated at the closest hospital. Crit Care. 2005;9(1):104–11.
9. D'Andrea SM, Goralnick E, Kayden SR. 2013 Boston Marathon bombings: overview of an emergency department response to a mass casualty incident. Disaster Med Public Health Prep. 2013 Apr;7(2):118–21.
10. Collaborative TBTCC. Boston Marathon bombings: an after-action review. J Trauma Acute Care Surg. 2014 Sep;77(3):501–3.
11. Service Médical du RAID. Tactical emergency medicine: lessons from Paris marauding terrorist attack. Crit Care. 2016 Feb 13;20(1):37.
12. Hirsch M, Carli P, Nizard R, Riou B, Baroudjian B, Baubet T, et al. The medical response to multisite terrorist attacks in Paris. Lancet. 2015 Dec;386(10012):2535–8.
13. Sauaia A, Moore FA, Moore EE, Moser KS, Brennan R, Read RA, et al. Epidemiology of trauma deaths: a reassessment. J Trauma. 1995 Feb;38(2):185–93.
14. Dorlac WC, DeBakey ME, Holcomb JB, Fagan SP, Kwong KL, Dorlac GR, et al. Mortality from isolated civilian penetrating extremity injury. J Trauma. 2005 Jul;59(1):217–22.
15. Tien HC, Spencer F, Tremblay LN, Rizoli SB, Brenneman FD. Preventable deaths from hemorrhage at a level I Canadian trauma center. J Trauma. 2007 Jan;62(1):142–6.
16. Mitra B, Cameron PA, Mori A, Fitzgerald M. Acute coagulopathy and early deaths post major trauma. Injury. 2012 Jan;43(1):22–5.
17. Jones AE, Aborn LS, Kline JA. Severity of emergency department hypotension predicts adverse hospital outcome. Shock. 2004 Nov;22(5):410–4.
18. MacLeod JBA, Lynn M, McKenney MG, Cohn SM, Murtha M. Early coagulopathy predicts mortality in trauma. J Trauma. 2003 Jul;55(1):39–44.
19. Davenport RA, Brohi K. Cause of trauma-induced coagulopathy. Curr Opin Anaesthesiol. 2016 Apr;29(2):212–9.
20. Neeki MM, Dong F, Toy J, Vaezazizi R, Powell J, Wong D, et al. Tranexamic acid in civilian trauma Care in the California Prehospital Antifibrinolytic Therapy Study. West J Emerg Med. 2018 Nov;19(6):977–86.
21. Stop The Bleed [Internet]. Stop the bleeding coalition. [cited 2019 Aug 26]. Available from https://stopthebleedingcoalition.org/
22. Curry N, Hopewell S, Dorée C, Hyde C, Brohi K, Stanworth S. The acute management of trauma hemorrhage: a systematic review of randomised controlled trials. Crit Care. 2011;15(2):R92.
23. Zwislewski A, Nanassy AD, Meyer LK, Scantling D, Jankowski MA, Blinstrub G, et al. Practice makes perfect: the impact of stop the bleed training on

hemorrhage control knowledge, wound packing, and tourniquet application in the workplace. Injury. 2019 Apr;50(4):864–8.
24. McPherson SW, Cook T, Sentamu J, Stone R. The Stephen Lawrence enquiry. Report of an inquiry. [Internet]. United Kingdom: The Stationery Office Ltd; 1999 Feb [cited 2020 May 15]. Available from https://webarchive.nationalarchives.gov.uk/20130814142658/http://www.archive.official-documents.co.uk/document/cm42/4262/4262.htm
25. Greater Glasgow and Clyde NHS Trust. Management of major Haemorrhage [Internet]. [cited 2020 May 8]. Available from https://handbook.ggcmedicines.org.uk/guidelines/resuscitation-and-anaphylaxis/management-of-major-haemorrhage/
26. ASA Committee on Blood Management. Massive transfusion protocol (MTP) For Hemorrhagic Shock [Internet]. American Society of Anesthesiologists; 2018 [cited 2020 May 9]. Available from https://www.asahq.org/search-results#q=MASSIVE%20TRANSFUSION%20PROTOCOL%20(MTP)%20FOR%20HEMORRHAGIC%20SHOCK&sort=relevancy
27. Norfolk D. United Kingdom blood services. Handbook of transfusion medicine. London: HMSO; 2013.
28. Hunt BJ, Allard S, Keeling D, Norfolk D, Stanworth SJ, Pendry K. A practical guideline for the haematological management of major haemorrhage. Br J Haematol. 2015;170(6):788–803.
29. I know it when I see it. In: Wikipedia [Internet]. 2020 [cited 2020 May 8]. Available from https://en.wikipedia.org/w/index.php?title=I_know_it_when_I_see_it&oldid=946560466
30. American College of Surgeons, Committee on Trauma. Advanced trauma life support: student course manual. 10th ed. Chicago, IL: American College of Surgeons; 2018.
31. Tan ECTH, Peters JH, Mckee JL, Edwards MJR. The iTClamp in the management of pre-hospital haemorrhage. Injury. 2016 May;47(5):1012–5.
32. Mckee JL, Mckee IA, Ball CG, Tan E, Moloff A, McBeth P, et al. The iTClamp in the treatment of pre-hospital craniomaxillofacial injury: a case series study. J Inj Violence Res. 2019 Jan;11(1):29–34.
33. Butler FK, Giebner S. Committee on tactical combat casualty care meeting: San Antonio, TX 5-6 September 2018 meeting minutes. J Spec Oper Med. 2019 Spring;19(1):136–45.
34. Life-Saving Hemorrhage Control by Tactical Police Using Tourniquets and the iTClamp [Internet]. JEMS. 2016 [cited 2020 May 21]. Available from https://www.jems.com/2016/12/22/life-saving-hemorrhage-control-by-tactical-police-using-tourniquets-and-the-iTClamp/
35. Committee on Tactical Combat Casualty Care. Tactical combat casualty care guidelines for medical personnel 1st August 2019.pdf [Internet]. 2019 [cited 2020 May 21]. Available from shorturl.at/bxBO5
36. McKee J, McKee I, Ball C, McBeth P, Bennett B, Filips D, et al. Subjective pain scores with the application and removal of the iTClamp in healthy volunteers. Can J Surg. 2017 Jun 1;60(3):S5–43.
37. Mckee JL, Lakshminarasimhan P, Atkinson I, LaPorta AJ, Kirkpatrick AW. Evaluation of skin damage from accidental removal of a hemostatic wound clamp (the iTClamp). Prehospital Disaster Med. 2017 Dec;32(6):651–6.
38. LaPorta A, Kirkpatrick AW, Mckee JL, Roberts DJ, Tien H, Beckett A, et al. Randomised controlled trial comparing marksmanship following application of a tourniquet or haemostatic clamp in healthy volunteers. BMJ Mil Health. 2017 Jun 1;163(3):177–83.
39. Harris T, Rice S, Watts B, Davies G. The emergency control of traumatic maxillofacial haemorrhage. Eur J Emerg Med. 2010 Aug;17(4):230–3.
40. Lockey DJ, Weaver AE, Davies GE. Practical translation of hemorrhage control techniques to the civilian trauma scene. Transfusion (Paris). 2013 Jan;53(Suppl 1):17S–22S.
41. Brown SN, Kumar D, James C, Mark J, Association of Ambulance Chief Executives (Great Britain), Joint Royal Colleges Ambulance Liaison Committee, et al. JRCALC clinical guidelines 2019 [Internet]. 2019 [cited 2020 May 15]. Available from https://search.ebscohost.com/login.aspx?direct=true&scope=site&db=nlebk&db=nlabk&AN=2293957
42. Scott I, Porter K, Laird C, Bloch M, Greaves I. The pre-hospital management of pelvic fractures: initial consensus statement. J Paramed Pract. 2014;6(5):248–52.
43. Chesser TJS, Cross AM, Ward AJ. The use of pelvic binders in the emergent management of potential pelvic trauma. Injury. 2012 Jun;43(6):667–9.
44. Hsu S-D, Chen C-J, Chou Y-C, Wang S-H, Chan D-C. Effect of early pelvic binder use in the emergency management of suspected pelvic trauma: a retrospective cohort study. Int J Environ Res Public Health. 2017;14(10):1217.
45. van Oostendorp SE, Tan ECTH, Geeraedts LMG. Pre-hospital control of life-threatening truncal and junctional haemorrhage is the ultimate challenge in optimising trauma care; a review of treatment options and their applicability in the civilian trauma setting. Scand J Trauma Resusc Emerg Med. 2016 Sep 13;24(1):110.
46. CRASH-2 Trial Collaborators. Effects of tranexamic acid on death, vascular occlusive events, and blood transfusion in trauma patients with significant haemorrhage (CRASH-2): a randomised, placebo-controlled trial. Lancet. 2010;376(9734):23–32.
47. Heddle NM, Cook RJ, Arnold DM, Liu Y, Barty R, Crowther MA, et al. Effect of short-term vs. long-term blood storage on mortality after transfusion. N Engl J Med. 2016 Nov 17;375(20):1937–45.
48. Sowers N, Froese P, Erdogan M, Green R. Impact of the age of stored blood on trauma patient mortality: a systematic review. Can J Surg. 2015 Oct 1;58(5):335–42.

49. Anand T, Ramnanan R, Skinner R, Martin M. Impact of massive transfusion and aging blood in acute trauma. Am Surg. 2016 Oct;82(10):957–9.
50. Douma MJ, O'Dochartaigh D, Brindley PG. Optimisation of indirect pressure in order to temporise life-threatening haemorrhage: a simulation study. Injury. 2016 Sep;47(9):1903–7.
51. Taylor DM, Coleman M, Parker PJ. The evaluation of an abdominal aortic tourniquet for the control of pelvic and lower limb hemorrhage. Mil Med. 2013 Nov;178(11):1196–201.
52. Smith S, White J, Wanis KN, Beckett A, McAlister VC, Hilsden R. The effectiveness of junctional tourniquets: a systematic review and meta-analysis. J Trauma Acute Care Surg. 2019 Mar;86(3):532–9.
53. Bonanno AM, Hoops HE, Graham T, Davis BL, McCully BH, Wilson LN, et al. Efficacy of the abdominal aortic junctional tourniquet-torso plate in a lethal model of noncompressible torso hemorrhage. J Spec Oper Med. 2018 Winter;18(4):106–10.
54. Welling DR, McKay PL, Rasmussen TE, Rich NM. A brief history of the tourniquet. J Vasc Surg. 2012 Jan;55(1):286–90.
55. Hawk AJ. How hemorrhage control became common sense. J Trauma Acute Care Surg. 2018;85:S13–7.
56. NICE. NICE Quality Standard 166: Trauma [Internet]. National Institute for Health and Clinical Excellence; 2018 [cited 2020 Jan 12]. Available from https://www.nice.org.uk/guidance/qs166/resources/trauma-pdf-75545603800261
57. Faculty of Pre-Hospital Care, Royal College of Surgeons of Edinburgh. Position Statement on the application of Tourniquets [Internet]. RCSEd; 2017 [cited 2020 May 15]. Available from https://fphc.rcsed.ac.uk/my-fphc/resources/position-statements
58. Beaucreux C, Vivien B, Miles E, Ausset S, Pasquier P. Application of tourniquet in civilian trauma: systematic review of the literature. Anaesth Crit Care Pain Med. 2018 Dec;37(6):597–606.
59. Yang B, Fung A, Pac-Soo C, Ma D. Vascular surgery-related organ injury and protective strategies: update and future prospects. Br J Anaesth. 2016;117(suppl_2):ii32–43.
60. Katseni K, Chalkias A, Kotsis T, Dafnios N, Arapoglou V, Kaparos G, et al. The Effect of Perioperative Ischemia and Reperfusion on Multiorgan Dysfunction following Abdominal Aortic Aneurysm Repair. BioMed Res Int [Internet]. 2015 [cited 2020 May 21];2015. Available from https://www.ncbi.nlm.nih.gov/pmc/articles/PMC4698535/
61. Iwama H, Kaneko T, Ohmizo H, Furuta S, Ohmori S, Watanabe K. Circulatory, respiratory and metabolic changes after thigh tourniquet release in combined epidural-propofol anaesthesia with preservation of spontaneous respiration. Anaesthesia. 2002 Jun;57(6):588–92.
62. TLai. Emergency tourniquet | Military and Pre-Hospital [Internet]. tourniquets.org. 2017 [cited 2020 May 21]. Available from https://tourniquets.org/military-and-pre-hospital-tourniquets/
63. Schwartz DS, Weisner Z, Badar J. Immediate lower extremity tourniquet application to delay onset of reperfusion injury after prolonged crush injury. Prehosp Emerg Care. 2015;19(4):544–7.
64. Sever MS, Vanholder R. Management of Crush Victims in mass disasters: highlights from recently published recommendations. Clin J Am Soc Nephrol. 2013 Feb 1;8(2):328–35.
65. Managing the Toxic Chemical Release that Occurs During a Crush Injury [Internet]. JEMS. 2018 [cited 2020 May 21]. Available from https://www.jems.com/2018/10/22/managing-the-toxic-chemical-release-that-occurs-during-a-crush-injury/
66. Percival TJ, Rasmussen TE. Reperfusion strategies in the management of extremity vascular injury with ischaemia. Br J Surg. 2012;99(S1):66–74.
67. Lee C, Porter KM. Tourniquet use in the civilian pre-hospital setting. Emerg Med J. 2007 Aug;24(8):584–7.
68. Lakstein D, Blumenfeld A, Sokolov T, Lin G, Bssorai R, Lynn M, et al. Tourniquets for hemorrhage control on the battlefield: a 4-year accumulated experience. J Trauma Acute Care Surg. 2003 May;54(5):S221.
69. Clifford CC. Treating traumatic bleeding in a combat setting. Mil Med. 2004;169(12 Suppl):8–10. 4
70. Cox ED, Schreiber MA, McManus J, Wade CE, Holcomb JB. New hemostatic agents in the combat setting. Transfusion (Paris). 2009 Dec;49:248S–55S.
71. McManus J, Hurtado T, Pusateri A, Knoop KJ. A case series describing thermal injury resulting from zeolite use for hemorrhage control in combat operations. Prehosp Emerg Care. 2007 Mar;11(1):67–71.
72. Wright JK, Kalns J, Wolf EA, Traweek F, Schwarz S, Loeffler CK, et al. Thermal injury resulting from application of a granular mineral hemostatic agent. J Trauma. 2004 Aug;57(2):224–30.
73. Smith AH, Laird C, Porter K, Bloch M. Haemostatic dressings in pre-hospital care. Emerg Med J. 2013 Oct 1;30(10):784–9.
74. Waibel KH, Haney B, Moore M, Whisman B, Gomez R. Safety of chitosan bandages in shellfish allergic patients. Mil Med. 2011 Oct;176(10):1153–6.
75. Bennett BL, Littlejohn L. Review of new topical hemostatic dressings for combat casualty care. Mil Med. 2014 May 1;179(5):497–514.
76. Welch M, Barratt J, Peters A, Wright C. Systematic review of pre-hospital haemostatic dressings. J R Army Med Corps. 2019 Feb;166(3):194–200.
77. Landsman TL, Touchet T, Hasan SM, Smith C, Russell B, Rivera J, et al. A shape memory foam composite with enhanced fluid uptake and bactericidal properties as a hemostatic agent. Acta Biomater. 2017;47:91–9.
78. Kollock RO, Hale D, Vogelpohl R, Kremer L, Horner J, Cox C, et al. The influence of body armor on balance and movement quality. Int J Exerc Sci. 2018 Jun 1;11(1):648–56.

79. Dempsey PC, Handcock PJ, Rehrer NJ. Impact of police body Armour and equipment on mobility. Appl Ergon. 2013 Nov;44(6):957–61.
80. Kotwal RS, Butler FK, Gross KR, Kheirabadi BS, Baer DG, Dubick MA, et al. Management of junctional hemorrhage in tactical combat casualty care: TCCC guidelines proposed change 13-03. J Spec Oper Med. 2013;13(4):85–93.
81. Kragh JF, Parsons DL, Kotwal RS, Kheirabadi BS, Aden JK, Gerhardt RT, et al. Testing of junctional tourniquets by military medics to control simulated groin hemorrhage. J Spec Oper Med. 2014;14(3):58–63.
82. Mueller GR, Pineda TJ, Xie HX, Teach JS, Barofsky AD, Schmid JR, et al. A novel sponge-based wound stasis dressing to treat lethal non-compressible hemorrhage. J Trauma Acute Care Surg. 2012 Aug;73(2 Suppl 1):S134–9.
83. National Institute for Health Research. XStat® Hemostatic Device for non-compressible junctional haemorrhage. Technol Alert. 2015 Jun;2.
84. Rall JM, Cox JM. Evaluation of Xstat and Combat Gauze in a Swine Model of Lethal Junctional Hemorrhage in Coagulopathic Swine [Internet]. 59th Medical Wing San Antonio United States; 2017 Mar [cited 2020 May 9]. Report No.: 17130. Available from https://apps.dtic.mil/docs/citations/AD1037122
85. Warriner Z, Lam L, Matsushima K, Benjamin E, Strumwasser A, Demetriades D, et al. Initial evaluation of the efficacy and safety of in-hospital expandable hemostatic minisponge use in penetrating trauma. J Trauma Acute Care Surg. 2019 Mar;86(3):424–30.
86. Sims K, Montgomery HR, Dituro P, Kheirabadi BS, Butler FK. Management of external hemorrhage in tactical combat casualty care: the adjunctive use of XStat™ compressed hemostatic sponges: TCCC guidelines change 15-03. J Spec Oper Med. 2016;16(1):19–28.
87. Stuart SM, Zarow G, Walchak A, McLean J, Roszko P. Pilot study of a novel swine model for controlling junctional hemorrhage using the iTClamp in conjunction with hemostatic agents. Mil Med. 2019;184(Supplement_1):367–73.
88. Glaser JJ, Fischer AD, Shackelford SA, Butler F, Rasmussen TE. A contemporary report on US military guidelines for the use of whole blood and resuscitative endovascular balloon occlusion of the aorta. J Trauma Acute Care Surg. 2019;87(1S):S22–7.
89. de Schoutheete JC, Fourneau I, Waroquier F, De Cupere L, O'Connor M, Van Cleynenbreugel K, et al. Three cases of resuscitative endovascular balloon occlusion of the aorta (REBOA) in austere pre-hospital environment—technical and methodological aspects. World J Emerg Surg. 2018 Nov 21;13(1):54.
90. Rees P, Waller B, Buckley AM, Doran C, Bland S, Scott T, et al. REBOA at role 2 afloat: resuscitative endovascular balloon occlusion of the aorta as a bridge to damage control surgery in the military maritime setting. BMJ Mil Health. 2018 May 1;164(2):72–6.
91. Reva VA, Hörer TM, Makhnovskiy AI, Sokhranov MV, Samokhvalov IM, DuBose JJ. Field and en route resuscitative endovascular occlusion of the aorta: a feasible military reality? J Trauma Acute Care Surg. 2017;83(1 Suppl 1):S170–6.
92. Rappold JF, Bochicchio GV. Surgical adjuncts to non-compressible torso hemorrhage as tools for patient blood management. Transfusion (Paris). 2016;56(Suppl 2):S203–7.
93. Kisat M, Morrison JJ, Hashmi ZG, Efron DT, Rasmussen TE, Haider AH. Epidemiology and outcomes of non-compressible torso hemorrhage. J Surg Res. 2013 Sep;184(1):414–21.
94. REVIVE: reducing exsanguination via in-vivo expandable foam – no study results posted – ClinicalTrials.gov [Internet]. [cited 2020 May 9]. Available from https://clinicaltrials.gov/ct2/show/results/NCT02880163
95. Chang JC, Holloway BC, Zamisch M, Hepburn MJ, Ling GSF. ResQFoam for the treatment of non-compressible hemorrhage on the front line. Mil Med. 2015 Sep;180(9):932–3.
96. Fitzpatrick GM, Cliff R, Tandon N. Thrombosomes: a platelet-derived hemostatic agent for control of non-compressible hemorrhage: lyophilized PDHA for hemorrhage control. Transfusion (Paris). 2013 Jan;53:100S–6S.
97. Thrombosomes (Lyophilized Platelets) Appear Safe in Phase 1 Trial [Internet]. [cited 2020 May 15]. Available from https://transfusionnews.com/2019/10/24/thrombosomes-lyophilized-platelets-appear-safe-in-phase-1-trial/
98. Hawksworth JS, Elster EA, Fryer D, Sheppard F, Morthole V, Krishnamurthy G, et al. Evaluation of lyophilised platelets as an infusible hemostatic agent in experimental non-compressible hemorrhage in swine. J Thromb Haemost. 2009;7(10):1663–71.
99. Inaba K, Barmparas G, Rhee P, Branco B, Fitzpatrick M, Okoye O, et al. Dried platelets in a swine model of liver injury. Shock. 2014 May;41(5):429–34.
100. Macko AR, Crossland RF, Cap AP, Fryer DM, Mitchell TA, Pusateri AE, et al. Control of severe intra-abdominal hemorrhage with an infusible platelet-derived hemostatic agent in a nonhuman primate (rhesus macaque) model. J Trauma Acute Care Surg. 2016 Apr;80(4):617–24.
101. Lashof-Sullivan MM, Shoffstall E, Atkins KT, Keane N, Bir C, VandeVord P, et al. Intravenously administered nanoparticles increase survival following blast trauma. Proc Natl Acad Sci. 2014 Jul 15;111(28):10293–8.
102. Shoffstall AJ, Everhart LM, Varley ME, Soehnlen ES, Shick AM, Ustin JS, et al. Tuning ligand density on intravenous hemostatic nanoparticles dramatically increases survival following blunt trauma. Biomacromolecules. 2013 Aug 12;14(8):2790–7.

103. Bertram JP, Williams CA, Robinson R, Segal SS, Flynn NT, Lavik EB. Intravenous hemostat: nanotechnology to halt bleeding. Sci Transl Med. 2009 Dec 16;1(11):11ra22.
104. Peng HT. Hemostatic agents for pre-hospital hemorrhage control: a narrative review. Mil Med Res. 2020 Mar 25;7(1):13.
105. Klein MK, Tsihlis ND, Pritts TA, Kibbe MR. Emerging therapies for prehospital control of hemorrhage. J Surg Res. 2020 Apr;248:182–90.
106. Chan LW, Wang X, Wei H, Pozzo LD, White NJ, Pun SH. A synthetic fibrin cross-linking polymer for modulating clot properties and inducing hemostasis. Sci Transl Med. 2015 Mar 4;7(277):277ra29.
107. Major haemorrhaging in the pre-hospital setting – NICE Pathways [Internet]. [cited 2020 May 15]. Available from https://pathways.nice.org.uk/pathways/trauma#path=view%3A/pathways/trauma/major-haemorrhaging-in-the-pre-hospital-setting.xml&content=view-node%3Anodes-circulatory-access-and-fluid-replacement
108. Spahn DR, Bouillon B, Cerny V, Duranteau J, Filipescu D, Hunt BJ, et al. The European guideline on management of major bleeding and coagulopathy following trauma: fifth edition. Crit Care. 2019 Mar 27;23(1):98.
109. Lyon RM, de Sausmarez E, McWhirter E, Wareham G, Nelson M, Matthies A, et al. Pre-hospital transfusion of packed red blood cells in 147 patients from a UK helicopter emergency medical service. Scand J Trauma Resusc Emerg Med. 2017 Feb 14;25(1):12.
110. RePHILL – University of Birmingham [Internet]. [cited 2020 May 21]. Available from https://www.birmingham.ac.uk/research/bctu/trials/portfolio-v/Rephill/index.aspx
111. Wise D, Davies G, Coats T, Lockey D, Hyde J, Good A. Emergency thoracotomy: 'how to do it'. Emerg Med J. 2005 Jan 1;22(1):22–4.
112. Lockey DJ, Lyon RM, Davies GE. Development of a simple algorithm to guide the effective management of traumatic cardiac arrest. Resuscitation. 2013 Jun;84(6):738–42.
113. Sherren PB, Reid C, Habig K, Burns BJ. Algorithm for the resuscitation of traumatic cardiac arrest patients in a physician-staffed helicopter emergency medical service. Crit Care Lond Engl. 2013 Mar 12;17(2):308.
114. Burlew CC, Moore EE, Moore FA, Coimbra R, McIntyre RC, Davis JW, et al. Western trauma association critical decisions in trauma: resuscitative thoracotomy. J Trauma Acute Care Surg. 2012 Dec;73(6):1359–63.
115. Deakin CD, Brown S, Jewkes F, Lockey D, Lyon RM, Moore F, et al. Pre-hospital resuscitation guidelines [Internet]. www.resus.org.uk. 2015 [cited 2020 May 20]. Available from https://www.resus.org.uk/resuscitation-guidelines/prehospital-resuscitation/
116. Leech C, Porter K, Steyn R, Laird C, Virgo I, Bowman R, et al. The pre-hospital management of life-threatening chest injuries: a consensus statement. Trauma. 2017;19(1):54–62.
117. Hughes M, Perkins Z. Outcomes following resuscitative thoracotomy for abdominal exsanguination, a systematic review. Scand J Trauma Resusc Emerg Med. 2020 Feb 6;28(1):9.
118. Goralnick E, Chaudhary MA, McCarty JC, Caterson EJ, Goldberg SA, Herrera-Escobar JP, et al. Effectiveness of instructional interventions for hemorrhage control readiness for laypersons in the public access and tourniquet training study (PATTS). JAMA Surg. 2018 Sep;153(9):791–9.
119. Zhao KL, Herrenkohl M, Paulsen M, Bulger EM, Vavilala MS, Moore M, et al. Learners' perspectives on stop the bleed: a course to improve survival during mass casualty events. Trauma Surg Acute Care Open. 2019 Jul 1;4(1):e000331.
120. Butler FK. Two decades of saving lives on the battlefield: tactical combat casualty care turns 20. Mil Med. 2017 Mar 1;182(3–4):e1563–8.
121. John HJ. Hinds on crack the chest-get crucified [Internet]. 2015 Jul 4 [cited 2020 May 20]. Available from https://emcrit.org/emcrit/john-hinds-on-crack-the-chest-get-crucified/
122. Cothren CC, Moore EE, Hedegaard HB, Meng K. Epidemiology of urban trauma deaths: a comprehensive reassessment 10 years later. World J Surg. 2007 Jul;31(7):1507–11.
123. Kauvar DS, Lefering R, Wade CE. Impact of hemorrhage on trauma outcome: an overview of epidemiology, clinical presentations, and therapeutic considerations. J Trauma. 2006 Jun;60(6 Suppl):S3–11.
124. Kauvar DS, Wade CE. The epidemiology and modern management of traumatic hemorrhage: US and international perspectives. Crit Care. 2005;9(Suppl 5):S1–9.

Fundamentals of Airway Management in Trauma

7

Peter Lax and Jonathan Veitch

- The importance of airway patency
- Why intubation may not always be the correct course of action
- Common reasons for airway intervention and underlying aims
- Basic manoeuvres, adjuncts and cervical spine injuries
- Supraglottic devices
- Needle and surgical airway techniques

Introduction

In many life support courses, "ABC" management emphasises the importance of airway management early, and in the MABCD sequence it is only trumped by the need for immediate control of life-threatening haemorrhage. If the patient does not have a patent airway of one description or another, hypoxia and cardiac arrest will ensue regardless of the presence or absence of other injuries.

Few subjects in trauma will raise as much debate as airway management and Rapid Sequence Induction (RSI)—who should be doing it, where, when, choice of drugs and equipment, checklists, use of cricoid pressure and the relative merits and drawbacks of video laryngoscopes versus standard laryngoscopes have all been debated *ad nauseam*. What follows is an overview of some of the fundamental principles, controversies and a set of recommendations that are as evidence-based as possible. The majority of manoeuvres outlined in this chapter can be performed on patients without drug administration if they are obtunded.

There will no doubt be disagreement or divergence from some of the material contained in these chapters, but those issues are largely for clinicians with advanced airway experience who may have increased personal or institutional familiarity with certain techniques. The bottom line is that a large amount of decision-making around the "best" method or technique of airway management is subjective, and depends on the balance of risk to the patient, their location, the skill of the individual operator and prevalent team dynamics [1].

The fundamental guiding principle at all points should be that ***oxygenation is the ultimate end goal*** and fixation on one particular method of achieving that goal by dismissing all others is likely to be harmful. There is not a minimum required concentration of plastic in the airway

P. Lax (✉)
Tactical Medical Wing, Royal Air Force, Brize Norton, Oxfordshire, UK
e-mail: p.lax@NHS.net

J. Veitch
Department of Anaesthesia, Nottingham University Teaching Hospitals NHS Trust, Nottinghamshire, UK

212 Field Hospital (Reserves), Sheffield, UK
e-mail: jveitch@doctors.org.uk

P. Lax (ed.), *Textbook of Acute Trauma Care*, https://doi.org/10.1007/978-3-030-83628-3_7

that is necessary for life, however there is a minimum oxygen requirement in the blood!

The Case Against Intubation

While it is easy for practitioners of all levels to become focused on intubation as the only method for airway management in trauma patients (and indeed it does have its benefits), it is not a risk-free procedure and should not be undertaken lightly.

Intubation is a skill with a learning curve in its acquisition and requires a degree of regular exposure to maintain competency. Exact case numbers for both acquisition and retention of skills are the subject of much debate [2–10] which is not helped by the lack of a clear consensus of what an acceptable rate of success should be. The minimum numbers suggested in the aforementioned papers range from 16 to 75 intubations to learn the skill, with "acceptable" success rates ranging from 71% to 90%. Whether a failure rate of (at best) one in ten patients for a high-stakes intervention is an acceptable standard is a matter for individual and organisational debate.

There is at least some acknowledgement in the evidence that location plays a part in success; Wang et al. [10] demonstrated that in the well-lit, spacious and well-resourced environment of the operating theatre with optimum patient positioning, the probability of success is much higher than in pre-hospital or intensive care settings. Whether learning these skills in optimum conditions translates to success in other environments is arguable. If intubation is learned in an operating theatre with skilled assistance, oversight and a perfect setup, is the practitioner likely to be competent enough to practice it in more demanding settings without additional checks or training? Does this give a false sense of security or lack of appreciation for how demanding it can be to perform the same skill in a different environment, even for experienced clinicians? The period of transitioning from awake to anaesthetised or vice versa represents a period where the airway reflexes are not fully intact and the airway is unprotected, and large amounts of training and resources are invested to make it as safe as possible. In other, more remote areas with patients who are physiologically more obtunded, who may have a full stomach and when help may not be immediately available, the decision to intubate may be more appropriately couched in terms of "should we?" rather than "*how* should we?".

All that has been mentioned thus far is the act of putting a tube in a hole; all of the other factors relating to improving outcomes around intubation such as providing adequate ventilation, post procedural care, adequacy of depth of anaesthesia etc further complicate the answer. A 6 year retrospective review by Lockey et al. [11] of survival of London HEMS trauma patients who could be intubated without drugs found only 1 survivor of 486 patients. This patient had a penetrating chest wound with cardiac tamponade and on-scene thoracotomy, myocardial suturing and return of spontaneous circulation so is not representative of the majority of trauma patients in the UK who require advanced airway management. The suggestion is that those patients who are likely to benefit most from intubation as the primary means of airway management in trauma need to be intubated early enough (i.e. those with a GCS greater than 3). This means the use of drug-assisted intubation rather than waiting until the patient's airway reflexes are so blunted that they can be intubated without drugs. In the UK, the current NICE Quality Standards in Trauma [12] state as their first quality marker:

> People with major trauma who cannot maintain their airway and/or ventilation have drug-assisted rapid sequence induction (RSI) of anaesthesia and intubation within 45 minutes of the initial call to the emergency services

This quality standard in conjunction with the evidence, logically leads to one of two courses of action; either take this capability closer to the point of injury (i.e. dedicated PHEM/HEMS teams) or move the patient to a location where they can have advanced airway management sooner. Depending on the incident location, the latter course of action may not be compatible with the drive to take seriously ill trauma patients to Major Trauma Centres (MTCs) directly. Though the extant guidelines do permit for "pit-stopping" at Trauma Units for airway management before onward transfer, this is usually logistically complex, very time-consuming and delays presentation at the MTC. If trauma networks are informed and regularly practiced in this procedure, then it is possible, though it currently tends to be the exception rather than the norm.

This therefore means that pre-hospital intubation for trauma should be a skill restricted to specialist practitioners who can provide anaesthesia in addition to intubation, but more importantly that intubation is not viewed as the only airway management option. This is also congruent with current guidelines on pre-hospital anaesthesia [13], with a strong emphasis on teaching and applying basic airway management skills well rather than focusing on an intervention which may only be possible without drugs in patients who, almost by definition, will not survive. Even in patients with a medical cause of cardiac arrest, intubation has not been proven to improve survival over other airway management techniques either in hospital [14] or in the pre-hospital [15, 16] environment.

Regarding morbidity and mortality around drug-assisted airway management, current evidence suggests that even a single, brief episode of hypotension in a patient with traumatic brain injury can worsen their neurological outcome [17], even if the intubation itself is successful. When the potentially deleterious side effects of positive pressure ventilation on hypovolaemic patients are considered, even in a technically perfect induction and intubation, there is still a subsequent post-procedure risk of hypotension that may catch out the unwary.

To sum the evidence up for intubation of trauma patients so far, if the patient is so sick they can be intubated without drugs they likely won't survive, unless they have a medical cause for their arrest before trauma (in which case intubation confers no additional survival advantage), and intubation with drugs if inexpertly performed may worsen neurological outcome if the patient is hypotensive for even a short period.

None of this is to say that trauma patients should not be intubated, but the emphasis on airway management should not be on intubation to the detriment of every other method. Airway management should not focus solely on the mechanical act of a procedure that involves putting a tube in a hole. Dynamic risk assessment and risk: benefit analysis is by its nature highly subjective and changes on a case to case basis. However, there should be good training, standardisation, peer review and quality assurance processes in place for any organisation or practitioner who may undertake this procedure. Intubation may be the wrong course of action in some cases and scenarios; the goal of any provider should always be adequacy of oxygenation and ventilation rather than focusing on the presence or absence of a plastic tube between the vocal cords.

Why Manage the Airway?

Airway compromise in the trauma situation can occur from a variety of causes; irrespective of pathology, actual or impending airway obstruction requires prompt management or patient deterioration and death will ensue.

All injuries above the level of the clavicles can potentially lead to airway compromise due to disruption of the airway itself. This may be from actual or impending swelling, soiling from blood or reduction in conscious level and consequent failure of protective airway reflexes. Obviously, these are factors commonly leading to loss of an airway in a matter of minutes, not hours. Therefore, this will affect the decisions made in how to manage the airway in the pre-hospital environment, as well as in hospital practice.

Trauma airway management can be a minefield, but practitioners must try to encourage not just a patient-centric process but an approach that considers the environment the patient occupies. In summary, an airway may need to be managed in the following situations:

- A primary airway compromise due to an injury
- A likely future airway compromise due to the expected course of other injuries sustained (e.g. head or chest injury with inadequate oxygenation and ventilation).
- As part of a treatment bundle to improve outcomes e.g. in head injury.

- To provide anaesthesia which allows for surgical procedures e.g. amputation.

To provide a more stable situation in which to assess, treat or transfer a patient.

-

Once again, the management of a situation will depend on the individual clinician's skillset and confidence in managing advanced airway and sedation techniques.

Airway Management Philosophy

As mentioned in the opening of this chapter, airway management does not always mandate intubation. When planning how to manage a patient's airway, the following questions must be asked:

- What would a perfect outcome look like?
- What would an acceptable outcome be?
- What would be the worst-case scenario?
- How likely are any of these things to occur and what mitigations can be put in place to affect them?
- How quickly and where does all this need to happen?

Good airway management begins before even encountering a patient. Each organisation and practitioner should have formal standardised operating procedures (SOPs) in place, and staff should be appropriately trained and qualified. The governance around airway management is an area that is probably not emphasised as often as it should be, though it is often scrutinised afterwards during investigations for bad outcomes. While there is a leadership and organisational responsibility to ensure an agreed and high level of practice, it is also each individual's responsibility to ensure they are adequately trained and prepared to undertake any work for which they may be tasked. While certain procedures such as surgical airways may never be used in a practitioner's career, they should always be trained for. Practitioners should be able to perform these rare procedures and know what equipment to use and procedure to follow. Performing an emergency procedure for the first time will always be stressful, but practitioners can minimise this stress by ensuring they are well-drilled as an individual and as a team.

While there are several different levels of professional expertise and roles within those who interact with patients, training should be complementary between levels. A senior practitioner should know what a more junior team member is capable of and what their limits are, and the corollary is also true. Junior members of the team may not be able to perform advanced interventions but should be able to know when they are indicated, how to summon help in a timely fashion, and how to make interventions easier (e.g. positioning and exposing a patient prior to the next tier of care arriving, setting up equipment etc). A bonus would be if they are able to assist in the intervention, though this would also require further standardised training. For some practitioners, certain interventions may be taught in a different order, or options omitted due to local working practices, locations or patient groups. For example, in recent conflicts in Iraq and Afghanistan, Combat Medical Technicians and General Duty (non-specialist) Medical Officers were taught to perform surgical airways. When needed, the intervention was required faster than most specialised medical teams could get to patients. Due to patterns of injury, the need for surgical airways was found to be approximately twice that in civilian practice [18], but the performance of these interventions by non-doctor and junior doctor staff was safe and effective with a 92% success rate [19]. Emergency anaesthesia and intubation was not an option in these cases, but performance of a surgical cricothyroidotomy is the same final end procedure regardless of the preceding failed technique. Surgical airways are a relatively simple technique to teach and use when indicated, however there is a large degree of anxiety over their use as they are often seen as a "failed" airway rather than a successful one.

Team Composition

In both hospitals and the pre-hospital environment it is rare that the same team will work together consistently. In the UK, junior doctors may rotate hospitals, PHEM schemes or departments every 6 months (or more frequently in some cases); an average paramedic crew may only see major trauma once a year so will be unlikely to work with the same PHEM team consistently. Even HEMS crews may rotate between different bases or platforms and not work with the same individuals consistently. All these issues combined, mean that SOPs and repeated simulation, feedback and adaptation, from both simulation and real-world cases, should be integral to airway management.

The below should be the basis for managing a patient, with escalation up the basic airway ladder (Fig. 7.1) balanced against providing the necessary standard in a fashion that minimises risk as much as possible. The decision to move further up the ladder should be based against the risks inherent in doing so, and the benefits to be gained. It may be that although current airway management isn't perfect, it is *good enough,* if adding to the complexity would increase risk to the patient based on the anticipated difficulty of the intended course of action.

Initial Airway Management and Causes of Airway Compromise

Diagnosing Airway Obstruction

In some cases, airway obstruction can be an obvious diagnosis if there are clear external signs such as severe facial or neck trauma. In other cases, signs of airway obstruction can initially be subtle and evolve over time without being picked up until almost complete obstruction occurs. At this point, airway management becomes much more difficult and there are potentially fewer options to choose from in a more pressured situation. For this reason, airway assessment has to be an active, interrogative process in all trauma patients who have the potential to deteriorate.

If a patient arrives and is speaking normally, there may be no initial rush to perform any interventions as their airway reflexes are sufficiently intact and whatever trauma they have suffered has not (yet!) affected their airway. Signs which may indicate impending airway obstruction include:

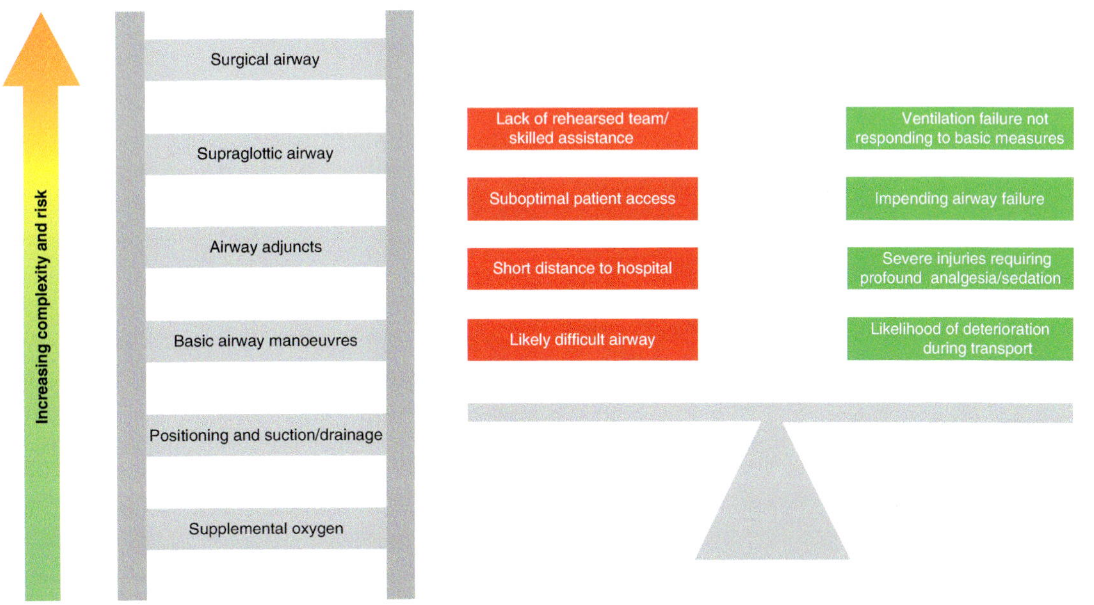

Fig. 7.1 The basic airway ladder and factors influencing decision to escalate

Sounds

- Gurgling from air flow through accumulated fluids at any point in the middle or upper airway, e.g. blood, vomit, saliva or airway secretions.
- Coughing—any irritation of the airway will cause protective reflexes to try and clear the obstruction by coughing.
- Snoring—loss of upper airway tone and reflexes can cause posterior displacement of the tongue and partial obstruction of the airway. This has the potential to progress on to complete obstruction. This is more likely in patients with sleep apnoea or in the obese.
- Stridor—an inspiratory high-pitched noise indicating obstruction around the level of the larynx or trachea.
- Stertor—a similar sounding noise to stridor but occurring in expiration and due to obstruction in the naso- or oropharynx.
- Hoarse or high-pitched voice due to laryngeal trauma, inflammation or swelling.
- Wheeze or shortness of breath—this can be from lower airway obstruction due to asthma, cardiac failure or inhalational damage to lungs from chemicals or hot gases.
- Absence of sound—all the above rely on the passage of air through a partially or completely open airway. If the airway is completely obstructed then no sound will be present.

Visual

- Bracing/"tripod" position—in an attempt to generate increased intrathoracic pressures by using the strap muscles of the neck, patients may brace their arms on a surface or their knees.
- Abdominal/"see-saw" breathing—complete or severe airway obstruction may present with a breathing pattern where the abdomen moves outwards in expiration and inwards during inspiration with little or opposite movement of the chest.
- Swelling of the lips/tongue—may indicate anaphylaxis or another cause of impending airway obstruction.
- Swelling of the neck/submandibular space—may indicate soft tissue infection or expansion of a haematoma from a bleeding vessel. May also indicate surgical emphysema (air accumulating under the skin from a hole in the airway. Surgical emphysema feels crunchy under the skin, like feeling breakfast cereal through a plastic packet or putting a hand into fresh snow).
- Cyanosis—this blue discolouration of mucus membranes, lips and nailbeds is a very late sign and indicates a significant degree of hypoxia.

These symptoms and signs may occur in isolation or concerto and may evolve over time. The key is to make an accurate baseline assessment and then keep re-assessing to see if there is any departure from this and take action as needed. This may be either in the form of handing over concerns when the patient goes to the next level of care, or actively intervening to perform an airway manoeuvre to deal with an obstruction.

Positioning, Basic Manoeuvres and C-Spine Injuries

Management of airways proceeds in a stepwise fashion and starts with patient assistance and positioning. In patients who have intact reflexes and have an airway obstruction due to a foreign body, they may be able to cough, and all that may be required is support or back blows to assist them expelling the obstruction. Patients with airway problems who do not have an impaired level of consciousness may put themselves in a position of comfort that helps maintain an airway spontaneously, such as on their side or sitting up in the tripod position as described above. If there is no other reason to alter their position and lay them flat (supine), the patient is best served by leaving them in their chosen posture. Supine positioning may cause a partial airway obstruction to become a complete one as well as increasing the work of breathing by putting the diaphragm at a mechanical disadvantage. When supine, the weight of the abdominal organs pushes against the diaphragm, increasing the force needed for inspiration and decreasing functional residual capacity of the lungs.

Other interventions which are sometimes seen as the hallmark of good trauma care, specifically application of a rigid cervical collar, may also worsen airway obstruction or increase work of breathing. Any decision about their application should be made on a case by case basis rather than a blanket rule for all patients. In the initial phases of resuscitation (and in certain situations as described in the tactical trauma chapter) the only possible airway manoeuvre in a semi- or unconscious patient may be to put them into a lateral or semi-prone position. The "recovery position" as taught in many first aid courses will allow the tongue to fall anterolaterally away from the posterior pharynx if airway reflexes are impaired. This is also true for any airway secretions, blood or vomit that may be in the airway, utilising gravity-assisted drainage to keep the airway clear. As well as positioning, an inspection should be made of the airway to ensure there are no foreign bodies or liquids present that could be aspirated or cause choking. Suctioning under direct vision with a Yankauer sucker, or removal of foreign bodies with a laryngoscope and Magill forceps should be attempted where possible. Some organisations are suggesting that laryngoscopy should be performed before LMA insertion to avoid the risk of displacing a foreign body further down the airway. This is largely reactionary and based on a coroners Regulation 28 recommendation following a case in London [20]. Any history of choking should alert the practitioner to the risk of a foreign body in the airway, and any problems with ventilation through an SGA should mean that they should be removed. Suspicion of a foreign body in the airway should mean an LMA should not be used until the foreign body has been removed or ruled out.

The first airway manoeuvres that are commonly taught are the head tilt/chin lift and the jaw thrust (see Fig. 7.2). Both manoeuvres deal with obstruction of the airway by the tongue and rely on the fact that the tongue is adherent to the mandible (lower jaw). By moving the mandible anteriorly and positioning the lower incisors anterior to the upper incisors, the posterior aspect of the tongue is moved anteriorly, and airway patency is restored. In the case of the jaw thrust, this is achieved by placing two fingers either side of the angle of the jaw and moving it anteriorly. For the head tilt/chin lift, the head is extended and one or two fingers placed under the chin to ensure the mandible is lifted, moving the tongue away from the posterior pharyngeal wall.

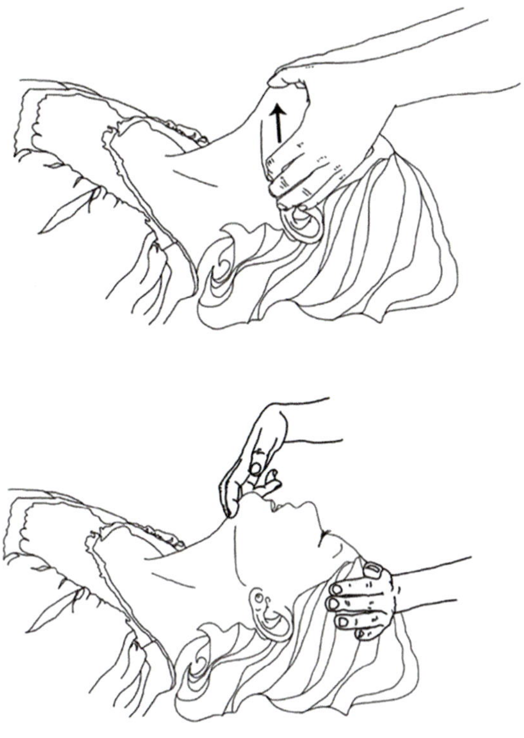

Fig. 7.2 Jaw thrust and head tilt chin lift (from Prasarn et al. [21])

Historically, in trauma patients jaw thrust has been preferred over the head tilt/chin lift due to concerns in moving the neck of patients who have potentially sustained a cervical spine injury. This was reviewed by the International Liaison Committee on Resuscitation in 2005, who found that both jaw thrust and head tilt/chin lift created similar, substantial degrees of cervical spine movement [22]. This degree of movement was not decreased by cervical collar application [23], whereas the effect of manual in-line stabilisation (MILS) had contradictory evidence, with some studies showing decreased range of movement with MILS [24, 25] and others showing no difference in movement [26]. A more recent publication based on degrees of motion in a cadaveric model with a surgically created C1-2 instability advocated the use of jaw thrust overhead tilt chin lift in the first instance [21]. The underlying principle remains the same no matter if cervical spine movement occurs with either method or not—**establishing and maintaining a patent airway always takes priority over minimising cervical spine movement in suspected or confirmed spinal injured patients.**

Spinal cord injuries are dealt with in the dedicated spinal chapter, but insofar as they affect perceptions around airway management, it is worth highlighting the excellent BJA editorial in 2000 by McLeod and Calder [27] which debunks many myths in these patients. It is still mandatory reading for any practitioner who deals with airway management in trauma patients, 20 years after its original publication.

A more recent review highlighted that 50% of all spinal cord injuries occur in the cervical region [28] and the most injured vertebra in the neck is C5. However, the majority of movements that occur during basic and advanced airway manoeuvres are at the occipito-atlanto-axial complex (C1-2), with minimal movement below C3, even during direct laryngoscopy [27].

Spinal cord injuries can be described in the same way as brain injuries; primary (occurring at the moment of impact) or secondary (the subsequent consequences of hypotension, hypoxia and impaired autoregulation). While compression of the spinal cord can and does cause injury, this is a primary injury before any airway interventions are attempted. Four main mechanisms of injury have been identified—impact plus persistent compression (e.g. bone or intervertebral disc fragments), impact with transient compression for a few seconds or less, distraction injury, and laceration or transection of the cord [29, 30]. If a spinal cord injury is due to the mechanical disruption of the cord then symptoms will appear almost instantaneously, but if the symptoms evolve over a period of time then this is due to secondary injury. Chief amongst the causes of secondary injury are hypoxia and vascular compromise of the cord, so maintaining an airway and good cord perfusion pressure (as well as urgent operative stabilisation) are key to minimising the extent of any neurological insult. **For the avoidance of doubt, if moving the patient's neck is essential to aid maintenance of an airway or to provide a view during laryngoscopy, the neck should be moved, but for the least amount of time and for the shortest distance possible.** The forces involved in laryngoscopy are also minor in comparison to the force required to fracture the neck and put the cord at risk in the first instance [31, 32]. Of note, the "protective" effect of MILS increases the forces required in direct laryngoscopy [33] and begs the question whether the application of MILS makes intubation safer or more risky. It should probably just act (predominantly) as a reminder to the person intubating, not to actively flex the neck and extend the head more than is absolutely necessary.

Basic Airway Adjuncts

While basic manoeuvres like a jaw thrust will move the tongue out of the airway, there are other basic adjuncts that can be used in airway management. The two most commonly employed are the Guedel or oropharyngeal (OP) airway and the nasopharyngeal (NP) airway, as demonstrated in Figs. 7.3, 7.4 and 7.5. Guedel airways are sized by putting the plastic flange at the level of the incisors and looking to see if the curve of the air-

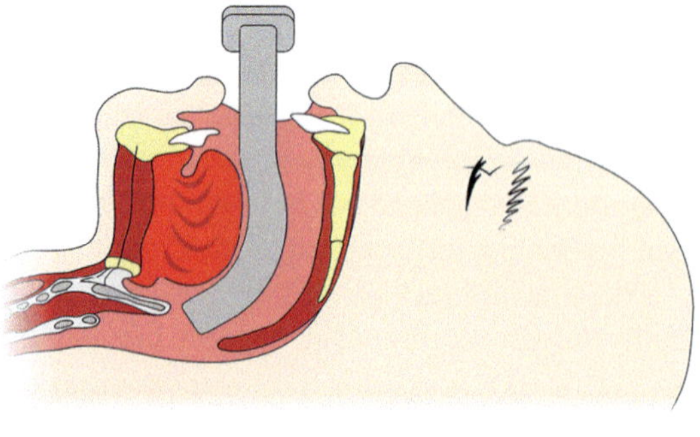

Fig. 7.3 Oropharyngeal (Guedel) airway in situ

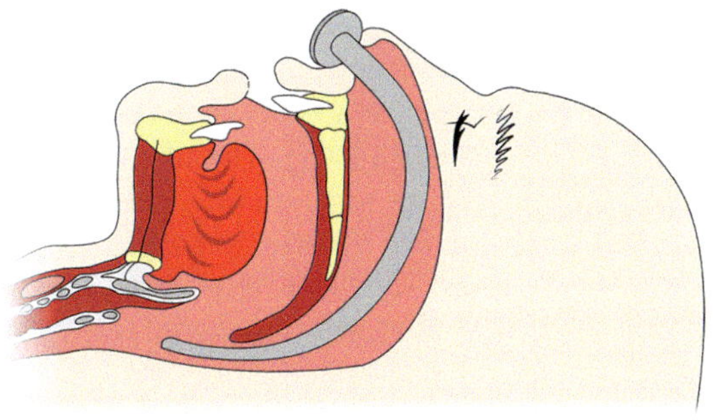

Fig. 7.4 Nasopharyngeal (NP) airway in situ

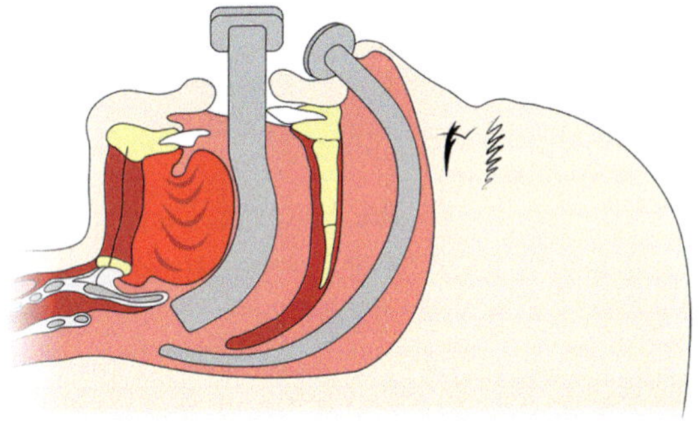

Fig. 7.5 Guedel and NP airways can be used together

way is appropriately sized—the curve should terminate just posterior to the angle of the jaw. Size 2 or 3 airways fit most adults—each manufacturer uses different sizes, so referring to them by colours can cause confusion. Guedel airways are initially inserted into the airway upside down to avoid pushing the tongue posteriorly and obstructing the airway, then rotated 180° to sit in the correct anatomical position. To tolerate a Guedel the patient's airway reflexes must be obtunded (either secondary to injury or drugs). In patients with intact reflexes, stimulation of the posterior pharynx by a Guedel will result in gagging and potentially vomiting. If a patient tolerates a Guedel then this should start to raise the question whether they require intubation, where that should take place and by whom. This is not always the case, as some treatments may obviate the need for intubation. For example, if a patient with an opiate overdose has suppressed airway reflexes and tolerates a Guedel the next correct treatment would be administration of naloxone either intravenously, intransally or intramuscularly. The rapid onset of the drug antagonises the effects of the opiates and restores the airway reflexes. Guedels can be useful as both a primary airway adjunct, and in intubated patients they can be used as a bite block to prevent patients biting and obstructing the ET tube if they suddenly wake from sedation.

The next most commonly used adjunct is the nasopharyngeal (NP) airway. Relatively (but not absolutely) contraindicated in basal skull fractures and in patients with coagulopathy because of the risk of epistaxis, the NP airway is otherwise well tolerated and can be used in patients who have intact airway reflexes. In patients who have signs of a basal skull fracture but who cannot have their jaw opened, NP airways can still be carefully used. Size 6 airways are commonly used in women and size 7 in men. The nasopharynx does not follow the angle of the nose, so NP airways should be lubricated with gel and inserted in a horizontal manner, parallel to the floor of the nasopharynx and aiming the tip towards the occiput. They should never be forced in; some patients may have a deviated septum so the NP may not fit down one nostril.

Suctioning of the airway can also be used in conjunction with positioning, or in isolation, to remove blood, secretions or vomit from the airway. In patients who are secured to a scoop stretcher or trauma board, they can be immediately turned 90° on their side if they vomit, and suction under direct vision performed. It is important to avoid inserting a hard Yankauer suction device blindly into the airway as it may cause trauma. Suction should be performed under direct vision wherever possible.

NP and OP airways can be used in conjunction, and this may make assisted ventilation with a bag-valve-mask (BVM) device easier. If BVM ventilation is performed at high pressure with poor airway opening, gastric distension with air can occur. This increases aspiration risk, and can potentially reduce venous return, resulting in decreased blood pressure, especially in paediatric resuscitation. Gastric distension can also cause diaphragmatic splinting and make it more difficult to ventilate the lungs; this usually leads to clinicians using more forceful ventilation which increases the risk of further gastric distension in a self-perpetuating cycle. Decompression of the stomach with a naso- or orogastric tube can be helpful in these patients.

Supraglottic Airway Devices

The original supraglottic airway (SGA) device was the Laryngeal Mask Airway (LMA). It was designed to sit in the oropharynx, above the glottic opening, using an inflatable cuff to hold soft tissues away from the channel through which the patient breathes. This allows a patent airway and either spontaneous or assisted ventilation without having to manually maintain airway patency. This revolutionised the administration of elective anaesthesia from the 1980s onwards [34, 35].

Since their introduction, various adaptations have been made to the basic design. Firstly a gastric drainage port was incorporated to reduce the aspiration risk and allow insertion of a gastric tube should this be required. There have also been variations providing narrower, flexible, tubing for intraoral surgery. They are available in a variety of sizes, including paediatric. The iGel is one of the most recent incarnations of the supraglottic airway. It has a preformed, non-inflatable, gel-like moulded end with a gastric channel. This reduces the steps required during insertion and also provides slightly increased protection to the glottic opening from refluxed gastric contents. However, it must be stressed that no commercially available supraglottic device can be considered to completely protect the lower airways from soiling. Only a cuffed endotracheal tube can provide that level of protection.

The use of supraglottic airways in the pre-hospital setting has been controversial. As discussed earlier in this chapter, intubation without drugs does not confer any survival advantage over SGA use in medical cardiac arrest, and intubation without drugs in trauma has an abysmal outcome. SGA's have been used successfully by personnel who have not been trained in intubation, either as the primary airway when laryngeal reflexes have been sufficiently depressed, allowing insertion without drugs, or where intubation attempts have failed [36–38]. The alternative in these cases would be basic airway manoeuvres and BVM ventilation. Use of SGA's has been found to decrease aspiration risk compared to BVM ventilation in cardiac arrest in both pre-hospital and hospital scenarios [39, 40], as well as being ergonomically easier to manage.

The question arises of whether ***drug-assisted*** use of SGA's may be useful in certain scenarios with specifically trained individuals, for example SGA use after administering drugs to a trapped patient with a head injury or trismus without necessary access to perform a rapid sequence induction and intubation.

The Faculty of Pre-Hospital Care brought together a group of stakeholders in 2014 in an attempt to provide guidance in this scenario. The resulting consensus statement on Pharmacologically Assisted Laryngeal Mask insertion (PALM) [41] has proved controversial. Despite the presence of the Royal College of Anaesthetists as part of the steering group, the RCoA felt unable to support the recommendations made by other parties. The consensus statement makes it clear that if considered, PALM should not be seen as an alternative to RSI and should only be performed by senior clinicians in rare and extreme circumstances. The consensus statement does not recommend specific drugs to facilitate PALM, but mentions ketamine and midazolam either as sole agents or in isolation. SGA insertion with agents other than propofol is more difficult as propofol depresses laryngeal reflexes profoundly. One study found that to obtain the laryngeal suppression that is equivalent to 2.5 mg/kg of propofol, a dose of 7 mg/kg thiopentone would be required [42]. Specific studies of propofol vs ketamine and/or midazolam as advocated in the guidelines have not been completed, but anecdotally SGA insertion with agents other than propofol (in elective anaesthesia at least) is incredibly difficult. Ketamine is usually chosen for sedation in pre-hospital care specifically because it preserves airway reflexes better than other agents, so its use in this particular patient cohort for this indication seems counter-intuitive. PALM has not found many proponents since its inception, and notably was not included as a suggested technique in the 2017 AAGBI guidelines on safter pre-hospital anaesthesia. It is a technique which would only rarely be required and appropriate, and as such the decision to use it should rest with individual clinicians and backed up with robust governance procedures rather than as a blanket recommendation.

Patients who have sufficient airway reflex suppression to tolerate oropharyngeal airways may tolerate SGA's, and insertion and ventilation via an SGA has a higher success rate than BVM ventilation with a Guedel airway [43]. SGA's have their place as a rescue device or as a temporising measure and occasionally as the primary airway device. Overall, SGA's are useful adjuncts, but it must be remembered that they are not a definitive airway.

Surgical Airways/Emergency Front of Neck Access (eFONA)

As previously mentioned, the mechanics of performing a surgical airway are relatively straightforward, however the decision-making around the procedure may build it up into something to be feared or viewed as a failure if performed [44]. This is not true—while the need for surgical airways is rare in civilian practice, when they are required and performed correctly, they are lifesaving procedures. They are included in the fundamental airway management section purposefully, as they can safely be performed by non-anaesthetic staff with appropriate training [19, 45]. The only truly failed airway is one where a surgical airway was indicated but not even attempted.

Cannula and Seldinger Techniques

These techniques are no longer routinely advocated. Traditionally, the use of needle cricothyroidotomy to allow emergency oxygenation was recommended as a first line technique, possibly reflecting anxiety around surgical techniques by non-surgeons. However, in the NAP 4 project, needle cricothyroidotomy had a 63% failure rate due to device misplacement, kinking or disconnection from the ventilating device [46]. The type of device attached to the needle and the type of needle itself are also important. A review of pre-hospital needle ventilation vs surgical airways found that the low-pressure systems set up in pre-hospital care became inadequate for ventilation within 60 s of insertion [47]. When jet ventilation is performed in hospital, specific high pressure ventilators such as the Sanders injector or Manujet are used, along with either a rigid bronchoscope or specific cannula designed to cope with high pressure rather than a standard intravenous cannula [48]. These jet devices and cannulae are not commonly available either pre-hospital or in the vast majority of emergency departments where a "Can't Intubate, Can't Oxygenate" (CICO) situation may occur in trauma airway management. For these reasons, needle cricothyroidotomy in adults has largely fallen out of practice in the context of emergency airway management in the UK. It has been replaced with surgical methods as a first line approach [49]. The situation in paediatrics is different, as the smaller airways in children mean that a surgical procedure is inherently more difficult. While current guidelines advocate needle cricothyroidotomy in children under 8 years [50], the broader picture is to avoid getting into the situation where one would be needed in the first instance, by doing the basics well. The threshold for increasingly complex intervention in paediatric airway management should be very high, and appropriately senior paediatric anaesthetic and ENT assistance should be sought whenever possible.

There are kits which will allow a Seldinger technique to be used to perform a cricothyroidotomy (e.g. Melker). While some cadaveric and manikin studies have suggested that familiarity with the Seldinger technique amongst anaesthetists may translate to increased success and shorter time to ventilation [51–53], this has not translated to significant difference in real-world applications [54–56]. There is also a significantly higher failure rate and longer placement time when Seldinger-based techniques are compared to surgical techniques, for providers with limited previous experience with either [57–59]. Most studies comparing methods have been cadaver or manikin based, which may fail to replicate some of the situational degradation in performance when this procedure is required on a live patient. The Seldinger technique relies on an initial needle puncture, threading a small guidewire through a needle, threading a dilator over the guidewire and finally threading the airway over the guidewire. Even in these cadaveric and manikin studies, steps have been omitted, guidewires have kinked making dilation difficult, and false passages have been created because of difficulties assessing needle placement. When considering how fine motor skills can degrade under stress [60–62], advocating a technique which involves more steps in total, with a higher requirement for fine motor skills and more opportunities for failure does not seem appropriate.

Surgical Techniques

The two principal methods of surgically accessing the airway are via tracheostomy or cricothyroidotomy. Tracheostomy is a longer procedure that can be performed by an open surgical approach or with a percutaneous kit and a modified Seldinger technique. The Seldinger method is common in intensive care when tracheostomies are placed electively for weaning in patients already intubated and with favourable anatomy. This is a procedure which is planned for and made as safe as possible with bronchoscopy through the ET tube. The many steps involved, and time taken is rarely appropriate or feasible in an emergency situation. Surgical tracheostomies for emergency airway management occasionally happen in hospital practice. These are largely due to infections or swelling making the upper airway inaccessible, such as epiglottitis or severe submandibular infections, rather than following trauma. Typically, they are performed by senior ENT or maxillofacial surgeons under local anaesthetic, with senior anaesthetic staff assisting (and occasionally providing some light sedation). The acute airway issue in these instances is usually the only pathology that the patient has, which means that factors such as patient positioning or compliance (which may be an issue in trauma) are less likely to be problematic. Surgical tracheostomy also involves direct visualisation of the trachea following sharp and blunt dissection along with haemostasis, in a surgically deeper area of the neck than the cricothyroid. It is a technically complex procedure that requires advanced anatomical knowledge of neck and thoracic structures in health as well as disease, in addition to a reasonable amount of surgical skill. For these reasons, it is a technique restricted to specifically trained surgeons.

Cricothyroidotomy, on the other hand, is a less complex procedure which can be taught relatively easily to both airway-competent and airway-naïve practitioners [63]. In an emergency, prominent anatomical landmarks are used (see Fig. 7.5). If there is time, adequate resources and a high risk of needing to perform a surgical airway (a so-called "surgically inevitable" airway [49]), ultrasound identification of the cricothyroid, and skin marking may be appropriate [64].

Surgical cricothyroidotomy is an emergency procedure that can be performed with a minimum amount of equipment (ideally a scalpel, artery forceps and a bougie) in an emergency. A demonstration of the anatomy relevant to this is technique is seen in Fig. 7.6. The cricothyroid membrane is bounded superiorly by the thyroid cartilage and by the cricoid cartilage inferiorly. These two cartilages form the palpable prominences used to identify the borders of the cricothyroid membrane, and provide a degree of protection by helping to prevent over-extending incisions too laterally and causing damage to the major vascular structures in the neck (i.e. the carotid artery and internal jugular vein). In most people, the cricothyroid membrane is directly palpable, however in the obese population the landmarks may not be as obvious. In these cases, a vertical incision in the midline of the neck should be made to expose the cricothyroid membrane, or at least make it palpable. At this point, the procedure is undertaken in the same manner as if the vertical incision had not been made.

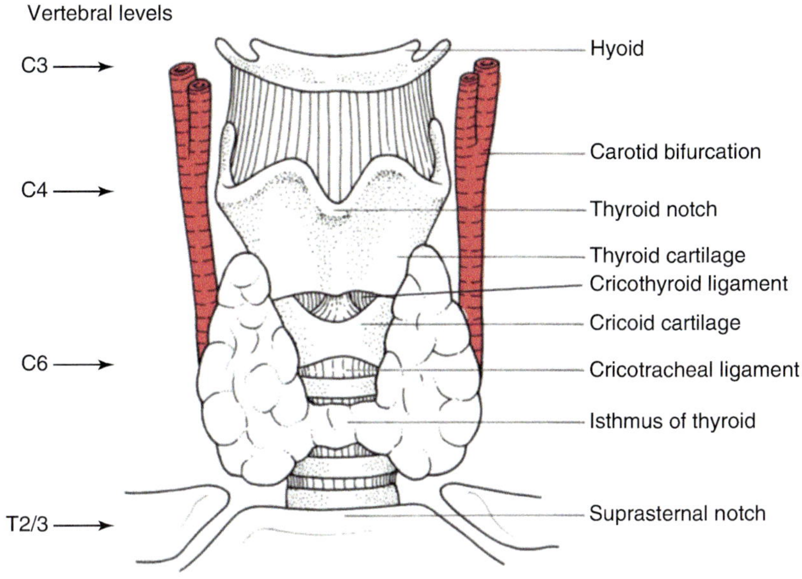

Fig. 7.6 Anatomy of the cricoid and trachea with corresponding vertebral levels on the left. Cricothyroidotomies are inserted via the cricothyroid membrane (aka cricothyroid ligament) and tracheotomies are inserted into the trachea, inferior to the cricoid cartilage (from Ellis and Mahadevan [65])

1. Identify the cricothyroid membrane
2. Make a single stab incision through the skin and cricothyroid with the scalpel held in a transverse orientation, and the incision extended to the lateral border of the cricothyroid.
3. Twist the scalpel 180° and extend the incision to the other lateral border of the cricothyroid.
4. Slide the artery forceps either side of the blade of the scalpel and open them to maintain the tract between the skin and the airway
5. Insert a bougie angulated towards the feet at a 30–45° angle into the airway
6. Railroad a size 5 or 6 ET tube over the bougie and inflate the cuff when it is inside the trachea
7. Remove the bougie and confirm effective ventilation by end tidal CO_2 measurement.

This is a mechanically simple procedure but the biggest delay when these cases are reviewed appears to be related to making the decision to perform it. This is why tools such as the Vortex approach and DAS guidelines (see following chapter) are useful as they emphasise surgical airways as the final step in CICO situations.

[External Video—https://www.youtube.com/watch?v=B8I1t1HlUac&t=276s]

Surgical Cricothyroidotomy technique

Conclusion

Trauma airway management is not all about intubations (though it may seem so). The myriad of methods taught to introduce a plastic tube into the airway are useful to know, but the bigger picture must not be forgotten. Oxygenation must always be the primary goal, and if the current management strategy is working, then any escalation from that point must be subject to a patient and situation specific risk assessment. Oftentimes, basics done well will obviate the need for advanced interventions in suboptimal conditions, or allow transport to a facility with more help and a higher chance of success.

Familiarity with the equipment, and its use, is essential in basic airway management. Simulation training and supervised clinical scenarios is an important part of training for all trauma practitioners. This reduces the possibility of a misplaced intervention worsening the situation. Well-practised technical skills, along with checklists, aid the clinician in maintaining situational awareness by reducing cognitive load.

Most importantly, getting the basics right first time can avoid the requirement for advanced airway manoeuvres and the complications that may arise from these.

Questions

1. The fundamental principle of airway management in trauma patients is:
   (a) Adequate CO_2 control
   (b) Adequate oxygenation
   (c) Avoidance of C-spine movement
   (d) Minimising aspiration risk
   (e) Intubating as many people as possible

2. Trauma patients who can be intubated without drugs have an overall survival of:
   (a) 0–5%
   (b) 5–10%
   (c) 10–20%
   (d) 30–40%
   (e) >40%

3. In patients with actual or suspected cervical spine injuries, airway manoeuvres:
   (a) Should never be undertaken
   (b) Should only be attempted after a cervical collar and three-point immobilisation has been applied
   (c) Should be used for normal indications and only move the neck as much as needed to ensure airway patency
   (d) Should only be undertaken by doctors
   (e) Have been shown to worsen outcomes from neurological injuries

4. In patients who require a surgical airway:
   (a) Tracheostomy should be the first course of action
   (b) Needle cricothyroidotomy is the gold standard intervention
   (c) Surgical cricothyroidotomy should only be performed by anaesthetic or surgical medical practitioners
   (d) Surgical airways should only be considered after trying and failing every other method to secure the airway
   (e) Surgical cricothyroidotomy performed by appropriately trained non-doctors and junior doctors has over a 90% success rate.

5. The use of Pharmacollogically Assisted Laryngeal Mask airways in pre-hospital care can be considered an alternative to rapid sequence induction and intubation.
   (a) True
   (b) False

Answers:

1. b
2. a
3. c
4. e
5. b

References

1. Brindley PG, Beed M, Law JA, Hung O, Levitan R, Murphy MF, et al. Airway management outside the operating room: how to better prepare. Can J Anaesth J Can Anesth. 2017;64(5):530–9.
2. Reed MJ. Intubation training in emergency medicine: a review of one trainee's first 100 procedures. Emerg Med J. 2007;24(9):654–6.
3. Konrad C, Schupfer G, Wietlisbach M, Gerber H. Learning manual skills in anesthesiology: is there a recommended number of cases for anesthetic procedures? Anesth Analg. 1998;86(3):635–9.
4. de Oliveira Filho GR. The construction of learning curves for basic skills in anesthetic procedures: an application for the cumulative sum method. Anesth Analg. 2002;95(2):411–6.
5. Savoldelli GL, Schiffer E, Abegg C, Baeriswyl V, Clergue F, Waeber J-L. Learning curves of the Glidescope, the McGrath and the Airtraq laryngoscopes: a manikin study. Eur J Anaesthesiol. 2009;26(7):554–8.
6. Komatsu R, Kasuya Y, Yogo H, Sessler DI, Mascha E, Yang D, et al. Learning curves for bag-and-mask ventilation and orotracheal intubation: an application of the cumulative sum method. Anesthesiology. 2010;112(6):1525–31.
7. Toda J, Toda AA, Arakawa J. Learning curve for paramedic endotracheal intubation and complications. Int J Emerg Med. 2013;6(1):38.
8. Je S, Cho Y, Choi HJ, Kang B, Lim T, Kang H. An application of the learning curve–cumulative summation test to evaluate training for endotracheal intubation in emergency medicine. Emerg Med J. 2015;32(4):291–4.

9. Rujirojindakul P, McNeil E, Rueangchira-urai R, Siripunt N. Learning curves of Macintosh laryngoscope in nurse anesthetist trainees using cumulative sum method. Anesthesiol Res Pract. 2014;2014:1–6.
10. Wang HE, Reitz SR, Hostler D, Yealy DM. Defining the learning curve for paramedic student endotracheal intubation. Prehosp Emerg Care. 2005;9(2): 156–62.
11. Lockey D, Davies G, Coats T. Survival of trauma patients who have prehospital tracheal intubation without anaesthesia or muscle relaxants: observational study. BMJ. 2001;323(7305):141.
12. NICE. NICE Quality Standard 166: Trauma [Internet]. National Institute for Health and Clinical Excellence; 2018. https://www.nice.org.uk/guidance/qs166/resources/trauma-pdf-75545603800261. Accessed 12 Jan 2020.
13. Lockey DJ, Crewdson K, Davies G, Jenkins B, Klein J, Laird C, et al. AAGBI: Safer pre-hospital anaesthesia 2017: Association of Anaesthetists of Great Britain and Ireland. Anaesthesia. 2017;72(3): 379–90.
14. Andersen LW, Granfeldt A, Callaway CW, Bradley SM, Soar J, Nolan JP, et al. Association between tracheal intubation during adult in-hospital cardiac arrest and survival. JAMA. 2017;317(5):494.
15. Stiell IG, Wells GA, Field B, Spaite DW, Nesbitt LP, De Maio VJ, et al. Advanced cardiac life support in out-of-hospital cardiac arrest. N Engl J Med. 2004;351(7):647–56.
16. Newell C, Grier S, Soar J. Airway and ventilation management during cardiopulmonary resuscitation and after successful resuscitation. Crit Care. 2018;22(1):190.
17. Manley G. Hypotension, hypoxia, and head injury: frequency, duration, and consequences. Arch Surg. 2001;136(10):1118.
18. Mabry RL. An analysis of battlefield cricothyrotomy in Iraq and Afghanistan. J Spec Oper Med Peer Rev J SOF Med Prof. 2012;12(1):17–23.
19. Kyle T, le Clerc S, Thomas A, Greaves I, Whittaker V, Smith JE. The success of battlefield surgical airway insertion in severely injured military patients: a UK perspective. J R Army Med Corps. 2016;162(6):460–4.
20. Hill H. Regulation 28 Report to prevent future deaths [Internet]. London Coroner; 2016. https://www.judiciary.uk/wp-content/uploads/2017/01/Dees-2016-0259.pdf. Accessed 4 Sep 2020.
21. Prasarn ML, Horodyski M, Scott NE, Konopka G, Conrad B, Rechtine GR. Motion generated in the unstable upper cervical spine during head tilt–chin lift and jaw thrust maneuvers. Spine J. 2014;14(4):609–14.
22. Part 2: Adult basic life support. Circulation. 2005;112(22 Suppl):III-5.
23. Aprahamian C, Thompson BM, Finger WA, Darinz JC. Experimental cervical spine injury model: evaluation of airway management and splinting techniques. Ann Emerg Med. 1984;13(8):584–7.
24. Majernick TG, Bieniek R, Houston JB, Hughes HG. Cervical spine movement during orotracheal intubation. Ann Emerg Med. 1986;15(4):417–20.
25. Lennarson PJ, Smith DW, Sawin PD, Todd MM, Sato Y, Traynelis VC. Cervical spinal motion during intubation: efficacy of stabilization maneuvers in the setting of complete segmental instability. J Neurosurg Spine. 2001;94(2):265–70.
26. Brimacombe J, Keller C, Künzel KH, Gaber O, Boehler M, Pühringer F. Cervical spine motion during airway management: a cinefluoroscopic study of the posteriorly destabilized third cervical vertebrae in human cadavers. Anesth Analg. 2000;91(5):1274–8.
27. McLeod ADM, Calder I. Editorial I: Spinal cord injury and direct laryngoscopy – the legend lives on. Br J Anaesth. 2000;84(6):705–9.
28. Alizadeh A, Dyck SM, Karimi-Abdolrezaee S. Traumatic spinal cord injury: an overview of pathophysiology, models and acute injury mechanisms. Front Neurol [Internet]. 2019. https://www.ncbi.nlm.nih.gov/pmc/articles/PMC6439316/. Accessed 10 Jun 2020.
29. Rowland JW, Hawryluk GWJ, Kwon B, Fehlings MG. Current status of acute spinal cord injury pathophysiology and emerging therapies: promise on the horizon. Neurosurg Focus. 2008;25(5):E2.
30. Dumont RJ, Okonkwo DO, Verma S, Hurlbert RJ, Boulos PT, Ellegala DB, et al. Acute spinal cord injury, Part I: Pathophysiologic mechanisms. Clin Neuropharmacol. 2001;24(5):254–64.
31. Carassiti M, Zanzonico R, Cecchini S, Silvestri S, Cataldo R, Agrò FE. Force and pressure distribution using Macintosh and GlideScope laryngoscopes in normal and difficult airways: a manikin study. BJA Br J Anaesth. 2012;108(1):146–51.
32. Russell T, Khan S, Elman J, Katznelson R, Cooper RM. Measurement of forces applied during Macintosh direct laryngoscopy compared with GlideScope® videolaryngoscopy. Anaesthesia. 2012;67(6):626–31.
33. Santoni BG, Hindman BJ, Puttlitz CM, Weeks JB, Johnson N, Maktabi MA, et al. Manual in-line stabilization increases pressures applied by the laryngoscope blade during direct laryngoscopy and orotracheal intubation. Anesthesiology. 2009;110(1):24–31.
34. Schmiesing CA, Brock-Utne JG. An airway management device: the laryngeal mask airway—a review. J Intensive Care Med. 1998;13(1):32–43.
35. van Zundert TCRV, Brimacombe JR, Ferson DZ, Bacon DR, Wilkinson DJ. Archie Brain: celebrating 30 years of development in laryngeal mask airways. Anaesthesia. 2012;67(12):1375–85.
36. Shavit I, Aviram E, Hoffmann Y, Biton O, Glassberg E. Laryngeal mask airway as a rescue device for failed endotracheal intubation during scene-to-hospital air transport of combat casualties. Eur J Emerg Med. 2018;25(5):368–71.
37. Jacobs P, Grabinsky A. Advances in prehospital airway management. Int J Crit Illn Inj Sci. 2014;4(1):57.
38. Bosch J, de Nooij J, de Visser M, Cannegieter SC, Terpstra NJ, Heringhaus C, et al. Prehospital use in

emergency patients of a laryngeal mask airway by ambulance paramedics is a safe and effective alternative for endotracheal intubation. Emerg Med J. 2014;31(9):750–3.

39. Flavell E, Boyle M. Which is more effective for ventilation in the prehospital setting during cardiopulmonary resuscitation, the laryngeal mask airway or the bag-valve-mask? A review of the literature. Australas J Paramed [Internet]. 2010;8(3). https://ajp.paramedics.org/index.php/ajp/article/view/94. Accessed 27 Jul 2020.
40. Stone BJ, Chantler PJ, Baskett PJF. The incidence of regurgitation during cardiopulmonary resuscitation: a comparison between the bag valve mask and laryngeal mask airway. Resuscitation. 1998;38(1):3–6.
41. Moss R, Porter K, Greaves I. on behalf of the consensus group, Faculty of Pre-Hospital Care. Pharmacologically assisted laryngeal mask insertion: a consensus statement. Trauma. 2015;17(1):73–6.
42. Amr YM, Amin SM. Comparison of two regimes of thiopental and propofol for I-gel supraglottic airway device insertion. Anesth Essays Res. 2010;4(1):25–8.
43. Alexander R, Hodgson P, Lomax D, Bullen C. A comparison of the laryngeal mask airway and Guedel airway, bag and facemask for manual ventilation following formal training. Anaesthesia. 1993;48(3):231–4.
44. Greenland KB, Acott C, Segal R, Goulding G, Riley RH, Merry AF. Emergency surgical airway in life-threatening acute airway emergencies–why are we so reluctant to do it? Anaesth Intensive Care. 2011;39(4):578–84.
45. Adams BD, Cuniowski PA, Muck A, De Lorenzo RA. Registry of emergency airways arriving at Combat Hospitals. J Trauma Inj Infect Crit Care. 2008;64(6):1548–54.
46. Cook T, Woodall N, Frerk C, Royal College of Anaesthetists (Great Britain), Difficult Airway Society (Great Britain). Major complications of airway management in the United Kingdom: report and findings. 4th National Audit Project of the Royal College of Anaesthetists and the Difficult Airway Society. NAP4 [Internet]. London: Royal College of Anaesthetists; 2011. 219 p. https://www.nationalauditprojects.org.uk/NAP4_home?newsid=463#pt. Accessed 4 Jul 2020.
47. Scrase I, Woollard M. Needle vs surgical cricothyroidotomy: a short cut to effective ventilation. Anaesthesia. 2006;61(10):962–74.
48. Evans E, Biro P, Bedforth N. Jet ventilation. Contin Educ Anaesth Crit Care Pain. 2007;7(1):2–5.
49. Price TM, McCoy EP. Emergency front of neck access in airway management. BJA Educ. 2019;19(8):246–53.
50. Black AE, Flynn PER, Smith HL, Thomas ML, Wilkinson KA. Development of a guideline for the management of the unanticipated difficult airway in pediatric practice. Pediatr Anesth. 2015;25(4):346–62.
51. Eisenburger P, Laczika K, List M, Wilfing A, Losert H, Hofbauer R, et al. Comparison of conventional surgical versus Seldinger technique emergency cricothyrotomy performed by inexperienced clinicians. Anesthesiol J Am Soc Anesthesiol. 2000;92(3):687–90.
52. Schaumann N, Lorenz V, Schellongowski P, Staudinger T, Locker GJ, Burgmann H, et al. Evaluation of Seldinger technique emergency cricothyroidotomy versus standard surgical cricothyroidotomy in 200 cadavers. Anesthesiol J Am Soc Anesthesiol. 2005;102(1):7–11.
53. Assmann NM, Wong DT, Morales E. A comparison of a new indicator-guided with a conventional wire-guided percutaneous cricothyroidotomy device in mannequins. Anesth Analg. 2007;105(1):148–54.
54. Langvad S, Hyldmo P, Nakstad A, Vist G, Sandberg M. Emergency cricothyrotomy – a systematic review. Scand J Trauma Resusc Emerg Med. 2013;21(1):43.
55. Paix BR, Griggs WM. Emergency surgical cricothyroidotomy: 24 successful cases leading to a simple 'scalpel-finger-tube' method: Scalpel-finger-tube cricothyroidotomy. Emerg Med Australas. 2012;24(1):23–30.
56. Hamaekers AE, Henderson JJ. Equipment and strategies for emergency tracheal access in the adult patient: Emergency tracheal access in the adult patient. Anaesthesia. 2011;66:65–80.
57. Schober P, Hegemann MC, Schwarte LA, Loer SA, Noetges P. Emergency cricothyrotomy—A comparative study of different techniques in human cadavers. Resuscitation. 2009;80(2):204–9.
58. Dimitriadis JC, Paoloni R. Emergency cricothyroidotomy: a randomised crossover study of four methods. Anaesthesia. 2008;63(11):1204–8.
59. Bruppacher HR, Naik VN, Bould MD, Friedman Z. Design flaw of Melker kit may compromise patient safety. Anaesthesia. 2009;64(10):1147.
60. Performance Under Pressure (how to manage stress) [Internet]. First10EM. 2017. https://first10em.com/performance-under-pressure/. Accessed 1 Aug 2020.
61. Grossman D, Christensen LW. On combat: the psychology and physiology of deadly conflict in war and in peace. 3. ed., [Nachdr.], 4. Nachdruck. Millstadt, IL: Warrior Science; 2008. 403 p.
62. Anderson GS, Di Nota PM, Metz GAS, Andersen JP. The impact of acute stress physiology on skilled motor performance: implications for policing. Front Psychol [Internet]. 2019. https://www.ncbi.nlm.nih.gov/pmc/articles/PMC6856650/. Accessed 1 Aug 2020.
63. Shetty K, Nayyar V, Stachowski E, Byth K. Training for cricothyroidotomy. Anaesth Intensive Care. 2013;41(5):623–30.
64. Weingart S. Surgical airway, cricothyrotomy, aka the emergent cric [Internet]. EMCrit Project. 2014. https://emcrit.org/emcrit/surgical-airway/. Accessed 1 Aug 2020.
65. Ellis H, Mahadevan V. Clinical anatomy: applied anatomy for students and junior doctors. 13th ed. Wiley-Blackwell: West Sussex; 2013. 477 p.

8 Drug Assisted Airway Management

Jonathan Veitch, Peter Lax, and Neil Roy

- Advanced airway assessment
- Decision making in the pre-hospital setting
- Rapid sequence induction of anaesthesia
- Pharmacology of commonly used anaesthetic agents
- The planning and management of the difficult airway
- Overview of analgesia and sedation in transfer

Introduction

Multiple and severe injuries will require analgesia, commonly with strong opiates or ketamine. Treatments including splinting of limbs and reductions of fractures can cause significant pain initially. These procedures will require analgesia, occasionally combined with sedation, and in normal circumstances the potential side effects of these drugs can include unwanted over-sedation and reduction in respiratory effort which may also require airway management. Those patients with cardiovascular instability, or head injuries, are more likely to suffer these effects and thereby require assistance in oxygenation and ventilation. Planning airway management in conjunction with providing good analgesia and sedation is of paramount importance.

While any practitioner should be able to perform basic airway assessment and management, as outlined in the fundamentals of airway management chapter, the use of drugs to facilitate airway management is currently a skill restricted to doctors, both in pre-hospital and hospital practice in the UK. Other countries have expanded the skill of pre-hospital RSI into paramedic practice.

Trauma airway management and the decision-making process around this also need to include situations where the airway itself is not the primary issue. Some of these factors are outlined in Fig. 8.1. Careful control of ventilation may be required in the immediate care of the head injured patient to maintain a normal carbon dioxide

J. Veitch
Department of Anaesthesia, Nottingham University Teaching Hospitals NHS Trust, Nottinghamshire, UK

212 Field Hospital (reserves), Sheffield, UK
e-mail: jveitch@doctors.org.uk

P. Lax (✉)
Tactical Medical Wing, Royal Air Force, Brize Norton, Oxfordshire, UK

The Air Ambulance Service (TAAS), Rugby, Warwickshire, UK
e-mail: p.lax@NHS.net

N. Roy
Department of Anaesthesia and Critical Care Medicine, Leeds General Infirmary, Leeds, UK
e-mail: neil.roy@nhs.net

P. Lax (ed.), *Textbook of Acute Trauma Care*, https://doi.org/10.1007/978-3-030-83628-3_8

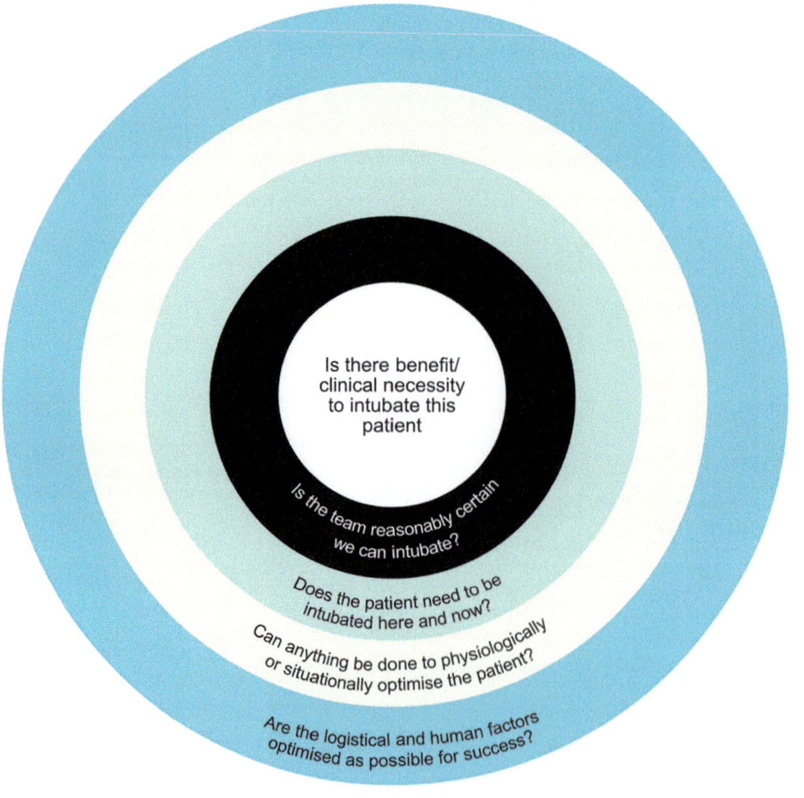
Is there benefit/
clinical necessity
to intubate this
patient
Is the team reasonably certain
we can intubate?
Does the patient need to be
intubated here and now?
Can anything be done to physiologically
or situationally optimise the patient?
Are the logistical and human factors
optimised as possible for success?

Fig. 8.1 Decision-making factors affecting intubation, most important factors are central and then subsequent decision s radiate from this

concentration in the blood and attempt to reduce intracerebral pressure. The most effective way of doing this in patients with a reduced conscious level is intubation and mechanical ventilation. The focus should not just be on putting a plastic tube in a hole, but also appropriate post-procedure sedation and anaesthesia. In patients with head injury, a single episode of hypotension can double mortality [1]. Hypoxia can also substantially worsen outcomes [2, 3] and the combined effects of hypoxia and hypotension together in these patients are synergistic rather than merely additive [4]. Decision-making around RSI should take into account logistical and human factors, as well as technical and pharmacological ones. It should also include plans for further management of the patient once the airway has been secured.

Along with the requirement for analgesia, the severity of injury itself may require sedation (or anaesthesia) of a patient on humanitarian grounds or on the basis of anticipated clinical course. Extraction from the site of injury to a medical centre will require transport by road or air, which inevitably causes discomfort to some extent. Rendering a patient unconscious for transport reduces their pain and distress, whilst removing the opportunity for the patient to become agitated during transfer.

This leads on to discussion on how to manage a patient who is already agitated and requires transfer for definitive care. This may be due to pre-injury reasons: intoxication, drugs, mental health issues, or due to head or other injuries sustained in the incident. Many will require some conscious sedation to enable assessment or treatment, and following this, a subset will require further anaesthesia and intubation. This is further covered in the sedation and field amputation chapter later in this textbook.

By now it is clear that the management of the trauma airway holds many caveats and the decision making can be both complex and nuanced. It can also be a significant distraction to the ongoing care of a multiply injured person. Without a secure airway, a clinician may be required to repeatedly reassess the airway or even tie up valuable personnel to maintain basic airway manoeuvres. With this in mind, safe intubation and sedation can free up the clinician's ability to manage the patient in their entirety, along with providing time to consider the non-clinical situation or the care of other casualties.

Airway Anatomy

The airway extends from the lips to the alveoli, but in the context of most management strategies, the areas of interest are from the mouth or nose to the trachea. Classically, the airway has been described as upper and lower, with the demarcation between the two being set at the level of the vocal cords, however there is now some interest in the concept of a "middle airway" [5]. This divides the airway into upper (nose to larynx), middle (larynx and trachea) and lower (bronchi and lungs) and may be of use when describing specific pathologies and symptoms. In health, the tongue and soft tissues of the upper airway are held open by muscular tone. Reflexes will detect the presence of foreign bodies or liquids and cause coughing to remove the obstruction. During trauma or after administration of some drugs, these reflexes and muscle tone may become diminished, and the soft tissues of the upper airway can fall back and cause obstruction. This can occur more readily in patients with sleep apnoea who can benefit from airway stabilisation with CPAP [6].

It is worth considering why intubation may be anatomically difficult. The fundamental principles that make obtaining a good view of the larynx during intubation are that light travels in a straight line, but the airway is curved. Ideas for optimising positioning for direct laryngoscopy were first discussed as far back as 1852, but it was not until 1936 that Magill formally described the "sniffing the morning air" position that is still taught today [7]. This was followed in 1944 by Bannister and Macbeth proposing the Three Axis Alignment Theory [8] which outlined the problem of having three distinct axes (oral, pharyngeal and laryngeal) that must be aligned to directly visualise the vocal cords. Magill's position aligned these axes well and explains why this position persists today.

When considering the use of direct laryngoscopy for intubation, positioning of the patient is

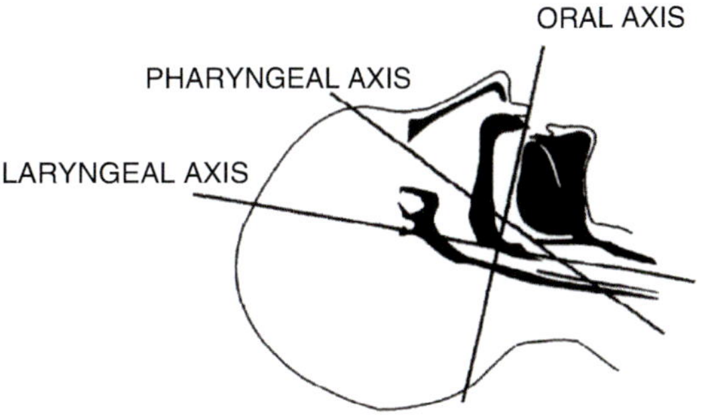

Fig. 8.2 Axial lines of sight in the neutral position. Courtesy of Dr Christine Whitten MD (www.airwayjedi.com)

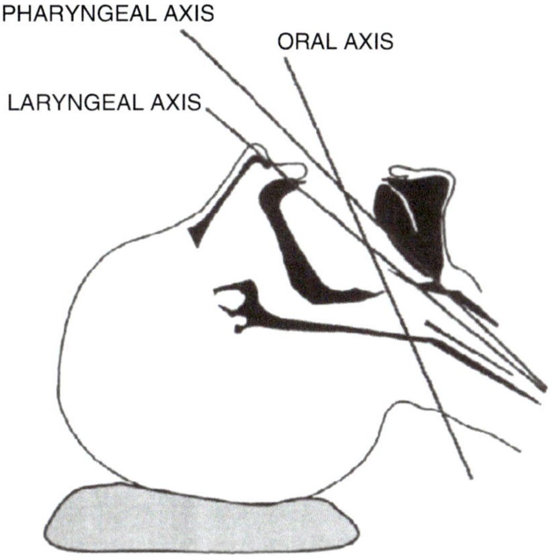

Fig. 8.3 Axial alignment in the sniffing position with the head extended. Courtesy of Dr Christine Whitten MD (www.airwayjedi.com)

paramount in order to create a direct line of sight through the patient's mouth, past the oropharynx to the glottic opening. The following diagrams demonstrate the line of sight in a neutral head position (Fig. 8.2) and a traditional "sniffing the morning air" position (Fig. 8.3).

There are many confounding factors that will interfere in gaining a direct view of the larynx, but it should be remembered that maintaining airway *patency and oxygenation,* with either basic airway adjuncts or supraglottic airways (SGAs), does not require a view of the larynx, nor alignment of these axes.

A great deal of time has been spent trying to predict the difficult airway using a variety of measurements and observations [9], however all of the discussion surrounding this has been carried out in the elective anaesthetic setting. In the field of pre-hospital (and occasionally in-hospital) trauma care, a full assessment is not possible and should not necessarily be attempted. It would be advisable to consider every trauma intubation as potentially a difficult airway and prepare accordingly. The predictors of difficult intubation that have been described (see Table 8.1) all predict difficulty in accessing the upper airway to the transition point at the level of the vocal cords.

In cases where there is direct laryngeal, tracheal or bronchial trauma, it may still be relatively easy to visualise the vocal cords, but trauma distal to them can still catch out the unwary. The larynx and cervical trachea can be injured by both blunt and penetrating mechanisms. In penetrating trauma, death is usually related to exsanguination from associated vascular injuries, rather than airway failure itself (though massive aspiration of blood causes significant mortality) [10]. Blunt injuries to the chest such as those sustained in vehicle collisions can cause vertical tears in the membranous part of the trachea or bronchi, usually (but not always) within 2.5 cm of the carina [11, 12]. Initial laryngoscopy may be easy but the passage of the tube distal to the cords and positive pressure ventilation may be impossible, or indeed may create a false passage if the false lumen of an airway tear is intubated inadvertently. Securing the airway distal to the defect is the correct course of action, but in injuries involving the cricothyroid or larynx, emergency tracheostomy inferior to this point may be the only option. Visualisation of the airway with a fibreoptic scope is necessary in these cases, using a smaller than normal ET tube (e.g. 6.0 mm). Many papers advocate induction of anaesthesia with volatile agents and a spontaneously breathing technique where possible [10, 13, 14]. Neuromuscular blockers should be avoided until the airway is secured, as loss of tone may cause complete collapse of an airway transection held open by accessory musculature.

Table 8.1 Airway assessment tools with areas that may give rise to difficulty (after CCAM website https://www.ccam.net.au/handbook/plan-a/)

Column	Potential difficulties	Assessment tools	Potential solutions
Posterior (spine and atlanto-occiptial joint)	● Cervical collar/MILS ● Halo application/fused neck ● Ankylosing Spondylitis ● Rheumatoid arthritis	● Range of neck flexion/extension	● Videolaryngoscope ± hyperangulated blade ● McCoy blade ● Fibreoptic scope ● Intubating SGA
Middle (airway)	● Foreign body (e.g. teeth) ● Epiglottitis ● Airway tumour	● History and examination findings ● Nasendoscopy (many not be possible in trauma) ● Imaging with CT or MRI if possible (rare in trauma)	● Standard Macintosh laryngoscope blade ● Videolaryngoscope ● McGill's forceps for foreign body ● Fibreoptic scope ● SGA with fibreoptic scope and Aintree exchange catheter
Anterior (soft tissues)	● Decreased volume of anterior triangle – Syndromes with micrognathia or macroglossia ● Decreased compliance of tissue – Expanding haematoma – Post-radiotherapy – Infection (e.g. Ludwig's angina) ● Protruding incisors ● Large tongue	● Short thyromental distance ● Impaired mouth opening ● Overbite ● Inability to protrude mandible anterior to maxilla ● Mallampati score	● Videoscope ● Fibreoptic scope with nasal intubation ● SGA with fibreoptic scope and Aintree exchange catheter

This was further reinforced in a systematic review by Mercer et al. in 2016 [15]. The nature of this injury and required specialist equipment, added to pre-hospital airway management being inherently more demanding, should raise the threshold for intervention in this environment for these injuries.

Two excellent articles by Greenland [16, 17] further describe a model explaining why there are difficulties in intubation. It considers curves, axes and complexes in the airway, and how they are affected by static positioning before intubation, and the dynamic movements during intubation. The model describes a posterior complex (the atlanto-occipital joint and spine), middle complex (the airway itself) and an anterior complex (soft tissues in the submandibular space including the tongue).

Greenland describes a primary curve (the oropharyngeal airway) and a secondary curve (the pharyngo-glotto-tracheal airway) that should be made as straight as possible by optimising positioning prior to administering drugs. Greenland refers to this as the static phase. Positioning into the sniffing position by extending the head at the atlanto-occipital joint and flexing the neck will straighten out the secondary (posterior) curve. When induction medications have been given and the laryngoscope introduced, the dynamic phase of intubation lifts the tongue and epiglottis anteriorly, straightening the primary (anterior) curve and exposing the vocal cords. Any factor which opposes the straightening of the two curves makes the manoeuvre more difficult, and when considering the factors associated with difficult intubation, they can be seen to interfere with one or both of these curves.

Pathology such as rheumatoid arthritis, ankylosing spondylitis, the presence of metalwork or a cervical collar may prevent head extension and neck flexion and impairs straightening of the posterior curve. Short mandibles, tongue swelling, short thyromental distances and difficulty in protruding the mandible all decrease the volume of the anterior complex, making compression of tissues and straightening of the primary curve more difficult (demonstrated in Figs. 8.4, 8.5 and 8.6).

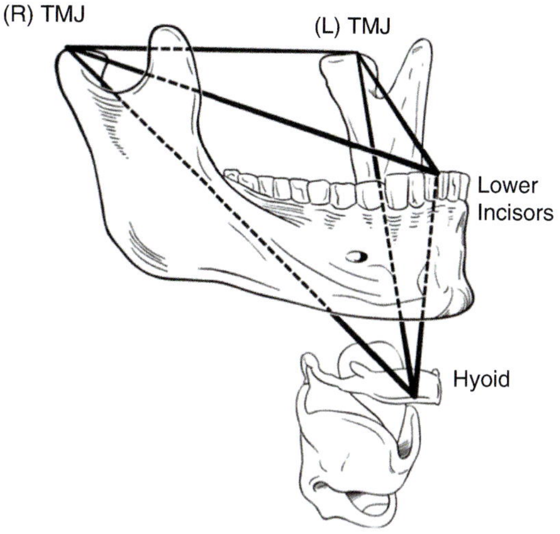

Fig. 8.4 Borders of the anterior complex (from "A proposed model for direct laryngoscopy and tracheal intubation" [17])

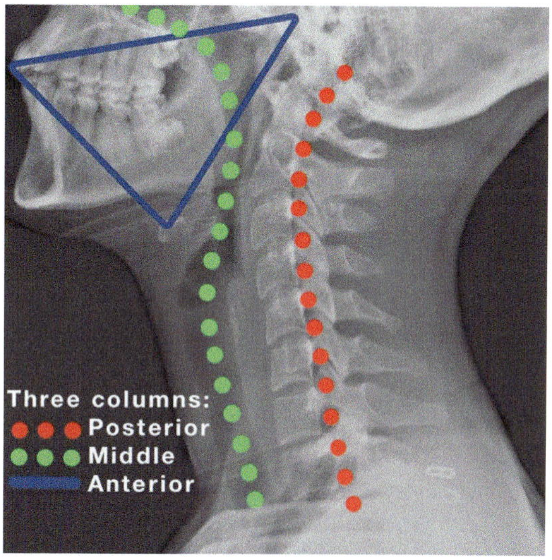

Fig. 8.5 Demonstration of the three columns approach. From CCAM Website (https://www.ccam.net.au/handbook/plan-a/)

Of the multiple clinical assessments in use, no individual marker has been proven to reliably and consistently predict difficulty [9], so multiple assessment methods should be considered. Returning to Greenland's work, a further paper groups these assessments by area that they effect—the posterior, middle or anterior complexes (See Table 8.1) [18]. These assessments

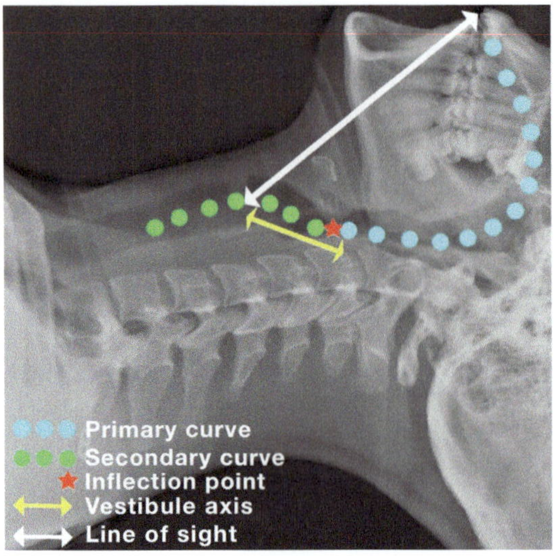

Fig. 8.6 Demonstration of the primary and secondary airway curves. From CCAM website (https://www.ccam.net.au/handbook/plan-a/)

and potential solutions are for general purposes only, and some investigations or methods may not be appropriate in trauma depending on the degree of urgency, fasting status and other logistical factors (e.g. location and availability of equipment).

As mentioned later, the use of videolaryngoscopes, with or without hyperangulated blades, may make intubation easier as they are not reliant on establishing a direct line of sight from vocal cords to mouth. They can (in effect) look around a corner, though manipulation of an ET tube may become more difficult, and usually requires the use of an adjunct such as a (steerable) gum elastic bougie or stylet to allow successful intubation. Issues with blood or secretions in the airway, cost and technical limitations mean videolaryngoscopes are unlikely to replace traditional direct laryngoscopy in entirety, but they can be useful in difficult airway management. Awake fibreoptic intubation (AFOI) can also occasionally be used for select indications in a minority of patients. Again, the same optical limitations that hamper videolaryngoscopes apply, in addition to the technical difficulties of anaesthetising a patient's airway adequately, potentially under pressure of time. AFOI is a slow procedure that requires patient cooperation and motivation, along with specialist assistance and equipment that is often only available in a dedicated area. It is rarely indicated in acute trauma that requires urgent intubation, though occasionally it may be used in cervical spine injuries in fasted patients, or extremely rarely in some cases of laryngotracheal disruption as previously described.

The question now remains, how should this information be assimilated into the practical aspects of emergency trauma anaesthesia? In the elective setting, the vast majority of intubations are achieved with successful direct laryngoscopy. This success is aided by a highly trained workforce, good lighting, and easy access to positioning aids, in order to maximise the chances of success. As the environment is never likely to be ideal in the pre-hospital setting, there is evidence to suggest that initial use of difficult airway equipment improves the chances of a successful first intubation attempt. One study showed that non-anaesthetists had a statistically higher chance of successful intubation in simple *and* difficult intubations when a bougie was used to pass through the glottic opening and the endotracheal tube was then railroaded over the top [19]. Most pre-hospital emergency anaesthesia protocols have followed this advice and incorporate use of the bougie as a first line piece of equipment [20].

Rapid Sequence Induction of Anaesthesia and Intubation

The standard of care for emergency intubation internationally, is rapid sequence induction of anaesthesia and tracheal intubation. This technique assumes the patient has a full stomach and is at risk of aspiration of gastric contents, so aims for a rapid procedure in order to minimise the risk of desaturation, gastric aspiration and to rapidly achieve a secure airway.

The medications chosen to facilitate a rapid sequence induction in a trauma situation, should have a rapid speed of onset, ease of use, and a wide therapeutic window, with minimal deleterious cardiovascular and intracerebral side effects. A "Classical" RSI technique, as taught to most anaesthetic trainees until relatively recently, is a period of 3 min of pre-oxygenation with a tight-fitting facemask, administration of thiopentone and suxamethonium without opiates, and application of cricoid pressure. The received wisdom is that the rapid onset and offset of these drugs would allow waking of the patient and recovery of airway reflexes in a short period if intubation was unsuccessful, with prevention of aspiration and a short apnoeic interval prior to intubation and ventilation. In reality, the procedure first described in 1970 by Stept and Safar [21] was a 15 step process involving insertion of NG tubes, pre-treatment with d-tubocurarine and placing the patient in a semi-sitting v-position. This is a prime example of the differences between what is taught as the "gold standard" for RSI from senior anaesthetists, versus what is actually in the paper. It is one of many myths that have entered practice on minimal evidence. The pre-treatment with d-tubocurarine in the original Stept and Safar method would have led to a partially paralysed but awake patient if the thiopentone had worn off; the concept of failed intubation or waking the patient up was never mentioned in their paper.

In trauma airway management, the idea of waking a patient after unsuccessful attempts at intubation is often not possible, either due to pathology, location or logistics. If a patient is being intubated for impending or actual airway failure in the context of trauma, then by definition their starting position is inadequate, otherwise why intubate in the first instance? Unlike elective or semi-elective anaesthesia, where waking patients up may be an option, many trauma patients cannot be woken, even in the event of difficulty. Before committing to taking over the airway in this group of patients, the possibility of a failed airway must be considered and mitigated against, without considering the ability to wake the patient up as a course of action.

Cricoid Pressure

Sellick's 1961 original description of cricoid pressure [22] has led to much controversy, and in recent years has come to be one of the most debated interventions in anaesthetic practice.

The anatomical theory behind the manoeuvre is that posterior displacement of the complete cricoid ring will obstruct the upper oesophagus and prevent passive regurgitation during induction of anaesthesia. In his Preliminary Communication paper, Sellick describes a single centre, non-randomised, non-blinded sequential case series of 26 patients who had an undefined amount of cricoid pressure (defined as "moderate" or "firm") applied by an assistant with minimal training ("The nurse or midwife accompanying the patient can be shown in a few seconds how to do it." [22]) in a head down position with the neck in extension. Whether this represents how it is currently employed is debatable. The patients in this case series predominantly presented with intestinal obstruction or oesophageal pathology, though there were two obstetric cases included (both forceps deliveries).

This technique (which was applied after the stomach had been emptied as much as possible by a Ryles tube and the tube then removed) allegedly prevented aspiration of gastric contents every time it was used. Sellick also claimed it would prevent gastric insufflation if ventilation during induction was performed, but provided no data to back up this assertation. This paper claims a 100% success rate for preventing regurgitation during emergency anaesthesia, without commenting on any difficulties with intubation. It also claims that both the absence of regurgitation during intubation and presence of regurgitation on release of cricoid pressure are proof of its success.

From this one paper, cricoid pressure has been incorporated into every major set of anaesthetic guidelines, and is commonly taught to new anaesthetists as the standard of care. However, the technique itself is taught in so many variations (one-handed vs two-handed techniques, amount and timing of compressive force used etc) that outside of the principle of compressing the oesophagus with the cricoid ring it is hard to ascertain what the "standard" technique is.

The use of cricoid pressure varies, and multiple observational, cadaveric and radiological techniques have been used to assess the application, effectiveness and downsides of the technique.

Replicated findings have been that: cricoid pressure often makes intubation by a variety of means more difficult [23–27], occlusion is very often difficult due to anatomical alignment [28–30], it may decrease lower oesophageal sphincter tone [31, 32], it may be ineffective even when correctly applied [33] (even in the pregnant population [34]), may cause oesophageal rupture [34], and can cause airway trauma or obstruction itself [35, 36].

The only double-blinded, randomised, controlled trial of cricoid pressure (The IRIS trial [37]) showed that a "sham" procedure failed to demonstrate noninferiority of the primary endpoint of aspiration. That is to say that the low numbers in both groups made it difficult to draw statistically significant conclusions regarding noninferiority. A commentary on this article mentions that while the sham procedure did not show noninferiority, no clinically different rate in aspiration was demonstrated when cricoid pressure was not used [38]. What was statistically significant however, was that both the grade of laryngoscopy and time taken for intubation were worse in the cricoid pressure group, in line with multiple other studies. It was also shown that the rate of aspiration is very low (0.5%), though pregnant patients and paediatrics were not included in this study.

The NAP4 audit [39] showed that deaths secondary to aspiration do still occur, and accounted for 50% of deaths related to anaesthesia (nine in total). However, when these data are interrogated further, it showed that the majority of these cases occurred when "ill advised" airway plans were enacted based on poor planning (e.g. using supraglottic airways when intubation was indicated or not performing RSI when indicated). Given the lack of intubation in the majority of airway-related complications reported in NAP4, it cannot be said that lack of cricoid pressure played a part in these aspiration-related deaths.

A full exploration of the issues around cricoid pressure are beyond the scope of this chapter, but a review article by Salem et al. [40] is recommended reading. It will ultimately be for the individual practitioner and their employing organisation to decide on whether or not to mandate the use of cricoid pressure. However, given the paucity of evidence of its effectiveness and evidence of harm, some organisations have started to remove it from their guidelines in recent years [41].

Choice of Induction Agents for Rapid Sequence Induction

Induction of anaesthesia is a necessary step to facilitate intubation, and the choice of agent will come down to several variables—patient pathological factors, operator familiarity, and agent availability amongst these. The key features of an ideal agent have been previously highlighted. No one agent fulfils all these criteria, and the modification of doses and agent selection will depend on the above-mentioned variables. Full discussion of all these agents are beyond the scope of this chapter, and overview papers by Sikorski et al. [42] and Hartmannsgruber et al. [43] are recommended for further information on the overall conduct of trauma anaesthesia. The four most commonly used agents worldwide for RSI are thiopentone, ketamine, propofol and etomidate. Though a "pure" RSI involves a precalculated dose of thiopentone as previously mentioned [21], modification with other induction agents is now common practice [44].

Thiopentone

Thiopentone is a barbiturate that was first used as an anaesthetic in the 1930s and was the first drug described for use in RSI. It is produced as a powder which must be reconstituted with water for injection. The induction dose for elective anaesthesia is 3–5 mg/kg (reduced in unstable patients), with a reliable end point of loss of eyelash reflex. Thiopentone is intrinsically neuroprotective as it decreases cerebral metabolic oxygen requirement ($CMRO_2$) and increases seizure thresholds [45]. Its offset is principally by redistribution to fat-rich tissues rather than metabolism, but it can accumulate if used in infusions and lead to long wake-up times. Infusions may be used in patients with intractable intracranial pressure or refractory seizures, but patients may then take days to wake up once the infusion has stopped if it has been administered over a period of hours to days [46]. Thiopentone's most often cited use in trauma anaesthesia was at the attack on Pearl Harbour in 1941, where it was said to have killed more US servicemen than the Japanese surprise attack [47]. This has been widely debunked, but the rumour still persists in some areas. Thiopentone can cause hypotension if given in higher doses, but if reduced doses are given in haemodynamically unstable patients, it will give good anaesthesia with minimal haemodynamic upset.

Thiopentone may cause a degree of histamine release and is contraindicated in patients with asthma and also those with porphyrias, as it may induce hepatic enzyme activity and precipitate a crisis. It can also cause vascular compromise if accidentally injected intra-arterially, leading to permanent disability or the need for surgery in extreme cases [48].

Thiopentone is not used any longer in the USA as the sole US manufacturer (Hospira) ceased production in 2010, and the EU and India prevented export to the USA on ethical grounds as thiopentone was being used as part of the cocktail to carry out the death penalty [49, 50].

Ketamine

Ketamine is a phencyclidine derivative and is the only induction agent which causes profound analgesia as well as anaesthesia [51]. Ketamine acts as an antagonist at NMDA receptors and causes dissociative anaesthesia; so titration to an end point is less precise than with other agents. Induction doses are 1–2 mg/kg IV, but unlike other agents, ketamine causes intrinsic catecholamine release and preserves systolic blood pressure, making it much more forgiving in haemodynamically unstable patients. Additionally, ketamine can safely be given either intransally [52–54] or intramuscularly for analgesia or sedation, if needed, in contrast to other induction agents (though the IM dose is much higher). IM ketamine can be a useful option to sedate combative patients and allow IV or IO access to be obtained before induction of anaesthesia. Ketamine also causes bronchodilation and is a useful agent in patients with severe asthma who require intubation [51].

Because of the potential for abuse, ketamine is currently classified as a class B drug in the UK. It is held under schedule 2 in storage, which requires the same precautions as morphine and methadone. This can make obtaining it in a hurry more difficult than other drugs such as thiopentone or propofol, and consequently experience of using ketamine is more limited in some areas. Ketamine can cause hallucinations on emergence when external stimuli are misinterpreted and amplified, so patients are best recovered in a dark room with minimal stimulation where possible and safe to do so. The evidence around addition of benzodiazepines to mitigate this risk is contentious; it has not been consistently proven that midazolam decreases the rate of emergence phenomena, and it may increase the rate of respiratory complications and prolong time to discharge [55–58].

Historically, ketamine was thought to increase intracranial pressure, but this has largely been disproven [59–61]. As ketamine preserves systolic blood pressure and hence oxygen delivery to the brain, it is considered safe (and often the agent of choice [62]) in patients with brain injury or polytrauma. It has also been shown to decrease ICP in clinical use [61, 63].

Propofol

Propofol is now the most commonly used drug for RSI in the UK (though this refers to all RSI's and not trauma specifically) [44, 64]. The standard dose range is from 2–3 mg/kg in elective practice but is reduced in haemodynamically unstable patients. Like thiopentone, its offset is principally by redistribution to fat-rich tissues rather than metabolism. The increase in use of propofol as an emergency induction agent most likely reflects familiarity with its use in elective anaesthesia rather than clinical superiority. In addition, there are not the practical impediments associated with its use, in comparison to other drugs. Thiopentone is becoming rarer in most anaesthetic rooms and has to be reconstituted from a powder before use; ketamine has to be signed out of a controlled drugs book or machine. Propofol can also be used for maintenance of anaesthesia or ongoing sedation post-induction, either by use of a specific target-controlled infusion pump or a normal syringe driver. It has also been associated with better intubating conditions due to increased laryngeal reflex suppression when used in combination with a lower dose of rocuronium than would otherwise be used [65].

While propofol is ubiquitous and production prices have dropped, it does not mean that it is the best choice for induction in trauma. On a dose equivalent basis, propofol is recognised as the induction agent that causes profound apnoea and the most marked fall in blood pressure [66], either when used in combination with other drugs, or in isolation [67–70] (nearly 40% of fit and well volunteers developed hypotension at 2 mg/kg in one study [71]). This is exacerbated when patients are already hypotensive prior to induction of anaesthesia (e.g. due to hypovolaemia or sepsis). This can be disastrous in patients with head injuries, as it may exacerbate secondary brain injury. In comparison to thiopentone, propofol has a less titratable end point for anaesthesia, a longer onset time, and is painful on injection. Reducing the dose to avoid haemodynamic instability, may lead to an insufficient dose for anaesthesia and a risk of awareness. Propofol can be used for induction of emergency anaesthesia in extremis, but its pharmacological profile means that there are other agents that may be preferable.

Etomidate

Etomidate is an imidazole derivative that works on GABA-A receptors to induce anaesthesia at a dose of 0.3 mg/kg. It provides relative cardiovascular stability in comparison to propofol and thiopentone, but can be painful on injection and cause involuntary movements/myoclonus that have occasionally been incorrectly labelled as seizures [72]. This is important as seizure activity may have non-medical implications, e.g. a patient may have to suspend their driving licence if they are told they had a seizure when given this drug. The principle reason that etomidate has fallen out of favour is that it has been shown to suppress corticosteroid synthesis by inhibiting 11b-hydroxylase in the adrenal cortex. When given in infusions (as was practice in ICU historically), etomidate caused excess deaths due to infections [73, 74]. However, post-hoc analysis of the CORTICUS trial data in 2008 showed that even a single dose of etomidate may be sufficient to cause increased deaths from infection in critically ill patients [75]. With the potential deleterious effects of etomidate outweighing benefits, etomidate has largely disappeared from practice in the UK over the last 12 years. Etomidate is still used in the USA, though publications suggest that perhaps it should not be, given its potential for harm [76].

Choice of Paralytic Agent

The two paralytic agents which can be used for RSI are rocuronium and suxamethonium.

Rocuronium

Rocuronium is a long-acting aminosteroid that causes non-depolarising neuromuscular blockade by competitive inhibition of the acetylcholine receptor. It is commonly used in elective anaesthesia and will provide good or excellent intubating conditions within 2 min at a standard dose of 0.5–0.6 mg/kg. This should be increased to 1–1.2 mg/kg for a rapid sequence induction. It is generally well tolerated, though can be painful on injection if the patient is not adequately anaesthetised. Its offset is via hepatic metabolism which usually requires 45–60 min in standard dosing, though the administration of a binding agent (Sugammadex) will rapidly reverse even high dose rocuronium administration faster than suxamethonium will naturally wear off [77] (though time must be allowed to draw it up).

Suxamethonium

Suxamethonium is a non-competitive agonist of acetylcholine and will provide good or excellent intubating conditions within 30–60 s. It is completely metabolised by plasma cholinesterase within 5–10 min in most patients. A small group of patients who have abnormal genes may develop a prolonged period of neuromuscular blockade lasting many hours [78]. For many years it was the only choice for rapid paralysis and intubation, and in a Cochrane review compared against rocuronium, suxamethonium was thought to provide superior intubating conditions [65]. However, the doses used for rocuronium in most of the trials analysed were typically lower than are currently advocated in RSI (0.6–0.7 mg/kg vs the current recommendations of 1–1.2 mg/kg). When the higher doses of 0.9–1.2 mg/kg of rocuronium were compared to suxamethonium, the intubating conditions were comparable. The review also noted that the accompanying induction agent played a part, as intubating conditions were better in combination with propofol than thiopentone, presumably due to the previously mentioned increased laryngeal reflex suppression from propofol.

Suxamethonium also causes myalgia, a short increase in intraocular and intracranial pressure, increased oxygen demand, and transient hyperkalaemia. The latter may cause arrhythmias in susceptible patients (e.g. burns >24 hours old, crush injuries, long term spinal injuries or renal failure with pre-existing hyperkalaemia). As a rare complication in susceptible patients it may also precipitate a malignant hyperthermia crisis [79]. For these reasons the use of high-dose rocuronium has increased in popularity over the last few years. The short offset time of suxamethonium was previously thought to be advantageous by allowing recovery of respiration as an "escape strategy" from a failed intubation.

If the final course of action in managing a failed airway in a patient who cannot be awoken is to perform a surgical airway, the conditions for success should be optimised. During the time it takes to progress through various airway plans, before deciding on a surgical airway, suxamethonium may have partially or completely worn off, and the patient may start to move. This may make a surgical airway more difficult and stressful, so the use of high dose rocuronium in these patients is advocated. Intubating conditions at 60 seconds post administration are comparable to suxamethonium, and the patient will not move if there is the need for a surgical airway. If there is the unlikely need for rapid reversal of paralysis, this is now also possible by using Sugammadex. Furthermore, the recent NAP6 audit project found that the rate of anaphylaxis in the UK population is lower with rocuronium than with suxamethonium (5.88 vs 11.1 cases per 100,000 administrations) [80]. However, a study in Anesthesiology reported a very similar incidence (40 vs 48 per 100,000 new patient exposures) [81]. Logistically, rocuronium is easier to manage as it has a longer shelf-life than suxamethonium when refrigerated (3 years vs 18 months), and rocuronium can be stored for up to 12 weeks at room temperature per manufacturers guidelines [82]. Some data suggests that suxamethonium may be equally stable [83], but its storage outside of a refrigerated environment contravenes manufacturer's instructions. For all the above reasons, while suxamethonium is still occasionally used its days may be numbered.

Protocolising Interventions

Many Pre-Hospital Services have an anaesthetic induction protocol to reduce errors from unfamiliarity and the impact of human factors in a high stress situation [84]. Most commonly, this centres around the combination of fentanyl, ketamine and rocuronium. This combination gives a relatively rapid onset, a wide therapeutic window and improved intubating conditions compared to other drugs [85]. In the most simplistic form, services use the 3:2:1 rule for fentanyl, ketamine and rocuronium. The dose is in micrograms per kilogram bodyweight for fentanyl and milligrams per kilogram for ketamine and rocuronium. In the haemodynamically stable patient, this provides appropriate analgesia, anaesthesia and excellent intubating conditions. It also reduces the likelihood of clinically significant hypertension associated with laryngoscopy. With experience, it can be modified to the clinical situation in the severely haemodynamically compromised patient (typically as a 1:1:1 ratio of drugs). In extreme cases the omission of fentanyl can be considered to further reduce the potential for hypotension. In the cardiovascularly compromised patient, there is rarely a clinically significant risk of extreme hypertension during laryngoscopy and therefore the addition of a strong opiate is not required. Severely injured patients are reliant on their sympathetic nervous system to maintain an adequate cardiac output in haemorrhagic shock. Induction of anaesthesia obtunds the sympathetic drive, and this can result in severe hypotension requiring vasoactive drugs to restore perfusion pressure to the brain. Hypotension may also result in a reduction in coronary artery perfusion that leads to ischaemia and cardiac arrest.

The practical use of these drugs requires an understanding of their pharmacodynamic effects and most importantly, time to onset. In the dosing protocol above, the administration of 3 mcg/kg of fentanyl is likely to cause significant respiratory depression in the trauma patient. This will happen faster than the published peak effect of 3–5 min following more conventional doses. This is due to the pharmacokinetic changes associated with a higher peak plasma concentration, and may be potentiated by having a smaller circulating volume due to blood loss. The onset of high dose rocuronium and ketamine are very similar, both clinically significant in 60 s. The importance of this becomes apparent when trying to maintain adequate oxygenation prior to intubation, whilst also ensuring adequate obtundation of the sympathetic response to laryngoscopy.

Planning for a rapid sequence induction is vital to ensure drugs, equipment and trained assistance are all prepared. This also extends to the location in which anaesthesia and intubation will be undertaken. It is important to have a safe location for the team and the casualty, along with good all-round access to the patient, warmth, good lighting and shelter from the elements. Understandably, compromises may have to be made in some of these areas depending on the situation faced. The planning stage should also include a briefing that includes the order of events, plans for airway or cardiovascular emergencies, and the sequence of events after intubation to ensure safe transfer to further medical care [86]. Roles should be allocated: intubator, airway assistant and drug administration. The person administering drugs can also monitor the patient's observations as they will be best placed to correct hypotension (usually with vasoconstrictors) should it occur. They would also be responsible for keeping the intubating team member informed if hypoxia is developing, and overseeing progression through the pathway of difficult intubation, should this be required. They are the least likely person to get task-focused and can maintain some oversight. A pre-agreed intubation checklist should be used to ensure that equipment is available and there are no errors of omission.

Prior to starting the process of anaesthesia and intubation, the following considerations should be made:

1. Is this an appropriate time and place to attempt this intervention?
2. Can anything else be optimised prior to induction?
3. How will the patient be pre-oxygenated and denitrogenation undertaken?
4. What is the airway plan should intubation turn out to be difficult, or impossible?

Table 8.2 Pre-intubation checklist (Courtesy of The Air Ambulance Service)

PHEA checklist	Expected response
Task allocation	Names and roles
Risk benefit agreed	Agreed
Environment optimised	Check
BVM and circuit assembled	Check
Pre-oxygenation, nasal oxygenation if possible, check O_2 supply	Check
Baseline observations including BM	Check
Suction positioned, working and spare	Check
IV/IO access, patency checked, second access	Check
Estimated weight	kg
Drugs to be given	Names, doses and volumes
Laryngoscope, Spare and McCoy	Size and check
Tube size and spare	Size and check
Bougie	Check
Syringe and tube holder	Check
Difficult airway plan	Agreed
Difficult airway equipment	Check
Thoracostomy post induction?	Yes/No
Collar off and MILS	Check

5. At what points will the team decide that intubation is difficult and declare a Can't Intubate, Can't Oxygenate (CICO) scenario and how likely is this?
6. What will be the action plan if the patient vomits?

Many services have developed their own checklists to aid the planning of intubation and ensure all team members have been briefed, and an example is seen in Table 8.2. There has been much discussion over the use of these and further reading is advised.

In the ideal situation, all patients should be pre-oxygenated for 3–5 min and to an end-tidal oxygen concentration of 80%, if this is measured. This should be undertaken with a tight fitting Mapleson C/Water's circuit with oxygen flow of 15 l/min. A non-rebreathe mask should not be used as it is not as efficacious as either an anaesthetic circuit or BVM device [87], and different BVMs may give different inspired oxygen concentrations in spontaneously ventilating patients so are suboptimal [88]. If end-tidal oxygen concentration measurement is not available, then reliance on time is adequate. During this period, it may be required to undertake basic airway manoeuvres to ensure a patent airway and oxygenation. Throughout the process of intubation, oxygenation of the patient should be the priority. In some circumstances it may not be possible to passively improve a patient's oxygen saturation due to poor respiratory drive, or simply poor peripheral perfusion resulting in inaccurate SpO_2. Recognition of these situations is important, as it will likely lead to a physiologically more unstable patient after intubation has been completed. Whilst the original RSI paper described above called for the avoidance of positive pressure ventilation to minimise the risk of gastric distension, this has to be balanced against the risks of hypoxia in these patients. If required, gentle positive pressure ventilation to maintain or improve saturations should be undertaken with 5–10 cmH_2O of Positive End Expiratory Pressure (PEEP) and airway adjuncts, as this maintains oxygen saturation, decreases the rate of significant desaturation and there is no difference in the rates of aspiration if patients are hand ventilated or left apnoeic [89]. A concept which has been suggested for optimising pre-oxygenation in agitated patients is "delayed sequence induction" [90, 91]. Essentially, this advocates using a small amount of procedural sedation to optimise pre-oxygenation with either non-invasive ventilation, or assisted ventilation with a BVM/Water's circuit setup. It relies on the person administering the sedation to be experienced enough to titrate sedation well enough to maintain some respiratory drive while allowing the airway operator to assist with ventilation. It has been employed in both adults and children with good results [92, 93], however both familiarity with the agent used and an ability to intervene if there is inadvertent over-sedation, are essential.

Once the administration of induction agents has commenced, pre-oxygenation should not cease until an intubation attempt is made. A mask with a good seal and high-flow oxygen has the ability to generate apnoeic oxygenation, thus decreasing the chances of desaturation between the onset of apnoea and intubation. Much research has been aimed at improving oxygen flow during apnoea. In elective hospital practice, Transnasal Humidified Rapid-Insufflation Ventilatory Exchange (THRIVE) has been shown to maintain oxygen saturation during periods of apnoea (Fig. 8.7) [94]. In the absence of the specialised humidification apparatus, high-flow through standard nasal cannulae can be used for short periods around induction [95]. THRIVE specifically works using high flow rates (up to 70 l/min) and data is from procedures on elective patients. Oxygenation with standard nasal cannulae has not been found to be as effective as THRIVE [96, 97]. This may be due to either lower flow rates, or the fact that if critically ill patients have atelectasis or partial lung collapse, the degree of shunt present (proportion of blood passing through the collapsed sections without picking up any oxygen) may be so large that it offsets the benefit of THRIVE in well recruited lungs. It may be that positive pressure ventilation during induction works by recruiting lungs, and the pressure effect is more important than the increased FiO_2 [98].

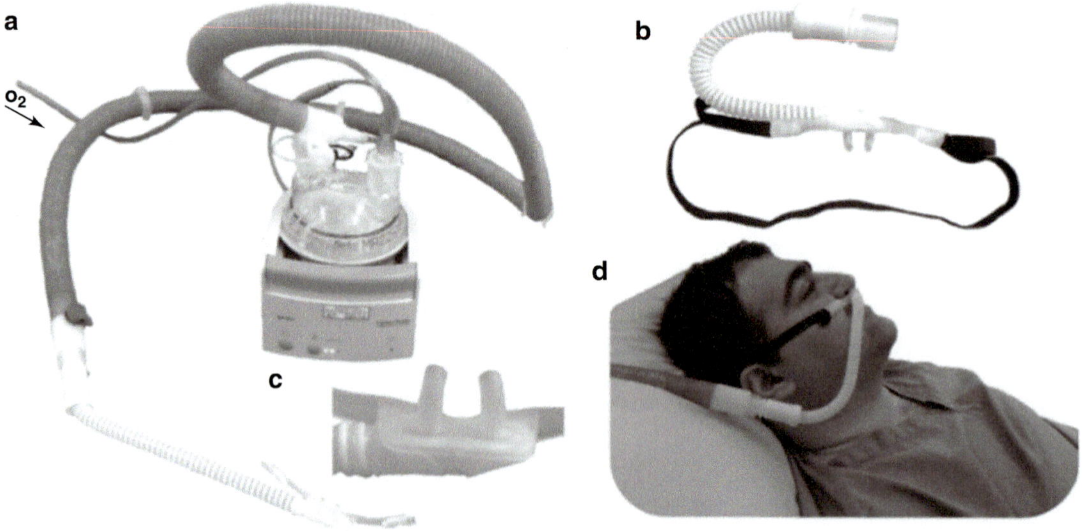

Fig. 8.7 THRIVE setup using the Optiflow system (from Patel and Nouraei [94]). The oxygen humidification unit (**a**) receives oxygen from a standard oxygen regulator and delivers humidified oxygen to a custom-build transnasal oxygen cannula (**b** and **c**) like a standard nasal oxygen cannula (**d**)

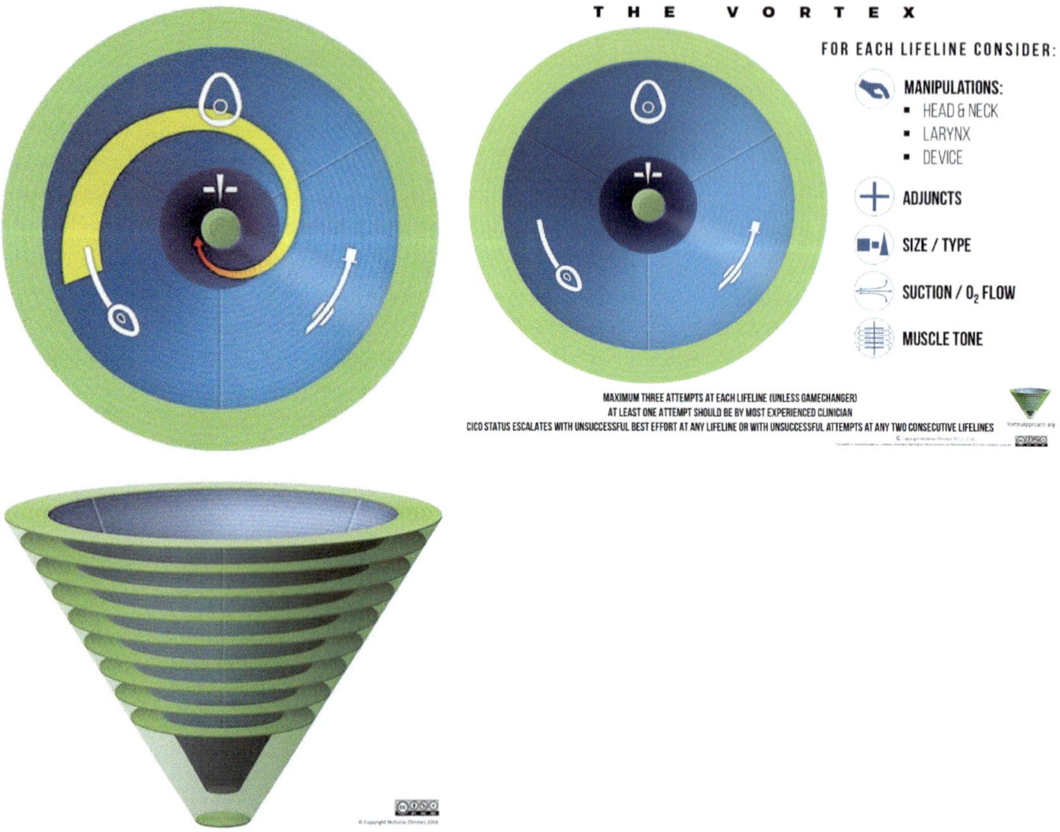

Fig. 8.8 Overview of the Vortex approach. Green zone is an area of successful oxygenation either with an awake patient or established airway on the outer ring, or after successful surgical airway in the inner spot. The blue zone represents the period after induction before an airway is established. Copyright Nicholas Chrimes. Used with permission

When intubating these patients, it is important that the first attempt at intubation should be the best attempt. If direct laryngoscopy fails, then each further attempt should include a change in technique. Do not continue to repeat the same technique, hoping for a different result! This principle has been codified in the Vortex approach to airway management, developed by Chrimes [99–101], and highlighted in Fig. 8.8. Vortex emphasises human factors and use of cognitive aids, so if difficulty is encountered during airway management then there are three strategies or "lifelines" that exist to promote oxygenation. No more than three attempts at each strategy is permitted, and a change in implementation must then be made. If oxygenation is still not possible, surgical airway management (or front of neck access—FONA—most commonly by surgical cricothyroidotomy) should be performed. This strategy aligns with the UK Difficult Airway Society guidelines [102] for the most part. However, the vortex approach de-emphasises a didactic flow through specified interventions and allows for individual expertise in different areas. Vortex has obvious advantages in terms of CRM as it sets out the options that may be available in their simplest forms, rather than trying to recall specific flowcharts in a time of crisis, e.g. paediatric, obstetric, adult etc. This is a strength, as at its core the key message of oxygenation is emphasised throughout airway management, and the idea of a surgical airway is made explicit if there is a failure to oxygenate.

Difficult Airways

In 2011, the Fourth National Audit Project by the Royal College of Anaesthetists [103] looked at all instances of complications from difficult intubation in the NHS over a 1 year period; a total of 2.9 million general anaesthetics. During this period, all cases of airway complications in hospital that led to death, brain damage, the need for an emergency surgical airway, unanticipated ICU admission or prolongation of ICU stay were reported and investigated. Pre-hospital cases and data from non-NHS hospitals were not included, but of the data reported there were 184 cases in total. This does not include previously identified difficult airways that were successfully managed, only complications from a mixture of anticipated and unanticipated difficult airways. While this relies on self-reporting, it is fair to say that the conduct of anaesthesia and airway management for the most part is safe, with only 16 reported deaths and three instances of brain damage; a mortality rate of 1 death per 5.6 million anaesthetics due to anaesthetic factors alone. When the data was interrogated further, it was revealed that there was a proportionally higher rate of complications when managing airways in the Emergency Department (ED) and ICU, in comparison to the anaesthetic room or theatre. This is congruent with the concept of physiologically and situationally difficult airways being more frequent in these environments as described later in this chapter. This is further borne out by the finding that only 14% of all incidents reported from an anaesthetic rooms/operating theatres led to death or brain damage, compared to 60% of incidents in ICU and 33% of incidents in ED. However, most instances of airway issues in ICU were in patients who already had a tracheostomy [104], and this potential risk had been recognised even before the NAP4 publication [105]. This higher rate of non-theatre intubation complications is also borne out in studies of the American Closed Claims Database [106]. One of the chief recommendations to come out of the NAP 4 report was the universal use of capnography to confirm successful intubation, but there were several factors around airway assessment, planning and human factors that are pertinent to managing any airway:

> Poor airway assessment contributed to poor airway outcomes... due to omission, incomplete assessment or a failure to alter the airway management technique in response to findings at assessment.
>
> Assessment to predict both potential airway difficulty and aspiration risk were equally important.
>
> Poor planning contributed to poor airway outcomes. When potential difficulty with airway management is identified a strategy is required. An airway plan suggests a single approach to management of the airway. A strategy is a co-ordinated, logical sequence of plans, which aim to achieve good gas exchange and prevention of aspiration.

Predicting a Difficult Airway

Every airway has the potential to be difficult—the degree of difficulty may vary with time, but it is never zero. Even in a purely elective setting with experienced providers, difficulties can be encountered—the well-publicised Elaine Bromiley case is a prime example of this [107–109]. While airway scoring grades and previous knowledge of difficulties may forewarn of impending problems, many difficult airways are unanticipated or difficult because of non-anatomical factors.

Specific Anatomical Difficulties

In addition to the factors outlined previously, several anatomical abnormalities linked to certain syndromes (e.g. Goldenhaar, Treacher-Collins, Pierre-Robin etc) are well known amongst anaesthetists approaching exams, and instantly will bring the potential for difficult airway management to the fore. Facial trauma may also increase anxiety about difficult intubation due to disrupted anatomy, blood in the airway or swelling and distortion of normal landmarks. Occasionally, trauma may actually make intubation easier e.g. in the case of a fractured mandible. Laryngoscopy may be easier as there is less mechanical force needed to lift the jaw and tongue anteriorly as broken mandibles are usually more mobile than intact ones. Facial fractures have the potential to bleed profusely due to their rich vascular supply, so bleeding into the airway may obscure the view. In these cases, the tactile feedback from a bougie as it "clicks" along tracheal rings, if correctly placed, can be invaluable. The use of a bougie has also been associated with increased first pass success for intubation when compared to stylets or

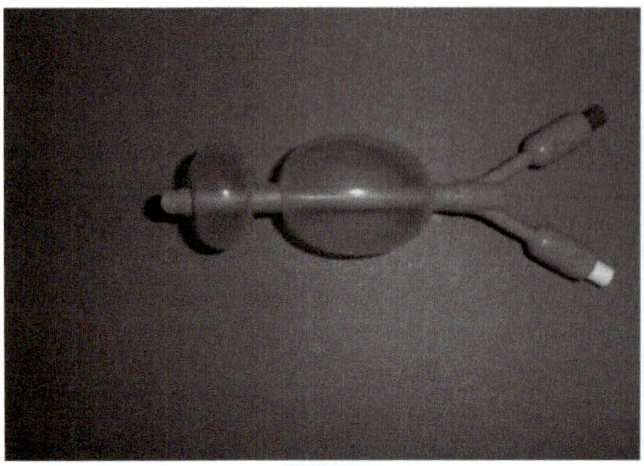

Epistat

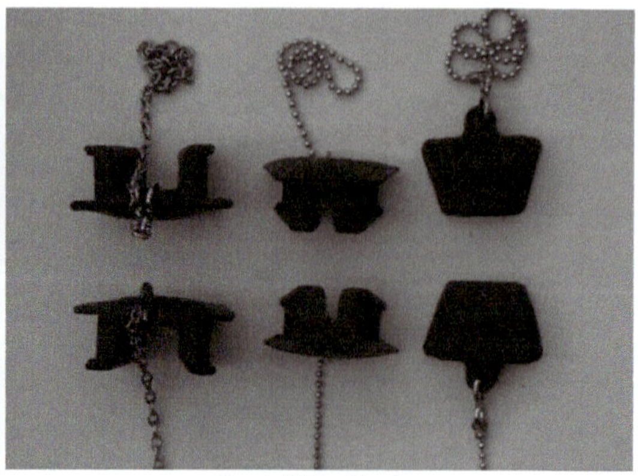

Dental bite blocks

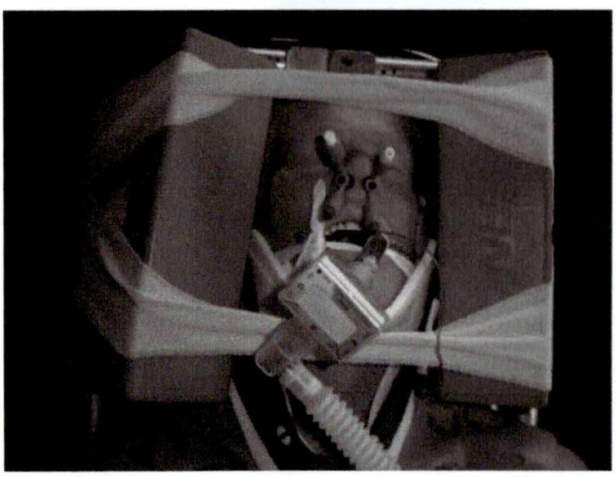

Complete kit *in situ.*

Fig. 8.9 Midface stabilisation and haemorrhage reduction. Reproduced from Harris et al. [114] by permission of Wolters Kluwer

use of no introducers [110–113]. There are also descriptions of "aiming for bubbles" in these scenarios, where air exits the vocal cords into pooled blood or fluid [110]. Intubation in these cases may be necessary for either primary airway management or for optimisation of an associated brain injury. Post intubation, temporary stabilisation of the midface is possible using two epistats, some bite blocks and a cervical collar to provide internal and external buttresses to support the fractures until definitive surgical fixation is possible (see Fig. 8.9) [114].

It is fair to say though that planning for difficult airway management is more common in patients where there is facial trauma or difficult associated syndrome than in those patients who appear to be relatively "normal". This is also true in areas where advanced airway management is relatively commonplace, such as an anaesthetic room or operating theatre. These locations also have the advantage of being well-lit, stocked with multiple airway devices, well-trained assistance and supportive colleagues. The approach to airway management in trauma, is evidently dependent not just on the anatomy of the patient, but also the environment, expertise, equipment available, location, anticipated course and team dynamics. These factors have previously been described by Brindley et al. as a "situationally difficult" airway [115].

Situationally Difficult Airways

While this generally refers to emergency intubations in hospital, the principles can be extended to pre-hospital care and may influence the decision to proceed with intubation [116]. Situationally difficult airways are largely untaught in most curriculae; however, it is arguable that they are the most commonly encountered. This is reinforced by the common experience of obtaining a better laryngoscopic view in theatres in hospital practice in optimum conditions when pre-hospital records showed a higher degree of difficulty. Even in hospital, rates of failed intubation or difficulties in intubation are higher outside of the operating theatre [103]. If there is a high degree of situational difficulty regardless of anatomical considerations, discretion may be the better part of valour and it may be more prudent to wait to perform advanced interventions in a safer environment if oxygenation is adequate.

It is virtually impossible to write a set of rules that will cover every situation, but some basic principles should be applied:

- Never forget that oxygenation is the primary goal.
- Never commit to a procedure or intervention from which a viable exit strategy has not been considered.
- Consider "*Is this the right time and place to be doing this? What is the likely course if intubation is delayed 5 or 10 min? Can the patient be transferred somewhere safer in this time with more support?*"
- Optimise the first attempt at any procedure and do not keep doing the same thing if it fails.
- Everyone will fail an intubation at some point in their career—the trick is recognising and declaring failure early and dealing with it.
- Airway management is a team endeavour. Do not assume the leader has all the answers and if there is a degree of hesitancy or concern before a course of action, ask "*Is this the right thing to do?*"
- Brief a plan and follow it—anticipate failure and plan how the team will collectively manage it.
- A surgical airway is a successful airway, not a consequence of a failed one. A patient who dies from airway issue without at least an attempt at front of neck access when indicated is the only true failed airway.
- Plan onward management and logistics—can the patient be moved after this intervention? Would intubation be easier if they were moved earlier? What is the plan for post intubation sedation and has this been prepared?

Video Laryngoscopy

There are many varieties of video laryngoscopes commercially available and it is beyond the scope of this book to discuss the pros and cons of each model. All have basic design similarities; curved blade, light source and fibreoptic systems attached to a video screen. The theory behind this design is that a direct line of sight is no longer required in order to intubate. Many video laryngoscopes have a blade which is less than 2 cm in breadth, thus aiding intubation when reduced mouth opening is a factor. Most models are easy to use with start-up times of only a few seconds and they can be kept readily available in case direct laryngoscopy fails.

The main disadvantage of video laryngoscopy is soiling of the camera with fluid in the airway. The presence of oral secretions, lubricant from an ET tube cuff, blood, mucus or gastric contents within the oropharynx can render visualisation of the larynx (and hence, intubation) impossible, requiring removal of the scope and cleaning of the lens.

There are many advantages of video laryngoscopy; already mentioned is the smaller blade size compared to a standard Macintosh blade. As the requirement for direct line of sight to the glottic opening is removed, it is possible to intubate the patient in a neutral head position with less force than direct laryngoscopy.

As video laryngoscopes largely bypass problems in the oropharynx, they can occasionally be used when soft tissue swelling or an engorged tongue may render a direct view of the glottis impossible. There have also been case reports of successful awake intubations with video laryngoscopes after local anaesthesia of the oropharynx [117–120]. Topical anaesthesia of the airway allows insertion of the videolaryngoscope until the glottis comes into view, further local anaesthetic can be administered under direct vision, directed at the vocal cords themselves. This is not a widely accepted or common technique, and should only be carried out by personnel with experience of awake intubations and the pitfalls that may present.

It is important to familiarise oneself with the type of video laryngoscopes used locally. Each has its own particular technique associated with it, some require a marked deviation from the 'normal' technique of direct laryngoscopy. This should be practised in a safe environment prior to use in emergency clinical situations. Proficiency with videolaryngoscopy is not a substitute for proficiency with direct laryngoscopy. Devices can fail, views may be tricky or impossible to obtain with videolaryngoscopes and pre-hospital services may operate in conditions outside of the functioning temperature and humidity parameters that manufacturers recommend. Videolaryngoscopy can be useful but will never fully replace direct laryngoscopy in trauma care [121].

Failed Intubation and Surgical Airways

Surgical airways have been covered in the previous chapter as they should be considered a fundamental skill in trauma rather than an advanced intervention. If basic manoeuvres, supraglottic airways and intubation have all failed to maintain oxygenation then a surgical airway is the next step. The performance of this intervention is simple and life-saving, but there is occasionally great hesitancy in performing it [122]. This may be due to a variety of factors including lack of confidence or experience, loss of situational awareness, anxiety around criticism of management thus far or task fixation on intubation above oxygenation.

On occasions when intubation fails, it is important to focus on oxygenation. The Vortex and DAS guidelines previously mentioned outline progression through various methods to ensure adequate oxygenation, and a surgical airway is the final step in CICO situations.

Sedation and Anaesthesia for Transfer

Once the airway has been secured, there is a need to provide adequate post-procedure care to optimise outcomes. This is as true for a transfer from a prehospital scene to hospital as it is for a transfer from the resuscitation bay to the CT scanner or the operating theatre. Both scenarios require planning, preparation and forethought, and the unwary practitioner can fall into many traps. There is occasionally a tendency to be less prepared during intra-hospital transfers [123–125] as help or further resources are closer to hand and the distances are shorter, though complications can occur at any stage in either environment [126–129].

Transfer of the intubated and ventilated patient requires sedation to allow tube tolerance, amnesia, and in many occasions, significant analgesia with general anaesthesia. This is true of all transfers, not just patients who have undergone a dramatic procedure such as an amputation. Most of the agents used to induce anaesthesia can be used to maintain anaesthesia. The most appropriate way to administer these is by infusion; this will reduce the cardiovascular instability that may occur with intermittent bolus techniques, and decrease the incidence of awareness [130]. The decision of which agent to use will be based on familiarity and the clinical situation encountered. Although propofol boluses can have a profound effect on cardiac output and blood pressure as previously described, infusions are tolerated much better by trauma patients. If there is any doubt regarding the haemodynamic stability of the patient, ketamine is a relatively safe agent to use in the minimal effective dose. It does not usually exhibit the cardiovascular depression associated with other agents, but will still provide dissociative anaesthesia and analgesia. This would also remove the requirement for a second analgesic agent, thus reducing complexity for transfer (e.g. a second infusion pump). Tachycardia, hypersalivation or dysphoria may occur, so the risk of this agent needs to be balanced against benefit in patients with a history of ischaemic heart disease or an unsecured airway. This may preclude certain methods of transport (e.g. a hallucinating, dysphoric patient may be a threat to flight safety so is not appropriate to fly in a helicopter unless fully sedated, paralysed and intubated). National guidelines exist in the UK for the minimum standards of the conduct of anaesthesia during transfer of patients and should be adhered to [131].

There is some controversy regarding using a mix of pharmaceutical agents in the same syringe to facilitate both anaesthesia and analgesia [132, 133]. Many combinations have been used in practise; propofol and ketamine, propofol and alfentanil, morphine and midazolam, all with a good deal of success. There are advantages to this approach, including simplifying the sedation regimen, reduction in equipment requirements and ensuring a combination of anaesthesia and analgesia. In austere environments, the military have used a combination of ketamine, midazolam and vecuronium in a single syringe driver with good results [134]. Care should be taken with the relative concentrations of each drug based on likely infusion rates, as low concentrations of anaesthetic agent with a high opiate dose may risk awareness.

Conclusion

Advanced airway management needs to incorporate planning for the technically, physiologically and situationally difficult airway. The clinical situation, along with operator experience, will dictate which techniques are utilised, and appropriate training is essential for consistently good outcomes. If a hospital is 5 min from the point of injury and it takes 10 min to perform a pre-hospital RSI, it is usually the wrong decision if the patient can be moved safely without intubation. A pre-alert to the receiving hospital allows for concurrent activity, and the hospital team can prepare for the procedure in a more permissive environment while the patient is being transported more quickly. If a pre-hospital anaesthetic is needed to facilitate transfer or for other reasons, the safety and monitoring standards must meet or exceed those found in hospital [135].

The decision-making in the situations described is paramount to successful treatment of the trauma patient. In addition, the process of dealing with difficulties and complications plays a vital role in advanced airway management. The focus should always be on adequate oxygenation [136], with secondary outcomes considered only if the situation and technical expertise allows.

These procedures and interventions should be considered in addition to the techniques described in the fundamentals chapter, rather than to replace them in their entirety. The skill-sets are complementary and overlapping, and just because interventions are technically possible, does not necessarily mean they should be undertaken. Once again, the utilisation of simulation, supervised clinical training and feedback into standardised procedures, whenever possible, cannot be overemphasised.

Questions

1. What is the main objective in airway management?
   (a) Oxygenation
   (b) Ventilation
   (c) Securing the airway

2. Intubating drug protocols should never be changed
   (a) True
   (b) False

3. Which is the most cardiovascularly stable induction agent?
   (a) Propofol
   (b) Ketamine
   (c) Thiopentone
   (d) Etomidate

4. Is a surgical airway a failed airway?
   (a) No
   (b) Yes

5. Transferring the intubated trauma patient requires
   (a) Anaesthesia and analgesia
   (b) Amnesia only
   (c) Analgesia only

Answers:

1. a
2. b
3. b
4. a
5. a

References

1. Manley G. Hypotension, hypoxia, and head injury: frequency, duration, and consequences. Arch Surg. 2001;136(10):1118.
2. Volpi PC, Robba C, Rota M, Vargiolu A, Citerio G. Trajectories of early secondary insults correlate to outcomes of traumatic brain injury: results from a large, single centre, observational study. BMC Emerg Med. 2018;18(1):52.
3. Yan EB, Satgunaseelan L, Paul E, Bye N, Nguyen P, Agyapomaa D, et al. Post-traumatic hypoxia is associated with prolonged cerebral cytokine production, higher serum biomarker levels, and poor outcome in patients with severe traumatic brain injury. J Neurotrauma. 2014;31(7):618–29.
4. Spaite DW, Hu C, Bobrow BJ, Chikani V, Barnhart B, Gaither JB, et al. The impact of combined prehospital hypotension and hypoxia on mortality in major traumatic brain injury. Ann Emerg Med. 2017;69(1):62–72.
5. Bardin PG, Johnston SL, Hamilton G. Middle airway obstruction—it may be happening under our noses. Thorax. 2013;68(4):396–8.
6. Hoffstein V. How and why should we stabilize the upper airway? Sleep. 1996;19(Suppl 9):S57–60.
7. Greenland KB, Eley V, Edwards MJ, Allen P, Irwin MG. The origins of the sniffing position and the three axes alignment theory for direct laryngoscopy. Anaesth Intensive Care. 2008;36(1 Suppl):23–7.
8. Bannister F, Macbeth R. Direct laryngoscopy and tracheal intubation. The Lancet. 1944;244(6325):651–4.
9. Crawley SM, Dalton AJ. Predicting the difficult airway. Contin Educ Anaesth Crit Care Pain. 2015;15(5):253–7.
10. Hurford WE, Peralta R. Management of tracheal trauma. Can J Anesth Can Anesth. 2003;50(S1):R17–22.
11. Carter R, Wareham EE, Brewer LA. Rupture of the bronchus following closed chest trauma. Am J Surg. 1962;104(2):177–95.
12. Bertelsen S, Howitz P. Injuries of the trachea and bronchi. Thorax. 1972;27(2):188–94.
13. Cicala RS, Kudsk KA, Butts A, Nguyen H, Fabian TC. Initial evaluation and management of upper airway injuries in trauma patients. J Clin Anesth. 1991;3(2):91–8.
14. Wei P, Yan D, Huang J, Dong L, Zhao Y, Rong F, et al. Anesthetic management of tracheal laceration from traumatic dislocation of the first rib: a case report and literature of the review. BMC Anesthesiol. 2019;19(1):149.
15. Mercer SJ, Jones CP, Bridge M, Clitheroe E, Morton B, Groom P. Systematic review of the anaesthetic management of non-iatrogenic acute adult airway trauma. BJA Br J Anaesth. 2016;117(Suppl 1):i49–59.

16. Greenland KB, Edwards MJ, Hutton NJ, Challis VJ, Irwin MG, Sleigh JW. Changes in airway configuration with different head and neck positions using magnetic resonance imaging of normal airways: a new concept with possible clinical applications. BJA Br J Anaesth. 2010;105(5):683–90.
17. Greenland KB. A proposed model for direct laryngoscopy and tracheal intubation. Anaesthesia. 2008;63(2):156–61.
18. Greenland KB. Airway assessment based on a three column model of direct laryngoscopy. Anaesth Intensive Care. 2010;38(1):14–9.
19. Sorbello M, Hodzovic I. Need to prepare our best shot for airway management in emergency department: when the going gets tough, the tough get going. J Emerg Crit Care Med [Internet]. 2019;3(0). http://jeccm.amegroups.com/article/view/5010. Accessed 18 Jun 2020.
20. Habig K, Reid C, Hanhrahan B. Greater Sydney Area HEMS Prehospital RSI Manual. Sydney: HEMS; 2011.
21. Stept WJ, Safar P. Rapid induction-intubation for prevention of gastric-content aspiration. Anesth Analg. 1970;49(4):633–6.
22. Sellick BA. Cricoid pressure to control regurgitation of stomach contents during induction of anaesthesia. The Lancet. 1961;278(7199):404–6.
23. Oh J, Lim T, Chee Y, Kang H, Cho Y, Lee J, et al. Videographic analysis of glottic view with increasing cricoid pressure force. Ann Emerg Med. 2013;61(4):407–13.
24. Allman KG. The effect of cricoid pressure application on airway patency. J Clin Anesth. 1995;7(3):197–9.
25. MacG Palmer JH, Ball DR. The effect of cricoid pressure on the cricoid cartilage and vocal cords: an endoscopic study in anaesthetised patients. Anaesthesia. 2000;55(3):263–8.
26. Smith CE, Boyer D. Cricoid pressure decreases ease of tracheal intubation using fibreoptic laryngoscopy (WuScope System). Can J Anaesth J Can Anesth. 2002;49(6):614–9.
27. Levitan RM, Kinkle WC, Levin WJ, Everett WW. Laryngeal view during laryngoscopy: a randomized trial comparing cricoid pressure, backward-upward-rightward pressure, and bimanual laryngoscopy. Ann Emerg Med. 2006;47(6):548–55.
28. Tsung JW, Fenster D, Kessler DO, Novik J. Dynamic anatomic relationship of the esophagus and trachea on sonography: implications for endotracheal tube confirmation in children. J Ultrasound Med. 2012;31(9):1365–70.
29. Smith KJ, Dobranowski J, Yip G, Dauphin A, Choi PT-L. Cricoid pressure displaces the esophagus: an observational study using magnetic resonance imaging. Anesthesiology. 2003;99(1):60–4.
30. Boet S, Duttchen K, Chan J, Chan A-W, Morrish W, Ferland A, et al. Cricoid pressure provides incomplete esophageal occlusion associated with lateral deviation: a magnetic resonance imaging study. J Emerg Med. 2012;42(5):606–11.
31. Chassard D, Tournadre JP, Berrada KR, Boulétreau P. Cricoid pressure decreases lower oesophageal sphincter tone in anaesthetized pigs. Can J Anaesth. 1996;43(4):414–7.
32. Garrard A, Campbell AE, Turley A, Hall JE. The effect of mechanically-induced cricoid force on lower oesophageal sphincter pressure in anaesthetised patients. Anaesthesia. 2004;59(5):435–9.
33. Brimacombe JR, Berry AM. Cricoid pressure. Can J Anaesth. 1997;44(4):414–25.
34. Fenton PM, Reynolds F. Life-saving or ineffective? An observational study of the use of cricoid pressure and maternal outcome in an African setting. Int J Obstet Anesth. 2009;18(2):106–10.
35. Ralph SJ, Wareham CA. Rupture of the oesophagus during cricoid pressure. Anaesthesia. 1991;46(1):40–1.
36. Hartsilver EL, Vanner RG. Airway obstruction with cricoid pressure. Anaesthesia. 2000;55(3):208–11.
37. Heath KJ, Palmer M, Fletcher SJ. Fracture of the cricoid cartilage after Sellick's manoeuvre. BJA Br J Anaesth. 1996;76(6):877–8.
38. Birenbaum A, Hajage D, Roche S, Ntouba A, Eurin M, Cuvillon P, et al. Effect of cricoid pressure compared with a Sham procedure in the rapid sequence induction of anesthesia: the IRIS randomized clinical trial. JAMA Surg. 2019;154(1):9–17.
39. Tisherman SA, Anders MG, Galvagno SM. Is 30 Newtons of prevention worth a pound of a cure?—Cricoid pressure. JAMA Surg. 2019;154(1):18.
40. Cook T, Woodall N, Frerk C, Royal College of Anaesthetists (Great Britain), Difficult Airway Society (Great Britain). Major complications of airway management in the United Kingdom: report and findings: 4th National Audit Project of the Royal College of Anaesthetists and the Difficult Airway Society: NAP4 [Internet]. London: Royal College of Anaesthetists; 2011. 219 p. https://www.nationalauditprojects.org.uk/NAP4_home?newsid=463#pt. Accessed 4 Jul 2020.
41. Salem MR, Khorasani A, Zeidan A, Crystal GJ. Cricoid pressure controversies: narrative review. Anesthesiol J Am Soc Anesthesiol. 2017;126(4):738–52.
42. Mayglothling J, Duane TM, Gibbs M, McCunn M, Legome E, Eastman AL, et al. Emergency tracheal intubation immediately following traumatic injury: an Eastern Association for the Surgery of Trauma practice management guideline. 2012;73(5):8.
43. Sikorski RA, Koerner AK, Fouche-Weber LY, Galvagno SM. Choice of general anesthetics for trauma patients. Curr Anesthesiol Rep. 2014;4(3):225–32.
44. Hartmannsgruber MWB, Gabrielli A, Layon AJ, Rosenbaum SH. The traumatic airway: the anesthesiologist's role in the emergency room. Int Anesthesiol Clin. 2000;38(4):87–104.

45. Sajayan A, Wicker J, Ungureanu N, Mendonca C, Kimani PK. Current practice of rapid sequence induction of anaesthesia in the UK – a national survey. Br J Anaesth. 2016;117:i69–74.
46. Khan KS, Hayes I, Buggy DJ. Pharmacology of anaesthetic agents I: intravenous anaesthetic agents. Contin Educ Anaesth Crit Care Pain. 2014;14(3):100–5.
47. Flower O, Hellings S. Sedation in traumatic brain injury. Emerg Med Int [Internet]. 2012. https://www.ncbi.nlm.nih.gov/pmc/articles/PMC3461283/. Accessed 30 Jun 2020.
48. Bennetts FE. Thiopentone anaesthesia at Pearl Harbor. Br J Anaesth. 1995;75(3):366–8.
49. Vangerven M, Delrue G, Brugman E, Cosaert P. A new therapeutic approach to accidental intra-arterial injection of thiopentone. Br J Anaesth. 1989;62(1):98–100.
50. Lethal injection challenges continue across the country [Internet]. https://www.americanbar.org/groups/committees/death_penalty_representation/project_press/2012/spring/li_challenges_continue/. Accessed 30 Jun 2020.
51. Staff Writer. Death penalty opposition: EU set to ban export of drug used in US executions. Der Spiegel [Internet]. International Edition. 2011. https://www.spiegel.de/international/europe/death-penalty-opposition-eu-set-to-ban-export-of-drug-used-in-us-executions-a-803238.html. Accessed 30 Jun 2020.
52. Pai A, Heining M. Ketamine. Contin Educ Anaesth Crit Care Pain. 2007;7(2):59–63.
53. Shaw BH, Ross M. Is intranasal ketamine safe and effective as a prehospital analgesic? CJEM. 2019:1–2.
54. Poonai N, Canton K, Ali S, Hendrikx S, Shah A, Miller M, et al. Intranasal ketamine for procedural sedation and analgesia in children: a systematic review. PLoS One. 2017;12(3):e0173253.
55. Reynolds SL, Bryant KK, Studnek JR, Hogg M, Dunn C, Templin MA, et al. Randomized controlled feasibility trial of intranasal ketamine compared to intranasal fentanyl for analgesia in children with suspected extremity fractures. Acad Emerg Med. 2017;24(12):1430–40.
56. BestBets: Midazolam use in children undergoing ketamine sedation to reduce emergence reaction [Internet]. https://bestbets.org/bets/bet.php?id=3044. Accessed 30 Jun 2020.
57. Akhlaghi N, Payandemehr P, Yaseri M, Akhlaghi AA, Abdolrazaghnejad A. Premedication with midazolam or haloperidol to prevent recovery agitation in adults undergoing procedural sedation with ketamine: a randomized double-blind clinical trial. Ann Emerg Med. 2019;73(5):462–9.
58. Wathen JE, Roback MG, Mackenzie T, Bothner JP. Does midazolam alter the clinical effects of intravenous ketamine sedation in children? A double-blind, randomized, controlled, emergency department trial. Ann Emerg Med. 2000;36(6):579–88.
59. Sener S, Eken C, Schultz CH, Serinken M, Ozsarac M. Ketamine with and without midazolam for emergency department sedation in adults: a randomized controlled trial. Ann Emerg Med. 2011;57(2):109–14.e2.
60. Filanovsky Y, Miller P, Kao J. Myth: Ketamine should not be used as an induction agent for intubation in patients with head injury. CJEM. 2010;12(02):154–7.
61. Chang LC, Raty SR, Ortiz J, Bailard NS, Mathew SJ. The emerging use of ketamine for anesthesia and sedation in traumatic brain injuries. CNS Neurosci Ther. 2013;19(6):390–5.
62. Zeiler FA, Teitelbaum J, West M, Gillman LM. The ketamine effect on ICP in traumatic brain injury. Neurocrit Care. 2014;21(1):163–73.
63. Morris C, Perris A, Klein J, Mahoney P. Anaesthesia in haemodynamically compromised emergency patients: does ketamine represent the best choice of induction agent? Anaesthesia. 2009;64(5):532–9.
64. Bar-Joseph G, Guilburd Y, Tamir A, Guilburd JN. Effectiveness of ketamine in decreasing intracranial pressure in children with intracranial hypertension. J Neurosurg Pediatr. 2009;4(1):40–6.
65. Sury MRJ, Palmer JHMG, Cook TM, Pandit JJ. The state of UK anaesthesia: a survey of National Health Service activity in 2013. Br J Anaesth. 2014;113(4):575–84.
66. Tran DT, Newton EK, Mount VA, Lee JS, Wells GA, Perry JJ. Rocuronium versus succinylcholine for rapid sequence induction intubation. Cochrane Database Syst Rev [Internet]. 2015; http://doi.wiley.com/10.1002/14651858.CD002788.pub3. Accessed 19 Jun 2020.
67. Lupton T, Pratt O. Intravenous drugs used for the induction of anaesthesia. 5.
68. Aggarwal S, Goyal VK, Chaturvedi SK, Mathur V, Baj B, Kumar A, et al. A comparative study between propofol and etomidate in patients under general anesthesia. Rev Bras Anestesiol. 2016;66(3):237–41.
69. Hino H, Matsuura T, Kihara Y, Tsujikawa S, Mori T, Nishikawa K. Comparison between hemodynamic effects of propofol and thiopental during general anesthesia induction with remifentanil infusion: a double-blind, age-stratified, randomized study. J Anesth. 2019;33(4):509–15.
70. Yang CY, Hsu JC, Lin CM, Huang SJ, Chung HS, Shyr MH. Hemodynamic responses of thiopental and propofol in different-aged patients during endotracheal intubation. Chang Gung Med J. 2001;24(6):376–82.
71. Möller Petrun A, Kamenik M. Bispectral index-guided induction of general anaesthesia in patients undergoing major abdominal surgery using propofol or etomidate: a double-blind, randomized, clinical trial. Br J Anaesth. 2013;110(3):388–96.
72. Farhan M, Hoda MQ, Ullah H. Prevention of hypotension associated with the induction dose of pro-

pofol: a randomized controlled trial comparing equipotent doses of phenylephrine and ephedrine. J Anaesthesiol Clin Pharmacol. 2015;31(4):526–30.
73. Scarth E, Smith S. Drugs in anaesthesia and intensive care. 5th ed. Oxford University Press; 2016. (Oxford Medical Publications; vol. 1).
74. Ledingham IM, Finlay WEI, Watt I, Mckee JI, Gemmell LW, Savege TM, et al. Etomidate and adrenocortical function. The Lancet. 1983;321(8339):1434.
75. Ledingham I. Influence of sedation on mortality in critically ill multiple trauma patients. The Lancet. 1983;321(8336):1270.
76. Sprung CL, Annane D, Keh D, Moreno R, Singer M, Freivogel K, et al. Hydrocortisone therapy for patients with septic shock. N Engl J Med. 2008;358(2):111–24.
77. Kulstad EB, Kalimullah EA, Tekwani KL, Courtney DM. Etomidate as an induction agent in septic patients: red flags or false alarms? West J Emerg Med. 2010;11(2):161–72.
78. Sørensen MK, Bretlau C, Gätke MR, Sørensen AM, Rasmussen LS. Rapid sequence induction and intubation with rocuronium–sugammadex compared with succinylcholine: a randomized trial. Br J Anaesth. 2012;108(4):682–9.
79. Martyn J, Durieux ME. Succinylcholine: New insights into mechanisms of action of an old drug. Anesthesiology. 2006;104(4):633–4.
80. Halsall PJ, Hopkins PM. Malignant hyperthermia. BJA CEPD Rev. 2003;3(1):5–9.
81. Anaesthesia, surgery and life-threatening allergic reactions. Report and findings of the Royal College of Anaesthetists' 6th National Audit Project: Perioperative Anaphylaxis [Internet]. London: NIAA Health Services Research Centre; 2018; p. 234. Report No.: 6. https://www.niaa.org.uk/NAP6Report. Accessed 18 Jun 2020.
82. Reddy JI, Cooke PJ, van Schalkwyk JM, Hannam JA, Fitzharris P, Mitchell SJ. Anaphylaxis is more common with rocuronium and succinylcholine than with atracurium. Anesthesiology. 2015;122(1):39–45.
83. Esmeron 10 mg/ml solution for injection – Summary of Product Characteristics (SmPC) – (emc) [Internet]. https://www.medicines.org.uk/emc/product/1345/smpc#SHELF_LIFE. Accessed 19 Jun 2020.
84. Adnet F, Le Moyec L, Smith CE, Galinski M, Jabre P, Lapostolle F. Stability of succinylcholine solutions stored at room temperature studied by nuclear magnetic resonance spectroscopy. Emerg Med J. 2007;24(3):168–9.
85. SOP-6.0-PHEA-2018.pdf [Internet]. https://www.magpas.org.uk/wp-content/uploads/2018/02/SOP-6.0-PHEA-2018.pdf. Accessed 17 Jun 2020.
86. McCourt KC, Salmela L, Mirakhur RK, Carroll M, Mäkinen M-T, Kansanaho M, et al. Comparison of rocuronium and suxamethonium for use during rapid sequence induction of anaesthesia. Anaesthesia. 1998;53(9):867–71.
87. Luck H, Morgan P. Prehospital emergency anaesthesia: considerations, pitfalls, and controversies. 2019;8.
88. Chrimes N. Not all bag-valve-mask devices are created equal: beware a possible lower FiO2 during spontaneous vetilation. Anaesth Intensive Care. 2014;42(2):276.
89. Casey JD, Janz DR, Russell DW, Vonderhaar DJ, Joffe AM, Dischert KM, et al. Bag-mask ventilation during tracheal intubation of critically ill adults. N Engl J Med. 2019;380(9):811–21.
90. Weingart SD. Preoxygenation, reoxygenation, and delayed sequence intubation in the emergency department. J Emerg Med. 2011;40(6):661–7.
91. Weingart SD, Trueger NS, Wong N, Scofi J, Singh N, Rudolph SS. Delayed sequence intubation: a prospective observational study. Ann Emerg Med. 2015;65(4):349–55.
92. Miescier MJ, Bryant RJ, Nelson DS. Delayed sequence intubation with ketamine in 2 critically ill children. Am J Emerg Med. 2016;34(6):1190.e1–e2.
93. Taylor JA, Hohl CM. Delayed sequence intubation: is it ready for prime time? Can J Emerg Med. 2017;19(1):68–70.
94. Patel A, Nouraei SR. Transnasal Humidified Rapid-Insufflation Ventilatory Exchange (THRIVE): a physiological method of increasing apnoea time in patients with difficult airways. Anaesthesia. 2015;70(3):323–9.
95. Gleason JM, Christian BR, Barton ED. Nasal cannula apneic oxygenation prevents desaturation during endotracheal intubation: an integrative literature review. West J Emerg Med. 2018;19(2):403–11.
96. Caputo N, Azan B, Domingues R, Donner L, Fenig M, Fields D, et al. Emergency department use of apneic oxygenation versus usual care during rapid sequence intubation: a randomized controlled trial (The ENDAO Trial). Acad Emerg Med Off J Soc Acad Emerg Med. 2017;24(11):1387–94.
97. Semler MW, Janz DR, Lentz RJ, Matthews DT, Norman BC, Assad TR, et al. Randomized trial of apneic oxygenation during endotracheal intubation of the critically ill. Am J Respir Crit Care Med. 2016;193(3):273–80.
98. Pulmonary SMF is the creator of P org H is an associate professor of, Vermont CCM at the U of. PulmCrit: is pure RSI a failed paradigm in critical illness? The primacy of pressure [Internet]. EMCrit Project. 2019. https://emcrit.org/pulmcrit/pressure-rsi/. Accessed 26 Jun 2020.
99. Chrimes N. The Vortex: a universal 'high-acuity implementation tool' for emergency airway management. BJA Br J Anaesth. 2016;117(Suppl 1):i20–7.
100. Chrimes N. The vortex approach to airway management. Australas Anaesth. 2019;2019:3.
101. Charco-Mora P, Urtubia R, Reviriego-Agudo L. The vortex model: a different approach to the difficult airway. Rev Esp Anestesiol Reanim Engl Ed. 2018;65(7):385–93.

102. Frerk C, Mitchell VS, McNarry AF, Mendonca C, Bhagrath R, Patel A, et al. Difficult Airway Society 2015 guidelines for management of unanticipated difficult intubation in adults. BJA Br J Anaesth. 2015;115(6):827–48.
103. Cook TM, Woodall N, Frerk C. Major complications of airway management in the UK: results of the Fourth National Audit Project of the Royal College of Anaesthetists and the Difficult Airway Society. Part 1: Anaesthesia. Br J Anaesth. 2011;106(5):617–31.
104. Cook TM, Woodall N, Harper J, Benger J. Major complications of airway management in the UK: results of the Fourth National Audit Project of the Royal College of Anaesthetists and the Difficult Airway Society. Part 2: Intensive care and emergency departments. Br J Anaesth. 2011;106(5): 632–42.
105. Thomas AN, McGrath BA. Patient safety incidents associated with airway devices in critical care: a review of reports to the UK National Patient Safety Agency. Anaesthesia. 2009;64(4):358–65.
106. Peterson GN, Domino KB, Caplan RA, Posner KL, Lee LA, Cheney FW. Management of the difficult airway: a closed claims analysis. Anesthesiology. 2005;103(1):33–9.
107. Harmer M. Independent Review on the care given to Mrs Elaine Bromiley on 29 March 2005 [Internet]. 2005; 18. https://emcrit.org/wp-content/uploads/ElaineBromileyAnonymousReport.pdf. Accessed 18 Jun 2020.
108. McClelland G, Smith M. Just a routine operation: a critical discussion. J Perioper Pract. 2016;26(5):114–7.
109. Bromiley M. The husband's story: from tragedy to learning and action. BMJ Qual Saf. 2015;24(7):425–7.
110. Howe D. Blowing bubbles helps intubation. Indian J Crit Care Med. 2017;21(10):710–1.
111. Driver BE, Prekker ME, Klein LR, Reardon RF, Miner JR, Fagerstrom ET, et al. Effect of use of a bougie vs endotracheal tube and stylet on first-attempt intubation success among patients with difficult airways undergoing emergency intubation: a randomized clinical trial. JAMA. 2018;319(21): 2179.
112. Driver B, Dodd K, Klein LR, Buckley R, Robinson A, McGill JW, et al. The bougie and first-pass success in the emergency department. Ann Emerg Med. 2017;70(4):473–8.e1.
113. Noguchi T, Koga K, Shiga Y, Shigematsu A. The gum elastic bougie eases tracheal intubation while applying cricoid pressure compared to a stylet. Can J Anesth Can Anesth. 2003;50(7):712–7.
114. Harris T, Rice S, Watts B, Davies G. The emergency control of traumatic maxillofacial haemorrhage. Eur J Emerg Med. 2010;17(4):230–3.
115. Brindley PG, Beed M, Law JA, Hung O, Levitan R, Murphy MF, et al. Airway management outside the operating room: how to better prepare. Can J Anesth Can Anesth. 2017;64(5):530–9.
116. Brindley PG, Beed M, Law JA, Hung O, Levitan R, Murphy MF, et al. Airway management outside the operating room: how to better prepare. Can J Anaesth J Can Anesth. 2017;64(5):530–9.
117. Gloria A, Melo A, Coutinho C, Magalhaes G, Fonseca C. Awake intubation with Airtraq® laryngoscope in patients with anticipated difficult airway. Eur J Anaesthesiol. | EJA [Internet]. 2008:247. https://journals.lww.com/ejanaesthesiology/fulltext/2008/05001/awake_intubation_with_airtraq__laryngoscope_in.799.aspx. Accessed 26 Jul 2020.
118. Gaszynski T. The use of the C-MAC videolaryngoscope for awake intubation in patients with a predicted extremely difficult airway: case series. Ther Clin Risk Manag. 2018;14:539–42.
119. Hodzovic I, Bedreag O. Awake videolaryngoscope – guided intubation – well worth adding to your skill-mix. Romanian J Anaesth Intensive Care. 2019;26(1):5–7.
120. Wilson WM, Smith AF. The emerging role of awake videolaryngoscopy in airway management. Anaesthesia. 2018;73(9):1058–61.
121. Hinds J. John Hinds defends prehospital direct laryngoscopy. [Internet]. Chicago: SMACCForce; 2015. https://www.youtube.com/watch?v=Z1YHmg_MBUs. Accessed 27 Jul 2020.
122. Greenland KB, Acott C, Segal R, Goulding G, Riley RH, Merry AF. Emergency surgical airway in life-threatening acute airway emergencies–why are we so reluctant to do it? Anaesth Intensive Care. 2011;39(4):578–84.
123. Gimenez FMP, Camargo WHB de, Gomes ACB, Nihei TS, Andrade MWM, Valverde ML de AFS, et al. Analysis of adverse events during intrahospital transportation of critically ill patients. Crit Care Res Pract. 2017;2017:1–7.
124. Parmentier-Decrucq E, Poissy J, Favory R, Nseir S, Onimus T, Guerry M-J, et al. Adverse events during intrahospital transport of critically ill patients: incidence and risk factors. Ann Intensive Care. 2013;3(1):10.
125. Knight PH, Maheshwari N, Hussain J, Scholl M, Hughes M, Papadimos TJ, et al. Complications during intrahospital transport of critically ill patients: focus on risk identification and prevention. Int J Crit Illn Inj Sci. 2015;5(4):256–64.
126. Barry PW, Ralston C. Adverse events occurring during interhospital transfer of the critically ill. Arch Dis Child. 1994;71(1):8.
127. Sablot D, Leibinger F, Dumitrana A, Duchateau N, Damme LV, Farouil G, et al. Complications during inter-hospital transfer of patients with acute ischemic stroke for endovascular therapy. Prehosp Emerg Care. 2019;0:1–7.
128. Valentin A, Schwebel C. Into the out: safety issues in interhospital transport of the critically ill. Intensive Care Med. 2016;42(8):1267–9.

129. Bourn S, Wijesingha S, Nordmann G. Transfer of the critically ill adult patient. BJA Educ. 2018;18(3):63–8.
130. NAP5: Accidental awareness during general anaesthesia in the UK and Ireland – National Audit Project [Internet]. https://www.nationalauditprojects.org.uk/NAP5home. Accessed 3 Jun 2020.
131. AAGBI. Interhospital transfer [Internet]. The Association of Anaesthetists of Great Britain and Ireland; 2009. https://anaesthetists.org/Home/Resources-publications/Guidelines/Interhospital-transfer-AAGBI-safety-guideline. Accessed 19 Jun 2020
132. Tafur-Betancourt LA. The hidden world of drug interactions in anesthesia. Colomb J Anesthesiol. 2017;45(3):216–23.
133. O'Connor S, Zhang YL, Christians U, Morrison JE, Friesen RH. Remifentanil and propofol undergo separation and layering when mixed in the same syringe for total intravenous anesthesia. Pediatr Anesth. 2016;26(7):703–9.
134. Restall J, Tully AM, Ward PJ, Kidd AG. Total intravenous anaesthesia for military surgery. A technique using ketamine, midazolam and vecuronium. Anaesthesia. 1988;43(1):46–9.
135. Lockey DJ, Crewdson K, Davies G, Jenkins B, Klein J, Laird C, et al. AAGBI: Safer pre-hospital anaesthesia 2017: Association of Anaesthetists of Great Britain and Ireland. Anaesthesia. 2017;72(3):379–90.
136. Groombridge C, Chin CW, Hanrahan B, Holdgate A. Assessment of common preoxygenation strategies outside of the operating room environment. Acad Emerg Med. 2016;23(3):342–6.

Breathing and Chest Trauma

9

Peter Lax

- Overview of applied thoracic anatomy
- Normal physiology of breathing
- Assessment of thoracic injuries
- Acute and subacute injuries and their management
- Escalation of respiratory care from basic to advanced
- Practical procedures—thoracostomy and chest drain insertion

Introduction

The third step in the MABCD assessment is breathing. Patients may sustain primary damage to their lungs or airways as a result of trauma or may suffer from respiratory complications as a result of trauma elsewhere, e.g. pulmonary fat embolus from femoral fractures, decreased respiratory drive from head injuries or abdominal pain causing diaphragmatic splinting and decreased effectiveness of the lungs. The most critical functions of the lungs are to dissolve oxygen into the blood and remove carbon dioxide (CO_2) from the body. These two functions are interlinked but separate, and the factors which affect oxygenation are not entirely the same as those which affect ventilation. The delivery of oxygen to tissues and cells is essential for life, and the removal of CO_2 is a crucial contributor to control of acid-base balance and is also important in regulating cerebral blood flow and pressure (see Chap. 11 - Disability head injury). Injuries to the thorax can create problems with oxygenation, ventilation, or both, in addition to bleeding or cardiac injuries. Before considering major aspects of thoracic trauma and how they present, it is crucial to have a basic understanding of the normal physiology of the lungs to comprehend how trauma can cause dysfunction and how our interventions can combat this.

Applied Anatomy and Common Pitfalls

This section is a very brief refresher of some of the thoracic structures, and it is worth consulting an anatomy textbook (or gaining some experience with a thoracic surgeon, physician or anatomist where possible) to understand the applied anatomy of the thorax further. A brief surface topography with underlying structures is available in Fig. 9.1 For practical purposes, consider the thorax as a bony cage which protects the lungs, heart and great vessels. Cardiac and mediastinal anatomy will be considered in greater

P. Lax (✉)
Tactical Medical Wing, Royal Air Force, Brize Norton, Oxfordshire, UK

The Air Ambulance Service (TAAS), Rugby, Warwickshire, UK
e-mail: p.lax@NHS.net

P. Lax (ed.), *Textbook of Acute Trauma Care*, https://doi.org/10.1007/978-3-030-83628-3_9

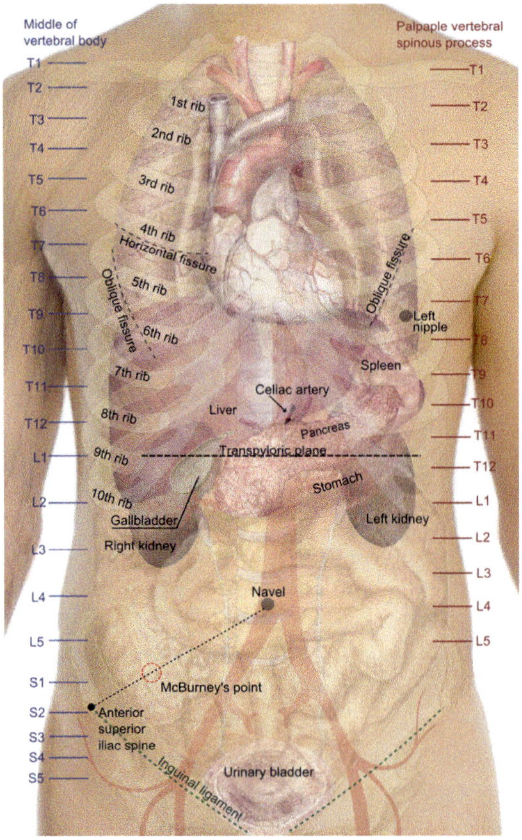

Fig. 9.1 Thoracoabdominal surface anatomy (Mikael Häggström via Wikimedia)

depth in Chap. 10 (Circulation); the emphasis of this section is on the thoracic cage and lungs.

There are 12 pairs of ribs which also act as the mechanical anchor points for the muscles of respiration (intercostals and diaphragm). Each rib has a neurovascular bundle (nerve, artery and vein) running under the inferior border of the rib. Knowledge of the location of this arrangement is relevant when considering interventions such as chest drain placement or thoracostomy, as improper placement may result in further injury. The ribs are joined anteriorly in the midline by the sternum at the inferior aspect and the manubrium superiorly, with the spinal column completing the ring posteriorly. The ribs are cartilaginous in childhood and progressively ossify throughout life to provide more protection as they harden. In the elderly, osteoporosis and decreased calcium content may cause the ribs to become more brittle. These age-related changes

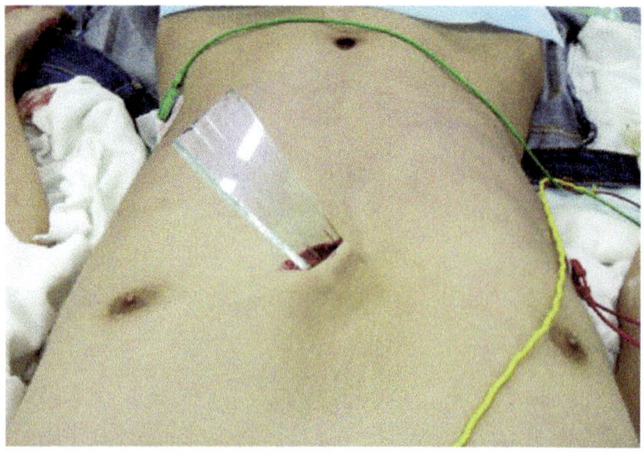

Fig. 9.2 Epigastric injuries can injure both abdominal and thoracic structures (Manabu Shiraishi from https://www.researchgate.net/publication/258994649_Successful_Surgical_Repair_of_Stabbing_Cardiac_Injury [under creative commons 3.0 license])

are important as in young children, the ability of the ribs to flex and bend may mean that significant damage to the underlying lungs may occur without visible external signs of trauma such as broken ribs.

Consequently, a higher degree of suspicion should be applied when assessing paediatric thoracic injuries. Conversely, in the elderly less force may be required to fracture ribs in comparison to paediatric and younger adult populations, and these fractures can have more deleterious effects. Even simple single rib fractures are notoriously painful, and more complex fracture patterns such as multiple fractured ribs and flail segments can intrinsically cause management challenges in terms of analgesia and respiratory mechanics regardless of if there is underlying pulmonary parenchymal injury or pre-existing disease. When considering the thorax as a structure, it is also essential to remain mindful that it does not exist in isolation. It is inferiorly bounded by the abdomen, so any injuries which can affect the abdomen can also potentially affect the thorax and vice versa, the classic example being an epigastric stab wound (such as the one seen in Fig. 9.2) which traverses the diaphragm and causes cardiac or pulmonary injury. When considering the ribs, surrounding structures and their interactions some observations can be made. The superior three ribs and scapulae are rarely fractured because of their location and protection from the surrounding shoulder girdle. When they are fractured, this should be a warning of a significant force transfer from impact, and potential for cervical spine or other significant injuries [1].

Similarly, the inferior three ribs protect some of the abdominal viscera, so consider if there could be an associated splenic or hepatic injury if ribs 10–12 have been fractured. Another common pitfall is inadequate exposure when assessing chest injuries. Do not forget to expose the back and axillae as small stab wounds in these areas are often missed, especially when patients are rapidly moved to CT scan or theatre due to instability before they have been log-rolled.

Physiology of Normal Breathing

Again, the whole of respiratory physiology is beyond the scope of this textbooks, and the below is a small primer or some of the key principles relevant in trauma that should be expanded on by study of dedicated textbooks. The lungs occupy the majority of the thoracic cage when expanded, and their normal expansion is dependent on the integrity of the thoracic cage. In normal breathing, the only way in or out of the thorax for air is the trachea via the mouth. As the diaphragm and intercostals contract, the ribs swing outward and the volume of the thorax increases, subsequently decreasing the pressure within the thoracic cavity. Normal intrapleural pressure is slightly lower than atmospheric, so when the thoracic cavity expands further, the lungs are pulled/sucked along with the thoracic wall and expand. As a result, at this point the external atmospheric pressure is higher than that within the respiratory tree, so air flows down the pressure gradient ending up at the alveoli for gas exchange. The lungs will expand until the point where the outward force of the slightly negative intrathoracic pressure is balanced by the inwards elastic recoil of the lung tissue. The degree of effort needed to expand the lungs is otherwise known as lung compliance. Compliance is decreased (i.e. it is more difficult to stretch the lungs) in conditions such as fibrosis, pneumonia and pulmonary contusions. There is also a mechanical extrathoracic contribution to overall compliance from pressure on the thoracic cage, pressure on the diaphragm and stiffness in the chest wall itself, all of which may be present in trauma.

Oxygenation

Oxygenation itself is an entirely passive process. The lungs are specialised organs with a fragile interface between gas in the alveoli and an abundant capillary blood supply. The three factors which will affect the rate of diffusion across a membrane are outlined in Fick's law (as outlined in Fig. 9.3); the rate of diffusion is proportional to concentration and surface area, and inversely proportional to the membrane thickness.

This explains one of the first therapeutic interventions that is performed in trauma—placing the patient on supplemental oxygen. Increasing the concentration gradient across the alveolar membrane and should increase the oxygen content blood that is delivered around the body. If, due to trauma, the surface area for oxygen diffusion decreases (e.g. in atelectasis) or the membrane thickness increases (e.g. pulmonary contusions, oedema or alveolar haemorrhage), the diffusion of oxygen will decrease as a consequence, so increasing the concentration gradient of oxygen is a practical measure to mitigate the other effects of injuries. Remember these three factors when assessing a hypoxic patient—their relevance in each of the major thoracic pathologies will be explained with each presentation later in this chapter.

Ventilation and V/Q Matching

Ventilation refers to the process by which carbon dioxide is eliminated through the body. There are some similarities with oxygenation in that it depends initially on the diffusion of a gas

$$\text{Diffusion} \propto \frac{\text{Concertration Gradient} \times \text{Surface Area}}{\text{Membrane Thickness}}$$

Fig. 9.3 Simplified mathematical representation of alveolar diffusion

across the alveolar membrane (albeit in the opposite direction), but the elimination of carbon dioxide depends on the total volume of air moved from the alveoli, out of the airways and into to the atmosphere per minute. This volume is calculated by the respiratory rate multiplied by the tidal volume, but also must take into account the volume of each breath which is not directly involved in gas exchange. This is known as the dead space and can be broken down into two components, anatomical and physiological. Anatomical dead space is the total volume of all of the airways from the mouth to the terminal bronchioles, and in most normal size adults is approximately 150 ml, though in intubated patients this can increase further with the addition of endotracheal tubes, connectors and other tubing. As gas exchange only takes place across the alveolar membrane and not in the trachea or bronchial tree (see Fig. 9.4), the composition of the volume of gas that is contained within these connecting airways at the end of inspiration remains the same as the inspired mixture. This gas does not contribute to either oxygenation or ventilation as it never reaches the alveoli but is a part of the volume of each breath. Physiological dead space refers to areas of the lung that are ventilated normally but are not perfused with blood, and this may be as a result of extreme hypovolaemia or pulmonary emboli, both of which can be seen in trauma. The overall relationship between alveolar ventilation and dead space is demonstrated in Fig. 9.5.

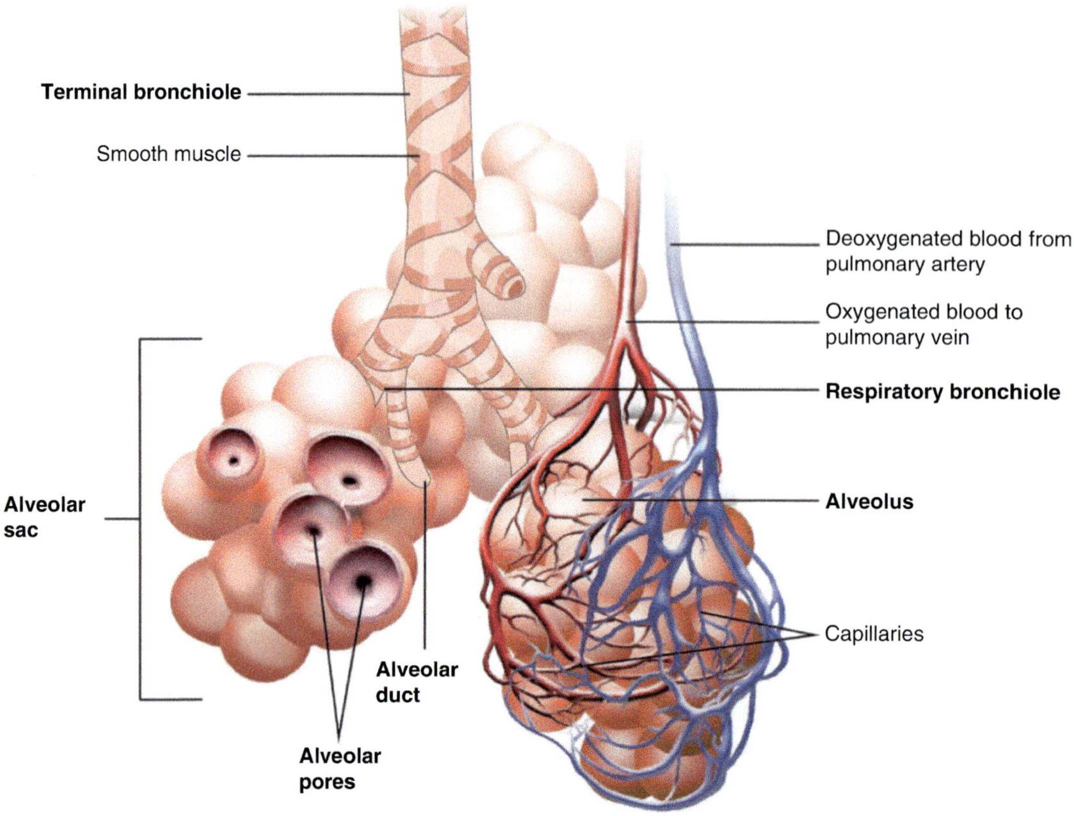

Fig. 9.4 Alveolar-capillary unit (© Openstax CNX/Rice University)

$$\textit{Alveolar ventilation} = (\textit{Tidal Volume} - \textit{Dead Space}) \times \textit{Respiratory Rate}$$

Fig. 9.5 Mathematical representation of alveolar ventilation

The corollary of this is where the lung is not ventilated but is adequately perfused, and blood passes from the right to the left side of the circulation without picking up oxygen as a consequence, which is referred to as shunt. An example of this in trauma is where there is a large pneumothorax where the volume of the lung is squashed and unable to transfer gas, but remains perfused initially.

The broad term for when ventilation and perfusion of lungs are not adequately paired is V/Q mismatch. The lungs are adapted for matching areas of ventilation to perfusion so that gas transfer is efficient as possible. The size of pulmonary arterioles and capillary beds will change in response to the presence of oxygen in alveoli so that more blood is sent to alveoli that have a higher oxygen content, and diverted from under-oxygenated areas. In patients with chronic severe lung disease, this balance may be on a knife edge. Changes to alveolar oxygen concentration may also paradoxically lead to retention of carbon dioxide in a very small subset of patients, but this is not the case in the vast majority of the population with or without Chronic Obstructive Pulmonary Disease (COPD). An excellent paper by Abdo and Heunks [2] explains the mechanism behind hypercarbic respiratory failure in COPD and dispels the often-heard myth of "hypoxic drive". To be clear—hypoxic drive does not exist in patients with COPD as it is commonly taught, and acutely restricting access to supplementary oxygen in patients with acute trauma should not be done over concerns of abolishing hypoxic drive.

Respiratory Failure

As oxygenation and ventilation are interlinked but separate processes, they can fail individually or together. Respiratory failure is essentially hypoxia, but it can be defined as type 1 failure (hypoxia only, low PaO_2) or type 2 failure (hypoxia with hypercarbia, low PaO_2 and high $PaCO_2$)—the simple way to remember this is that type 1 failure involves one gas, and type 2 failure involves two gasses. The treatment will depend on the underlying cause, but it is important to acknowledge that one can exist without the other. A key point to remember is that a therapeutic intervention may mitigate a type of respiratory failure, but the underlying cause needs to be adequately addressed before it is said to be resolved. I.e. if a patient has a low PaO_2 with a normal $PaCO_2$ and has supplemental oxygen applied to bring them back to a normal PaO_2, they still have type 1 respiratory failure as they have an ongoing supplementary oxygen requirement. A clinical example in trauma would be a patient with a pneumothorax displaying signs of hypoxia requiring supplemental oxygen. They may have a normal PaO_2 and oxygen saturation whilst on oxygen, but they still have underlying hypoxia—type one respiratory failure. If the pneumothorax progresses, or the patient tires and their $PaCO_2$ rises if their minute volume drops, then this is type 2 respiratory failure.

Another example of type 2 respiratory failure in trauma is where a patient may have significant compression of their chest, e.g. entrapped in a vehicle in a road traffic collision or crush injury with weight on their chest. As such, they may be unable to generate significant tidal volumes above their dead space, resulting in a decreased proportion of each breath being involved in gas exchange. This then causes hypercarbia and hypoxia, aka type 2 respiratory failure. A mathematical example of this is if a person has a 500 ml average breath and 150 ml of that volume is dead space, the alveolar ventilation (volume per minute involved in gas transfer) is 350 ml or 70%. If the same person has impairment of chest expansion and can only generate a 300 ml tidal volume, the effective volume involved in gas transfer is 150 ml or 50%. With less efficient breathing it is not difficult to see why hypercarbia develops. This is both a mathematical and physiological effect; efficiency of each breath drops and the amount of effort needed to draw breath (the work of breathing) increases. With increased effort comes increased oxygen requirement and CO_2 production, and when patients tire further the tidal volume will fall further still. The dead space remains constant, resulting in an even lower efficiency per breath and increasing difference between oxygen supply and demand, and

CO_2 production and ventilation. This downward spiral results in increasing hypercarbia and worsening type 2 respiratory failure. Another cause is patients with a high cervical spine injury resulting in loss of the nerve supply to the intercostals and diaphragm. If the muscles are effectively paralysed, then the chest cannot expand and ineffective ventilation will again occur via the same mathematical principles.

When patients are intubated and ventilated it is especially important to review blood gas results as improper ventilator settings may result in isolated hypoxia, isolated hypercarbia or both simultaneously. There is increasing evidence that hyperoxia may also be deleterious and should be avoided [3].

Assessment of Chest Injuries

As part of the primary survey, chest assessment begins with the observation of the patient on the initial approach—do they appear calm and breathing normally or are they struggling to breathe? Do they appear cyanosed and peri-arrest or are they well perfused and comfortable? Are they able to speak normally or are they unable or have auditory signs of airway obstruction such as choking, stridor or stertor? Putting a pulse oximeter on a patient at the earliest opportunity will give a wealth of information quickly on cardiorespiratory function and guide subsequent action. If the patient looks unwell in this first 5 second assessment, place them on supplementary oxygen while continuing to assess them. Remember that the chest has a back as well as a front—make sure that the patient is both adequately exposed and rolled or positioned to assess all areas of the chest, including the axillae, neck and upper abdomen to account for pathology in areas that may be missed or cross the diaphragm. While in the pre-hospital environment hypothermia is a real concern, but so is missing an injury. Ensure that exposure and examination are thorough enough not to miss anything but rapid enough to avoid exposing the patient to the elements for longer than is necessary. Several mnemonics can be used to assess chests, but they all revolve around the standard inspection, palpation, percussion and auscultation sequence taught in clinical training. One such mnemonic is FLAPSS which stands for Feel, Look, Auscultate, Percuss and Search Side and back. This is often taught with TWELVE for neck examination as an extension of the respiratory exam for other findings (Tracheal deviation, Wounds, Emphysema, Laryngeal crepitus, Venous distension and Everything else). This is a useful starting point as most pathology will have some signs that will be picked up by the above examination if done correctly.

Feel begins with apparent areas of pain on palpation—is this due to rib fractures, bruising or abrasions? It is worth starting away from the painful area to elucidate injuries which may be missed if the obvious areas are focussed on initially. One should also make a conscious effort to assess for the crunchy sensation of surgical emphysema in the chest, highly suggestive of a pneumothorax. Surgical emphysema feels like the crunch of putting fingers in snow or feeling cereal through a plastic bag even if there are no visual clues to its presence. It can be quite dramatic and spread a considerable distance subcutaneously; however, it will usually resolve in a few days when the underlying cause is addressed. In trauma, the most common cause of surgical emphysema is an air leak from the respiratory tract, though it can occur in infections with gas producing organisms such as clostridium perfringens. The click or step deformity of rib fractures may also be felt, in addition to a provoked pain response to damaged tissue that is pressed.

Look for areas of noticeable bruising, swelling, paradoxical movement or asymmetry. Compare both sides of the chest to see if there are signs of hyper-expansion raising the suspicion of pneumothorax, paradoxical chest wall movement in flail chest or incised or sucking wounds in an open pneumothorax. If possible, a respiratory rate should be obtained at this point as a baseline measure to assess for either improvement or deterioration later on in conjunction with other vital signs. Respiratory rate can be a sensitive predictor of deterioration [4], however there is evidence that despite this it is often poorly assessed or documented [5]—do not fall into this trap, assess rate properly!

Auscultation is a favourite examination of medical professionals the world over but is of limited use in the noisy pre-hospital environment (and occasionally in the hospital too). The rest of the examination should not be rushed through or abbreviated in order to put a stethoscope on a chest, as the sum of the other steps may be more reliable than auscultation alone. There is also an experience-related difference in the sensitivity and specificity of certain examination signs [6–8], so auscultation in isolation is not as useful as one may think. Indeed, a review of the literature from 1966 to 2009 published in the Journal of General Internal Medicine in 2010 concluded that there has long been concern about the poor reliability and sensitivity of physical examination signs in respiratory examination overall [9]. However, the article states that the use of physical examination to explore a diagnostic hypothesis remains a cornerstone of clinical practice. That is to say, examining a chest to build a hypothesis from what is heard is less likely to be useful than taking in all the other data available, and then listening with an idea of which signs to look for specifically to confirm or refute a suspected diagnosis. Specific signs that may be useful are decreased air entry in the context of haemo- or pneumothorax, and wheeze or crepitations in the case of airway narrowing or cardiac failure.

Percussion can be useful to assess for hyper-resonance or dullness in the case of fluid or air in the hemithorax respectively, but it is often as much as a tactile examination as it is an auditory one. The feel of a hyper-resonant chest is different from that of a normal one, as is the dullness associated with intrapleural fluid. A search of the axillae, neck, upper abdomen and back for any injuries that may have been missed concludes the physical examination and is arguably one of the most critical parts—do not neglect it.

Ultrasonography is rapidly gaining more support in the assessment of both trauma and medical patients who present with breathlessness or shock. Specific protocols such as BLUE [10] and RUSH [11] have standardised the approach to using ultrasound in these situations and decreased variability in its application. The ubiquity, decreased size and costs of ultrasound machines also make this modality an attractive option, as well as the increasing evidence of superior sensitivity in comparison to plain x-ray assessment of the chest when looking for specific pathology such as pneumothorax [12] or pneumonia [13]. Ultrasonography is gaining increased popularity even in pre-hospital care, with evidence of appropriate short training courses upskilling providers who have had no previous ultrasound experience [14]. However a note of caution should be applied—in the same way that physical examination is improved when thought is put into its interpretation to confirm or refute a pre-existing pathological hypothesis, ultrasound must be similarly interpreted. If there is a lack of lung sliding on ultrasound examination, is this because there is a pneumothorax or because an endotracheal tube has advanced into the contralateral main bronchus and the lung is no longer moving? Before undertaking any intervention based on physical exam or ultrasound, clinicians should ask themselves "does this fit with the current mental model or am I missing something?". Do not be afraid to re-assess or ask for a second opinion before embarking on a course of treatment where there is reasonable doubt that it is the correct one. Ultrasound is undoubtedly going to take on more of a prominent role in thoracic diagnostics in the future, but it must be subject to data capture and peer review in the same way as radiographic studies, and an image is not a surrogate or replacement for an engaged brain!

Diagnoses of Immediately Life-Threatening Chest Trauma

Trauma can lead to the disruption of the normal anatomical or physiological arrangements outlined above, or cause pain sufficient to cause respiratory failure. The six immediately life-threatening and treatable conditions are outlined below with a pathophysiological explanation and advised treatment. They are best remembered using the mnemonic **ATOM FC**. It is essential to point out that these conditions can occur in isolation or together, so assessment and treatment may involve multiple methods.

A: Airway Obstruction

Airway obstruction can occur at any point in the respiratory tree, and the more proximal and complete the obstruction, the more severe it can be. A completely obstructed trachea is rapidly fatal, whereas a partially obstructed distant bronchus may cause a degree of respiratory failure but can be compensated for or mitigated against for a period. Causes of airway obstruction in trauma are numerous; inhaled foreign bodies from primary choking or damaged and aspirated teeth from facial trauma are examples that are commonly seen and are treated by removing the obstruction. However, airway obstruction can also be caused by posterior displacement of the tongue if protective airway reflexes are lost as a result of head trauma, intoxication, sedation or use of paralytic drugs such as rocuronium. The mucosa of the airway can also become swollen or inflamed due to inhalational burns from hot gasses, corrosive chemicals or in anaphylaxis. If the swelling is severe enough then the entire airway can become obstructed at any level. If this occurs proximally, endotracheal intubation may overcome upper airway injuries, but more distal airway burns or swelling can be fatal if extensive and distal enough.

Airway obstruction and management is covered more fully in the dedicated chapters, but it must be remembered that the airway includes all structures from the lips to the terminal bronchioles, so the majority of structures are intrathoracic. Airway obstruction kills by causing a decreased concentration gradient of oxygen across the alveolar membrane and subsequent hypoxia and shunt. Distal airway burns from heated gases can also cause sloughing of cells, capillary leak and ultimately lead to hypoxia by increased membrane thickness in addition to decreased flow of oxygen to the alveoli. Airway obstruction may also cause hypercarbia by proportionally increasing shunt fraction. Patients will present with hypoxia and physical signs consistent with the underlying cause—absent air entry/silent chest in the case of complete obstruction, localising crepitations/wheeze if there is an inhalational burn.

T: Tension Pneumothorax

A tension pneumothorax is a pneumothorax that continues to increase in size with each inspiration to a point where the affected lung completely collapses (Fig. 9.6). Beyond this point, the pressure in one hemithorax continues to increase and cause twisting of mediastinal structures into the opposite hemithorax. In spontaneously breathing patients, this is mitigated by the increasingly negative intrathoracic pressure in the unaffected side

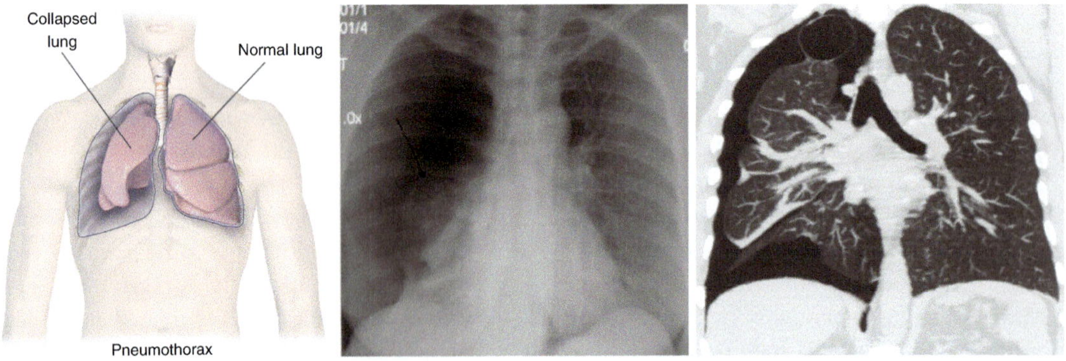

Fig. 9.6 Right sided pneumothorax demonstrated conceptually and clinically on x-ray and coronal CT (Wikipedia/Blausen.com staff (2014). "Medical gallery of Blausen Medical 2014". WikiJournal of Medicine & http://clinicalcases.blogspot.com/2004/02/tension-pneumothorax.html & Robertolyra)

(caused by increasing respiratory effort) aiding venous return to the heart, but in ventilated patients this is not the case. As well as causing respiratory failure, tension pneumothorax in ventilated patients will cause circulatory failure by decreasing the venous return to the heart. The intrathoracic pressure equals or exceeds the venous return pressure to the heart from both the inferior vena cava in the abdomen and the superior vena cava in some cases. This combined cardiorepiratory insult causes hypotension and shock which may mimic hypovolaemia. Two points are to be remembered regarding this presentation: firstly, a true tension pneumothorax in a patient who is spontaneously breathing is vanishingly rare—they are much more common in patients who are being positively pressure ventilated. Secondly, the classic signs of tension pneumothorax that are often cited (distended jugular veins, tracheal deviation away from the affected side and hyper-resonance to percussion) are not universal and are ominously late signs if they occur at all. Leigh-Smith and Harris's paper in Chest [15] gives an excellent overview of the "classical" signs of tension pneumothorax and the frequency of their presentation in both spontaneously breathing and ventilated patients and should be required reading for any trauma clinician. The correct treatment of a tension pneumothorax is urgent decompression to allow the build-up of pressure in the affected hemithorax to be released and the lung to re-expand. In an emergency, this has historically often been by the use of needle decompression in the first instance. Taking a large cannula and inserting it perpendicular to the skin, over the superior margin of the second rib in the mid-clavicular line is often cited as the correct emergency management of this condition. Recent studies based on the chest wall thickness on CT's, case reports and series have revealed an alarmingly high failure rate [16], and an 8cm needle may be needed to ensure success rather than a standard 3.2 or 4.5 cm IV cannula [17]. An adaptation to this approach is to use the needle in the fifth intercostal space, mid-axillary line where a chest drain would traditionally be inserted, or anterior axillary line. The chest wall is thinner in these locations, so there is a higher chance of penetration into the intrapleural space and subsequent release of gas. There are specific devices which have been developed to overcome the issues with high failure and complication rates of needle decompression [18] such as the ThoraQuik. These devices have their own issues, amongst them cost and potential for injury to the underlying lung and small numbers presented in initial assessment data [19]. The "gold standard" procedure would be to perform a thoracostomy, followed by the insertion of an intercostal (chest) drain as outlined above. This procedure is both diagnostic and therapeutic as by inserting a finger into the thoracic cavity it can be determined whether the lung is collapsed or not ("lung down" or "lung up") and creates a larger hole for air to escape from than a small needle. It also allows for an assessment of blood in the thoracic cavity, allows for intrathoracic adhesion breakdown and assessment of the presence of cardiac motion if a left-sided thoracostomy is performed. In a patient who is intubated, there is less physiological urgency to insert a formal drain post thoracostomy for a pneumothorax. In these patients, air is being forced into the lungs by the ventilator (positive pressure ventilation) as opposed to relying on an intact thoracic cage to generate sufficient negative pressure to draw air in during normal respiration (negative pressure ventilation). This is useful to remember, as patients who are rapidly deteriorating and need to be transported urgently to hospital, CT or theatre can have thoracostomies performed without having to insert an intercostal drain immediately. Formal drain insertion can be time consuming and make the onward transfer more logistically challenging in the presence of chest tubes and bottles. In the event of deterioration, a finger can be re-inserted into these holes to check for reaccumulation and release of air or blood. Tissue planes may close over the track created from the outside to the inside of the thoracic cavity and pneumothoraces may re-accumulate in the presence of an ongoing air leak from damaged lung, or blood if there is significant ongoing bleeding. The creation and "re-fingering" of a thoracostomy should be undertaken with appropriate caution and made as clean as possible without causing significant delay. The published risk of subsequent empyema/infection can be as high as 25% of intercostal drain insertions even when sterile precautions are taken [20]. This is a serious complication and may necessitate multiple surgeries to treat if there is a severe infection. There is also a risk to the operator of contracting a blood-borne virus if there is an iatrogenic sharps injury due to haste, or the patient has multiple broken ribs and a fragment injures the operator. Care should be taken whenever this procedure is performed for those reasons, and where possible the drain should be inserted away from palpable fractures/flail segments though this is not always practical. Adequate local analgesia to the skin and pleura is be required to perform this procedure safely in an awake patient, and occasionally systemic analgesia or sedation may also be required.

In patients who are spontaneously breathing, performance of a thoracostomy is essentially converting a tension or simple pneumothorax into a small open pneumothorax and should be managed appropriately as the situation dictates. This may either be by immediate insertion of an intercostal drain or by sealing and monitoring with an appropriate dressing such as an Asherman dressing or Russell chest seal. Tension pneumothorax causes hypoxia by decreasing surface area for gas transfer, and in ventilated patients may cause cardiac arrest via the combination of hypoxia and decrease in venous return to the heart. In spontaneously breathing patients, tension pneumothorax presents with chest pain and respiratory distress, with tachycardia and decreased air entry in 50–75% of cases, hypoxia, hypotension and tracheal deviation in less than 25% of cases and cyanosis, hyper-resonance, decreased level of consciousness and chest hyperexpansion in less than 10% of cases. In ventilated patients, tension pneumothorax universally presents with sudden onset and progressive hypoxia and a reduction in cardiac output and blood pressure. In approximately 33% of cases there may be high ventilator pressures, chest hyperexpansion or decreased air entry. The occurrence of venous distension and surgical emphysema is rare, occurring in only 20% of cases [15].

O: Open Pneumothorax

[https://www.youtube.com/watch?v=sfk6dqxMvNI]

Video: Treatment of an open chest injury

If there is a large wound in the chest, air may preferentially enter the chest through the wound rather than through the mouth when the respiratory muscles contract and intrathoracic pressure drops. This leads to air surrounding the lung in the pleural space and collapsing it, rather than being inside the alveoli/lung parenchyma and available for gas transfer. Entrainment of air through a wound requires a hole of sufficient diameter to be present ($\frac{2}{3}$ the diameter of the trachea or greater) in order for air to preferentially be entrained in the wound rather than by the normal route via the respiratory tract. These chest injuries are relatively simple to manage, as the major pathology can be treated in one of two main ways. In the first instance, seal the open pneumothorax with an occlusive dressing, converting it to a simple pneumothorax which can be addressed with an intercostal drain. If the patient requires emergency anaesthesia and positive pressure ventilation for another reason (e.g. head injury), or if the wound is too large to seal in this manner and causing respiratory failure, the act of intubation and positive pressure ventilation will lead to re-expansion of the lung. There are apocryphal stories of defibrillator pads being used or credit cards being taped across open pneumothoraces and occluded on three sides to create a one-way valve system, but there are so many devices that are commercially available and inexpensive that there is no excuse for not having one available in services which regularly deal with trauma. The main principle of these devices is that they will completely occlude the wound and allow air under pressure to escape via a one-way flutter valve mechanism so that the lung will re-expand. Open pneumothoraces should not be occluded entirely without a route for air escape as this may potentially convert an open pneumothorax to a pneumothorax which may tension [21]. Some wounds may be larger than the available dressings, and in those circumstances, anaesthesia and intubation is the appropriate management of this condition. There are some modifications of a traditional chest drain bottle system which may be used in the case of pneumothorax to make the system more portable, but in the event of haemothorax these systems have the potential to clot with blood and prevent the escape of air, potentially causing a tension haemopneumothorax. They are rarely appropriate acutely but may form part of ongoing ambulatory management if the patient has a persistent air leak.

Untreated, open pneumothorax causes hypoxia by decreasing surface area for gas transfer and may cause hypercarbia by proportionally increasing dead space. The presenting findings are usually an open wound that may be sucking or gurgling and a patient who is hypoxic and in respiratory distress.

M: Massive Haemothorax

Haemorrhage is the leading preventable cause of death in trauma, and there are a large number of vascular structures in the thorax which can cause significant bleeding (Fig. 9.7). Some injuries such as a major aortic transection are almost universally unsurvivable and will cause death within seconds to minutes of injury, but some bleeds may be significant while accumulating at a slower rate. Blood can fill the intrapleural space from rib fractures as each rib has an artery and vein running under its inferior border which can be damaged. Blood can also accumulate from several other sources including the great vessels, lung parenchyma or internal mammary and subclavian arteries. Patients with massive haemothorax may present with signs of respiratory failure, circulatory compromise or both. Resuscitation with large volumes of blood products may be necessary, as may formal thoracotomy if insertion of chest drains and tamponade of the lung after reinflation is insufficient to stop bleeding. Bleeding from parenchymal injuries usually settles with a chest drain as these bleeds are from low-pressure systems and easily tamponaded, but more substantial bleeds should mandate referral to a thoracic surgeon for consideration of interventional radiology or an urgent or emergency thoracotomy. This is defined as 1500 ml drain output on the first insertion of the drain, 1500 ml total drain output in 24 hours or more than 200 ml/h blood drainage for three consecutive hours [22]. Traditional teaching which is still occasionally mentioned was to clamp chest drains in the setting of large volume output. This approach is a fallacy without merit, as bleeding will not stop and there is an inadequate tamponade effect; if a bleed rapidly accumulates it is unlikely to be small venous ooze which could be adequately addressed by tamponade alone. Also it causes a false sense of security—just because the blood is not pouring into drains does not mean it remains in the circulation! This has been evaluated in animal models, and clamping the drain worsened gas exchange, but the amount of hypotension, bleeding and mortality rate were unchanged after clamping vs conventional management [23]. The advent of cell salvage technology (taking blood that has been lost during surgical procedures, washing it and returning it to the patient [24] has led to the creation of some chest drains systems as the atrium device, which may enable re-

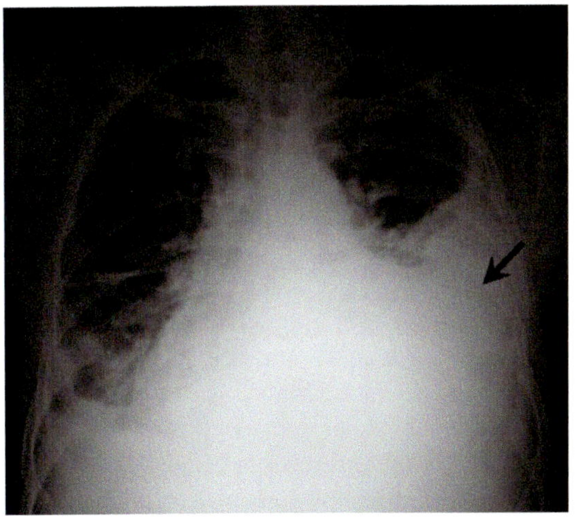

Fig. 9.7 Massive haemothorax (https://openi.nlm.nih.gov/detailedresult.php?img=PMC2567296_1757-1626-1-225-2&query=hemothorax&lic=by&req=4&npos=52 via wikimedia under Creative Commons Attribution 2.0 Generic license)

transfusion of blood that has been lost into the drains. There are several caveats to using cell salvage, aside from the obvious training and cost implications (which remain contentious with contradictory studies from different populations [25–28]). Patients who have a malignancy, infectious contaminants or have had certain medications applied such as topical clotting agents or some irrigation solutions should not routinely have cell salvage used. There is an excellent review article from Blood Transfusion in 2011 [29] that provides an overview of this technique.

The longer-term management of patients with retained intrapleural blood clots is still contentious, but most centres are leaning towards increased intervention earlier to remove retained clot. Currently, the two main strategies are either a formal VATS procedure (Video Assisted Thorascopic Surgery—keyhole surgery of the chest) within 72 hours to 7 days, or further chest drain insertion to manage any residual clot [30, 31]. The late complications of haemothorax are either infection (leading to empyema) or scarring and fibrosis of the pleura (fibrothorax). Both can be debilitating and require multiple operations or interventions to treat, so should be avoided where possible by appropriately aggressive early treatment. In patients who are too frail for surgery and have failed to resolve a hemothorax after a second drain insertion, there is some data supporting the use of intrapleural thrombolytics outside of the immediate phase of resuscitation and stabilisation [31, 32]. However, this data refers to haemothorax and non-trauma loculated pleural effusions so should be interpreted with caution.

Massive haemothorax causes hypoxia and hypercarbia by decreasing surface area for gas transfer and also decreasing lung perfusion which causes a physiological increase in dead space. It may also lead to cardiac arrest due to hypovolaemia if untreated. The presenting physical signs are tachycardia, hypoxia, dull percussion note and potentially hypotension depending on the degree of blood loss. Massive haemothoraces can also present with tension physiology if blood in the hemithorax is under enough pressure [33, 34].

F: Flail Segment

[https://www.youtube.com/watch?v=k78yENIpmFE]

Video: Clinical appearances of a flail chest

A flail segment is defined as two or more consecutive ribs that are broken in two or more places and is a clinical diagnosis (though it is increasingly made on radiological grounds). As previously mentioned, the mechanical integrity of the chest is essential for generating negative pressure to breathe normally. When a rib is broken in one place, each end of the rib remains attached to one side of the sternum or the vertebra, and while painful, expansion can still occur. If the same rib is broken in two or more places, there will be a free-floating segment that is not anchored to the axial skeleton at any point and the mechanical stability of the chest is lost in that area.

Flail segments cause issues for multiple reasons—they are a marker of significant energy transfer, reflect a large degree of damage to the underlying lung, can cause significant bleeding from the neurovascular bundle underlying the rib causing a haemothorax, or the sharp ends of the fractures can pierce the pleura and lung parenchyma causing a pneumothorax. All these issues (while important) are secondary to the major pathology in flail chest—loss of the ability to effectively expand the lung while spontaneously breathing. The cardinal sign of a flail chest is paradoxical chest movement. When the patient is spontaneously breathing, the intact section of the chest will expand outwards with contraction of the external intercostals and diaphragm, whereas the free-floating section will move inwards towards the lower pressure of the thorax. Conversely, when the patient breathes out by increasing their intrathoracic pressure via contracting their internal intercostals, the intact segment is pulled inwards whereas the higher intrathoracic pressure forces the flail segment outwards. Management of this condition acutely usually involves the induction of general anaesthesia and intubation to manage incipient respiratory failure, as well as insertion of a chest drain to manage the complications alluded to above. Flail segments need to be mechanically fixed, and early intervention has been proven to decrease length of time on a ventilator and hospital stay [35] as well as improve both functional outcomes in terms of return to work and spirometry scores at 6 month follow up [36–40]. While in the UK, there is NICE guidance for the fixation of flail segments, there is some evidence that fixation of more straightforward rib fractures may also benefit patients in terms of improved pain scores, reduction of length of stay and decreased complications such as pneumonia [41]. May et al. produced an excellent educational overview of rib fracture management from an anaesthetic perspective, including operative management and analgesic options and it is recommended reading for those who may deal with rib fractures regularly [42].

Flail chest causes decreased tidal volumes by both severe pain and loss of mechanical integrity. The subsequent lack of expansion causes decreased surface area for gas exchange and increased proportional anatomic dead space, leading to hypercarbia. This is in addition to any other associated pathology such as pulmonary contusions or pneumothorax having an additive effect. The pathognomic sign is of paradoxical chest movement, and the patient will also present with respiratory distress and other signs related to any co-existing chest pathology.

C: Cardiac Tamponade

Tamponade is discussed more fully in Chaps. 10 (Circulation) and 12 (Traumatic cardiac arrest). Accumulation of blood in the pericardial sac can cause compression of the right ventricle and cardiac failure (Fig 9.8). Needle pericardiocentesis in the context of trauma has a high failure rate, as aspiration of more viscous clotted blood rather than more thin fluid associated with pericardial effusions due to medical causes is inherantly more difficult. Cardiac tamponade may cause respiratory failure by shunt (decreasing the amount of blood pumped to the lungs) but is not a primary lung pathology. Some of the signs classically described in cardiac tamponade may mimic tension pneumothorax (moribund looking patient, distended neck veins and low blood pressure), so it is important to consider alternative diagnoses when treating either of these conditions.

Other Serious Pathology: The Subacute Six

While the above six pathologies are the leading reversible causes of death or severe disability from thoracic trauma which may present immediately on assessment, the below six pathologies can be just as lethal but can be harder to diagnose and may be more insidious in their development. Maintaining a high degree of clinical suspicion based on the mechanism of injury, presenting pathology and imaging results is often the key to diagnosing these injuries. The majority of these

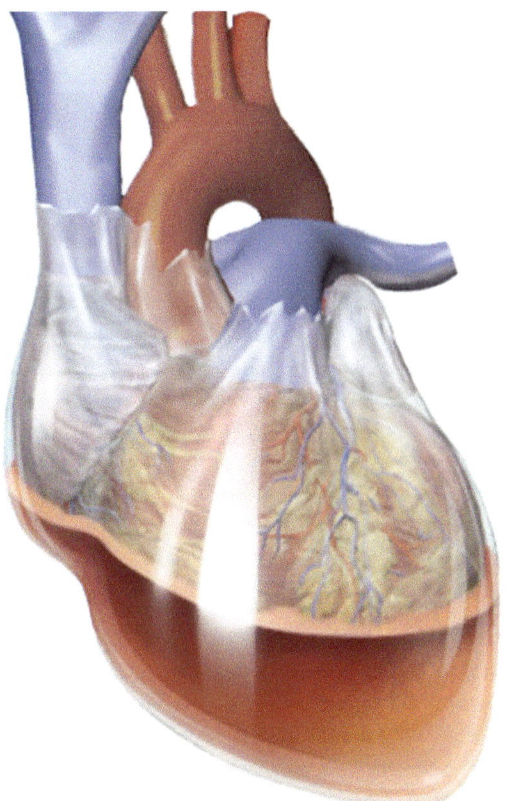

Fig. 9.8 Cardiac tamponade (Blausen.com staff (2014). *WikiJournal of Medicine*. DOI:https://doi.org/10.15347/wjm/2014.010)

conditions may develop or worsen after the first 24 h of acute care when the patient is on a trauma ward or intensive care. Prompt recognition and treatment are essential for a good outcome. As they will require further thought and reading around to appreciate fully, a useful mnemonic to remember these six injuries is **GOT CPD**.

G: Great Vessel Injury

The thorax has several large vessels which can become injured in blunt or penetrating trauma, and while a severe injury can rapidly prove fatal, occasionally major vessels can be damaged without failing catastrophically. While specific arteries may require specific surgical approaches and management of severe bleeding, the principles are mostly the same as arterial repairs elsewhere in the body. It is worth explicitly mentioning aortic and vena cava injuries as they can be rapidly fatal and there are multiple options for management.

Aortic Injuries

The most common survivable example of this would be aortic dissection or disruption which is incomplete—complete aortic dissection is fatal within seconds or minutes from the point of injury. During rapid deceleration injuries (or occasionally penetrating trauma) the aorta can shear around its attachments to the posterior thoracic wall. These anchoring points are the aortic isthmus/ligamentum arteriosum just distal to the origin of the left subclavian artery distally, and the aortic root proximally. This shearing can give rise to an aortic dissection where blood is forced between the innermost layers of the aortic wall (the intima and media) and the high pressure in the aorta hydrodissects the layers apart, creating a false lumen. This dissection can follow the direction of blood flow away from the point of intimal rupture (anterograde dissection) or track back proximally (retrograde dissection).

For this reason, dissections can involve either just the descending aorta (Stanford type B or DeBakey III), just the ascending aorta (DeBakey II or Stanford type A) or both the ascending and descending aorta (DeBakey I or Stanford type A). Understanding the different classifications is vital because it influences the likely management strategy; lesions involving the ascending aorta or arch (Stanford A) are almost exclusively managed surgically with cardiopulmonary bypass and replacement of the aortic arch and occasionally the aortic valve. Lesions which begin distally to the left subclavian and extend inferiorly (Stanford B) are more amenable to either conservative/non-surgical management. This may be with blood pressure lowering agents such as intravenous beta blockers or GTN, interventional radiology procedures such as TEVAR (Thoracic Endovascular Aortic Repair), or both. TEVAR is a minimally invasive endovascular procedure which allows the stenting of the aorta and occlusion of a dissection flap and false lumen through a small incision in the groin. It is much less invasive than open surgery, has faster recovery time and much less associated morbidity and mortality acutely. It is more dependent on patient's having relatively straightforward anatomy, as tortuous vessels may be too ectatic to allow for adequate placement of the TEVAR device. This may lead to re-intervention in approximately 15% of cases [43], additional need for acute pharmacotherapy or an open repair if there are serious complications or failure of initial management. Because of the comparatively recent development of this procedure, long term follow up data is scarce, though there are a few small case series and meta-analyses [44] with favourable results and a planned Cochrane systematic review [45]. In computer modelled studies of patients with complicated type B dissections, the predicted morbidity and mortality overall from TEVAR compared with open repair is less. This is predominantly due to acute operative complications of open procedures [46], and it will be interesting to see how these results compare to the systematic review once complete.

[https://www.youtube.com/watch?v=Hlhezm-a9E4&t=215s]

Video: TEVAR repair of a blunt aortic injury

Vena Cava Injuries

Vena cava injuries are very rare and have a high mortality even after arriving in hospital (approximately 70–90%) [47]. The vena cava is challenging to access surgically in an emergency, and vena cava injuries rarely occur in isolation, commonly being seen concomitantly with liver injuries. If the patients do not exsanguinate and the leak seals spontaneously then conservative management is advised, though this is pragmatic mainly due to surgical difficulties with access and high perioperative mortality during a repair. Only 39 cases of vena cava injury and aneurysm have been reported in the medical literature, so there is little published data on which to base a consensus approach. The current approach of conservative management is caveated with the fact that follow up CT venography should be performed at 30 days, 6 months and a year to assess the growth of vena cava aneurysms or further leak, or if the patient becomes symptomatic, then they should be urgently imaged.

O: Oesophageal Injury

Oesophageal injuries are rare and tend to present late (usually with mediastinitis) in the context of blunt trauma. Occasionally there will be an obvious mechanism which predisposes the patient to oesophageal injury, for example, ingestion of a caustic substance such as concentrated acid or alkali. Specifically in the case of caustic ingestion, treatment is initially supportive. This can include extensive washout of the oesophagus and stomach to minimise further damage, systemic treatment with broad-spectrum antibiotics to minimise the effect of bacterial translocation from the breakdown of the gastrointestinal mucosa, and gastric acid suppression with PPI's, parenteral nutrition and the patient rendered nil by mouth. The oesophagus remains friable for the first couple of weeks, and anything other than life-saving surgery should be discouraged until the initial inflammatory storm has settled and the integrity of oesophageal tissue improves. Depending on the site, degree of damage and damage to the stomach, surgical repair (if necessary) may be possible by pulling part of the stomach into the chest to create a neo-oesophagus, or in severe cases there have been reports of free colonic grafts being used for the same purpose.

In the context of oesophageal perforation from either blunt or penetrating trauma, the management follows along similar lines. The diagnosis is made on clinical suspicion leading to formal upper GI endoscopy and then management as appropriate by specialist upper GI teams in conjunction with intensive care resources. The morbidity and mortality is largely from infective complications, so a low threshold for investigation and empirical antibiotic coverage is advised. For a fuller explanation of the diagnosis and management of traumatic oesophageal injury, the article by Mubang and Stawicki is recommended [48].

T: Tracheobronchial Injury

This refers to any injury to the airway from below the level of the cricoid cartilage to the level of the first segmental bronchi. This is a rare condition, with upper tracheobronchial injuries commonly being the result of penetrating trauma to the neck and lower tracheobronchial injuries as a result of blunt trauma/barotrauma. Occasionally they can present as a result of inhalational injuries (e.g. chlorine or hot gases causing inflammation, swelling and mucosal breakdown and subsequent perforation or scarring), or iatrogenically from violent intubation or as a complication of tracheostomy. If these injuries are not immediately apparent on presentation from the mechanism they are usually diagnosed by flexible bronchoscopy early. The persistence of an air leak despite adequate size and number of chest drains being placed to drain a pneumothorax in late-presenting cases should raise the suspicion of tracheobronchial injury (Fig. 9.9). Occasionally, tracheobronchial injury can present as a pneumomediastinum. The management of these injuries depends on their site, size and physiological impact and can range from observation with a chest drain in situ and minimising airway pressure, continuing through the use of tracheobronchial stents to support the airway, and occasionally surgery up to and including lobectomy or

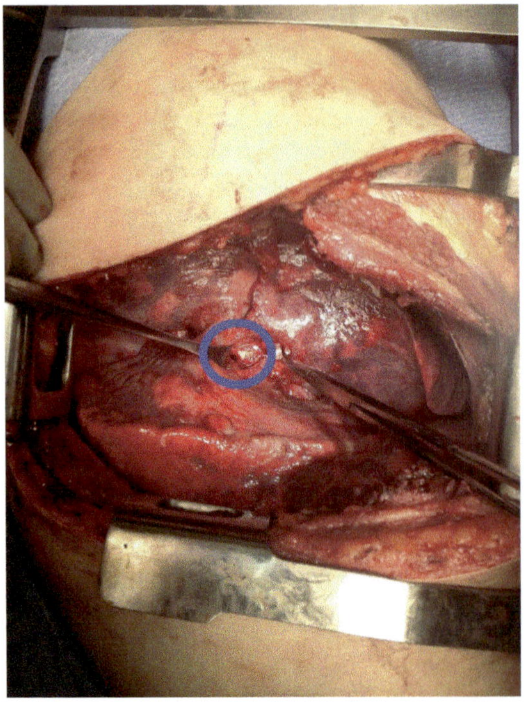

Fig. 9.9 Right main bronchus injury at thoracotomy (ringed). The patient's head is at the top of the image. This defect had not closed with standard chest drain management and required a muscle patch across it for definitive closure. The patient recovered well and chest drains were removed a week later

pneumonectomy in the most severe cases. Pneumonectomy is avoided wherever possible in favour of wedge resections or tractotomy due to the high morbidity and mortality of the procedure (approaching 60% overall and 80% if the underlying mechanism is blunt trauma [49]). If a repair of a bronchial lesion is necessary, then it is usually performed with sutures and a pericardial, pleural or muscle tissue patch fashioned around the defect. These injuries may be challenging to manage in the postoperative period as they can occur concomitantly with pulmonary contusions, and while higher airway ventilator pressures may be beneficial to recruit areas of the lung for gas exchange, these high airway pressures may prove deleterious to the integrity of the patch repair. Excellent overviews of the management of these injuries and some of their complications are available from Karmy-Jones & Wood [50] and Matsushima et al. [49]. Late complications of tracheobronchial injuries are related to scarring and fibrosis and may include airway stenosis and difficulty in breathing. Due to their cartilaginous nature, tracheal injuries are notoriously difficult to repair as they do not heal quickly if at all.

C: Cardiac Contusion

Blunt cardiac injuries can cause bruising and damage to the heart, causing a release of troponin similar to that seen in myocardial infarction. Damage to the heart is often seen in road traffic collisions if there is a significant frontal collision, and any patient who presents with a fractured sternum should be considered at risk from developing a cardiac contusion. This injury can present a spectrum of severity, from a minor troponin raise with no clinical sequelae to gross cardiovascular instability requiring inotropes and invasive monitoring in a critical care area. A baseline ECG, echocardiography and telemetric monitoring should be considered for susceptible patients, and there should be a lower threshold for admission to hospital or critical care for those patients who have pre-existing cardiac disease presenting with cardiac contusions. One common difficulty to negotiate is the situation where the mechanism of injury may suggest a cardiac condition which could have contributed to the trauma. In patients with arrhythmia or troponin rise, always consider an arrhythmia causing loss of consciousness and control of the vehicle before attributing the cardiac abnormality as the result of contusions. This can be a difficult diagnosis to make, and prehospital professionals who highlight this as a potential concern from "reading the scene" should be taken seriously, and the threshold for cardiac investigation and intervention should be appropriately lowered. Cardiac contusions will typically improve over 3–5 days with appropriate supportive care and monitoring, and in the absence of other injuries it may be appropriate to take these patients to a coronary care unit rather than a formal trauma ICU or ward. All patients with cardiac contusions require consultation from a cardiologist in addition to normal trauma team management, and a decision should be made on individual basis on the risk:benefit profile of certain medications (such as anti-platelet agents) if recommended.

P: Pulmonary Contusion

As previously mentioned, the lung parenchyma is a highly specialised functional tissue that allows diffusion of gasses and its function is governed by the factors described above in Fick's law. If the lung parenchyma is damaged and bruised, swelling can occur as in any other tissue. This swelling can affect the smaller airways or alveolar interface itself and there may also be a degree of bruising or bleeding. The cumulative effect of this is that more effort may be needed to overcome airway resistance and move air to and from the alveoli (increased work of breathing) and there may be a decreased efficiency in gas transfer due to a combination of increased membrane thickness and decreased surface area. The subsequent swelling can also cause decreased chest compliance and a necessity for higher airway pressures if ventilated. Pulmonary contusions when considered in isolation can be severe, but they often occur in conjunction with other pathology that may also impact on work of breathing or effective gas exchange. However, it is rare that pulmonary contusions occur in isolation, except for some blast injuries or inhalational injury. It is also notable that pulmonary contusions may only appear mild on initial presentation, but they can blossom over the first 72 h of injury and render patients profoundly hypoxic. X-ray findings tend to lag behind the clinical picture (Fig. 9.10), and the diagnosis is most sensitively made with chest CT. The effects of pulmonary contusions may also be worsened by injudicious or excessive administration of fluids or blood products causing endothelial activation and varying degrees of compromise from mild hypoxia to the development of fulminant adult respiratory distress syndrome (ARDS) [51]. Treatment is supportive and there is no specific cure other than time, avoidance of fluid overload, chest physiotherapy as needed and lung protective settings if mechanically ventilated (limiting tidal volume to less than 6 ml/kg, avoiding high peak pressures) [52]. The degree of support and ventilator strategies are discussed later in the chapter, but in rare cases may include advanced methods only available in some super-regional centres such as ECMO.

D: Diaphragmatic Rupture

Diaphragmatic rupture occurs with either direct injury in penetrating trauma or when the abdominal viscera are suddenly and violently compressed during blunt trauma, causing tearing of the diaphragm and herniation of abdominal contents into the thoracic cavity. This causes respiratory compromise through the dual actions of compressing the lung and reducing the surface area available for gas transfer, as well as causing mechanical disruption and inability to generate negative pressure during spontaneous respiration. The chest x-ray of these patients is unusual and has been mistaken for pneumothorax in some patients (Fig. 9.11), so caution is advised before inserting a chest drain. This is another reason why a finger sweep is important as part of inserting a chest drain, as abdominal viscera can be differentiated from the sponge-like texture of lung before inserting a chest drain into an abdominal organ. Acute management mainly involves respiratory support and escalation as needed, then repair when the patient is physiologically stable enough to tolerate surgery [53]. Diaphragmatic rupture itself is unlikely to be fatal, but the associated respiratory compromise may be. By treating the consequences acutely and then the underlying pathology when possible, the patients have the best chance of a good outcome. Left sided diaphragmatic ruptures are more common

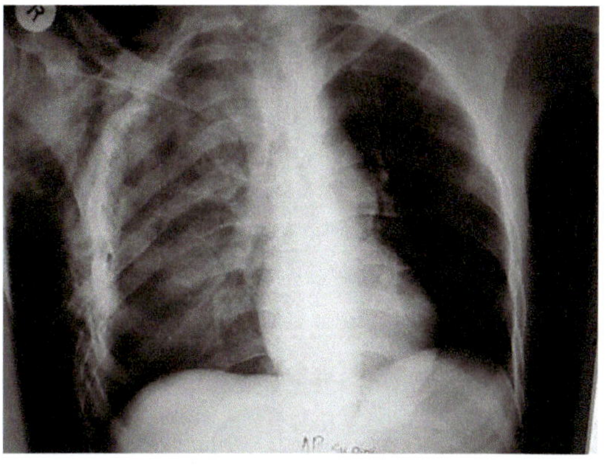

Fig. 9.10 Pulmonary contusions on chest x-ray. Note surgical/subcutaneous emphysema over the right shoulder and neck (trauma.org (http://www.trauma.org/index.php/main/image/32/) via Wikimedia under Creative Commons Attribution-Share Alike 3.0 Unported license)

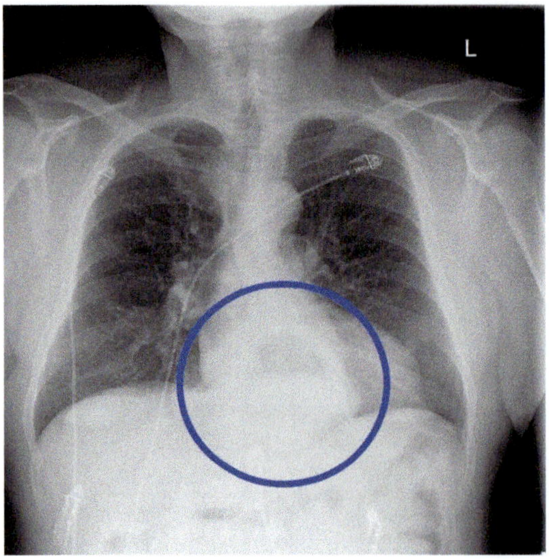

Fig. 9.11 Diaphragmatic hernia with fluid level projected over the mediastinum. Note this is a hiatus (non-traumatic) hernia, but diaphragmatic rupture can present with a similar fluid level or bowel contents visible in the chest on x-ray (Ahmed Farhat and Daryn Towle via Wikimedia [Under CC-BY 4.0 license])

than right sided ones as the mass of the liver tends to provide a degree of diaphragmatic protection in abdominal trauma. All defects should be repaired as even small tears can potentially cause incarceration of any abdominal viscera which herniate through if left unrepaired. A repair can be effected from either side of the diaphragm (thoracic or abdominal) and either by laparo/thoracoscopic means or open repair, usually concurrently with other surgical procedures if necessary. The location of the liver means that right sided repairs are technically easier via a VATS or thoracotomy in the case of large or complex defects.

Escalation of Respiratory Support from Basics to Advanced Critical Care

Patients with any of the above chest injuries can present challenges to anyone from a first responder to a professor of intensive care medicine, but the underlying principles remain the same—ensure adequate oxygenation and ventilation while dealing with the underlying pathology and protect the lungs as much as possible. There are a large number of strategies that can be employed depending on the severity of the injury and the available resources. This section aims to illustrate the progression from simple measures to advanced intensive care intervention that may only be available in super specialised centres. The number of patients that require these interventions decreases as they become more advanced, as simple interventions performed early enough may prevent the patient from requiring more advanced care. A consequence of this is that because there are fewer patients that have to undergo advanced procedures, the evidence surrounding them and how we implement them is not as abundant. Some of the controversies or limitations of our current understanding have been included in the advanced intervention section. Patients should have therapy directed towards the underlying cause—if there is a significant pneumothorax, drain it; if there is airway obstruction, remove it. The below escalation strategy assumes that the underlying cause has been treated as best possible, but the patient continues to deteriorate. It is also important to emphasise that this should prompt re-assessment, as additional pathology may have evolved or there may be a recurrence of the primary issue. One example of this is respiratory deterioration in a patient with a chest drain in situ that has become displaced or obstructed and needs clearing or repositioning to address a re-accumulated pneumothorax.

Basic Principles and Baseline Care

Although there are a large number of pathologies which may affect breathing, a stepwise approach to maintaining oxygenation and ventilation should be applied in each case, with each subsequent step building on the previous. It may occasionally be appropriate to escalate immediately to a higher level of intervention either due to significant chest pathology or because of coexisting pathology outside the thorax requiring intervention. For example, a patient with hypoxia due to mild pulmonary contusions may not require immediate intubation for their chest injury, but they may have a coexisting head injury which requires intubation. To start with, positioning or extrication may be all that is needed to improve both oxygenation or ventilation. Patients who are mechanically trapped in vehicles or with weight on their chest may develop respiratory failure due to crush/asphyxiation but have normal lungs. It is vital that when assessing patients in both pre- and in-hospital practice that the importance of positioning is not forgotten. Healthy patients who are laying flat on their back have a decreased vital capacity compared to when they are sitting up. The weight of their abdominal viscera presses against their diaphragm and can cause minor compression and atelectasis of their underlying lung after a while. The work of the diaphragm is also less efficient in this position, as it must contract against abdominal pressure in inspiration to generate negative intrathoracic pressure. Patients who have chest injuries, abdominal pain or pathology or any neurological injury that may affect breathing will have this positional disadvantage exacerbated. When unrestrained, patients will typically assume the most comfortable position that minimises their work of breathing, and they should be supported in assuming this position where possible. Pulse oximeters are invaluable devices as they give information about oxygen saturation, pulse rate and a degree of insight into tissue perfusion and cardiac output by extension. Applying a pulse oximeter early gives a good baseline to judge improvement or deterioration from, and the units can be quite small and self-contained to avoid getting in the way at a busy resuscitation. If the patient is hypoxic, the next intervention would be to provide supplemental oxygen via a face mask or nasal cannula depending on the degree of hypoxia, likely clinical course and other injuries. The British Thoracic Society has created guidelines for the use of oxygen in a variety of situations including emergencies and acute trauma. The current iteration recommends high flow oxygen at 15 l/min for trauma resuscitation but advises decreasing it to target an oxygen saturation of 94–98% as soon as possible [54]. It is also essential to give appropriate analgesia to these patients, as this may aid oxygenation and ventilation compromised by pain such as in rib fractures. Analgesia may be pharmacological, non-pharmacological (such as splinting) or both. Chapter 13 (Analgesia) has several suggestions on appropriate agents, doses or other regional techniques which may be appropriate depending on location and setup.

Intermediate Options

If respiratory failure is still an issue despite the above measures, giving respiratory support via CPAP (Continuous Positive Airway Pressure) or non-invasive ventilation (NIV, occasionally called BiPAP for Bilevel Positive Airway Pressure) is the next step (Fig. 9.12). This usually requires a dedicated machine, but some newer transport ventilators such as the Hamilton T1 or Oxylog 3000+ have the facility to be used as an NIV machine. In this mode, an airtight oxygen mask is placed on the patient's face and when the machine senses the patient attempting to inhale, they are given support in the form of a positive airway pressure boost. This decreases the work of breathing of the patient and allows them to ventilate more efficiently. When the patient exhales, the airway pressure does not fall to atmospheric but stays slightly above (usually starting at

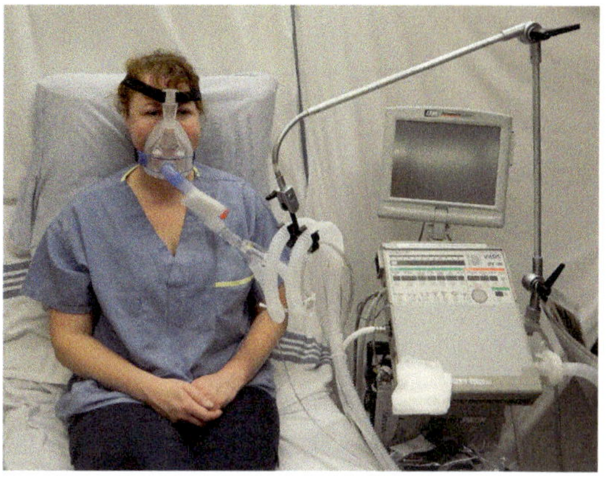

Fig. 9.12 A patient on a BiPAP machine. CPAP externally appears the same, but does not provide inspiratory support (James Heilman, MD via Wikimedia [under CC SA4.0 license])

5 cmH_2O and increasing as needed) to help hold the smaller airways open and improve oxygenation. This is known as either PEEP (Positive End Expiratory Pressure) if the patient is invasively ventilated, or alternately P_{Low} or P_{Exp} if using BiPAP/NIV. CPAP is a similar system, but only provides the resistance to exhalation to improve oxygenation—the patient does all the work themselves during inhalation.

In summary, both BiPAP/NIV and CPAP can improve oxygenation by splinting open the lower airways (and hence increasing alveolar surface area). However, BiPAP/NIV will aid in CO_2 clearance in addition to this by decreasing the work of breathing and increasing tidal volumes by supporting the patient during inspiration too. It is also important to note that due to the airtight nature of the mask that oxygen concentration can be titrated accurately too. Although patients are often said to be breathing 100% oxygen when being given 15 l/min via a non-rebreather mask, this is not true. They will entrain air from the outside of the mask, and the actual fraction of inspired O_2 (FiO_2) is not known. Systemic reviews and meta-analysis of NIV in trauma have described positive benefits in terms of improved oxygenation, decrease in intubation rates and associated complications [55].

NIV is not an entirely benign procedure, but it has a far higher chance of success when initiated early rather than waiting for patients to deteriorate and being administered with clear goals set at the start of treatment. A plan for managing common complications (e.g. siting a nasogastric tube before commencing NIV to decrease gastric distension), as well as endpoints for weaning or escalating NIV, should be formulated so that improvement or deterioration can be acted on appropriately. Adequate and significant analgesia should be given to optimise the patient for success, but anxiolytics should be avoided where possible as they do not contribute to analgesia and may increase the rate of complications. Per the British Thoracic Society/Intensive Care Society guidelines for the ventilatory management of acute hypercapnic respiratory failure in adults [56] anxiolytics must be administered in an intensive care or high dependency unit with 1:1 or 2:1 nursing support if used at all.

Absolute contraindications to NIV include untreated pneumothorax, gastric/laryngeal or oesophageal injury, patients with a decreased level of consciousness or apnoeic spells, lack of protective airway reflexes or significant maxillofacial injuries. NIV should be initiated with low pressures to begin with to allow the patient to acclimatise to the sensation of the machine, but support and PEEP should be increased incrementally until adequate (but not necessarily normal) oxygenation and ventilation is achieved. Again, these acceptable goals should be defined a priori and subsequent management plans defined. Care should be given to set the trigger appropriately (the amount of patient effort necessary to instigate a machine supported breath). Too high a trigger may mean the patient feels suffocated as they have to generate significant negative pressure before they have a supported breath, but too low a trigger may mean the patient is continually being given an assisted breath when they instigate the smallest movement of air (e.g. when rolling in bed). Similar care should be used when setting a ramp (the speed at which inspiratory flow goes from zero to maximum). For a more full overview of the practicalities of non-invasive ventilation, an article from Thorax by Rabec et al. [57] is recommended, and for more evidence on NIV across a range of presentations, an article by Scala and Pisani is a good starting point [58].

Advanced Interventions Available Commonly

If NIV is not an option due to lack of equipment or the patient has failed a trial of NIV, the next step on the airway escalator is intubation and ventilation. The procedure, risks and benefits of intubation have been covered in the airway chapters, so please refer there for a fuller discussion. Once the airway has been secured there are several ways in which hypoxia can be treated, but they all revolve around Fick's law as described above—increase the concentration gradient (FiO_2), increase the surface area (PEEP or mean airway pressure), and decrease the membrane thickness (usually diuretics, chest physiotherapy, suctioning or antibiotics in the case of infection). Remember that patients' lungs do not exist in isolation from the rest of their body, and what might be an appropriate or desirable intervention to improve their respiratory function (e.g. increasing their PEEP) may have deleterious effects elsewhere (e.g. increasing intracranial pressure or decreasing venous return and subsequently decreasing blood pressure in a hypovolaemic patient). This is where experience and risk:benefit balance inherent in critical care come into play.

Several modes can be used with different ventilators, and a full explanation of these is outside the scope of this text. Each mode will either be volume or pressure controlled, allow/support the patient taking spontaneous breaths or not and will have a minimum background respiratory rate. The vast amount of proprietary names, trademarks and acronyms from various manufacturers has made discussions around ventilators unnecessarily complex and occasionally confusing. The vast majority of conventional ventilation modes can be broken down into some combination of the above three parameters, and the settings understood by referring to first principles once it is understood what the ventilator is trying to achieve and how. An excellent handbook from the Intensive Care Society [59] is available for free for anyone with interest in demystifying ventilators and is recommended reading.

If the patient still has respiratory failure while on conventional ventilation, despite increasing FiO_2, surface area and decreasing membrane thickness the next evidence-based options involve proning patients. This involves changing positions from lying on their back to their front every few hours to maximise perfusion to sections of the lungs which may be better recruited and hence improve V/Q matching. The PROSEVA Trial [60] in 2014 showed an improvement in both oxygenation and mortality when this strategy is implemented, but the units involved were experienced in the use of the proning procedure and it is not without risks. These risks mainly involve tube dislodgement and pressure area damage due to improper care during and after positioning. Some patients may not be suitable for proning despite requiring it, e.g. patients with unstable cervical spine or pelvic injuries with an ex-fix system in situ. Options in these cases include infusions of paralytic drugs to improve oxygenation, though again this is not without risk. For an overview of the risk/benefit ratio of paralytics in severe respiratory distress, the article by Bourenne et al. [61] is a good starting point. There are some ventilator modes which may be of assistance, such as airway pressure release ventilation (APRV), and some recent trials have suggested that this may be a useful rescue technique if applied early enough [62], though it is still a contentious area [63]. Historically, high-frequency oscillatory ventilation (HFOV) had been used to treat refractory hypoxia, but two recent trials have triggered a move away from HFOV. In the OSCAR trial [64], no benefit was shown above standard therapy, and the OSCILLATE trial [65] showed that HFOV may increase mortality when compared to standard therapy. As a result, HFOV is no longer a recommended treatment strategy for refractory hypoxia in adults, though it is still sometimes employed in neonates and paediatrics.

Super-Specialised Centre Options

[https://www.youtube.com/watch?v=FiETnE4as5M]

Video: Explanation of ECMO

In patients who have refractory respiratory failure despite all the above treatments the prognosis is poor, but there are some other options which may be useful in super-specialist regional centres. These involve improving oxygenation and CO_2 removal with extra-corporeal devices while resting the lungs and allowing them time to recover. The technique is called ECMO (Extra-Corporeal Membrane Oxygenation) and is similar in principle to how a cardiac bypass machine works (Fig. 9.13). Blood is continuously taken from the body after the patient has been anticoagulated, passed through a fine membrane which allows the uptake of oxygen and removal of CO_2 across concentration gradients and returned to

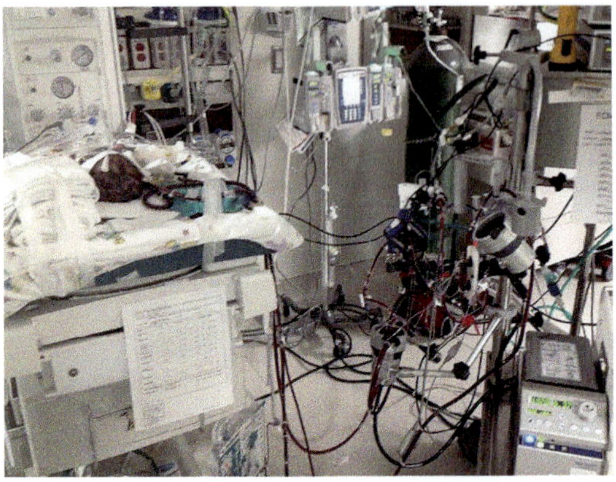

Fig. 9.13 ECMO circuit in use on a small baby

the patient. ECMO can be performed by either veno-venous circuits (blood taken from a vein, cycled through the EMCO machine and returned to another vein) or veno-arterial circuits (taken from a vein, returned to an artery) depending on the indications for the procedure. For pure respiratory failure V-V ECMO is all that is necessary, but for patients with cardiac failure V-A ECMO can provide additional support. This is a highly complicated, labour intensive and expensive procedure so is not available in every centre. Regional referral networks have sprung up in the UK to make the system as efficient and affordable as possible. Trauma patients may have relative contraindications to ECMO as they need to be anticoagulated, so any active bleeding or bleeding in a perilous area which is currently contained but cannot be addressed is cause for concern (e.g. brain parenchymal bleeds). The only absolute contraindications are unsurvivable injury or concomitant comorbid conditions (e.g. terminal cancer), or vascular disease which means that ECMO cannulae cannot be placed [66]. Each centre will have its own acceptance criteria after referral, so it is worth locating the nearest centre and learning them before referring a patient for the first time.

One option that may be employed outside super-specialist centres if hypoxia can be mitigated to a degree is a process known as $ECCO_2R$ (Extra-Corporeal CO_2 Removal). This depends on the patients' lungs being sufficient to maintain an arterial PO_2 of 8 kPa, and the ongoing issue is primarily CO_2 clearance. $ECCO_2R$ devices such as the Novolung take blood from the femoral artery, pass it along a membrane with a fresh oxygen flow across it and return it to the venous side of the circulation. The oxygenation capacity of this device will not provide adequate compensation for failing lungs, and the oxygen "sweep" is purely to ensure the maintenance of a CO_2 concentration gradient across the membrane. As CO_2 is more soluble than O_2, there needs to be a higher concentration gradient to remove CO_2 from the circulation. The device also uses the difference between the patient's arterial and venous blood pressures to drive blood flow—there are no pumps involved unlike ECMO. In some units, $ECCO_2R$ can be incorporated into haemofiltration circuits [67], so if a patient requires renal replacement therapy in addition to $ECCO_2R$ then this can be incorporated into the same system without the risks of additional line placement. This may also allow the use of lung protective ventilation strategies using small tidal volumes or APRV, without the potentially deleterious effects of hypercapnia. This is the premise of the current REST Trial which is recruiting in the UK.

Practical Procedures: Thoracostomies and Insertion of Chest Drains

A thoracostomy is the formation of a tract from the thoracic cavity to the outside environment to allow the release of air, blood or fluid contained in the thoracic cavity. It should be a sterile procedure when possible, but occasionally (such as in the case of traumatic cardiac arrest or peri-arrest patients), it is necessary to sacrifice an element of sterility for speed.

For spontaneous pneumothorax, there is current guidance that Seldinger-type drains are appropriate to use [68], and some small studies have suggested that their failure rate is comparable to formal surgical drains in traumatic pneumothorax [69]. In patients who are stable and are found to require a chest drain for haemothorax 24 h post injury, there is some evidence that even small 14F Seldinger drains may be appropriate here too [70]. Whilst the formal surgical drain insertion technique is still seen by many as the gold standard, there is an evolving and growing role for Seldinger-based techniques which may be more familiar and less daunting to some practitioners. It must be noted that Seldinger techniques are not complication free, with the National Patient Safety Agency reporting 12 deaths and 15 cases of serious harm directly attributable to Seldinger chest drain insertion between January 2005 and March 2008 as highlighted in a 2010 editorial in Thorax [71]. Drain size has previously been studied, with some advocating large (36–40F) drains for haemothorax. The current literature does not support the "bigger is better" argument, with multiple studies suggesting that 28–32F drains are just as effective and less painful for the patient [72, 73], and one study suggesting a potential use of central venous catheters as a replacement for some chest drains [74]! Whilst a novel use of a central venous catheter, this approach is not recommended when there is appropriate and tested equipment available to perform the procedure.

It would seem reasonable therefore, to suggest that a 32F drain should be the biggest drain used acutely, and that patients who are otherwise stable and do not require immediate drainage should have a Seldinger system considered rather than mandating a formal surgical drain for all. However, the skill of performing a thoracostomy in its own right, and subsequently insertion of a formal surgical drain is still mandatory for anyone involved in trauma care. Thoracostomy is also one of the first steps in performing a resuscitative thoracotomy, and in patients who require emergency decompression of their chest has a lower failure rate than needle-based techniques as previously described.

Insertion Technique

[https://www.youtube.com/watch?v=IdmMR8JxmFo]

Video: guide to chest drain insertion

The preferred site for thoracostomy insertion is anterior to the mid-axillary line in or above the fifth intercostal space (fourth or sixth are acceptable alternatives), over the superior margin of the rib, and posterior to the lateral border of pectoralis major. This area is commonly referred to as the "triangle of safety" as it avoids the posterior-lying long thoracic nerve, stays above the diaphragm and avoids going through the potentially thick pectoralis muscle. Whilst counting the rib spaces down from the manubriosternal joint is one method of locating the correct space, it is often difficult and time consuming in an acute trauma situation. Visual estimation of the correct site for drain insertion without identifying the space via any method very often leads to drains being inserted below the diaphragm, even in experienced hands; drains inserted in the correct space very often appear to be high. An Australian paper in 2017 [75] suggested the use of the mid arm point as a sensitive and specific marker for identifying the correct insertion point, with 86% of insertion points being located in the fifth intercostal space, and none lower than the sixth. This technique uses the patients' adducted arm and finds the midpoint between the tip of the acromion and the olecranon to use as the insertion point. This is a quick, patient specific and reproducible measurement which could easily be implemented in patient care, however there must be a caveat that it should not be used in patients with shoulder or humeral fractures, or patients with suspected shoulder dislocations.

Once appropriate insertion point has been identified, the site should be cleaned and sterile precautions taken as much as possible depending on the speed necessary for drain insertion. As a minimum, chlorhexidine or iodine skin prep should be used and sterile gloves even in an emergency. Where possible, full prep and draping should be used with surgical scrubbing and gowning. The skin and subcutaneous tissue over the site of insertion should be anaesthetised with lignocaine or other appropriate rapid onset local anaesthetic in non-anaesthetised patients. Effort should also be made to numb the parietal pleura, as its perforation is frequently cited as the most painful part of chest drain insertion. Local anaesthetic can be injected into the thoracic cavity before insertion, or flushed via the chest tube for post procedure analgesia. Consideration should be given to some form of procedural sedation in most patients undergoing formal surgical drain insertion. The person performing the procedure should not be the same person administering the sedative agent. Ketamine is a good option for this procedure as it gives a good combination of rapid onset analgesia and dissociation, but may make a patient overly euphoric and cause problems with intra-procedural compliance if improperly dosed.

A 3–4 cm incision should be made over the top of the rib through the anaesthetised skin and blunt dissection with artery forceps or similar should be used through the subcutaneous tissue, muscles and down to pleura. The forceps should be inserted in a closed position through the pleura, opened and retracted to create a path for the chest tube to pass along. It may also be useful (though painful) to close the forceps, re-insert them through the pleural defect, rotate 90 degrees and re-open and re-retract them to create a bigger, cruciform tract for drain insertion. Before withdrawing the forceps from the tract a finger should be inserted to check that the pleura has been breached and the lung is palpable (it should feel like a wet sponge), if there are any adhesions that need breaking down and if there is any air or blood in the thoracic cavity. This finger sweep can also be used to increase tract size, and in ventilated patients it may assist the evacuation of air from the thoracic cavity. At this point, the thoracostomy is complete and it may be appropriate to end the procedure here if formal drain insertion is not required immediately at this point (e.g. ventilated patient about to go to CT scan or operating theatre for instability). The whole procedure until now should take 60 seconds or less, and the part of the procedure which extends this time is invariably insertion, connection and securing of a drain. If it is not immediately required in an unstable patient, don't do it.

If drain insertion is to be performed at this point, using the little finger of the non-dominant hand to insert along the track to the pleura has the advantage that it does not sacrifice dexterity for the next part of the procedure by keeping the index finger and thumb of the non-dominant hand free. This depends on the length and strength of the operators finger and the distance from skin to pleura (largely determined by the patient's BMI).

An appropriately sized drain should be selected and the artery forceps inserted in the lateral hole at the top of the drain (Fig. 9.14). Trocars should not be used for insertion due to the high rate of visceral injury associated with their use and no apparent advantages. One clinical pearl is to have a second pair of forceps clamping the drain closed at the inferior end during the insertion process until the underwater drain is attached in order to avoid rapid expulsion of blood or fluid onto the operator or the rapid entrainment of air into the spontaneously breathing patient.

Once loaded onto the forceps, the tube should be passed along the tract which is being held open by the operator's finger into the pleural space (Fig. 9.15). An appropriate length of tube should be inserted into the thoracic cavity, ensuring that all holes in the head of the tube are intrathoracic by 2 cm, and the external end of the tube securely connected to an appropriately filled underwater drainage system. At this point, the second set of forceps can be unclamped and the drain should start bubbling (if air is present), draining blood or fluid, and the fluid meniscus

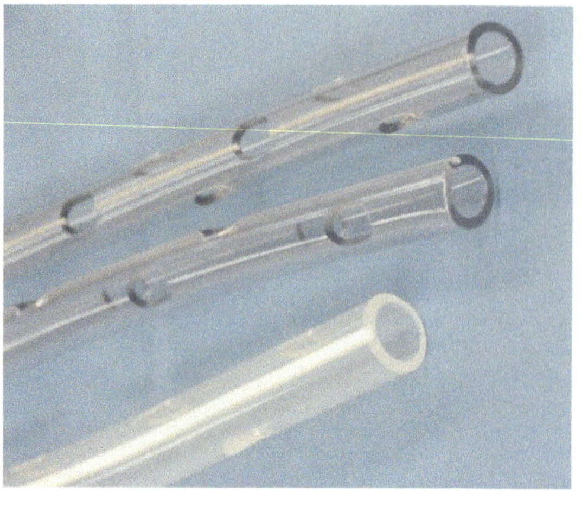

Fig. 9.14 Chest drains with drainage holes (Bentplate84 via Wikimedia [CC SA3.0])

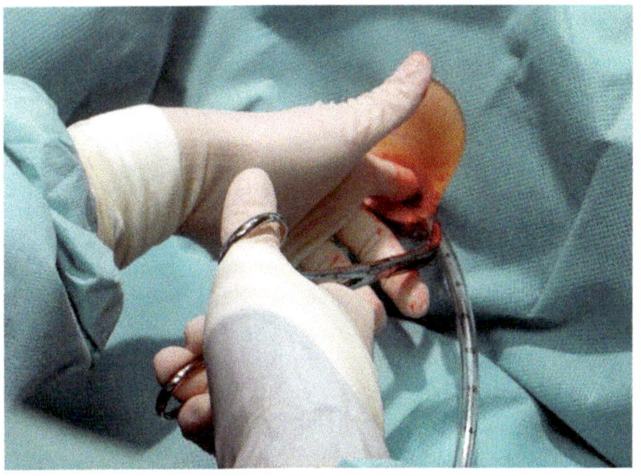

Fig. 9.15 Chest drain insertion after thoracostomy

should start swinging with changes in the patient's intrathoracic pressure.

All that is left now is to secure and dress the drain. There are a multitude of suggestions on how to complete this, but the most important thing is that it does not migrate or fall out. Some concerns with cosmesis and use of purse string sutures are not a major consideration at this point, as if they are truly causing problems when the patient is rehabilitated then a scar can be revised. Securing the defect with some sort of mattress suture in isolation in preparation for drain removal is sensible, and it would be prudent to have a second stitch in situ to take the weight of the drain rather than putting the closure stitch under tension and risk losing it or cutting through. Two transparent dressings such as a tegaderm are useful to sandwich together over the drain site so the depth of insertion can be easily seen and confirmed, and make identification of migration or signs of infection easier to identify than having to remove multiple dressings. Adhesive dressings can also be used, in addition to padding around the tube for patient comfort as needed. As long as the drain doesn't fall out, all other considerations are secondary!

Conclusion

Thoracic trauma is a significant cause of morbidity and mortality, and the majority of treatment strategies are easily understood in terms of restoring normal cardiorespiratory physiology. Whilst this section has covered some fundamentals, specific textbooks such as West's Respiratory Physiology: The Essentials are highly recommended to understand the baseline physiology of how the lungs work. In addition, there are several textbooks which can de-mystify ventilators such as the Intensive Care Society ebook and Pilbeam's Mechanical Ventilation—physiological and clinical applications. In common with a lot of trauma principles, fundamentals done well early and efficiently can negate the need for advanced therapies later on, so thorough and efficient early examination and management are advocated.

Questions

1. Injuries outside of the thoracic cavity cannot lead to respiratory compromise
   (a) True
   (b) False

2. Most patients are at risk of loss of hypoxic drive and should not be given supplementary oxygen as a routine
   (a) True
   (b) False

3. Analgesia for rib fractures should be withheld to decrease the risk of opiate toxicity and further respiratory compromise
   (a) True
   (b) False

4. Traumatic injuries are an absolute contraindication to ECMO
   (a) True
   (b) False

5. Chest drains should be placed above the fifth intercostal space on the effected side
   (a) True
   (b) False

Answers:

1. b
2. b

3. b
4. b
5. a

References

1. Sammy IA, Chatha H, Lecky F, Bouamra O, Fragoso-Iñiguez M, Sattout A, et al. Are first rib fractures a marker for other life-threatening injuries in patients with major trauma? A cohort study of patients on the UK Trauma Audit and Research Network database. Emerg Med J [Internet]. 2017;34(4):205–11. https://emj.bmj.com/content/34/4/205. Accessed 11 May 2019
2. Abdo WF, Heunks LM. Oxygen-induced hypercapnia in COPD: myths and facts. Crit Care [Internet]. 2012;16(5):323. http://ccforum.biomedcentral.com/articles/10.1186/cc11475. Accessed 7 May 2019.
3. Horncastle E, Lumb AB. Hyperoxia in anaesthesia and intensive care. BJA Educ [Internet]. 2019;19(6):176–82. https://linkinghub.elsevier.com/retrieve/pii/S2058534919300447. Accessed 10 May 2019
4. Mochizuki K, Shintani R, Mori K, Sato T, Sakaguchi O, Takeshige K, et al. Importance of respiratory rate for the prediction of clinical deterioration after emergency department discharge: a single-center, case–control study. Acute Med Surg [Internet]. 2016;4(2):172–8. https://www.ncbi.nlm.nih.gov/pmc/articles/PMC5667270/. Accessed 11 May 2019
5. Cretikos MA, Bellomo R, Hillman K, Chen J, Finfer S, Flabouris A. Respiratory rate: the neglected vital sign. Med J Aust [Internet]. 2008;188(11):657–9. https://onlinelibrary.wiley.com/doi/abs/10.5694/j.1326-5377.2008.tb01825.x. Accessed 11 May 2019
6. Xavier G, Melo C, Gaio E, Amado V. Accuracy of lung auscultation to detect abnormal respiratory mechanics: A cross-sectional diagnostic study. Eur Respir J [Internet]. 2014;44(Suppl 58):P4333. https://erj.ersjournals.com/content/44/Suppl_58/P4333. Accessed 11 May 2019.
7. Ramsay CF. An evaluative study of breath sounds teaching. 1.
8. Newnham M, Jones E, Wall D, Mukherjee R. P186 The reliability of the respiratory physical examination. Thorax [Internet]. 2011;66(Suppl 4):A143. https://thorax.bmj.com/content/66/Suppl_4/A143.2. Accessed 11 May 2019
9. Benbassat J, Baumal R. Narrative Review: Should teaching of the respiratory physical examination be restricted only to signs with proven reliability and validity? J Gen Intern Med [Internet]. 2010;25(8):865–72. https://www.ncbi.nlm.nih.gov/pmc/articles/PMC2896600/. Accessed 11 May 2019
10. Lichtenstein DA. BLUE-protocol and FALLS-protocol: two applications of lung ultrasound in the critically ill. Chest. 2015;147(6):1659–70.
11. Ghane MR, Gharib M, Ebrahimi A, Saeedi M, Akbari-Kamrani M, Rezaee M, et al. Accuracy of early rapid ultrasound in shock (RUSH) examination performed by emergency physician for diagnosis of shock etiology in critically ill patients. J Emerg Trauma Shock [Internet]. 2015;8(1):5–10. https://www.ncbi.nlm.nih.gov/pmc/articles/PMC4335159/. Accessed 11 May 2019
12. Ebrahimi A, Yousefifard M, Mohammad Kazemi H, Rasouli HR, Asady H, Moghadas Jafari A, et al. Diagnostic accuracy of chest ultrasonography versus chest radiography for identification of pneumothorax: a systematic review and meta-analysis. Tanaffos [Internet]. 2014;13(4):29–40. https://www.ncbi.nlm.nih.gov/pmc/articles/PMC4386013/. Accessed 11 May 2019
13. Amatya Y, Rupp J, Russell FM, Saunders J, Bales B, House DR. Diagnostic use of lung ultrasound compared to chest radiograph for suspected pneumonia in a resource-limited setting. Int J Emerg Med [Internet]. 2018;11. https://www.ncbi.nlm.nih.gov/pmc/articles/PMC5845910/. Accessed 11 May 2019.
14. Noble VE, Lamhaut L, Capp R, Bosson N, Liteplo A, Marx J-S, et al. Evaluation of a thoracic ultrasound training module for the detection of pneumothorax and pulmonary edema by prehospital physician care providers. BMC Med Educ [Internet]. 2009;9(1):3. https://bmcmededuc.biomedcentral.com/articles/10.1186/1472-6920-9-3. Accessed 7 May 2019.
15. Leigh-Smith S, Harris T. Tension pneumothorax–time for a re-think? Emerg Med J [Internet]. 2005;22(1):8–16. http://emj.bmj.com/cgi/doi/10.1136/emj.2003.010421. Accessed 7 May 2019
16. Laan DV, Vu TDN, Thiels CA, Pandian TK, Schiller HJ, Murad MH, et al. Chest wall thickness and decompression failure: a systematic review and meta-analysis comparing anatomic locations in needle thoracostomy. Injury [Internet]. 2016;47(4):797–804. https://linkinghub.elsevier.com/retrieve/pii/S0020138315007688. Accessed 7 May 2019
17. Ball CG, Wyrzykowski AD, Kirkpatrick AW, Dente CJ, Nicholas JM, Salomone JP, et al. Thoracic needle decompression for tension pneumothorax: clinical correlation with catheter length. Can J Surg [Internet]. 2010;53(3):184–8. https://www.ncbi.nlm.nih.gov/pmc/articles/PMC2878990/. Accessed 11 May 2019
18. Wernick B, Hon H, Mubang R, Cipriano A, Hughes R, Rankin D, et al. Complications of needle thoracostomy: a comprehensive clinical review. Int J Crit Illn Inj Sci [Internet]. 2015;5(3):160. http://www.ijciis.org/text.asp?2015/5/3/160/164939. Accessed 10 May 2019.
19. Rathinam S, Quinn DW, Bleetman A, Wall P, Steyn RS. Evaluation of ThoraQuik: a new device for the treatment of pneumothorax and pleural effusion. Emerg Med J [Internet]. 2011;28(9):750–3. http://emj.bmj.com/cgi/doi/10.1136/emj.2009.082297. Accessed 10 May 2019

20. Stawicki Stanislaw PA, Kwiatt M, Tarbox A, Seamon Mark J, Swaroop M, Cipolla J, et al. Thoracostomy tubes: A comprehensive review of complications and related topics. Int J Crit Illn Inj Sci [Internet]. 2014;4(2):142. http://www.ijciis.org/text.asp?2014/4/2/142/134182. Accessed 7 May 2019.
21. Butler FK, Holcomb JB, Shackelford S, Montgomery HR, Anderson S, Cain JS, et al. Management of suspected tension pneumothorax in tactical combat casualty care: TCCC Guidelines Change 17-02. J Spec Oper Med Peer Rev J SOF Med Prof. 2018;18(2):19–35.
22. Karmy-Jones R. Timing of urgent thoracotomy for hemorrhage after trauma: a multicenter study. Arch Surg [Internet]. 2001;136(5):513. http://archsurg.jamanetwork.com/article.aspx?doi=10.1001/archsurg.136.5.513. Accessed 7 May 2019.
23. Ali J, Qi W. Effectiveness of chest tube clamping in massive hemothorax. J Trauma. 1995;38(1):59–62. discussion 62-63
24. Kuppurao L, Wee M. Perioperative cell salvage. Contin Educ Anaesth Crit Care Pain [Internet]. 2010;10(4):104–8. https://linkinghub.elsevier.com/retrieve/pii/S1743181617302111. Accessed 7 May 2019
25. Brown CVR, Foulkrod KH, Sadler HT, Richards EK, Biggan DP, Czysz C, et al. Autologous blood transfusion during emergency trauma operations. Arch Surg [Internet]. 2010;145(7):690–4. https://jamanetwork.com/journals/jamasurgery/fullarticle/406120. Accessed 8 May 2019
26. Odak S, Raza A, Shah N, Clayson A. Clinical efficacy and cost effectiveness of intraoperative cell salvage in pelvic trauma surgery. Ann R Coll Surg Engl [Internet]. 2013;95(5):357–60. https://www.ncbi.nlm.nih.gov/pmc/articles/PMC4165140/. Accessed 8 May 2019
27. McLoughlin C, Roberts TE, Jackson LJ, Moore P, Wilson M, Hooper R, et al. Cost-effectiveness of cell salvage and donor blood transfusion during caesarean section: results from a randomised controlled trial. BMJ Open [Internet]. 2019;9(2):e022352. https://bmjopen.bmj.com/content/9/2/e022352. Accessed 8 May 2019.
28. Bilgili MG, Erçin E, Peker G, Kural C, Başaran SH, Duramaz A, et al. Efficiency and cost analysis of cell saver auto transfusion system in total knee arthroplasty. Balk Med J [Internet]. 2014;31(2):149–53. https://www.ncbi.nlm.nih.gov/pmc/articles/PMC4115923/. Accessed 8 May 2019
29. Esper SA, Waters JH. Intra-operative cell salvage: a fresh look at the indications and contraindications. Blood Transfus [Internet]. 2011;9(2):139–47. https://www.ncbi.nlm.nih.gov/pmc/articles/PMC3096856/. Accessed 8 May 2019
30. Karmy-Jones R, Holevar M, Sullivan RJ, Fleisig A, Jurkovich GJ. Residual hemothorax after chest tube placement correlates with increased risk of empyema following traumatic injury. Can Respir J. 2008;15(5):255–8.
31. DuBose J, Inaba K, Demetriades D, Scalea TM, O'Connor J, Menaker J, et al. Management of post-traumatic retained hemothorax: a prospective, observational, multicenter AAST study. J Trauma Acute Care Surg. 2012;72(1):11–22. discussion 22-24; quiz 316
32. Heimes J, Copeland H, Lulla A, Duldulao M, Bahjri K, Zaheer S, et al. The use of thrombolytics in the management of complex pleural fluid collections. J Thorac Dis [Internet]. 2017;9(5):1310–6. https://www.ncbi.nlm.nih.gov/pmc/articles/PMC5465141/. Accessed 10 May 2019
33. Brunckhorst O, Guidozzi NM, Warren LR, Peters CJ. Tension haemothorax from a bleeding branch of the renal artery following isolated penetrating thoracic trauma: a rare presentation. Case Rep [Internet]. 2018;2018:bcr-2018-225678. https://casereports.bmj.com/content/2018/bcr-2018-225678. Accessed 11 May 2019.
34. Tan J, Alvarez JM. Tension haemothorax: an uncommon life-threatening complication. ANZ J Surg. 2002;72(1):72–4.
35. Jayle CPM, Allain G, Ingrand P, Laksiri L, Bonnin E, Hajj-Chahine J, et al. Flail chest in polytraumatized patients: surgical fixation using stracos reduces ventilator time and hospital stay. BioMed Res Int [Internet]. 2015;2015. https://www.ncbi.nlm.nih.gov/pmc/articles/PMC4331314/. Accessed 8 May 2019.
36. Hasenboehler EA, Bernard AC, Bottiggi AJ, Moghadamian ES, Wright RD, Chang PK, et al. Treatment of traumatic flail chest with muscular sparing open reduction and internal fixation: description of a surgical technique. J Trauma. 2011;71(2):494–501.
37. Qiu M, Shi Z, Xiao J, Zhang X, Ling S, Ling H. Potential benefits of rib fracture fixation in patients with flail chest and multiple non-flail rib fractures. Indian J Surg [Internet]. 2016;78(6):458–63. https://www.ncbi.nlm.nih.gov/pmc/articles/PMC5218931/. Accessed 8 May 2019
38. Bemelman M, de Kruijf MW, van Baal M, Leenen L. Rib fractures: to fix or not to fix? An evidence-based algorithm. Korean J Thorac Cardiovasc Surg [Internet]. 2017;50(4):229–34. https://www.ncbi.nlm.nih.gov/pmc/articles/PMC5548197/. Accessed 8 May 2019
39. Alfaro M, Skinner R, Pakula A. Improved outcomes after surgical stabilization of rib fractures in patients with polytrauma and associated chest wall fractures. https://clinmedjournals.org/articles/tcr/trauma-cases-and-reviews-tcr-4-058.php?jid=tcr. Accessed 8 May 2019.
40. Doben AR, Eriksson EA, Denlinger CE, Leon SM, Couillard DJ, Fakhry SM, et al. Surgical rib fixation for flail chest deformity improves liberation from mechanical ventilation. J Crit Care. 2014;29(1):139–43.
41. Moya M de, Nirula R, Biffl W. Rib fixation: who, what, when? Trauma Surg Acute Care Open [Internet]. 2017;2(1):e000059. https://tsaco.bmj.com/content/2/1/e000059. Accessed 8 May 2019.

42. May L, Hillermann C, Patil S. Rib fracture management. BJA Educ [Internet]. 2016;16(1):26–32. https://academic.oup.com/bjaed/article/16/1/26/2463139. Accessed 8 May 2019
43. Hsu H-L, Shih C-C. Re-intervention after thoracic endovascular aortic repair is high, but we should keep optimistic. J Thorac Dis [Internet]. 2017;9(2):E162–3. https://www.ncbi.nlm.nih.gov/pmc/articles/PMC5334088/. Accessed 8 May 2019
44. Moulakakis KG, Mylonas SN, Dalainas I, Kakisis J, Kotsis T, Liapis CD. Management of complicated and uncomplicated acute type B dissection. A systematic review and meta-analysis. Ann Cardiothorac Surg [Internet]. 2014;3(3):234–46. https://www.ncbi.nlm.nih.gov/pmc/articles/PMC4052408/. Accessed 8 May 2019.
45. Fitzgibbon B, Jordan F, Hynes N, McGarry JP, Kavanagh EP, McHugh P, et al. Endovascular versus open surgical repair for complicated chronic type B aortic dissection. Cochrane Database Syst Rev [Internet]. 2018;(4). https://www.cochranelibrary.com/cdsr/doi/10.1002/14651858.CD012992/full. Accessed 8 May 2019.
46. Hogendoorn W, Hunink MGM, Schlösser FJV, Moll FL, Sumpio BE, Muhs BE. Endovascular vs. open repair of complicated acute type B aortic dissections. J Endovasc Ther Off J Int Soc Endovasc Spec. 2014;21(4):503–14.
47. Cheaito A, Tillou A, Lewis C, Cryer H. Management of traumatic blunt IVC injury. Int J Surg Case Rep [Internet]. 2016;28:26–30. https://www.ncbi.nlm.nih.gov/pmc/articles/PMC5037255/. Accessed 8 May 2019
48. Mubang RN, Stawicki SP. Esophageal trauma. StatPearls [Internet]. Treasure Island, FL: StatPearls Publishing; 2019. http://www.ncbi.nlm.nih.gov/books/NBK470161/. Accessed 10 May 2019.
49. Matsushima K, Aiolfi A, Park C, Rosen D, Strumwasser A, Benjamin E, et al. Surgical outcomes after trauma pneumonectomy: revisited. J Trauma Acute Care Surg. 2017;82(5):927–32.
50. Karmy-Jones R, Wood DE. Traumatic injury to the trachea and bronchus. Thorac Surg Clin [Internet]. 2007;17(1):35–46. https://linkinghub.elsevier.com/retrieve/pii/S1547412707000151. Accessed 7 May 2019
51. Bakowitz M, Bruns B, McCunn M. Acute lung injury and the acute respiratory distress syndrome in the injured patient. Scand J Trauma Resusc Emerg Med [Internet]. 2012;20:54. https://www.ncbi.nlm.nih.gov/pmc/articles/PMC3518173/. Accessed 8 May 2019.
52. Ganie FA, Lone H, Lone GN, Wani ML, Singh S, Dar AM, et al. Lung contusion: a clinico-pathological entity with unpredictable clinical course. Bull Emerg Trauma [Internet]. 2013;1(1):7–16. https://www.ncbi.nlm.nih.gov/pmc/articles/PMC4771236/. Accessed 8 May 2019
53. Simon LV, Burns B. Diaphragm rupture. StatPearls [Internet]. Treasure Island, FL: StatPearls Publishing; 2019. http://www.ncbi.nlm.nih.gov/books/NBK470214/. Accessed 10 May 2019
54. O'Driscoll BR, Howard LS, Earis J, Mak V. British Thoracic Society Guideline for oxygen use in adults in healthcare and emergency settings. BMJ Open Respir Res [Internet]. 2017;4(1):e000170. https://bmjopenrespres.bmj.com/content/4/1/e000170. Accessed 8 May 2019.
55. Chiumello D, Coppola S, Froio S, Gregoretti C, Consonni D. Noninvasive ventilation in chest trauma: systematic review and meta-analysis. Intensive Care Med. 2013;39(7):1171–80.
56. Davidson C, Banham S, Elliott M, Kennedy D, Gelder C, Glossop A, et al. British Thoracic Society/Intensive Care Society Guideline for the ventilatory management of acute hypercapnic respiratory failure in adults. BMJ Open Respir Res [Internet]. 2016;3(1). https://www.ncbi.nlm.nih.gov/pmc/articles/PMC4800170/. Accessed 11 May 2019.
57. Rabec C, Rodenstein D, Leger P, Rouault S, Perrin C, Gonzalez-Bermejo J, et al. Ventilator modes and settings during non-invasive ventilation: effects on respiratory events and implications for their identification. Thorax [Internet]. 2011;66(2):170–8. http://thorax.bmj.com/cgi/doi/10.1136/thx.2010.142661. Accessed 11 May 2019
58. Scala R, Pisani L. Noninvasive ventilation in acute respiratory failure: which recipe for success? Eur Respir Rev [Internet]. 2018;27(149):180029. https://err.ersjournals.com/content/27/149/180029. Accessed 11 May 2019.
59. Camporota L, Montgomery H, Dlouhy P, editors. Handbook of mechanical ventilation [Internet]. London: Intensive Care Society; 2015. 192 p. http://www.ics.ac.uk/AsiCommon/Controls/BSA/Downloader.aspx?iDocumentStorageKey=cc84e8ce-ddf8-4fba-8912-1e602af0656f&iFileTypeCode=PDF&iFileName=Ventilation%20handbook. Accessed 5 Sep 2019.
60. Guérin C, Reignier J, Richard J-C, Beuret P, Gacouin A, Boulain T, et al. Prone positioning in severe acute respiratory distress syndrome. N Engl J Med [Internet]. 2013;368(23):2159–68. http://www.nejm.org/doi/10.1056/NEJMoa1214103. Accessed 9 May 2019
61. Bourenne J, Hraiech S, Roch A, Gainnier M, Papazian L, Forel J-M. Sedation and neuromuscular blocking agents in acute respiratory distress syndrome. Ann Transl Med [Internet]. 2017;5(14):291. http://atm.amegroups.com/article/view/15714/15783. Accessed 9 May 2019
62. Zhou Y, Jin X, Lv Y, Wang P, Yang Y, Liang G, et al. Early application of airway pressure release ventilation may reduce the duration of mechanical ventilation in acute respiratory distress syndrome. Intensive Care Med. 2017;43(11):1648–59.
63. Mireles-Cabodevila E, Dugar S, Chatburn RL. APRV for ARDS: the complexities of a mode and how it affects even the best trials. J Thorac Dis [Internet]. 2018;10(Suppl 9):S1058–63. https://www.ncbi.nlm.

nih.gov/pmc/articles/PMC5949414/. Accessed 9 May 2019

64. Young D, Lamb SE, Shah S, MacKenzie I, Tunnicliffe W, Lall R, et al. High-frequency oscillation for acute respiratory distress syndrome. N Engl J Med [Internet]. 2013;368(9):806–13. https://doi.org/10.1056/NEJMoa1215716. Accessed 9 May 2019
65. Hand L. The OSCILLATE trial: implications for respiratory therapists then and now. Can J Respir Ther CJRT Rev Can Thérapie Respir RCTR [Internet]. 2014;50(3):74–5. https://www.ncbi.nlm.nih.gov/pmc/articles/PMC4456840/. Accessed 9 May 2019
66. Zonies D, Codner P, Park P, Martin ND, Lissauer M, Evans S, et al. AAST Critical Care Committee clinical consensus: ECMO, nutritionExtracorporeal membrane oxygenation (ECMO)Nutrition. Trauma Surg Acute Care Open [Internet]. 2019;4(1):e000304. https://tsaco.bmj.com/content/4/1/e000304. Accessed 9 May 2019.
67. Morelli A, Del Sorbo L, Pesenti A, Ranieri VM, Fan E. Extracorporeal carbon dioxide removal (ECCO2R) in patients with acute respiratory failure. Intensive Care Med. 2017;43(4):519–30.
68. Laws D, Neville E, Duffy J, Pleural Diseases Group, Standards of Care Committee, British Thoracic Society. BTS guidelines for the insertion of a chest drain. Thorax. 2003;58(Suppl 2):ii53–9.
69. Kulvatunyou N, Vijayasekaran A, Hansen A, Wynne JL, O'Keeffe T, Friese RS, et al. Two-year experience of using pigtail catheters to treat traumatic pneumothorax: a changing trend. J Trauma Inj Infect Crit Care [Internet]. 2011;71(5):1104–1107. https://insights.ovid.com/crossref?an=00005373-201111000-00002. Accessed 10 Sep 2019.
70. Kulvatunyou N, Joseph B, Friese RS, Green D, Gries L, O'Keeffe T, et al. 14 French pigtail catheters placed by surgeons to drain blood on trauma patients: is 14-Fr too small? J Trauma Acute Care Surg [Internet]. 2012;73(6):1423–7. http://content.wkhealth.com/linkback/openurl?sid=WKPTLP:landingpage&an=01586154-201212000-00014. Accessed 10 Sep 2019
71. Maskell NA, Medford A, Gleeson FV. Seldinger chest drain insertion: simpler but not necessarily safer. Thorax [Internet]. 2010;65(1):5–6. http://thorax.bmj.com/cgi/doi/10.1136/thx.2009.117200. Accessed 10 Sep 2019
72. Rivera L, O'Reilly EB, Sise MJ, Norton VC, Sise CB, Sack DI, et al. Small catheter tube thoracostomy: effective in managing chest trauma in stable patients. J Trauma Inj Infect Crit Care [Internet]. 2009;66(2):393–399. https://insights.ovid.com/crossref?an=00005373-200902000-00014. Accessed 10 Sep 2019.
73. Inaba K, Lustenberger T, Recinos G, Georgiou C, Velmahos GC, Brown C, et al. Does size matter? A prospective analysis of 28–32 versus 36–40 French chest tube size in trauma: J Trauma Acute Care Surg [Internet]. 2012;72(2):422–7. https://insights.ovid.com/crossref?an=01586154-201202000-00016. Accessed 10 Sep 2019.
74. Yi J, Liu H, Zhang M, Wu J, Yang J, Chen J, et al. Management of traumatic hemothorax by closed thoracic drainage using a central venous catheter. J Zhejiang Univ Sci B [Internet]. 2012;13(1):43–8. http://www.springerlink.com/index/10.1631/jzus.B1100161. Accessed 10 Sep 2019
75. Bing F, Fitzgerald M, Olaussen A, Finnegan P, O'Reilly G, Gocentas R, et al. Identifying a safe site for intercostal catheter insertion using the mid-arm point (MAP). J Emerg Med Trauma Acute Care [Internet]. 2017;2017(1):3. http://www.qscience.com/doi/10.5339/jemtac.2017.3. Accessed 10 Sep 2019.

Circulation

10

Peter Lax

- Physiology of normal blood pressure and its determinants
- Definition, classification and causes of shock
- Signs and assessment of shock
- Hypotension in trauma
- Historic and current treatment of hypovolaemia
- Practical aspects of massive blood transfusion

Introduction

The cardiovascular system has evolved to deliver oxygenated blood and nutrients to the tissues and vital organs of the body while removing waste products to the liver and kidney for excretion. A simplified overview of this system is that there is a pump, a series of connecting pipes and a fluid which is necessary for the correct functioning of all other body systems. In trauma, any one of these components can fail in isolation or conjunction with each other and lead to morbidity or mortality.

P. Lax (✉)
Tactical Medical Wing, Royal Air Force, Brize Norton, Oxfordshire, UK

The Air Ambulance Service (TAAS), Rugby, Warwickshire, UK
e-mail: p.lax@NHS.net

Gross Physiology of Circulation and Blood Pressure

Blood pressure is regulated by the balance between the sympathetic and parasympathetic nervous system on both the heart and vessels. The degree of vasoconstriction or vasodilatation (otherwise known as the systemic vascular resistance or SVR) and the cardiac output (the amount of blood ejected from the left ventricle per minute) can both be increased or decreased by an intact nervous system or by certain hormones such as adrenaline.

Figure 10.1 gives an overview of the common factors that combine or can be manipulated to influence blood pressure and circulation. The cardiac output is the product of the heart rate and the stroke volume. In order to increase cardiac output, there either needs to be more beats per minute or each beat has to eject more blood. This leads to the first compensatory mechanism that can be observed in patients with shock—mounting a tachycardic response to increase blood flow around the body. If there is not enough blood returning to the heart, then the heart speeds up to try and offset decreased stroke volume by increasing its rate. This brings us onto stroke volume, which is itself controlled by three factors—preload (volume of blood in the ventricle just before it contracts), contractility (the amount of strength the heart muscle can contract with) and afterload (the amount of resistance to blood being ejected from the heart, for example by a tight aortic valve

P. Lax (ed.), *Textbook of Acute Trauma Care*, https://doi.org/10.1007/978-3-030-83628-3_10

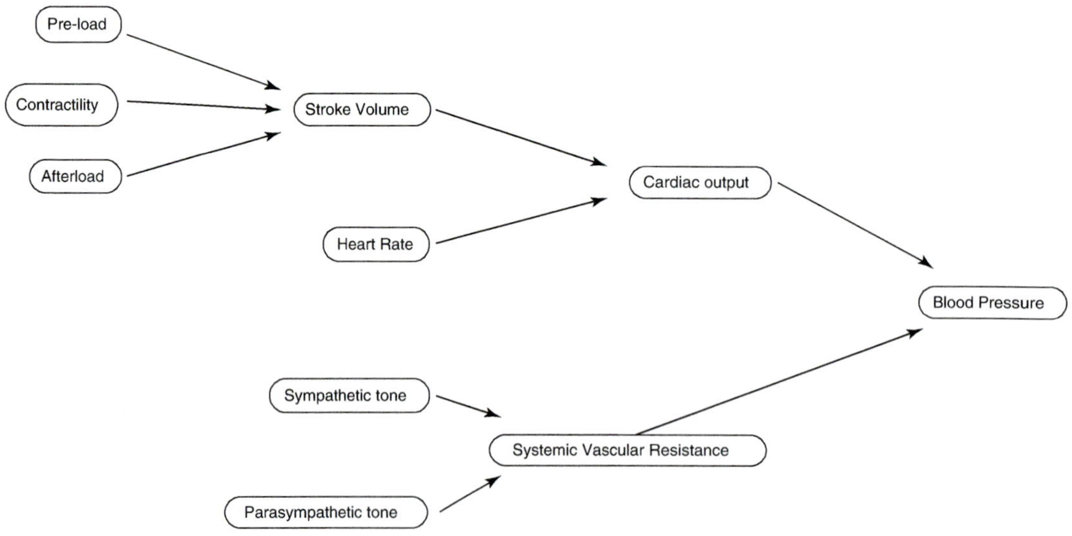

Fig. 10.1 Gross overview of physiological parameters and their relation to blood pressure

or high SVR). By increasing the amount of blood returning to the heart, the fibres in cardiac muscle are increasingly stretched and will contract with more force up to a point when they become overstretched and less efficient. Beyond this point, although the amount of filling of the heart increases, the contractility and volume of blood ejected per beat decreases. This ultimately leads to a lower cardiac output and ventricular failure with pulmonary oedema and is known as the Frank-Starling law. This rarely happens in trauma, but occasionally, patients who are given large volumes of blood products or fluid and have an underlying cardiac condition may develop acute heart failure via this mechanism.

Decreases in contractility can be seen in patients who have developed cardiac contusions as a result of blunt chest trauma, or alternately patients who have suffered a cardiac event which has subsequently led to trauma. An example of this may be the patient who has a myocardial infarction or arrhythmia and subsequently blacks out and crashes their car. Depending on the underlying nature of the injury, decreases in contractility can be mitigated against by judicious use of inotropes to increase myocardial work. However, this is a complicated area of management as the failing heart may subsequently fail altogether if it is pushed too hard pharmacologically. It may be possible, or even preferable in some cases, to tolerate a slightly lower than normal blood pressure or to use small fluid boluses to see if the heart will cope with additional preload if there are no other considerations such as ongoing bleeding.

Shock

Shock is simultaneously very simple to define but very difficult to quantify objectively on occasion. On a systemic level, any state where there is an imbalance between the body's demands for delivery of blood and oxygen to the vital organs and its supply is termed shock. This usually is because the circulatory system's output has fallen below demand, but occasionally the imbalance is due to increasing demand rather than dropping supply, and this is termed high output cardiac failure. This occurs in conditions such as beriberi, severe hyperthyroidism and morbid obesity. The types of shock are defined by their underlying mechanism (distributive, obstructive, cardiogenic or hypovolaemic), but ultimately the result is the same—inadequate blood and oxygen delivery. When considering shock, it should be conceptualised in the basic terms explained above if the problem is with the pump, the pipes or the fluid. All treatments of shock are targeted against treating the underlying cause or mitigating the effects that it causes.

Distributive Shock

Distributive shock is where the heart is functioning well, and there is sufficient blood or fluid in the body, but it is not in the correct location, i.e. a problem with the pipes. The classic examples of this are anaphylaxis, septic shock and neurogenic shock. It should be noted that neurogenic shock and spinal shock are two different things—neurogenic shock can be a cardiovascular consequence of spinal shock, but spinal shock is a specific injury to the spinal cord. Spinal shock is a sensorimotor phenomenon, usually caused by hyperextension or hyperflexion of the neck—this is covered more in Chap. 32 (Spinal and neurological trauma). In distributive shock, the vasomotor tone (amount of constriction in the arterial and venous systems) is decreased, and the effective volume that the normal circulating volume has had to fill is vastly increased as a consequence. Imagine a bucket that has a capacity of 5 litres and contains 4 litres of water initially. If the pressure of the water at the bottom of the bucket is measured, it is directly related to the vertical height of water above it. If the same 4 litres of water remain but the diameter of the bucket is doubled, the pressure of the water at the bottom of the bucket will be much lower as the volume it has to fill is larger, and hence the vertical height reduced. The volume of water in the bucket is the same both times and is an analogy for the circulating volume of blood. By changing the capacitance of the bucket (increasing vasodilation—increasing the capacity of the pipes in the circulatory system), the pressure is lowered.

Anaphylaxis

In anaphylaxis, vasomotor tone is lost due to histamine release from mast cells, causing sudden and profound vasodilation. There is also increasing porosity of the circulatory system so that fluid can leak out of the capillary system

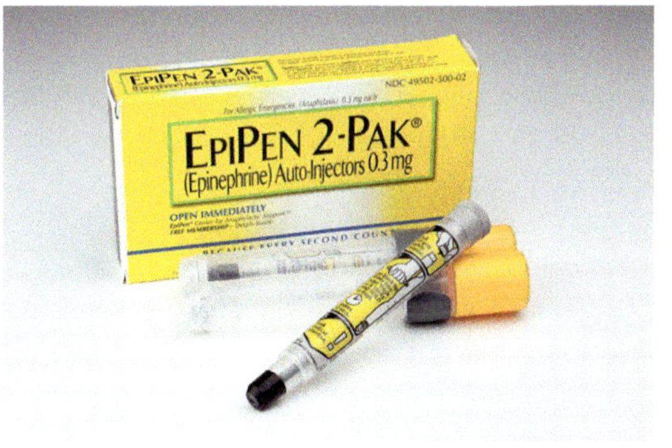

Fig. 10.2 Epipen autoinjector box. IM adrenaline is the first line treatment for anaphylaxis in the community

and not re-enter into the venous side of the circulation as it would under normal circumstances. This is known as capillary leak and adds an element of hypovolaemia to the picture (i.e. the fluid component of the circulatory system is also decreased). This leads to a hyperdynamic circulation with the widespread vasodilation leading to profound hypotension, warm peripheries, a sudden onset erythematous rash and a compensatory tachycardia. In severe cases, this can also cause a large amount of tissue swelling, which if it affects the airway, can be rapidly fatal. The vasodilation itself can cause cardiac collapse and arrest without airway involvement. Anaphylaxis in trauma is rare, but potentially any drug that a patient receives can cause an allergic reaction and anaphylaxis is the worst-case scenario. The immediate treatment of anaphylaxis is with adrenaline/epinephrine, usually given by an intramuscular injection (e.g. with an EpiPen as seen in Fig. 10.2), but in patients with IV access, small aliquots of intravenous adrenaline can be given by those with appropriate expertise.

Sepsis

Similarly to anaphylaxis, sepsis is a combination of both high output failure and vasodilation, but also may have an element of increased oxygen demand. The body's basal metabolic rate increases as it attempts to mount an immune response to invading pathogens and so it requires enhanced oxygen delivery. At the same time, bacterial toxins and cytokines are released, which cause peripheral vasodilation and a drop the systemic vascular resistance. There may also be capillary leak as described in anaphylaxis. In both these cases, the correct treatment is to address the underlying cause, and provide organ support, usually by giving additional vasoactive medications (such as noradrenaline, vasopressin or adrenaline) to counteract the vasodilation and increase SVR. In anaphylaxis, this may only require a short treatment for a few minutes while the histamine release has been counteracted, but in sepsis, the administration of vasoactive drugs may be required for days. Successful treatment involves controlling the source of infection by either surgery, antibiotics or both while counteracting direct effects of the pathogen and the body's immune response. The increased oxygen requirement may also induce an element of high output failure as described above.

Neurogenic Shock

Neurogenic shock is where there is a high thoracic or cervical cord lesion, which decreases the vasomotor tone of the cardiovascular system. The degree of vasoconstriction or vasodilation usually is held in balance by the opposing forces of the sympathetic and parasympathetic nervous system. The main outflow of the sympathetic nervous system is in the thoracolumbar spinal cord, whereas the parasympathetic system originates in the cranial, cervical and sacral nerves (see Fig. 10.3). If an injury to the cord occurs above the level of T3-4 (the upper limits of sympathetic innervation), then the balance is lost, and the parasympathetic nervous system dominates. This leads to vasodilation and increased capacitance of all the circulatory vessels (but without capillary leak as described in anaphylaxis). However, there is also a compounding cardiac response.

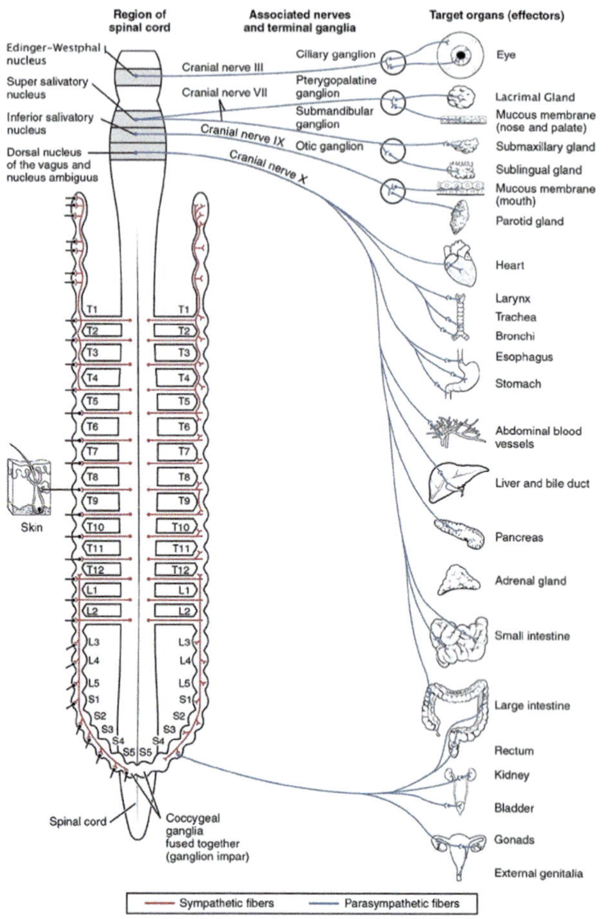

Fig. 10.3 Outflow of the sympathetic and parasympathetic nervous systems (Craniosacral outflow, Wikimedia under the Creative Commons Attribution 3.0 Unported license)

In the same way that vasomotor tone is balanced by sympathetic and parasympathetic innervation, the heart is equally dual innervated. The sympathetic cardio-acceleratory fibres originate from T2-T4, and parasympathetic cardioinhibitory fibres arise from a branch of the vagus nerve, the 10th cranial nerve. If the level of the injury is higher than the cardio-acceleratory fibres, then in addition to the distributive hypotension caused by vasodilation the body is unable to mount a compensatory tachycardia. Indeed, unopposed vagal stimuli will cause worsening bradycardia and subsequent decrease in cardiac output and compound the hypotension further. The correct treatment of neurogenic shock involves infusions of vasopressors such as noradrenaline, vasopressin, phenylephrine or metaraminol to maintain blood pressure and cord perfusion. If the injury is above T2-T4 then directly acting cardiac inotropes/chronotropes may be needed in addition to vasopressors. Isoprenaline may be sufficient if added to a vasopressor or alternatively adrenaline may be used initially to act as a combined inotrope/chronotrope and vasopressor. By maintaining this perfusion pressure to the damaged cord (and the rest of the vital organs), the risk of secondary injury is minimised.

Obstructive Shock

Stressing the heart by increasing the afterload significantly can cause the heart to fail. Due to the way that the heart has evolved, the right ventricle does not need to be as strong as the left as it only pushes blood through the low-pressure circulatory system of the lungs. The left ventricle, in contrast, has to supply the whole body so needs to be able to generate more forceful contractions. Consequently, it is easier to cause the right side of the heart to fail than the left. The common trauma scenarios in which this is seen are pulmonary embolus and tension pneumothorax.

Pulmonary Embolus

In pulmonary embolus, a large blood clot or fat embolus obstructs the pulmonary artery and increases the right ventricular afterload, causing impairment of blood flow to the lungs and increased dead space. This causes both hypoxia and hypotension, as obstruction of blood flow to the left ventricle causes decreased preload and subsequent decrease in cardiac output. Depending on the nature and size of the embolus and other factors associated with trauma such as bleeding risk, the options for treatment may vary [1, 2]. These can range from observation only, anticoagulation to reduce the risk of the clot increasing in size, thrombolytic drugs to break down the clot with enzymes, removal of the embolus with interventional radiology guidance or open surgery with cardiac bypass to remove large, life-threatening clots. Each step grows particularly more aggressive and increases the risk of side effects, so each case requires an individualised approach.

Tension Pneumothorax

While pulmonary embolus causes increased afterload on the right ventricle from inside the circulation, external compression of the lung and pulmonary artery by a tension pneumothorax causes the same issues. This is compounded by hypoxia and decreased venous return caused by twisting of the mediastinum—please refer to Chap. 9 (Breathing and chest trauma) for more details.

Cardiogenic Shock

Cardiogenic shock is when the heart itself cannot generate sufficient force to pump blood effectively, despite having adequate blood volume returned to it and no problems with afterload. This may be due in broad terms as a result of intrinsic heart diseases such as cardiomyopathies, an arrhythmia such as supraventricular tachycardia or a myocardial infarction; these causes of failure are outside the scope of this text. The two leading causes in trauma are as a result of cardiac contusions as described in Chap. 9 (Breathing and chest trauma), or rarely as a result of cardiac tamponade.

Cardiac Tamponade

The heart is surrounded by a tight, fibrous sack called the pericardium. This structure has evolved to keep the heart in place in the mediastinum, is filled with fluid to decrease friction on surrounding structures when the heart contracts and is a physical barrier against infection. As it is a fibrous structure, it does not stretch when the pressure inside it increases. Because the pericardium is so inflexible and closely opposed to the heart, if fluid accumulates between the heart and the pericardium, then it will compress the heart from the outside and decrease the ventricular volume available to fill with blood (see Fig. 10.4). This decreases the stroke volume in both ventricles, though it affects the right more than the left due to the previously mentioned weakness of the right ventricle compared to the left. Any fluid that accumulates in the pericardium can compress the ventricle, but in trauma, it is most commonly blood. In cases of patients presenting with penetrating chest or upper abdominal trauma, the heart may have been pierced, and blood may leak from the injured chamber or vessel into the pericardium. This is an emergency and requires surgical intervention. If the patient arrests, this may need to be by a resuscitative thoracotomy (see Chap. 12 - Traumatic cardiac arrest). There is no role for needle aspiration of pericardial blood (needle pericardiocentesis) in trauma as blood tends to clot quickly and become too viscous to aspirate through a needle. There is also the risk of missing the collection altogether and causing further cardiac injury if using a blind technique, and even ultrasound-guided techniques are not guaranteed to succeed [3].

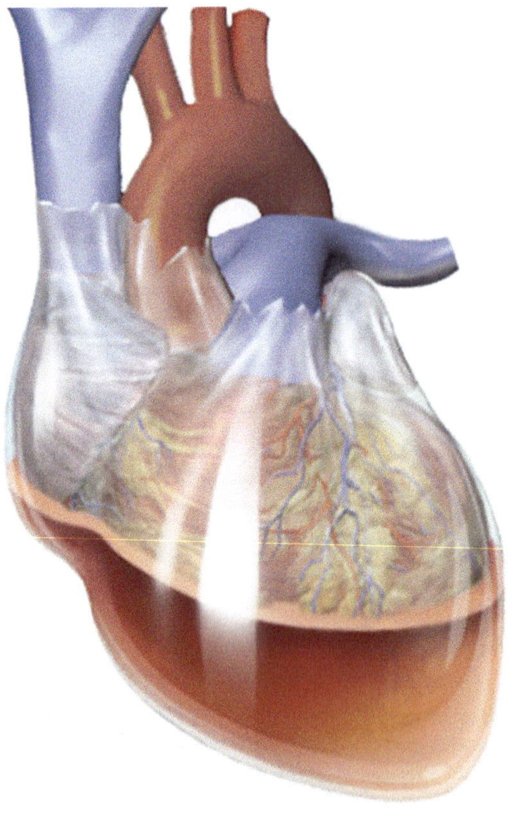

Fig. 10.4 Cardiac tamponade—blood fills the pericardial space and prevents diastolic filling (Blausen.com staff (2014). "Medical gallery of Blausen Medical 2014". WikiJournal of Medicine 1 (2). DOI:10.15347/wjm/2014.010. ISSN 2002-4436)

Tamponade itself is not an intrinsic cardiac muscular problem, but the mechanism by which it produces shock is due to pump failure as opposed to fluid or pipe failure; hence its inclusion in this section. There is an element of obstruction to filling, but the mechanism of failure is different from those pathologies listed in the Obstructive Shock section. With tamponade, the issue is with the heart filling whereas, with pure obstructive shock, the pathological mechanism is impairment of the heart emptying.

Hypovolaemic Shock

The final mechanism of shock is hypovolaemia. This is by far the most common cause of shock in trauma as the principal cause is bleeding. A cardinal maxim is that all shock in trauma should be considered to be hypovolaemic until conclusively proven otherwise. More than one pathology can coexist, so clinicians must aggressively search for haemorrhage before concluding that shock is not due at least in part to hypovolaemia.

Failure to Identify Active Bleeding

Typically this is occult bleeding into a major body cavity which, if not appreciated from the mechanism of injury or developing signs, will result in rapid deterioration or death. These patients typically need rapid transport to a hospital which can manage such bleeds (which usually means surgery or angiography, e.g. in the case of splenic

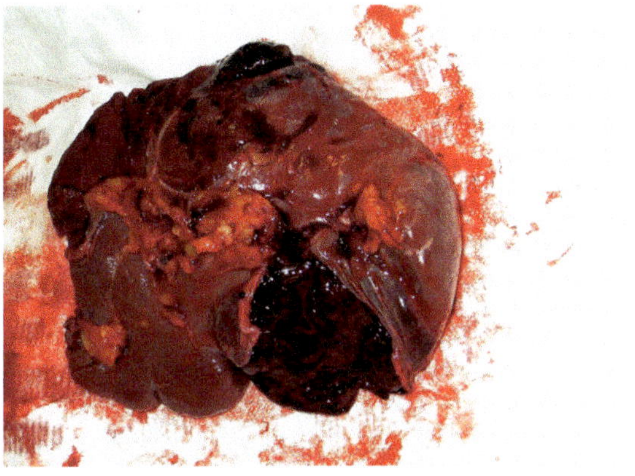

Fig. 10.5 A ruptured spleen such as this example can cause significant hypovolaemia. Current practice is to try and preserve the spleen and treat with interventional radiology measures, but a severely shattered spleen with ongoing bleeding needs surgical intervention (Thomas Zimmerman via Wikimedia under the Creative Commons Attribution-Share Alike 3.0 Germany license)

bleeds as in Fig. 10.5) but could also include REBOA or resuscitative thoracotomy with cross-clamping of the descending aorta. The latter course of action is not recommended except in extremis due to increased morbidity and extremely high mortality when performed for extra-thoracic causes of hypovolaemia. Management before this point should concentrate on active volume replacement with blood and rapid access to facilities to obtain definitive haemostatic control.

Failure to Control Active Bleeding

There is no excuse for not trying to manage external bleeding. Every drop of blood is precious circulating volume for that patient, and transfusion or intravenous fluids are not equivalent replacements. Every possible effort should be made to preserve circulating volume where possible. This concept of circulation preservation is now a fundamental part of bleeding and shock management and is far more effective than relying on replacement strategies. The bottom line is that at present, the patient's own blood is the best substance to be circulating in their vessels. Circulation preservation may be as simple as a pressure dressing, tourniquet or may be as involved as urgent laparotomy or angiography for internal bleeding.

In the MABCD assessment, if there is no visible massive external haemorrhage, move on but be aware of the signs of more occult bleeding during the assessment of other systems such as A-airway and B-breathing and inevitably C-circulation and D-disability.

Key Points

Typical features that may be identified include:

- Rapid, shallow breathing. Increased respiratory rate is the best single indicator or sign of an unwell patient. This could be from many causes and not just shock, but should never be ignored. In shock, the reduced tissue perfusion and metabolic acidosis which occur result in signs of 'air hunger'. Casualties may appear to be distressed or gasping to get their breath as they hyperventilate to compensate in respiratory terms for the metabolic acidosis and rising lactate. Whilst it is a sensitive sign, it is unfortunately not highly specific for any one pathology.
- The oxygen saturation may be difficult to obtain, due to lack of perfusion causing a low signal and generalised peripheral shut down. It may also be genuinely low as a result of increasing ventilation/perfusion mismatching in the lungs.
- Confusion, agitation or anxiety may occur as cerebral perfusion drops and blood supply to the brain is reduced. This may lead to feeling faint and ultimately to a falling conscious level and responsiveness

Remember these are also features which may suggest a pneumothorax. Hopefully, this has been excluded as part of the respiratory assessment, but the possibility of a significant pneumothorax should be considered in trauma patients presenting with cardiovascular compromise.

The management of hypovolaemia has changed over many years as the understanding of traumatic haemorrhage has evolved. This is driven primarily from military experience in war, and some lessons are re-learned at the start of each new conflict. The three principles that should be adhered to are 1) preserving circulation whenever possible (e.g. with the use of tourniquets and other devices and techniques described in Chap. 6 (Massive haemorrhage control), 2) achieving haemostatic control as soon as possible and 3) employing a damage control resuscitation strategy. Definitive haemostasis can be either via surgical or radiological means or both [4], and resuscitative radiology is becoming more advanced as time passes. It has several advantages including specific targeting of individual vessels without the morbidity of some surgical approaches, for example some pelvic arterial bleeding can be controlled by minimally invasive arteriography and coiling rather than a laparotomy to access the vessels and may decrease the time to definitive haemostasis [5].

"Classical" Clinical Signs of Shock

As previously stated, shock is easy to define but can be hard to quantify. As the body attempts to compensate for blood loss, adaptive physiological changes include increased heart rate to compensate for decreased stroke volume, increasing diastolic blood pressure to maintain perfusion pressure and diversion of blood from the periphery to vital organs. This means that patients may feel peripherally cool to the touch, have a prolonged capillary refill time and look pale on clinical examination. As blood pressure decreases further, the end organs become less perfused, and other clinical signs may become apparent. These include decreased urine output as the kidneys attempt to retain circulating volume or become hypoperfused, and confusion or unconsciousness if cerebral perfusion is not maintained.

The ATLS classification of hypovolaemic shock has been graded from level 1 to 4 depending on ranges of heart rate, blood pressure and Glasgow Coma Scale (GCS) with approximate blood loss inferred from these three signs. This has been part of the ATLS course since 1980, but the validity of this concept (while attractive based on first principles) has not been established. A paper by Little et al. [6] from 1995 first explained why these measurements are imperfect in practice, and a more recent paper by Mutschler et al. [7] retrospectively reviewed the German Trauma Register and the UK TARN database with these measurements. They concluded that only 9.3% of all trauma patients could be allocated to one of the ATLS classifications based on their vital signs. Further, this classification may overestimate the degree of tachycardia and underestimate the degree of GCS impairment associated with hypovolaemic shock; i.e. patients may have lost more than the 40% of their circulating volume that classifies them as category 4 shock, but their vital signs are not as deranged as the ATLS classification suggests they should be. Young, fit patients may be more hypovolaemic than their vital signs suggest. This is before any other confounding factors are taken into consideration such as medications, age and other comorbidities, which may mean that patients have "abnormal" vital signs before they have any trauma inflicted on them. Classically ATLS and other courses teach that tachycardia is shock until proved otherwise and this is true. However, the corollary is not true—the absence of tachycardia does not mean the absence of shock. Consider an elderly, bleeding patient on regular beta-blockers who may be unable to mount a tachycardia or a triathlete with a very low resting heart rate. Both may be bleeding and in shock but have a heart rate of less than an arbitrarily defined 100 BPM. Thankfully there are other useful clinical signs of developing shock and failure of compensation mechanisms such as skin colour, capillary refill time and level of consciousness. For more information on this concept and specific examples, please refer to Chap. 37 (Silver Trauma).

Conscious level is particularly useful as a practical indicator of the level of brain perfusion. Tachycardia may be present and signify blood loss, but if the patient is coherent and not confused, then they are adequately perfusing their brain at present and may not warrant fluid resuscitation immediately, especially with crystalloids. This was the basis for US forces pre-hospital fluid resuscitation in recent conflicts in Iraq and Afghanistan. If the patient could recite their name, date of birth and serial number when asked, they were deemed to be adequately perfusing their brain and not given any fluids.

While previous editions of the ATLS course manual have given specific values for specific classes of shock, the 10th edition [8] has done away with these but retained a table illustrating the features associated with progressive shock. Other courses such as the European Trauma Course have done away with the classification altogether, and advocate multi-factorial assessment of shock on clinical, physiological and biochemical grounds such as lactate, pH and base deficit on arterial or venous blood gas analysis [9]. This is more in keeping with current practice, as the arbitrary division of patients into four groups which are not supported by data adds little if anything to their management. What is very clear is that while tachycardia is one indicator of shock, it should no longer be considered a 'target for resuscitation'. In other words, for a bleeding patient with a high heart rate, the traditional approach was to continue fluid resuscitation and avoid anaesthesia until the tachycardia has resolved, indicating that the patient was then "resuscitated". This approach is fundamentally flawed when a patient is still actively bleeding, and the high volumes of fluid required to "treat the tachycardia" will create even more severe problems and could even be fatal.

Another proposal which appeals to first principles is that as patients become progressively more hypotensive, peripheral pulses become impalpable at specific blood pressures. This is often quoted as a radial pulse requires a pressure of ≥80 mmHg, femoral ≥70 mmHg and carotid ≥60 mmHg. The presence of a palpable peripheral or central pulse in itself is a reasonable generalised indicator of adequate perfusion [10, 11] and the radial > femoral > carotid pressures appear to hold clinically. However there is no reproducible evidence that the presence of a specific pulse equates to a specific blood pressure, and this approach may overestimate blood pressure [12, 13].

Metabolic Assessment of Shock

While clinical signs may give a trend of decline or response to therapy and extreme values may be useful in defining severe forms of shock, as discussed, vital signs are not entirely reliable in assessing some patients. The metabolic consequences of shock may be apparent before clinical signs develop, or before young and fit patients (who make up a large proportion of trauma patients) exhaust their reserve and start to decompensate. No one test will accurately, consistently and infallibly predict major haemorrhage, shock, the need for mass transfusion or adequate resuscitation early [14]. While the below tests, their basis, merits and current evidence are discussed, having multiple data points to correlate and interpret in the context of both mechanism of injury and physiological signs is far more useful.

pH and Base Excess/Deficit

Base excess is defined as the relative amount of acid or alkali that must be added to each litre of fully oxygenated blood to return the pH to 7.40 at a temperature of 37 °C once the effect of carbon dioxide dissolved in the blood has been accounted for and normalised to 5.3 kPa [15]. Carbon dioxide is an acidic gas which dissociates into H^+ and HCO_3 in water in a reaction catalysed by carbonic anhydrase, so changes in the amount of CO_2 in the blood will subsequently cause a change in pH. The more CO_2 present, the more dissociation occurs and the lower the pH, purely from the effect of CO_2. Of course, CO_2 is not the only contributor to pH, and metabolic acids and alkalis may have a more significant role depending on how much is present. By calculating the amount of H^+ present due to CO_2 dissociation and subtracting it from the total acid burden, whatever remains must be the degree of acidity or alkalinity which is due to metabolic rather than respiratory causes. The usual range of base excess or deficit is +2.0 to −2.0 MEq/l, and values below −2 indicate an excess of metabolic acids, and values above +2 indicate an excess of alkali (base).

To be explicit, base deficit and base excess are corollary measurements of the same thing—a negative base excess means that there is more metabolic acid present and is the same as a positive base deficit. This occasionally is not clear from reading some physiology textbooks and has been a cause of some confusion when teaching this subject clinically. For the avoidance of confusion, this text will refer to base excess only when discussing this area.

In trauma, base excess is used as a surrogate marker of perfusion, as hypoperfusion (assumed to be from haemorrhage and/or tissue ischaemia) causes the production of acidic metabolites. The use of base excess to quantify hypoperfusion and infer haemorrhage has been studied in several papers and found to have better discriminatory value than the physiological parameters described in ATLS [16]. Whilst purists will state that base excess must be drawn from an arterial sample (which may be more challenging in hypovolaemic trauma patients), there are data that base excess calculated from venous samples is at least as sensitive (if not better) than arterial samples as a marker of shock and predictor of survival [17]. It has been hypothesised that this is due to post-capillary acid-base balance being a better marker of tissue perfusion than arterial measurements [18], and also that changes occur earlier (at least in animal models) in the venous circulation in haemorrhage than in the arterial [19]. The more severe the hypoperfusion, the larger the base deficit. The Mutschler paper referenced above stratified patients into four groups based on base excess—no shock (BE $\leq$ 2.0), mild shock (BE > 2–6.0), moderate shock (BE > 6–10.0) and severe shock (BE > 10). These groups showed a linear progression in terms of transfusion requirements, lactate levels, morbidity and mortality when their outcomes and length of ICU and hospital stay were followed up. This is an important paper as it was a retrospective analysis of over 16,000 patients in the German Trauma Register, which correlated with similar findings from the UK TARN database.

While there is a role for arterial blood gasses in the assessment of the adequacy of oxygenation and ventilation in trauma [20], a venous blood gas taken at the time of initial venipuncture can give reliable and actionable prognostic results in minutes. Clinical pitfalls in interpretation are similar to those around lactate measurement as described below, but also other causes of an increased base deficit can interfere with clinical interpretation.

A comparatively recent change in the understanding of pH is the Stewart model of acid-base balance [21] which looks at the concentration of strong and weak ions in a solution and their effect on pH. A full explanation of this model is impractical in this textbook, suffice to say that the contribution of ions other than H^+ and OH^- are essential in determining pH and subsequently base excess. Amongst these strong ions are Cl^-, Na^+, lactate, Ca^{2+}, proteins, Mg^{2+}, K^+ and albumin—all of which may be deranged or administered at some point in resuscitation and consequently have a knock-on effect on pH and base deficit. For example, giving “normal” 0.9% or hypertonic saline will increase the concentration of Cl^- ions, which under the Stewart model will lower the strong ion difference and subsequently cause a hyperchloraemic metabolic acidosis [22, 23]. This has been verified in clinical publications [24] and a corresponding decrease in this effect when balanced salt solutions such as Plasmalyte, Hartmann’s solution or Ringer’s Lactate are used [25]. It has been suggested that this translates to an increased rate of adverse effects such as blood transfusion requirement and ventilator days in at least one meta-analysis [26]. While base deficit may be an accurate reflection of perfusion on admission, if large volumes of saline are given, then this may lead to clinical decisions being made on iatrogenic complications rather than evolving pathology. This is yet another argument against crystalloid resuscitation generally, but thoughtless administration of saline solutions specifically. While there is a role for hypertonic saline in the role of brain-injured patients (see Chap. 11 - Disability and head injury), in a well-resourced centre there is no role for 0.9% saline as a resuscitation fluid for acute trauma. In more austere environments where blood and blood products are not readily available, 0.9% saline could be considered in the minimum amount necessary in accordance with permissive hypotension and damage control strategies if it is all that is available [27]. One redeeming feature is that while Hartmann’s and Ringer’s solutions are mildly hypotonic and could theoretically worsen cerebral oedema in brain-injured patients, 0.9% saline is theoretically isotonic so should not cause this issue.

Lactate

As tissue perfusion becomes impaired, oxygen-starved tissues may revert to anaerobic respiration and produce lactate as a result. The initial lactate on presentation has been found to correlate with mortality and the need for operative intervention, and the subsequent clearance of lactate at 6 h is an independent predictor of mortality [28, 29]. Lactate in itself is a misunderstood entity at times; high serum lactate levels are occasionally the source of concern for many healthcare staff, but lactate is an intrinsically biologically useful molecule. It can be used as an energy substrate by the brain, heart and kidneys and may act to mitigate against acidosis by acting as a "shuttle" to mop up hydrogen ions in anaerobic tissue and transfer them to aerobic tissue, where ATP can be produced more efficiently than by glycolysis [30]. Lactate has been found to improve cardiac output [31] in addition to being the primary energy substrate of injured brain and may be neuroprotective [32, 33]. Lactate has also been shown to be superior to the base deficit when assessing the initial severity of trauma [34]. Caution is advised though as high lactate levels automatically equating to hypoperfusion is not a universal truth; specific pathology, normal physiology and some therapeutic agents can raise lactate levels. For example, a runner who falls and twists his ankle may have a high lactate level from exercise if it is checked acutely—he is a trauma patient who is not bleeding but will have a high lactate. Similarly, patients who have brain parenchymal injury or high brain glucose usage may have slightly raised lactate as a consequence of acute lactate release from an outward brain: blood lactate gradient, though this effect is more likely to be localised and small [35]. Finally, patients who have been given beta-agonists such as salbutamol or adrenaline will also have a raised lactate due to the pharmacological action of these agents—it does not mean they are hypoperfused.

Haemoglobin

Traditional teaching is that haemoglobin does not correlate with acute blood loss as the blood that is lost has the same haemoglobin concentration as the blood that stays in the body, i.e. the total volume of blood decreases but the measured haemoglobin concentration remains the same because whole blood is lost. This is undoubtedly true in hyperacute haemorrhage at the initial point of injury and the immediate post-injury minutes, but physiological compensation may have started by the time the pre-hospital team reach the patient. A study by Bruns et al. [36] looked at the initial haemoglobin concentration taken within 30 min of arrival in the emergency department and correlated this with physical and biochemical signs of blood loss and ultimately the need for urgent interventions to stop haemorrhage. There was a small but statistically significant difference in average presenting haemoglobin concentrations in patients who required urgent intervention compared to those who did not (mean of 12 g/dl ± 2 g/dl in those requiring intervention versus 13 g/dl ± 2 g/dl in those who did not). What was noted was that a presenting haemoglobin concentration of less than 10 g/dl was associated with over a threefold increase in the need for haemostatic intervention. A similar (but more extensive and multi-centre) study was undertaken in France in 2018 by Figureiredo et al. [37]. Enrolling over 6400 patients, this study went further and compared sequential pre-hospital and in-hospital blood results on the point of care testing machines with against a formal laboratory sample on arrival in hospital. The volume of crystalloid given (which may have contributed to an iatrogenic dilutional anaemia) was taken into account in the analysis, and again similar results were found. A pre-hospital haemoglobin concentration of less than 12 g/dl in women or 13 g/dl in men was modestly predictive for significant haemorrhage (defined as requiring ≥ four units of blood or death within 24 h attributable to exsanguination). In hospital, the same point of care test could discriminate between those who had a significant haemorrhage, though the cut off points dropped to 10 g/dl for women and 12 g/dl for men. This is presumably as a result of a combination of ongoing haemorrhage, physiological compensation by drawing fluid from the periphery into the circulating volume and as a result of crystalloid administration. Of note, the point of care device was as sensitive as a formal laboratory result but without the wait for processing. A drop in haemoglobin concentration between pre- and in-hospital point of care testing of 2 g/dl or more was also predictive of significant haemorrhage. Patients who required IV fluids for hypotension with significant haemorrhage were also compared to those who were hypotensive and also required IV fluids but did not meet the definition of significant haemorrhage. It was found that for the same amount of fluid administration, there was a significantly higher drop in the haemoglobin concentration of those who had significant haemorrhage than those who were not bleeding as severely.

Other Biomarkers

There has been much interest in the use of biomarkers in conditions such as sepsis to identify and treat patients early, and trauma is no different. Most research has been done in animal models and identified specific proteins or other biomarkers which may be up- or down-regulated in response to trauma, and potential treatments such as valproic acid [38, 39]. What is not known is whether these markers are specific for trauma, whether treatment is effective for mitigating the underlying cause of the rise, whether they will have cross-species validity or whether they would be part of a practical and timely laboratory test that could be used to guide management in these patients. It has not stopped early development and patent applications for the use of these biomarkers [40]. There are currently no other specific predictive biomarkers in routine clinical use other than the ones explored above, though this may be an area for development in the future.

Hypotension in Trauma

While hypotension is a manifestation of shock, the modality of treatment of hypotension can have significant impacts on mortality. While the idea of having a specific number to target seems appealing, several factors interact to make this a complex treatment decision. Should hypotension be treated at all? If so, with fluids or vasopressors? Which ones and when? Is there a role for antifibrinolytic agents such as tranexamic acid?

History of Permissive Hypotension

Permissive hypotension is a concept which appears to have been rediscovered at the start of every major conflict in the twentieth century, but thankfully is now being accepted as the standard of care in trauma. W B Cannon first described it in World War One [41], amongst many other fascinating discoveries that seem to have been largely forgotten for the better part of a century. Cannon also described acidosis in hypoperfused states, observations on raised blood pressure in severe head injuries that are consistent with current interpretations of cerebral perfusion pressure and the deleterious effects of hypothermia on trauma patients [42]. A professor of physiology at Harvard University, Cannon volunteered to be a field investigator at a casualty clearing station in Bethune, France and was appointed the president of the Red Cross medical research society in November 1917. He was a shrewd observer and documenter of observations and encouraged the publication of case reports as a learning tool. In his 1918 paper The Preventive Treatment of Wound Shock [42], he advised caution in administering IV fluids to shocked patients without the facility to achieve surgical haemostasis:

> Injection of a fluid that will increase blood pressure carries danger in itself. Haemorrhage in the case of shock may not have occurred to a large degree because the blood pressure is too low, and the flow too scant to overcome the obstacle offered by a clot. If the pressure is raised before the surgeon is ready to check any bleeding that may take place, blood that is sorely needed may be lost.

This lesson was forgotten after the war but re-emerged with the advent of World War 2 and further combat casualties. Lt Col Henry Beecher in his 1945 publication Preparation of Battle Casualties for Surgery [43] argued that a systolic blood pressure of 85 mmHg was adequate and that the minimum amount of plasma should be given to achieve this aim. He also advanced the idea that resuscitation should continue during

surgery rather than operate late (as was the preferred French and Italian model at the time)—a concept integral to what we now consider Damage Control Resuscitation. Again, this lesson appeared to be lost after the conflict ended. Patients who presented to medical treatment facilities during the Vietnam and Falklands conflicts often survived for prolonged periods with low blood pressure, before being "resuscitated" with large volumes of crystalloid and dying of their injuries. It was not until 1994 when Bickell et al. published a prospective trial showing improved survival, fewer complications and decreased length of hospital stay in patients who had delayed fluid resuscitation while hypotensive from penetrating abdominal trauma [44]. From then, the direction of research and current practise has been to understand what blood pressure to tolerate before intervention, what intervention to perform and when.

Permissive Hypotension as a Concept

A baseline understanding of the first principles and pathophysiology of bleeding is essential when discussing strategies for treating haemorrhage-induced hypotension. If bleeding occurs and a significant amount of circulating volume is lost, the ventricular pre-load drops. In turn, this drops the stroke volume, and the cardiac output is initially maintained or slightly increased by a compensatory tachycardia. Eventually, if there is enough blood loss and decompensation occurs, the cardiac output will drop and the blood pressure will also decrease (even if circulating catecholamines cause an increase in the SVR). This low blood pressure reduces the flow of blood to peripheral tissues, and the hypoperfusion causes the raised lactate referred to earlier (with the already expressed caveats).

At this point, the hydrostatic pressure of the blood in the vessels drops, and circulating factors may be able to form a clot over the bleeding vessel temporarily sealing it. Two important points need highlighting—firstly, this clot has formed under the best possible circumstances in terms of the amount of available circulating clotting factors, temperature, pH and presence of cofactors such as calcium. Secondly, at this point the clot is immature and vulnerable to breakdown by either rough handling of the patient or further increases in the hydrostatic pressure in the injured vessel, e.g. by administering fluids. The ethos behind permissive hypotension is to protect this clot while it matures and prevents further bleeding while maintaining an acceptable degree of end-organ perfusion. To reiterate—while the patients' blood pressure is not normal, if there is adequate perfusion to vital organs then this should be tolerated until definitive haemostasis can be assured. If the pressure continues to fall, then the resuscitative target should be to restore an adequate blood pressure only, not a normal one. This is usually defined as a systolic pressure of approximately 80–90 mmHg and is mostly pragmatic and based on entrance criteria of trials of liberal vs restrictive fluid resuscitation in trauma. An editorial on the concept of permissive hypotension from Nevin and Brohi appeared in Anaesthesia in December 2017 and is well worth reading for a more comprehensive overview [45].

More recent work has looked at the effect of permissive hypotension over a prolonged period and concluded that (in animal models at least) prolonged permissive hypotension can lead to increased morbidity and mortality. The approach trialled in animal models by Doran et al. is 'Hybrid' or 'targeted' resuscitation [46]. This aims to offer the best compromise between prolonged hypotension and overly aggressive resuscitation. It is based on the principle that it is not blood pressure that matters, but rather blood 'flow' and perfusion of tissues as described above.

The following recommendations were made:

- Maintain a Systolic BP of 80 mmHg for the first hour of care
- Increase the systolic BP to 110 mmHg after this period even if definitive haemostasis has not been achieved
- Then fully restore normotension with blood and blood products once definitive control has been secured.

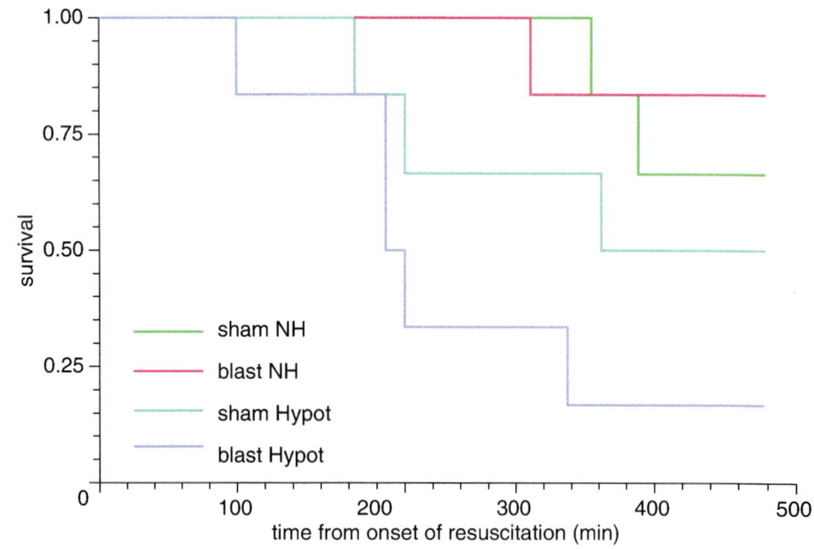

Fig. 10.6 Effect of Novel Hybrid resuscitation compared to hypotensive resuscitation (From *Kirkman E, Watts S, Cooper G. Blast injury research models. Philos Trans R Soc Lond B Biol Sci. 2011 Jan 27;366(1562):144–59*)

By doing this the overall extent of the shock is reduced, base deficit improved, the degree of coagulopathy and systemic inflammation reduced and this may well be the kind of best compromise approach that will be adopted in future years.

When this approach was applied to a blast model in rats [47], survival was significantly improved in the group that had a short period of permissive hypotension followed by slow resuscitation to normotension (Blast NH), rather than prolonged hypotensive resuscitation (Blast Hypot), until bleeding was adequately controlled (see Fig. 10.6).

Whether or not this can be applied to human cases is still not clear, but the animal work does suggest promising results. However, this further confirms that the shorter the period of hypotensive 'hit' the better, but this has to be balanced against how it is corrected. Merely filling the actively bleeding casualty with any available resuscitation fluid is potentially a greater risk.

This is a complicated picture requiring some compromises and caution, and a single definitive solution is unlikely ever to exist. When considering the other effects of shock, the picture becomes even more complicated. However, some interventions have been demonstrated to worsen outcome and should be avoided:

- Excessive volumes of resuscitation fluid while still bleeding
- Delays in achieving control of bleeding
- Prolonged or extreme shock

Cyclic Hyper-resuscitation and Crystalloids

Before permissive hypotension was accepted, traditional teaching was to aggressively treat hypotension by the administration of a fluid challenge—usually 2000 ml of a crystalloid solution such as Hartmann's or Ringer's lactate. The thinking behind this approach was that by restoring a normal blood pressure, the flow of blood to the vital organs would be restored and the patient stabilised so they were in the best possible condition for an operative prcedure. In some cases, the timing of operations would depend on whether the patient was a responder or non-responder to the initial administration of fluids. From the perspective of having an endpoint to target and assess against, it is easy to see why this approach was undertaken. It does, however, have several flaws which have been discovered as research has progressed. Consider the above emphasis on clot protection and preservation—by increasing the blood pressure with crystalloids, hydrostatic pressure increases and stress on any clot which has formed increases. This may cause the clot to rupture and cause further bleeding and hypotension (sometimes referred to colloquially as "pop-

ping the clot"). Once the blood pressure decreases to its previous level, a clot may form again to prevent further haemorrhage. However, the problem with this is that the second clot that forms may not be as strong as the first for several reasons. Firstly, the initial clot was formed under the best conditions with the highest number of clotting factors available, and many of these factors and cofactors may have been consumed in the production of the first clot. As a result, the formation of a subsequent clot (if possible) may start with 50% or less of the available clotting factors used in the first purely from a consumptive perspective. Secondly, the action of giving a 2000 ml crystalloid bolus will dilute the remaining clotting factors and cofactors that are present further and impair their effectiveness. Thirdly, as a result of further bleeding from the clot being disrupted (and more often than not the 2000 ml bolus not being as warm as body temperature), the patients' temperature falls, decreasing the efficiency of the enzymatic systems involved in forming a clot. Finally, as crystalloid has no oxygen-carrying capacity it cannot intrinsically improve the delivery of oxygen to tissues (other than by a transient rise in stroke volume/cardiac output which is subsequently offset by deleterious effects), and so hypoperfusion and acidosis worsen, causing a decrease in plasma pH which adds a second hit to the function of enzymatic-dependent clotting.

If the patient is fortunate enough to be able to form a second clot despite being replete of coagulation factors, cold, acidotic and having suffered further bleeding, they will be hypotensive. This may trigger further crystalloid resuscitation and the downward spiral continues in the same manner until no clot can be formed, with the patient bleeding to death if surgical control cannot be achieved. This repeated pattern of hypotension, crystalloid administration and further bleeding has been termed cyclic hyper-resuscitation and should be avoided [48]. Even if the patient survives to the intensive care unit, administration of large volumes of crystalloid has been associated with the development of Adult Respiratory Distress Syndrome (ARDS), abdominal compartment syndrome and the worsening of pulmonary contusions if present [49–54]. Another paper by Sharpe et al. [55] compared high and low ratios of crystalloid to blood products in resuscitation acutely and concluded that there was no appreciable difference between the strategies in terms of mortality. This paper raises a couple of methodological questions, as the range of crystalloid doses in the high ratio group (1000–11,000 ml, mean of 4000 ml) compared to the low group (500–8200 ml mean of 1300 ml) does not appear significantly different and the low ratio group had a higher amount of HES administered in their initial resuscitation. The volumes of crystalloids given in both groups appear at first glance to be excessive, but even in this paper there is a statistically significant difference in the rate of development of ARDS!

Fluid Therapy in Trauma

While some patients may develop hypotension, form a clot and maintain an acceptable blood pressure, many may not and will require some degree of fluid resuscitation in order to get to the point of definitive haemorrhage control. The question then becomes "which fluid should be given"? Crystalloid solutions do not transport oxygen and excess administration causes further bleeding, hypothermia, dilution of clotting factors and ARDS as previously described, so the alternatives become colloids or blood products.

Colloids

Colloids are large molecules that exert an osmotic pressure and theoretically stay in the circulation and exert their effects for longer than crystalloids. The most common colloids in recent clinical use are dextrans, modified gelatine or starches. Blood is technically a colloid, but in this textbook, blood is considered a separate entity and the use of the word "colloid" refers exclusively to non-blood, non-crystalloid resuscitative solutions.

An often-quoted rule from historic ATLS teaching is "3:1"—students are often told that giving a bolus of colloid is the equivalent of giving three times the amount of crystalloid for the same haemodynamic effect. In terms of mitigating the effects of excessive volume, this would seem a good solution between the deleterious effects of crystalloid and the risks and expense of blood transfusion if it is not necessary. The problem lies in the fact that this is an urban myth—the actual ratio is only somewhere between 1:1.3 and 1:1.6 [27, 56–60]. Moreover, a Cochrane review [61] showed no evidence of benefit in using colloids over crystalloids in the resuscitation of patients following burns, trauma or surgery and that the use of hydroxyethyl starch (HES) may increase mortality in these patients. A further review which excluded papers which had been retracted because of research fraud further condemned HES as it showed an increase in mortality and acute kidney injury in comparison to other resuscitation solutions [62]. As some colloids are modified gelatine proteins they also carry a risk of provoking anaphylaxis in susceptible patients [63]. They are also more expensive to produce than crystalloids, and with no overall benefit demonstrated, it is difficult to justify their continued use in clinical practice.

Synthetic Oxygen Carriers

An off-the-shelf, oxygen-carrying solution which does not need to be cross-matched, stored under certain constrictive conditions, is cheap to produce and with few serious side effects is considered the Holy Grail of trauma resuscitation fluids. The morbidity and mortality from blood transfusions like acute transfusion reactions, mismatched blood groups, the passage of blood-borne diseases before the advent of effective screening and immunologically mediated problems such as Transfusion Related Acute Lung Injury is not insignificant. Because of the lack of an alternative solution, these complications remain a risk of this life-saving therapy. Efforts have rightly been made to reduce the risk by focussing on systems and reporting to minimise it as much as possible. If a synthetic drug were produced that could perform the same function as even just haemoglobin as opposed to the clotting aspects of blood, that would be game-changing. The current mortality in the USA from a blood transfusion in isolation is currently estimated as 2.3 deaths for every 1 million component units transfused [64]. Some improvements have been made due to the evolution of reporting networks such as the annual SHOT (Serious Hazards of Transfusion) report in the UK [65] and subsequent changes in practice. One example is the use of male-only FFP in transfusions in the UK due to a recognised increase in immune-mediated complications when female plasma is used. However, sidestepping these issues altogether with a synthetic product would be much preferred.

There has been much research done on synthetic haemoglobins and perfluorocarbons over the last 25–30 years, but the results have not been promising. Only one perfluorocarbon has been approved for use in humans by the FDA since research began (Fluosol-DA-20 in 1989), but it was withdrawn 5 years later due to side effects ranging from transient hypertension to myocardial infarction, arrhythmias and death. Notably, one of the main drivers for the development of haemoglobin substitutes was for patients with haemoglobinopathies such as sickle cell disease rather than trauma, and there has yet to be any agents approved for use internationally for any indication.

Hemopure has been approved in South Africa for treatment of acutely anaemic adult surgical patients, but despite trials in other countries, it has not been accepted into mainstream practice. There have been some phase three clinical trials of using synthetic haemoglobins in trauma or emergency surgery that were small scale but initially positive [66, 67], though these were conducted by the product manufacturers (PolyHeme from Northfield Laboratories). A recent review by Ferenz and Steinbicker [68] has highlighted many of the outstanding issues with synthetic haemoglobins from clinical and pre-clinical trials from 2013 to 2018. It is an interesting article, highlighting issues around the short lifespan of products, side effects, inflammatory reactions, difficulties in either loading or unloading oxygen appropriately and different approaches to solving these problems. The takeaway message, however, is that while research in this field is ongoing and making some progress, it will likely be many years before these products make it to market, or the medical literature advances much beyond case studies and small trial series. An alternate source of blood may be from mass production or manufacture from stem cells. There is work in progress at DARPA, though the cost is currently prohibitively high to scale up. Currently, each unit of blood costs £30,000 to produce [69] in comparison to £120–150 per unit of cross-matched blood in the UK. Twenty-five years in the future this may be an option as production costs decrease and scale increases, but it is not yet a viable option.

Blood Transfusions in Trauma

Blood has a distinct advantage over all other transfusion fluids in that it delivers oxygen to tissues in addition to expanding volume. While red blood cells will increase oxygen-carrying capacity, if given in isolation, then they will also dilute clotting factors that are present. Interestingly, more and more research has shown that red blood cells themselves are essential components in haemostasis due to their adhesion to endothelial cells and platelets and their ability to generate thrombin [70, 71], with anaemia increasing bleeding times [72]. A full discussion of the role of blood transfusion in trauma and the management of trauma-associated coagulopathy is found in Chap. 15 (Haemostasis and coagulopathy) later in this textbook. Suffice it to say the best strategy is to preserve as much of the patient's blood as possible (including the use of cell salvage where possible), and replace blood with blood—either by units of whole blood or balanced component therapy. Ultimately, blood transfusion aims to promote the delivery of oxygen to tissues (otherwise known as DO_2). This is dependent on two factors—the cardiac output and the oxygen content of arterial blood that reaches the tissues.

Oxygen Content of Blood

This content is principally due to the amount of haemoglobin present in the blood, but there is also a small amount of oxygen dissolved in plasma itself. The overall formula for calculating DO_2 is, therefore:

$$DO_2 = CO \times CaO_2$$

Where CO is cardiac output and CaO_2 is the oxygen content of arterial blood that is being delivered to the tissues. This can be expanded into individual components further by examining what constitutes the oxygen content of the blood.

The fully expanded equation is seen if Fig. 10.7, where:

- [Hb] = Concentration of haemoglobin in grams per deciliter (g/dl)
- 1.34 = Hüfner's constant—the amount of oxygen carried by fully saturated haemoglobin (1.39 ml O_2/g Hb is the theoretical maximum, but in direct measurement, the maximum is 1.34)
- SpO_2 = Percentage arterial O_2 saturation
- PaO_2 = arterial oxygen tension in kilopascals (kPa)
- 0.023 = amount of oxygen in ml dissolved per 100 ml of plasma per kPa

It can be seen that the most significant determinant of oxygen content in the blood is haemoglobin concentration. The amount of oxygen dissolved in plasma is itself a minor contributor, and assuming a patient is on 100% dry oxygen, with maximum efficiency in metabolism with a normal $PaCO_2$ of 5 kPa, the theoretical maximum amount of oxygen that could be dissolved is only 2.19 ml O_2/100 ml plasma In contrast, by increasing the haemoglobin concentration by only 1.6 g by the administration of just over 1 unit of blood to an average adult, the same raise in CaO_2 can be achieved while still breathing room air. The dissolved concentration of oxygen rarely makes a

$$DO_2 = CO \times (([Hb] \times 1.34 \times SpO_2 \times 0.01) + PaO_2 \times 0.023)$$

Fig. 10.7 The oxygen delivery equation

significant contribution to DO_2 overall, as physiologically a PaO_2 of 11–13 is a normal value, giving a dissolved oxygen concentration of 0.25 ml O_2/100 ml blood, in comparison to 1 g of 100% oxygenated blood which transports 1.34 ml O_2/100 ml blood, i.e. 5.36 times more. This dissolved fraction only tends to be physiologically significant when there is severe lung damage or exceptionally high oxygen demand, and a high FiO_2 is required.

Cardiac Output, Blood Pressure and Flow

As previously discussed, cardiac output is the product of the stroke volume and heart rate. When this is combined with systemic vascular resistance, it determines the blood pressure. While physiological first principles are sound and give a good mental model of how the circulatory system works, there are a few other factors to consider when discussing oxygen delivery to tissues outside of gross systemic models. The flow of oxygenated blood to tissues is the important measure, and there are a couple of factors which may affect flow rather than blood pressure. Examining the mathematical model described at the start of the chapter, by increasing SVR (causing vasoconstriction) blood pressure is increased. While blood pressure is a driving force for perfusion, downstream vasoconstriction may decrease the flow of blood in hypovolaemic states and subsequently decrease DO_2. The reason for this is that the Hagen-Poiseuille equation governs laminar flow:

$$Q \propto \frac{\Delta P \pi r^4}{8 \eta l}$$

Where:

Q = Flow
P = Driving pressure
r = radius of the tube
η = Viscosity
l = length of tubing

As the factor with the greatest influence in terms of flow is the radius of the tube (as it is raised to the fourth power), it is therefore obvious why peripheral vasoconstriction decreases flow. Mathematically, doubling the radius of the tube (or in this case, blood vessel) and keeping everything else the same will increase flow by a factor of 16 times. This relationship is also why having short, large-bore IV access in patients who may require large amounts of blood products is preferable to smaller access. The rest of the equation is also important to consider. There needs to be a driving pressure (P) in order to have flow into a vessel, so in most cases adequate filling is necessary to achieve this by increasing preload and stroke volume. Flow rate is inversely proportional to viscosity, so thicker solutions such as FFP and red blood cells may not be as quickly transfused as crystalloids through the same IV access due to this. There is also a slight evolutionary advantage, however. When a patient bleeds and their haemoglobin levels fall, the blood becomes less viscous and flow improves as a consequence. As flow improves, DO_2 must also become more efficient, and this may possibly be why management in ICU of patients with a haemoglobin level of 7 g/dl is sufficient. Current practice is to avoid transfusion above this threshold unless there is a history of ischaemic heart disease [73, 74]. It must be pointed out that this strategy in acute blood loss does not work—if a patient presents with a haemoglobin of 7 g/dl before intervention, then they are bleeding and require resuscitation with blood and blood products, not crystalloid. After achieving definitive haemostasis and restoring an adequate circulating volume with blood products, there may be a role for crystalloids on ICU. One pitfall to point out is that when a patient arrives in ICU, they may not be adequately resuscitated and still have an ongoing requirement for blood products to catch up. This is not the time to employ a restrictive transfusion strategy or to use vasopressors/inotropes to correct a low blood pressure caused by undertreated hypovolaemia. Inappropriate use of vasopressors in this group of patients may increase mortality by at least 200% [75–78].

Blood Components or Warm Fresh Whole Blood?

As blood is usually split into its component fractions (red blood cells, fresh frozen plasma and platelets) once it has been donated and cold-stored, there has been much debate over the effectiveness of how best to use blood. Questions posed include the optimum ratio of blood products to administer to patients who are acutely bleeding [79], whether there is a difference in outcomes in patients administered blood stored for longer or shorter periods [80–82] and whether using warm fresh whole blood (WFWB) is superior to individual component therapy. The military experience of using warm fresh whole blood (WFWB) to resuscitate patients (i.e. taking a unit of blood from a walking donor panel and administering it without fractionation to a bleeding casualty [83]) has generally been positive. Small series reports and trial data have shown increased survival and decreased transfusion volume requirements over 24 h compared to component therapy [84–86]. The exact reasons for this are not entirely understood and this approach also throws up many questions on the effectiveness of troops who have donated blood whilst on deployment (though marksmanship [87] and cognitive performance [88] have been reported as being preserved or improved). Is WFWB intrinsically superior to fractionated components? Is the process of buddy-buddy donation between non-medically trained personnel safe? There are many aspects which need further consideration and research, not only in medical but also military spheres.

Practical Aspects of Blood Transfusion

A full exploration of the current state of evidence behind blood transfusion ratios is available in Chap. 15 (Haemostasis and coagulopathy), but there are some practical points which are worth following in managing blood transfusions in major trauma. Firstly, the time to review a mass transfusion policy is not the first time it is needed—a thorough stress testing of the policy should be undertaken well in advance of it being used in vivo. Simulation (and specifically in situ simulation) is a readily available tool to assess the weak points of policies. If a blinded exercise is undertaken by the people who may be expected to use a mass transfusion policy in real-time, there may be some surprising results. Unanticipated chokepoints can be elucidated [89], explored and improved on, and there are several ready-made scenarios which can be implemented to test departmental responses [90]. Investing a couple of hours in simulation and debriefing will pay dividends in the event of the mass transfusion policy being enacted. It is also vital to let blood bank know where to send products; if a mass transfusion has been declared and the patient moves from the emergency department to interventional radiology or the operating theatre then blood bank and portering staff should be made aware. If issues are identified in simulation, then these should be fed into the live organisational reporting system—no patients have been harmed but risks/problems may be identified which could lead to future harm. If these problems are not captured, they may well lead to actual morbidity or mortality in a live patient in future.

Secondly, make sure IV access is adequate and appropriate for what is needed. Per the Hagen-Poiseuille equation already mentioned, flow is optimum in wide and short tubes so IV access should be established with this in mind. When comparing flow rates through different devices in vitro in a paper by Khoyratty et al. [91] the Hagen-Poiseuille equation predicts the salient points. Peripheral access outperforms central lines of the same width, the use of a needle-free access device decreases flow rates in cannulae of 16G or larger (with or without pressured infusion), Rapid Infusion Catheters (RIC) are superior to 14G cannulae, and flow is improved when a pressure system is used to increase the rate in all devices. These findings are similar to papers by Reddick et al. from 2011 [92] and Wrenn et al. from 2017 [93], reinforcing the basic principle of IV access being short, wide and peripheral in the first instance.

Third, several mnemonics can be used to prepare a patient and team for a mass transfusion and trauma anaesthetic (see TRAUMATIC and POLYTRAUMAS examples, above in Figs. 10.8 and 10.9 respectively). Use of cognitive aids should be encouraged as any tool which can increase the use of evidence-based practice and the available cognitive bandwidth to deal with complex trauma are undoubtedly a good thing [94, 95]. It is crucial, however, to consider how

Major Trauma?
Major Haemorrhage? Then...

T	**Tranexamic Acid**	• Initial 1g bolus: • Often already given pre-hospital • Otherwise, administer only if within 3 hours of injury or ongoing hyperfibrinolysis • Do not delay, every minute counts • Subsequent 1g infusion over 8 hours
R	**Resuscitation**	• Activate Major Haemorrhage Protocol • Initial Transfusion Ratio 1:1:1 and consider: • Rapid infuser and cell salvage • Time limited hypotensive resuscitation • Pelvic binder / splint fractures / tourniquet • Avoid any crystalloid use
A	**Avoid Hypothermia**	• Target temperature > 36°C • Increase ambient theatre temperature • Remove wet clothing and sheets • Warm all blood products & irrigation fluids • Warm the patient using forced-air warming device / blanket / mattress
U	**Unstable? Damage Control Surgery**	• If unstable, coagulopathic, hypothermic or acidotic, perform damage control surgery of: • Haemorrhage control, decompression, decontamination and splintage • Time surgery aiming to finish < 90mins and conduct Surgical Pauses at least every 30mins
M	**Metabolic**	• Perform regular blood gas analysis • Base excess and lactate guide resuscitation • Adequate resuscitation corrects acidosis • If lactate > 5mmol/L or rising, consider stopping surgery, splint and transfer to ICU • Haemoglobin results are misleading
A	**Avoid Vasoconstrictors**	• Use of vasoconstrictors doubles mortality • However, use may be required in cases of spinal cord or traumatic brain injury • Anaesthetic induction - Suggest Ketamine • Maintenance - When BP allows, titrate high dose Fentanyl and consider Midazolam
T	**Test Clotting**	• Check clotting regularly to target transfusion: • Laboratory or point of care (TEG / ROTEM) • Aim platelets > 100×10^9/L • Aim INR & aPTTR ≤ 1.5 • Aim fibrinogen > 2g/L
I	**Imaging**	• Consider: • CT. Most severely injured / haemodynamically unstable patients gain most from CT • Interventional radiology
C	**Calcium**	• Maintain ionised Calcium > 1.0 mmol/L • Administer 10mls of 10% Calcium Chloride over 10 minutes, repeating as required • Monitor Potassium and treat hyperkalaemia with Calcium and Insulin / Glucose

Fig. 10.8 TRAUMATIC Aide Memoire for acute haemorrhage resuscitation (© L May, A Kelly and M Wyse, University Hospitals Coventry and Warwickshire)

Leeds Major Trauma Centre

CODE RED SURGERY

Actions to take when the decision has been made in the Emergency Department to transfer a POLYTRAUMA patient to the Operating Theatre for immediate surgery (CEPOD Category 1 Case).

P	**PREPARATION**	• Inform theatre team (surgeons, anaesthetic, Scrub Team, ODP, radiographer, runners, portering staff). Hold initial team brief. • Inform relevant staff of potential injuries and procedures that may occur • Surgical team to confirm which equipment/instruments required • Complete WHO Safter surgical checklist as able
O	**OSI TABLE**	• Identify appropriate OSI table with arm extensions to move to theatre
L	**LOCATION**	• Identify a suitable currently empty theatre if possible or next available theatre for list break if required. • Notify operating theatre to be utilised • Communicate destination theatre to Emergency Department, MTS nurse, blood bank and theatre team. • Inform ICU Bed Manager of need for post op bed (Bleep 2244)
Y, (I)	**INFUSIONS**	• 4 Infusion pumps with chargers to be made available in theatre • Rapid infuser to be set up and primed with minimal amount of warm saline • Set up large central access kit (Swan sheath, Vascath or trialysis line) and insertion pack • Run through a double transducer for arterial and central lines • Prepare a TXA maintenance infusion, 1g in 500ml 0.9% NaCl • Prepare 50ml 2% propofol infusion for post op transfer to ICU
T	**TEMPERATURE**	• Warm up theatre (Max T°C) • Locate and set up forced air warming system (Bair Hugger or equivalent) • Locate and turn on under body warming mattress (Inditherm or equivalent) • Ensure temperature probe (oesophogeal) is available
R	**RADIOLOGY**	• PACS Monitor logged on and relevant imaging displayed • If image intensifier required, contact radiographer (Bleep 1624/Extension 28356)
A	**AIRWAY**	• Prepare for in-theatre RSI if patient not intubated already • Difficult airway trolley available if required
U	**ULTRASOUND/ URINARY**	• Set up urinary catheter insertion kit • Ensure ultrasound available for lines etc if required
M	**MAJOR HAEMORRHAGE**	• Ensure blood bank is aware of patient if MH protocol has been/likely to be activated. • If MH in progress, ensure blood bank know which theatre to send blood to. • Aim for 1:1:1 transfusion and set up area for storing blood products and empty bags in theatre • Set up and allocate staff member to operate cell salvage system • Check coagulation - TEG and ABG every 30 minutes • Check tourniquet integrity prior to draping if in use, consider conversion to orthopaedic pneumatic tourniquets • Locate a box of 10% Calcium Chloride in the anaesthetic room and aim to administer 10ml for every 4 units of PRBC administered/maintain ionised Ca++ > 1.0
A	**ANAESTHESIA/ DRUGS**	• Anaesthetists to prompt SURGICAL PAUSE every 30 minutes to assess whether physiology permissive for further operating time. No damage control surgery should extend beyond 60-90 minutes operating time (including closure) • Have ketamine/rocuronium/fentanyl/thiopentone available • Draw up 10mg metaraminol in 20ml 0.9% NaCl • Consider appropriate antibiotics dependent on surgery
S	**SURGICAL EQUIPMENT**	• Set up surgical trolleys so kit readily accessible if required • Ligaclips and haemostatic agents (quick clot/Hemcon) available • Abdominal packs and warmed wash (12 x 0.9% NaCl) prepared

PLEASE SEE CODE RED FILE AND TRAUMATIC MNEMONIC FOR FURTHER DIRECTION

Fig. 10.9 POLYTRAUMAS Aide Memoire for ED-Theatre communication for emergency surgery (© B Rippin, K Lowery, P Lax, N Kanakaris, Leeds Teaching Hospitals NHS Trust)

these aids are designed as a poorly thought out tool may decrease performance [96]. NASA have produced guidelines on how to produce checklists which are based on experience and sound research methodology [97, 98], and work best when internally designed by the people who will use them rather than being externally imposed [99].

Fourth, having a dedicated clinician managing the mass transfusion is exceptionally useful [100, 101]. Due to the time needed for checking of blood, ensuring correct ratios of plasma, platelets, PRBCs and calcium, a dedicated anaesthetist or emergency medicine physician should be tasked to keep track of blood products administered as well as the practicalities of running a mass transfusion device such as a Belmont or Level 1. Practically, a count is best maintained by either a tally chart or keeping bags of transfused products in a set space and separating them by type for later documentation. Some centres have included a check box system in the blood boxes that are issued from the lab for units to be ticked off when administered to keep track. This allows the lead anaesthetist to concentrate on other aspects of resuscitation and request volume boluses as needed without having the additional cognitive burden of ensuring compliance with transfusion protocols.

Fifth, ensure that adequate amounts of calcium are given. A general rule of thumb is to try and keep the ionised calcium above 1.0 mmol/l on ABG testing. In cases where product administration is rapid due to ongoing loss and ABG's cannot be checked, give 10 ml of 10% calcium chloride for every four units of PRBCs or FFP that are administered. This should counteract the leaching effect of the sodium citrate that is used to preserve red blood cells and FFP, and an adequate calcium level is essential to ensure clotting. Calcium is also a positive inotrope and may contribute to increased blood pressure by increasing stroke volume. Calcium gluconate is not an ideal substitute in comparison to calcium chloride as it has approximately one-third of the amount of elemental calcium of calcium chloride, so three times the volume would be required for the same clinical effect [102]. Higher levels of calcium are also cardioprotective when dealing with hyperkalaemia which may be associated with muscle damage from trauma or massive transfusion itself [103, 104].

Sixth, give a 1 g tranexamic acid (TXA) bolus early, or 15 mg/kg in children—the same dose as paracetamol/acetaminophen. The CRASH-2 [105] and MATTERS [106] trials have been widely accepted as proof of decreased morbidity and mortality from bleeding if TXA is given within 3 h of injury. There have been a few unconvincing post-hoc analyses which have attempted to show an increase in thrombotic complications, but these mainly refer to administration outside the 3-h window or are methodologically flawed. The source data from CRASH-2 is open for public scrutiny and analysis. Professor Brohi has offered to collaborate and publish an analysis of the data with groups sceptical of the effect of TXA as long as he had a right of reply in the paper but has not yet been taken up on this offer.

Seventh, make use of near-patient testing of coagulation such as ROTEM or TEG devices where available. Both will give real-time indications of coagulation and may guide further blood product administration, and have been associated with lower overall transfusion requirements and may lead to improved mortality [107–109]. This is covered in more detail in the Chap. 15 (Haemostasis and coagulopathy).

Active Management of Circulatory Failure

In light of the complex state of the evidence base, some contradictory research and uncertainty on how to proceed, Revell, Porter and Greaves proposed a new UK consensus statement in 2002 [110] regarding the pre-hospital management of hypotension in trauma.

They stated that:

- Trauma victims with a radial pulse do not require fluid until haemostasis is achieved

- If a radial pulse is absent, then a 250 ml bolus of normal saline is given
- In penetrating torso trauma, the presence of a major pulse, e.g. femoral, is considered adequate

They went on to explain that this approach must be combined with rapid transfer to theatre or control of bleeding, but they did also identify some exceptional situations:

- Head injuries—they were unsure of what best evidence to recommend.
- Children—titration to a brachial pulse was recommended.

Shock is a pathological, abnormal physiological state, and every patient has varying degrees of tolerance of it. Even advocates of hypotensive resuscitation/delayed fluid resuscitation will accept that the limits of this strategy are not only defined by the level of the blood pressure, but also the duration of the shock.

In-Hospital On-Going Care

In-hospital, many of the fundamental principles remain the same such as the importance of rapid control of bleeding and preservation of circulating volume. The Task Force for Advanced Bleeding in Trauma was established in 2004 and publishes regular updates to the latest evidence, with the fifth edition published in 2019 [111].

The first iteration of the guidelines made some key recommendations, with the main beneficial factor that they identified in cases of severe haemorrhage was to achieve the shortest time to theatre.

They also highlighted the importance of circulation preservation with measures such as:

- Use of a damage control approach
- Early recognition of bleeding
- Pelvic stabilisation
- Consideration of early angiography and embolisation for pelvic bleeding
- A multi-disciplinary approach.

The latest critical messages from the 2019 guidelines are:

- Traumatically injured patients should be transported quickly and treated by a specialised trauma centre whenever possible.
- Measures to monitor and support coagulation should be initiated as early as possible and used to guide a goal-directed treatment strategy.
- A damage-control approach to surgical intervention should guide patient management.
- Coagulation support and thromboprophylaxis strategies should consider trauma patients who have been pre-treated with anticoagulants or platelet inhibitors.
- Local adherence to a multidisciplinary, evidence-based treatment protocol should serve as the basis of patient management and undergo regular quality assessment

Continuing the same key principles started in the pre-hospital arena, external bleeding should be controlled, excessive crystalloids should be avoided, and rapid assessments should be made before making decisions about ongoing care and moving forward to CT, theatre or interventional radiology.

Circulation preservation remains a key priority by whatever means necessary, and at this point, it should be noted that immobilisation devices such as pelvic binders or traction splints are considered part of 'C' for circulation management. Their application can significantly reduce ongoing blood loss and also reduce fracture movement and pain.

Finally, do not forget that simple measures such as 'gentle patient handling' can also have profound effects in terms of minimising further blood loss. The increased use of the scoop stretcher to reduce bleeding from log-rolling has little firm supporting evidence, but anecdotally it may reduce sudden internal blood loss and pain by avoiding the need for a full log-roll if appropriately used. If used badly with poor technique, however, it can result in two log-rolls in opposite directions to introduce the two halves of the scoop.

Others would argue that a 'log-roll' will have to be performed at some point to check the back of the patient thoroughly, and it can be performed without compromise once the pelvis is strapped. This is also controversial, as those that actively promote limited movement would suggest that the traditional rolling and checking of the back offers very little unless searching for wounds. Major trauma casualties almost invariably going through the CT scanner regardless, which should pick up back injuries far more effectively than simple examination.

As it stands at present, the scoop is favoured over the long-board by UK ambulance services, but there are concerns that this is being proposed as better in terms of its 'pressure area' risk when in reality, it is just another hard plastic board. Ultimately, a vacuum mattress or "vac-mat" is probably a far better device than both of these for the casualty, but this does have both cost and practical limitations. Movement of patients onto a vac-mat from a scoop when they arrive in hospital is possible and may minimise other additional movements before and during CT scan. It can also be used to minimise heat loss if the vac-mat is wrapped securely and has a heating or warmed blanket enclosed next to the patient's skin where possible.

Throughout the early time in the hospital, it is essential to look for any signs of ongoing uncontrolled bleeding. If identified, then this should be managed quickly and effectively to preserve the patient's circulation. Practitioners should not be over-reliant on the lab and transfused blood, as transfused blood will never be as good as the patient's own.

Brain Injury and Permissive Hypotension

Neurosurgeons would like normotension (or perhaps slight hypertension) and rapid delivery to their care within 4 h to optimise their outcome (see disability and head injury chapter for more information). The application of permissive hypotension in patients with concomitant brain injury is a compromise at best, and there is still no precise data to guide this approach despite several reviews and meta-analyses [112]. The best approach would undoubtedly be to deal with both severe haemorrhage and surgically amenable brain injury at the same operative sitting in a damage control approach, but outside a few centres of excellence in the world, this is rarely possible. Conventional wisdom is that active haemorrhage takes precedence over brain injury, but once bleeding is controlled, then blood pressure should be increased to maintain a cerebral perfusion pressure of 50–60 mmHg. The Brain Trauma Foundation Guidelines [113] are discussed in the disability and head injury chapter and form the mainstay of current treatment.

Damage Control Resuscitation

A damage control resuscitation and damage control surgical approach should be adopted, and the bleeding arrested in the shortest time possible. Once control has been achieved, circulating volume can be restored and the shock and hypoperfusion addressed (typically correcting the base deficit and lactate).

During damage control surgery, other factors will help to minimise further blood loss, including the use of a cell saver system, anti-fibrinolytic agents and other blood products such as FFP, platelets and cryoprecipitate.

In theatre during surgery, the temptation exists to reach for many of the numerous clinical devices traditionally associated with assessing resuscitation, cardiac output and hydration. In reality, few if any of these offer much value until bleeding is controlled and coagulopathy corrected.

Even relatively simple monitors such as arterial lines (often erroneously considered immediately essential) can delay transfer and definitive control of bleeding. Therefore, much as in in the pre-hospital domain, every action must be considered; is it appropriate and necessary to perform a procedure right now or will it introduce unnecessary delay?

Failure to Respond to Resuscitation

For some patients, attempts to maintain an ideal target MAP may fail, there may be continued deterioration and absence of a normal response to filling with blood or other fluids. Similarly, even after haemorrhage is controlled, it may remain difficult to improve the shocked state of the patient. This may be as a result of such rapid and massive bleeding that the volume loss has not been adequately replaced, there may be myocardial damage that is starting to manifest or the patient may be still falling further behind as a result of concealed or occult ongoing bleeding. There may be no response, inadequate response or even deterioration to any filling and then the prospect of a missed injury or intervention should be considered. These may include

Conditions which may mimic hypovolaemic shock

- Tension pneumothorax—ultrasound is quick and sensitive
- Cardiac tamponade—ultrasound could quickly reveal a tamponade
- Adrenal insufficiency or crisis—consider a dose of hydrocortisone
- Hypocalcaemia—especially after massive transfusion of stored blood and FFP/cryoprecipitate
- Hypoglycaemia—always check a blood sugar
- Spinal injury—mechanism, history, examination, CT

Summary

Shock and fluid resuscitation seem so simple if the circulation is merely considered as an empty bucket that needs re-filling, or a simple system of a pump, a fluid and connecting pipes. While it is an excellent theoretical analogy to understand the basic concepts of the circulatory system, it is a gross oversimplification in practice.

Filling patients to a normal blood pressure while still bleeding risks not only further bleeding, but also producing a wide range of severe side effects from the large volumes of resuscitation fluids, no matter what type is chosen. Every casualty will cope with blood loss and shock differently, and this is not merely down to cardiovascular fitness but a far broader concept of 'shock tolerance'.

Blood pressure is a poor marker in this respect as patients may have low blood pressure, but with adequate blood flow maintained. They may display few signs of under-perfusion while others may demonstrate worsening acidosis and increasing base deficit with minimal blood loss and no drop in blood pressure. The focus must still be circulation preservation and rapid haemostasis, usually with surgery or interventional radiology. Until this is achieved, permissive hypotension, minimal crystalloid use, blood and possibly hybrid resuscitation will all help to minimise complications and achieve the best chances of survival.

As yet, no synthetic alternative to blood has proved itself to a satisfactory degree, but they may be a panacea in future. Stem cell-produced blood cells or fresh whole blood are currently likely to offer better alternatives but are prohibitively expensive or unavailable in everyday practice.

Damage control resuscitation is a hugely complex challenge and requires excellent diagnostic and decision skills and continuous ongoing evaluation of patient physiology. It is not just filling a bucket, and there is a very challenging balance to achieve despite the large amount of research that has been completed.

Questions

1. Patients who present with a normal blood pressure by definition cannot have suffered significant hypovolaemia
   (a) True
   (b) False
2. Synthetic haemoglobins are commonly used in current practice
   (a) True
   (b) False

3. Permissive hypotension means actively lowering a patient's blood pressure to stop bleeding
   (a) True
   (b) False
4. The most important determinant of flow through resuscitative IV access is its diameter
   (a) True
   (b) False
5. All trauma patients should be given a 2000 ml fluid challenge as part of standard resuscitation
   (a) True
   (b) False

Answers

1. b
2. b
3. b
4. a
5. b

References

1. Lapner ST, Kearon C. Diagnosis and management of pulmonary embolism. BMJ. 2013;346:f757.
2. Yamamoto T. Management of patients with high-risk pulmonary embolism: a narrative review. J Intensive Care. 2018;6(1):16.
3. Kumar R, Sinha A, Lin MJ, Uchino R, Butryn T, O'Mara MS, et al. Complications of pericardiocentesis: a clinical synopsis. Int J Crit Illn Inj Sci. 2015;5(3):206–12.
4. Otsuka H, Sato T, Sakurai K, Aoki H, Yamagiwa T, Iizuka S, et al. Importance of the capability for complete resuscitative treatment combining surgery and interventional radiology for potentially lethal multiple injuries: a case report. Trauma Case Rep. 2017;11:13–7.
5. Chakraverty S, Zealley I, Kessel D. Damage control radiology in the severely injured patient: what the anaesthetist needs to know. Br J Anaesth. 2014;113(2):250–7.
6. Little RA, Kirkman E, Driscoll P, Hanson J, Mackway-Jones K. Preventable deaths after injury: why are the traditional 'vital' signs poor indicators of blood loss? Emerg Med J. 1995;12(1):1–14.
7. Mutschler M, Paffrath T, Wölfl C, Probst C, Nienaber U, Schipper IB, et al. The ATLS® classification of hypovolaemic shock: a well established teaching tool on the edge? Injury. 2014;45:S35–8.
8. American College of Surgeons, Committee on Trauma. Advanced trauma life support: student course manual. 10th ed. Chicago, IL: American College of Surgeons; 2018.
9. Goode P, Mountain A, Thies K, editors. The European Trauma Course Manual. 4.0. European Trauma Course Organisation; 2019. 164 p.
10. Duchesne JC, McSwain NE, Cotton BA, Hunt JP, Dellavolpe J, Lafaro K, et al. Damage control resuscitation: the new face of damage control. J Trauma Inj Infect Crit Care. 2010;69(4):976–90.
11. McManus J, Yershov AL, Ludwig D, Holcomb JB, Salinas J, Dubick MA, et al. Radial pulse character relationships to systolic blood pressure and trauma outcomes. Prehospital Emerg Care Off J Natl Assoc EMS Physicians Natl Assoc State EMS Dir. 2005;9(4):423–8.
12. Deakin CD. Accuracy of the advanced trauma life support guidelines for predicting systolic blood pressure using carotid, femoral, and radial pulses: observational study. BMJ. 2000;321(7262):673–4.
13. Poulton TJ. ATLS paradigm fails. Ann Emerg Med. 1988;17(1):107.
14. Porter JM, Ivatury RR. In search of the optimal end points of resuscitation in trauma patients: a review. J Trauma. 1998;44(5):908–14.
15. Kibble JD, Halsey CR. The big picture medical physiology [Internet]. New York: McGraw-Hill Medical; 2009. http://site.ebrary.com/id/10346923. Accessed 22 May 2019
16. Mutschler M, Nienaber U, Brockamp T, Wafaisade A, Fabian T, Paffrath T, et al. Renaissance of base deficit for the initial assessment of trauma patients: a base deficit-based classification for hypovolemic shock developed on data from 16,305 patients derived from the TraumaRegister DGU®. Crit Care. 2013;17(2):R42.
17. Wijaya R, Ng JH, Ong L, Wong ASY. Can venous base excess replace arterial base excess as a marker of early shock and a predictor of survival in trauma? Singapore Med J. 2016;57(2):73–6.
18. Rudkin SE, Kahn CA, Oman JA, Dolich MO, Lotfipour S, Lush S, et al. Prospective correlation of arterial vs venous blood gas measurements in trauma patients. Am J Emerg Med. 2012;30(8):1371–7.
19. Oropello JM, Manasia A, Hannon E, Leibowitz A, Benjamin E. Continuous fiberoptic arterial and venous blood gas monitoring in hemorrhagic shock. Chest. 1996;109(4):1049–55.
20. Schmelzer TM, Perron AD, Thomason MH, Sing RF. A comparison of central venous and arterial base deficit as a predictor of survival in acute trauma. Am J Emerg Med. 2008;26(2):119–23.
21. Stewart PA. Modern quantitative acid-base chemistry. Can J Physiol Pharmacol. 1983;61(12):1444–61.
22. Thomas R, Power KJ. Interpreting the base deficit. Anaesthesia. 2000;55(7):696–7.
23. Handy JM, Soni N. Physiological effects of hyperchloraemia and acidosis. Br J Anaesth. 2008;101(2):141–50.

24. Scheingraber S, Rehm M, Sehmisch C, Finsterer U. Rapid saline infusion produces hyperchloremic acidosis in patients undergoing gynecologic surgery. Anesthesiology. 1999;90(5):1265–70.
25. McFarlane C, Lee A. A comparison of Plasmalyte 148 and 0.9% saline for intra-operative fluid replacement. Anaesthesia. 1994;49(9):779–81.
26. Krajewski ML, Raghunathan K, Paluszkiewicz SM, Schermer CR, Shaw AD. Meta-analysis of high- versus low-chloride content in perioperative and critical care fluid resuscitation. Br J Surg. 2015;102(1):24–36.
27. Wise R, Faurie M, Malbrain MLNG, Hodgson E. Strategies for intravenous fluid resuscitation in trauma patients. World J Surg. 2017;41(5):1170–83.
28. Odom SR, Howell MD, Silva GS, Nielsen VM, Gupta A, Shapiro NI, et al. Lactate clearance as a predictor of mortality in trauma patients. J Trauma Acute Care Surg. 2013;74(4):999–1004.
29. Parsikia A, Bones K, Kaplan M, Strain J, Leung PS, Ortiz J, et al. The predictive value of initial serum lactate in trauma patients. Shock. 2014;42(3):199.
30. Handy J. Lactate—The bad boy of metabolism, or simply misunderstood? Curr Anaesth Crit Care. 2006;17(1–2):71–6.
31. Nalos M, Leverve XM, Huang SJ, Weisbrodt L, Parkin R, Seppelt IM, et al. Half-molar sodium lactate infusion improves cardiac performance in acute heart failure: a pilot randomised controlled clinical trial. Crit Care. 2014;18(2):R48.
32. Glenn TC, Martin NA, Horning MA, McArthur DL, Hovda DA, Vespa P, et al. Lactate: Brain fuel in human traumatic brain injury: a comparison with normal healthy control subjects. J Neurotrauma. 2015;32(11):820–32.
33. Patet C, Suys T, Carteron L, Oddo M. Cerebral lactate metabolism after traumatic brain injury. Curr Neurol Neurosci Rep. 2016;16(4):31.
34. Raux M, Manach YL, Gauss T, Baumgarten R, Hamada S, Harrois A, et al. Comparison of the prognostic significance of initial blood lactate and base deficit in trauma patients. Anesthesiol J Am Soc Anesthesiol. 2017;126(3):522–33.
35. Dienel GA. Brain lactate metabolism: the discoveries and the controversies. J Cereb Blood Flow Metab. 2012;32(7):1107–38.
36. Bruns B, Lindsey M, Rowe K, Brown S, Minei JP, Gentilello LM, et al. Hemoglobin drops within minutes of injuries and predicts need for an intervention to stop hemorrhage. J Trauma. 2007;63(2):312–5.
37. Figueiredo S, Taconet C, Harrois A, Hamada S, Gauss T, Raux M, et al. How useful are hemoglobin concentration and its variations to predict significant hemorrhage in the early phase of trauma? A multicentric cohort study. Ann Intensive Care. 2018;8(1):76.
38. Li Y, Liu B, Dillon ST, Fukudome EY, Kheirbek T, Sailhamer EA, et al. Identification of a novel potential biomarker in a model of hemorrhagic shock and valproic acid treatment. J Surg Res. 2010;159(1):474–81.
39. Abassi ZA, Okun-Gurevich M, Salah NA, Awad H, Mandel Y, Campino G, et al. Potential early predictors for outcomes of experimental hemorrhagic shock induced by uncontrolled internal bleeding in rats. PLoS One. 2013;8(11):e80862.
40. Alam HB, Li Y. Biomarkers of hemorrhagic shock [Internet]. US9435813B2, 2016. https://patents.google.com/patent/US9435813B2/en. Accessed 22 May 2019.
41. Horne S. WB Cannon: a trauma pioneer. Trauma. 2004;6(1):79–81.
42. Cannon WB, Fraser J, Cowell EM. NATURE AND TREATMENT OF WOUND SHOCK AND ALLIED CONDITIONS. J Am Med Assoc. 1918;70(8):520–35.
43. Beecher HK. Preparation of battle casualties for surgery. Ann Surg. 1945;121(6):769–92.
44. Bickell WH, Wall MJ, Pepe PE, Martin RR, Ginger VF, Allen MK, et al. Immediate versus delayed fluid resuscitation for hypotensive patients with penetrating torso injuries. N Engl J Med. 1994;331(17):1105–9.
45. Nevin DG, Brohi K. Permissive hypotension for active haemorrhage in trauma. Anaesthesia. 2017;72(12):1443–8.
46. Doran CM, Doran CA, Woolley T, Carter A, Male K, Midwinter MJ, et al. Targeted resuscitation improves coagulation and outcome. J Trauma Acute Care Surg. 2012;72(4):835–43.
47. Kirkman E, Watts S, Cooper G. Blast injury research models. Philos Trans R Soc Lond B Biol Sci. 2011;366(1562):144–59.
48. Mattox KL. Timing of transfusion in trauma. Vox Sang. 2004;87(s2):222–6.
49. Kasotakis G, Sideris A, Yang Y, de Moya M, Alam H, King DR, et al. Aggressive early crystalloid resuscitation adversely affects outcomes in adult blunt trauma patients: an analysis of the Glue Grant Database. J Trauma Acute Care Surg. 2013;74(5):1215–22.
50. Marik PE. Iatrogenic salt water drowning and the hazards of a high central venous pressure. Ann Intensive Care. 2014;4:21.
51. Malbrain MLNG, Roberts DJ, Sugrue M, De Keulenaer BL, Ivatury R, Pelosi P, et al. The polycompartment syndrome: a concise state-of-the-art review. Anaesthesiol Intensive Ther. 2014;46(5):433–50.
52. Marik PE, Monnet X, Teboul J-L. Hemodynamic parameters to guide fluid therapy. Ann Intensive Care. 2011;1(1):1.
53. Hahn RG, Bergek C, Gebäck T, Zdolsek J. Interactions between the volume effects of hydroxyethyl starch 130/0.4 and Ringer's acetate. Crit Care. 2013;17(3):R104.
54. Strunden MS, Heckel K, Goetz AE, Reuter DA. Perioperative fluid and volume management: physiological basis, tools and strategies. Ann Intensive Care. 2011;1:2.

55. Sharpe JP, Magnotti LJ, Croce MA, Paulus EM, Schroeppel TJ, Fabian TC, et al. Crystalloid administration during trauma resuscitation: does less really equal more? J Trauma Acute Care Surg. 2014;77(6):828–32. discussion 832
56. Lira A, Pinsky MR. Choices in fluid type and volume during resuscitation: impact on patient outcomes. Ann Intensive Care. 2014;4:38.
57. Myburgh JA, Finfer S, Bellomo R, Billot L, Cass A, Gattas D, et al. Hydroxyethyl starch or saline for fluid resuscitation in intensive care. N Engl J Med. 2012;367(20):1901–11.
58. Perner A, Haase N, Guttormsen AB, Tenhunen J, Klemenzson G, Åneman A, et al. Hydroxyethyl starch 130/0.42 versus Ringer's acetate in severe sepsis. N Engl J Med. 2012;367(2):124–34.
59. Annane D. Effects of fluid resuscitation with colloids vs crystalloids on mortality in critically ill patients presenting with hypovolemic shock: the CRISTAL randomized trial. JAMA. 2013;310(17):1809.
60. Guidet B, Martinet O, Boulain T, Philippart F, Poussel JF, Maizel J, et al. Assessment of hemodynamic efficacy and safety of 6% hydroxyethylstarch 130/0.4 vs. 0.9% NaCl fluid replacement in patients with severe sepsis: The CRYSTMAS study. Crit Care. 2012;16(3):R94.
61. Perel P, Roberts I, Ker K. Colloids versus crystalloids for fluid resuscitation in critically ill patients. Cochrane Database Syst Rev [Internet]. 2013;(2). https://www.cochranelibrary.com/cdsr/doi/10.1002/14651858.CD000567.pub6/full. Accessed 20 May 2019.
62. Zarychanski R, Abou-Setta AM, Turgeon AF, Houston BL, McIntyre L, Marshall JC, et al. Association of hydroxyethyl starch administration with mortality and acute kidney injury in critically ill patients requiring volume resuscitation: a systematic review and meta-analysis. JAMA. 2013;309(7):678–88.
63. Apostolou E, Deckert K, Puy R, Sandrini A, Leon MPD, Douglass JA, et al. Anaphylaxis to Gelofusine® confirmed by in vitro basophil activation test: a case series*. Anaesthesia. 2006;61(3):264–8.
64. Vamvakas EC, Blajchman MA. Transfusion-related mortality: the ongoing risks of allogeneic blood transfusion and the available strategies for their prevention. Blood. 2009;113(15):3406–17.
65. NHS Blood and Transplant. Serious hazards of transfusion home page [Internet]. Serious Hazards of Transfusion. https://www.shotuk.org/. Accessed 22 May 2019.
66. Gould SA, Moore EE, Hoyt DB, Ness PM, Norris EJ, Carson JL, et al. The life-sustaining capacity of human polymerized hemoglobin when red cells might be unavailable. J Am Coll Surg. 2002;195(4):445–52.
67. Gould SA, Moore EE, Hoyt DB, Burch JM, Haenel JB, Garcia J, et al. The first randomized trial of human polymerized hemoglobin as a blood substitute in acute trauma and emergent surgery. J Am Coll Surg. 1998;187(2):113–20.
68. Ferenz KB, Steinbicker AU. Artificial oxygen carriers—past, present, and future—a review of the most innovative and clinically relevant concepts. J Pharmacol Exp Ther. 2019;369(2):300–10.
69. Lee N. The Lancet technology: pharming blood. The Lancet. 2016;387(10037):2496.
70. Litvinov RI, Weisel JW. Role of red blood cells in haemostasis and thrombosis. ISBT Sci Ser. 2017;12(1):176–83.
71. Tombak A. Red blood cells and relation to thrombosis. Transfus Med Sci Dev [Internet]. 2017. https://www.intechopen.com/books/transfusion-medicine-and-scientific-developments/red-blood-cells-and-relation-to-thrombosis. Accessed 20 May 2019.
72. Valeri CR, Cassidy G, Pivacek LE, Ragno G, Lieberthal W, Crowley JP, et al. Anemia-induced increase in the bleeding time: implications for treatment of nonsurgical blood loss. Transfusion (Paris). 2001;41(8):977–83.
73. Hébert PC, Wells G, Blajchman MA, Marshall J, Martin C, Pagliarello G, et al. A multicenter, randomized, controlled clinical trial of transfusion requirements in critical care. Transfusion Requirements in Critical Care Investigators, Canadian Critical Care Trials Group. N Engl J Med. 1999;340(6):409–17.
74. Hébert PC. The TRICC Trial: a focus on the subgroup analysis. Vox Sang. 2002;83(s1):387–96.
75. Aoki M, Abe T, Saitoh D, Hagiwara S, Oshima K. Use of vasopressor increases the risk of mortality in traumatic hemorrhagic shock: a nationwide cohort study in Japan. Crit Care Med. 2018;46(12):e1145–51.
76. Tsuneyoshi I, Onomoto M, Yonetani A, Kanmura Y. Low-dose vasopressin infusion in patients with severe vasodilatory hypotension after prolonged hemorrhage during general anesthesia. J Anesth. 2005;19(2):170–3.
77. Gupta B, Garg N, Ramachandran R. Vasopressors: Do they have any role in hemorrhagic shock? J Anaesthesiol Clin Pharmacol. 2017;33(1):3–8.
78. Sperry JL, Minei JP, Frankel HL, West MA, Harbrecht BG, Moore EE, et al. Early use of vasopressors after injury: caution before constriction. J Trauma Inj Infect Crit Care. 2008;64(1):9–14.
79. McQuilten ZK, Crighton G, Brunskill S, Morison JK, Richter TH, Waters N, et al. Optimal dose, timing and ratio of blood products in massive transfusion: results from a systematic review. Transfus Med Rev. 2018;32(1):6–15.
80. Anand T, Ramnanan R, Skinner R, Martin M. Impact of massive transfusion and aging blood in acute trauma. Am Surg. 2016;82(10):957–9.
81. Sowers N, Froese P, Erdogan M, Green R. Impact of the age of stored blood on trauma patient mortality: a systematic review. Can J Surg. 2015;58(5):335–42.
82. Heddle NM, Cook RJ, Arnold DM, Liu Y, Barty R, Crowther MA, et al. Effect of short-term vs. long-term blood storage on mortality after transfusion. N Engl J Med. 2016;375(20):1937–45.

83. Olszewski A, Korzeniewski K, Lass A. Selected epidemiological aspects of fresh whole blood application in the Polish Field Hospital in Afghanistan. Int Marit Health. 2014;65(1):23–7.
84. Cotton BA, Podbielski J, Camp E, Welch T, del Junco D, Bai Y, et al. A randomized controlled pilot trial of modified whole blood versus component therapy in severely injured patients requiring large volume transfusions. Ann Surg. 2013;1.
85. Jones AR, Frazier SK. Increased mortality in adult patients with trauma transfused with blood components compared with whole blood. J Trauma Nurs. 2014;21(1):22–9.
86. Spinella PC, Perkins JG, Grathwohl KW, Beekley AC, Holcomb JB. Warm fresh whole blood is independently associated with improved survival for patients with combat-related traumatic injuries. J Trauma. 2009;66(4 Suppl):S69–76.
87. Strandenes G, Skogrand H, Spinella PC, Hervig T, Rein EB. Donor performance of combat readiness skills of special forces soldiers are maintained immediately after whole blood donation: a study to support the development of a prehospital fresh whole blood transfusion program. Transfusion (Paris). 2013;53(3):526–30.
88. Eliassen HS, Hervig T, Backlund S, Sivertsen J, Iversen VV, Kristoffersen M, et al. Immediate effects of blood donation on physical and cognitive performance–A randomized controlled double-blinded trial. J Trauma Acute Care Surg. 2018;84(6S Suppl 1):S125–31.
89. Langston A, Downing D, Packard J, Kopulos M, Burcie S, Martin K, et al. Massive transfusion protocol simulation: an innovative approach to team training. Crit Care Nurs Clin North Am. 2017;29(2):259–69.
90. Kamerer JL. Massive transfusion protocol simulation: compound femur fracture and hypovolemic shock. Simul Healthc. 2012;7(3):196.
91. Khoyratty SI, Gajendragadkar PR, Polisetty K, Ward S, Skinner T, Gajendragadkar PR. Flow rates through intravenous access devices: an in vitro study. J Clin Anesth. 2016;31:101–5.
92. Reddick AD, Ronald J, Morrison WG. Intravenous fluid resuscitation: was Poiseuille right? Emerg Med J. 2011;28(3):201–2.
93. Wrenn EA, Wohlers R, Montgomery MH, Cobb H, Condra J, Tharpe S. Comparison of flow dynamics of peripherally and centrally inserted intravenous catheters using a rapid infusion system (ThermaCor 1200). Am Assoc Nurse Anaesth. 2017;85(4):256–60.
94. Marshall SD, Sanderson P, McIntosh CA, Kolawole H. The effect of two cognitive aid designs on team functioning during intra-operative anaphylaxis emergencies: a multi-centre simulation study. Anaesthesia. 2016;71(4):389–404.
95. Long E, Fitzpatrick P, Cincotta DR, Grindlay J, Barrett MJ. A randomised controlled trial of cognitive aids for emergency airway equipment preparation in a Paediatric Emergency Department. Scand J Trauma Resusc Emerg Med. 2016;24(1):8.
96. Marshall S. The use of cognitive aids during emergencies in anesthesia: a review of the literature. Anesth Analg. 2013;117(5):1162–71.
97. Degani A, Wiener EL. Cockpit checklists: concepts, design, and use. Hum Factors J Hum Factors Ergon Soc. 1993;35(2):345–59.
98. Schultz C. Here are NASA's top 19 typography tips [Internet]. Smithsonian. https://www.smithsonianmag.com/smart-news/here-are-nasas-top-19-typography-tips-180947788/. Accessed 26 May 2019
99. Gawande A. The Checklist Manifesto: how to get things right. London: Profile Books Ltd: [distributor] TBS The Book Service Ltd; 2011.
100. Mercer SJ, Whittle CL, Mahoney PF. Lessons from the battlefield: human factors in defence anaesthesia. BJA Br J Anaesth. 2010;105(1):9–20.
101. Mercer SJ, Tarmey NT, Woolley T, Wood P, Mahoney PF. Haemorrhage and coagulopathy in the Defence Medical Services. Anaesthesia. 2013;68(s1):49–60.
102. Cote' CJ, Drop LJ, Daniels AL, Hoaglin DC. Calcium chloride versus calcium gluconate: comparison of ionization and cardiovascular effects in children and dogs. Anesthesiology. 1987;66(4):465–70.
103. Raza S, Ali Baig M, Chang C, Dabas R, Akhtar M, Khan A, et al. A prospective study on red blood cell transfusion related hyperkalemia in critically ill patients. J Clin Med Res. 2015;7(6):417–21.
104. Vraets A, Lin Y, Callum JL. Transfusion-associated hyperkalemia. Transfus Med Rev. 2011;25(3):184–96.
105. CRASH-2 Trial Collaborators. Effects of tranexamic acid on death, vascular occlusive events, and blood transfusion in trauma patients with significant haemorrhage (CRASH-2): a randomised, placebo-controlled trial. The Lancet. 2010;376(9734):23–32.
106. Morrison JJ. Military application of tranexamic acid in trauma emergency resuscitation (MATTERs) study. Arch Surg. 2012;147(2):113.
107. Gonzalez E, Moore EE, Moore HB. Management of trauma-induced coagulopathy with thrombelastography. Crit Care Clin. 2017;33(1):119–34.
108. Spahn DR, Bouillon B, Cerny V, Coats TJ, Duranteau J, Fernández-Mondéjar E, et al. Management of bleeding and coagulopathy following major trauma: an updated European guideline. Crit Care. 2013;17(2):R76.
109. Schöchl H, Maegele M, Solomon C, Görlinger K, Voelckel W. Early and individualized goal-directed therapy for trauma-induced coagulopathy. Scand J Trauma Resusc Emerg Med. 2012;20(1):15.
110. Revell M. Fluid resuscitation in prehospital trauma care: a consensus view. Emerg Med J. 2002;19(6):494–8.

111. Spahn DR, Bouillon B, Cerny V, Duranteau J, Filipescu D, Hunt BJ, et al. The European guideline on management of major bleeding and coagulopathy following trauma: fifth edition. Crit Care. 2019;23(1):98.
112. Kudo D, Yoshida Y, Kushimoto S. Permissive hypotension/hypotensive resuscitation and restricted/controlled resuscitation in patients with severe trauma. J Intensive Care. 2017;5(1):11.
113. Carney N, Totten AM, O'Reilly C, Ullman JS, Hawryluk GWJ, Bell MJ, et al. Guidelines for the management of severe traumatic brain injury, Fourth EditionNeurosurgery. 2016;1.

11 Disability and Head Injury

Richard J. Gould and Peter Lax

1. Understand and differentiate between primary and secondary brain injury
2. Understand common neuroprotective strategies for minimising secondary brain injury
3. Be able to make a referral for neurosurgical intervention with salient points from history, examination and radiological results

Introduction

Identification of head injuries forms part of the 'Disability' section of the MABCD assessment. Some injuries may immediately be apparent, but many require advanced imaging to diagnose. The brain is an incredibly complex organ, much of which we are yet to understand fully, and injury sustained at the scene cannot be directly treated during the initial assessment. The focus of management is to stop further injury by preventing physiological conditions that are harmful to brain perfusion and expedite transfer to a hospital where definitive surgical treatment can occur if needed. To understand how to do this, it is crucial to appreciate how blood flow to the brain functions in health.

Primary Versus Secondary Brain Injury

Patients with head injuries are affected by both primary and secondary brain injuries. A primary brain injury is the damage done at the initial point of injury and cannot be reversed or modified as it represents acute destruction of brain tissue and cannot be repaired. The only treatment for primary brain injury is prevention. Schemes such as increasing helmet usage amongst bikers and motorcyclists are crucial to decreasing morbidity and mortality in this area.

Secondary brain injuries, in contrast, are preventable and can be minimised or avoided altogether by prompt treatment and attention to detail. Chief amongst the insults that cause secondary brain injury and worsen neurological outcome are hypoxia, hypotension (both leading to impaired oxygen delivery to vulnerable tissues [1]), hypo-

The original version of this chapter was revised. The correction to this chapter can be found at https://doi.org/10.1007/978-3-030-83628-3_45

R. J. Gould (✉)
Department of Anaesthesia and Critical Care Medicine, Leeds General Infirmary, Leeds, UK
e-mail: richardgould@nhs.net

P. Lax
Tactical Medical Wing, Royal Air Force, Brize Norton, Oxfordshire, UK

The Air Ambulance Service (TAAS), Rugby, Warwickshire, UK
e-mail: p.lax@NHS.net

P. Lax (ed.), *Textbook of Acute Trauma Care*, https://doi.org/10.1007/978-3-030-83628-3_11

glycaemia and hypercarbia. These factors are all identifiable and treatable, and the attentive practitioner should be alert to aggressively excluding or treating them as part of the primary survey and ongoing critical care management.

Applied Anatomy

While a detailed review of neuroanatomy is beyond the scope of this book, a basic understanding of the anatomy is essential to appreciating the mechanisms by which brain injury occurs.

The brain is protected by the cranium (or skull). The cranium is divided into those bones that form the cranial vault and those that comprise the facial bones (Fig. 11.1). The bones that encase the brain are the left and right parietal and temporal bones, plus the frontal, occipital, sphenoid and ethmoid bones.

The rounded top of the cranium, the calvaria (or 'skull cap'), is predominately composed of the two parietal bones and the frontal bone. These bones join (but do not articulate) at the suture lines. The coronal suture runs from side to side and attached the frontal bone to the parietal bones. The sagittal suture unites the left and right parietal bones. A lambdoid suture attaches the occipital bone to the parietal bones. The temporal bones form the skull's lateral sides and join the parietal bones at the squamous suture. These sutures are incomplete in neonates and young

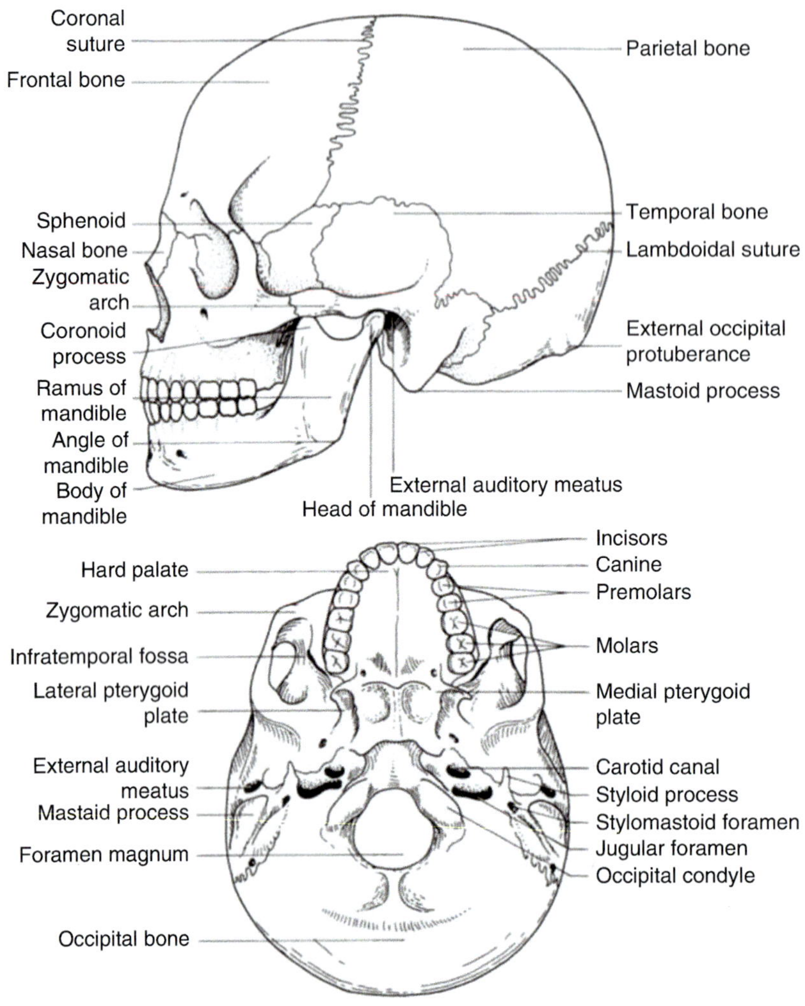

Fig. 11.1 Bony anatomy of the skull (from Ellis [2])

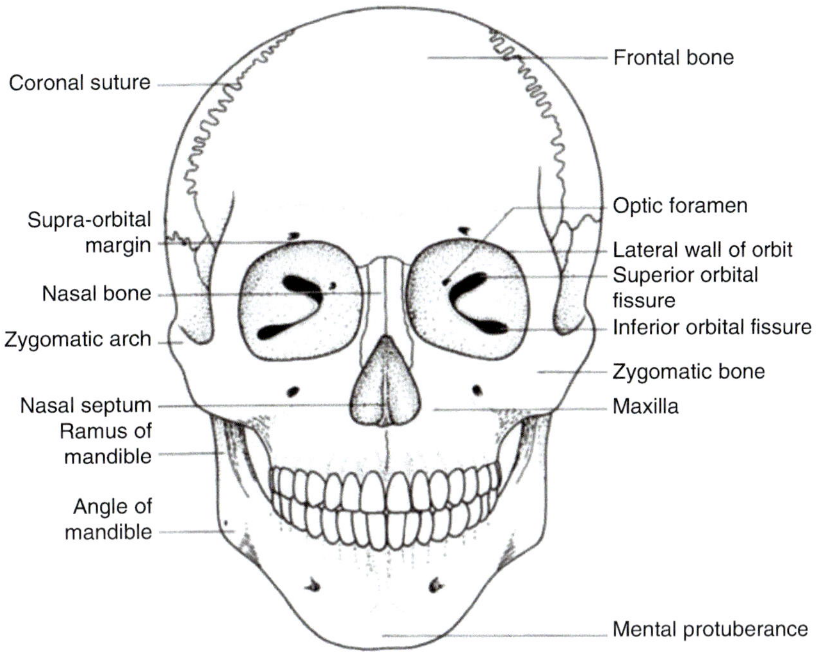

Fig. 11.1 (continued)

children, only closing at around the age of two years in most cases. This degree of laxity (amongst other factors) means that very young children have a more considerable degree of compensation for changes in intracranial volume and pressure than older children and adults [3].

The frontal, parietal and temporal bones join with the sphenoid bone at a point on the side of the skull called the pterion. This intersection is the weakest part of the skull. It is located approximately 3 cm superior to the zygomatic arch—the part of the zygomatic bone that forms the prominent 'cheek line'. Directly behind the pterion sits the middle meningeal artery. Due to its close relationship with the skull, this vessel is often injured in trauma and the brisk arterial bleeding results in the formation of an extradural haematoma. Extradural haematomas are primary skull injuries, but they will cause a secondary brain injury if left unchecked.

The meninges provide a protective covering for the brain. The dura mater is the thick, outmost layer. It supports the arachnoid layer deep to it, which itself contains the cerebrospinal fluid (CSF). The subdural space also contains numerous veins and sinus that are responsible for venous drainage of the brain. The veins are only thin-walled structures; they are easily damaged and

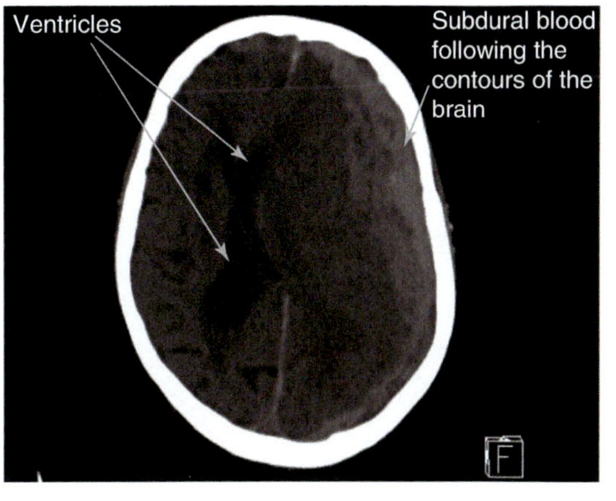

Fig. 11.2 Left subdural haematoma with mass effect (the "slice" is viewed from the position of looking up from the patient's feet towards their head). Note the lighter grey collection of blood on the patient's left (right side of the image), causing the ventricles to collapse and be pushed across to the other side

can rupture in response to only very mild trauma, especially if stretched. As age-related cerebral atrophy occurs, these veins become weaker as the arachnoid layer is increasingly separated from the dura. A rupture of a dural vein is referred to as a subdural haemorrhage. It can form part of a head injury or be found incidentally on imaging undertaken for a different reason (Fig. 11.2).

With the skull cap and brain removed, the floor of the cranial cavity is exposed. Known as the base of the skull, this complex structure is formed by the fusion of the frontal, ethmoid, sphenoid, temporal and occipital bones. Functionally, it is thought of as three depressions (or fossae) which each seat different intracranial structures.

The largest part of the brain is the cerebrum, and easily the most identifiable part of the central nervous system. It is divided into left and right hemispheres and then into lobes whose names correspond with the overlying bone. The cerebrum's external appearance is dominated by ridges and grooves referred to as the gyri and sulci. Deeper sulci separate the lobes. The frontal lobe rests in the anterior cranial fossa, and the temporal lobes sit in the middle cranial fossa.

Beneath the occipital lobe is the cerebellar tentorium. This extension of the meninges forms a tough membrane that separates the cerebrum from the cerebellum beneath it. The cerebellum (literally translates into 'little brain') occupies most of the posterior cranial fossa. Also within the posterior fossa are the brainstem structures—namely the medulla oblongata, pons and midbrain. The brainstem is responsible for autonomic controls essential to life (e.g. breathing and cardiovascular functions), and insults in this region are often life-threatening. The presence of the tentorium limits the potential space available to accommodate an increase in volume, so the pressure effect of blood or tumour in the posterior fossa can rapidly compress these structures.

Physiology

The cranium forms an inherently rigid box that is only in communication with the vertebral canal. The normal pressure inside this 'box' is 3–10 mmHg and is referred to as the intracranial pressure (ICP). The ICP value results from a dynamic relationship between the volumes of the various intracranial contents (see Figs. 11.3, 11.4, 11.5, 11.6 and 11.7, below).

Figures 11.3, 11.4, 11.5, 11.6, and 11.7 demonstrating physiological and pathophysiological fluid volumes in head trauma (reproduced courtesy of TeachMeSurgery.com and Rose Ingleton).

Because this container is rigid, a rise in one component's volume must be compensated by a fall in one of the others, or the pressure will rise. This is the Monro-Kellie Doctrine [4]. In health, the cranium will contain intravascular blood, CSF and brain tissue. Only the volumes of intravascular blood and CSF inside the head can be regarded as reducible. If a pathological blood clot or excess oedema occurs, CSF can be displaced into the spinal subarachnoid space, but once this compensation is exhausted, pressure can rise very quickly.

The volume of intracranial intravascular blood is primarily determined by cerebral

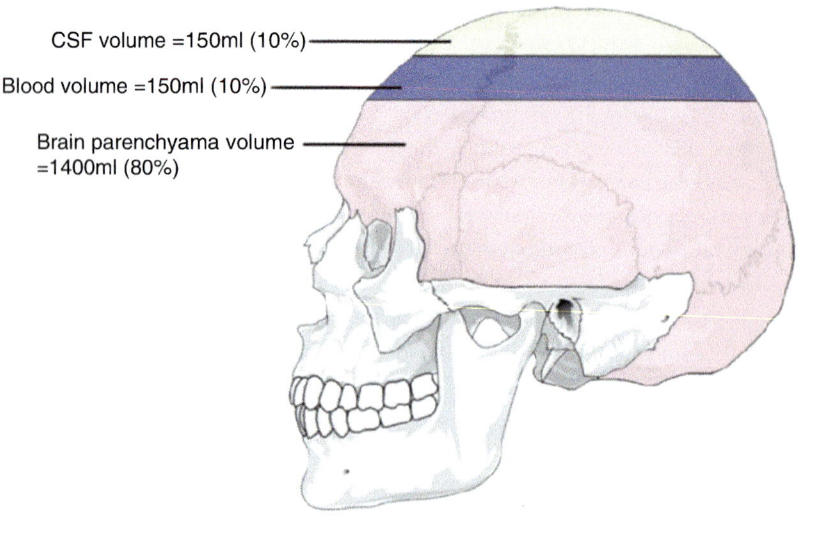

Fig. 11.3 The intracranial components and their respective volumes

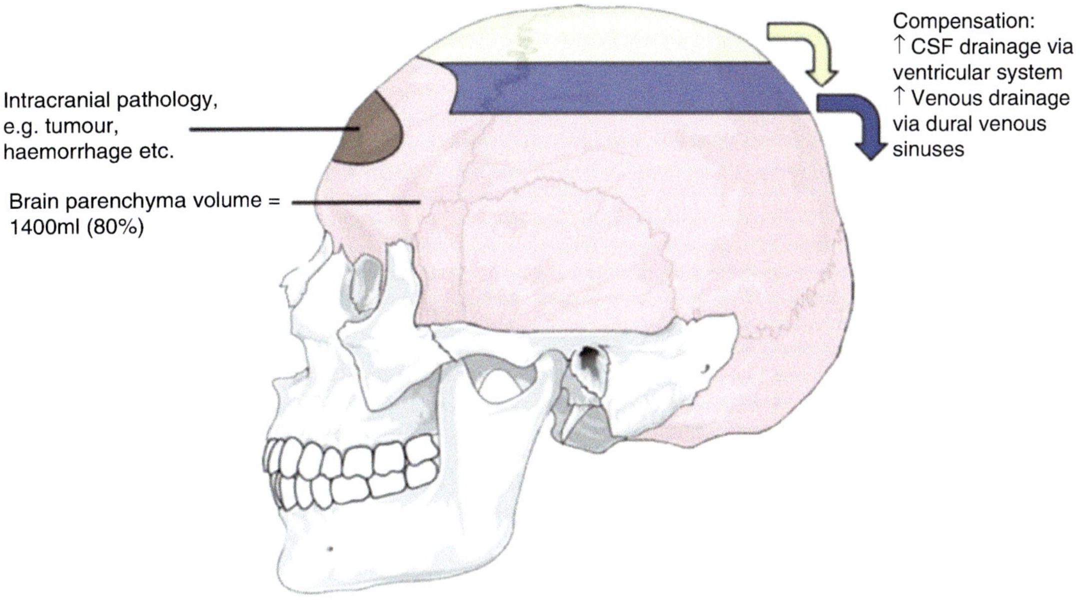

Fig. 11.4 Intracranial compensation in the presence of pathology to maintain a normal intracranial pressure

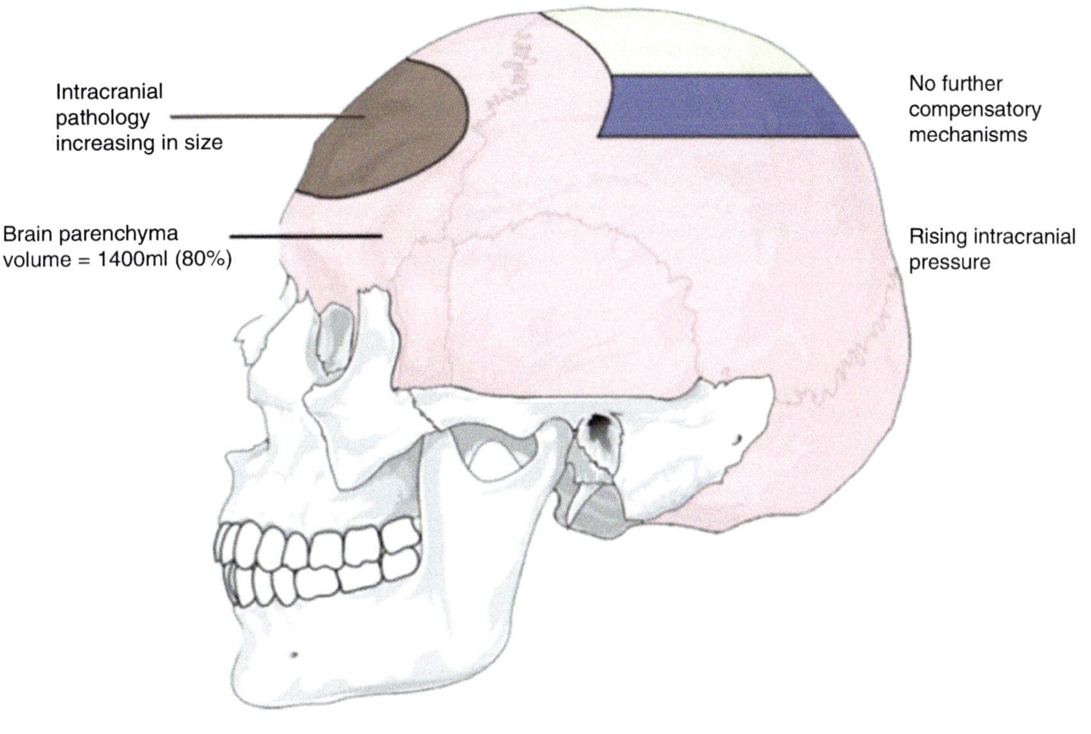

Fig. 11.5 Intracranial decompensation in the presence of pathology causing a rise in intracranial pressure

blood flow (CBF). The body can autoregulate this in health to match the metabolic demands of the brain. There are important modifiable factors that can profoundly influence CBF, and these are significant in the context of head injury.

The partial pressure of CO_2 in the arterial blood is a major regulating factor in cerebral vasodilatation and constriction. A rise in $PaCO_2$ causes cerebral vasodilation and increased intracranial pressure in a linear relationship. As expected, a reduction in $PaCO_2$ will cause vasoconstriction and correspond with a fall in CBF and, therefore, ICP. However, excessive vasoconstriction (and consequent decreased CBF) decreases the delivery of oxygen to brain tissue, consequently worsening secondary brain injury. Control of $PaCO_2$ is a fundamental principle in managing severe head injuries, and mechanical ventilation is commonly employed to achieve this. However, arterial oxygenation (PaO_2) also has an essential role in regulating cerebral blood flow. Hypoxia itself will cause cerebral vasodilation in an effort to promote arterial oxygen delivery. This physiological adaptation also obtunds the vasoconstrictive effects of hypocarbia in hyperventilation if the patient is hypoxic [5, 6].

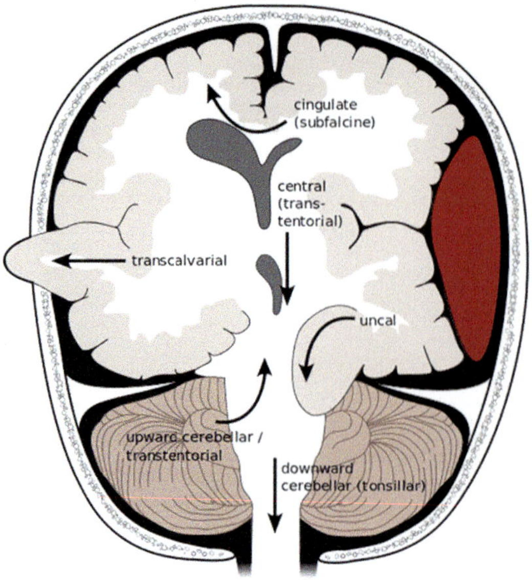

Fig. 11.6 Types of Herniation

The clinical implications of this are that in patients with documented hypoxia or hypotension, the proportion of poor outcomes (death or persistent vegetative state) rises alarmingly. Poor outcomes are proportional to both the depth and duration of hypoxia and hypotension in patients with susceptible brain injuries [1]. The aim of management in these patients must be to maintain normal levels of oxygenation and an adequate Cerebral Perfusion Pressure (CPP). Preventing excessive arterial oxygen levels may be as important as preventing hypoxia. One large retrospective study of ventilated stroke patients [7] found a worsening mortality rate in those exposed to hyperoxia (defined as a PaO_2 higher than 40 kPa or 300 mmHg). This finding was replicated in a prospective study of stroke patients after mechanical thrombectomy, where the definition of hyperoxia was tightened to greater than 16 kPa or 120 mmHg [8]. Those exposed to greater oxygen levels had higher mortality and

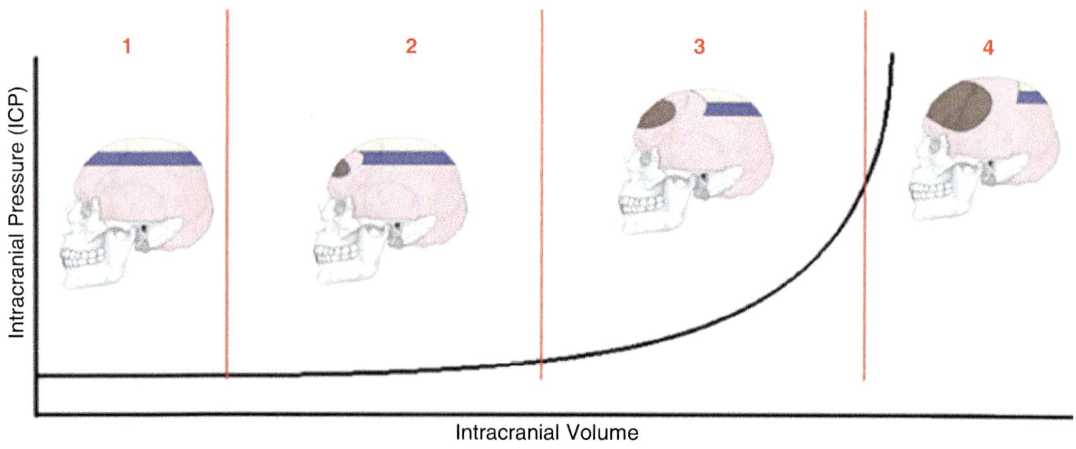

Fig. 11.7 The intracranial volume-pressure curve (1) No pathology (2) Small volume pathology in a compensated state with normal ICP (3) Large volume pathology in a decompensated state with elevated ICP (4) Very large volume pathology with a significantly elevated ICP and brain herniation

worse functional outcome after multiple regression analysis. This is not a phenomenon explicitly limited to stroke patients, as worse outcomes with hyperoxia have been reported in post-cardiac arrest patients, those with sepsis and in patients with traumatic brain injury [9]. For this reason, normoxia rather than hyperoxia should be the target when reliable measurements of PaO_2 are available, but for brief periods hypoxia is more likely to be harmful than hyperoxia.

CPP is defined as the difference between Mean Arterial Pressure (MAP) and Intracranial Pressure (ICP):

$$CPP = MAP - ICP.$$

While it is quite easy to obtain a reliable estimate of any patient's mean arterial pressure at any time in hospital as it is calculated by 2/3 diastolic pressure +1/3 systolic pressure, measurement of intracranial pressure requires specialist invasive equipment. In the early stages of resuscitation and management of these patients, therefore, it is imperative to assume that any patient with a head injury who has a depressed level of consciousness or neurological deficit may have raised intracranial pressure. This presents a problem in patients with head and other concurrent severe injuries and bleeding. The correct strategy for managing a head injury is to increase the MAP and hence CPP to minimise secondary injury. In contrast, the initial management of bleeding polytrauma patients favours permissive hypotension. Tolerating a low blood pressure may help avoid further bleeding, but may be disastrous for a patient with a significant head injury. Assuming an ICP of 25–30 mmHg in patients with a mechanism and clinical signs of a head injury (as outlined below) is a reasonable starting point if ICP is not directly measured. While many management strategies have focused on the contribution of CSF volumes and control of CO_2 to effect changes in the arterial side of the cerebral circulation, there is renewed interest in the venous components and their contribution to ICP. A paper by Wilson [10] outlines how impairment to venous drainage from a variety of sources can lead to increased ICP despite adequate perfusion pressure and CO_2 control. For this reason, strategies to minimise the obstruction to venous drainage are vital. Practical measures outside an intensive care setting include the removal of cervical collars, use of ET tube tapes instead of ties around the neck, raising the head of the bed to 30° where possible and decreasing ventilator pressures and PEEP. Various guidelines offer suggestions for target blood pressures and cerebral perfusion pressures as a "one size fits all" approach. The European Brain Injury Consortium guidelines [11] advocate a MAP of >90 mmHg; the AAGBI [12] recommend a systolic of >110 mmHg and a MAP of >90 mmHg, and the Brain Trauma Foundation [13] advise a systolic BP of >100 or > 110 mmHg depending on patient age.

While these models quite possibly simplify the complex dynamics in brain injury, they provide a reasonable starting point for individualising treatment [14]. However, multiple factors may interact with each other and complicate the picture.

Assessment of Head Injuries

Unfortunately, it is occasionally impossible to obtain a history from the patient with a head injury, and therefore the focus should be on obtaining as much collateral information as possible. Bystanders, other patients, first responders and paramedics may all be considered useful sources.

Important information to obtain will include a description of the nature of the incident (including details of the mechanism) and the patient's clinical condition at the scene. This is particularly important if the patient has been sedated and ventilated before transfer to the trauma centre.

The cause of severe head injuries varies with the age of the victims [15–17]. In the young adult population, road traffic accidents predominate as the cause, either as pedestrians or occupants of a vehicle. Assaults are also common in this age group, and over 50% of these patients will have other extracranial injuries that should be identified on assessment. In the elderly, falls are the primary cause of head injury.

As with all clinical handovers, details regarding the patient's stability during transfer, treatment, and drugs administered should also form part of the assessment. If available, any information regarding the patient's health and pre-existing medical conditions may aid the assessment. Chronic alcohol abuse and patients taking antiplatelet or blood-thinning medications are significant related factors, and injuries may be related to relatively minor trauma and separated from a hospital presentation by a significant period (especially in the elderly).

As previously discussed, disorders of ventilation and circulation can profoundly affect brain perfusion, with the risk of further injury being sustained. Therefore, the initial assessment of the head-injured patient must follow the MABCD methodology. Problems identified during this assessment should be corrected (e.g. securing a compromised airway) before proceeding to the next step. Readers are encouraged to refer to the appropriate chapters in this book for details of these interventions.

The specific neurological assessment can be considered as having three essential constituents:

- Level of Consciousness
- Pupil size and reactivity
- Focal neurological assessment for gross deficits

Level of Consciousness

This is perhaps the broadest assessment of cerebral function but is recognised for its ability to provide useful information to triage and prognosticate the patient with a head injury. Repeated assessment over time allows clinical decisions to be based upon trends in a patient's score.

The most straightforward system in use is the AVPU scale [18] (Alert, responds to Voice, responds to Pain, Unresponsive to stimuli). This four-point scale is easy to remember and utilise. It forms part of routine nursing observations and can be taught to all those with even basic first aid training. In some places where the NEWS2 system is employed, this is being superseded by ACVPU, with confusion being used as a marker of neurological deterioration between alert and responding to voice [19]. Confusion can be challenging to quantify, especially in the presence of alcohol or other drugs. However, as a general rule, patients who become more confused or drowsy should be managed with a high index of suspicion for serious injury and investigated promptly with CT scanning.

The Glasgow Coma Scale (GCS) [20] is a more detailed measure of a patient's level of consciousness. It is the sum of the scores from three areas of assessment: eye-opening, verbal response and best motor response. The lowest score is 3, the highest 15 (Table 11.1).

Using the GCS is more complex than AVPU but is believed to allow for a more descriptive neurological assessment. When assessing the motor score, it is essential to remember that it is the best response that is recorded. To correctly assess the motor score, a painful stimulus must be applied within the distribution of the cranial nerves and the response of the upper limbs used to generate the motor score. A painful stimulus applied to other parts of the body (such as the feet) could cause a spinal cord generated 'with-

Table 11.1 Classical Glasgow coma scale

Best eye response	Best verbal response	Best motor response	Score
		Obeys commands	6
	Normally conversant and orientated	Localises to a painful stimulus	5
Spontaneously open	Conversant but confused	Withdraws from a painful stimulus	4
Opens to verbal stimulus	Inappropriate words	Abnormal flexion to pain (decorticate response)	3
Opens to a painful stimulus	Incomprehensible sounds	Abnormal extension to pain (decerebrate response)	2
No response	No response	No response	1

drawal' reflex, which is not an assessment of cerebral function and can even occur in patients with no brain activity [21]. To minimise these errors and the inter-operator variability of values, the GCS assessment is often performed by two practitioners who will confer and agree on a score.

It is crucial to accurately score the GCS as it is used to categorise both the severity of the head injury and to determine treatment [22]:

- GCS ≤8 Severe Head Injury
- GCS 9–12 Moderate Head Injury
- GCS 13–15 Mild Head Injury

Patients in a coma are defined as having a GCS of 8 or less per ATLS guidelines [23]. The threshold of 8 has historically been believed to be important for the initial management of head injuries. Below this value, it is believed that most patients cannot adequately protect their airway and are at risk of gastric aspiration. However, GCS has not been validated as a predictor of the need for intubation despite the persistence of the maxim that all patients with a GCS of 8 or less should be intubated [24, 25].

As many patients with a severe head injury will have been intubated at the scene, the receiving hospital clinicians will frequently be unable to perform their own GCS assessment due to the continuous sedation the patient will be receiving. It is, therefore, crucial to get an accurate handover from the transfer team to ascertain (i) the initial GCS, (ii) the best GCS post-injury and (iii) the GCS immediately before anaesthesia. The most sensitive predictor of the degree of primary brain injury within the GCS breakdown (and the likelihood of good functional recovery if a secondary brain injury is avoided) is the best motor score since the point of injury.

Problems with GCS

Despite the Glasgow Coma Scale becoming the accepted international measure of level of consciousness since its inception in 1974, the use of GCS in its current form is not without problems. A 2011 article by Green [26] best outlines the issues, but to briefly describe them:

- It can be difficult to calculate/remember even by experienced personnel [27]. One study showed that 23.6% of UK Emergency Departments and 40% of Neurosurgical units were using an old version of the GCS nearly 27 years after it was updated [28]. There have been subsequent updates in both 2014 and 2018, which are not widely known about.
- Inter-operator variability is high in both clinical and written assessments (when assessing patients, two consultant level Emergency physicians graded GCS the same only 38% of the time in one study [29], and Neurosurgeons 56% in another [27]).
- The original authors [30] did not advise the summation of three components to give a single score, and there are 120 possible combinations of scores from the three elements with varying prognostic significance. A GCS of 4 predicts a 48% mortality if calculated as E1V1M2, 27% if calculated as E1V2M1 and 19% if calculated as E2V1M1 [31].
- Positive predictive value for individual patients is poor, and either individual elements (such as motor score only [31–34]) or simpler systems [35, 36] perform just as well.

However, it is unlikely that the GCS will fall out of clinical use in the immediate future despite these problems.

Pupils

Pupils are assessed for their size, shape and response to bright light. Their speed of response must be recorded. Unequal pupil sizes of 1 mm or less may be normal, but any greater difference requires further assessment. If the larger pupil is either sluggish to respond to light or is fixed, then this suggests a significantly raised ICP with a local mass lesion on the side of the dilated pupil.

Bilaterally fixed dilated pupils may be an ominous sign of critically raised ICP and brain stem compression. If urgent investigation does not demonstrate pathology that would be amenable to surgical intervention to reduce the ICP, the prognosis in these patients is very poor. If the pathology is rapidly treated by surgical intervention, then even patients who present with fixed pupils can make a good recovery. A meta-analysis of patients with fixed pupils due to an extradural haematoma demonstrated that if surgical evacuation was performed, over 50% made a good recovery [37].

There are several potential pitfalls to be aware of when assessing the pupils. Small 'pinpoint' pupils can result from opioid administration, and atropine can cause pupillary dilatation. It can be challenging to determine whether a small pupil is reactive or not, but small, unresponsive pupils can be associated with midbrain pathology. Patients who have had lens implantation surgery to correct cataracts will have irregular pupils that are often unresponsive to light. In these patients, the value of pupillary assessment is therefore limited.

Focal Neurological Deficit

While it is often not practical to conduct a full assessment of all motor and sensory groups in the limbs during trauma resuscitation, it is vital to observe and assess whether any motor response is equal on both sides.

If there is no spontaneous movement, then painful stimuli must be applied as part of the GCS assessment. If there is a suggestion of a difference, then this may need to be repeated to confirm. A clear difference on one side may indicate a localised brain injury, such as an evolving intracranial bleed. It is crucial to quickly examine the patient and document any gross lateralising signs before induction of anaesthesia; once the patient is intubated and ventilated, the opportunity for examination is lost.

Treatment and Principles of Care

Initial Treatment

As has been emphasised previously, preventing secondary injury should be the priority of initial treatment. A structured approach is essential, and this should be the familiar MABCD protocol used in all trauma patients.

Early intubation and ventilation are recommended to prevent aspiration and optimise gas exchange (PO_2 and PCO_2). In patients with a GCS of 8 or less on admission, this should be considered urgently, but is often required in patients with higher scores too. Many patients with head injury are agitated or combative and require anaesthesia and intubation to facilitate transfer and investigation, or prevent them from sustaining further injuries.

Patients with head injury often have associated maxillo-facial injuries. These can cause problems with intubation due to blood in the airway or possibly restricted mouth opening. All patients with a head injury must also be suspected of having a cervical spine injury, and manual in-line stabilisation should be considered during intubation. Although early intubation may be required, the medical team must be satisfied that they have the correct experience and skills to deal with these potential problems. Failed intubation attempts will result in hypoxia and hypercarbia and potentially worsen the degree of brain injury.

There is always likely to be variation amongst clinicians regarding the choice of drugs used to induce anaesthesia and maintain muscle relaxation for intubation. Rapid-sequence induction (RSI) is recommended due to the risk of aspiration. The use of suxamethonium is associated with a short rise in ICP, although the clinical importance of this is unclear. Rocuronium does not cause an increase in ICP and is often preferred. However, the emphasis should be on using drugs that the practitioner is familiar with and avoiding the deleterious effects of hypotension and hypercarbia. A more detailed discussion of airway management can be found in the drug assisted airway management chapter.

Optimising ventilation should occur next. This should initially consist of instituting mechanical ventilation and ensuring an end-tidal CO_2 ($ETCO_2$) waveform is present. Obtaining an arterial blood gas will confirm that oxygenation and ventilation are adequate. It is recommended to keep PaO_2 above 13 KPa and $PaCO_2$ between 4.5 and 5.0 KPa. If unable to achieve these targets, then further investigation is needed. Potential reasons may include the presence of chest trauma (such as an untreated pneumothorax), blood and secretions in the airway (requiring endotracheal suctioning or bronchoscopy) or 'fighting the ventilator' due to inadequate sedation and muscle relaxation. All ventilatory issues should be addressed, and further details and advice can be found in the Ventilation chapter.

In situations where there is concern regarding impending tonsillar herniation and brainstem compression, a short-term reduction in ICP can be achieved by hyperventilation. This lowers the $PaCO_2$ and reduces the intravascular cerebral blood volume at the expense of decreasing blood flow and oxygen delivery. Reducing the $PaCO_2$ to 3.5 KPa can allow enough time for transfer and definitive management. If neurological assessment shows improvement (such as the return of pupillary function), it may suggest that further medical and neurosurgical intervention should be expedited. It is important to remember that the acute effect of hyperventilation is transient, and prolonged hyperventilation will be ineffective and will worsen brain injury [38].

Maintenance of an adequate blood pressure is required to prevent further brain injury, but in complex trauma patients there are often competing problems such as haemorrhage. Aggressive fluid loading, vasopressor use and aiming for hypertension to treat a head injury before achieving haemostasis may prove harmful. Ultimately this approach may worsen cardiovascular instability and increase morbidity and mortality. An initial target systolic blood pressure of 110 mmHg is a reasonable compromise. This can usually be achieved with fluid boluses—ideally blood or blood products if hypotension is due to haemorrhage. Early insertion of an arterial line to permit continuous monitoring is also prudent, but should not delay the patient in getting a diagnostic CT scan.

If haemorrhage is not present or has been controlled, blood pressure should be raised to achieve a CPP of 60–70 mmHg. As previously explained, this is a calculated figure based on subtracting the ICP from the MAP. Although the ICP may not be known at this stage, it is reasonable to assume a value above normal, and 30 mmHg is often considered an approximation in patients with a severe head injury. It therefore follows that the target MAP should be 90–100 mmHg.

Achieving a MAP of 90 mmHg can be a challenge in these patients. They may be hypovolaemic from their injuries, cold from exposure and have reduced cardiac output and vasodilation due to sedation. A thorough assessment of fluid status should be performed, and boluses given if needed. Most patients will require some form of vasopressor or inotrope to improve their blood pressure. This is initially commenced with peripheral agents until central venous access has been obtained. There is no optimum agent to use if a vasopressor is required in the context of an isolated head injury. As long as the drug is employed quickly and the clinician is familiar with its use, minimising the duration and depth of any hypotension is more important than using a specific drug [39].

Other essential parts of the initial treatment can include actions to temporarily reduce ICP in order to stabilise a patient before imaging or neurosurgical treatment. Hyperventilation has previously been discussed, but other pharmacological options also exist. There are no set rules as to when these agents are used. Evidence of impending brainstem compression (such as unilateral unresponsive pupil) or a worsening neurological assessment are often cited as indications for a trial of these agents. In reality, it is a multidisciplinary decision made by the treating clinicians.

Mannitol is an osmotic diuretic that also acts as a free radical scavenger [40]. It does not cross the blood-brain barrier and is thought to reduce cerebral oedema by drawing free water out of brain tissue, reducing cerebral volume and consequently pressure. It will raise the serum osmolarity and produce a diuresis. This diuresis can cause a fall in blood pressure if the patient is hypovolaemic, and hypovolaemia should be corrected before mannitol administration. A urinary catheter is also essential when considering the administration of mannitol to prevent distention of the bladder, which can result in sympathetic stimulation.

Hypertonic saline solutions (HSS) are another option to lower ICP. These often consist of 30% Saline in a 10 ml volume. A bolus of this can 'dehydrate' brain tissue and reduce ICP. The hypertonic action also results in interstitial fluid being drawn into the intravascular compartment, and the associated rise in blood pressure is often also advantageous. With their small volumes and ease of administration, HSS has replaced mannitol as the first-line ICP lowering agent in many centres [41]. Its small volume and portability, in addition to the fact it will not crystallise at low temperatures (unlike mannitol), lends itself well to use in pre-hospital practice.

Continued Management

For patients with isolated head injuries, further investigation and management are directed by a protocol based on their initial and subsequent performance in repeated neurological assessments. Patients with multiple severe or life-threatening injuries must undergo resuscitation and stabilisation before any transfer for imaging can take place. This may include going to theatre for life-saving surgery (e.g. laparotomy and arrest of severe bleeding) if they are too unstable to go to CT initially. However, it may be that these patients have the most to gain from CT scan [42, 43], and modern scanners can complete the process in under a minute. It is usually logistical factors that prolong the process rather than technical limitations nowadays.

CT Scanning

All patients in a coma and those with focal neurology or with open injuries will require CT scanning. Intra-hospital transfers to the scanner should be regarded in the same way as transfers out of the hospital and carefully planned. Full anaesthetic monitoring should be applied to the patient in line with local and national guidelines. During the scan, the anaesthetist must be positioned to see patient monitoring clearly. Restless or agitated patients may not tolerate scanning without sedation to keep them still, and this should be considered an indication for intubation and ventilation.

Neurosurgical Consultation

Following the results of scanning, all patients with severe head injuries will require consultation with a neurosurgeon. The duty neurosurgeon will need as complete a picture as possible about the patient, and a successful consultation will require a telephone history containing the following elements:

- Basic patient details (age/sex etc.)
- Very brief relevant past medical history
- History of incident
- GCS at the scene (if available)
- GCS on admission, pupils, focal neurology
- Other injuries
- Initial Management
- Basic investigation results (bloods, gases, c/spine films)
- CT scan results
- Current neurological status
- If possible, transmit the CT images to the neurosurgical centre as soon as they are available (most District General Hospital x-ray departments can do this).

Diagnosis and Management of Specific Pathologies

So far, this chapter has focused on the general management of the patient with a head injury. Little can be done initially to correct the direct damage caused by the first impact on the head, and the focus is on preventing secondary brain damage. The effects of secondary insults can be reduced by focusing on the prevention of hypoxia, hypercarbia and hypotension, as has been explained previously.

Once CT imaging has been acquired, the nature of the primary injury can be identified. Apart from superficial damage to the scalp, head injuries include: skull fractures, focal brain injuries, diffuse brain injuries, and secondary brain damage. If there are lesions amenable to surgery, this should be expedited as a priority. The longer that surgery is delayed from the time of deterioration, the worse the outcome.

Skull Fractures

Skull fractures are common but do not cause neurological disability in themselves. They do, however, provide an indicator of the force of impact and thus identify patients at higher risk of significant neurological damage (Fig. 11.8). If the fracture is compound, it may be associated with a CSF leak and the risk of air and bacterial entry into the skull. Any base of skull fracture, CSF leak or penetrating brain injury should trigger the question of whether vaccination against pneumococcus should be given to minimise the risk of pneumococcal meningitis. There is no good evidence for the routine use of prophylactic antibiotics in base of skull fractures (even with CSF leaks) [44], though penetrating brain injuries should be covered with co-amoxiclav to minimise the risk of meningitis.

Focal Brain Injuries

These are classified as lesions where macroscopic damage occurs in a localised area. They comprise contusions and haematomas. Emergency surgery may be required because of the mass effects of these lesions. 30% of patients with a head injury (who are in a coma/ and GCS <8) have an intracranial haematoma [45].

Contusions

Contusions are caused by contact between the surface of the brain and the interior ridges of the skull. The brain is usually well protected against

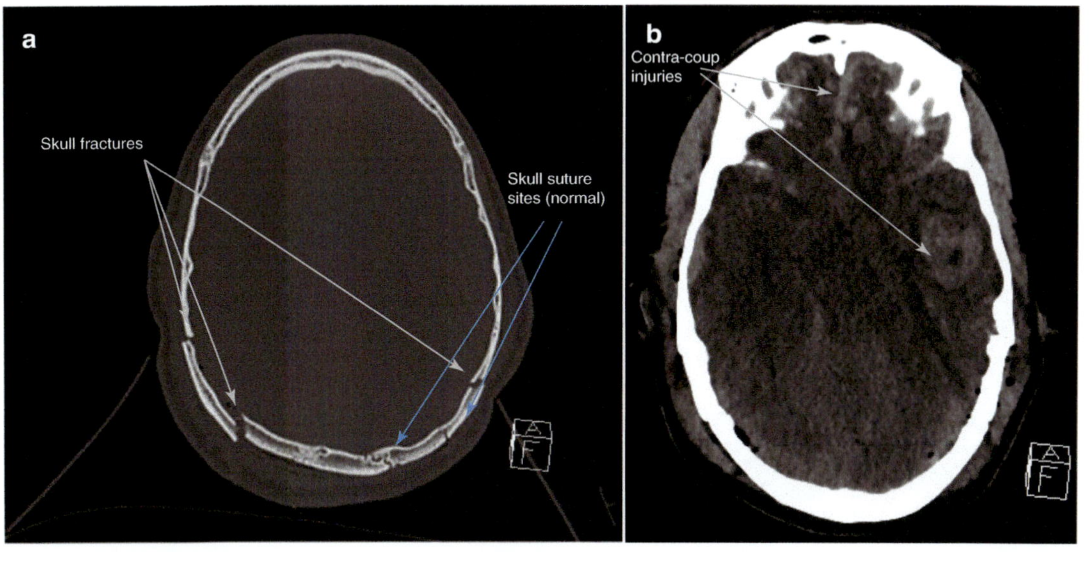

Fig. 11.8 Skull fracture and associated contra-coup injury. (**a**) CT scan of the brain demonstrating multiple skull fractures. Depressed fractures usually require surgery if compound, or if displaced more than 1 cm inwards; (**b**) CT scan from the same patient demonstrating associated contra-coup injury

these impacts by the CSF's cushioning effect; the brain's weight (1200 g) is reduced to effectively only 50 g by floating in the fluid. Rapid accelerations caused by impacts to the head or decelerations from falls, RTCs or similar mechanisms will result in shock waves travelling through the soft substance of the brain. This leads to contusions under the site of impact or remote from it (coup and contra-coup injuries).

Extradural Haematomas

Extradural haematomas are almost always associated with a tear in a dural artery, usually the middle meningeal (Fig. 11.9). Primary brain damage can be minimal, and evacuation without delay minimises secondary problems from cerebral compression. Studies have shown that about one-third of patients with fatal head injuries were talking at some time after their injury. 75% of such patients have been found to have an intracranial haematoma at post mortem [46].

The classical presentation of an extradural haematoma is of a loss of consciousness followed by a 'lucid period'. This is followed by a lapse back into unconsciousness associated with the development of an ipsilateral dilated pupil and contralateral hemiparesis. Unfortunately, only about 45% of extradural haematomas present like this.

It has been consistently demonstrated in acute extradural haematomas that operating within four hours of deterioration in conscious level leads to less death and disability (though even shorter delays were associated with better outcomes—Fig. 11.10) [47–51]. As previously mentioned, this is a skull injury that becomes a secondary brain injury if not promptly treated. It is important to note that patients with an extradural haematoma who develop fixed dilated pupils before craniotomy, if treated promptly, can still return to independent living or have minor disability only [37]. Extradural haematomas are evacuated by formal flap craniotomy and haemostasis of the meningeal artery as needed.

Acute Subdural Haematomas

More common than extradural haematomas, these lesions are caused by the rupture of veins that bridge the space between the cerebral cortex and the dura. Increasing cerebral atrophy with advancing age and chronic alcohol abuse tends to open up this space, making these lesions more

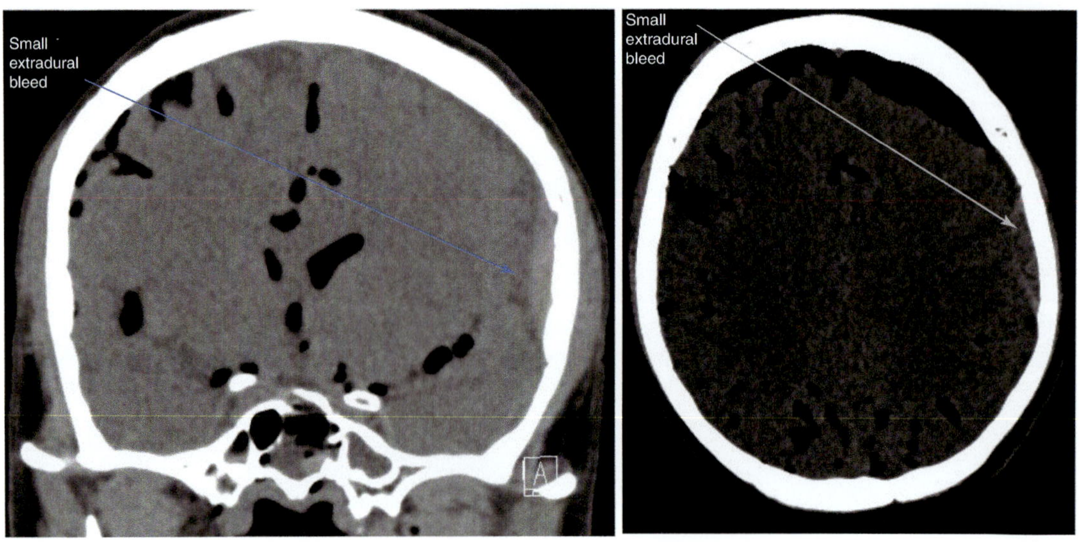

Fig. 11.9 CT scan of left sided extradural haematoma in sagittal (bottom) and coronal (top) slices

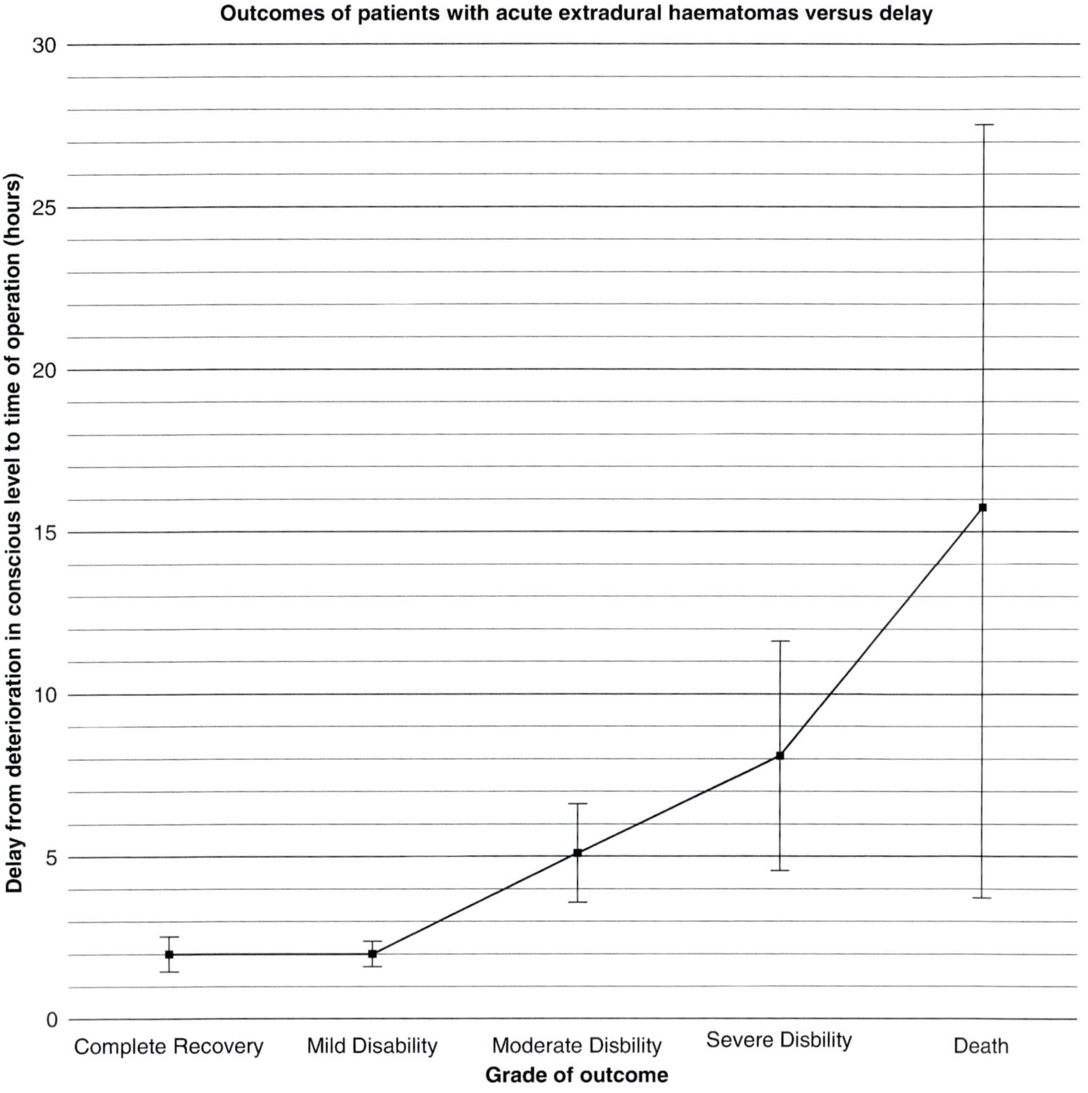

Fig. 11.10 Effect in delay on extradural evacuation on outcome (based on data from Mendelow et al. [47])

common in the elderly. In the young, associated primary brain injury is often more severe, resulting in a coma from the outset. Early evacuation (within 4 h of injury) has been shown to improve outcomes if these patients have symptoms because of mass effect (Fig. 11.11) [52]. In elderly patients, subdural haematomas may present with a variety of symptoms—these range from incidental findings in well patients to acute confusion or loss of consciousness. The management of these is consequently dependent on the degree of compromise. Small bleeds that are not progressing will benefit from a later operation when they have coagulated more and are easier to remove. Early operation in small bleeds which are not causing compromise may result in difficulties in haemostasis and subsequent re-accumulation [53]. Hence, a period of observation and re-imaging in non-compromised patients is a reasonable strategy [54, 55]. This is especially true if patients are on anticoagulant or antiplatelet medication, which can be reversed or stopped to ensure adequate postoperative haemostasis. Subdural haematomas are evacuated via Burr

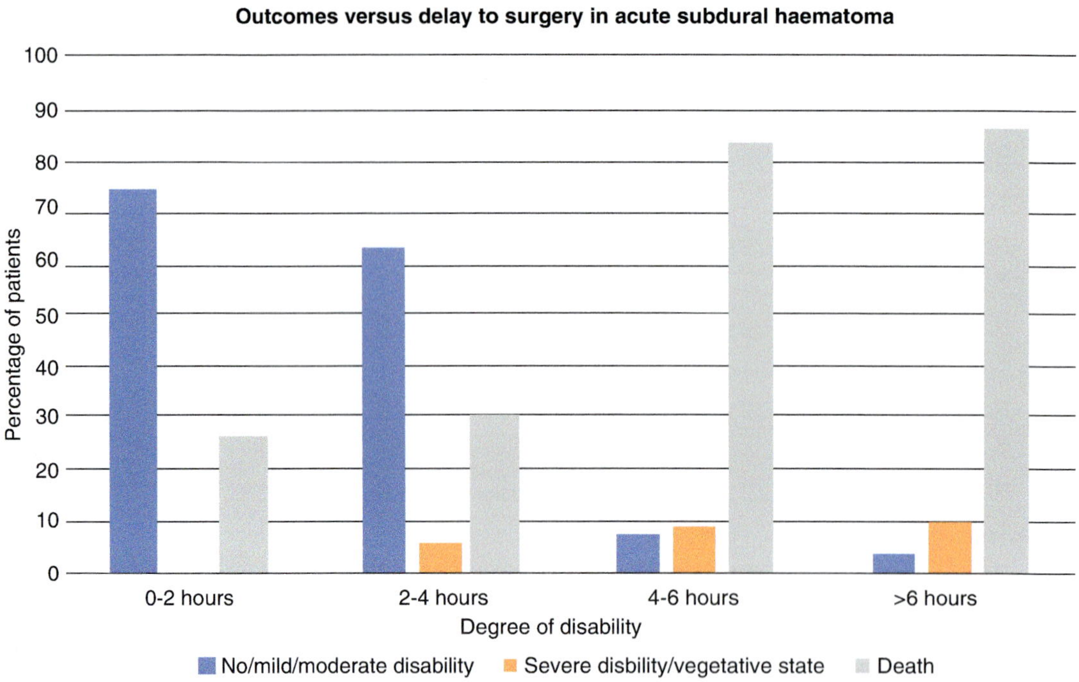

Fig. 11.11 Effect of delay in subdural evacuation on outcome (based on data from Seelig et al. [52])

hole craniotomy. The operation itself is relatively minor, though the patient group requiring these procedures may have other co-morbidities that could make anaesthesia and postoperative care challenging.

Diffuse Brain Injuries

The rapid acceleration forces transmitted to the brain following an impact to the head result in pressure waves travelling through the brain substance. These can cause stretching and tearing of axonal tracts resulting in widespread disruption of brain function. Mild forms of this, usually termed concussion, may result in temporary unconsciousness and amnesia—severe and diffuse axonal injury results in a prolonged coma. Little can be seen at a macroscopic level, even with sophisticated imaging. Post-mortem, however, microscopic examination of the brain reveals widespread tearing of the tracts within the white matter. Cerebral oedema is an inevitable accompaniment to this type of injury, giving the characteristic appearance of a swollen brain on CT scan. The progressive development of oedema leads to a rise in intracranial pressure that may cause severe secondary injury or death [56]. There is no surgical option for managing the primary injury, though decompressive craniectomy may be considered in a few select cases for management of intractably raised ICP. However, this has its problems (see later section).

Neuro Intensive Care

If not taken directly to the operating theatre, patients with a severe traumatic brain injury should be admitted to the ICU. The principles of care here are to prevent further brain injury and allow optimum physiological conditions for recovery. As initial stabilisation will have already taken place, the focus of management needs to be guided by the ICP. Therefore, all comatose patients with a head injury should be considered for insertion of an intracranial pressure monitor [57–59]. The most common variety is an intracranial 'bolt' that introduces a sensor wire through a small hole in the skull. The wire sits in the subdural space and reflects intracranial pressure. The site chosen for the monitor should be away from any focal contusion or swelling to give an accurate reading. Once continuous ICP monitoring has been established, ICP-directed therapy can be used to minimise raised ICP and ensure adequate CPP.

Several interventions can be performed in ICU to treat elevated ICP. Standards of care include ensuring the patient is 30 degrees head up without tight tube ties around the neck, and any cervical collar is removed. The rationale is not to obstruct but instead encourage venous drainage from the cerebral circulation. This, in turn, will prevent the ICP from rising [10].

Ongoing ventilation settings are based on the same principles as explained previously, avoiding hyperoxia and hypoxia, hypercarbia and hypocarbia. Very often, $PaCO_2$ targets between 4.5–5 kPa (33–37.5 mmHg) and PaO_2 of 13 kPa (97 mmHg) are chosen as acceptable parameters. If the treating physicians set targets, in the UK, the bedside ICU nurses are empowered to adjust ventilator settings to achieve this. This is also true when aiming for a CPP of 60–70 mmHg through the combination of intravenous fluid and vasopressor drugs as previously described.

Adequate pharmacological sedation is required to reduce cerebral oxygen consumption and the associated increase in blood flow. Analgesia will also be required to prevent discomfort associated with injuries and the interventions being performed. The presence of an endotracheal tube can cause considerable distress, with tachycardia and hypertension that may be undesirable. It is usual for ICU patients to be sedated with a combination of drugs. The primary sedative agent is propofol. Propofol is an intravenous anaesthetic agent that reduces cerebral blood flow (CBF), blood pressure, and cardiac output. While the reduction in CBF is desirable, the fall in cardiac output is not. Therefore, patients receiving propofol often require additional medication to ensure adequate blood pressure. If central venous access is present, the most commonly used vasopressor is noradrenaline, and this is likely the most appropriate agent [14]. Peripherally administered alpha agonists such as phenylephrine or metaraminol are also commonly used either as a temporising measure before central access has been established or if central access is not otherwise desirable [39]. The dose of propofol required can be reduced if it is co-administered with an analgesic agent. Infusions of potent, short-acting opioids are used in conjunction with a sedative. Alfentanil and fentanyl are the most commonly used drugs. As well as providing analgesia, these opioids work synergistically with the sedative agents, meaning that a smaller dose of each is required when they are given in combination.

Propofol has several undesirable side effects. The most concerning of these is the Propofol Related Infusion Syndrome (PRIS) [60–62]. While poorly understood, the development of worsening metabolic acidosis combined with cardiac arrhythmias, liver and renal dysfunction is observed in patients sedated with propofol infusions at high doses (generally thought to be greater than 4 mg/kg/h. for more than 48 h). If not detected early, multi-organ failure can develop, and without any specific treatments available, the outcome can often be fatal. As patients with traumatic brain injuries are often young and otherwise fit, with a requirement for more considerable amounts of sedation, the incidence of PRIS is thought to be higher in neurosurgical ICUs.

To prevent this complication, an alternative sedative can be used in addition to or substituted for propofol. Midazolam is often used for this purpose. Midazolam is a short-acting benzodiazepine frequently used for procedural sedation. It can cause respiratory depression but is generally more cardiovascularly stable than propofol. It is a potent anticonvulsant and decreases cerebral blood flow and metabolism. The liver metabolises the drug, and the kidneys then excrete its active metabolites. As a result, accumulation of midazolam can present a clinical problem following an infusion in the presence of organ failure. Most hospital laboratories can analyse serum for midazolam levels. While helping in the assessment of patients who are slow to wake up, the assay often takes several days to be performed. Because of this limitation, midazolam is often reserved as a second-line therapy for patients with refractory ICP in whom a more extended period of sedation is anticipated.

Sedation should be titrated to ensure that the brain is as relaxed as possible, particularly in the initial management phase or if the ICP is elevated. The Richmond Agitation-Sedation Scale (RASS) [63] is one scoring system used by ICU staff to adjust infusion rates. A RASS score of −5 (the most sedated score) is required when managing raised ICPs.

If ICP remains elevated despite the addition of a third sedative agent and hypertonic therapies have been tried, and no surgical option exists (or is thought inappropriate), a final rescue option exists in the form of a barbiturate coma [64, 65]. Barbiturates are chemically similar to benzodiazepine, and both can cause profound suppression of brain activity. Given as a single bolus, a short-acting agent such as Thiopentone can induce anaesthesia for around 10–15 min [66]. When given by infusion in the ICU, the drug rapidly accumulates and results in a prolonged period of sedation, even after discontinuation of the infusion. This accumulation is due to the long half-life (around 12 h) and the likelihood for metabolic pathways to become saturated and zero-order kinetics to predominate. Thiopentone is such a potent agent at suppressing cortical activity it is not uncommon for it to cause an isoelectric EEG (see below), giving the potential to misdiagnose brain death.

Thiopentone infusions are associated with many complications in the ICU patient. These are generally related to the depth of sedation produced. It is common to see gastroparesis and hypotension on induction of the coma. As the hypothalamus is affected, loss of thermoregulation occurs. There is also evidence to suggest that immune dysfunction occurs and there is a risk of nosocomial infections. Of particular concern to ICU clinicians are disorders of potassium, with hypokalaemia during the infusion and rebound hyperkalaemia on emergence both requiring identification and management [67, 68].

As well as the assessment of conscious level by ICU staff, continuous monitoring of brain activity can be performed by a variety of bedside devices [69–71]. Although their exact details differ, they are all based on the electroencephalogram (EEG). It is comparable to the cardiac ECG in that it is obtained by placing electrodes on the skin to record electrical impulses beneath. Usually, ten channels are recorded simultaneously. Interpretation of the full EEG is complex and usually done by a neurophysiologist, but several systems exist that process EEG data to produce a more user-friendly output. A cerebral function monitor (CFM) obtains information from scalp electrodes but produces a simplified EEG recording that focuses on the amplitude or 'strength' of brain activity. By monitoring the amplitude over hours or days, sedation can be adjusted to ensure deep sedation (identified as a 'burst suppressed' pattern). Monitoring can also detect the development of subclinical seizures. Another more processed monitor is the Bispectral Index (BIS). This monitor averages EEG values over time to give a single reading between 0 (an isoelectric 'flat' EEG) to 100. It has been shown that general anaesthesia results in a BIS between 40 and 60, but it is unclear what the target BIS should be in neuroprotective ICU management. Some treatment modifications are possible based on BIS monitoring, such as decreasing the dose of thiopentone infusions and, subsequently, fewer dose-related complications [72].

Coughing is another spontaneous response to the presence of an endotracheal tube and can be induced during endobronchial suctioning in mechanically ventilated patients. While suctioning is required, the cough response is associated with an increase in ICP, and it is often desirable to reduce it. Opioids can partly suppress the reflex, but a bolus or continuous infusion of non-depolarising muscle relaxants are also employed for this purpose.

It is no surprise that a traumatic brain injury can result in seizure activity. These seizures can increase cerebral metabolic activity, blood flow and subsequently ICP, which will result in worsening secondary injury. While a generalised tonic-clonic seizure is usually quickly identified and treated, much time can be spent trying to identify subclinical seizures in the neurosurgical patient as a cause of failure to wake from sedation or wean from invasive ventilation. Clinical signs such as dilated (but reactive) pupils or abnormal postures, combined with associated changes in heart rate or blood pressure, should lead to a suspicion of seizure activity. An elevated ICP without changes on CT scan should also raise the question of seizures. A formal EEG may also confirm this diagnosis but is rarely available before treatment should be initiated.

The management of seizures in a patient with a head injury should follow that in other settings. A dose of a short-acting benzodiazepine may be both diagnostic and therapeutic, and a loading dose followed by a maintenance regime of an anticonvulsant is then commenced. If the seizure activity is refractory to first-line therapies, treatments can be escalated with the addition of further anticonvulsants or aiming for a higher plasma concentration of established therapies. Other options include using the anticonvulsant properties of sedative agents (particularly midazolam and thiopentone) to terminate seizure activity. While treating or preventing seizures using sedative infusions may allow time to introduce other therapies, the associated loss of ability to monitor consciousness and record GCS should limit its use to short-term only.

As seizures can result in further brain injury and worse outcomes, there has been interest in using anticonvulsants as prophylactic therapy. Anticonvulsants have also been thought to offer a neuroprotective effect beyond seizure control, perhaps by preventing the calcium-induced neurotoxicity seen after neuronal hypoxia. Phenytoin has been the most studied drug for this purpose and has been shown to reduce the incidence of seizures in the first seven days following injury [73]. After this period, the prophylactic use of anticonvulsants has not been demonstrated to prevent seizures. Therefore, it is considered a standard of care for an anticonvulsant to be prescribed to patients for the first week following a traumatic brain injury. While phenytoin is still widely used, levetiracetam (Keppra) has similar efficacy, mechanism of action and more favourable pharmacodynamic properties. For these reasons, it is used as an alternative in many centres [74–77].

As much of the focus of pharmacological therapy is to suppress brain activity, it is no surprise that there has been much interest in non-pharmacological treatments to produce the same results. Inducing hypothermia, either prophylactically or therapeutically, has been the subject of research for many decades. Therapeutic hypothermia, now often referred to as 'Targeted Temperature Management' (TTM) has shown promising results in patients who have suffered a hypoxic brain injury following cardiac arrest. Several studies have demonstrated improved neurological outcomes in patients whose temperature was maintained at or below 36 degrees for the first 72-hours following their event [78]. While the mechanism is not clear, animal models have shown that hypothermia reduces free radical formation, cellular metabolism and inflammation, all of which may prevent the progression to apoptosis.

When the same principles have been applied to the traumatically injured brain, the results have been more variable. While many laboratory studies have confirmed that lowering core temperature is associated with a slowing of brain activity, these have not been reliably translated into clinical studies [79]. Large, international trials have explored cooling in a variety of patients and clinical scenarios, but none have demonstrated an improvement in survival or outcomes [80]. There could be many reasons for this, but it is generally accepted that the heterogeneous nature of traumatic brain injuries, and the ongoing insult that these injuries produce, make a simple comparison with post-cardiac arrest patients unreliable. Additionally, it has been shown that inducing hypothermia in traumatic brain injury patients prolongs their length of ICU stay and results in a higher incidence of pneumonia. Currently, it is not possible to recommend the routine use of hypothermia to treat traumatic brain injury. While hypothermia is not currently proven to be neuroprotective, hyperthermia (or pyrexia) has been shown to worsen outcome in both human and animal studies [81–84]. Fever can be a primary neurogenic response, part of the SIRS response or as part of an incidental infection. Whatever its basis, pyrexia should be aggressively treated and normal body temperature restored.

Even with multiple interventions, ICP often remains high and refractory to medical management. As untreated raised ICP will result in brain stem compression and death, one surgical option is to create space for the swelling brain tissue with a craniectomy. A decompressive craniectomy is an operation that involves removing a large area of the skull (often bifrontal or frontotemporal) in an attempt to prevent cerebral herniation. While this is often successful in preventing brain stem death, there has been much debate whether patients recover with good functional outcomes. One of the challenges in managing patients with TBI is to provide ongoing support to those patients in whom rehabilitation and some recovery are expected. The most extensive study looking at craniectomy as a rescue treatment (RESCUEicp) [85] showed that surgery improved survival. However, the probability of being in a vegetative state at six months was four times higher, and more patients remained dependent on others at 12 months. Compared with the DECRA trial [86] looking at medical vs surgical intervention for refractory intracranial hypertension, the cutoff points for favourable vs unfavourable outcomes were different, confounding the analysis. When the data from both trials were analysed with the same cutoff points used for outcomes employed in DECRA, there was no difference in favourable vs unfavourable outcomes, whether medical or surgical management was chosen [87]. The results from this and similar trials demonstrate the challenges in decision making in such situations.

Summary

In patients with a head injury, the initial resuscitation targets are summarised in the below table:

	Primary	Secondary
Blood Pressure	>110 mmHg systolic	CPP 60–70
Oxygenation	$SpO_2 > 95\%$	$PaO_2 > 13$ kPa
Ventilation	Clinically Adequate	$PaCO_2$ 4.5 kPa

Head injuries can be challenging to treat, whether in isolation or as part of a polytrauma patient. It is not helped by the fact that neurosurgical ICUs are regionalised resources, and patients may present to non-specialist centres before being transferred onwards. Improved outcomes are not just due to surgical intervention. Patients with neurological injuries that are cared for on specialist neurosurgical critical care units have better outcomes than neurologically injured patients treated on conventional critical care units [88]. The whole multi-disciplinary team contributes to this, rather than one particular intervention. Improved speed of access to surgery when indicated, minimising delays in treatment or transfer, and attention to detail in managing these patients will all reap dividends. Initial management, as always, is driven by the MABCD approach and is directed towards the prevention of secondary brain injury once the primary brain injury has occurred.

Questions

1. The Monroe-Kelly Doctrine describes:

    (a) The severity of brain injury
    (b) Assessment of conscious level following TBI
    (c) The intracranial relationship between pressure and volume
    (d) The relationship between cerebral perfusion and ventilation
    (e) Indications for decompressive craniectomy

2. A patient is found at the scene of a road traffic collision. He makes no response to a verbal stimulus. His eyes open on supra-orbital pressure, and his right elbow bends so that his hand is at the shoulder level. There is no verbal response throughout. What best describes his neurological assessment?

    (a) GCS 6 - E2, V1, M3
    (b) GCS 7 - E2, V1, M4
    (c) GCS 7 - E3, V1, M4

(d) GCS 8 - E2, V1, M5
(e) GCS 8 - E3, V1, M5

3. Cerebral Perfusion Pressure (CPP) is dependent on:

(a) SBP and ICP
(b) SBP and CVP
(c) MAP and ICP
(d) MAP and DBP
(e) ICP and TCD

4. The following statement about an epidural haematoma is correct:

(a) The onset of symptoms is slow, over hours or days
(b) Bleeding occurs between the dura and arachnoid mater
(c) The bleeding is venous in origin
(d) Non-operative management is most commonly employed
(e) The bleeding is between the cranium and dura.

5. Which of the following is NOT a method to reduce ICP on ICU patients:

(a) Head-up positioning
(b) Prophylactic anticonvulsants
(c) Prevention of pyrexia
(d) RASS score of +5
(e) CSA monitoring

Answers

1. c
2. b
3. c
4. e
5. d

References

1. Reilly P, Bullock R, editors. Head injury: pathophysiology and management. 2nd ed. New York: Hodder Arnold; 2005. distributed in the USA by Oxford University Press; 501 p
2. Ellis H. Clinical anatomy: a revision and applied anatomy for clinical students. 11th ed. Blackwell: Malden; 2006. p. 439.
3. Figaji AA. Anatomical and physiological differences between children and adults relevant to traumatic brain injury and the implications for clinical assessment and care. Front Neurol [Internet]. 2017 [cited 2020 July 16]: [8 p.]. Available from: https://www.ncbi.nlm.nih.gov/pmc/articles/PMC5735372/
4. Mokri B. The Monro-Kellie hypothesis: Applications in CSF volume depletion. Neurology. 2001;56(12):1746–8.
5. Borgström L, Jóhannsson H, Siesjö BK. The relationship between arterial po2 and cerebral blood flow in hypoxic hypoxia. Acta Physiol Scand. 1975;93(3):423–32.
6. Ogoh S. Cerebral blood flow regulation during hypoxia. Exp Physiol. 2015;100(2):109–10.
7. Rincon F, Kang J, Maltenfort M, Vibbert M, Urtecho J, Athar MK, et al. Association between Hyperoxia and mortality after stroke: a multicenter cohort study*. Crit Care Med. 2014;42(2):387–96.
8. López HV, Vivas MF, Ruiz RN, Martínez JR, Navaridas BG-V, Villa MG, et al. Association between post-procedural hyperoxia and poor functional outcome after mechanical thrombectomy for ischemic stroke: an observational study. Ann Intensive Care [Internet]. 2019 [cited 2020 July 17]: [9 p.]. Available from: https://www.ncbi.nlm.nih.gov/pmc/articles/PMC6534627/
9. Vincent J-L, Taccone FS, He X. Harmful effects of Hyperoxia in postcardiac arrest, sepsis, traumatic brain injury, or stroke: the importance of individualised oxygen therapy in critically Ill patients. Can Respir J [Internet]. 2017 [cited 2020 July 17]: [2017 p.]. Available from: https://www.ncbi.nlm.nih.gov/pmc/articles/PMC5299175/
10. Wilson MH. Monro-Kellie 2.0: The dynamic vascular and venous pathophysiological components of intracranial pressure. J Cereb Blood Flow Metab. 2016;36(8):1338–50.
11. Maas AI, Dearden M, Teasdale GM, Braakman R, Cohadon F, Iannotti F, et al. EBIC-guidelines for management of severe head injury in adults. European Brain Injury Consortium. Acta Neurochir. 1997;139(4):286–94.
12. Nathanson MH, Andrzejowski J, Dinsmore J, Eynon CA, Ferguson K, Hooper T, et al. Guidelines for safe transfer of the brain-injured patient: trauma and stroke, 2019. Anaesthesia. 2020;75(2):234–46.
13. Carney N, Totten AM, O'Reilly C, Ullman JS, GWJ H, Bell MJ, et al. Guidelines for the management of severe traumatic brain injury. Fourth Edn Neurosurg. 2016;80:1.
14. Myburgh JA. Driving cerebral perfusion pressure with pressors: how, which, when? Crit Care Resusc. 2005;7(3):200–5.
15. TARN - Major Trauma in Older People [Internet]. The Trauma Audit and Research Network; 2017 [cited 2019 Dec 30] [40 p.]. Available from: https://

www.tarn.ac.uk/content/downloads/3793/Major%20Trauma%20in%20Older%20People%202017.pdf
16. TARN. Severe Injury in Children January 2015–December 2016 [Internet]. The Trauma Audit and Research Network; 2016 [cited 2019 Dec 9] [37 p.]. Available from: https://www.tarn.ac.uk/content/downloads/3572/SevereInjuryinChildren15-16.pdf
17. National Institute for Health and Care Excellence. Head Injury Quality Standard [Internet]. 2014 [cited 2020 July 17]. Available from: https://www.nice.org.uk/guidance/qs74
18. Romanelli D, Farrell MW. AVPU (Alert, Voice, Pain, Unresponsive). In: StatPearls [Internet]. Treasure Island (FL): StatPearls Publishing; 2020 [cited 2020 July 17]. Available from: http://www.ncbi.nlm.nih.gov/books/NBK538431/
19. Williams B. The national early warning score and the acutely confused patient. Clin Med (Lond). 2019;19(2):190–1.
20. Teasdale G, Maas A, Lecky F, Manley G, Stocchetti N, Murray G. The glasgow Coma scale at 40 years: standing the test of time. Lancet Neurol. 2014;13(8):844–54.
21. Beckmann Y, Çiftçi Y, Incesu TK, Seçil Y, Akhan G. Spinal reflexes in brain death. Acta Neurol Belg. 2014;114(4):303–6.
22. Mena JH, Sanchez AI, Rubiano AM, Peitzman AB, Sperry JL, Gutierrez MI, et al. Effect of the modified Glasgow coma scale score criteria for mild traumatic brain injury on mortality prediction: comparing classic and modified Glasgow coma scale score model scores of 13. J Trauma. 2011;71(5):1185–93.
23. American College of Surgeons, Committee on Trauma. Advanced trauma life support: student course manual. 10th ed. Chicago, IL: American College of Surgeons; 2018.
24. Rotheray KR, Cheung PSY, Cheung CSK, Wai AKC, Chan DYS, Rainer TH, et al. What is the relationship between the Glasgow coma scale and airway protective reflexes in the Chinese population? Resuscitation. 2012;83(1):86–9.
25. Duncan R, Thakore S. Decreased Glasgow Coma Scale Score does not mandate endotracheal intubation in the emergency department. J Emerg Med. 2009;37(4):451–5.
26. Green SM. Cheerio, Laddie! Bidding Farewell to the Glasgow coma scale. Ann Emerg Med. 2011;58(5):427–30.
27. Bassi S, Buxton N, Punt J, O'Reilly G. Glasgow coma scale: a help or hindrance. Br J Neurosurg. 1999;13(526):2.
28. Wiese MF. British hospitals and different versions of the Glasgow coma scale: telephone survey. BMJ. 2003;327(7418):782–3.
29. Gill MR, Reiley DG, Green SM. Interrater reliability of Glasgow coma scale scores in the emergency department. Ann Emerg Med. 2004;43(2):215–23.
30. Teasdale G, Jennett B, Murray L, Murray G. Glasgow coma scale: to sum or not to sum. Lancet. 1983;2(8351):678.
31. Healey C, Osler TM, Rogers FB, Healey MA, Glance LG, Kilgo PD, et al. Improving the Glasgow coma scale score: motor score alone is a better predictor. J Trauma. 2003;54(4):671–8. discussion 678–680
32. Fortune P-M, Shann F. The motor response to stimulation predicts outcome as well as the full Glasgow Coma Scale in children with severe head injury: Pediatr Crit Care Med. 2009;1.
33. Ross SE, Leipold C, Terregino C, O'Malley KF. Efficacy of the motor component of the Glasgow coma scale in trauma triage. J Trauma. 1998;45(1):42–4.
34. Al-Salamah MA, McDowell I, Stiell IG, Wells GA, Perry J, Al-Sultan M, et al. Initial emergency department trauma scores from the OPALS study: the case for the motor score in blunt trauma. Acad Emerg Med. 2004;11(8):834–42.
35. Gill M, Steele R, Windemuth R, Green SM. A comparison of five simplified scales to the out-of-hospital Glasgow Coma Scale for the prediction of traumatic brain injury outcomes. Acad Emerg Med. 2006;13(9):968–73.
36. Gill M, Windemuth R, Steele R, Green SM. A comparison of the Glasgow coma scale score to simplified alternative scores for the prediction of traumatic brain injury outcomes. Ann Emerg Med. 2005;45(1):37–42.
37. Scotter JM, Hendrickson SA, Marcus HJ, Wilson MH. Prognosis of patients with bilateral fixed dilated pupils secondary to traumatic extradural or subdural haematoma who undergo surgery: a systematic review and meta-analysis. Emerg Med J: EMJ. 2015;32(8):654–9.
38. Curley G, Kavanagh BP, Laffey JG. Hypocapnia and the injured brain: more harm than benefit. Crit Care Med. 2010;38(5):1348–59.
39. Lax P, Dagal A. Recent advances in the use of vasopressors and inotropes in Neurotrauma. Curr Anesthesiol Rep. 2018;8(1):86–93.
40. Shawkat H, Westwood M-M, Mortimer A. Mannitol: a review of its clinical uses. Contin Educ Anaesth Crit Care Pain. 2012;12(2):82–5.
41. Mangat HS, Wu X, Gerber LM, Schwarz JT, Fakhar M, Murthy SB, et al. Hypertonic saline is superior to mannitol for the combined effect on intracranial pressure and cerebral perfusion pressure burdens in patients with severe traumatic brain injury. Neurosurgery [Internet]. 2019 [cited 2019 May 7]; Available from: https://academic.oup.com/neurosurgery/advance-article/doi/10.1093/neuros/nyz046/5381832
42. Ordoñez CA, Herrera-Escobar JP, Parra MW, Rodriguez-Ossa PA, Mejia DA, Sanchez AI, et al. Computed tomography in hemodynamically unstable severely injured blunt and penetrating trauma patients. J Trauma Acute Care Surg. 2016;80(4):597–603.
43. Huber-Wagner S, Biberthaler P, Häberle S, Wierer M, Dobritz M, Rummeny E, et al. Whole-body CT in haemodynamically unstable severely injured patients – a retrospective, multicentre study. PLoS One [Internet]. 2013 [cited 2019 Aug 26];8(7).

Available from: https://www.ncbi.nlm.nih.gov/pmc/articles/PMC3722202/
44. Ratilal BO, Costa J, Pappamikail L, Sampaio C. Antibiotic prophylaxis for preventing meningitis in patients with basilar skull fractures. Cochrane Datab Syst Rev [Internet]. 2015 [cited 2020 July 17];(4). Available from: https://www.cochranelibrary.com/cdsr/doi/10.1002/14651858.CD004884.pub4/full
45. Schmidt WU, Ploner CJ, Lutz M, Möckel M, Lindner T, Braun M. Causes of brain dysfunction in acute coma: a cohort study of 1027 patients in the emergency department. Scand J Trauma Resusc Emerg Med [Internet]. 2019 [cited 2020 July 29]: [27 p.]. Available from: https://www.ncbi.nlm.nih.gov/pmc/articles/PMC6836468/
46. Alexis RJ, Jagdish S, Sukumar S, Pandit VR, Palnivel C, Antony MJ. Clinical profile and autopsy findings in fatal head injuries. J Emerg Trauma Shock. 2018;11(3):205–10.
47. Mendelow AD, Karmi MZ, Paul KS, Fuller GA, Gillingham FJ. Extradural haematoma: effect of delayed treatment. Br Med J. 1979;1(6173):1240–2.
48. Chowdhury NK, Raihan M, Chowdhury F, Ashadullah A, Sarkar M, Hossain S. Surgical management of traumatic extradural haematoma: experiences with 610 patients and prospective analysis. Indian J Neurotrauma. 2008;5(2):75–9.
49. Lobato RD. Acute epidural hematoma: an analysis of factors influencing the outcome of patients undergoing surgery in coma. J Neurosurg. 1988;68:10.
50. Cheung PSY, Lam JMY, Yeung JHH, Graham CA, Rainer TH. Outcome of traumatic extradural haematoma in Hong Kong. Injury. 2007;38(1):76–80.
51. Paterniti S, Fiore P, Macrì E, Marra G, Cambria M, Falcone F, et al. Extradural haematoma. Acta Neurochir. 1994;131(3):207–10.
52. Seelig JM, Becker DP, Miller JD, Greenberg RP, Ward JD, Choi SC. Traumatic acute subdural hematoma: major mortality reduction in comatose patients treated within four hours. N Engl J Med. 1981;304(25):1511–8.
53. Jang KM, Choi HH, Mun HY, Nam TK, Park YS, Kwon JT. Critical depressed brain volume influences the recurrence of chronic subdural hematoma after surgical evacuation. Sci Rep. 2020;10(1):1145.
54. Yadav YR, Parihar V, Namdev H, Bajaj J. Chronic subdural hematoma. Asian J Neurosurg. 2016;11(4):330–42.
55. Karnjanasavitree W, Phuenpathom N, Tunthanathip T. The optimal operative timing of traumatic intracranial acute subdural hematoma correlated with outcome. Asian J Neurosurg. 2018;13(4):1158–64.
56. Mesfin FB, Gupta N, Hays Shapshak A, Taylor RS. Diffuse axonal injury (DAI). In: StatPearls [Internet]. Treasure Island (FL): StatPearls Publishing; 2020 [cited 2020 July 17]. Available from: http://www.ncbi.nlm.nih.gov/books/NBK448102/
57. Intracranial Pressure Monitoring - Indications - Types [Internet]. TeachMeSurgery. [cited 2020 July 17]. Available from: https://teachmesurgery.com/neurosurgery/flow-and-pressure/icp-monitoring/
58. Munakomi SM, Das J. Intracranial Pressure Monitoring. In: StatPearls [Internet]. Treasure Island (FL): StatPearls Publishing; 2020 [cited 2020 July 17]. Available from: http://www.ncbi.nlm.nih.gov/books/NBK542298/
59. Le Roux P. Intracranial pressure monitoring and management. In: Laskowitz D, Grant G, editors. Translational research in traumatic brain injury [Internet]. Boca Raton (FL): CRC Press/Taylor and Francis Group; 2016 [cited 2020 July 17]. (Frontiers in Neuroscience). Available from: http://www.ncbi.nlm.nih.gov/books/NBK326713/
60. Loh N-HW, Nair P. Propofol infusion syndrome. Contin Educ Anaesth Crit Care Pain. 2013;13(6):200–2.
61. Mirrakhimov AE, Voore P, Halytskyy O, Khan M, Ali AM. Propofol infusion syndrome in adults: a clinical update. Crit Care Res Pract [Internet]. 2015 [cited 2020 July 17];2015. Available from: https://www.ncbi.nlm.nih.gov/pmc/articles/PMC4410753/
62. Hemphill S, McMenamin L, Bellamy MC, Hopkins PM. Propofol infusion syndrome: a structured literature review and analysis of published case reports. Br J Anaesth. 2019;122(4):448–59.
63. Sessler CN, Gosnell MS, Grap MJ, Brophy GM, O'Neal PV, Keane KA, et al. The richmond agitation–sedation scale: validity and reliability in adult intensive care unit patients. Am J Respir Crit Care Med. 2002;166(10):1338–44.
64. Kim Y-I, Park S-W, Nam T-K, Park Y-S, Min B-K, Hwang S-N. The effect of barbiturate coma therapy for the patients with severe intracranial hypertension: a 10-year experience. J Korean Neurosurg Soc. 2008;44(3):141–5.
65. Cordato DJ, Herkes GK, Mather LE, Gross AS, Finfer S, Morgan MK. Prolonged thiopentone infusion for neurosurgical emergencies: usefulness of therapeutic drug monitoring. Anaesth Intensive Care. 2001;29(4):339–48.
66. Scarth E, Smith S. Drugs in Anaesthesia and Intensive Care. 5th ed. Oxford University Press; 2016. (Oxford Medical Publications; vol. 1).
67. Ng SY, Chin KJ, Kwek TK. Dyskalaemia associated with thiopentone barbiturate coma for refractory intracranial hypertension: a case series. Intensive Care Med. 2011;37(8):1285–9.
68. Kim TK, Lim Y-J, Ju J-W, Kim JW, Park H-P. The effects of propofol and thiopental continuous infusion on serum potassium disturbances in neurosurgical patients. J Korean Neurosurg Soc. 2015;57(3):197–203.
69. Smith M. Multimodality neuromonitoring in adult traumatic brain injury a narrative review. Anesthesiology. 2018;128(2):401–15.
70. Jones S, Schwartzbauer G, Jia X. Brain monitoring in critically neurologically impaired patients. Int

J Mol Sci [Internet]. 2016 Dec 27 [cited 2020 July 17]:18(1). Available from: https://www.ncbi.nlm.nih.gov/pmc/articles/PMC5297678/

71. Matz PG, Pitts L. Monitoring in traumatic brain injury. Clin Neurosurg. 1997;44:267–94.
72. An H-S, Cho B-M, Kang J-H, Kim M-K, Oh S-M, Park S-H. Efficacy of low dose barbiturate coma therapy for the patients with intractable intracranial hypertension using the bispectral™ index monitoring. J Korean Neurosurg Soc. 2010;47(4):252–7.
73. Temkin NR, Dikmen SS, Wilensky AJ, Keihm J, Chabal S, Winn HR. A randomised, double-blind study of phenytoin for the prevention of post-traumatic seizures. N Engl J Med. 1990;323(8):497–502.
74. Jones KE, Puccio AM, Harshman KJ, Falcione B, Benedict N, Jankowitz BT, et al. Levetiracetam versus phenytoin for seizure prophylaxis in severe traumatic brain injury. Neurosurg Focus. 2008;25(4):E3.
75. Harris L, Hateley S, Seemungal B. P22 Phenytoin versus levetiracetam for post traumatic brain injury seizure prophylaxis; a retrospective study at a UK major trauma centre. J Neurol Neurosurg Psychiatry. 2019;90(3):e31.
76. Zhao L, Wu Y-P, Qi J-L, Liu Y-Q, Zhang K, Li W-L. Efficacy of levetiracetam compared with phenytoin in prevention of seizures in brain injured patients: a meta-analysis. Medicine. 2018;97(48):e13247.
77. Helmy T, Tamam H, Mahmoud M. Comparison between levetiracetam and phenytoin for seizure prophylaxis in patients with traumatic brain injury. Res Opin Anesth Intensive Care. 2018;5(4):307.
78. Nielsen N, Wetterslev J, Cronberg T, Erlinge D, Gasche Y, Hassager C, et al. Targeted temperature management at 33°C versus 36°C after cardiac arrest. N Engl J Med. 2013;369(23):2197–206.
79. Dietrich WD, Bramlett HM. Therapeutic hypothermia and targeted temperature management in traumatic brain injury: clinical challenges for successful translation. Brain Res. 1640;2016:94–103.
80. Lewis SR, Evans DJ, Butler AR, Schofield-Robinson OJ, Alderson P. Hypothermia for traumatic brain injury. Cochrane Datab Syst Rev [Internet]. 2017 [cited 2020 July 17]: [9 p.]. Available from: https://www.cochranelibrary.com/cdsr/doi/10.1002/14651858.CD001048.pub5/full
81. Li J, Jiang J. Chinese head trauma data bank: effect of hyperthermia on the outcome of acute head trauma patients. J Neurotrauma. 2012;29(1):96–100.
82. Sakurai A, Atkins CM, Alonso OF, Bramlett HM, Dietrich WD. Mild hyperthermia worsens the neuropathological damage associated with mild traumatic brain injury in rats. J Neurotrauma. 2012;29(2):313–21.
83. Thompson HJ, Pinto-Martin J, Bullock MR. Neurogenic fever after traumatic brain injury: an epidemiological study. J Neurol Neurosurg Psychiatry. 2003;74(5):614–9.
84. Mrozek S, Vardon F, Geeraerts T. Brain temperature: physiology and pathophysiology after brain injury. Anesthesiol Res Pract. 2012;2012:1–13.
85. Hutchinson PJ, Kolias AG, Timofeev IS, Corteen EA, Czosnyka M, Timothy J, et al. Trial of decompressive craniectomy for traumatic intracranial hypertension. N Engl J Med. 2016;375(12):1119–30.
86. Cooper DJ, Rosenfeld JV, Murray L, Arabi YM, Davies AR, D'Urso P, et al. Decompressive craniectomy in diffuse traumatic brain injury. N Engl J Med. 2011;364(16):1493–502.
87. Cooper DJ, Nichol A, Hodgson C. Craniectomy for traumatic intracranial hypertension. N Engl J Med. 2016;375(24):2401–4.
88. Kurtz P, Fitts V, Sumer Z, Jalon H, Cooke J, Kvetan V, et al. How does care differ for neurological patients admitted to a neurocritical care unit versus a general ICU? Neurocrit Care. 2011;15(3):477–80.

12 Traumatic Cardiac Arrest

Matthew O'Meara and Peter Lax

- Epidemiology of traumatic cardiac arrest
- Reversible causes of cardiac arrest in trauma
- Managing medical cardiac arrests in trauma patients
- Resuscitative thoracotomy in traumatic cardiac arrest
- Human factors in traumatic cardiac arrest
- Other causes of arrest relevant to trauma

Introduction

Traumatic cardiac arrest is the final common pathway of several pathologies, often resulting in high mortality.

M. O'Meara (✉)
EMRTS Wales, Llanelli, UK

Deprtment of Anaesthesia and Critical Care Medicine, University Hospital of North Staffordshire, Stoke, UK
e-mail: Matthew.OMeara@doctors.org.uk

P. Lax
Tactical Medical Wing, Royal Air Force, Brize Norton, Oxfordshire, UK

The Air Ambulance Service (TAAS), Rugby, Warwickshire, UK

Epidemiology

Office of National Statistics data highlights that trauma causes approximately 20,000 deaths per year in the UK, out of 500,000 deaths overall (4% of all deaths), but that it disproportionately affects certain age groups (10% of all deaths in those of working age) [1]. Survival rates of up to 4% have been reported in traumatic cardiac arrest, but may be higher in specific situations and for specific underlying conditions.

Out-of-hospital cardiac arrest accounts for 0.5% of all calls to the UK ambulance service, of which traumatic aetiology accounts for 10% of these (1:20,000) calls overall. There are approximately ten million calls to the service each year, yielding the total number of traumatic arrests as 5000 per annum. Up to 50% of these patients will be beyond help and will not have resuscitation commenced, in line with ambulance service guidelines [2].

If these patients were distributed equally across the trauma system, each network would see one potentially treatable patient in traumatic cardiac arrest every 4 days. Thus, it is a comparatively rare event for most healthcare practitioners across the system [3].

Presentation

Reversible traumatic cardiac arrest may occur in the presence of the team caring for the patient or

P. Lax (ed.), *Textbook of Acute Trauma Care*, https://doi.org/10.1007/978-3-030-83628-3_12

on hospital arrival of a patient who has been pre-alerted as being peri-arrest by prehospital teams.

It is possible for patients to be assumed to be peri-arrest but to have actually arrested. This emphasises the importance of situational awareness, especially during critical phases of care, such as during handover. Pulse checks are therefore vital, especially in those with agonal breathing.

Management

Cardiopulmonary Resuscitation

Two theoretical principles exist concerning closed chest compressions during CPR. The cardiac pump theory purports that compression between the bony thorax expels blood into the aorta, as would be the case if the heart was beating natively. The thoracic pump theory relates changes in intra- and extrathoracic pressure to changes in pressure in the vascular system [4].

The role of closed-chest massage has been questioned in the management of traumatic cardiac arrest. Evidence to support or refute its use is weak on both sides of the argument. Therefore, CPR should be initiated and performed (especially if there is a possibility of a medical cause of cardiac arrest) unless it is impeding the performance of other procedures of a higher priority, such as intubation, thoracic decompression, resuscitative thoracotomy (where indicated) or the administration of resuscitative fluids [5–9].

Trauma patients in cardiac arrest are much more likely to present in non-shockable rhythms [10, 11]. In patients who are extremely hypovolaemic but have arterial pressure monitoring in situ, there may be no palpable pulse, but an arterial waveform remains. This indicates a severely compromised but present cardiac output. However, under traditional ALS teaching, this state would be considered Pulseless Electrical Activity (PEA) and managed according to standard cardiac arrest guidelines. Most patients will not have arterial lines in situ unless they arrest in hospital. Still, echocardiography in prehospital care and emergency departments has been used to demonstrate "low-flow" as opposed to "no-flow" states. If echocardiography indicates effective myocardial contraction but severe hypovolaemia, the correct treatment would be aggressive resuscitation with blood and source control of bleeding instead of the administration of adrenaline and CPR [6, 11]. If there is an inadequate circulating volume to the point where pulses cannot be palpated, even the most effective CPR will not correct this.

Reversing the Reversible

The reversible causes of traumatic cardiac arrest vary from those of medical arrest subtly. They can be remembered using the mnemonic HOTT (Hypovolaemia, Oxygenation, Tension pneumothorax and tamponade) [5, 6].

Hypovolaemia

Where traumatic cardiac arrest occurs in the context of hypovolaemia, the chances of survival are reduced as compared with traumatic cardiac arrest from other mechanisms (except for severe neurotrauma) [11].

Hypovolaemia in trauma must always be assumed to be secondary to bleeding. This can occur externally or internally. External blood loss should be aggressively treated with direct pressure, dressings, tourniquets, staples or sutures as mentioned in the massive haemorrhage chapter. Internal haemorrhage from fractures should be managed with manual traction and splintage before surgical fixation. The pelvis should be bound to limit further bleeding into the pelvic cavity. Non-compressible thoracic or abdominal haemorrhage is only controllable surgically, or via interventional radiological means in select cases.

Surgical methods to control haemorrhage include the need to perform a thoracotomy or laparotomy, with packing, clamping or repair of bleeding vessels. In the short term, a thoracotomy performed in the resuscitation room with aortic cross-clamping may buy valuable time to assess and address distal bleeding sites. This procedure should only be performed in the right environment with the right equipment and team and with a viable exit strategy for the next phase of care as discussed later in this chapter.

Current guidelines recommend resuscitative thoracotomy in the event the resuscitation team witnesses the patient arrest, or the patient has had signs of life and CPR within the previous 10 min (blunt trauma) or 15 min (penetrating trauma), with a suspected or confirmed cause that may be amenable to surgical treatment [12]. The indications for resuscitative thoracotomy may change depending on available expertise and resources, as non-specialist surgeons or non-surgical practitioners are able to treat fewer pathologies in comparatively austere environments compared to trained trauma surgeons in an operating theatre [5, 12].

Endovascular techniques have been employed since the 1950s to control excessive haemorrhage in trauma [13, 14]. Modern balloon technology allows for an endovascular balloon to be placed into one of the three zones of the aorta to arrest haemorrhage distal to that site. The occlusion is thought to be temporising while the balloon is inflated. However, it may also be temporarily therapeutic in itself since a reduction in pressure in bleeding vascular beds may facilitate clot formation. Zone three REBOA is reserved for pelvic/lower extremity bleeding. Zone one occlusion (above the diaphragm) is likely to be more appropriate for cases of witnessed or near-witnessed traumatic cardiac arrest where haemorrhage is thought to be the primary aetiology. Once the balloon is inflated, it is imperative to have strict protocols to minimise inflation time, and the patient should be transferred for definitive management to either the interventional radiology suite or operating theatre. When source control has been achieved, effective communication is needed between the surgeon/interventionalist and anaesthetist regarding deflating the balloon to manage the cardiovascular effects of reperfusion. This may lead to cardiovascular instability as cold, acidic and potassium-rich blood is returned into the central circulation at the same time as the volume of the circulation is increased.

Vascular access can be achieved by several methods. The need for short, large bore vascular access for aggressive and ongoing fluid resuscitation is essential. Peripheral access may be possible and adequate, but is frequently challenging (if possible at all) in severe hypovolaemia. Failure of the rapid establishment of adequate peripheral access dictates the placement of central access, ideally with a Swan sheath introducer or another large-bore device (e.g. Vascath or MAC line). Standard central lines are too narrow to provide adequate flow rates for resuscitation (Fig. 12.1). If peripheral access is going to be placed, it should be 16G or larger in the first instance. However, devices such as the Rapid Infusion Catheter (RIC) sets can be used to upsize smaller cannulae via a Seldinger technique.

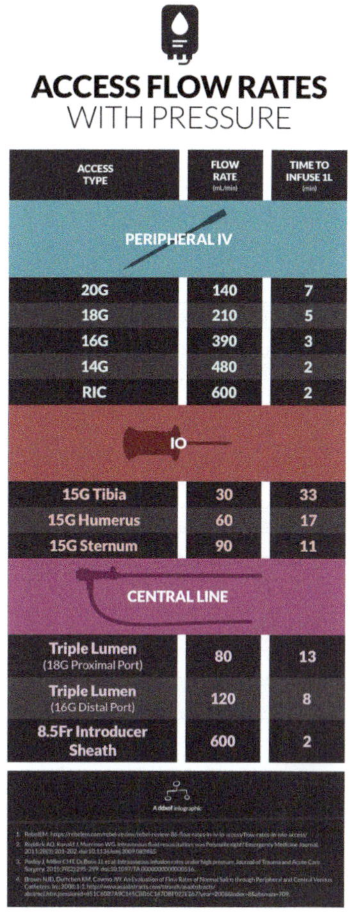

Fig. 12.1 Flow rates through various vascular access devices (from ddxof.com [15])

Central access can be achieved in the internal jugular, subclavian or femoral veins [16, 17]. The subclavian vein is often preferred for several reasons. Logistically, the chest is accessible for intervention without impeding the airway operator if a concurrent procedure such as intubation is ongoing. There is also no requirement to move the neck, which may also have a cervical collar applied, rendering the internal jugular veins inaccessible. Anatomically, the subclavian vein is held open by the clavipectoral fascia and therefore easier to cannulate in hypovolaemic patients, allowing large volume resuscitation straight into the superior vena cava. Compared to other central access sites, subclavian lines carry the lowest risk of infection [18–21], and when secured is more comfortable for the patient than an internal jugular or femoral line [22]. The subclavian route additionally avoids the risk of fluids or drugs not getting to the central circulation due to an interrupted vascular supply (e.g. iliac vein or IVC injury) in the case of femoral lines.

Intra-osseous (IO) access can be helpful for drugs administration and can be used for fluid resuscitation; however, if not appropriately guarded, they are easily displaced. Even when working well, IO lines often require high pressure to ensure flow. This makes them appropriate for drug bolus administration, but for ongoing large volume resuscitation they are impractical and central (or large peripheral) access is preferred.

Fluid resuscitation for bleeding trauma patients is covered in the Circulation Chap. 10 and should follow principles of haemostatic and blood resuscitation where possible. Whole blood, initially used in World War One, is a promising solution as compared with mixed ratios of blood, plasma and platelets. Fibrinogen levels fall early in hypovolaemic shock (especially in traumatic cardiac arrest) and should be replaced with cryoprecipitate or reconstituted fibrinogen [23, 24]. Electrolytic abnormalities, especially hypocalcaemia and hyperkalaemia, are a feature of large volume product transfusion and should be actively sought and excluded in the event traumatic arrest occurs on the operating table [25–28]. All blood products should be warmed to mitigate against hypothermia caused by the administration of refrigerated blood products.

In the context of a traumatic arrest, universal donor blood products should be brought from the blood bank as part of an ongoing major haemorrhage protocol. This ensures a steady and smooth flow of products to the patient. Early tests of coagulation and coagulopathy should be sent, including the use of thromboelastography.

Oxygenation

Hypoxia occurs in traumatic cardiac arrest from a variety or combination of pathologies. Asphyxia occurs when the airway is occluded from any cause—in blunt trauma, the most common cause is a head injury with secondary airway obstruction. There may be a direct injury to the structures of the airway or the neck as a result of blunt or penetrating trauma, which may entirely or partially occlude the airway or limit ventilation and contribute to asphyxia.

Failure to deliver oxygen occasionally occurs due to depletion of portable cylinders or supply lines in a medical context, and constant surveillance for low FiO_2 should be kept whilst managing patients suffering from a traumatic cardiac arrest.

The inspiration of oxygen-deplete air occurs with smoke inhalation and will be associated with toxicity, for example of carbon monoxide or cyanide and will result in histotoxic hypoxaemia.

Failure of the respiratory system to adequately oxygenate the blood can occur due to indirect or direct injury. High cord injuries result in paralysis of the phrenic or intercostal nerves resulting in failure of nerve impulse transmission to the diaphragm or intercostal muscles. Ventilation is impaired and may cease altogether with resulting hypoxia and hypercarbia. Classic mechanisms include those resulting in high cervical spinal injuries from neck hyperflexion or hyperextension, such as diving into shallow water or cycling injuries. Once hypoxia is corrected, a return of spontaneous circulation (ROSC) usually follows. Spinal precautions are essential in these incidents.

Thoracic injury causes damage to the lungs or pleura which may impede ventilation, resulting in hypoxic cardiac arrest—see the Breathing Chap. 9 for more information.

Airway Management

The airway should be managed according to standard protocols. This usually means that the patient should be intubated when possible and the practitioner appropriately trained. This affords optimal ventilation, oxygenation and airway protection, though as described in the fundamentals of airway management chapter, it has not been associated with an increased rate of ROSC in cardiac arrest from medical causes. If a well-seated supraglottic airway is providing effective ventilation and there is no other immediate advantage, there is no immediate need to convert to an endotracheal (ET) tube. This may change if a resuscitative thoracotomy is to be performed, or there is significant chest trauma which may mean that a supraglottic device is inadequate or ineffective to ensure oxygenation and ventilation. Where a cervical spinal injury is thought to co-exist, the patient should be intubated with manual in-line stabilisation of the cervical spine wherever possible, acknowledging that securing the airway takes priority over ensuring spinal immobilisation. Videolaryngoscopy offers some advantage in terms of reduced spinal movement; however, it may be difficult if the airway is significantly contaminated with blood or other liquid debris. Locally agreed protocols should limit intubation attempts, and a failed intubation drill should be followed in the event it proves impossible.

Ventilation

Once intubated, the cuff of the ET tube should be inflated and the patient connected to a ventilator delivering 100% oxygen in the first instance. The exact mode of ventilation matters less than the observance of the principles of lung-protective ventilation, in which the volumes the lungs are exposed to are limited to 6 ml tidal volume per Kg body weight to reduce volutrauma and barotrauma. End-tidal CO_2 monitoring via waveform capnography is mandatory to confirm ET tube placement. It may give a gross marker of cardiac output or adequacy of CPR in the peri-arrest or arrested patient [29–31]. If the patient is successfully resuscitated then a low-normal end-tidal value (approximately 4.5 kPa/34 mmHg) should be targeted to minimise secondary brain injury.

Traumatic Asphyxia

If the patient has been crushed in the thoracic area, ventilation will be impaired, often to the point of cardiac arrest. Patients usually appear plethoric, with petechial haemorrhage visible to the upper torso/face and subconjunctival haemorrhages. Oxygenation will reverse cardiac arrest if delivered early enough [32, 33] (Fig. 12.2).

Impact Brain Apnoea

Traumatic arrest may present secondary to impact brain apnoea syndrome [34]. In this condition, historically referred to as commotio medullaris, the respiratory centre is transiently paralysed by a

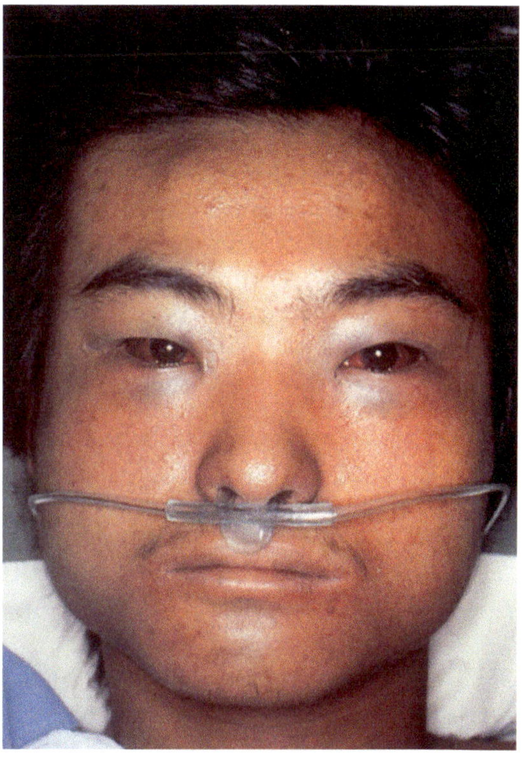

Fig. 12.2 Features of traumatic asphyxia include cervicofacial cyanosis with multiple petechiae and subconjunctival haemorrhage (From Lee et al. [32])

blunt force injury in the absence of demonstrable structural brain injury. When laypeople call the emergency services, they usually describe the patient as not conscious and not breathing after a traumatic event (e.g. assault with a head injury). CPR advice is usually given, and the patient may present to the emergency services or hospital as a traumatic arrest. Current dispatcher-advised CPR advises compression-only CPR, which will not reverse the underlying pathology, namely the need to ventilate and oxygenate the patient. CT scans and postmortem data from these patients reveal a hypoxic brain injury pattern without other parenchymal injuries. Many of these patients may have survived with basic airway management and effective oxygenation during the apnoeic period.

Spinal Injury

High (C1–C3) spinal cord injury can result in traumatic cardiac arrest at the scene by the mechanism described above and is often reversed by oxygenation. Following the return of spontaneous circulation, the patient may develop some respiratory effort, but this will be significantly limited by the injury. Neurogenic shock and bradycardia are usually features, and doses of vasopressors or inotropes are required to raise blood pressure. Cord perfusion and cerebral perfusion (and hence oxygen delivery) are reliant on an appropriate blood pressure. A comprehensive search for other injuries is essential to avoid missing concomitant hypovolaemic shock. Excessive fluid resuscitation in these patients will result in pulmonary oedema, and cardiac output monitoring may be helpful in the early phases of management (see circulation chapter for further discussion).

Tension Pneumothorax

Air in the pleural cavity can build up due to blunt or penetrating trauma, particularly if the patient is undergoing positive pressure ventilation. It is essential to decompress the pleural cavity of all patients presenting with suspected traumatic cardiac arrest. Chest examination is not reliable enough to rule out this treatable and straightforward injury [35].

Decompression should be done according to skill-set and may be by needle or surgical techniques. However, needle decompression has a high failure rate, and surgical methods are strongly preferred (see breathing chapter for further discussion). In an emergency, it is not necessary to place chest drains; simple finger thoracostomies will adequately release tension pathophysiology; intercostal drains can be placed later in the patient care pathway.

Significant air leak may reveal the diagnosis of injury to the bronchial tree. Selective right or left main stem bronchial intubation may be required. This can be done with a bronchial blocker, double-lumen endotracheal tube, or simply advancing the endotracheal tube further, ideally under bronchoscopic guidance in the first instance. In cases of acute massive air leak, pleural air will re-accumulate unless adequately drained.

Tamponade

The heart sits in a tough, fibrous sack (the pericardium) that provides separation from other thoracic structures, allows protection against ventricular dilatation, and facilitates ventricular interdependence and atrial filling. There is usually a small volume of pericardial fluid present to allow lubrication and low friction movement of the heart within the pericardium. Because the volume is so small (usually 10–50 ml in health), the lack of distensibility of the pericardium does not cause a problem with compression of the heart.

Cardiac tamponade occurs when blood fills the pericardium. The thin-walled right atrium and ventricle will become compressed by blood or other fluid between the pericardium and the heart. This impedes the filling of the right side of the heart and forward flow of blood into the lungs and left ventricle. Cardiac output is reduced, and ultimately the patient will suffer a cardiac arrest. The condition is a dynamic and physiological diagnosis, i.e. cardiovascular compromise / traumatic arrest in the face of known or suspected pericardial fluid (usually blood). The pericardium is rich in tissue factor and blood quickly clots. Volumes of blood as small as 200 ml can cause cardiac tamponade if they accumulate rapidly enough. Patients stabbed through the pericardium may bleed into it from a hole in one of the heart's chambers, from the myocardium itself or a pericardial vessel. Similarly, blunt traumatic injuries to the chest may result in a laceration to the pericardium.

Treatment consists of the evacuation of pericardial blood via a thoracotomy and haemostasis of bleeding vessels or chambers; surgical haemostasis can be achieved with sutures or staples. If performed expeditiously, survival rates of 10–35% have been reported (far higher than those from medical cardiac arrest), most of whom will be neurologically intact [11, 36].

For medical causes of cardiac tamponade where fluid other than blood may accumulate (pericarditis, auto-immune or infective causes commonly), needle pericardiocentesis may be an option. This involves inserting a needle into the pericardium under ultrasound guidance and draining the accumulated fluid. This is not appropriate in trauma for two main reasons; firstly, blood will clot quickly, and a needle-based technique will not remove clotted blood. Secondly, there will still be an underlying defect that may still be bleeding and require repair. Without exploration and repair via a thoracotomy, bleeding may continue and the tamponade may re-accumulate.

Resuscitative Thoracotomy in Traumatic Cardiac Arrest

Several international guidelines exist concerning the performance of resuscitative thoracotomy in traumatic cardiac arrest. There is broad agreement that this aggressive intervention should be performed if the patient suffers a cardiac arrest in front of the assembled trauma team, where the skill-set exists. Contraindications to this procedure in this context are primarily relative, and would include excessive time since cardiopulmonary arrest or the presence of other unsurvivable injuries (such as massive head injury).

Risk to Clinicians

Resuscitative thoracotomy is a high-stakes, low-occurrence procedure with significant risks to staff and bystanders, primarily due to potential exposure to bloodborne viruses or psychological sequelae [37]. Patient selection is paramount when deciding to perform this procedure, not only in terms of patient benefit but also in justifying risk to practitioners. Historical US data suggests a 4–8 times higher rate of HIV, hepatitis B or C virus infection risk in the urban trauma population, compared to the trauma population as a whole [38]. With more community awareness and better treatments, new diagnoses have dropped. However, patients live longer with these diseases, so the absolute number of cases has increased [39, 40]. A more recent study has confirmed that approximately 9% of patients who sustained penetrating trauma in one US centre were positive for one of these diseases, many without knowing themselves [38]. This is further supported by a Canadian study that confirmed a three-fold higher rate of hepatitis C prevalence in trauma patients than the background population [41]. Considering that the rates of sharp and needlestick injuries are higher during emergency procedures than elective surgery [42, 43], and that the risk of seroconversion of these diseases is higher with deeper contamination or injury from hollow needles or broken ribs [44], this is a procedure with significant risk to the provider. Prospective multi-centre data shows 7.2% of participants (22 staff members) from 305 emergency department thoracotomies suffered a sharps injury—but only 15 patients survived [45]. The procedure mandates universal precautions to make it as safe as possible. However, there must be a realistic *a priori* prospect of the patient benefitting from the intervention to justify performing it due to the risk to staff.

Patient Selection

Survival is dependent on indication (blunt mechanisms have a worse outcome than penetrating trauma) and time to performance. Again, for patients presenting with penetrating thoracic trauma in cardiac arrest, survival rates up to 10% have been recorded in traumatic cardiac arrest, with most of these patients leaving hospital neurologically functional [36]. The rate may further be increased if resuscitative thoracotomy is undertaken for patients before they arrest, and with specific injury patterns (up to 35% in some case series of patients with penetrating cardiac injuries [12, 46]).

As previously described, the decision to proceed with resuscitative thoracotomy is dependent on a multitude of factors, including the operator, location, likely pathology and time since patient arrest. If a patient is not about to arrest immediately and can be transferred to the operating theatre for the procedure, they should be. This frequently may not be possible, and patients in cardiac arrest already (with appropriate indications) should have a resuscitative thoracotomy in the Emergency Department rather than being transferred to the operating theatre in cardiac arrest with ongoing CPR.

Indications to perform a resuscitative thoracotomy are a penetrating injury to the chest or epigastrium, with the arrest occurring in the presence of the treating team or a thoracotomy commencing within 15 min of arrest. This is also predicated on having a team with appropriate experience and an appropriately permissive environment with good all-round access (either in the emergency department or prehospital). Factors that are associated with better outcomes in Emergency Department (ED) thoracotomy are the presenting pathophysiology causing arrest and timing [47–50]:

- Treatment of tamponade has the best outcome of all causes of traumatic arrest
- Cardiac causes are more amenable to treatment than lung injuries
- Right ventricular injuries are more accessible and treatable than left ventricular injuries
- Single chamber injuries have better outcomes than multiple chamber injuries
- Prehospital arrests survive less frequently than those who arrest during transfer, and the highest survival is in those who arrive at the ED with some vital signs and then subsequently arrest.

There is not universal mortality amongst blunt chest trauma patients who undergo thoracotomy. While blunt mechanisms have poorer outcomes, the increased use of ultrasound scanning in prehospital medicine and emergency departments has meant that pathologies amenable to a resuscitative thoracotomy may be more easily identified. If there is an obvious tamponade following blunt trauma, a resuscitative thoracotomy would be justified, and there are now case reports of survivors with this pathology in the published literature [51]. Some would perform resuscitative thoracotomy for blunt trauma (even if the cause is not clear) on the grounds that it would allow compression of the aorta and internal cardiac massage whilst replacing blood. This depends on local practice, experience and logistics, and a blanket recommendation for or against this is not possible based on current evidence.

Outcomes from resuscitative thoracotomy can be better than cardiac arrest in the general population in some subgroups (e.g. penetrating chest injury, treated immediately before, or just after arrest). This may reflect differences in pathophysiology, resource investment and baseline population differences. As is often highlighted, trauma tends to affect younger people disproportionately and is the leading cause of death in adults under 40 years old. Extrapolating from this, one may theorise that the majority of patients who suffer a traumatic cardiac arrest from penetrating injuries are likely to be younger. Consequently, they may have more physiological reserve, less cardiorespiratory comorbidity and be thought more salvageable than a patient who is elderly and has had a "medical" cardiac arrest. Extrapolating this line of thought further, the younger trauma patient potentially may have a higher level of prehospital or in-hospital healthcare resources allocated to them. Any individual or combination of these variables may account for the differences in survival, though there is currently a paucity of data looking at this phenomenon.

Surgical Technique

The principles of resuscitative thoracotomy are to access the thoracic cavity, assess for reversible pathology and address it. A secondary aim may be to compress the descending aorta. This has two benefits: Firstly, it ensures maximal perfusion of coronary and cerebral circulations. Secondly, it decreases or removes perfusion pressure to subdiaphragmatic organs. This will reduce or stop bleeding in these structures (for example, major pelvic bleeding) in addition to temporarily decreasing the effective volume that is attempting to be perfused. However, from the moment of applying aortic compression, distal organs become ischaemic and this will rapidly cause significant physiological derangement. This ischaemic burden will continue to accumulate with time until reperfusion. Surgical control of any bleeding must be achieved urgently, transferring the patient rapidly to theatre for ongoing damage control resuscitation and surgery.

All other aspects of resuscitation must be performed simultaneously as part of a well-led trauma response to achieve success—airway management, oxygenation & ventilation, vascular access and blood resuscitation. Good lighting and suction are essential.

Clamshell vs Anterolateral Approach

In the resuscitative situation, the thoracic cavity can be accessed by a left lateral or clamshell incision. There has been much discussion regarding the "best" approach to resuscitative thoracotomy, with proponents of both the left anterolateral and clamshell approach. Ultimately, the "best" procedure is the one that works and will primarily be dependent on the skill of the individual operator and experience within the care system. For trained thoracic or trauma surgeons, the anterolateral approach may be more familiar and safer in their hands. For non-thoracic surgeons or non-surgeons, a clamshell approach provides optimal access quickly for the potentially reversible causes that they can treat and is easily taught [52, 53]. A recent prospective study in US trauma centres has indicated that the clamshell approach does not cause additional systemic or thoracic complications when compared to an anterolateral approach [54].

Further, a recent prospective randomised crossover trial of emergency physicians performing both procedures on cadavers showed a higher success rate using the clamshell approach [55]. This trial also showed a lower rate of procedural iatrogenic injuries and greater physician preference and is congruent with other published research [56]. When considering the need to perform this procedure pre-hospitally, the clamshell approach may be preferable as the environment is more austere compared to the emergency department. The superior exposure afforded by a clamshell incision may mitigate against difficulties caused by less than perfect lighting or space afforded to the practitioner.

Clamshell Thoracotomy

A 2004 article by Wise et al. provides a succinct stepwise guide to performing a clamshell thoracotomy [52]. Preparation for thoracotomy should begin with pre-alert information, and the potential (or actual) need for a resuscitative thoracotomy should be discussed before first seeing the patient. Roles should be allocated, and the procedure discussed to minimise time wasted and prepare the team mentally before proceeding [57]. Once the decision made to proceed to thoracotomy, the patient should be positioned supine with their arms abducted to 90° whilst the airway and vascular access are secured. Bilateral finger thoracostomies should be performed in the fifth intercostal space. An assessment made at this point to see if there has been any return of circulation following any of the interventions so far (Fig. 12.3). These are IV fluid challenge to correct **h**ypovolaemia, intubation and correction of hyp**o**xia, and thoracostomies to treat **t**ension pneumothorax—**HOT**. If the assessment reveals the return of circulation, based on the effective intervention and physiological state, the decision must be made regarding the next step. This may be to continue to thoracotomy (Figs. 12.4, 12.5, 12.6, and 12.7) if there is pathology requiring immediate treatment, or may be transferring the patient to the CT scanner or operating theatre (or hospital if the procedure is carried out in prehospital care).

If there is no return of circulation, the next step is to join the two thoracostomies across the chest in a "swallowtail" shape cut following the line of the rib in the intercostal space (Fig. 12.4).

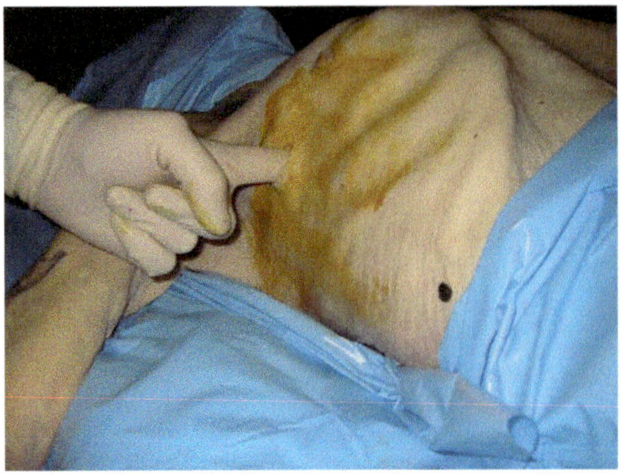

Fig. 12.3 Finger thoracostomy. (Figures 12.3, 12.4, 12.5, 12.6, and 12.7 reproduced from Voiglio EJ, Coats TJ, Baudoin YP, Davies GD, Wilson AW. Thoracotomie transverse de réanimation. Annales de Chirurgie. 2003 Dec;128(10):728–33)

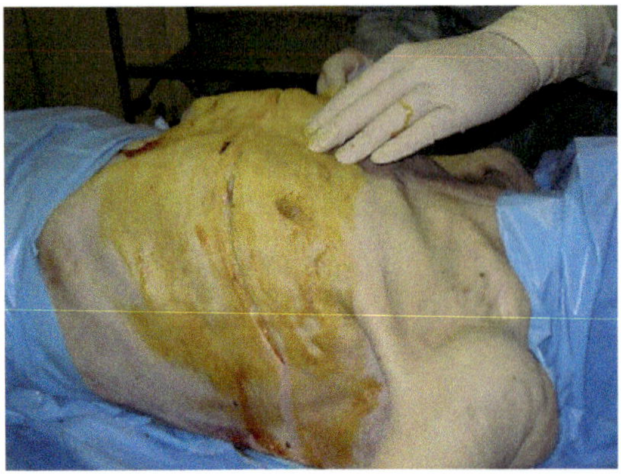

Fig. 12.4 Joining of thoracostomies

The skin and underlying fat should be cut down to the muscle layer. Scissors can then be placed through the thoracostomies, deep to the innermost intercostal muscles. The muscle layers can then be cut through, following the rib line up to the sternum. This is performed bilaterally, and the sternum is subsequently divided with a large pair of scissors or a Gigli saw (Fig. 12.5).

Once access is achieved, it should be maintained using rib spreaders in the right hemithorax (if available) or an assistant to retract the sternum superiorly (Fig. 12.6).

This incision allows full access to the thoracic structures. On opening the chest, the anterior pericardium may be adherent to the posterior sternum and can be liberated by simple blunt finger dissection. The superior pericardium should

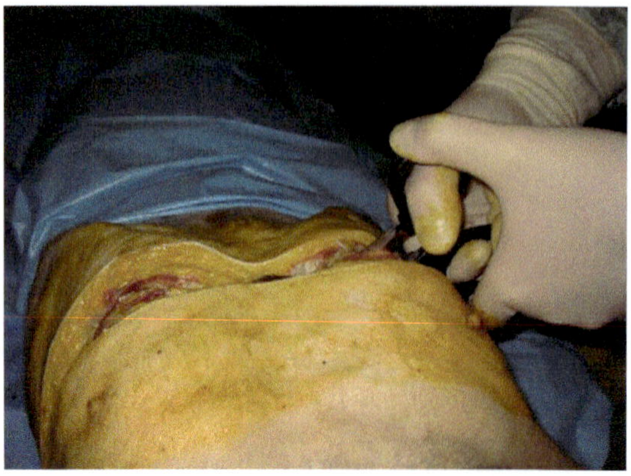

Fig. 12.5 Cutting through the sternum with trauma shears

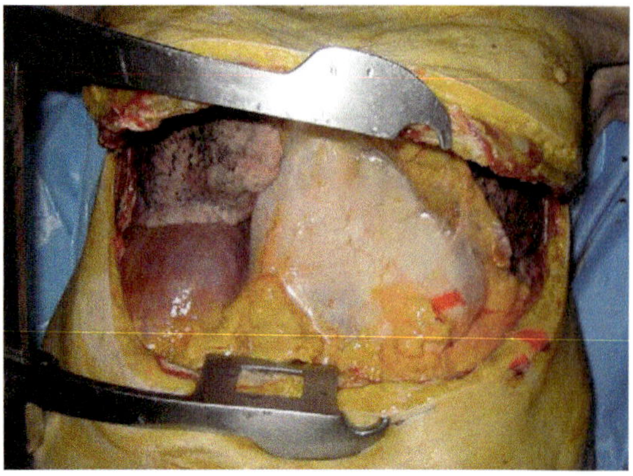

Fig. 12.6 Rib spreader in situ with good visualisation of thoracic structures from above

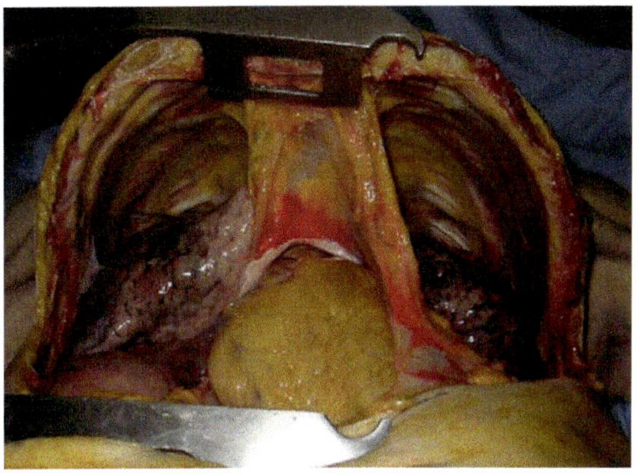

Fig. 12.7 The delivered heart. Note the incised pericardium at the top of the heart and the right atrial appendage in view

be held up with heavy forceps and cut open with a pair of scissors, starting at the cranial aspect and continuing caudally. It may be necessary to extend this incision laterally at the caudal aspect in the so-called "inverted T" incision. This avoids damage to the phrenic nerves, which run laterally along the pericardium, and care should be taken to avoid injuring the coronary vessels. The heart should then be delivered through the pericardium and inspected for wounds, even if there is no overt evidence of tamponade on first opening the chest (Fig. 12.7).

In the event of penetrating trauma, wounds can be temporarily occluded with a finger, secured with mattress sutures or staples, or in extremis, a Foley catheter can be inserted into the defect. If a Foley is used, then the lumen should be occluded to prevent bleeding, and the balloon gently inflated to occlude the hole. This is not the first choice intervention as it may cause further damage to the myocardium if overinflated, and the balloon may decrease chamber volume and impair cardiac output if circulation is returned. For non-surgeons, cardiac staples may be challenging to place, and mattress sutures may cut through muscle if they are pulled too tight. A small section of the pericardium may be used as a pledget or buttress to guard against this in the acute setting. Again, care should be taken to avoid inadvertently suturing any of the coronary vessels. The posterior aspect of the heart should be inspected, but care should be taken to avoid lifting the heart and kinking the great vessels as this will compromise cardiac output. Swabs can be inserted behind the heart (starting from the apex and moving superiorly) to lift the heart anteriorly for inspection without kinking the vessels. Internal cardiac massage should be performed using a two-handed technique. One hand is inserted behind the heart and kept flat while the other lies anteriorly. These then compress the heart in a "clapping" manner from the apex to the superior aspect in an attempt to mimic normal cardiac ejection. This is an efficient manner to improve cardiac output and allows a degree of assessment of circulating volume. Fluid resuscitation (ideally with blood) should continue at this point.

The patient may develop ventricular fibrillation—this can be treated by either "flicking" the heart or by internal defibrillation paddles set to deliver a 10 J shock. If these are not available, the chest can be closed, and standard external pads can be used at normal energy settings.

Once haemostasis is achieved and massage has continued, the patient may develop a return of spontaneous circulation and even wake up. The team should be prepared for this and administered sedation/anaesthesia as required. Dividing the sternum also divides the internal mammary arteries, which should be clamped or tied off at both ends to prevent further bleeding once a cardiac output is restored. The patient should be rapidly transferred to theatre for definitive surgical control of wounds/bleeding / other injuries.

Other Manoeuvres

In the event of damage to lung structures, bleeding can be controlled by performing hilar twisting or clamping. The inferior pulmonary ligament (anchoring the posterior aspect of the lung and the hilum to the posterior thoracic cavity) must be divided in order to twist the lung, bronchial and pulmonary vascular structures around the hilum. An endotracheal tube tie or foley catheter can be used to tie the whole of the hilum off temporarily.

Control of the descending aorta can be achieved by following the posterior ribs on the left side and manually placing the hand against the soft structures lateral to the spinal column and pressing back against it. Surgical cross-clamping requires dissection of the descending aorta from within its fascial plane—this is best done by those specifically trained to do so. Once dissected, a Satinsky clamp can be applied to ensure temporary hands-free control of defending aortic blood flow. Occlusion of the aorta may be a temporising measure to buy time in hospital. However, it may not be feasible to maintain following prehospital thoracotomy during transfer depending on distance and transport modality. The use of REBOA in patients with non-thoracic haemorrhage is discussed more fully in the dedicated chapter.

Resuscitation should continue until reversible causes have been reversed. In the event the patient does not achieve a return of spontaneous circulation, resuscitation should stop. As a dramatic and rarely performed procedure, the team should debrief where possible.

Medical Confounders

When accidents are reported to emergency services, the full history of antecedent events is rarely known. Patients often crash cars or fall down stairs due to co-existing medical conditions such as cardiac, respiratory or renal disease. The key is usually in eliciting a history from bystanders or family members, which is not always possible in the early phases of arrest. These patients must be treated according to standard resuscitative guidelines, with uninterrupted CPR, defibrillation and drugs as appropriate to the situation.

Human Factors in Traumatic Cardiac Arrest

The nature of resuscitation often involves an impromptu formed team of varying levels of experience and understanding. Thus, good followership and leadership are essential components of a well-functioning team, which will be crucial in the optimal treatment of a patient having suffered a traumatic cardiac arrest [58]. Resuscitative thoracotomy is a damage control procedure, and the decision making around it is more fully explored in Chap. 29.

Given the comparative rarity of traumatic arrest as presented to healthcare teams, teams must regularly rehearse and practice together where possible. Most centres have pre-drawn up algorithms/standard-operating procedures (SOPs) to assist in managing traumatic arrest, including when and when not to perform aggressive resuscitative procedures. Cognitive aids such as these assist in decision-making and the expeditious execution of a traumatic cardiac arrest algorithm. It is helpful that each team member understands their own and others roles in the management of traumatic cardiac arrest. Various courses, such as the American College of Surgeons Advanced Trauma Life Support (ATLS) or the European Trauma Course (ETC) provide guidance and help individuals prepare for managing a patient in traumatic cardiac arrest.

In hospital practice, the Trauma Team Leader (usually an emergency medicine consultant in the UK) has a critical role. The role of the TTL is to remain "hands-off" the patient to retain overall situational awareness while coordinating several other clinicians. This leadership role begins even before the patient arrives with pre-briefing based on the ambulance pre-alert, assignment of roles and setting expectations of likely courses of action [57]. Whilst the TTL is an experienced clinician who should be able to perform resuscitative thoracotomy if required, they should limit themselves to directing others rather than get involved in the procedure itself. Should they be the only person capable of performing the procedure, they should formally hand off the role of TTL to another clinician who can retain oversight and situational awareness while the ED consultant performs the procedure.

Given the high mortality rate and the dramatic nature of presentation and treatment, the welfare of the team should be considered in the aftermath of managing a patient with traumatic cardiac arrest, in addition to that of the patient and their family. Debriefing is an essential part of processing such events and should be offered, both hot and cold. Hot debriefs are conducted as near to the incident as possible, in time terms, whereas cold debriefs are conducted some time later. They offer a crucial opportunity for questions to be raised, issues addressed and individual and organisational learning.

Other Causes of Arrest Relevant to Trauma

The following special circumstances of traumatic cardiac arrest are discussed since they are included in most trauma registries as traumatic death.

Commotio Cordis

Commotio Cordis is a condition in which the sudden application of blunt force to the chest, usually over the manubrium, results in the transmission of that force to the mediastinum, pericardium and the heart within [59]. The putative mechanism is that mechanical energy is converted into electrical energy within the heart's conducting system. If the energy is delivered in such a way to interfere with normal sinus rhythm (for example, by inducing an R on T phenomenon), it may put the patient into a malignant arrhythmia such as ventricular fibrillation or pulseless ventricular tachycardia. Much of this mechanism is speculative or derived from animal studies since it is impossible to contrive a situation in which a patient suffering blunt chest trauma is ECG monitored at the time of injury.

Treatment consists of standard resuscitation protocols, including the use of defibrillation and anti-arrhythmic drugs as appropriate. If successfully resuscitated, the patient should be ECG monitored, have myocardial enzymes or troponin levels sent and be admitted for observation. Discussion with cardiology should be initiated as appropriate. The patient rarely requires any long term follow up. The diagnosis is more often made postmortem if a sudden blunt force to the chest has caused cardiac arrest in the absence of any underlying post mortem findings. A slight myocardial contusion may be apparent, but this is unusual.

Lightning

Several thousand people are struck by lightning worldwide each year. Some bodies provide advice about what to do if caught in a storm, but most of this is based on expert opinion and conjecture. Electrical injuries are more fully considered in the Burns section of this textbook (Chap. 40).

Lightning causes injuries due to the passage of high voltage, high current electricity through the body. The electricity passes through the body for fractions of a second, which may go some way to explain the high survival rate. The body may be thrown some distance, causing secondary blunt force injury, and burns over the skin may also be visible. There is usually an entry and an exit wound apparent, as with all electrical injuries. Where the skull is struck, severe cranial injury is likely reducing the chance of survival. If the patient is standing, the exit wound is often on the foot. Traumatic cardiac arrest usually follows respiratory arrest, most probably as a result of paralysis of the respiratory centre. Consequently, cardiac arrest will ensue in the absence of artificial respiration. Most authorities comment on the need for prolonged resuscitative attempts, with some case reports advocating the use of extracorporeal support. A full trauma response, appropriate diagnostic workup and transport to critical care are crucial to survival.

The science of lightning injuries, "Keraunomedicine" (from the Greek for lightning/thunderbolt), flags up some interesting clinical phenomena. Keraunoparalysis is a transient clinical syndrome observed in most lightning strike victims. The patients often report being unable to get up/move after the event and of paraesthesia and paralysis of the limbs. It bears all the hallmarks of an acute spinal cord injury, with lower motor neurone findings on examination and a spinal level. The limbs may appear acutely pale and pulseless as if suffering from severe vascular compromise. This finding has led most authors to conclude that the pathophysiology of the neurological findings are caused by acute vasospasm to the cord. As with other forms of vasospasm, the syndrome is reversible, and in most patients it resolves over the next 12 h.

Lichtenberg phenomena occur as a result of charged particles becoming discoloured within the skin. They often occur in the form of unusual patterns (e.g. the appearance of trees or leaves—"arborialisation"), giving the appearance of a photograph of the environment the patient was standing in at the time of the strike. This has led the science of keraunomedicine to be surrounded in mystique and folklore over the ages. These phenomena are usually transient and disappear within 24 h.

The patient may have other acute and severe burns which require consultation with burns and plastics teams. The burns are often full thickness and may involve deeper structures such as muscle and bone, requiring early surgical management and observation for complications such as rhabdomyolysis and compartment syndrome.

The heart may be affected, however in survivors this is usually transitory.

In summary, those presenting to a hospital who have been struck by lighting usually have a good prognosis and, even in traumatic arrest, extensive resuscitative efforts should be offered.

Electrocution

Electrocution occurs when the patient contacts a suitable source. It may be classified as high voltage (usually industrial) or low voltage (domestic).

In the context of high voltage electrocution, as may occur secondary to industrial or railway accidents, the patient usually suffers severe burns, which can be of high percentage. Traumatic arrest is thought to occur secondary to respiratory arrest or disturbance to cardiac rhythm, but incineration of the patient by secondary burning can occur. These patients have a poor prognosis.

Domestic power usually arises from alternating current at a power of less than 400 volts and a frequency of 50–60 Hz. The peculiarity of this frequency is that it the exact frequency to induce tetany in the muscles. Thus, the patient may touch the source and then be unable to let go, prolonging the electrocution injury.

Rescue efforts must focus on safety to the rescuers before extrication of the casualty. Early application of defibrillators alongside conventional life support algorithms is the mainstay of treatment. In the event of a return of spontaneous circulation, the patient should be transferred to critical care for ongoing management. If the patient regains consciousness quickly, they should be ECG monitored for a suitable period before hospital discharge to exclude any underlying cardiac injury or rhythm disturbance.

Hypothermia

Hypothermia is discussed more fully in the immersion and submersion and burns and thermal injuries chapters (39 and 40). Severe hypothermia is classified as anyone with a body temperature of less than 32 °C. The confounding problem is trying to elucidate whether a patient has gone into cardiac arrest because of hypothermia, or whether they have been in cardiac arrest for a while and become cold. As the body cools down, the basal metabolic rate of oxygen consumption decreases (approximately 10% per degree of cooling). As the body cools, physiological functions are affected, respiration decreases, arrhythmias including AF, VF, and bradycardia can all occur, resulting in cardiac arrest.

Treatment should include active and passive rewarming. In the context of cardiac arrest, several points are worth considering. Firstly, resuscitative protocols alter, including the sequence of the delivery of cardioversion and the use of resuscitative drugs. Pulses may be challenging to feel, and the use of ultrasound may elucidate some cardiac activity.

There have been case reports of successful resuscitation with full neurological recovery with aggressive resuscitation depending on the degree and speed of cooling. Extracorporeal membraneous oxygenation (ECMO) and cardiopulmonary bypass may be utilised where facilities are available. These are often only needed for short periods to provide oxygenation to the organs and warm the patient. Some guidelines incorporate potassium as part of the prognostic workup, with patients having serum potassium of greater than 8 mmol/l being beyond help.

Hanging/Strangulation

There are two categories of hanging: Judicial and non-judicial. Whilst traumatic cardiac arrest secondary to judicial hanging is unlikely to present to healthcare practitioners, patients attempting to commit suicide may do so following the same mechanism, i.e. a long drop with a noose tied anteriorly around the neck with a thick rope. This has the effect of the weight of the body pulling on the neck and hyperextending it, injuring the upper cervical vertebrae and brain stem. This results in near-instant cardiac arrest due to high cord lesions, brain stem effects or severe internal vascular damage to the vertebrobasilar and carotid vessels. Careful handling, immobilisation of the neck and imaging for spinal injuries is essential in patients who have unsuccessfully attempted suicide via this mechanism.

Injuries from non-judicial hanging usually occur secondary to an impairment of blood flow to the brain due to compression of the vessels in the neck or hypoxia from occlusion of the trachea. Compression of the veins results in raised ICP as the hanging ensues and may present as petechiae or subconjunctival haemorrhage. The hyoid bone may be fractured, and there may be damage to the carotid vasculature. Ligature marks are often present externally on the neck, and it is good practice to note their presence.

As cerebral hypoxia ensues, the patient often starts to fit. This may be reported by rescuers or be witnessed by emergency medicine services arriving on scene quickly after the event.

If presenting in cardiac arrest, these patients frequently develop a sustained return of spontaneous circulation once oxygenation resumes, for example, following endotracheal intubation. Airway management is usually straightforward in the early phase of this injury. Whilst ROSC may ensue, survival with a favourable neurological outcome is less common. The vessels in the neck should be imaged to exclude injury/dissection. Hanging injuries which present as short drops and asphyxia are incredibly unlikely to have unstable neck injuries. In a 2014 literature review of 2,795 patients, cervical fracture occurred in approximately 2% of all fatal and non-fatal hangings, and more harm may be caused by a blanket rule advocating the application of a cervical collar to these patients [60]. If the patient has had a true "judicial style" hanging, they will suffer an irreversible cardiac arrest almost instantaneously due to severe vascular and or neural trauma. If the patient shows signs of life when prehospital practitioners arrive, it is highly unlikely that they are in this group. Given that the primary pathology is asphyxia, these patients do not require transfer to a major trauma centre and can be well managed at any hospital with intensive care facilities.

Forensic Aspects

A traumatic cardiac arrest will have been caused as a direct result of an intentional or unintentional act by way of assault or accident. In most jurisdictions, there will follow an investigatory process, which will fall to the police and coronial services.

In the UK, all deaths and injuries which occur in the workplace are reportable under the Health hand Safety law via the Reporting of Injuries, Diseases, and Dangerous Occurrences Regulations 2013 (RIDDOR). This places a legal duty on employing organisations to file an initial report if a person dies or is incapacitated for more than 7 days. Whilst it is not the immediate responsibility of the healthcare team to form a report, it can be helpful to advise the patient/relatives or employers of the need to report. In addition, the follow-up investigation is likely to require a report from the healthcare team to help inform the level of harm and risk of the incident to other people in the workplace.

The Coroner is a judicial appointment by the local council (or other unitary area) under the Coroners and Justice Act 2009. The key responsibility of the Coroner is to investigate any death which is unexpected or unexplained. There is a further list of specific situations which must be discussed with or reported to the Coroner. These include deaths that were sudden, violent or unnatural (including accidents and suspected suicides or murders). All traumatic cardiac arrests should be discussed and referred to the coroner. Those occurring outside the hospital will be reported to the police initially, who may take on the role of 'Coroner's Officers', particularly out of hours. Most ambulance services have established reporting relationships with the local coroner to assist in these out of hospital situations. In-hospital reporting is usually undertaken the next working day by a senior member of the healthcare team. The body will have been taken to the mortuary.

After death, "last offices" are administered. This is the process of respectful treatment of the body per the religious or cultural wishes of the patient as and when they are known. There are some crucial forensic aspects to consider in the context of traumatic cardiac arrest. First and practically, injuries or incisions from medical procedures may continue to bleed. Medical procedures may involve the placement of cannulae, catheters, endotracheal tubes, for example. Although coroners vary in the extent to which they mandate drips and lines stay in, it is usually good practice to discuss these requirements with the local coroner, their officer or the pathologist/mortuary who will ultimately carry out the post mortem. If medical devices are removed, this should be carefully documented in the notes to assist in the subsequent post mortem examination.

There are various types of post mortem examinations carried out In the event of traumatic death. The coroner ultimately decides on whether or not a post mortem examination is required. In the event of a traumatic cardiac arrest, it would be unusual not to request some form of post mortem. In cases of multiple casualty events or major incidents, virtual or computer-reconstructive post mortem examinations have been used to arrive at the cause of death. It is more common for the coroner to request a standard "Virchov" post mortem examination, in which a pathologist reviews the notes and makes an examination of the body before arriving at a cause of death. The cause is often recorded as "multiple injuries" in such cases. If there is a criminal investigation pending, the police may well commission a forensic post mortem. These are undertaken by independent pathologists and comprise a thorough review of injuries, illnesses, interventions and the antecedent history of events. Second post mortem examinations may be requested by a defendant as some of the findings may be subsequently challenged. There is increasing use of scanning technology (CT or MRI) to elucidate injuries after death, and some faith groups favour this. Advantages include an accurate radiographic description of injuries and the ability to carry out limited dissection of the body. Although increasingly popular, their validity compared with classic post mortem techniques is currently the subject of ongoing research. Samples of blood, hair, vitreous humour may be taken for toxicological analysis as part of the post mortem.

When providing evidence concerning those suffering a traumatic injury, whether deceased or alive, several principles are worth bearing in mind. Firstly, the healthcare team providing treatment should stick to simple descriptions of injuries and interventions such that a layperson can understand the information. Excessive medical jargon within statements or verbal evidence is likely to lead to further questioning/extended requests for evidence. Opinion about causation or fault should be avoided. Police and hospitals usually have standard a standard pro forma to help in writing statements. It must be signed and dated. Numbering any paragraphs helps with subsequent requests.

The patient still has a right to confidentiality which extends after death. Each healthcare practitioner must be familiar with the relevant guidance outlining the circumstances in which information can be disclosed, particularly to outside agencies. If information is disclosed, it is good practice to note down what has been revealed, why, and to whom in the patient's notes.

Conclusion

Traumatic cardiac arrest can be from many causes, and the treatment varies depending on the suspected mechanism. Patients may have been in cardiac arrest from medical causes before they suffered trauma, and their treatment is different from patients who have suffered a cardiac arrest *because* of trauma. While some patients with particular injury patterns may benefit from invasive treatments conducted early (e.g. penetrating chest injury with tamponade physiology requiring resuscitative thoracotomy), this is not a universal fact. The presenting pathology and time since arrest are more likely to determine the likelihood of successful resuscitation than a specific mechanism, though certain mechanisms make certain pathologies more apparent. The risks to staff from the procedure are not insignificant, so there must be a reasonable expectation of success rather than performing resuscitative thoracotomies on patients where it is clearly inappropriate.

Questions

1. All patients in traumatic cardiac arrest are candidates for resuscitative thoracotomy.
   (a) True
   (b) False
2. Thoracotomy for penetrating thoracic injuries has a better outcome than for blunt injuries.
   (a) True
   (b) False
3. Flow rates through peripheral 18G cannulae are higher than those through centrally placed 18G cannulae.
   (a) True
   (b) False
4. Hypokalaemia is a commonly encountered cause of traumatic cardiac arrest
   (a) True
   (b) False
5. Patients who present following a hanging must be taken to a major trauma centre as they are highly likely to have a cervical spinal injury.
   (a) True
   (b) False

Answers

1. b
2. a
3. a
4. b
5. b

References

1. Office of National Statistics. Leading causes of death, UK: 2001 to 2018 [Internet]. 2020 [cited 2020 Oct 17]. Available from: https://www.ons.gov.uk/peoplepopulationandcommunity/healthandsocialcare/causesofdeath/articles/leadingcausesofdeathuk/2001to2018
2. Clinical Audit and Research Unit. Cardiac Arrest Annual Report 2018/19 [Internet]. London Ambulance Service NHS Trust; 2019 [cited 2020 Oct 17]. Available from: https://www.londonambulance.nhs.uk/wp-content/uploads/2020/01/Cardiac-Arrest-Annual-Report-2018-2019.pdf
3. London Ambulance Service NHS Trust - Annual Report & Accounts 2018–19. Annu Rep.:128.
4. Redberg RF, Tucker KJ, Cohen TJ, Dutton JP, Callaham ML, Schiller NB. Physiology of blood flow during cardiopulmonary resuscitation. A transesophageal echocardiographic study. Circulation. 1993;88(2):534–42.
5. Lockey DJ, Lyon RM, Davies GE. Development of a simple algorithm to guide the effective management of traumatic cardiac arrest. Resuscitation. 2013;84(6):738–42.
6. Smith JE, Rickard A, Wise D. Traumatic cardiac arrest. J R Soc Med. 2015;108(1):11–6.
7. Leis CC, Hernández CC, Blanco MJG-O, Paterna PCR, Hernández RE, Torres EC. Traumatic cardiac arrest: should advanced life support be initiated? J Trauma Acute Care Surg. 2013;74(2):634–8.
8. Pickens JJ, Copass MK, Bulger EM. Trauma patients receiving CPR: predictors of survival. J Trauma Injury Infect Crit Care. 2005;58(5):951–8.
9. Sherren PB, Reid C, Habig K, Burns BJ. Algorithm for the resuscitation of traumatic cardiac arrest patients in a physician-staffed helicopter emergency medical service. Crit Care Lond Engl. 2013;17(2):308.
10. Morrison JJ, Poon H, Rasmussen TE, Khan MA, Midwinter MJ, Blackbourne LH, et al. Resuscitative thoracotomy following wartime injury. J Trauma Acute Care Surg. 2013;74(3):825–9.
11. Harris T, Masud S, Lamond A, Abu-Habsa M. Traumatic cardiac arrest: a unique approach. Eur J Emerg Med. 2015;22(2):72–8.
12. Moore EE, Knudson MM, Burlew CC, Inaba K, Dicker RA, Biffl WL, et al. Defining the limits of resuscitative emergency department thoracotomy: a contemporary Western trauma association perspective. J Trauma Injury Infect Crit Care. 2011;70(2):334–9.

13. Hughes CW. Use of an intra-aortic balloon catheter tamponade for controlling intra-abdominal hemorrhage in man. Surgery. 1954;36(1):65–8.
14. Napolitano LM. Resuscitative endovascular balloon occlusion of the aorta: indications, outcomes, and training. Crit Care Clin. 2017;33(1):55–70.
15. Editor. Differential Diagnosis of Infographic: Access Flow Rates [Internet]. Differential Diagnosis of. 2019 [cited 2020 Oct 17]. Available from: https://ddxof.com/infographic-access-flow-rates/
16. Scalea TM, Sinert R, Duncan AO, Rice P, Austin R, Kohl L, et al. Percutaneous central venous access for resuscitation in trauma. Acad Emerg Med Off J Soc Acad Emerg Med. 1994;1(6):525–31.
17. Joy MA, Marciniak D, Rubin KP. Establishing vascular access in the trauma patient. In: Smith CE, Como JJ, editors. Trauma Anesthesia [Internet]. 2nd ed. Cambridge: Cambridge University Press; 2015. [cited 2020 Oct 17]: [79–92 p.]. Available from: https://www.cambridge.org/core/product/identifier/9781139814713%23c03826-5-0/type/book_part.
18. Nagashima G, Kikuchi T, Tsuyuzaki H, Kawano R, Tanaka H, Nemoto H, et al. To reduce catheter-related bloodstream infections: is the subclavian route better than the jugular route for central venous catheterisation? J Infect Chemother Off J Jpn Soc Chemother. 2006;12(6):363–5.
19. Lorente L, Henry C, Martín MM, Jiménez A, Mora ML. Central venous catheter-related infection in a prospective and observational study of 2,595 catheters. Crit Care. 2005;9(6):R631–5.
20. Ruesch S, Walder B, Tramèr MR. Complications of central venous catheters: internal jugular versus subclavian access--a systematic review. Crit Care Med. 2002;30(2):454–60.
21. Merrer J, De Jonghe B, Golliot F, Lefrant JY, Raffy B, Barre E, et al. Complications of femoral and subclavian venous catheterisation in critically ill patients: a randomised controlled trial. JAMA. 2001;286(6):700–7.
22. Tan BK, Hong SW, Huang MH, Lee ST. Anatomic basis of safe percutaneous subclavian venous catheterisation. J Trauma. 2000;48(1):82–6.
23. Holcomb JB, Tilley BC, Baraniuk S, Fox EE, Wade CE, Podbielski JM, et al. Transfusion of plasma, platelets, and red blood cells in a 1:1:1 vs a 1:1:2 ratio and mortality in patients with severe trauma: the PROPPR randomized clinical trial. JAMA. 2015;313(5):471.
24. Janelle GM, Shore-Lesserson L, Smith CE, Levy JH, Shander A. What is the PROPPR transfusion strategy in trauma resuscitation? Anesth Analg. 2016;122(4):1216–9.
25. Webster S, Todd S, Redhead J, Wright C. Ionised calcium levels in major trauma patients who received blood in the emergency department. Emerg Med J. 2016;33(8):569–72.
26. Wilson RF, Binkley LE, Sabo FM, Wilson JA, Munkarah MM, Dulchavsky SA, et al. Electrolyte and acid-base changes with massive blood transfusions. Am Surg. 1992;58(9):535–44. discussion 544–545
27. Sihler KC, Napolitano LM. Complications of massive transfusion. Chest. 2010;137(1):209–20.
28. Clevenger B, Kelleher A. Hazards of blood transfusion in adults and children. Contin Educ Anaesth Crit Care Pain. 2014;14(3):112–8.
29. Touma O, Davies M. The prognostic value of end tidal carbon dioxide during cardiac arrest: a systematic review. Resuscitation. 2013;84(11):1470–9.
30. Kolar M, Krizmaric M, Klemen P, Grmec S. Partial pressure of end-tidal carbon dioxide successful predicts cardiopulmonary resuscitation in the field: a prospective observational study. Crit Care Lond Engl. 2008;12(5):R115.
31. Deakin CD, Sado DM, Coats TJ, Davies G. Prehospital end-tidal carbon dioxide concentration and outcome in major trauma. J Trauma. 2004;57(1):65–8.
32. Lee M-C, Wong S-S, Chu J-J, Chang J-P, Lin P-J, Shieh M-J, et al. Traumatic asphyxia. Ann Thorac Surg. 1991;51(1):86–8.
33. Eken C, Yıgıt O. Traumatic asphyxia: a rare syndrome in trauma patients. Int J Emerg Med. 2009;2(4):255–6.
34. Wilson MH, Hinds J, Grier G, Burns B, Carley S, Davies G. Impact brain apnoea – a forgotten cause of cardiovascular collapse in trauma. Resuscitation. 2016;105:52–8.
35. Roberts DJ, Leigh-Smith S, Faris PD, Blackmore C, Ball CG, Robertson HL, et al. Clinical presentation of patients with tension pneumothorax: a systematic review. Ann Surg. 2015;261(6):1068–78.
36. Lockey D, Crewdson K, Davies G. Traumatic cardiac arrest: who are the survivors? Ann Emerg Med. 2006;48(3):240–4.
37. Søreide K, Petrone P, Asensio JA. Emergency thoracotomy in trauma: rationale, risks, and realities. Scand J Surg. 2007;96(1):4–10.
38. Sloan EP, McGill BA, Zalenski R, Tsui P, Chen EH, Duda J, et al. Human immunodeficiency virus and hepatitis B virus Seroprevalence in an urban trauma population. J Trauma Injury Infect Crit Care. 1995;38(5):736–41.
39. Centres for Disease Control and Prevention. CDC Fact Sheet - Today's HIV/AIDS Epidemic [Internet]. US Department of Health and Human Services; 2016 [cited 2020 Oct 17]. Available from: https://www.cdc.gov/nchhstp/newsroom/docs/factsheets/todaysepidemic-508.pdf
40. van den Berg CHSB, Smit C, Bakker M, Geskus RB, Berkhout B, Jurriaans S, et al. Major decline of hepatitis C virus incidence rate over two decades in a cohort of drug users. Eur J Epidemiol. 2007;22(3):183–93.
41. Xeroulis G, Inaba K, Stewart TC, Lannigan R, Gray D, Malthaner R, et al. Human immunodeficiency virus, hepatitis B, and hepatitis C Seroprevalence in a Canadian trauma population. J Trauma Injury Infect Crit Care. 2005;59(1):105–8.
42. Adams S, Stojkovic SG, Leveson SH. Needlestick injuries during surgical procedures: a multidisciplinary online study. Occup Med. 2010;60(2):139–44.
43. Elder A, Paterson C. Sharps injuries in UK health care: a review of injury rates, viral transmission and

potential efficacy of safety devices. Occup Med. 2006;56(8):566–74.
44. US Public Health Service. Updated US Public Health Service Guidelines for the Management of Occupational Exposures to HBV, HCV, and HIV and Recommendations for Postexposure Prophylaxis. MMWR Recomm Rep Morb Mortal Wkly Rep Recomm Rep. 2001;50(RR–11):1–52.
45. Nunn A, Prakash P, Inaba K, Escalante A, Maher Z, Yamaguchi S, et al. Occupational exposure during emergency department thoracotomy: a prospective, multi-institution study. J Trauma Acute Care Surg. 2018;85(1):78–84.
46. Burlew CC, Moore EE, Moore FA, Coimbra R, McIntyre RC, Davis JW, et al. Western trauma association critical decisions in trauma: resuscitative thoracotomy. J Trauma Acute Care Surg. 2012;73(6):1359–63.
47. Henderson VJ, Smith RS, Fry WR, Morabito D, Peskin GW, Barkan H, et al. Cardiac injuries: analysis of an unselected series of 251 cases. J Trauma. 1994;36(3):341–8.
48. Seamon MJ, Shiroff AM, Franco M, Stawicki SP, Molina EJ, Gaughan JP, et al. Emergency department thoracotomy for penetrating injuries of the heart and great vessels: an appraisal of 283 consecutive cases from two urban trauma centers. J Trauma. 2009;67(6):1250–7. discussion 1257–1258
49. Codner PA, Brasel KJ. Emergency department thoracotomy: an update. Curr Trauma Rep. 2015;1(4):212–8.
50. Molina EJ, Gaughan JP, Kulp H, McClurken JB, Goldberg AJ, Seamon MJ. Outcomes after emergency department thoracotomy for penetrating cardiac injuries: a new perspective. Interact Cardiovasc Thorac Surg. 2008;7(5):845–8.
51. Rogerson T, Efstratiades T, Von Oppell U, Davies G, Curtin R. Survival after prehospital emergency clamshell thoracotomy for blunt cardiac rupture. Injury. 2020;51(1):122–3.
52. Wise D, Davies G, Coats T, Lockey D, Hyde J, Good A. Emergency thoracotomy: "how to do it". Emerg Med J. 2005;22(1):22–4.
53. Puchwein P, Sommerauer F, Clement HG, Matzi V, Tesch NP, Hallmann B, et al. Clamshell thoracotomy and open heart massage—a potential life-saving procedure can be taught to emergency physicians. Injury. 2015;46(9):1738–42.
54. DuBose JJ, Morrison J, Moore LJ, Cannon JW, Seamon MJ, Inaba K, et al. Does clamshell thoracotomy better facilitate thoracic life-saving procedures without increased complication compared with an anterolateral approach to resuscitative thoracotomy? Results from the American Association for the Surgery of Trauma aortic occlusion for resuscitation in trauma and acute care surgery registry. J Am Coll Surg. 2020; S107275152032322X
55. Newberry R, Brown D, Mitchell T, Maddry JK, Arana AA, Achay J, et al. Prospective randomised trial of standard left anterolateral thoracotomy versus modified bilateral clamshell thoracotomy performed by emergency physicians. Ann Emerg Med. 2020; S019606442030439X
56. Flaris AN, Simms ER, Prat N, Reynard F, Caillot J-L, Voiglio EJ. Clamshell incision versus left anterolateral thoracotomy. Which one is faster when performing a resuscitative thoracotomy? The tortoise and the hare revisited. World J Surg. 2015;39(5):1306–11.
57. Reid C, Brindley P, Hicks C, Carley S, Richmond C, Lauria M, et al. Zero point survey: a multidisciplinary idea to STEP UP resuscitation effectiveness. Clin Exp Emerg Med. 2018;5(3):139–43.
58. Marsch SCU, Müller C, Marquardt K, Conrad G, Tschan F, Hunziker PR. Human factors affect the quality of cardiopulmonary resuscitation in simulated cardiac arrests. Resuscitation. 2004;60(1):51–6.
59. Link Mark S. Commotio Cordis. Circ Arrhythm Electrophysiol. 2012;5(2):425–32.
60. Chikhani M, Winter R. Injury after non-judicial hanging. Trauma. 2014;16(3):164–73.

13 Pain Management in Trauma

Bhavana Yalamuru, Tejinder S. Swaran Singh, and Peter Lax

- The stress response after multiple trauma is far greater than after elective surgery3 and includes cytokine and acute phase reactant release, impaired coagulation and immune response and accounts for a large portion of mortality in trauma patients. Provision of good pain relief will decrease the stress response and long term psychological sequelae of injury [1].
- Acute pain during trauma may progress to chronic pain. Effective early intervention may prevent or minimise the development of chronic pain, and appropriate psychological support and non-pharmacological means of treatment have a vital role to play [2].
- Non pharmacological measures such as splinting, reduction of fractures, irrigation of burns and covering burns and raw areas with saran wrap might help minimize pain.
- Analgesic agents can be administered via multiple routes- IV, IO, IM, Intranasal, Subcutaneous, Transdermal, Oral, oral transmucosal and inhalational.
- Ketamine is a useful adjunct to patient controlled analgesia regimens [3, 4]. There are now consensus guidelines available on the use of IV ketamine for acute pain management from the American Society of Regional Anesthesia and Pain Medicine, the American Academy of Pain Medicine, and the American Society of Anesthesiologists [5]
- There are multiple regional anesthetic techniques outlined in the chapter that can be utilized to provide analgesia to the trauma patient. Brachial plexus blocks for upper extremity analgesia, femoral and sciatic nerve blocks for lower extremity analgesia, fascial plane blocks (serratus anterior, erector spinae, paravertebral) and thoracic epidural for thoracic trauma.
- There is currently no evidence to suggest that regional anaesthesia prevents the diagnosis of compartment syndrome or delays its diagnosis if the patient is appropriately examined, though many surgeons still believe this to be the case [6–10]

B. Yalamuru
Department of Anesthesiology and Perioperative Medicine, University of Massachusetts Memorial Medical Group, Worcester, MA, USA
e-mail: Bhavana-yalamuru@umassmemorial.org

T. S. Swaran Singh (✉)
Department of Anesthesiology, University of Iowa Healthcare, Iowa City, IA, USA
e-mail: tejindersingh-swaransingh@uiowa.edu

P. Lax
Tactical Medical Wing, Royal Air Force, Brize Norton, Oxfordshire, UK

The Air Ambulance Service (TAAS), Rugby, Warwickshire, UK

P. Lax (ed.), *Textbook of Acute Trauma Care*, https://doi.org/10.1007/978-3-030-83628-3_13

- An assessment of pre-existing nerve function should be performed and recorded before any block is attempted.
- For patients in severe pain and or unable to tolerate oral medication, an IV analgesic regimen in the form of patient controlled analgesia (PCA) can be initiated. Prior to initiating patient controlled analgesia consider age, ability to comprehend instructions, physical ability to use the infusion pump and comorbidities.

While the need to treat pain for humanitarian and physiological reasons is entirely obvious, the evidence is that pain is managed poorly and disjointedly at every stage of a trauma patient's journey [11]. Who is responsible for pain management now? Who is responsible for pain management in the next few hours? Who is responsible for ongoing pain management? Is there an overriding plan and will any interventions now limit analgesic options later (e.g. anticoagulation and regional anaesthesia)?

Assessing Pain

Pain, according to the International Association for the Study of Pain, is defined as an unpleasant sensory and emotional experience associated with actual or potential tissue damage or described in terms of such damage. There are multiple modalities of pain relief which can be utilised. However, the trauma patient poses some particular challenges that may limit how we can employ them.

The dogma that analgesia should not be given [12] lest it mask subtle surgical signs or cause gross haemodynamic instability has been debunked and is not supported by the current evidence base; however it is still a view held by some clinicians. The stress response after multiple trauma is far greater than that after elective surgery [13]. This response, includes cytokine and acute phase reactant release such as elevated levels of catecholamines, cortisol, growth hormone, and adrenocorticotropic hormone. It also causes activation of the rennin angiotensin system, impairment of coagulation and an altered immune response, and accounts for a large portion of the mortality in trauma patients. In several studies, inadequately treated acute pain has been shown to increase this response, resulting in higher morbidity [14]. The provision of not just adequate, but good pain relief is not only a humane aim but also will decrease the stress response and the long term psychological sequelae of injury [1].

The requirement for analgesia may also vary between injuries and between individuals; there may be up to a tenfold inter individual difference in the required doses of opioid analgesics such as morphine leading to a reluctance to give larger doses despite having a patient that is very much awake and still in pain. This is aside from concerns around long term issues such as addiction. The differences are because of physiological or pharmacological aspects (e.g. some patients will be ultra-rapid, rapid, slow or even non-metabolisers of some drugs such as codeine) and the psychological suppression or down-regulation of pain pathways depending on the context of the injury [15–18].

The anticipated duration of severe pain also plays a part in agent choice—e.g. for a short but painful procedure such as relocating a joint or fracture/dislocation, potent agents are needed to provide good analgesia for a short period. Once realignment has been achieved however, the amount of pain from the injury dramatically decreases. If a potent, long-acting analgesic and/or sedative is given (e.g. morphine and midazolam), then once the painful stimulus is removed there may be a rebound over-sedation or increased rate of side effects and complications such as respiratory depression.

The measurement of pain is essential in targeting the appropriate treatment, and as previously mentioned each individual's perception of pain will differ depending on circumstance. There may be a hyperacute suppression of what looks like a catastrophic injury—for example, the injured soldier missing an arm in the middle of a firefight but who declines analgesia. At the other end of the spectrum is what appears to be a minor injury that ultimately requires multiple modalities of treatment, as is seen in chronic regional pain syndrome (previously known as Sudeck's atrophy, reflex sympathetic dystrophy or causalgia).

The time from injury and surrounding psychological issues also play an important role. Although the primary concern with pain in trauma is acute, this may progress to chronic pain. Consequently, the treatment goals may change from the complete alleviation of pain where possible in the acute phase, to strategies aimed at coping with pain on a day to day basis to allow a return of as much function as possible. Effective early intervention may prevent or minimise the development of chronic pain, and appropriate psychological support and non-pharmacological means of treatment have a vital role to play [2].

Firstly, an assessment must be made of the magnitude of pain as this will guide the level of intervention needed. A patient with a pain score of 1/10 will not require strong opiates, and conversely, a patient with a 10/10 rating will require more than paracetamol! Multiple systems can be used, but a 0-10 scale is the most commonly used in the UK with 0 representing no pain and 10 being the worst pain imaginable. Other indices are available (e.g. 0-3 scale, mild/moderate/severe rating, "smiley faces", FLACC scoring) and the clinician should ultimately use whichever one they are most familiar with and can be most easily understood by the patient; certain pain scores have been optimised for certain patient populations (e.g. FLACC for children and PAINAD for patients who have dementia). Potential pitfalls include patients who cannot speak either due to injury, age, language barriers or mental disturbance, or patients who are intubated and assumed to have an adequate degree of analgesia.

With the exception of ketamine [19], none of the standard anaesthetic induction agents or benzodiazepines have any analgesic action. Whilst anaesthesia may be considered as a highly invasive form of analgesia for humane reasons in some extreme circumstances, induction and maintenance of anaesthesia will not provide analgesia to obtund the physiological responses to pain. An intravenous opiate or opioid should be considered in these patients to treat pain even when anaesthetised. Opiates are naturally occurring compounds, i.e. morphine and diamorphine, whereas opioids refer to both the natural opiates and also the synthetically created compounds based on opiates, e.g. fentanyl, alfentanil, pethidine, etc.

A reassessment of pain after an intervention is always required as the clinician may be tempted to try and give repeated doses of drugs which are not indicated and run the risk of increased side effects without clinical benefit, or possibly not give more analgesia when it is needed. The likely clinical course of a patient should also be considered when selecting and implementing an analgesic strategy. An extreme example would be a patient who is trapped by their leg in a motor vehicle accident and currently complains only of 3/10 pain. If the scene becomes unsafe or a patient deteriorates drastically and there is a need for amputation for rescue purposes, ketamine analgesia/anaesthesia would be appropriate in this case. A less extreme example would be the same patient who is about to be extricated with a severe compound fracture of the leg. Although they may complain of 3/10 pain at the moment, moving the car and hence the fracture fragments which may be relatively splinted by the vehicle position will be painful. Either fentanyl, morphine, ketamine or some other analgesic reserved for severe pain may be indicated in anticipation of this.

The following segments of this chapter will be directed at specific analgesia modalities in certain kinds of trauma but it is far from comprehensive. Familiarity with drugs is paramount, as acute traumatic patients represent several management problems and it would not be appropriate to use a new drug or technique on these patients unsupervised for the first time. Existing experience with specific techniques (such as regional anaesthesia) or medications (such as ketamine) is essential before being tried in the trauma arena, as liability for the use of said techniques lies with the individual practitioner.

Pre-hospital practitioners may be faced with a large number of problems in the undifferentiated trauma patient, and good analgesia may make their subsequent management easier. Initial management with reassurance and simple splintage will provide a degree of relief which may be sufficient on its own; however several other options can be employed.

Non-Pharmacological Treatments

Splinting

Splinting not only provides analgesia when the patient is still but may also provide a degree of pain relief when the casualty is moved by preventing fracture ends from rubbing together. The reduction of fractures back into their normal anatomical alignment also decreases bleeding and the risk of fat embolus from long bone fractures. Specific devices may be used (e.g. Kendrick splints for lower limb fractures), or splints may be improvised (e.g. using a bed sheet or triangular bandage for an improvised pelvic splint) if a bespoke device is not available.

Reduction

The management of dislocations also relies on splinting techniques, and the dislocated limb should be splinted in the position it is found in if that is comfortable for the patient and there are no contraindications. An assessment of distal neuromuscular status should be made before and after moving the limb. Following a radiological assessment, limbs should be reduced into the neutral position and splinted in place with further orthopaedic input as needed for ongoing management.

Limbs that are ischaemic secondary to dislocation require urgent reduction; this may be in the pre-hospital environment without the benefit of access to x-rays pre-procedure. Reduction in these instances provides significant pain relief almost instantly. Be very cautious of using long-acting opioids before reduction, as over-analgesia post reduction can occur with a potential for complications such as respiratory failure, nausea and vomiting.

Irrigating

Burns should be cooled and irrigated with normal saline prior to dressing. In the case of chemical irritation, dry chemicals should be brushed away, followed by copious irrigation to dilute the irritated area. The inflamed area should be dried and be managed according to local burns protocols as needed.

Covering

Covering of raw, exposed tissue protects from further irritation from both friction and air moving across exposed nerve endings. Plain cling film (aka Saran wrap) is immensely useful in the pre-hospital and early emergency department management of such pain, particularly following burns.

Routes of Drug Administration

An ideal analgesic agent has high patient satisfaction with few adverse events and effects. Some drugs can be given by more than one route, e.g. diamorphine, fentanyl and ketamine can all be given intranasally as well as intravenously. The following is a very brief overview of the different routes available for administration.

Intravenous (IV)

The most frequent route of administration of drugs for rapid onset and most familiar to acute healthcare providers. It requires a cannula that is working and an intact vascular supply to the central circulation for onward distribution. Medications may be given in the form of a bolus, infusion or as patient controlled analgesia for narcotic pain medication.

Interosseous (IO)

The interosseous route was popular historically in paediatrics and is becoming more and more practised in the adult population with the development of devices like the EX-IO (Fig. 13.1), FAST-1, FAST-Responder and BIG (Bone Injection Gun). The IO route has all the advantages of IV access, is less likely to become dislodged and has few drawbacks on first assessment [20–23]. It is increasingly used in both military and civilian practice, with the caveat that the IO should be removed as soon as is reasonably practical (i.e. when reliable IV access has been secured). It should not be left in for more than 24 h, and depending on the device used it may render some military personnel non-deployable for up to 1 year regardless of other injuries.

The risks associated with IO access are misplacement, joint injury and osteomyelitis, though these complications are rare if the device is used correctly. There are very few contraindications to IO use, and these are all relatively self-evident—overlying skin infection, fracture proximal to the site of insertion (e.g. femoral or pelvic if tibial site used, humeral if humeral head used, sternal fracture or previous sternotomy if FAST-1 used) overlying burns, inability to locate anatomical landmarks, previous joint replacement at the insertion site or patient refusal.

The insertion of various devices has not been described as unduly painful, but the initial flushing and overpressure of the marrow cavity of the bones has been reported as transiently very painful and lasts a couple of seconds. There has been the suggestion of flushing the IO device with 2% lignocaine, and various protocols exist regarding insertion. However, in the severely obtunded patient, this is probably unnecessary.

Various sites of insertion have been described (medial malleolus, medial tibia, distal femur, pelvic crest, distal radius and humeral head), and whichever site is chosen must be cleaned and inspected for contraindications before insertion of the needle. All acute drugs that are given IV (with the exception of bretylium, a historical antiarrhythmic agent no longer commonly used) may be given through an IO needle. The speed of access has been reported to be faster than establishing IV access in some cases [23, 24], and the IO device has also been recommended in ALS guidelines for use in cardiac arrest due to ease of use and decrease in time to establish access in the arrested patient. The increased use of the IO route has led to several recent papers comparing the merits and drawbacks of each site. In an animal

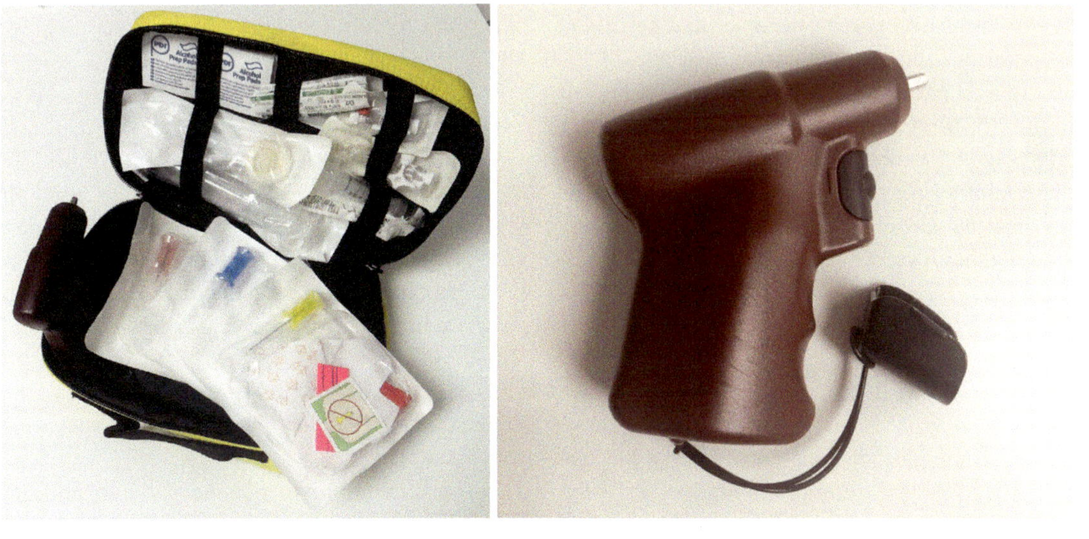

Fig. 13.1 EZ-IO needles and driver. This is one of the most commonly used IO systems in use

model, sternal and humeral routes outperformed tibial in terms of producing higher mean maximal plasma concentrations of adrenaline in cardiac arrest, with the tibial route leading to a statistically significant lower plasma concentration when compared with the IV route. This difference was not seen with other IO routes, however the time taken to reach maximal concentrations was lower in the tibial group than other IO sites, and even lower than the IV route [25]. This may be significant, as a subgroup analysis of the Continuous Chest Compression trial showed that IO access was significantly associated with a lower rate of return of spontaneous circulation (ROSC) than IV access, despite marginally faster times to initial drug administration. There was no overall effect on mortality, or survival with favourable neurological outcome after adjusting for population variances [26].

Speed of establishing access is important when considering various IO routes in comparison to IV. A randomised controlled trial by Reades et al. [27] showed a higher first pass success rate with a lower time to initial success when using the tibial route compared to humeral IO or peripheral IV access, with tibial IO access is less likely to dislodge. In the FAST-1 sternal IO device, the time of spread to the central circulation has been shown with dye testing to be the same as drugs given via a central line [28].

Whilst IO access may be faster and perceived as easier in some cases, they are still not infallible. In a recent paediatric post-mortem study, up to 30% of IO devices were found to be improperly placed (i.e. not intramedullary) [29]. Whilst these findings may not be generalisable to adults (as the trial has not been done) they do serve as a warning that IO access may not be as easy as first thought.

Intramuscular (IM)

The IM route has been used historically, but due to unquantifiable differences in muscle perfusion in trauma has fallen out of favour. The speed of absorption of drugs from IM injections is highly variable and unreliable, and if the patient is hypovolaemic and not perfusing their muscles, then the drug may not reach the circulation to have an effect. This may be further compounded by multiple doses being given to achieve an effect, and when the patient is resuscitated and normal perfusion restored, a large amount of drug may suddenly be dumped centrally causing an overdose. There is a current trial in the design phase (The Trauma INtramuscular Tranexamic Acid Clinical Trial (TraumaINTACT)) [30] to use intramuscular tranexamic acid auto-injectors in trauma, where the skill of IV access is not available such as forward military units. Occasionally, tetanus toxoid immunisations are given IM in trauma, but this is the only routine use for the IM route in trauma patients.

Intranasal (IN)

Intranasal administration is a popular route in paediatrics and becoming more popular in adults. Ketamine, diamorphine, fentanyl and dexmedetomidine (Precedex) have been used with a mucosal atomiser for analgesia and anxiolysis. Drugs given by this route benefit from fast onset speeds and good bioavailability, with few if any contraindications and a bonus that naloxone can also be given intranasally if an opiate overdose is suspected. It is very good for children who are in pain and needle-phobic [31–34].

Subcutaneous (SC)

Subcutaneous injections are no longer used in acute trauma care (with the exception of giving prophylactic low molecular weight heparin for DVT prophylaxis), but subcutaneous drugs can be given in palliative care via syringe drivers.

Transdermal

The transdermal route can be used in chronic pain with fentanyl or buprenorphine patches, but these are inappropriate in the emergency setting as the onset time of medications given by this route is measured in hours which precludes their use in acute trauma. However it is essential to look for patches that the patient may have been wearing at the time of their injury as this could cause either an overdose of opioid if left in position, or potentially an underdosing in acute pain if the patient is extremely opiate tolerant and a "normal" dose is ineffective in relieving acute distress.

Oral

This can be a useful route of drug administration in the ICU, and in minor trauma. However absorption from the GI tract may take a prolonged period in trauma due to hypoperfusion and shunting of blood away from the gut in hypovolaemia. Some drugs which are useful in managing subacute or chronic pain (e.g. amitriptyline, gabapentin, pregabalin) may have to be given orally as there is no IV alternative.

Oral Transmucosal

Transmucosal administration of fentanyl can be achieved via either "lollipop" or lozenges that are held between the lip and gum and is of use if immediately available as the patient is in control of their level of analgesia. American military practice [35] suggests taping the stick of the lollipop to the patient's finger so if they become obtunded then they will remove the lollipop when their hand drops out of their mouth. The relatively shorter half-life of fentanyl in these patients means that the duration of respiratory depression is less than with morphine. Once the drug source has been removed and the systemically absorbed fraction starts to redistribute, the patient will start to wake up. This practice has also crossed over into some civilian centres with good results [36]. However, there can be problems of dependence if used longer term which is why they are rarely used in UK.

The availability of fentanyl lollipops in the UK is less than on deployed operations, and unfortunately, they are not available in the JRCALC formulary at the time of writing, so their use is restricted to independent prescribers.

Inhalational

Entonox is a gas containing 50% nitrous oxide and 50% oxygen. It is a good analgesic, with a rapid onset and offset (approximately 6–8 breaths at either end). It requires a patient who can cooperate, but it reduces the inhaled fraction of oxygen from around 85% on a non-rebreathe mask to 50% on a mouthpiece, and so is not suitable for patients with shock or severe injury and a high FiO_2 requirement. It is, however, a useful agent for some patients and should not be forgotten, especially in pre-hospital care. It is contraindicated in chest trauma until a pneumothorax has been excluded and where the effect of nitrous oxide diffusing into air-filled spaces would be deleterious (for example, pneumocephalus). It is also contraindicated after SCUBA diving and in decompression illness. One practical point is that the pseudo-critical temperature of entonox (the temperature at which it separates into its individual components of O_2 and N_2O) is −6 °C. This means that around or below this temperature the cylinder should be repeatedly inverted to ensure an adequate mixture of the two chemicals. Failure to do this results initially in the oxygen rising to the top of the cylinder and no N_2O, and hence no analgesia, being given. This is followed by 100% N_2O being delivered when the O_2 has been preferentially inhaled first, and thus a hypoxic mixture is delivered.

Penthrox (methoxyflurane) is an inhalational agent which has been popularly used in Australasia for many years and has recently been marketed in the UK for adults. This may present a useful alternative to entonox as it does not suffer from the same logistical challenges and some contraindications, and has been found to be non-inferior to entonox in a recent review [37], though inferior to intranasal fentanyl and intravenous morphine [38]. Early experience has been largely positive, and the concentrations used provide analgesia without causing renal failure—the reason penthrox was withdrawn as an anaesthetic gas in the first instance. Some studies and reviews in the paediatric population have shown safety and efficacy [39, 40], but it is still considered an off license medication for children.

Brief Pharmacological Comparison of Analgesics

Opiates (Oral, IV, IM, IO, Transmucosal, Intranasal)

Traditionally the gold standard analgesia in trauma but best used in conjunction with other techniques if possible. The standard opiate in UK practice is morphine and it is given at a dose of 0.1 mg/kg via the IV or IO route as an initial bolus in severe pain. However, a more practical approach may be to give a 3 mg bolus and repeat every 5 min until adequate analgesia is attained, as the wide variance in tolerance that has previously been described may lead to an inadvertent overdose in some instances. As a rule of thumb, it is always easier to give more opiate than it is to take opiate out of the patient that has overdosed! Of note is that the pharmacokinetics and pharmacodynamics of morphine means it does not reach its peak analgesic effect until 30 minutes after administration due to hepatic metabolism of the more potent morphine-6-glucuronide.

The antagonist to opioid overdose (naloxone) is a useful and rapid-acting drug. However, the half-life of naloxone is shorter than that of morphine. In practical terms this means an episode of secondary respiratory depression or unconsciousness may occur after the naloxone has worn off and before the morphine has been metabolised. Traditional teaching was to give both an IM and IV dose of naloxone as it was thought that the IM dose would be absorbed more slowly and thus have a more prolonged effect, but this has not been born out in clinical practice [41]. Naloxone can also be given intranasally [42] or subcutaneously with equal efficacy, or via an endotracheal tube in intubated patients.

Paracetamol/Acetaminophen (Oral, IV, Rectal)

N-acetyl-para-aminophenol, otherwise known as paracetamol or acetaminophen is a commonly used analgesic worldwide. It is available in a licensed IV preparation for management of acute pain. It should be given regularly instead of a PRN basis as it forms the foundation of the analgesic ladder and has been shown to decrease opiate requirement. This effect has been increased when IV paracetamol has been given in anticipation of a painful stimulus [43] (e.g. surgical incision) rather than as a reactionary medication.

The benefits of IV versus oral or rectal paracetamol are:

- a shorter time until maximum availability
- a higher dose bioavailability (by definition the IV dose is 100% bioavailable in comparison to 60% oral and 40% via rectal routes)
- less hepatic damage (the paracetamol is given systemically rather than being absorbed and metabolised by the liver via the portal circulation)
- less dependence on gut blood flow, which may be altered in trauma, or the patient may be strict nil-by-mouth in the case of some bowel injuries.

Despite the above, a recent study and systematic review found no clinical benefit of IV over oral forms of paracetamol in patients who were able to take oral doses [44, 45]. Maximal doses should be 4 g in 24 h for adults or one dose of 15 mg/kg every 6 h for paediatric patients or adults under 50 kg. Paracetamol administration should be documented in the patients drug chart, especially if given in theatre as there is the potential for inadvertent overdose if multiple administrations from different areas is not recorded in one chart. There is also the potiential for iatrogenic injury if preparations containing paracetamol and another drug are not identified as such (e.g. co-codamol, co-proxamol, co-dydramol), and paracetamol is prescribed in addition to these. Paracetamol overdose is treated with N-acetylcysteine (Parvolex) to reduce toxicity of the toxic metabolite NAPQI and is given as a series of three IV infusions over 1, 4 and 16 h respectively. Oral dosing is possible, but IV is preferred.

NSAIDs (Oral, IV, IM)

NSAIDs inhibit prostaglandin synthesis in the arachidonic acid pathway producing clinical anti-inflammatory and analgesic effects. However, the inhibition of certain prostaglandins also causes a decrease in production of COX I and COX 2 which are gastroprotective, as well as decreased bicarbonate and mucus secretion in the stomach. Care is needed with renal function in hypovolaemia and in patients with pre-existing renal disease, but NSAIDs are very useful if the patient is normovolaemic with no ongoing bleeding. Caution is also advised in asthmatics, as up to 20% of patients with susceptible asthma may experience an acute asthma attack [46]. Typically, these patients will also suffer from allergic rhinitis and nasal polyps, and children with asthma also appear to be susceptible to this effect [47]. Depending on other injuries (renal, orthopaedic, GI bleeding) there may be relative contraindications to NSAID use, but where possible they should be used as they are well tolerated and opiate sparing. The "safest" NSAID in terms of GI side effect profile is ibuprofen (400 mg three times a day) as this has the least anti-inflammatory effect, but not the least analgesic effect. If this is insufficient, naproxen may be the next agent to consider [48]. Other NSAIDs such as diclofenac, meloxicam and ketorolac have the advantage that they are also available in an IV form, so may be used if the patient is nil by mouth for any reason. However, even when taking IV NSAIDS, patients at risk of GI bleeding should be given proton pump inhibitors [49] as the GI side effects are as a result of systemic absorption, not local toxicity.

Ketamine and S-Ketamine

Ketamine is a phencyclidine derivative and a racemic mixture of two optical enantiomers. The R- form is responsible for approximately 30% of the analgesic activity of the mixture and has been implicated in the side effect profile more than the S- form. In Europe, the S- form (often referred to as esketamine) is available as a purified preparation but is more expensive than the racemic form. However, the usage of s-ketamine has not crossed into mainstream UK or US practice in comparison to the relative resurgence of racemic ketamine in recent years, though it is gaining popularity as a rapid acting antidepressant [50]. Historical concerns about the deleterious effects of ketamine have made some clinicians wary of using it, but these fears have been proven ill-founded, and the evidence that these concerns were based on has proven to be of poor quality. Ketamine is enjoying a resurgence in both pre- and in-hospital trauma use for analgesia and induction of general anaesthesia [19]. It may be a useful adjunct to patient controlled analgesia regimens [3, 4]. There are now consensus guidelines available on the use of IV ketamine for acute pain management from the American Society of Regional Anesthesia and Pain Medicine, the American Academy of Pain Medicine, and the American Society of Anesthesiologists [5].

Neuropathic Pain Modulating Agents

Gabapentin/Pregabalin

Gabapentin is an anti-seizure medication that has been used in the treatment of chronic pain thought to be neuropathic in origin. It was thought to be a GABA analogue (hence its name), but further investigation has revealed that gabapentin does not have any effects on GABA receptors. The mechanism of action is not fully understood and thought to have some direct inhibition of calcium channel-medicated neurotransmitter release, but even this has been questioned as gabapentinoids do not consistently reduce calcium currents in laboratory studies [51]. Although its mechanism is not fully appreciated, it is an effective agent but it was initially thought to take several days if not weeks to exert an analgesic effect. However, more recent data suggests that it may also have a role to play in acute pain and be opiate sparing. Some studies have concluded that gabapentin may not be any more effective than carbamazepine in neuropathic pain [52], is equally effective as pregabalin but cheaper [53] and may be effective in treating complex regional pain syndrome [54]. Its main side effects are dizziness, drowsiness and peripheral oedema, with an increase in depression, and suicidal ideation. Gabapentin should not be stopped abruptly as it may cause a withdrawal-like syndrome, potentially resulting in seizures. Pregabalin was released as a competitor to gabapentin, and the two drugs are structurally similar, however pregabalin is more potent, absorbed faster and has higher bioavailability [55]. It is also marketed for the treatment of neuropathic pain and post herpetic neuralgia, whereas this is an off-license indication for gabapentin. The dose of gabapentin is increased over the course of a week and if problems with dizziness, somnolence, insomnia or other side effects are experienced, the dose held at that particular level until tolerance is achieved.

Amitriptyline

Amitriptyline is a tricyclic antidepressant which has been used in the treatment of neuropathic pain for many years but also can be used in the treatment of post-traumatic stress disorder and insomnia related to this. A typical dose for neuropathic type pain is 25–50 mg at night as tolerated. The main side effects are anticholinergic symptoms such as dry mouth, blurred vision, urinary retention, nausea, increased sweating, constipation and prolongation of QTc. In relatively low doses it is well tolerated and has a synergistic effect with gabapentin.

Regional Anaesthesia

Systemic analgesia requires the administration of medications via one of the above routes and may cause unwanted side effects depending on the drugs used. One other potential method of analgesia would be a peripheral nerve block, if possible.

General principles of nerve blockade include ensuring that the standard of monitoring used when performing these blocks is the same as in patients undergoing general anaesthesia [56]. Patients should also be screened for coagulation defects which may present a relative or absolute contraindication for regional or neuraxial anaesthesia. Guidelines exist from the Association of Anaesthetists of Great Britain and Ireland (AAGBI) [57] and the American Society for Regional Anesthesia (ASRA) [58] which outline the accepted standards for testing, risks, limits and contraindications to performing peripheral and central nerve blocks in these patients. Occasionally there may be a patient who on risk:benefit analysis falls outside of these guidelines, they are largely the standard to which practitioners will be held and are essential reading.

There have been several case reports of regional anaesthesia used in the pre-hospital environment [59–61], and depending on the indication for use and the transit time to hospital, it may be an appropriate modality to use. Indeed, for secondary transfer or aeromedical evacuation, the supplementation or replacement of parenteral analgesia has many attractive advantages. It diminishes the risk of respiratory depression which may be deleterious at altitude, as well as the potential eu- or dysphoria of ketamine, it allows the patient to remain awake, promotes orientation and allows assessment of the casualty when they are awake. Regional anaesthesia should not be employed if it delays time to definitive care but is a useful tool in the analgesic armamentarium. The introduction of hand-held ultrasound machines has made regional anaesthesia pre-hospital more available than in previous years, and the Royal Flying Doctor Service of Australia has employed this technique on many occasions, and some regional anaesthesia is taught as part of their standard operating procedures. Landmark techniques are possible (and regional nerve blocks are also being increasingly used in emergency departments for certain patient groups (e.g. neck of femur fractures) with good results [62, 63]), but in some cases the use of a nerve stimulator or preferentially an ultrasound machine is mandatory (e.g. supra- or infraclavicular blocks). It is worth explicitly stating that pre-hospital regional anaesthesia may preclude a repeat regional anaesthetic procedure for surgery (e.g. due to maximum dosing and risk of local anaesthetic toxicity) or make a proper surgical neurovascular exam difficult so should be chosen with care.

Compartment Syndrome

Orthopaedic surgeons are rightly concerned about the development of compartment syndrome. This is where increased pressure within a fascial compartment of a limb (classically following nailing of the tibia) increases due to muscle swelling. This swelling increases to a point where the venous drainage of the affected compartment is not possible, thus causing more swelling. The limb still has pulses as arterial pressure is much higher than venous pressure, but necrosis of the muscle begins, and the patient requires a fasciotomy (an operation to cut the fibrous band that separates compartments in the limb). The hallmark of compartment syndrome is pain out of proportion to the injury, with worsening pain on a passive muscular stretch.

> *There is currently no evidence to suggest that regional anaesthesia prevents the diagnosis of compartment syndrome or delays its diagnosis if the patient is appropriately examined, though many surgeons still believe this to be the case* [6–10].

The diagnosis of compartment syndrome is mainly clinical and relies to a large degree on clinical suspicion and examination, as a normal compartment pressure measured by manometry does not exclude compartment syndrome completely. Recent work has looked at probes which measure localised tissue pH or infrared spectroscopy as an indicator of hypoperfusion in suspected compartment syndrome and may prove more reliable in future [64–67].

Specific Regional Anaesthetic Techniques

There are fundamental key blocks which theoretically may be employed in- or in some cases pre-hospitally for limb trauma. The exact details of how to perform these blocks are beyond the scope of this text, but there are many resources (such as the NYSORA website) for the interested practitioner to learn from with appropriate senior supervision and oversight.

It must again be reinforced that these blocks should be done in as aseptic a fashion as possible, and should not increase scene time or time to definitive care if performed pre-hospital. They may be appropriate in only an extremely small number of scenarios, usually when a prolonged transfer is anticipated, or other analgesic options are not practical. An assessment of pre-existing nerve function should be performed and recorded before any block is attempted, as well as any subsequent block performed, the time and dose of any agent given.

The peripheral nerve blocks outlined can also be utilised as a primary anaesthetic technique in some instances for surgery in appropriate patients, or more commonly are used to supplement general anaesthesia for postoperative pain relief. Either a single shot injection or a continuous nerve catheter [68] can be placed to allow for infusion of local anaesthetic for a prolonged analgesic effect [69]. These catheters if appropriately cared for can be left in situ for over four weeks [70], and have the added advantage they can be bolused for procedures such as bedside dressing changes, which may otherwise require further sedation or general anaesthesia.

The techniques outlined in this chapter can all be employed effectively, as can epidural analgesia/anaesthesia for lower limb injuries. The only difference in epidurals used in lower limb injuries compared to those in use for thoracic pain is that the catheter is inserted in the lumbar spine rather than at a thoracic level. The chances of nerve injury and profound hypotension are less, though the rate of post-dural puncture headache changes with type of needle used and procedure [71]. Primary anaesthesia for lower limb fractures can also be achieved with a spinal or subarachnoid block, though this can cause profound cardiovascular changes (hypotension and vasodilatation after injection) and is limited to operative procedures less than 2 h in length. However, in the same way as adding opioids to an epidural potentiates its effects, intrathecal opiates can give up to 12 h postoperative relief. Although surgical anaesthesia is limited to 90–120 min with a single shot spinal, there is a degree of postoperative analgesia that may persist for up to 8 h or beyond in some patients. The use of intrathecal opiates in the elderly population is not without complications, and a more full discussion is available in the Silver Trauma chapter.

Spinal anaesthesia is not appropriate in the hypovolaemic, under-resuscitated patient, the coagulopathic or the patient requiring a prolonged procedure. However, in a small group of patients with longstanding and severe respiratory disease it may be considered an alternative to general anaesthesia for certain operations.

NB, hyperlinks in the following section will take the reader to videos demonstrating ultrasound-guided regional anaesthesia. The following section details the associated anatomy and describes the risks associated with each of the blocks. Readers are advised to be cognisant of the serious associated side effects. These nerve blocks are best performed under ultrasound guidance and by appropriately trained personnel.

Upper Limb Blocks

Brachial Plexus Anatomy

The brachial plexus is formed by union of anterior primary rami of C5-T1 nerves (Fig. 13.2). There may be occasional minor contributions from C4 and T2. As the nerve roots emerge from the intervertebral foramina, they converge to form trunks, divisions, cords, branches and terminal nerves. Three trunks (superior, middle and inferior) are formed between the anterior and middle scalene muscles. The trunks divide into anterior and posterior divisions. These fibres combine again under the clavicle to form three cords—lateral, medial and posterior (based on their relationship to the axillary artery). Each of the cords gives off branches before ending as a terminal nerve.

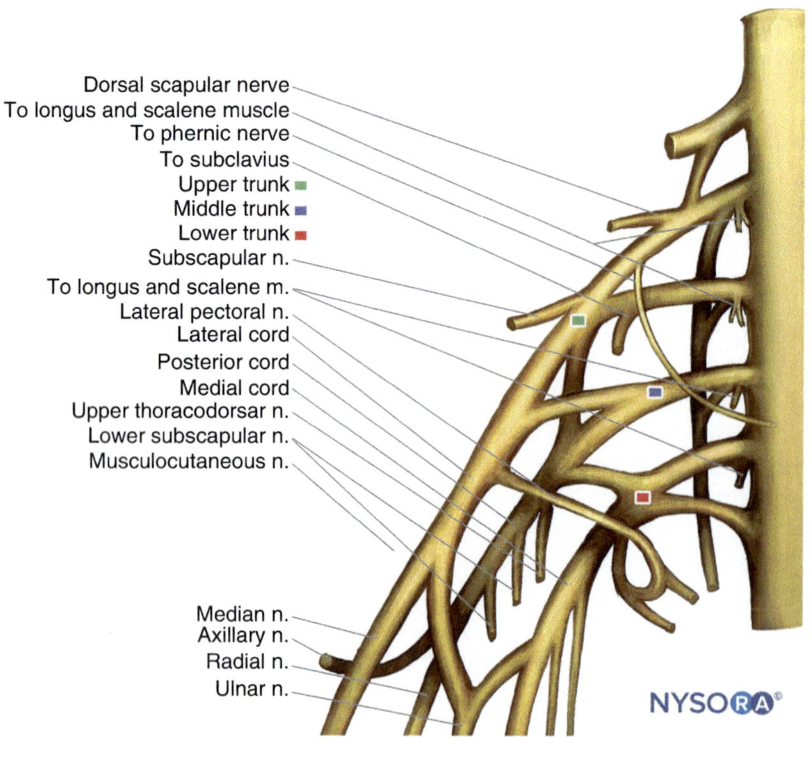

Fig. 13.2 Brachial plexus (Courtesy of NYSORA.com)

Interscalene Block

Video: Interscalene block [https://www.youtube.com/watch?v=OhFs-batCSY].

This block is indicated for procedures involving the shoulder and upper arm. The roots of C5-7 are usually more densely blocked and C8 and T1 are spared (ulnar sparing). Contraindications to the block include: Patient refusal, coagulopathy, local infection, allergy to local anaesthetics. The complications specifically associated with an interscalene block include ipsilateral phrenic nerve paralysis and pneumothorax, so caution must be used in patients with severe pulmonary disease or contralateral phrenic nerve palsy. Horners syndrome (due to proximal tracking of the local anaesthetic and blockade of the sympathetic fibres to the cervico-thoracic ganglion), vertebral artery injection, spinal or epidural injection and recurrent laryngeal nerve blockade have also been reported.

Supraclavicular Block

Video: Supraclavicular block [https://www.youtube.com/watch?v=9vW1uo7mKDc].

The supraclavicular block is at the level of the divisions of the brachial plexus. It is performed under ultrasound guidance and provides analgesia for upper limb, forearm and hand as well as the shoulder. There can be sparing of the ulnar nerve and it does not reliably anaesthetise the axillary and suprascapular nerves. Complications are similar to those for interscalene blocks and infraclavicular blocks. It is a suboptimal site for a continuous catheter because they can be easily displaced due to lack of muscle mass. Supraclavicular blocks are more commonly performed in the UK than infraclavicular blocks.

Infraclavicular Block

Video: Infraclavicular block [https://www.youtube.com/watch?v=Z9woYkyJl_U].

This block must not be performed without ultrasound. This block relies on depositing local anaesthetic under the clavicle and around the subclavian/axillary artery. This envelops the lateral, posterior and medial cords of the brachial plexus where they run in close continuity with the artery. Complications include inadvertent arterial puncture, bleeding, local anaesthetic toxicity and pneumothorax due to the proximity of the pleura. This block is suitable for anaesthesia or analgesia distal to the mid humerus for the distal upper limb.

Axillary Block

Video: Axillary block [https://www.youtube.com/watch?v=GaH-CO6OrV0].

Axillary blocks provide similar coverage to the infraclavicular block, however the point of injection is the medial humerus, thus avoiding the risk of pneumothorax. The traditional technique called for a trans-arterial puncture, but with the development of ultrasound-guided regional anaesthesia, it is no longer necessary to puncture the vessel as the nerves can be visualised. There is the potential to spare the musculocutaneous nerve as it is usually inferoposterior to the artery and occasionally difficult to visualise.

Lower Limb Blocks

Lumbar and Sacral Plexus Anatomy

The lumbosacral plexus provides innervation to the lower extremity (Figs. 13.3 and 13.4). The lumbar plexus is formed by ventral rami of L1-4. The femoral (L2-4), lateral femoral cutaneous nerve (L1-3) and obturator nerve (L2-4) arise from the lumbar plexus and provide motor and sensory innervation to the anterior thigh and sensory innervation to the medial leg.

The sacral plexus arises from L4-5 and S1-4. The posterior thigh and most of the leg and foot are innervated by the tibial and peroneal component of the sciatic nerve.

The possible complications associated with lower extremity peripheral nerve blocks

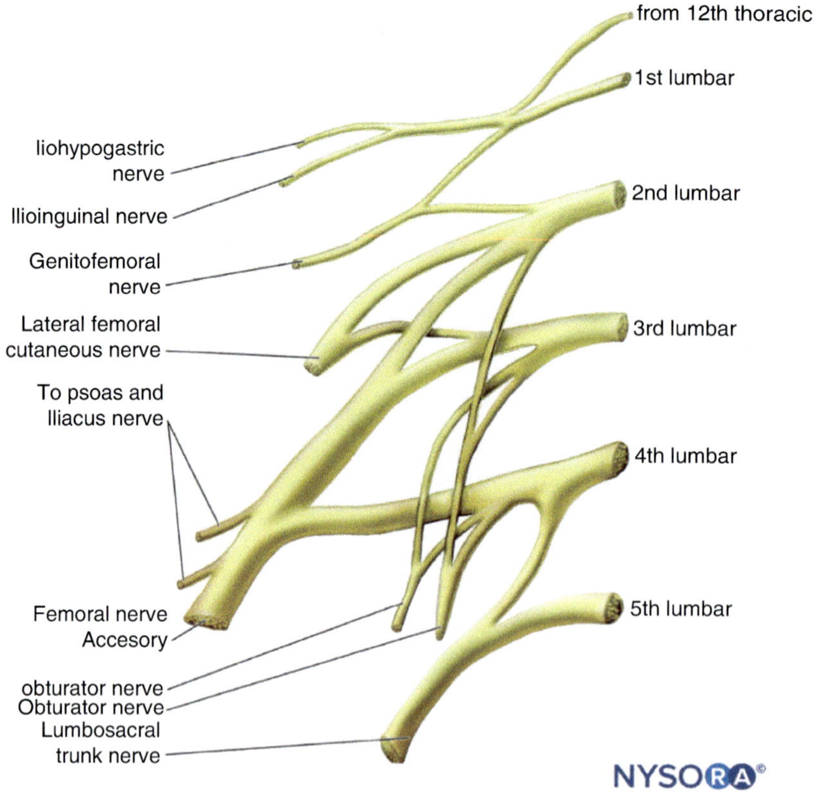

Fig. 13.3 Lumbar Plexus (Courtesy of NYSORA.com)

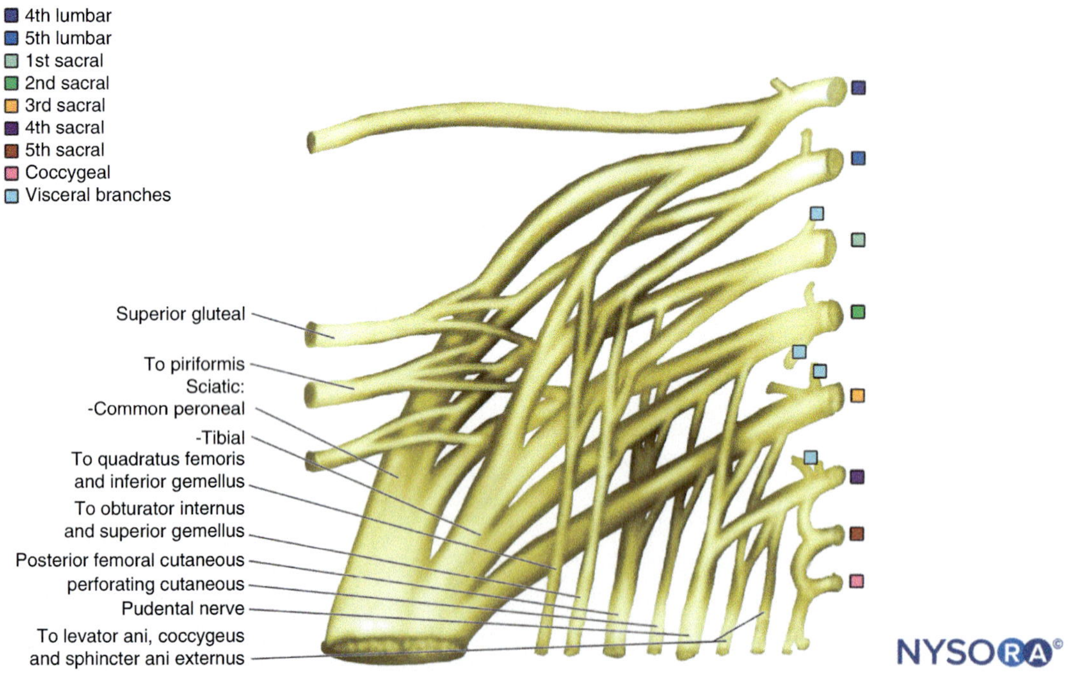

Fig. 13.4 Lumbarsacral plexus (Courtesy of NYSORA.com)

include infection, nerve damage, accidental intravascular injection, local anaesthetic systemic toxicity and allergic reactions to the local anaesthetic.

Femoral Block

Video: Femoral nerve block [https://www.youtube.com/watch?v=DwtvZ0tC9ng].

This block can be performed by a landmark technique as well as under ultrasound guidance and provides suitable analgesia for femoral fractures. The femoral artery is palpated as proximally as possible in the leg, and a needle is inserted 1–2 cm lateral to the pulse until two fascial pops are felt. The local anaesthetic is then slowly injected after negative aspiration unless resistance or pain on injection is felt. A variant on this, the fascia iliaca block, can be used in neck of femur fractures.

Video: Fascia Iliaca block [https://www.youtube.com/watch?v=p6X0IiYolIk].

Saphenous Block

Video: Saphenous nerve block [https://www.youtube.com/watch?v=C_Xmlqrn68Q].

The saphenous nerve is a branch of the femoral nerve which supplies some knee joint sensation and a small area of skin on the medial aspect of the leg below the knee. It is identified with ultrasound by tracing the femoral artery down the anteromedial thigh to the point where the artery starts to disappear (typically at the lower third). Look for the fascial "corner" just above the artery and infiltrate local anaesthetic to give excellent pain relief to the knee, but without quadriceps motor block.

Sciatic Block

Video: Anterior sciatic nerve block [https://www.youtube.com/watch?v=h14Ee2yAmUU].

Video: Popliteal sciatic nerve block [https://www.youtube.com/watch?v=qYM2sft8R2I].

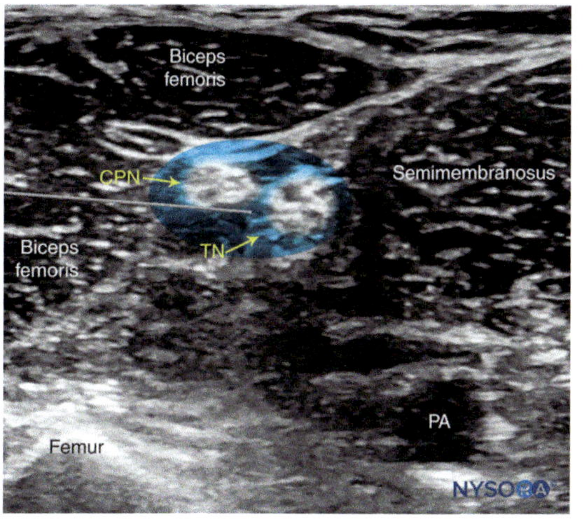

Fig. 13.5 Simulated needle path and local anesthetic distribution to block the sciatic nerve (at the level of bifurcation into the Tibial Nerve and Common Peroneal Nerve) in the popliteal fossa using the lateral approach. PA, popliteal artery (courtesy of NYSORA.com)

Video: Subgluteal sciatic nerve block [https://www.youtube.com/watch?v=rl8rZOEMveE].

The sciatic nerve supplies sensation to the knee joint and all the structures distal to the knee, (except the small strip of skin over the medial malleolus innervated by the saphenous nerve as described above). The sciatic can be blocked high at the buttock, sub-gluteally in the anterior thigh or in the popliteal fossa (Fig. 13.5).

Analgesia for Thoracic Trauma

Case Study

The patient is an 80-year-old male with a history of chronic atrial fibrillation on warfarin, hypertension, smoking and chronic obstructive pulmonary disease on home oxygen and spinal stenosis on opioids. He was involved in a motor vehicle accident and sustained left sided fractures of ribs 3-10, pulmonary contusions and a pneumothorax. He is admitted to the ICU and is complaining of severe pain and is unable to take a deep breath. What would be your analgesic plan?

As identified in the respiration and chest trauma chapter, the causes of perioperative morbidity and mortality in patients with thoracic trauma are airway obstruction, respiratory failure and haemorrhage. The anaesthetist is ideally suited and trained to deal with the problems of airway control, ventilatory and circulatory resuscitation, and adequate analgesia in all phases from pre-hospital care, through the operating room and ICU and eventually into the pain clinic in some cases. However, good analgesia is not the sole responsibility of anaesthetic staff—all clinicians who deal with trauma should have at least a basic understanding of common agents and techniques.

Pain from musculoskeletal trauma to the chest is a significant contributor to the failure of normal respiratory dynamics as previously highlighted. Inadequately controlled pain may cause hypoxic and/or hypercapnoeic respiratory failure. The inability to deep breathe and cough adequately leads to sputum retention, atelectasis and collapse/consolidation of lung tissue, which potentially may lead to superadded infection. This exacerbates hypoxia and leads to progressive respiratory failure which may result in a need for invasive ventilation if not addressed rapidly and effectively. The best way to avoid this predictable deterioration is to provide adequate analgesia from the first presentation of the patient.

The method and magnitude of analgesia required will depend more on the amount of pain suffered and baseline respiratory reserve than on the type and degree of injury sustained in many cases. A single lateral rib fracture in an elderly smoker with COPD may precipitate respiratory failure whereas multiple posterior rib fractures in a young fit person may be relatively well tolerated.

Key Points

Effective analgesia reduces stress, helps stabilise cardiovascular function, reduces oxygen requirements and allows early mobilisation. Analgesia is best achieved with a multi-modal approach combining several different drug types rather than relying on one technique alone and minimises the potential for side effects. Suitable analgesic components include:

Non-pharmacological Methods

Splinting, e.g. "Cough Lock" Support with Median Sternotomy

- Splinting by hand may offer some temporary relief, but binding or strapping may result in increased respiratory complications
- Surgical fixation of ribs may reduce pain, morbidity, mortality and length of stay [72–74]

Regional Anaesthesia

Single Shot or Infusion Catheter

- Intercostal Block
- Intrapleural/paravertebral blocks
- Thoracic epidurals (± epidural opiates/opioids)
- Serratus anterior plane block

Systemic Analgesia

- Simple analgesia with paracetamol or NSAIDs
- Opioids
- Low dose ketamine infusion
  - 5–10 mg IV loading dose followed by 0.5–2 mcg/kg/min infusion in a monitored High Dependency Unit (HDU) environment with 10–20 mg boluses as required 11. Confusion or agitation should be managed by reducing the dose of the infusion. Ketamine infusions are very useful in combination with any or all of the above techniques.

Regional Techniques for Thoracic Trauma

These can produce excellent analgesia with no sedation when performed well and allow almost normal chest movement with respiration. The technique chosen depends on experience and equipment available in addition to any contraindications and local agreements (e.g. site-specific requirement for HDU level care for all patients with epidurals). However, particularly high blocks may reduce the function of the intercostal muscles and cause respiratory insufficiency on their own, so caution is advised with their implementation. With certain techniques (e.g. thoracic epidural) there may also be deleterious cardiovascular effects including hypotension secondary to sympathetic blockade causing vasodilatation and bradycardia if the cardio-acceleratory fibres are blocked and unopposed vagal tone predominates. If appropriately implemented and monitored then these techniques have a high success rate. In order to avoid complications then good nursing care and appropriate monitoring are as important as medical technical proficiency. Thus, placement of an epidural catheter may require a high dependency or ITU setting if ward staff are unfamiliar with epidural management or not exposed to epidural care on a regular basis.

Intercostal and intra-pleural blocks have the potential for local anaesthetic toxicity due to the relatively rapid uptake of drug from the pleural and intercostal spaces, as well as the risk of pneumothorax. The insertion of these blocks may be done before or after an operation while the patient is under general anaesthesia, or potentially awake in a sitting position if no operation is planned. However, the positioning required for these blocks in some patients may preclude them being done due to restrictions on movement (e.g. pelvic ex-fix in situ or unstable spinal fracture awaiting fixation) or severe pain. In the latter case, if the patient can be positioned or spontaneously move when they are awake for an intercostal or intrapleural block then they usually will not require one. Intrapleural catheters can be placed under direct vision at the time of operation if surgeons perform a thoracotomy.

Intercostal Block

Video: Intercostal block [https://www.youtube.com/watch?v=JVLZoxxthTY].

This block requires multiple injections, one for each rib fracture plus one segment above and below. The needle is placed just over the lower border of the rib at the angle of the rib with the injection of 5 ml of bupivacaine 0.25% at each site. The limited duration of action of each injection necessitates repeated injections. Good analgesia with bupivacaine or ropivacaine typically only lasts about 4 h. Single shot techniques therefore require repeated injections at multiple levels and is not practical for upper rib or posterior rib fractures. Therefore, this block is included for completion, but in practical terms is of limited value.

Intra/Inter-Pleural Block

Video: Interpleural block [https://www.youtube.com/watch?v=HBupyAtEkHw].

Insertion of an epidural catheter via a 16 g Touhy needle into the pleural space allows repeated or continuous injection of local anaesthetic. Various techniques have been reported for detecting the pleural cavity and rely on negative pressure within the space. 20 ml of 0.25% bupivacaine will produce several hours of good analgesia and may be repeated every few hours. It is effectively an intercostal block from inside the thoracic cavity, and the patient should be positioned during the bolus administration to allow the local anaesthetic to pool in the paravertebral gutter on the affected side. The intercostal nerve at this point is separated from the pleural space by the thin posterior intercostal membrane through which the local anaesthetic solution diffuses rapidly. This provides excellent analgesia for unilateral rib fractures or unilateral thoracotomy with bolus administration of local anaesthetic, and only requires one needle insertion into the chest wall. A catheter technique may be used for several days, but it does not work well in the presence of pleural fluids or pleural adhesions. In addition, the presence of a chest drain may result in local anaesthetic being lost from pleural space and an ineffective block.

Paravertebral Block

Video: Paravertebral block [https://www.youtube.com/watch?v=l97p0mbOv1E].

This block may be performed with either a continuous catheter technique to avoid repeated

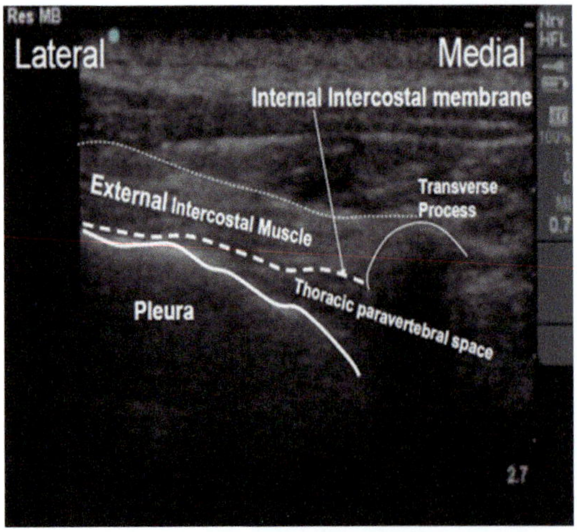

Fig. 13.6 Paravertebral space seen on ultrasound (Courtesy of NYSORA.com)

injections or as a single shot technique. Unfortunately, there is a less definite end point detected on insertion in comparison to epidural techniques (ultrasound image in Fig. 13.6). Drawbacks include the potential for LA toxicity, potential for sympathetic blockade, risk of pneumothorax and possible injection into a dural sleeve resulting in total or high spinal anaesthesia. Significant sympathetic blockade to the lung may predispose to bronchospasm and production of tenacious secretions.

Thoracic Epidural (+/− Opioid)

A midline or paramedian approach to the epidural space can be used and analgesia provided with a continuous infusion of local anaesthetic with or without opioid supplementation. Repeated bolus administration of local anaesthetic can be beneficial if a continuous infusion is not a practical proposition though this is rare. It is an excellent technique for unilateral and bilateral fractures of the middle and lower ribs. Epidural blockade may be used for several days but is not as effective for upper rib fractures, which would require very high blockade, increasing the likelihood of previously mentioned cardiovascular complications. This technique is contraindicated with thoracic vertebral injuries, other unstable spinal injuries, spinal cord injuries, overlying skin infection and in the presence of coagulopathy. A typical infusion regime is using 0.125% bupivacaine with 2 mcg/ml fentanyl at 6 ml/hour with a 6 ml bolus infusion with a 20-minute bolus lockout. If large numbers of boluses are demanded and the catheter is technically positioned correctly, the background infusion rate can be increased. Epidural solutions can be pre-made by pharmacy or reconstituted with strict aseptic technique on a volume by volume basis. The addition of opioids to an epidural has the effect of covering a less than perfect block, as epidural/spinal opioid receptors can be stimulated at lower doses than would be required systemically. This also has the effect of reducing (but not eliminating) the incidence of opioid side effects, namely nausea, vomiting, decreased level of consciousness and constipation.

One other potential complication of epidural analgesia is inadvertent dural puncture (estimated at 1% by the Royal College of Anaesthetists of all epidurals performed). This may cause a post dural puncture headache, or in severe cases an injury to the spinal cord in the thoracic region which may result in a permanent sensory or motor defect. Even in a perfectly placed epidural there is still the risk of infection and spinal abscess. Meticulous attention to asepsis and technique is essential. If there is any suggestion of spinal cord abscess or infection around the site then the infusion should be stopped, the epidural discontinued, and an urgent MRI requested regardless of the time of day or night. Unless caught and operated on early, spinal abscesses and haematomas have a very poor prognosis, so a high degree of clinical suspicion and a low threshold for intervention must be maintained. This is also why an epidural is contraindicated if there are overlying skin breaks, infections or systemic sepsis as the epidural and intrathecal spaces are sterile under normal conditions, and seeding of infection into them is a purely iatrogenic complication.

Serratus Anterior Plane Block

Blanco et al. [75] first described the regional anaesthetic technique of serratus anterior plane block in 2013. Local anaesthetic medication deposited superficial to the serratus anterior muscle and can provide analgesia to the hemithorax. It has been used in patients with rib fractures or following lateral thoracotomy as an excellent alternative to thoracic paravertebral blocks and thoracic epidurals in patients who have appropriate rib fractures and cannot be repositioned from a supine position. In certain patients who are intubated and have rib fractures, serratus anterior catheters can be placed prior to reducing sedation to provide effective analgesia and aid weaning from the ventilator [76–80]. If the rib fractures are lateral or anterior, then a serratus anterior block will likely be effective, but it will not provide analgesia for posterior rib fractures.

Local Anaesthetic Systemic Toxicity

Local anaesthetic systemic toxicity (LAST) results in CNS and cardiovascular symptoms [81–83]. The CNS symptoms include tinnitus, dizziness, blurred vision, paraesthesias, perioral numbness, seizures, agitation or restlessness. Eventually this can culminate in CNS depression, respiratory depression and cardiac arrhythmias. If toxicity is not treated at this point, further cardiac symptoms include ventricular dysrhythmias, ventricular fibrillation, myocardial depression and cardiac arrest (Fig. 13.7).

The Algorithm for Management of LAST Includes

1. Stop injecting local anaesthetic
2. Get Help:
   a. Consider Lipid emulsion therapy (intralipid) at the first sign of LAST
   b. Call for LAST rescue kit
   c. Alert nearest facility with Cardio-Pulmonary Bypass if appropriate
3. Airway management: Ventilate with 100% oxygen/avoid hyperventilating
4. Control seizures
5. Treat Hypotension and bradycardia

Cardiac arrest following LAST may be responsive to prolonged advanced life support with some adaptations to the universal ALS algorithm [84]. The ASRA recommendations are outlined in Fig. 13.8, below:

IV access and appropriate resuscitation facilities are mandated (including access to lipid rescue therapy) before commencing any form of regional anaesthesia under, the ASRA [85] and the AAGBI [86] guidelines for treatment of local toxicity. The same standard of monitoring should be applied to patients whether they are having a general or local/regional anaesthetic [56]. A more comprehensive discussion on local anaesthetic toxicity treatment is available on the www.lipidrescue.org educational website.

Analgesia for Neuro-Trauma

There are no specific treatment modalities for neurotrauma, the only caveat that must be born in mind is that specific treatments may cause neurological symptoms. For example, high doses of opioids can decrease the patient's level of consciousness and cause pinpoint pupils via stimulation of the Edinger-Westphal nucleus, both of which may alter findings in a neurological exam. Another example is ketamine, which has both pro- and anticonvulsant properties, so any focal neurological examination should ideally take place with the patient as free from impediment as possible. Frequently, the initial responder may have the most reliable examination findings as the patient may need high doses of analgesia, or even general anaesthesia before arriving at the hospital and the attention of a neurosurgeon or critical care team. It is important therefore to examine as thoroughly as possible and document clearly the highest GCS since injury and any lateralising neurological signs in the limbs or eyes before induction of general

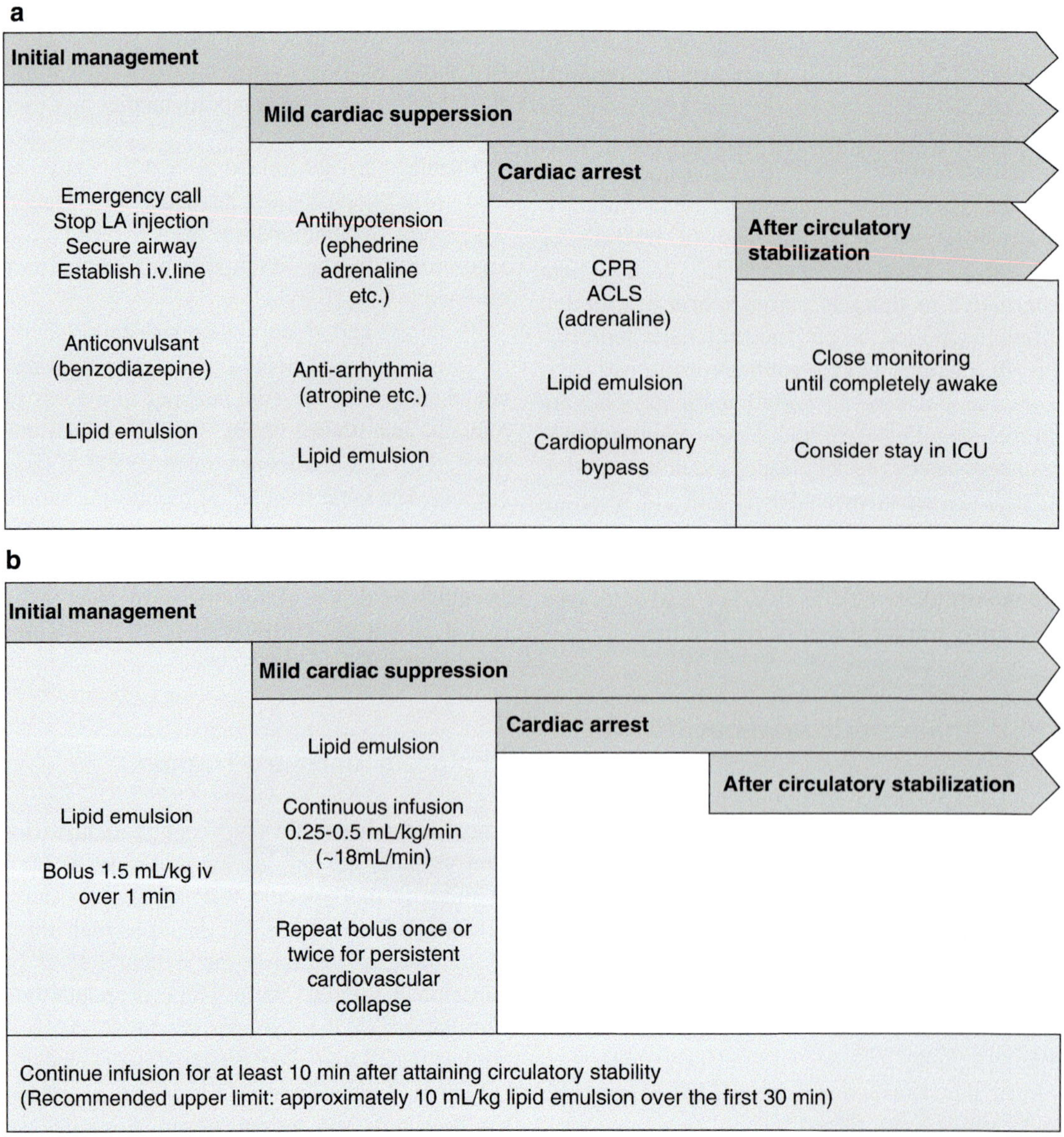

Fig. 13.7 Management of acute local anaesthetic toxicity. (**a**) Sequence of symptoms and required treatments. (**b**) Sequence of symptoms and program of lipid emulsion (20%) infusion. ACLS, advanced cardiac life support, CPR, cardiopulmonary resuscitation, ICU, Intensive Care Unit. From Sekimoto et al. [84]

anaesthesia or sedation. A focused neurological examination ("move your arms, your legs, close your eyes, where are you, what is your name, what day/week/month is it") will give a baseline to work from in hospital. It is also important to note the time of administration and dose of any neuromuscular blockers or other drugs which could change neurological examination findings in hospital.

It is essential to provide adequate analgesia to patients who are intubated and ventilated as pain may cause or substantially contribute to a raised intracranial pressure. Awareness under anaesthesia and coughing can also cause raised ICP, so assessment and maintenance of an adequate plane of anaesthesia even when not in the operating room (i.e. during CT scan, transfer inter- or intra-hospitally) are of vital importance.

Fig. 13.8 From Sekimoto et al. [84]

Table 3. Special considerations in cardiac life support for patients with local anesthetic-induced cardiac arrest†

1) If epinephrine is used, small initial doses (10 –100 μg boluses in adults) are preferable
2) Vasopressin is not recommended
3) Avoid calcium channel blockers and bete-blockers
4) If ventricular arrhythmias develop, amiodarone is preferable
5) In patients with cardiac toxicity avoiding the use of lidocaine and related class IB antidysrhythmic agents (e.g., mexiletine, tocainide) is crucial because they may worsen toxicity. Lidocaine has been used successfully bupivacaine-induced dysrhythmias, but its additive central nervous system toxicity is still a major concern.
6) In patients who do not respond to standard resuscitative measures, cardiac pacing and cardiopulmonary by pass may be introduced to improve the outcome. Cardiopulmonary by pass may serve as a bridging therapy until tissue levels of the local anesthetic have cleared.

†Adapted from ASRA guidelines.[4]

Clinical Pearls in the Management of Acute Pain in a Patient Following Trauma

It is important to perform a comprehensive assessment of the extent of trauma and injury, severity of pain, history of chronic pain, narcotic use and other comorbidities in the patient prior to initiating an analgesic plan in the acute period. Consider using regional anaesthetic techniques (peripheral nerve blockade or neuraxial techniques such as epidural analgesia) if the patient is an appropriate candidate. This assessment must take into account type, location and extent of injury, coagulation parameters, haemodynamics, allergies, infection, neurovascular injury and other comorbidities including cardiac and respiratory disease. A multimodal analgesic regimen should be initiated based on individual patient characteristics (severity of pain, allergies, contraindications to specific drugs). This regimen may incorporate several agents including paraceatamol (acetaminophen), non- steroidal anti-inflammatory medications, neuropathic agents (gabapentinoids, tricyclic antidepressants), opioids analgesics, adjuvants like intravenous ketamine and lidocaine infusions. The WHO analgesic ladder (Fig. 13.9) provides a good outline for initiating therapy based on pain severity, though this approach was initially developed for treating pain due to cancer and is considered outdated by some.

Initiating Patient Controlled Analgesia in the Acute Setting for Pain Management

For patients in severe pain and or unable to tolerate oral medication, an IV analgesic regimen in the form of patient controlled analgesia (PCA) can be initiated. Prior to initiating patient controlled analgesia consider age, ability to comprehend instructions, physical ability to use the

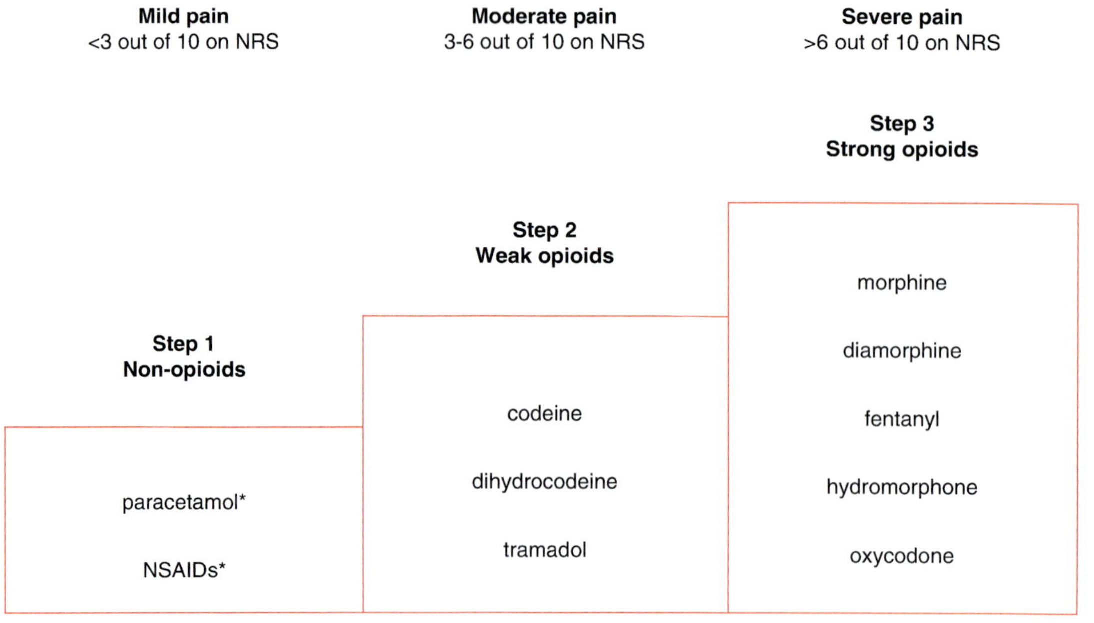

Fig. 13.9 WHO analgesic ladder

Table 13.1 Typical IV PCA setting for opioids

Analgesic	Typical Bolus Dose	Lockout period (minutes)
Morphine	1–2 mg	5–10 min
Fentanyl	10–50 mcg	5–10 min
Hydromorphone	0.2–0.5 mg	5–10 min
Remifentanil	0.5 mcg/kg	2 min

infusion pump and comorbidities. Comorbidities that increase the risk of respiratory depression include sleep apnoea, severe obesity, head injury, respiratory failure, renal failure (accumulation of potent metabolites like Morphine-6 glucuronide) and concurrent use of other synergistic medications such as benzodiazepines. Monitoring of patients using PCAs should include monitoring of sedation, respiratory rate and pulse oximetry. Medications used in PCA regimens include morphine, hydromorphone and fentanyl. Dosing strategy for PCA includes a bolus dose and a lockout period (Table 13.1). A bolus dose should be able to provide significant analgesia but should not cause respiratory depression. An appropriate lockout interval prevents repeat administration until a predetermined time period has elapsed. Even though the patient presses the demand button during this interval, medication is not administered. Lockout periods are tailored based on the drugs pharmacokinetics. Basal infusions should not be initiated in opioid naive patients and additionally have shown no improvement in analgesic effect, but instead are associated with higher risk of respiratory depression and side effects [87, 88].

Transitioning from PCA to an oral regimen is the next step in the acute pain management of a patient admitted for trauma. It is necessary to calculate the patients total daily opioid requirement. The first step is to assess the frequency of demands vs supply from the PCA machine to ensure the patient is not requesting analgesia greatly in excess of that delivered. Assuming that the doses are reasonably concordant with demands, add up the total dose of opioids given by the PCA in the last 24 h period and covert to oral equivalency of the new agent (typically oral morphine). This basal requirement is divided in two and given as a long acting analgesic twice a day. A bolus dose of 10–15% of the total requirement calculated is prescribed as a short acting opioid as needed for breakthrough pain. After the next 24 h the process is repeated again, looking at the total opioid dose given as basal dosing and adding the total dose of breakthrough boluses. If there are only one or two breakthrough episodes, then the regime should remain unchanged. If there are multiple doses given for breakthrough pain, the basal oral dose is recalculated in the same way as previously for the IV requirement. Does should be tapered down as able over a few days as pain subsides in the acute period.

For example, a PCA shows that 70 mg of morphine has been used in the last 24 h and the pain specialist decides to transition to oral medications. The total dose is divided in half (70/2 = 35) and prescribed as a twice daily long acting opioid (oxycontin 35 mg BD) and 10 mg as a PRN dose of oxynorm for breakthrough pain. Analgesia should be given well in advance of anticipated painful procedures or physiotherapy sessions so patients can participate and achieve maximal benefit. This must be balanced against risk of over-sedation and inability to engage with the session, so feedback and a multi-disciplinary approach are needed.

When rotating between opioids, it is prudent to perform a dose reduction to account for cross tolerance. At the authors'institution some commonly used oral opioids in the acute setting include oxycodone, hydromorphone and morphine.

There are several apps, policies and methods which can be used for conversion between doses and drugs, and a paper by Nielson et al. [89] found general consensus amongst the recommended conversion factors internationally.

Chronic Pain After Trauma

Chronic post-surgical or post traumatic pain as defined by the International Association for Study of Pain is chronic pain that develops or increases in intensity after tissue trauma (surgical or accidental) and persists beyond three months [90]. The incidence of chronic pain after polytrauma ranges from 46 to 85% [91] and after burns is between 18 and 52% [92, 93]. Comparatively, chronic pain after injury to muscles, bones, joints (aka post traumatic arthritis) is about 18.7%. Chronic pain after trauma is often under recognised and poorly treated. Several studies [94, 95] have identified the following risk factors which are predictive of patients developing chronic pain;

- female sex
- injury mechanism
- injury regions (brain-brainstem- cerebellum, disc- vertebra, thorax/ skeletal, face, abdominal, spinal cord, thorax, upper extremity)
- previous history of alcoholism, anxiety or depression
- two or more rib fractures
- mild traumatic brain injury
- spinal cord injury
- back and spine problems.

It is important to recognise chronic pain after trauma and to attempt to identify the primary mechanism which may be nociceptive. This could be musculoskeletal or neuropathic (including sympathetically-maintained), and the physician should initiate appropriate multidisciplinary management. For nociceptive pain this will include opioids, while for neuropathic pain this also includes use of medications like neuropathic agents (gabapentinoids, tricyclic antidepressants), antidepressants (duloxetine, SSRIs and SNRIS), muscle relaxants (baclofen, tizanidine, cyclobenzaprine), non-steroidal anti-inflammatory medications and paracetamol. Consideration should be given to early initiation of physiotherapy and interventional management like sympathetic blocks for complex regional pain syndrome (CRPS) and peripheral nerve blocks for pain due peripheral nerve mononeuropathy. Cognitive behavioural therapy can be useful in appropriate patients, and a multidisciplinary approach should be taken to chronic pain management in trauma patients.

In patients with chronic pain which is neuropathic in origin and associated with a diagnosis of complex regional pain syndrome, failed back surgical syndrome with radicular pain and phantom limb pain secondary to amputation, implantable neuromodulatory devices like spinal cord stimulators may be considered in the treatment algorithm in the longer term. It is beyond the scope of this chapter to cover the mechanisms and placement of neurostimulators for chronic pain, and review articles by Moisset et al. [96], Rokyta and Fricova [97] or Jeon [98] give good oversight.

Summary

Treatment of pain is one of the most important interventions that can be undertaken by any personnel involved in trauma. While there are many drugs with complex pharmacological actions and interactions that can be used, basic principles should not be forgotten in the acute phase. Treating pain can be an end in itself but can also have impact on patients physiology and outcomes, so it is important to get it right for a multitude of reasons. The development of complex pain syndromes following trauma can be as debilitating as the biomechanical or tissue effects of the injury itself, and chronic pain management is as much about assisting patients to cope with the impact of their pain as it is alleviating it. By giving appropriate treatment early enough, the development of chronic pain syndromes may be prevented.

Questions

1. Which of the following nerve blocks has the highest likelihood of ipsilateral phrenic nerve paralysis?
   a. Intercostal nerve block
   b. Interscalene nerve block
   c. Supraclavicular nerve block
   d. Suprascapular nerve block
2. Which of the following should be avoided in management of local anesthestic system toxicity?
   a. Use of intralipid
   b. Epinephrine
   c. Vasopressin
   d. Benzodiazepenes
3. The advantages of IV paracetamol over other routes of administration include all of the following except:
   a. shorter time until maximum availability
   b. higher dose bioavailability
   c. less hepatic damage
   d. Significant clinical benefit over other routes of administration.
4. Which of the following nerve blocks cannot provide analgesia to patient with thoracic trauma:
   a. Intercostal nerve block
   b. Interscalene nerve block
   c. Intrapleural nerve block
   d. Serratus anterior plane block
5. Which of the following regional anesthetic techniques has the highest systemic absorption of local anesthetic?
   a. Epidural
   b. Axillary
   c. Intercostal
   d. Femoral

Answers

1. b. Interscalene nerve block
2. c. Vasopressin is avoided in the management of LAST. Calcium channel blockers and Betablockers are to be avoided as well in treating arrthymias in the setting LAST
3. d. A recent study and systematic review found no clinical benefit of IV over oral forms of paracetamol in patients who were able to take oral doses [44, 45]
4. b. Interscalene Nerve block provides analgesia to the shoulder and upper arm
5. c. Intercostal nerve block has the highest systemic absorption of local anesthetic

Acknowledgement The authors would like to acknowledge the assistance of Dr. Amy Pearson, MD in the preparation of this chapter.

References

1. Joshi GP, Ogunnaike BO. Consequences of inadequate postoperative pain relief and chronic persistent postoperative pain. Anesthesiology Clinics of North America [Internet]. 2005 [cited 2019 Nov 14];23(1):21–36. Available from: https://linkinghub.elsevier.com/retrieve/pii/S0889853704001270
2. Tick H, Nielsen A, Pelletier KR, Bonakdar R, Simmons S, Glick R, et al. Evidence-based non-pharmacologic strategies for comprehensive pain care. Explore [Internet]. 2018 [cited 2020 Feb 23];14(3):177–211. Available from: https://linkinghub.elsevier.com/retrieve/pii/S1550830718300223

3. Chazan S, Buda I, Nesher N, Paz J, Weinbroum AA. Low-dose ketamine via intravenous patient-controlled analgesia device after various transthoracic procedures improves analgesia and patient and family satisfaction. Pain Manage Nurs [Internet]. 2010 [cited 2020 Jan 25];11(3):169–76. Available from: https://linkinghub.elsevier.com/retrieve/pii/S152490420900068X
4. Carstensen M, Møller AM. Adding ketamine to morphine for intravenous patient-controlled analgesia for acute postoperative pain: a qualitative review of randomized trials. Br J Anaesth [Internet]. 2010 [cited 2020 Jan 25];104(4):401–6. Available from: https://linkinghub.elsevier.com/retrieve/pii/S0007091217336413
5. Schwenk ES, Viscusi ER, Buvanendran A, Hurley RW, Wasan AD, Narouze S, et al. Consensus guidelines on the use of intravenous ketamine infusions for acute pain management from the American Society of Regional Anesthesia and pain medicine, the American Academy of Pain Medicine, and the American Society of anesthesiologists. Reg Anesth Pain Med [Internet]. 2018 [cited 2020 Jan 26];1. Available from: https://rapm.bmj.com/lookup/doi/10.1097/AAP.0000000000000806
6. Klucka J, Stourac P, Stouracova A, Masek M, Repko M. Compartment syndrome and regional anaesthesia: critical review. Biomed Pap Med Fac Univ Palacky Olomouc Czech Repub [Internet]. 2017 [cited 2019 Nov 14];161(3):242–51. Available from: http://biomed.papers.upol.cz/doi/10.5507/bp.2017.025.html
7. Lönnqvist P-A, Ecoffey C, Bosenberg A, Suresh S, Ivani G. The European society of regional anesthesia and pain therapy and the American society of regional anesthesia and pain medicine joint committee practice advisory on controversial topics in pediatric regional anesthesia I and II: what do they tell us? Curr Opin Anaesthesiol [Internet]. 2017 [cited 2019 Nov 14];30(5):613–20. Available from: http://Insights.ovid.com/crossref?an=00001503-201710000-00017
8. Johnson DJG, Chalkiadis GA. Does epidural analgesia delay the diagnosis of lower limb compartment syndrome in children? Pediatr Anesth [Internet]. 2009 [cited 2019 Nov 14];19(2):83–91. Available from: http://doi.wiley.com/10.1111/j.1460-9592.2008.02894.x
9. Erdös J, Dlaska C, Szatmary P, Humenberger M, Vécsei V, Hajdu S. Acute compartment syndrome in children: a case series in 24 patients and review of the literature. International Orthopaedics (SICOT) [Internet]. 2011 [cited 2019 Nov 14];35(4):569–75. Available from: http://link.springer.com/10.1007/s00264-010-1016-6
10. Walker BJ, Noonan KJ, Bosenberg AT. Evolving compartment syndrome not masked by a continuous peripheral nerve block: evidence-based case management. Reg Anesth Pain Med [Internet]. 2012 [cited 2019 Nov 14];37(4):393–7. Available from: https://rapm.bmj.com/lookup/doi/10.1097/AAP.0b013e31824df1ac
11. Dißmann PD, Maignan M, Cloves PD, Gutierrez Parres B, Dickerson S, Eberhardt A. A review of the burden of trauma pain in emergency settings in Europe. Pain Ther [Internet]. 2018 [cited 2020 Feb 23];7(2):179–92. Available from: http://link.springer.com/10.1007/s40122-018-0101-1
12. Thomas SH, Silen W, Cheema F, Reisner A, Aman S, Goldstein JN, et al. Effects of morphine analgesia on diagnostic accuracy in emergency department patients with abdominal pain: a prospective, randomized trial. J Am Coll Surg [Internet]. 2003 [cited 2019 Nov 14];196(1):18–31. Available from: https://linkinghub.elsevier.com/retrieve/pii/S1072751502014801
13. Cohen SP, Christo PJ, Moroz L. Pain management in trauma patients. Am J Phys Med Rehabil [Internet]. 2004 [cited 2020 Jan 24];83(2):142–61. Available from: http://content.wkhealth.com/linkback/openurl?sid=WKPTLP:landingpage&an=00002060-200402000-00011
14. Gan TJ. Poorly controlled postoperative pain: prevalence, consequences, and prevention. JPR [Internet]. 2017 [cited 2020 Feb 23];10:2287–98. Available from: https://www.dovepress.com/poorly-controlled-postoperative-pain-prevalence-consequences-and-preve-peer-reviewed-article-JPR
15. Hayhurst CJ. Differential Opioid Tolerance and Opioid-induced Hyperalgesia.: 6.
16. Rivat C, Ballantyne J. The dark side of opioids in pain management: basic science explains clinical observation. PAIN Rep [Internet]. 2016 [cited 2020 Feb 23];1(2):e570. Available from: http://journals.lww.com/01938936-201608300-00003
17. Yam M, Loh Y, Tan C, Khadijah Adam S, Abdul Manan N, Basir R. General pathways of pain sensation and the major neurotransmitters involved in pain regulation. IJMS [Internet]. 2018 [cited 2020 Feb 23];19(8):2164. Available from: http://www.mdpi.com/1422-0067/19/8/2164
18. Boadas-Vaello P, Castany S, Homs J, Álvarez-Pérez B, Deulofeu M, Verdú E. Neuroplasticity of ascending and descending pathways after somatosensory system injury: reviewing knowledge to identify neuropathic pain therapeutic targets. Spinal Cord [Internet]. 2016 [cited 2020 Feb 23];54(5):330–40. Available from: http://www.nature.com/articles/sc2015225
19. Pai A, Ketamine HM. Continuing Education in Anaesthesia. Crit Care Pain [Internet]. 2007 [cited 2019 Nov 14];7(2):59–63. Available from: https://linkinghub.elsevier.com/retrieve/pii/S1743181617305012
20. Atkins DL, Chameides L, Fallat ME, Hazinski MF, Phillips B, Quan L, et al. Resuscitation science of pediatrics. Ann Emerg Med [Internet]. 2001 [cited 2019 Nov 14];37(4):S41–8. Available from: https://linkinghub.elsevier.com/retrieve/pii/S0196064401161524
21. Waisman M, Waisman D. Bone marrow infusion in adults. J Trauma Injury Infect Crit Care [Internet]. 1997 [cited 2019 Nov 14];42(2):288–93. Available from: https://insights.ovid.com/crossref?an=00005373-199702000-00019
22. Lowther A. Intraosseous access and adults in the emergency department. Nurs Stand [Internet].

2011 [cited 2019 Nov 14];25(48):35–8. Available from: http://rcnpublishing.com/doi/abs/10.7748/ns2011.08.25.48.35.c8647
23. Byars DV, Tsuchitani SN, Erwin E, Anglemyer B, Eastman J. Evaluation of success rate and access time for an adult sternal intraosseous device deployed in the prehospital setting. Prehosp Disaster Med [Internet]. 2011 [cited 2019 Nov 14];26(2):127–9. Available from: https://www.cambridge.org/core/product/identifier/S1049023X11000057/type/journal_article
24. Petitpas F, Guenezan J, Vendeuvre T, Scepi M, Oriot D, Mimoz O. Use of intra-osseous access in adults: a systematic review. Crit Care [Internet]. 2016 [cited 2019 Nov 14];20(1):102. Available from: http://ccforum.biomedcentral.com/articles/10.1186/s13054-016-1277-6
25. Burgert JM, Johnson AD, O'Sullivan JC, Blalock WJ, Duffield BC, Albright BP, et al. Pharmacokinetic effects of endotracheal, intraosseous, and intravenous epinephrine in a swine model of traumatic cardiac arrest. Am J Emerg Med [Internet]. 2019 [cited 2020 Jan 24];37(11):2043–50. Available from: https://linkinghub.elsevier.com/retrieve/pii/S0735675719301226
26. Mody P, Brown SP, Kudenchuk PJ, Chan PS, Khera R, Ayers C, et al. Intraosseous versus intravenous access in patients with out-of-hospital cardiac arrest: Insights from the resuscitation outcomes consortium continuous chest compression trial. Resuscitation [Internet]. 2019 [cited 2020 Jan 24];134:69–75. Available from: https://linkinghub.elsevier.com/retrieve/pii/S0300957218310669
27. Reades R, Studnek JR, Vandeventer S, Garrett J. Intraosseous versus intravenous vascular access during out-of-hospital cardiac arrest: a randomized controlled trial. Ann Emerg Med [Internet]. 2011 Dec [cited 2020 Jan 24];58(6):509–16. Available from: https://linkinghub.elsevier.com/retrieve/pii/S0196064411013369
28. Hoskins SL, Do Nascimento P, Lima RM, Espana-Tenorio JM, Kramer GC. Pharmacokinetics of intraosseous and central venous drug delivery during cardiopulmonary resuscitation. Resuscitation [Internet]. 2012 [cited 2019 Nov 14];83(1):107–12. Available from: https://linkinghub.elsevier.com/retrieve/pii/S0300957211005016
29. Bolster F, Ali Z, Fowler D, Daly B. Imaging of resuscitation and emergency resuscitation devices—Lessons learned from post mortem computed tomography. J Forensic Radiol Imaging [Internet]. 2019 [cited 2020 Jan 24];17:23–30. Available from: https://linkinghub.elsevier.com/retrieve/pii/S2212478019300383
30. London School of Hygeine and Tropical Medicine. The Trauma INtramuscular Tranexamic Acid Clinical Trial (TraumaINTACT) [Internet]. ClinicalTrials.gov. 2020 [cited 2020 Feb 23]. Available from: https://clinicaltrials.gov/ct2/show/NCT03875937
31. Sin B, Wiafe J, Ciaramella C, Valdez L, Motov SM. The use of intranasal analgesia for acute pain control in the emergency department: a literature review. Am J Emerg Med [Internet]. 2018 [cited 2019 Nov 14];36(2):310–8. Available from: https://linkinghub.elsevier.com/retrieve/pii/S0735675717309518
32. Reynolds SL, Bryant KK, Studnek JR, Hogg M, Dunn C, Templin MA, et al. Randomized controlled feasibility trial of intranasal ketamine compared to intranasal fentanyl for analgesia in children with suspected extremity fractures. Miner JR, editor. Acad Emerg Med [Internet]. 2017 [cited 2019 Nov 14];24(12):1430–40. Available from: http://doi.wiley.com/10.1111/acem.13313
33. Poonai N, Canton K, Ali S, Hendrikx S, Shah A, Miller M, et al. Intranasal ketamine for procedural sedation and analgesia in children: a systematic review. Ma Z-L, editor. PLoS ONE [Internet]. 2017 [cited 2019 Nov 14];12(3):e0173253. Available from: https://dx.plos.org/10.1371/journal.pone.0173253
34. Shaw BH, Ross M. Is intranasal ketamine safe and effective as a prehospital analgesic? CJEM [Internet]. 2019 [cited 2019 Nov 14];1–2. Available from: https://www.cambridge.org/core/product/identifier/S1481803519004330/type/journal_article
35. Wedmore IS, Kotwal RS, McManus JG, Pennardt A, Talbot TS, Fowler M, et al. Safety and efficacy of oral transmucosal fentanyl citrate for prehospital pain control on the battlefield. J Trauma Acute Care Surg [Internet]. 2012 [cited 2019 Nov 14];73:S490–5. Available from: http://content.wkhealth.com/linkback/openurl?sid=WKPTLP:landingpage&an=01586154-201212005-00019
36. Singh R, Choubey S, Mehra R. Efficacy of oral transmucosal fentanyl citrate for premedication in patients for surgery under general anesthesia. Anesth Essays Res [Internet]. 2017 [cited 2020 Jan 24];11(4):854. Available from: http://www.aeronline.org/text.asp?2017/11/4/854/211949
37. Rahman SM, Quinn E. BET 1: Green or blue for you? Methoxyflurane (Penthrox) or nitrous oxide/oxygen 50% mixture (Entonox) for the management of acute pain in the ED. Emerg Med J [Internet]. 2019 [cited 2019 Nov 14];36(8):506–8. Available from: http://emj.bmj.com/lookup/doi/10.1136/emermed-2019-208777.1
38. Middleton PM, Simpson PM, Sinclair G, Dobbins TA, Math B, Bendall JC. Effectiveness of morphine, fentanyl, and methoxyflurane in the prehospital setting. Prehosp Emerg Care [Internet]. 2010 [cited 2019 Nov 14];14(4):439–47. Available from: http://www.tandfonline.com/doi/full/10.3109/10903127.2010.497896
39. Porter KM, Dayan AD, Dickerson S, Middleton PM. The role of inhaled methoxyflurane in acute pain management. OAEM [Internet]. 2018 [cited 2019 Nov 14];10:149–64. Available from: https://www.dovepress.com/the-role-of-inhaled-methoxyflurane-in-acute-pain-management-peer-reviewed-article-OAEM
40. Hartshorn S, Dissmann P, Coffey F, Lomax M. Low-dose methoxyflurane analgesia in adolescent patients with moderate-to-severe trauma pain: a subgroup analysis of the STOP! study. JPR [Internet]. 2019 [cited 2019 Nov 14];12:689–700. Available from: https://

www.dovepress.com/low-dose-methoxyflurane-analgesia-in-adolescent-patients-with-moderate-peer-reviewed-article-JPR

41. Kelly A-M, Kerr D, Dietze P, Patrick I, Walker T, Koutsogiannis Z. Randomised trial of intranasal versus intramuscular naloxone in prehospital treatment for suspected opioid overdose. Med J Aust. 2005;182(1):24–7.
42. Robertson TM, Hendey GW, Stroh G, Shalit M. Intranasal naloxone is a viable alternative to intravenous naloxone for prehospital narcotic overdose. Prehosp Emerg Care [Internet]. 2009 [cited 2019 Nov 14];13(4):512–5. Available from: http://www.tandfonline.com/doi/full/10.1080/10903120903144866
43. Arici S, Gurbet A, Türker G, Yavaşcaoğlu B, Sahin S. Preemptive analgesic effects of intravenous paracetamol in total abdominal hysterectomy. Agri. 2009;21(2):54–61.
44. Bright H, Carey R. Intravenous or oral paracetamol: Which is better in the emergency department? Curr Med Issues [Internet]. 2018 [cited 2020 Jan 24];16(1):16. Available from: http://www.cmijournal.org/text.asp?2018/16/1/16/231366
45. Jibril F, Sharaby S, Mohamed A, Wilby KJ. Intravenous versus Oral Acetaminophen for Pain: Systematic Review of Current Evidence to Support Clinical Decision-Making. CJHP [Internet]. 2015 [cited 2020 Jan 24];68(3). Available from: http://www.cjhp-online.ca/index.php/cjhp/article/view/1458
46. Jenkins C, Costello J, Hodge L. Systematic review of prevalence of aspirin induced asthma and its implications for clinical practice. BMJ [Internet]. 2004 [cited 2019 Nov 14];328(7437):434. Available from: http://www.bmj.com/lookup/doi/10.1136/bmj.328.7437.434
47. Lo P-C, Tsai Y-T, Lin S-K, Lai J-N. Risk of asthma exacerbation associated with nonsteroidal anti-inflammatory drugs in childhood asthma: A nationwide population-based cohort study in Taiwan. Medicine [Internet]. 2016 [cited 2019 Nov 14];95(41):e5109. Available from: http://Insights.ovid.com/crossref?an=00005792-201610110-00032
48. Ong CKS, Lirk P, Tan CH, Seymour RA. An evidence-based update on nonsteroidal anti-inflammatory drugs. Clin Med Res [Internet]. 2007 [cited 2020 Jan 24];5(1):19–34. Available from: http://www.clinmed-res.org/cgi/doi/10.3121/cmr.2007.698
49. Kim TJ, Kim ER, Hong SN, Kim Y-H, Lee YC, Kim HS, et al. Effectiveness of acid suppressants and other mucoprotective agents in reducing the risk of occult gastrointestinal bleeding in nonsteroidal anti-inflammatory drug users. Sci Rep [Internet]. 2019 [cited 2020 Feb 23];9(1):11696. Available from: http://www.nature.com/articles/s41598-019-48173-6
50. Jauhar S, Morrison P. Esketamine for treatment resistant depression. BMJ [Internet]. 2019 [cited 2020 Jan 25];l5572. Available from: http://www.bmj.com/lookup/doi/10.1136/bmj.l5572
51. Chincholkar M. Analgesic mechanisms of gabapentinoids and effects in experimental pain models: a narrative review. Br J Anaesth [Internet]. 2018 [cited 2020 Feb 24];120(6):1315–34. Available from: https://linkinghub.elsevier.com/retrieve/pii/S0007091218302344
52. Wiffen PJ, Collins S, McQuay HJ, Carroll D, Jadad A, Moore RA. Anticonvulsant drugs for acute and chronic pain. Cochrane Pain, Palliative and Supportive Care Group, editor. Cochrane Datab Syst Rev [Internet]. 2010 [cited 2019 Nov 14]; Available from: http://doi.wiley.com/10.1002/14651858.CD001133.pub3
53. Finnerup NB, Sindrup SH, Jensen TS. The evidence for pharmacological treatment of neuropathic pain: Pain [Internet]. 2010 [cited 2019 Nov 14];150(3):573–81. Available from: http://content.wkhealth.com/linkback/openurl?sid=WKPTLP:landingpage&an=00006396-201009000-00031
54. Tran DQH, Duong S, Bertini P, Finlayson RJ. Treatment of complex regional pain syndrome: a review of the evidence. J Can Anesth [Internet]. 2010 [cited 2019 Nov 14];57(2):149–66. Available from: http://link.springer.com/10.1007/s12630-009-9237-0
55. Dauri M, Faria S, Gatti A, Celidonio L, Carpenedo R, Sabato A. Gabapentin and pregabalin for the acute post-operative pain management. A systematic-narrative review of the recent clinical evidences. CDT [Internet]. 2009 [cited 2019 Nov 14];10(8):716–33. Available from: http://www.eurekaselect.com/openurl/content.php?genre=article&issn=1389-4501&volume=10&issue=8&spage=716
56. Checketts MR, Alladi R, Ferguson K, Gemmell L, Handy JM, Klein AA, et al. Recommendations for standards of monitoring during anaesthesia and recovery 2015: Association of Anaesthetists of Great Britain and Ireland. Anaesthesia [Internet]. 2016 [cited 2020 Jan 26];71(1):85–93. Available from: http://doi.wiley.com/10.1111/anae.13316
57. Membership of the Working Party, Harrop-Griffiths W, Cook T, Gill H, Hill D, Ingram M, et al. Regional anaesthesia and patients with abnormalities of coagulation: the association of Anaesthetists of Great Britain & Ireland the obstetric anaesthetists' association regional anaesthesia UK. Anaesthesia [Internet]. 2013 [cited 2020 Jan 27];68(9):966–72. Available from: http://doi.wiley.com/10.1111/anae.12359
58. Horlocker TT, Vandermeulen E, Kopp SL, Gogarten W, Leffert LR, Benzon HT. Regional anesthesia in the patient receiving antithrombotic or thrombolytic therapy: American society of regional anesthesia and pain medicine evidence-based guidelines (Fourth Edition). Reg Anesthesia Pain Med [Internet]. 2018 [cited 2020 Jan 27];43(3):263–309. Available from: https://rapm.bmj.com/lookup/doi/10.1097/AAP.0000000000000763
59. Lopez S. Fascia iliaca compartment block for femoral bone fractures in prehospital care. Reg Anesth Pain Med [Internet]. 2003 [cited 2019 Nov 14];28(3):203–7. Available from: https://rapm.bmj.com/lookup/doi/10.1053/rapm.2003.50134
60. Hards M, Brewer A, Bessant G, Lahiri S. Efficacy of prehospital Analgesia with Fascia Iliaca compartment block for femoral bone fractures: a system-

atic review. Prehosp Disaster med [Internet]. 2018 [cited 2019 Nov 14];33(3):299–307. Available from: https://www.cambridge.org/core/product/identifier/S1049023X18000365/type/journal_article
61. Büttner B, Mansur A, Kalmbach M, Hinz J, Volk T, Szalai K, et al. Prehospital ultrasound-guided nerve blocks improve reduction-feasibility of dislocated extremity injuries compared to systemic analgesia. A randomized controlled trial. Eller K, editor. PLoS ONE [Internet]. 2018 [cited 2019 Nov 14];13(7):e0199776. Available from: https://dx.plos.org/10.1371/journal.pone.0199776
62. Rashid A, Beswick E, Galitzine S, Fitton L. Regional analgesia in the emergency department for hip fractures: survey of current UK practice and its impact on services in a teaching hospital. Emerg Med J [Internet]. 2014 [cited 2020 Jan 25];31(11):909–13. Available from: http://emj.bmj.com/lookup/doi/10.1136/emermed-2013-202794
63. Ketelaars R, Stollman JT, van Eeten E, Eikendal T, Bruhn J, van Geffen G-J. Emergency physician-performed ultrasound-guided nerve blocks in proximal femoral fractures provide safe and effective pain relief: a prospective observational study in The Netherlands. Int J Emerg Med [Internet]. 2018 [cited 2020 Jan 25];11(1):12. Available from: https://intjem.biomedcentral.com/articles/10.1186/s12245-018-0173-z
64. Challa ST, Hargens AR, Uzosike A, Macias BR. Muscle microvascular blood flow, oxygenation, pH, and perfusion pressure decrease in simulated acute compartment syndrome. J Bone Joint Surg [Internet]. 2017 [cited 2020 Jan 25];99(17):1453–9. Available from: http://Insights.ovid.com/crossref?an=00004623-201709060-00005
65. Garr JL, Gentilello LM, Cole PA, Mock CN, Matsen FA. Monitoring for compartmental syndrome using near-infrared spectroscopy: a noninvasive, continuous, transcutaneous monitoring technique. J Trauma Injury Infect Crit Care [Internet]. 1999 [cited 2020 Jan 25];46(4):613–8. Available from: https://insights.ovid.com/crossref?an=00005373-199904000-00009
66. Schmidt AH. Novel modalities to diagnose and prevent compartment syndrome. In: Mauffrey C, Hak DJ, Martin III MP, editors. Compartment syndrome [Internet]. Cham: Springer; 2019. [cited 2020 Jan 25]. p. 169–76. Available from: http://link.springer.com/10.1007/978-3-030-22331-1_17.
67. Gumbs S. Acute compartment syndrome: a literature review and updates. Clin J Surg. 2019;2(2):1–5.
68. Hughes S, Birt D. Continuous peripheral nerve blockade on OP Herrick 9. J Royal Army Med Corps [Internet]. 2009 [cited 2019 Nov 14];155(1):57–8. Available from: http://jramc.bmj.com/lookup/doi/10.1136/jramc-155-01-18
69. Devonport L, Edwards D, Edwards C, Aldington D, Mahoney P, Wood P. Evolution of the role 4 UK military pain service. J Royal Army Med Corps [Internet]. 2010 [cited 2019 Nov 14];156(Suppl_4):S398-401. Available from: http://jramc.bmj.com/lookup/doi/10.1136/jramc-156-04s-22
70. Buckenmaier CC, Shields CH, Auton AA, Evans SL, Croll SM, Bleckner LL, et al. Continuous peripheral nerve block in combat casualties receiving low-molecular weight heparin. Br J Anaesth [Internet]. 2006 [cited 2019 Nov 14];97(6):874–7. Available from: https://linkinghub.elsevier.com/retrieve/pii/S0007091217353424
71. Turnbull DK, Shepherd DB. Post-dural puncture headache: pathogenesis, prevention and treatment. Br J Anaesth [Internet]. 2003 [cited 2020 Jan 25];91(5):718–29. Available from: https://linkinghub.elsevier.com/retrieve/pii/S0007091217363080
72. Qiu M, Shi Z, Xiao J, Zhang X, Ling S, Ling H. Potential benefits of rib fracture fixation in patients with flail chest and multiple non-flail rib fractures. Indian J Surg [Internet]. 2016 [cited 2019 May 8];78(6):458–63. Available from: https://www.ncbi.nlm.nih.gov/pmc/articles/PMC5218931/
73. Doben AR, Eriksson EA, Denlinger CE, Leon SM, Couillard DJ, Fakhry SM, et al. Surgical rib fixation for flail chest deformity improves liberation from mechanical ventilation. J Crit Care. 2014;29(1):139–43.
74. de Moya M, Nirula R, Biffl W. Rib fixation: who, what, when? Trauma Surg Acute Care Open [Internet]. 2017 [cited 2019 May 8];2(1):e000059. Available from: https://tsaco.bmj.com/content/2/1/e000059
75. Blanco R, Parras T, McDonnell JG, Prats-Galino A. Serratus plane block: a novel ultrasound-guided thoracic wall nerve block. Anaesthesia [Internet]. 2013 [cited 2020 Jan 26];68(11):1107–13. Available from: http://doi.wiley.com/10.1111/anae.12344
76. López-Matamala B, Fajardo M, Estébanez-Montiel B, Blancas R, Alfaro P, Chana M. A new thoracic interfascial plane block as anesthesia for difficult weaning due to ribcage pain in critically ill patients. Medicina Intensiva [Internet]. 2014 [cited 2019 Nov 18];38(7):463–5. Available from: https://linkinghub.elsevier.com/retrieve/pii/S0210569113002222
77. Madabushi R, Tewari S, Gautam SK, Agarwal A, Agarwal A. Serratus anterior plane block: a new analgesic technique for post-thoracotomy pain. Pain Phys. 2015;18(3):E421–4.
78. Okmen K, Okmen BM, Uysal S. Serratus anterior plane (SAP) block used for thoracotomy analgesia: a case report. Korean J Pain [Internet]. 2016 [cited 2019 Nov 18];29(3):189. Available from: https://synapse.koreamed.org/DOIx.php?id=10.3344/kjp.2016.29.3.189
79. Moll V, Groff R, Budhrani G, Sathiyakumar A, McKenzie-Brown AM. 1945: Bilateral Serratus Anterior Plane Block Facilitates Ventilator Weaning in Patient With Rib Cage Pain. Crit Care Med [Internet]. 2016 [cited 2019 Nov 18];44:561. Available from: http://content.wkhealth.com/linkback/openurl?sid=WKPTLP:landingpage&an=00003246-201612001-01902

80. Foley E, Bashir F, Gaber M, Kumar V, Castresana M. 1592: Ultrasound-guided serratus plane block analgesia for blunt thoracic trauma. Crit Care Med [Internet]. 2018 [cited 2019 Nov 18];46:780. Available from: http://Insights.ovid.com/crossref?an=00003246-201801001-01545
81. Christie LE, Picard J, Weinberg GL. Local anaesthetic systemic toxicity. BJA Educ [Internet]. 2015 [cited 2019 Nov 19];15(3):136–42. Available from: https://linkinghub.elsevier.com/retrieve/pii/S2058534917301543
82. El-Boghdadly K, Pawa A, Chin KJ. Local anesthetic systemic toxicity: current perspectives. LRA [Internet]. 2018 [cited 2019 Nov 19];11:35–44. Available from: https://www.dovepress.com/local-anesthetic-systemic-toxicity-current-perspectives-peer-reviewed-article-LRA
83. Neal JM, Woodward CM, Harrison TK. The American Society of regional anesthesia and pain medicine checklist for managing local anesthetic systemic toxicity: 2017 version. Reg Anesth Pain Med [Internet]. 2018 [cited 2019 Nov 19];43(2):150–3. Available from: https://rapm.bmj.com/lookup/doi/10.1097/AAP.0000000000000726
84. Sekimoto K, Tobe M, Saito S. Local anesthetic toxicity: acute and chronic management. Acute Med Surg [Internet]. 2017 [cited 2020 Jan 26];4(2):152–60. Available from: http://doi.wiley.com/10.1002/ams2.265
85. Neal JM, Barrington MJ, Fettiplace MR, Gitman M, Memtsoudis SG, Mörwald EE, et al. The Third American Society of regional anesthesia and pain medicine practice advisory on local anesthetic systemic toxicity: executive summary 2017. Reg Anesth Pain Med [Internet]. 2018 [cited 2020 Jan 26];43(2):113–23. Available from: https://rapm.bmj.com/lookup/doi/10.1097/AAP.0000000000000720
86. Cave DG, Harrop-Griffiths DW, Harvey DM, Meek DT, Picard DJ, Short DT, et al. Management of severe local anaesthetic toxicity [Internet]. The Association of Anaesthetists of Great Britain and Ireland; 2010 [cited 2020 Jan 26]. Available from: https://www.anaesthetists.org/Home/Resources-publications/Guidelines/Management-of-severe-local-anaesthetic-toxicity
87. Ginsberg B, Gil KM, Muir M, Sullivan F, Williams DA, Glass PSA. The influence of lockout intervals and drug selection on patient-controlled analgesia following gynecological surgery: Pain [Internet]. 1995 [cited 2020 Jan 13];62(1):95–100. Available from: http://content.wkhealth.com/linkback/openurl?sid=WKPTLP:landingpage&an=00006396-199507000-00011
88. Mather L, Woodhouse A. Pharmacokinetics of opioids in the context of patient controlled analgesia. Pain Rev. 1997;4:20–32.
89. Nielsen S, Degenhardt L, Hoban B, Gisev N. A synthesis of oral morphine equivalents (OME) for opioid utilisation studies: oral morphine equivalents. Pharmacoepidemiol Drug Saf [Internet]. 2016 [cited 2020 Jan 24];25(6):733–7. Available from: http://doi.wiley.com/10.1002/pds.3945
90. Schug SA, Lavand'homme P, Barke A, Korwisi B, Rief W, Treede R-D. The IASP classification of chronic pain for ICD-11: chronic post-surgical or posttraumatic pain. PAIN [Internet]. 2019 [cited 2020 Jan 24];160(1):45–52. Available from: http://Insights.ovid.com/crossref?an=00006396-201901000-00006
91. Gross T, Amsler F. Prevalence and incidence of longer term pain in survivors of polytrauma. Surgery [Internet]. 2011 [cited 2020 Jan 24];150(5):985–95. Available from: https://linkinghub.elsevier.com/retrieve/pii/S0039606011001644
92. Browne AL, Andrews R, Schug SA, Wood F. Persistent pain outcomes and patient satisfaction with pain management after burn injury. Clin J Pain [Internet]. 2011 [cited 2020 Jan 24];27(2):136–45. Available from: https://insights.ovid.com/crossref?an=00002508-201102000-00007
93. Dauber A, Osgood PF, Breslau AJ, Vernon HL, Carr DB. Chronic persistent pain after severe burns: a survey of 358 burn survivors. Pain Med [Internet]. 2002 [cited 2020 Jan 24];3(1):6–17. Available from: https://academic.oup.com/painmedicine/article-lookup/doi/10.1046/j.1526-4637.2002.02004.x
94. Crombie IK, Davies HT, Macrae WA. Cut and thrust: antecedent surgery and trauma among patients attending a chronic pain clinic. Pain. 1998;76(1–2):167–71.
95. Daoust R, Paquet J, Moore L, Émond M, Gosselin S, Lavigne G, et al. Early factors associated with the development of chronic pain in trauma patients. Pain Res Manag [Internet]. 2018 [cited 2020 Jan 24];2018:1–8. Available from: https://www.hindawi.com/journals/prm/2018/7203218/
96. Moisset X, Lanteri-Minet M, Fontaine D. Neurostimulation methods in the treatment of chronic pain. J Neural Transm [Internet]. 2019 [cited 2020 Jan 26]; Available from: http://link.springer.com/10.1007/s00702-019-02092-y
97. Rokyta R, Fricova J. Noninvasive neuromodulation methods in the treatment of chronic pain. In: Racz GB, Noe CE, editors. Pain and treatment [Internet]. InTech; 2014 [cited 2020 Jan 26]. Available from: http://www.intechopen.com/books/pain-and-treatment/noninvasive-neuromodulation-methods-in-the-treatment-of-chronic-pain
98. Jeon YH. Spinal cord stimulation in pain management: a review Korean J Pain [Internet]. 2012 [cited 2020 Jan 26];25(3):143. Available from: https://synapse.koreamed.org/DOIx.php?id=10.3344/kjp.2012.25.3.143

Further Reading

Regional Anaesthesia

www.nysora.com
www.neuraxiom.com

IO Access

http://www.jems.com/article/intraosseous/pain-management-use-io
http://bestbets.org/bets/bet.php?id=2515
http://reference.medscape.com/article/80431-overview

Intransal Drug Administration

http://www.lmana.com/pwpcontrol.php?pwpID=6359

Part III

Haemostatic Interventions in Trauma

14 Initial Approach to Damage Control Resuscitation

Peter Lax

- Non-medical examples of damage control
- Philiosophy of damage control in trauma
- History of damage control surgery
- Damage control anaesthesia and resuscitation
- Other examples of damage control resusitation

What Is Damage Control?

Damage control is a concept that comes from Naval warfare and was first implemented by the German Navy at the battle of Jutland in World War One [1]. It was subsequently adopted and refined by the US Navy and came to prominence in the Battle of the Coral Sea and the Battle of Midway in World War Two with the efforts of the USS Yorktown to stay afloat after taking heavy damage [2]. When a ship is damaged in combat, if it is still under fire then simultaneous activity must take place to concurrently fix the damage that has been caused while maintaining the ability to fire and manoeuvre, and "take the fight to the enemy". A balance must be struck in the division of labour in these two areas; sufficient manpower should be assigned to repair damage threatening to sink the ship without compromising combat effectiveness. The idea is that only damage which is an immediate threat to the ship is addressed via quick interventions. Definitive repairs are not performed, as what is needed in the acute situation is to keep the ship afloat and functional. Temporising techniques such as sealing compartments which are flooding, putting bands of metal around ruptured pipes and sealing them with clamps, and removal of floodwater are used in preference to definitive repairs. These measures are temporising, and all Naval personnel are commonly trained and assessed in their application before a vessel and her crew are certified as seaworthy.

A more commonly known example of a damage control approach is the Apollo 13 mission, in which an explosion mid-way into the flight to the moon crippled the Command and Service module, threatening the lives of the three astronauts on board. By minimising consumption of oxygen, power and water, and use of the Lunar Excursion Module as a lifeboat (as well as many novel procedures from Mission Control), the damage was mitigated, and the astronauts returned safely to Earth. This took a well-led, well-coordinated and well-understood effort to achieve the ultimate goal. This brings forward an essential parallel

P. Lax (✉)
Tactical Medical Wing, Royal Air Force, Brize Norton, Oxfordshire, UK

The Air Ambulance Service (TAAS), Rugby, Warwickshire, UK
e-mail: p.lax@NHS.net

P. Lax (ed.), *Textbook of Acute Trauma Care*, https://doi.org/10.1007/978-3-030-83628-3_14

between damage control on ships, spacecraft and in medicine: there has to be a systemic awareness, appreciation and application of the approach rather than personnel working in isolation for it to be optimally effective. There needs to be a whole team working together to the same end rather than individual practitioners in silos, else the approach will be uncoordinated, haphazard and ultimately counterproductive.

Similarly, a second parallel is that the damage control in both medical and mechanical terms does not emphasise a return to normality, but aims for prompt action to prevent further damage and restore essential (rather than complete) function. To compare Naval and medical approaches, a damaged ship is made waterproof and then returns to port for repairs before a new coat of paint is applied; painting is not essential to survival but needs doing at some point. A damage control laparotomy deals with bleeding and source control, but not forming stomas in the first instance; they need doing but are not a survival priority in the first operation.

Philosophy of Damage Control Resuscitation

While the acute stress of surgery has long been recognised as a potential contributor to morbidity and mortality, previous paradigms of care emphasised early, definitive operative intervention [3]. The theory behind this was that by performing all necessary surgical interventions early, the chances of recovery were optimised as there was only one significant "hit" for the patient to get over. The prevailing idea was to adequately resuscitate the patient before surgery and then do everything in one sitting. While the thought process behind this course of action is understandable, what it led to was patients arriving post-operatively in the ICU who were cold, acidotic, often under-resuscitated and in severe metabolic derangement despite the best efforts of staff in the operating theatre. This approach, unfortunately, led to significant morbidity and mortality. As our understanding of trauma-induced coagulopathy, haemostasis and surgical decision making has changed, so too has the approach to the sickest and most complex patients.

Damage control resuscitation is a group of complementary approaches in resuscitation, surgery, anaesthesia and critical care. This culminates in an early and intense focus on expeditious surgery to arrest haemorrhage and prevent contamination, resuscitation with balanced ratios of blood products and aggressive treatment of acidosis, hypothermia, hypocalcaemia and coagulopathy. It is explicitly not definitive surgery, it is not the required approach for every trauma patient, nor is it limited to a particular surgical speciality; damage control options exist in abdominal, thoracic and orthopaedic injuries. Once the initial surgery has been performed, some time for stabilisation is allowed on ICU. When the patient is optimised, they can return for definitive surgical procedures.

History and Concepts Around Damage Control Surgery

Damage control surgery is defined as a multi-step operative intervention, which includes a brief initial surgical procedure that aims to control mechanical bleeding, a massive air leak, and/or gross contamination [4]. The concept of damage control surgery has evolved from multiple military and civilian surgical concepts over the last 100 years. The first reports of techniques that could be broadly described as Damage Control were from cases in 1902 by Pringle [5], in which he described supra-hepatic liver packing for control of haemorrhage which was not amenable to primary ligation. This technique fell in and out of favour over many years as other surgical options developed for managing liver trauma, but it is still a useful technique which is employed in certain circumstances today. The first publication which espoused damage control principles was by Stone et al. in 1983 [6]. This paper advocated early termination of surgery when it was recognised that patients were developing a coagulopathy during surgery due to hypothermia, acidosis and bleeding. This coagulopathy was exacerbated by prolonged surgery and was recognised as potentially contributing to morbidity and mortality. This led to the development of the "staged laparotomy" concept in which a short initial procedure was followed by a period of resuscitation on ICU and then a return to theatre for definitive surgery. If a patient was identified as suffering from a coagulopathy intraoperatively, the protocol advocated techniques which we now consider part of damage control surgery. These included "…immediate termination of the operation; repair of only those vessels vital to survival, with ligation of all others; ligation of bowel ends… The spleen and kidney, if bleeding, were removed unless the renal injury was bilateral, for which the kidneys were packed. Ureteral wounds were managed by simple ligation, while the bladder was closed with a one-layered purse-string suture. If the pancreas had been resected, the stump was ligated with an umbilical tape. Gallbladder wounds were closed by a purse-string suture, yet major bile duct injuries were merely isolated by laparotomy pack" [6].

This approach was refined further and formally termed Damage Control Surgery in a publication by Rotondo and Schwab in 1993 [7]. Rotondo was an ex-Navy surgeon who appreciated the parallels between this surgical approach and strategies to keep ships afloat during battle. Further publications from their surgical group refined the concept of damage control into three distinct stages—initial operation (DC1), ICU resuscitation (DC2) and definitive surgery (DC3). Subsequent definitive abdominal closure in cases where the abdomen was left open for a prolonged period was termed DC4, and resuscitation before initial surgery was subsequently termed damage control ground zero (DC0) [8]. What is notable in Rotondo's publications is that he identifies explicitly that there is no mortality benefit in applying damage control principles to patients who do not require it. Specifically, there is no benefit in applying damage control principles to patients who have less severe injuries as opposed to a definitive laparotomy as the initial treatment. However, in those who have a significant vascular injury AND two or more visceral injuries, the survival rate in the damage control group was 77% compared to 11% in those who had definitive surgery at the time of their first operation [7].

The hallmark of damage control surgery is that it only addresses issues which may be fatal or pose a severe threat to life within the first 72 hours. Acute haemorrhage control and revascularisation, as well as prevention of gross contamination and subsequent infection, are the main principles. For patients who require immediate or urgent intervention, the initial surgery should last no more than 1 hour from incision to closing. Examples of strategies employed in this initial phase for haemorrhage control would include primary splenectomy (if needed), cautery or use of clotting agents on large, raw areas of bleeding such as liver edges, and use of packs on areas which ooze and which can be left in situ for 48–72 hours. A true trauma laparotomy will mandate a "second-look" operation within 48–72 hours to address any outstanding issues and remove these intentionally retained packs. Acutely, packing may prove life-saving for ongoing non-compressible haemorrhage. However, blood is a perfect culture medium, so packs need to be removed before they start to become a potential source of infection. Due to this, occasionally abdomens are left open with the use of a silastic pouch or Bogota bag as a temporary mechanism of closure which may also decrease the incidence of acute abdominal compartment syndrome [9, 10].

Bowel injuries are also not definitively managed, insofar as formal ileostomies or colostomies should not be formed at the initial operation. Bowel and mesenteries should be examined, and any perforations that are amenable to oversewing should be quickly closed. For more extensive damage, removal of the affected segment should be performed with stapled ends, and the two blind ends not rejoined at the initial surgery. In the initial period, higher than normal circulating levels of catecholamines (whether endogenous or therapeutic) may divert blood from the alimentary tract and cause a threefold risk of anastomotic leak or breakdown [11]. The time taken to form an anastomosis or stoma is also not inconsiderable, and given that neither is an essential or acutely life-saving procedure they should not be undertaken during the initial surgery as part of the damage control strategy. A similar thought process applies to the acute formation of tissue flaps by plastic surgery. While they may be required subsequently, temporary coverage should be applied until the patient is adequately resuscitated and able to tolerate a prolonged procedure. Performing flap or graft surgery at the first damage control operation will ultimately prove deleterious to the patient; it will unacceptably prolong operative time, have a high chance of the flap failing and eliminate a donor site for tissue coverage that may be more appropriate to use in 72 hours or thereafter. Temporary closure or use of a vacuum system at the end of initial surgical debridement is usually appropriate in these cases unless there are contraindications such as the presence of fistulae [10].

Damage control orthopaedic surgery has also been well described [12, 13], and the first surgical approach usually consists of external fixation of fractures rather than definitive repair. In common with abdominal damage control surgery, the rationale is to maintain or restore the integrity of blood supply to the limb or pelvis, provide a degree of fracture stabilisation for analgesia and to minimise the early risk of further bleeding or fat embolus. Intramedullary nailing or plating should not be performed in these patients acutely, but be deferred until physiological stability has been achieved.

For a more thorough overview of damage control surgery, refer to the relevant decision making and surgical chapters later in this textbook.

Damage Control Anaesthesia

Anaesthesia for acutely injured patients can be challenging, as many agents in common use have undesirable and dose-related side effects (such as hypotension) which may cause further morbidity and mortality. Patients requiring damage control resuscitation are usually unfasted and may be unable to give any information that may affect the choice of anaesthetic. In addition, they will invariably be bleeding, may have injury patterns requiring different anaesthetic strategies (e.g. permissive hypotension for bleeding, but with a concurrent head injury requiring normo/hypertension) and yet there will be little (if any) time for optimisation. These patients are some of the most challenging that an anaesthetist can deal with, and often require two or more clinicians to ensure optimum care. The general principle in these patients is to ensure that they have adequate circulating volume and blood pressure to perfuse vital organs and ensure adequate oxygen delivery. Once that has been achieved, amnesia, analgesia and anaesthesia can then be prioritised.

Multiple strategies have been employed; however, an excellent paper by Sikorski et al. [14] outlines the various options. In terms of ensuring cardiostability, amnesia, analgesia and anaesthesia, a strategy of periodic boluses of high dose opioids is advised, with large doses of fentanyl given at increments as permitted by blood pressure. This has the advantage of blunting the intrinsic catecholamine response, preserving microvascular flow, limiting damage to the glycocalyx (which has been implicated in the development of trauma-induced coagulopathy) and avoiding vasodilation with inhalational agents. Techniques such as propofol TIVA (total intravenous anaesthesia) by infusions are unreliable as computed models of vascular compartments and subsequent distribution of drugs are not valid when there is sizeable circulating volume loss or replacement. This is in addition to propofol's unfavourable pharmacodynamic profile in these patients. In patients who are sick enough to require a damage control approach, waking at the end of an operation is not usually a consideration. These patients will universally require admission to intensive care and will usually be kept sedated until they have had definitive surgery after adequate resuscitation. It is common to give 20–30 μg/kg of fentanyl in total to these patients, if not more (the author has used up to 5 mg in total in some cases). The restoration of microvascular flow in conjunction with blood product volume replacement rapidly assists in resolving acidosis and restoring base deficit to normal by improving perfusion and oxygen delivery.

The typical division of labour in these cases between anaesthetists involves one clinician managing blood transfusion and large venous access, and the other administering drugs and monitoring oxygenation/ventilation parameters and adequacy of anaesthesia. The transfusion anaesthetist should ensure an appropriate ratio of blood products is given, ideally with monitoring of response both clinically and in terms of using near-patient testing such as TEG or ROTEM to guide further product administration. Asking surgeons if patients are forming clots in the surgical field may give a broad indication as to the overall haemostatic picture. The transfusion anaesthetist should also be responsible for liaising with the blood bank, haematologists and the administration of agents such as tranexamic acid and calcium as needed. The second anaesthetist should monitor response to transfusion, ensure communication with the surgical teams, ensure an adequate balance between depth of anaesthesia/analgesia and adequate blood pressure, liaise with ICU to arrange postoperative care and ensure other relevant drugs such as antibiotics are administered. This was the general approach that was developed and modified in Camp Bastion during the Afghanistan conflict [15, 16] and was one of the factors which saw massive improvements in survival from injuries previously thought to be unsurvivable [17]. Several mnemonics or aide memoirs can be used in civilian practice, and the TRAUMATIC mnemonic developed by the University Hospital of Coventry and Warwickshire in the UK is an excellent example (see Fig. 14.1).

When to Start Damage Control Resuscitation: Indications

As mentioned above, damage control resuscitation is a systemic approach to trauma. Consequently, there needs to be a systemic acknowledgement that this is the strategy which is being employed. In terms of triggers to use damage control, there are several factors which can prompt the team to consider adopting this approach at various stages.

The first indications that a patient may require damage control resuscitation can be from the initial physiological observations or mechanism of injury. When dealing with pre-hospital trauma care in the UK, trauma triage tools have been implemented to identify patients who will benefit from transport to Major Trauma Centres (MTC) versus those who can safely be dealt with at local Trauma Units (TU) or smaller hospitals. The absolute triggers for transfer to an MTC are primarily based on physiological data such as systolic blood pressure less than 90 mmHg, GCS less than 13 or extremes of respiratory rate following trauma. However, in some areas, mechanism of injury can also be used as absolute based on anatomical considerations (e.g. penetrating trauma to head, neck or torso mandate MTC transfer) or relative indications (e.g. fall from more than 20 ft, ejection from a vehicle in the case of road traffic collisions or death in the same vehicle). An example of this is the West Midlands Major Trauma tool (Fig. 14.2).

Any triage tool that may be used will not be absolute, and clinical discretion is needed to avoid both under- and over-triaging patients to MTC care, hence the involvement of senior clinicians on the regional trauma desk. As discussed in the mechanism of injury chapter, some trauma systems (e.g. London) are moving away from using non-anatomical mechanism of injury factors when deciding on destination hospital based on locally gathered audit data (Fig. 14.3). When the patient arrives in hospital, a rapid reassessment of the casualty takes place, and similar vital signs to those outlined in the PHEM trauma tool or other significant deterioration may also prompt the adoption of a damage control strategy.

Damage Control Resuscitation in PHEM

The first clinician with a patient may be the best placed to highlight and initiate the need for damage control practices. The presenting physiology and the context in which the patient has been injured are likely to be the most apparent, and how the pre-hospital teams work will set the tempo for subsequent care. This is not only a medical matter, as the speed of extrication and patient handling by firefighters can also be considered as part of the damage control paradigm. If the patient is visibly deteriorating, the balance

Major Trauma?
Major Haemorrhage? Then...

T	**Tranexamic Acid**	• Initial 1g bolus:
		  • Often already given pre-hospital
		  • Otherwise, administer only if within 3 hours of injury or ongoing hyperfibrinolysis
		  • Do not delay, every minute counts
		• Subsequent 1g infusion over 8 hours

R	**Resuscitation**	• Activate Major Haemorrhage Protocol
		• Initial Transfusion Ratio 1:1:1 and consider:
		  • Rapid infuser and cell salvage
		  • Time-limited hypotensive resuscitation
		  • Pelvic binder / splint fractures / tourniquet
		• Avoid any crystalloid use

A	**Avoid Hypothermia**	• Target temperature > 36^{0}C
		  • Increase ambient theatre temperature
		  • Remove wet clothing and sheets
		  • Warm all blood products & irrigation fluids
		  • Warm the patient using forced-air warming device / blanket / mattress

U	**Unstable? Damage Control Surgery**	• If unstable, coagulopathic, hypothermic or acidotic, perform damage control surgery of: • Haemorrhage control, decompression, decontamination and splintage • Time surgery aiming to finish < 90mins and conduct Surgical Pauses at least every 30mins
M	**Metabolic**	• Perform regular blood gas analysis • Base excess and lactate guide resuscitation • Adequate resuscitation corrects acidosis • If lactate > 5mmol/L or rising, consider stopping surgery, splint and transfer to ICU • Haemoglobin results are misleading
A	**Avoid Vasoconstrictors**	• Use of vasoconstrictors doubles mortality • However, use may be required in cases of spinal cord or traumatic brain injury • Anaesthetic induction - Suggest Ketamine • Maintenance - When BP allows, titrate high dose Fentanyl and consider Midazolam
T	**Test Clotting**	• Check clotting regularly to target transfusion: • Laboratory or point of care (TEG / ROTEM) • Aim platelets > 100x10^{9}/L • Aim INR & aPTTR ≤ 1.5 • Aim fibrinogen > 2g/L

I	**Imaging**	• Consider:
		  • CT:
		  Most severely injured / haemodynamically unstable patients gain most from CT
		  • Interventional radiology

C	**Calcium**	• Maintain ionised Calcium > 1.0 mmol/L • Administer 10mls of 10% Calcium Chloride over 10 minutes, repeating as required • Monitor Potassium and treat hyperkalaemia with Calcium and Insulin / Glucose

Fig. 14.1 TRAUMATIC Mnemonic for Trauma Anaesthesia

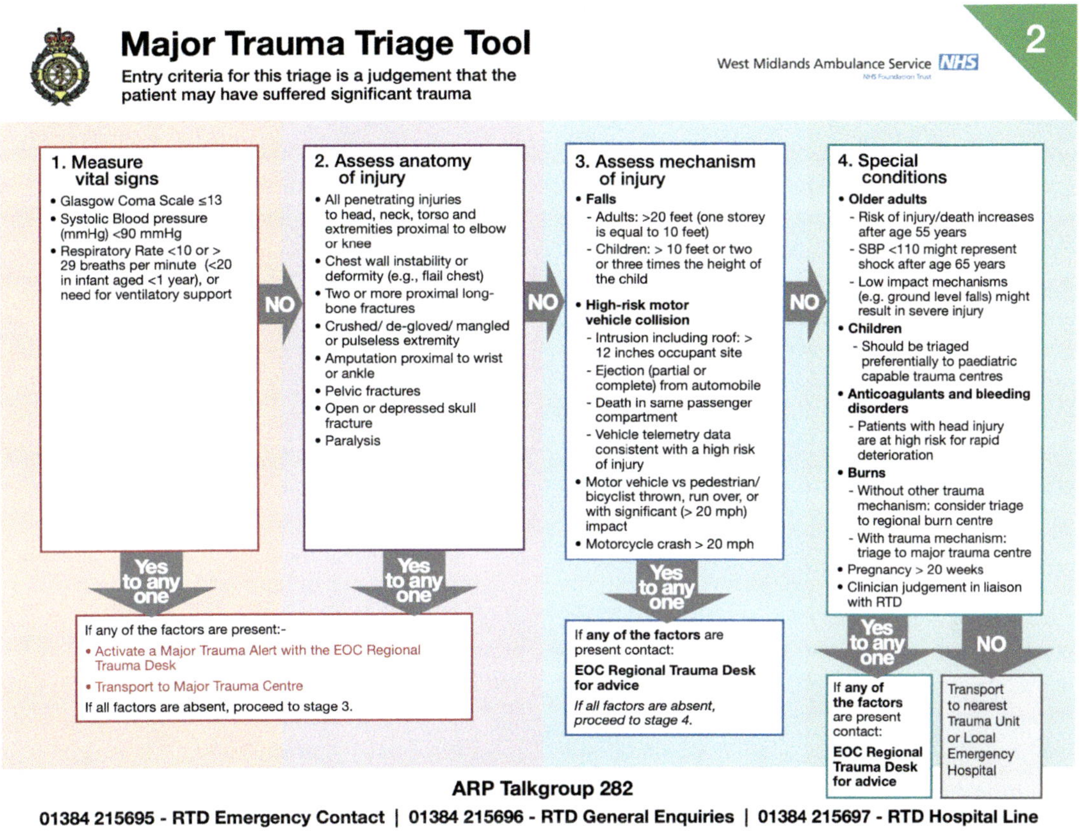

Fig. 14.2 West Midlands Major Trauma Triage Tool (Reproduced thanks to West Midlands Ambulance Service)

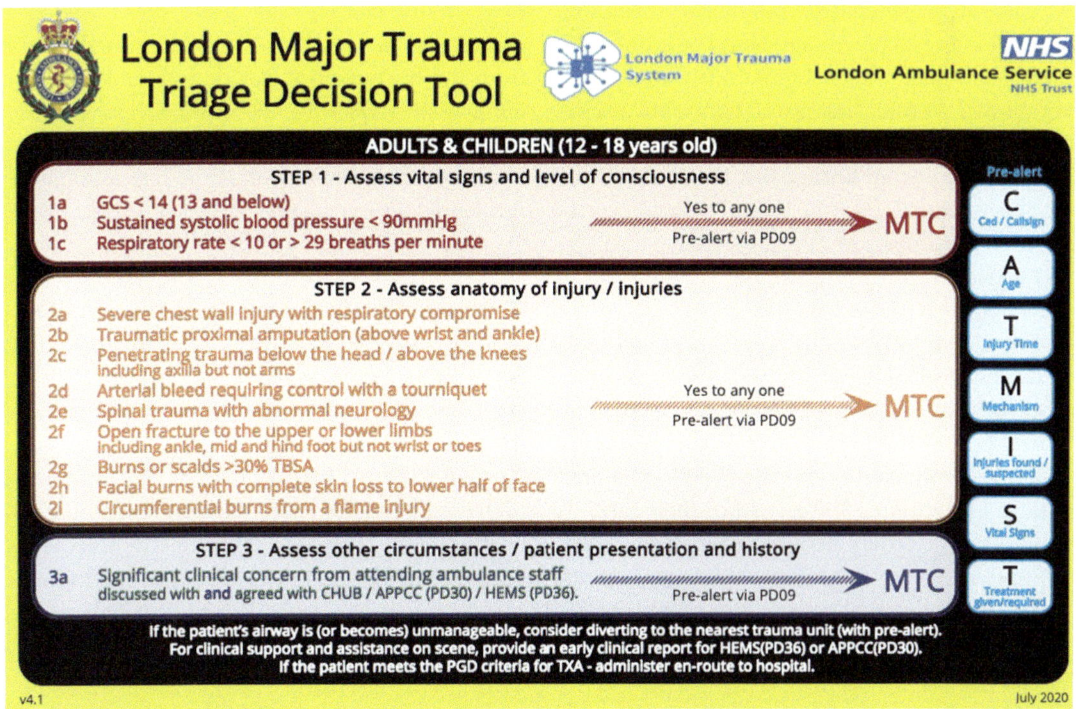

Fig. 14.3 New London Major Trauma tool, de-emphasising mechanism of injury as a screening criteria

between minimising movement and maximising speed for access to the patient and treatment may shift so that the compromise between the two favours speed over finesse. The often-quoted dichotomy of "Scoop and run vs stay and play " [18, 19] is a false one. Meaningful interventions should be undertaken on scene that maximise the chance of a good patient outcome without delaying transport to hospital and other life-saving interventions. This balance can change depending on patient injury pattern, level of pre-hospital response, distance to hospital et cetera, but a general rule is that major haemorrhage control, airway and breathing interventions should be performed on scene with everything else done en route.

PHEM damage control measures are targeted primarily at circulation preservation and ensuring adequate oxygenation and ventilation. These interventions include the application of tourniquets, pelvic binders and occasionally femoral traction splints, airway measures appropriate to the level of clinician and patient need, and establishing sufficient respiratory support. Beyond this, measures such as blood or fluid administration, advanced analgesia etc. can be accomplished on the way to the hospital. Even during transfer, damage control principles should be applied. For example, fluids should be withheld if there is adequate blood pressure (in line with a permissive hypotension/novel hybrid resuscitation strategy) and tranexamic acid should be given to help avoid fibrinolysis of the first clots that have formed. Patients should also be kept as warm as possible by minimising passive heat loss and actively heating fluids or the environment in the ambulance where possible.

The caveat to "A and B on scene, C and D en route" is when drug or blood administration is required to safely facilitate the management of an airway or breathing problem (e.g. administration of a unit of blood to a hypotensive head-injured patient who requires RSI as part of their care). A second instance may also be when scene times are prolonged due to entrapment or other immediately insurmountable factors preventing patient transport. In those cases, additional scene time should not be wasted, and the emphasis should still be on minimising delays while enhancing patient care and decreasing the time to surgery and ICU beyond.

Ensuring that activity is continuous, complementary and running in parallel while the factors that are causing the delay are dealt with is the hallmark of good pre-hospital care. The ability of pre-hospital teams to think three steps ahead of where they are now is an essential requirement; even if they are incapable of performing advanced interventions themselves, they can set the conditions to minimise scene times. This spectrum of activity must also include extrication, so only necessary interventions and monitoring should be performed in order to avoid impeding firefighters and increasing scene times further. An example of good crew management decreasing scene times might be a technician level ambulance crew arriving first on scene at a remote accident and identifying a patient who requires RSI for a head injury. After requesting appropriate backup and performing a primary survey to deal with any immediate life-threatening injuries within their scope of practice, the first crew should appropriately expose and position the patient on a stretcher in an area with good all-round access. When their backup arrives, the patient can be anaesthetised much more quickly and leave the scene in a shorter period than if the backup crew had to start from the beginning of positioning and exposing the patient. Improving all-round access to facilitate a rapid further assessment, performing any necessary interventions on scene and minimising further delays assists everyone.

Damage Control Resuscitation in ED

As well as being a guide to patient dispersal (MTC vs TU) for pre-hospital clinicians, the initial pre-alert/report from scene can prompt in-hospital teams to prepare for a patient who has a high likelihood of needing damage control resuscitation. At a systemic level in the emergency department, this can lead to the activation of a mass transfusion protocol before the patient arrives, drawing up emergency anaesthesia drugs, preparing invasive monitoring or ensuring that the CT scanner or operating theatre is ready to receive an urgent patient. Sharing a mental model and conducting a "Zero point survey" [20] is a useful way to ensure that each member of the team is expecting to manage the patient in the same manner (see Fig. 14.4). This involves briefing and preparing the in-hospital team and facilities before the arrival of the patient based on the information from the pre-alert.

On arrival of the patient, the MABCD assessment will begin again to confirm the injuries that have been suspected in the pre-hospital phase and monitor any progression of physiology. In addition to a reassessment of vital signs and calculation of the shock index [21] (ratio of systolic blood pressure to heart rate), there are several additional diagnostic point of care tests that can be performed in ED that may not be available pre-hospital. These can aid in the assessment of shock, triggering a damage control approach and include blood gas analysis for pH, lactate levels and haemoglobin. The evidence behind these tests is considered in the circulation chapter, and an excellent article by Petrosniak and Hicks [22] discusses how they can be integrated into ED to optimise resuscitation. One pitfall to avoid is false reassurance from an apparently normal blood pressure on arrival in the ED in a previously hypotensive patient. Patients with isolated hypotension in the pre-hospital phase of their care which resolves spontaneously in ED have been found to have higher injury severity scores, higher rates of admission to ICU with longer lengths of stay, a nearly four-fold increase in the need for blood transfusion in the first 24 h and increased mortality [23, 24].

In the same way that PHEM damage control aims to preserve the patients' own circulating volume, avoid heat loss and ensure quick transport, the goals of ED damage control are mostly similar. Patients should be rapidly assessed and a decision made whether to image the patient with CT or ultrasound, to take the patient straight to the operating theatre, or even to operate in the ED. The emergency department is better equipped and has more personnel than the pre-hospital environment (usually), so the occasional temptation in this scenario is for personnel to perform multiple procedures which may not be strictly necessary and ultimately slow the progression of care. An example may be siting an arterial line in a head-injured patient—it is likely to be unnecessary before a CT and may ultimately delay time to diagnosis. Similarly, in an intubated patient a thoracostomy may be necessary for pneumothorax. However, formal intercostal drain insertion

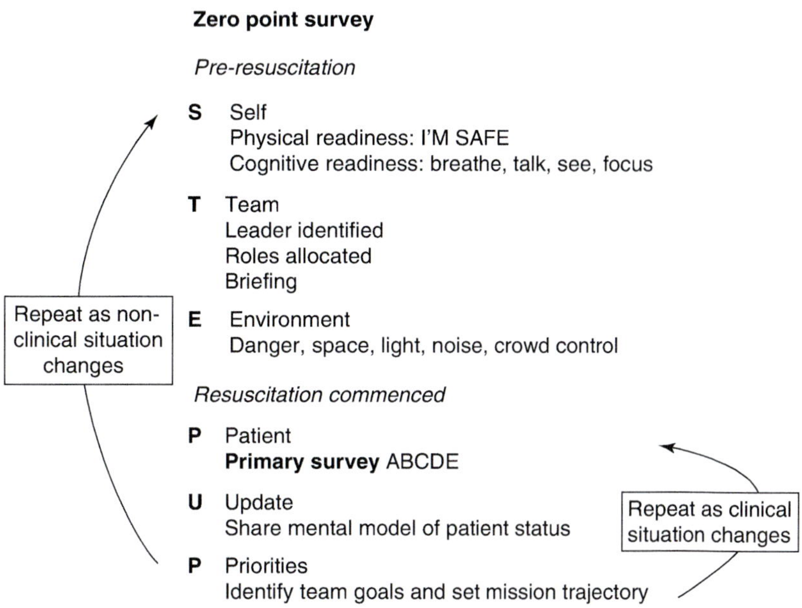

Fig. 14.4 Zero point survey from Reid et al. [20]

is a time-consuming process that puts the patient further away from definitive diagnostics and treatment. Perform the thoracostomy if necessary but do not put the drain in until the patient has been to CT—time that is wasted during insertion, and the logistics of moving a patient with a chest drain in situ are more troublesome than one with a simple thoracostomy. A final example is tranexamic acid infusions; give the 1 g bolus in ED if it has not been given pre-hospital, but there is little benefit (and potential logistical challenges) in commencing the subsequent 8-hour infusion via a syringe driver before the patient has been to CT.

The second-order effects of an intervention should also be considered in the sequence of events; if the patient requires intubation, it is rarely so urgent that it needs to be done as soon as they arrive in the department. An assessment of their haemodynamic state and injury pattern may change the order in which interventions are performed. For example, a hypotensive trauma patient with a chest injury, suspected pneumothorax and decreasing GCS has competing management priorities and may require intubation. The team leader should take an overall view and prioritise; resuscitate with blood products, prepare for a thoracostomy and once the patient has been optimised then induce anaesthesia with a reduced dose of induction agents. If a rigid, historical "vertical" ABCD sequence of interventions was followed, inducing anaesthesia and managing the airway without any of the other interventions could result in worsening hypotension due to the effects of positive pressure ventilation on an under-filled patient with evolving chest pathology. Parallel actions rather than sequential ones are the key to smooth and efficient care.

Consider ED damage control resuscitation to be a prime example of marginal gains theory [25, 26]—multiple small changes can lead to a substantial overall improvement in the standard of care. Once immediately life-threatening injuries have been identified and temporised as needed, the decision comes as to what the appropriate disposition of the patient is. Do they require ongoing damage control in theatre? Do they need to be admitted to ICU or HDU, or has their treatment been sufficient to allow them to be monitored on a ward level?

Damage Control: More Than Surgery

Damage control is a paradigm, not an operation. It requires a large group of people all with the same understanding and mindset to achieve necessary but not definitive care and an understanding that perfect may be the enemy of good. By implementing strategies which allow appropriately selected patients to be diagnosed and resuscitated as rapidly as possible, then allowing ongoing resuscitation on critical care before definitive surgery, outcomes have demonstrably improved.

Questions

1. Damage control surgery should be used for *all* trauma patients who require an operation.
   (a) True
   (b) False
2. Critically unwell patients who require skin grafts or tissue flaps to cover soft tissue loss should have these procedures deferred until they have been adequately resuscitated and stable for >24 h.
   (a) True
   (b) False
3. Patients who have had a damage control procedure will usually require post-operative care in an Intensive Care Unit
   (a) True
   (b) False
4. Once a decision has been made to perform damage control or a definitive procedure, it cannot be changed
   (a) True
   (b) False
5. Triage tools may be overridden by clinical judgement of staff to divert patients to or away from Major Trauma Centres
   (a) True
   (b) False

Answers

1. b
2. a
3. a
4. b
5. a

References

1. Toghil G. The Battle of Jutland: The Largest Naval Clash of World War One [Internet]. History Hit. 2019 [cited 2019 June 19]. Available from: https://www.historyhit.com/the-battle-of-jutland-the-largest-naval-clash-of-world-war-one/
2. Bergeron DL. Fighting for Survival: USS Yorktown (CV5) Damage Control Experiences in 1942 [Internet]. University of New Orleans; 2016 [cited 2019 June 19]. Available from: https://scholarworks.uno.edu/cgi/viewcontent.cgi?article=3224&context=td
3. Brohi K. TRAUMA.ORG: Damage Control Surgery [Internet]. trauma.org. 2000 [cited 2019 June 19]. Available from: http://www.trauma.org/archive/resus/DCSoverview.html
4. Roberts DJ, Ball CG, Feliciano DV, Moore EE, Ivatury RR, Lucas CE, et al. History of the innovation of damage control for management of trauma patients: 1902–2016. Ann Surg. 2017;265(5):1034–44.
5. Pringle JH. Notes on the arrest of hepatic hemorrhage due to trauma. Ann Surg. 1908;48(4):541–9.
6. Stone HH, Strom PR, Mullins RJ. Management of the major coagulopathy with onset during laparotomy. Ann Surg. 1983;197(5):532–5.
7. Rotondo MF, Schwab CW, McGonigal MD, Phillips GR, Fruchterman TM, Kauder DR, et al. 'Damage control': an approach for improved survival in exsanguinating penetrating abdominal injury. J Trauma. 1993;35(3):375–82. discussion 382–383
8. Johnson JW, Gracias VH, Schwab CW, Reilly PM, Kauder DR, Shapiro MB, et al. Evolution in damage control for exsanguinating penetrating abdominal injury. J Trauma. 2001;51(2):261–9. discussion 269–271
9. Malbrain MLNG, Roberts DJ, Sugrue M, De Keulenaer BL, Ivatury R, Pelosi P, et al. The polycompartment syndrome: a concise state-of-the-art review. Anaesthesiol Intensive Ther. 2014;46(5):433–50.
10. Huang Q, Li J, Lau W. Techniques for abdominal wall closure after damage control laparotomy: from temporary abdominal closure to early/delayed fascial closure—a review [Internet]. Gastroenterol Res Pract 2016 [cited 2019 Aug 2]. Available from: https://www.hindawi.com/journals/grp/2016/2073260/
11. Zakrison T, Nascimento BA, Tremblay LN, Kiss A, Rizoli SB. Perioperative vasopressors are associated with an increased risk of gastrointestinal anastomotic leakage. World J Surg. 2007;31(8):1627–34.
12. Scalea TM. Optimal timing of fracture fixation: have we learned anything in the past 20 years? J Trauma Injury Infect Crit Care. 2008;65(2):253–60.
13. Roberts CS, Pape H-C, Jones AL, Malkani AL, Rodriguez JL, Giannoudis PV. Damage control orthopaedics: evolving concepts in the treatment of patients who have sustained orthopaedic trauma. JBJS. 2005;87(2):434.
14. Sikorski RA, Koerner AK, Fouche-Weber LY, Galvagno SM. Choice of general Anesthetics for trauma patients. Curr Anesthesiol Rep. 2014;4(3):225–32.
15. Mercer SJ, Whittle CL, Mahoney PF. Lessons from the battlefield: human factors in defence anaesthesia. Br J Anaesth. 2010;105(1):9–20.
16. Buckenmaier C, Mahoney PF, United States, Borden Institute (US), editors. Combat anesthesia: the first 24 hours. Falls Church, Virginia: Fort Sam Houston, Texas: Office of the Surgeon General, United States Army; Borden Institute; 2015. 571 p. (TMM series).
17. Penn-Barwell JG, Roberts SAG, Midwinter MJ, Bishop JRB. Improved survival in UK combat casualties from Iraq and Afghanistan: 2003–2012. J Trauma Acute Care Surg. 2015;1
18. Deakin CD. Scoop and run versus stay and play: strategies in pre-hospital care. In: Gullo A, editor. Anaesthesia, Pain, Intensive Care and Emergency Medicine — APICE [Internet]. Milano: Springer Milan; 2003 [cited 2019 July 23]: [1019–26 pp.]. Available from: http://link.springer.com/10.1007/978-88-470-2215-7_31
19. Smith RM, Conn AKT. Pre-hospital care - scoop and run or stay and play? Injury. 2009;40(Suppl 4):S23–6.
20. Reid C, Brindley P, Hicks C, Carley S, Richmond C, Lauria M, et al. Zero point survey: a multidisciplinary idea to STEP UP resuscitation effectiveness. Clin Exp Emerg Med. 2018;5(3):139–43.
21. Mutschler M, Nienaber U, Münzberg M, Wölfl C, Schoechl H, Paffrath T, et al. The shock index revisited – a fast guide to transfusion requirement? A retrospective analysis on 21,853 patients derived from the TraumaRegister DGU®. Crit Care. 2013;17(4):R172.
22. Petrosoniak A, Hicks C. Resuscitation resequenced: a rational approach to patients with trauma in shock. Emerg Med Clin North Am. 2018;36(1):41–60.
23. Damme CD, Luo J, Buesing KL. Isolated pre-hospital hypotension correlates with injury severity and outcomes in patients with trauma. Trauma Surg Acute Care Open [Internet]. 2016 Aug 12 [cited 2019 July 24];1(1). Available from: https://www.ncbi.nlm.nih.gov/pmc/articles/PMC5891702/
24. Codner P, Obaid A, Porral D, Lush S, Cinat M. Is field hypotension a reliable indicator of significant injury in trauma patients who are normotensive on arrival to the emergency department? Am Surg. 2005;71(9):768–71.

25. Lemer C, Cheung R, Klaber R, Hibbs N. Understanding healthcare processes: how marginal gains can improve quality and value for children and families. Arch Dis Child Educ Pract. 2016;101(1):31–7.
26. Pentecost C, Richards DA, Frost J. Amalgamation of marginal gains (AMG) as a potential system to deliver high-quality fundamental nursing care: a qualitative analysis of interviews from high-performance AMG sports and healthcare practitioners. J Clin Nurs. 2018;27(11–12):2387–402.

Haemostasis and Coagulopathy

15

Robert A. Sikorski, Shaun C. Moeller, and Ryan Fransman

- Review of the "classical" model of the clotting cascade
- Overview of trauma induced coagulopathy (TIC)
- Competing models to explain TIC
- Hyperfibrinolysis
- The role of platelets in TIC and haemostasis
- Haemostasis and resuscitation
- Tranexamic acid
- Clincical applications and physiological approach to the bleeding patient

Introduction

Trauma remains the leading cause of death in North America in those 40 years of age and younger [1], and those 35 years and younger globally [2]. On a global scale severe trauma contributes to approximately one in ten deaths across all ages accounting for more than 5.8 million fatalities per year [3, 4]. Death due to haemorrhage remains the primary cause in about 40% of these potentially preventable deaths [5], and trauma induced coagulopathy (TIC) develops in about ten to 25% of these patients (Fig. 15.1). The presence of acute traumatic coagulopathy (ATC), a component of TIC, increases the odds ratio towards mortality almost nine-fold, and is unrelated to transfusion practice [6]. These patients also have a higher incidence of multi-system organ failure, prolonged hospital and intensive care stay as well as increased blood

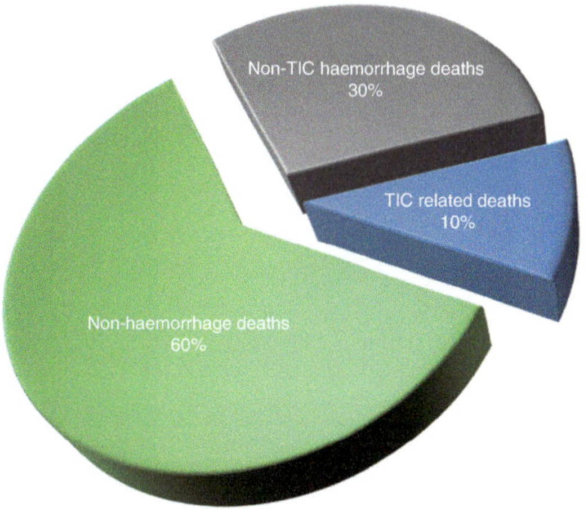

Fig. 15.1 Haemorrhage as a cause of preventable trauma deaths, and subset who developed TIC

The original version of this chapter was revised. The correction to this chapter can be found at https://doi.org/10.1007/978-3-030-83628-3_45

R. A. Sikorski (✉) · S. C. Moeller
Department of Anesthesiology and Critical Care Medicine, The Johns Hopkins Hospital, Baltimore, MD, USA
e-mail: rsikors2@jhmi.edu; smoelle4@jhmi.edu

R. Fransman
Surgical Department, The Johns Hopkins Hospital, Baltimore, MD, USA
e-mail: rfansm1@jhmi.edu

P. Lax (ed.), *Textbook of Acute Trauma Care*, https://doi.org/10.1007/978-3-030-83628-3_15

utilisation [7–9]. Death from exsanguination occurs within 2–3 h (median time) after presentation and accounts for nearly 50% of trauma death [5, 10, 11]. Early recognition and treatment of TIC, along with massive transfusion guidelines, represent an opportunity to improve outcomes in trauma resuscitation [6].

The "Classical" Clotting Cascade

The blood clotting cascade and use of Roman numerals associated with various factors as described in the below diagram was finally agreed on in 1962 by a committee that would go on to become the International Committee on Thrombosis and Haemostasis [12]. As with other areas of medicine, advances in research have changed our understanding of how this complex system works. However, the fundamental pathways are still taught to undergraduate and postgraduate students despite there being many other factors which influence clot formation (Fig. 15.2). Subsequent work based on this model such as the cell based scheme of coagulation [13] shows that some of the assumptions made above fall apart under closer scrutiny (e.g. why do Haemophiliac patients bleed if their intrinsic pathway is intact?). The fundamental principles that are useful from this schemata are that the system is enzyme dependent; changes in pH and temperature can effect the efficiency of the system, and some reactions require co-factors such as calcium to complete. While what follows represents our current understanding of coagulopathy in trauma, the finer points may change further with subsequent research. As with our understanding of coagulation generally, the general management principles outlined at the end of the chapter may have more longevity than the specific mechanisms outlined below.

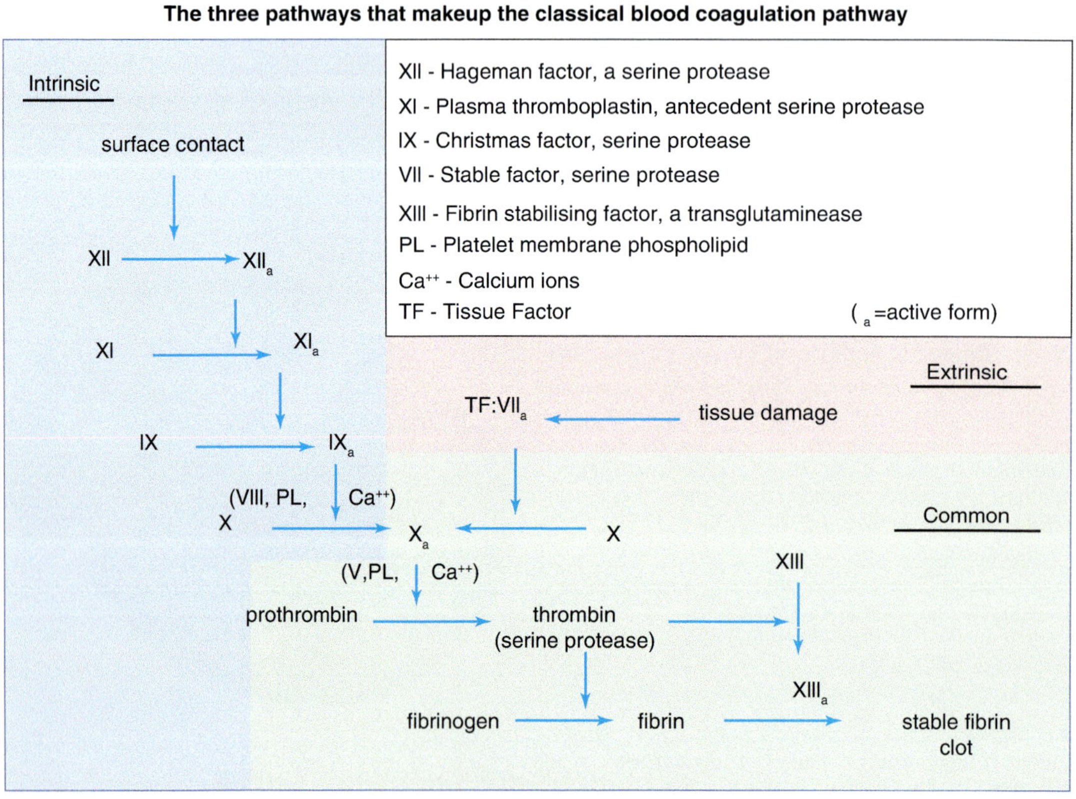

Fig. 15.2 The "Classical" clotting cascade (by Dr. Graham Beards via Wikimedia under Creative Commons 3.0 license)

Trauma Induced Coagulopathy

Most cases of traumatic bleeding are not caused by coagulopathy, either innate or iatrogenic. The majority of traumatic bleeding is caused by a primary injury or disruption of the large blood vessels (arteries and veins) and not the coagulopathy caused by the failure to form adequate clots at the level of the capillary beds/the microcirculation. Bleeding at the level of the capillary beds is extremely difficult, if not impossible, to control by conventional surgical methods such as diathermy, suturing or packing [10]. The extent of this coagulation deficit at the level of the capillary bed appears to be dependent on the extent of tissue damage, degree of hypoperfusion and injury to the endothelial surface layer, all of which are dependent on degree of blood loss and subsequent shock. Without a bleeding source to begin with, TIC should not develop. The perturbations at the microcirculatory level will be aggravated further by acidosis, hypothermia and the use of crystalloids in resuscitation. Trauma patients with TIC as well as large vessel injury must be taken to the operating room without delay. Hence, damage control surgery (DCS) and damage control resuscitation (DCR) must occur in parallel in order to address the immediate causes of bleeding (Fig. 15.3).

In order to understand the pathophysiology of trauma induced coagulopathy one must define the process. Trauma induced coagulopathy begins between the time of injury and approximately 30 min post injury. It has been described by Davenport and Brohi as a "multifactorial, global failure of the coagulation system to sustain adequate haemostasis after major trauma haemorrhage" [15].

Part of the confusion that arises when discussing trauma induced coagulopathy can be attributed to the vast number of acronyms and descriptions of pathological processes, some of which are describing the same process with a different name. As an overview, TIC is comprised of two pathophysiologic processes, the coagulopathy caused by severe shock and traumatic injury (Acute Traumatic Coagulopathy (ATC)) and a dilutional coagulopathy or "iatrogenic traumatic coagulopathy" (ITC). ATC describes the pathological process that occurs due to bleeding, whereas ITC refers to the negative iatrogenic effects of suboptimal resuscitation (e.g. haemodilution due to crystalloid use or hypothermia if cold fluids are used). These iatrogenic factors

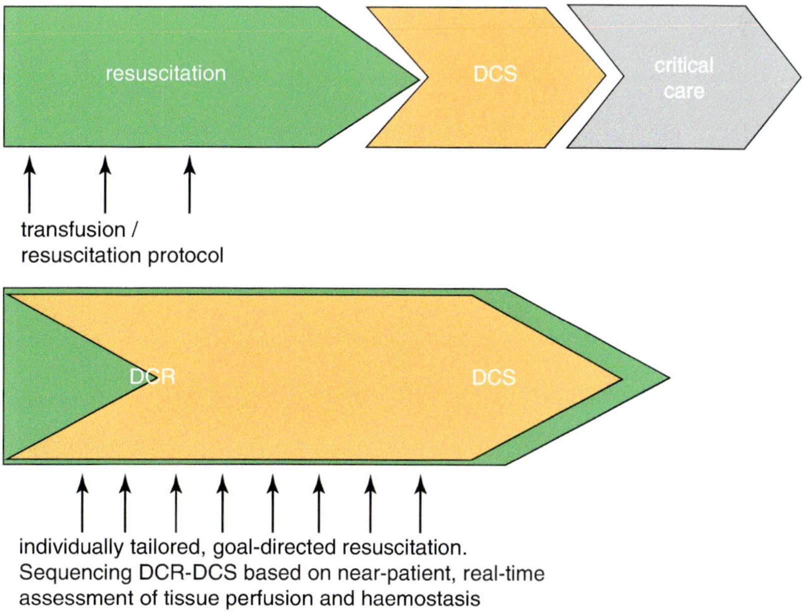

Fig. 15.3 The top scheme represents Classical damage control resuscitation -damage control surgery sequence. The lower scheme represents "integrated" damage control resuscitation-damage control surgery sequencing [14].

have also been referred to as systemic acquired coagulopathy (SAC) or resuscitation associated coagulopathy (RAC) [14, 16]. To avoid confusion, in this chapter any factors that are associated with iatrogenic problems will be henceforth referred to as ITC (Fig. 15.4).

Moore and colleagues demonstrated that the multivariate predictors of coagulopathy included the severity of trauma as defined by the Injury Severity Score (ISS), but not base deficit or lactate. The often quoted risk factors for iatrogenically induced coagulopathy such as hypothermia and acidosis were found to *contribute* to the development of ITC but they were poor *predictors* of patients who develop ITC. Hypothermia, defined as a temperature of 34 °C or lower, as well as a low transfusion ratio (low number of units of platelets and FFP in comparison to units of red blood cells) have been implicated in an increased mortality from coagulopathy [17]. The only relevant multivariate predictor of ITC was crystalloid volumes in the setting of shock. Clinically relevant cut-offs ranged from 2 liters (l) to greater than 4 l. Patients that received less

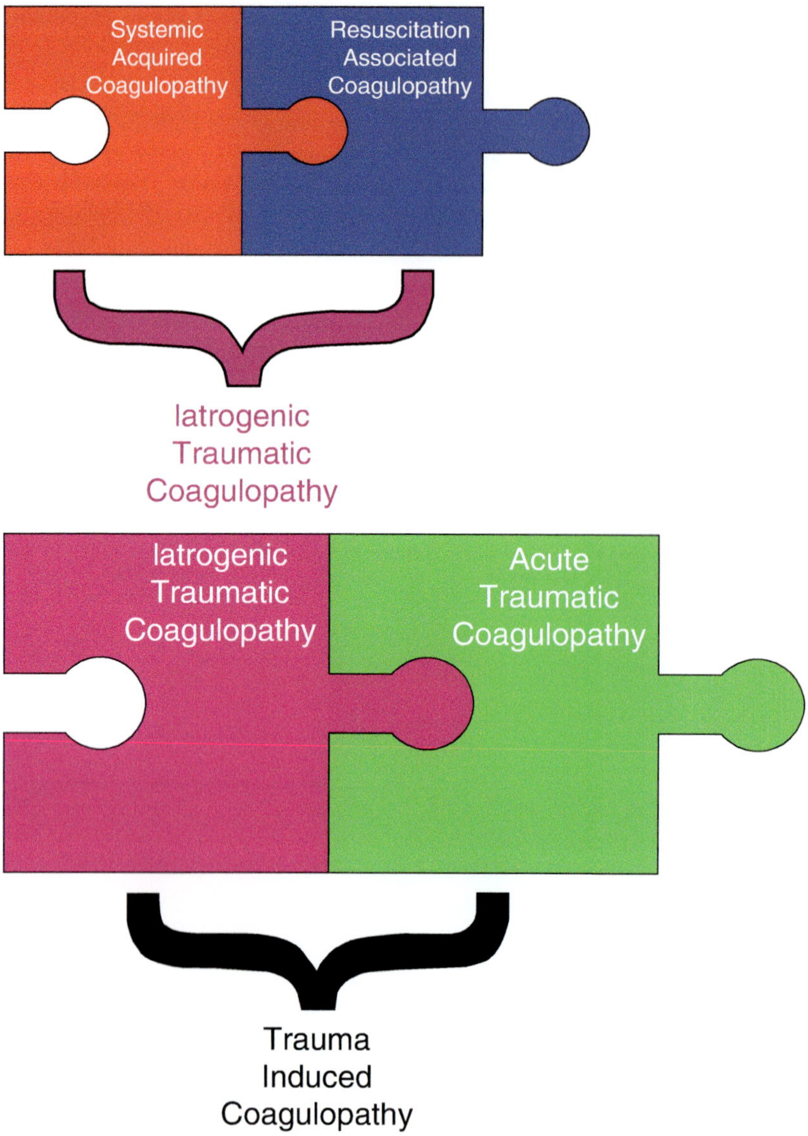

Fig. 15.4 Relationship between TIC, ATC, ITC, RAC and SAC

than 2 l of crystalloid pre-hospital were unlikely to become coagulopathic regardless of admission lactate. Patients who received between 2 and 4 l of crystalloid were at risk for coagulopathy only if their arrival lactate was elevated. Patients who received greater than 4 l of prehospital crystalloid elevated the risk for coagulopathy regardless of arrival lactate. This provides yet more validation for the concept of permissive hypotension, as not only does increasing systolic blood pressure with crystalloids increase the risk of mechanically "popping the clot", but this evidence shows that the risk of subsequent morbidity and mortality due to acquired coagulopathy is increased too.

Haemorrhage control, correction of hypovolaemia and hypotension via a product balanced resuscitation or fresh whole blood (FWB), avoiding the phenomenon of dilution coagulopathy, as well as a detailed approach in the prevention and correction of TIC is paramount. In DCR organ perfusion may be marginally sacrificed (permissive hypotension) in the face of severe haemorrhage during the early phase of DCS. Once achieving haemostasis, attention may then be shifted to a goal of optimal organ perfusion [18, 19].

Functionally, TIC may be defined by the use of viscoelastic monitoring as well as standard laboratory testing (prothrombin time, INR, activated partial thromboplastin time, fibrinogen, etc.). The two most common viscoelastic monitoring devices are the Thromboelastogram (TEG®) and the ROTEM®. A sample of blood is taken and injected into a receptacle with reagents to accelerate clot formation in specific pathways. Into this is placed a pin connected to a strain gauge on the device, and the sample is rotated until clot begins to form. As the clot matures and strengthens, the resistance to movement of the pin increases and this is plotted against time on a graph to give a visual representation of clot formation time, strength and degradation (Fig. 15.5). These devices can be used for near patient testing in areas such as the emergency department or operating theatre and can provide useable results within 10 min, much quicker than results are typ-

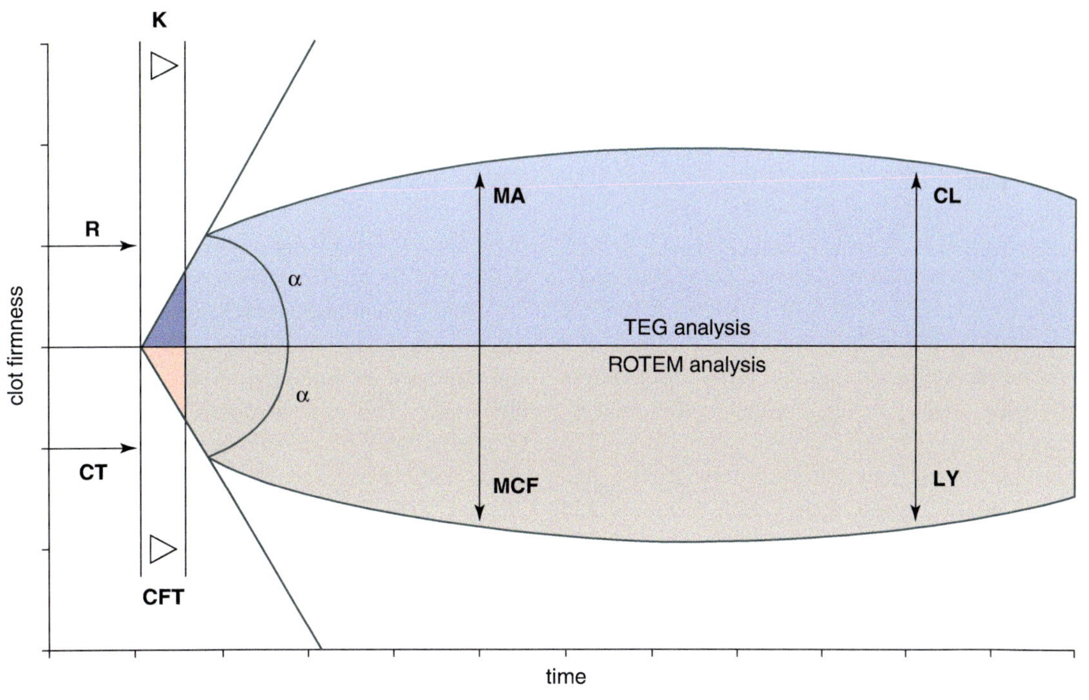

Fig. 15.5 TEG and ROTEM tracing. TEG parameters: *R* reaction time, *k* kinetics (Fibrin), ∝ alpha angle, *MA* maximum amplitude, *CL* clot lysis. ROTEM parameters: *CT* clotting time, *CFT* clot formation time, ∝ alpha angle, *MCF* maximum clot firmness, *LY* clot lysis. (from Sankarankutty et al. [23])

ically available from haematology labs. These whole blood clotting tests define the relationship between laboratory based abnormalities and clinically relevant bleeding more closely than standard laboratory testing [20–23].

TIC: Pathophysiology and Mechanism

TIC is a complicated multi-faceted pathophysiologic state that has not been fully elucidated [24]. TIC may be identified clinically by its presentation related to the timing and severity (defined by ISS) of the traumatic injury. The mechanisms and hypotheses used to explain TIC are much less clear and overlapping. The hypotheses are not mutually exclusive of each other either. The hypotheses were elegantly described by Dobson et al. These are

1. The DIC-fibrinolysis hypothesis
2. The activated protein C hypothesis
3. The glycocalyx hypothesis
4. The "fibrinogen-centric" hypothesis [18]/theory of hypofibrinogenaemia

The Theory of DIC-Fibrinolysis

The DIC-fibrinolysis hypothesis proposes that coagulopathy is closely related to tissue hypoperfusion, shock, endothelial activation and endothelial injury. This sequence of events leads to a prolonged prothrombin time (PT), a picture of a consumptive type process (i.e. the clotting factors are being used up in a pathological inflammatory process that seems to meet the criteria for DIC), low fibrinogen and anti-thrombin levels, and increased fibrinogen degradation products and D-dimer levels. The disproportionate increase in plasmin levels relative to the activation of thrombin is thought to be the cause for the hyperfibrinolytic state [25]. Plasmin is a thrombolytic enzyme which breaks down blood clots whereas fibrin is a clotting factor (Factor 1a) which promotes clot formation. In health, these proteins are held in balance so when levels of thrombin increase, plasmin increases too in order to ensure clots are formed only where needed and not in widespread distal areas of the body. In response to major trauma, the theory of DIC-fibrinolysis suggests that there is an over-activation of plasmin relative to the levels of thrombin so all clots are broken down. As the stimulus for clot formation has not been removed, the coagulation system still attempts to form thrombi and uses up additional clotting factors in the process. These factors are then subsequently broken down by thrombin in a downwards spiral. This model proposes a similar mechanism of coagulopathy as is seen in Disseminated Intravascular Coagulation (DIC), a coagulopathy with medical causes as opposed to trauma (e.g. sepsis, certain malignancies, vasculopathies or liver failure). The International Society of Thrombosis and Haemostasis (ISTH) have developed scoring systems and guidelines for the diagnosis, classification and treatment of DIC [26], however these guidelines are not valid in TIC. As described by Rizoli et al. [27] within the first 24 h after traumatic injury almost all severely injured trauma patients (ISS > 16) have an ISTH score of "overt DIC" or "suggestive of non-overt DIC" (Fig. 15.6). There is a paucity of evidence that suggests thrombus formation in the microcirculation of trauma patients and consumption of clotting factors and platelets (thrombocytopenia).

The authors also reported that upon autopsy or organs/tissues removed surgically that no evidence was found to support evidence of DIC at the microcirculatory level in patients with TIC. However, this initial fibrinolytic phase may subsequently be followed by a DIC-thrombotic phenotype. This second phase may be initiated by a high level of plasminogen activator inhibitor-1 (PAI-1) from both the endothelium and platelets. Tissue plasminogen activator (tPA) is inhibited causing an inhibition in fibrinolysis. This process may begin as early as 3–4 h post injury and continue for up to 24–48 h post trauma [20, 28, 29]. This *may* be the same mechanism involved in fibrinolysis shutdown, but it occurs later on in trauma and is part of the reactive phase of coagulation when patients become prothrombotic and show an increased rate of VTE. It is

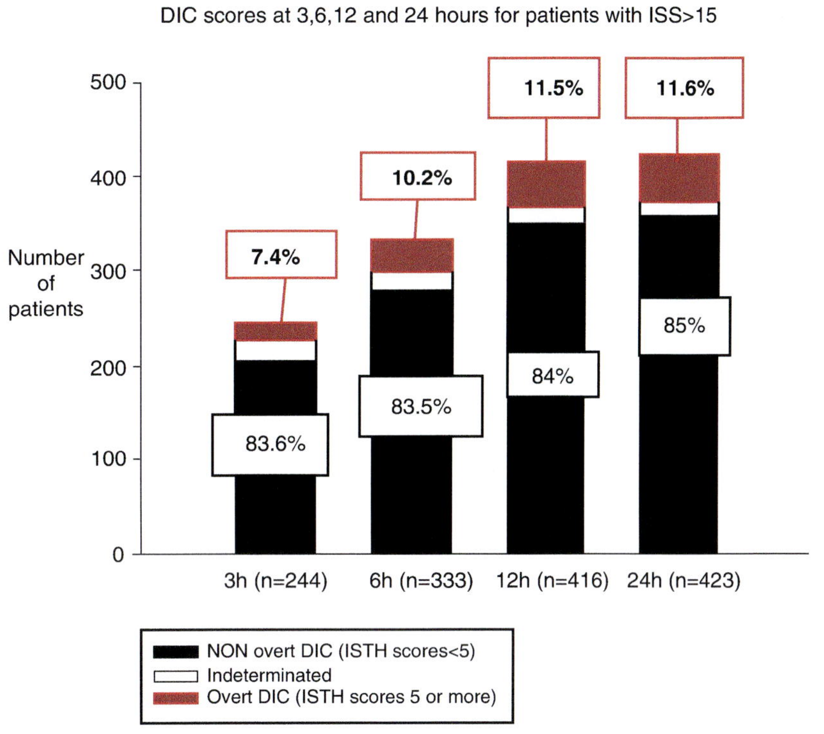

Fig. 15.6 DIC scores at 3, 6, 12, and 24 h for all adult trauma patients with severe trauma (ISS > 16) [27]

unclear when one mechanism ends and the other begins, and what the implications for VTE prophylaxis are.

The Theory of Activated Protein C

Tissue hypoperfusion is the driving force behind the endogenous hypo-coagulable state of TIC. This theory suggests that the hypo-coagulable state is mediated primarily by the activation of protein C (aPC). In the presence of intact endothelium when thrombin binds to thrombomodulin, protein C (PC) is activated in combination with protein S (PS) and causes a proteolytic cleaving of activated factor V (aV) and activated factor VIII (aVIII) reducing ongoing thrombin generation (Fig. 15.7). Tissue factor pathway inhibitor (TFPI) and antithrombin (AT) bind to the uninjured, intact endothelium, and inhibit the action of procoagulant proteases. TFPI and AT will circulate in a low concentration, but levels are substantially increased after Tissue Factor is released. Confusingly, Tissue Factor is also present in the circulation, but it is a different subset of Tissue Factor from that released following trauma. Intact endothelium is essential in preventing further thrombin generation in the absence of vascular injury [30–33]. In the presence of vascular injury, circulating protein C undergoes activation by binding to the endothelial protein C receptor in the presence of protein S and the thrombin-thrombomodulin complex. The binding of thrombin by thrombomodulin depletes the availability of thrombin necessary for clot formation [10]. Thrombomodulin is a receptor present on the endothelium in usual homeostasis, but when it complexes with thrombin it then activates protein C (with protein S as a co-factor). Once protein C has been activated, this causes an anticoagulant effect by inactivating Factors Va and VIIIa to stop thrombin generation, and inhibiting PAI-1, which consequently means more tPA is available for clot breakdown (i.e. hits it from both sides). At the same time the thrombomodulin-thrombin complex also decreases the amount of circulating thrombin which decreases clot formation. Brohi and colleagues showed a significant relationship between thrombomodulin activity, tissue hypoperfusion,

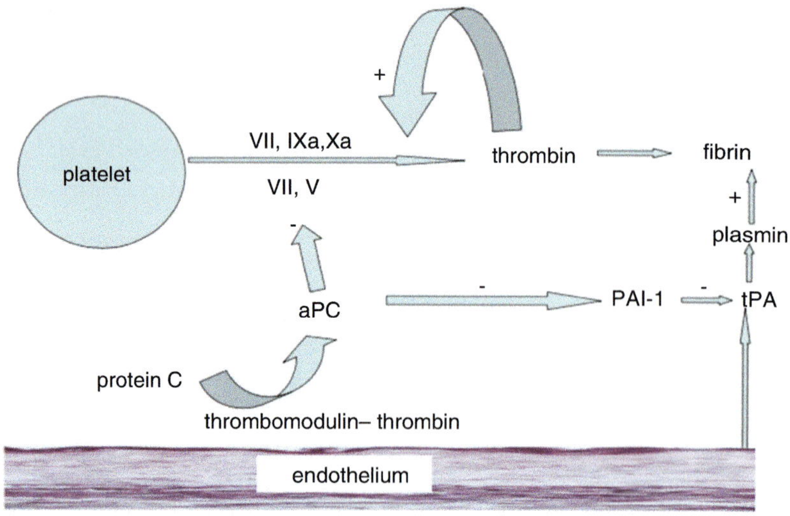

Fig. 15.7 Acute Traumatic Coagulopathy: activated protein C (aPC) mediated sequencing [14]

prolonged measurements of coagulation, fibrinolytic activity and decreased levels of protein C. The authors postulated an upregulation of thrombomodulin leading to the lower levels of protein C (i.e. protein C levels are lower because it is being activated; aPC levels are increased and this is reflected in a lower PC assay) [10, 25, 34, 35]. Cohen, et al. reported that coagulopathy and fibrinolysis correlated strongly with elevated activity of aPC. This correlation was noted only when associated with the presence of hypoperfusion (base deficit >6) and severe injury (Injury Severity Score (ISS) > 15) [36]. Protein C, a serine protease, has both anticoagulant as well as cytoprotective functions. During the onset of sepsis it has been shown that aPC has a beneficial effect on organ injury and mortality. This has been demonstrated in both experimental and clinical investigations. The resultant reduction in aPC seen in severe sepsis may contribute to endothelial cell dysfunction and a prothrombotic state. The evidence, as previously mentioned, does not support a procoagulant state at the microcirculatory level. The depletion of aPC may result in a cytoprotective loss and subsequently increased end organ damage in severe trauma [36–39]. Platelet activation occurs through the proteolytic activation of factors V and VIII to Va and VIIIa. The proteolytic *deactivation* of Va and VIIIa with protein S as a cofactor, leads to a depletion of PAI-1 as well as an inhibition of thrombin activatable fibrinolysis inhibitor. Fibrinolysis proceeds unchecked leading to increased activity of tPA and products of clot breakdown (D-dimers).

The presence of hypoperfusion and shock with the subsequent activation of protein C has been implicated as the driver of TIC. This hypothesis has come under question recently. Researchers have shown that in the absence of hypoperfusion and shock, coagulopathy occurred in blunt traumatic injury. Coagulopathy was present in isolated blunt traumatic brain injury and pulmonary contusion [40]. Protein C levels or activity of aPC were not measured in these studies [10, 41]. A negative correlation between the activity of clotting factors Va and VIIIa and the degree of hypoperfusion was demonstrated by investigators, perhaps implicating that the proteolytic deactivation of Va and VIIIa in shock states are not solely responsible for driving TIC [42, 43]. Chapman et al. found the overwhelming release of tPA not the lack or degradation of PAI-1 was the cause of hyperfibrinolysis in trauma patients [44]. This has biological concordance with the historic use of tPA as a thrombolytic medication used to treat myocardial infarctions, pulmonary emboli and ischaemic strokes. The contribution of aPC to TIC was studied by Campbell et al. The in *vitro study* found that physiologic concentrations of aPC had no significant effect on the depletion of Va (plasma or platelet-derived). They also demonstrated that fibrinolysis was not induced by aPC in the presence or absence of tPA. The authors were aware and acknowledge that there were some *ex vivo* limitations to the study [43, 45].

Moore and colleagues demonstrated an increased mortality in trauma patients with a procoagulant, prothrombotic, non-hyperfibrinolytic phenotype. The phenotypes were classified by Ly30—clot lysis 30 min after the maximum amplitude (MA) by thromboelastography (TEG). This was termed "fibrinolysis shutdown" and shown to be an independent predictor of morbidity and mortality (Fig. 15.8).

The theory of Glycocalyx injury

The breakdown of the endothelial surface layer related to hypoperfusion, shock and endothelial injury is partly addressed by this theory. The glycocalyx is an endothelial luminal surface layer, which in humans has a thickness which varies from 0.5 to 5.0 μm. The glycocalyx consists of glycosaminoglycans (GAG), proteoglycans (PG), and associated plasma proteins in which approximately one third of the total volume of plasma proteins reside. It serves as a protective barrier to vascular permeability [46]. The main subtype of PG found in the glycocalyx is syndecan-1. The proteoglycans are considered "core proteins" which are attached to the intraluminal surface of the endothelial cells and it is to the PG that the GAG are covalently bound. The GAG chains that are bound to the PG are comprised of primarily heparan sulphate, dermatan sulphate and chondroitin sulphate. The sulphated GAGs are negatively charged enabling the interaction with plasma proteins. There are numerous proteins which interact with the GAGs. Included in these are fibrinogen fibronectin, albumin, thrombomodulin, antithrombin III as well as various cell adhesion molecules [47].

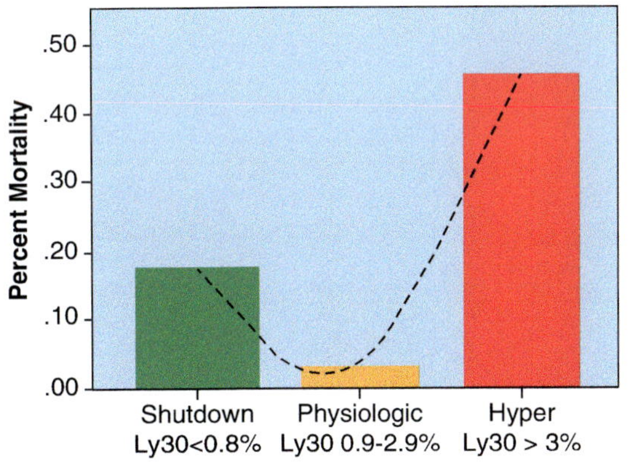

Fig. 15.8 U-shaped distribution of mortality related to fibrinolysis phenotype. The y axis represents the percentage of mortality per phenotype. There is a U-shaped distribution of mortality, with a nadir in mortality identified in the physiologic group (Ly30 between 0.9% and 2.8%). Percentage of Ly30 higher and lower than this range had statistical increases in mortality. Hyper, hyperfibrinolysis; Ly30, percentage of fibrinolysis 30 min after reaching maximum amplitude measured by thromboelastography; Physiologic, physiologic fibrinolysis; Shutdown, fibrinolysis shutdown [29]. Moore et al. Page 12 J Trauma

Products of glycocalyx shedding (primarily syndecan-1) have been detected in trauma, sepsis and chronic inflammatory states. Catecholamine levels have also been implicated in the rate of glycocalyx shedding [48, 49]. This has been described as shock induced endotheliopathy of trauma [50]. Components of the glycocalyx which have anticoagulant properties are of particular interest in TIC. Heparan sulphate (HS) and chondroitin sulphate (CS), which augment the efficiency of antithrombin III and thrombomodulin leading to a potential auto-heparinization effect at the microcirculatory level. This phenomenon may be a component of TIC, or perhaps be necessary in order to provide an improved red cell flow in the microcirculation during hypoperfused states [25, 51]. Both HS and CS have been shown to be crucial in maintaining membrane integrity [52–54].

The Theory of Hypofibrinogenaemia

There is much renewed interest in the role of fibrinogen loss as the primary responsible factor for the development of TIC. Fibrinogen loss leads to a reduction in clot tensile strength and clot amplitudes by viscoelastic monitoring, with high levels of clot breakdown as demonstrated by high levels of fibrin degradation products and d-dimers [55, 56]. The hypofibrinogenaemia seen in severe trauma is related to the rate of breakdown as compared to the synthesis and is directly related to the degree of injury as well as methods of resuscitation [57]. This has led to the use of antifibrinolytics such as tranexamic acid (TXA), fibrinogen concentrates and fibrinogen replacement with cryoprecipitate to correct hypofibrinogenaemia in an attempt to reverse hyperfibrinolysis and reduce bleeding (Fig. 15.9) [58–62].

The Role of Platelets

Platelets and associated platelet derived microparticle (PMPs) are critical for clot genesis and clot strength. Both are necessary for coagulation especially in traumatic injury and the prevention of TIC. PMPs are procoagulant and have been implicated in the genesis of prothrombotic states in trauma [63, 64]. Platelets contribute to over 60% of clot strength primarily in coagulopathy and resuscitation [65]. They provide a network for clot structure and provide the environment necessary for thrombin burst. Although lower platelet counts are related to mortality in coagulopathy and resuscitation, platelet function is also related to inadequate clot formation and clot strength. Investigators found that platelet "hypo-function" related to four different agonists; adenosine diphosphate (ADP), arachidonic acid (AA), thrombin receptor activating peptide and collagen. Platelet hypo-function related to these agonists was present on 45% of patients on admission and 90% of patients at some point during their ICU stay compared to healthy controls. Platelet function can be measured in isolation as part of the clotting cascade, and platelet dysfunction on admission increases mortality tenfold despite adequate platelet numbers. In this study, inhibition related to AA and collagen stimulation was predictive of mortality [66]. Solomon et al. found that ADP and thrombin receptor activating peptide pathway inhibition was associated with mortality as well [67]. Stalker described "location dependent differential platelet activation" referring to the location of activated platelets in relation to the centre of

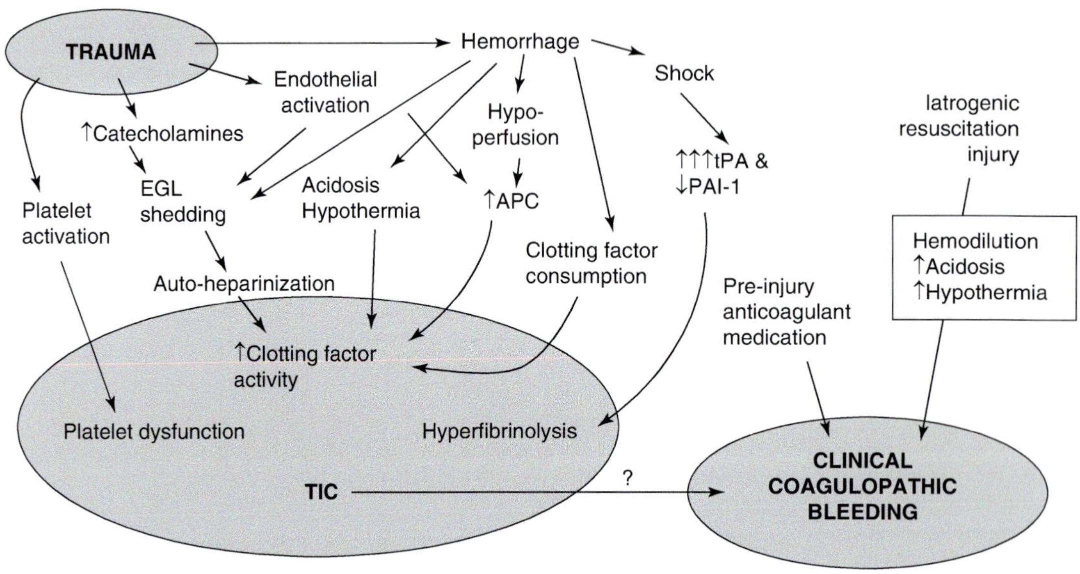

Fig. 15.9 Schematic overview of TIC. Trauma induces a laboratory-evident coagulopathy through a variety of different pathways, which is likely modulated by baseline patient factors such as genetics and comorbidities. Unfortunately, few causative relationships are currently known. TIC is a separate entity from iatrogenic causes of coagulopathy including haemodilution and pre-injury anticoagulant therapy. Currently, the literature only identifies TIC based on laboratory abnormalities, and its relationship to true clinical coagulopathic bleeding is unknown [10]

the clot. A combination of confocal intravital imaging, genetically engineered mice and antiplatelet agents following intravascular injury were used to determine the hierarchical structure of a haemostatic plug as related to the activation of platelets and fibrin accumulation. Two types of penetrating injuries were produced in the mice, however one was produced with a laser and introduced a heat induced variable to the injury pattern. Both types of injury produced a hierarchical structure which had a core of closely packed "irreversibly activated" platelets overlaid by a loosely packed minimally activated platelets. Thrombin was shown to be generated close to the site of injury and close to the core of the thrombus. ADP release from platelet dense granules extends throughout the core and throughout the outer shell. This study demonstrated the various states of platelet activation and response in injury and haemostatic plug formation [65, 68, 69]. Moore et al. demonstrated a sex dependent signalling and cellular activation. Females tend toward hypercoagulability and have shown a survival benefit in TIC [70]. Native platelets may also undergo a downregulation via a signalling process from plasma of trauma patients; in platelets that are otherwise normal, exposure to proteins that are released into the plasma in trauma patients causes downregulation of ADP and collagen receptors (Glycoprotein VI) expressed on the platelet surface. These platelets also showed a decrease in calcium mobilization when exposed to the plasma. Approximately one-third demonstrated a return of calcium mobilization at 120 h, but not fully returning to baseline. Similarly, infusion of healthy donated platelets into a trauma patient may cause the platelets to become unresponsive when exposed to the trauma patient's plasma [66].

Trauma induced coagulopathy is a multifactorial, global process induced by hypoperfusion and shock. It is characterised by an imbalance of haemostasis, protein C activation, cellular dysfunction, hypofibrinogenaemia, endothelial surface layer degradation and shedding, plasma mediated inhibitory effects on platelet signalling pathways and fibrinolysis. The extent of shock and hypoperfusion determines the severity of the trauma induced coagulopathy [15].

Haemostasis and Resuscitation

The previous section detailed the mechanisms and results of TIC. The identification and rapid treatment of the patient with TIC often determines the immediate and long term outcomes of these patients [6]. Several methods and scoring systems have been implemented with varying degrees success for both pre hospital and in hospital prediction for the need to activate a massive transfusion event [71–79].

The Assessment of Blood Consumption (ABC) by Cotton et al. [72] was a comparative, retrospective study looking at trauma admissions to a Level 1 trauma centre. The ABC score was assigned based on four non-weighted parameters: penetrating mechanism, positive focused assessment sonography for trauma (FAST) scan, arrival systolic blood pressure of 90 mm Hg or less, and arrival heart rate >120 bpm. The Trauma-Associated Severe Haemorrhage (TASH) as well as the McLaughlin scores were calculated in addition, but both TASH and McLaughlin require laboratory and radiology results to complete calculations. Comparatively, the area under the receiver operator curves (AUROC) between all three were statistically similar as predictors of massive transfusion. An ABC score of 2 or greater was 75% sensitive and 86% specific for predicting the need for MTP (correctly classifying 85%) [71, 72]. The Shock Index (SI) is calculated by dividing the heart rate by the blood pressure with a normal range of 0.5 to 0.7 in healthy adults. SI had a significantly greater sensitivity ($P = 0.035$), but a significantly weaker specificity ($P < 0.001$) compared to ABC score [78]. Sensitivity is a measure of the true positive predictive value of the test, i.e. if the patient requires a massive transfusion, how likely is the test to pick this up? Sensitivity is the corollary of this—if the test indicates the patient does not require a massive transfusion, what is the accuracy of this negative prediction?

There is no consensus on a specific or perfect scoring system in both the civilian and military populations. El-Menyar et al. [80] performed a systematic search yielded 241 articles and 24 different scoring systems. Key words used were "massive transfusion," "score," "model," "trauma," and "haemorrhage" in different combinations. Many of the scores are complex requiring difficult calculation and time consuming lab tests whereas some were simple and easy to remember using physiologic parameters, injury characteristics, and/or simple procedures done as point of care. At present, despite the various scoring systems implemented, there remains either an institutional based system or a reliance on treating physician "gestalt" to activate/implement a massive transfusion protocol [81]. The need for adopting a consensus score or merging several scoring systems to better predict the need for a life-saving massive transfusion must be addressed [80]. Unnecessary blood product administration is accompanied by an increased incidence of acute renal failure, acute lung injury and nosocomial infection. Being correct in predicting which patients that will need massive transfusion early will aid in the treatment and ultimately favourable outcome in those patients with TIC [8, 82].

Tranexamic Acid

As mentioned in this chapter, early recognition and treatment is essential. The need for prehospital treatment early may determine survival in trauma patients with haemorrhage. This begins with the prevention and reversal of the hypofibrinogenemia and fibrinolysis that accompanies traumatic shock. The use of the antifibrinolytic, TXA, prehospital and on arrival to the trauma centre has been a matter of investigation and discussion for many years. Several studies in favour of early administration have shown a decrease in mortality or a decrease in blood product administration.

The CRASH-2 trial, over 20,000 patients at risk for haemorrhage who received TXA versus placebo, showed a decrease in death due to haemorrhage with the early administration (<1 h) of TXA. The subgroup analysis showed an increase survival benefit in patients with severe shock and a systolic blood pressure of <75 mmHg. TXA administered greater than 3 h after injury was shown to increase mortality. One of the major limitations of the CRASH-2 trial is the difficulty in extrapolating the results to major trauma systems and centres [83]. Military studies such as the MATTERS and MATTERS-II trial showed and significant decrease in death due to haemorrhage more evident in the cohort receiving massive resuscitation. Twenty four hour and 30 day mortality were reduced in both groups and further reduced in the MATTERS-II trial when cryoprecipitate was given in addition to TXA. In both trials there was a suggestion of the anti-inflammatory effects of TXA administration in trauma. In a univariate model patients treated with TXA trended toward an increase in thrombotic events but there was no statistical difference in a multivariate model [60, 61]. The results of the TAMPITI trial are eagerly awaited [84]. This trial is a randomized placebo controlled prehospital trial to define the effects of TXA on the immune system, its mechanism of action, pharmacokinetic data, and efficacy as well as safety data for the use of TXA in severely injured trauma patients. The patients will be randomized into pre-hospital placebo, 2 g or 4 g doses of TXA within 2 h of injury. Primary outcome measures will be the portion of activated monocytes between the 3 treatment arms through 72 h after admission. Secondary outcome measures between the three arms will be cytokine measurements, leukocyte function, plasma drug availability, rate of thromboembolic events, incidence of seizures and all adverse events in total. This may have clinical implications in terms of the anti-inflammatory response versus complication rate, and may change dosage recommendations if it has an impact on immunomodulation.

In patients with traumatic brain injury (TBI) the CRASH-3 trial examined the effects of TXA on patients, with a GCS of 12 or less, with isolated intracranial bleeding compared to placebo. The risk of head injury-related death was reduced with tranexamic acid in patients with mild-to-moderate head injury (RR 0·78 [95% CI 0·64–

0·95]) but not in patients with severe head injury (0·99 [95% CI 0·91–1·07]; p value for heterogeneity 0·030). The authors demonstrated that the incidence of thrombotic events as well as seizures were similar between the TXA and placebo group [85]. The American College of Surgeons Committee on Trauma [86], European Task Force for Advanced Bleeding Care in Trauma [87, 88], and UK National Institute for Health and Care Excellence [89] all recommend administering TXA for hospitalized trauma patients as soon as possible if within 3 h of injury [90]. Care must be given to all trauma patients in terms of receiving TXA in this author's opinion. Those patients who arrive at a trauma centre should undergo viscoelastic monitoring prior to receiving TXA. Moore et al. elegantly described the phenomenon of fibrinolysis shutdown and the associated mortality associated with a Lys30 < 0.9% and the association with TXA administration and physiologic fibrinolysis [91]. In hospital TXA should be reserved for those in hyperfibrinolysis (Lys30 > 3%) [92, 93]. In the pre-hospital setting where testing is not available it is in the discretion of the pre-hospital personnel to administer TXA at their discretion solely if it is within their purview to do so.

In the California Pre Hospital Antifibrinolytic Therapy Study (CalPAT) [94], investigators compared 724 patients in 2 groups—those who received TXA and those who did not (control group). Both groups were similar in ISS, age and mechanism of injury. It was determined by the first responders that the patients exhibited signs of shock and were candidates for TXA administration. TXA administration in the pre-hospital setting showed a reduced mortality at 28 days which was statistically more evident in the most severely injured patients. The study group reported no increase in incidence of untoward effects in the TXA group. It was concluded that TXA may be used safely in the pre-hospital setting. The use of pre-hospital TXA was reviewed and analyzed in the German Trauma Registry. They propensity score matched two similar groups of patients, those who were administered TXA and those who were not. TXA was associated with prolonged time to death and significantly improved early survival. The difference was more pronounced in those who were more severely injured [95]. El-Menyar, et al. performed a meta-analysis on the efficacy of pre-hospital TXA. Only two out 92 referenced studies met their inclusion criteria. 24 h, 30 day mortality and thromboembolic events were the searched outcomes for the analysis. Prehospital TXA appears to reduce early mortality in trauma patients. The pooled analysis also showed a trend toward lower 30-day mortality and reduced risk of thromboembolic events [96]. The administration of TXA during aeromedical transport showed no survival benefit between pre and in-hospital administration of TXA [97]. In this author's opinion, trauma patients with prolonged transport in haemorrhagic shock, with the current available evidence, TXA should be administered in the pre hospital setting.

Historical Evolutions

Historically speaking, trauma resuscitation was performed with large volumes of crystalloid, low ratio of red cells to thawed plasma as well as the addition of inotropes to optimise oxygen delivery by increasing cardiac output [98]. In 2007, Borgman et al. demonstrated that early aggressive high ratio resuscitation of red blood cells to thawed plasma in a 1:1 ratio improved survival in a combat setting [99]. Later Holcomb et al. showed that not only RBC:Plasma ratios improved survival but a high Platelet:RBC ratio improved survival as well [100].

In the same year it was shown that an increasd fibrinogen to RBC ratio improved survival in military personnel needing a massive transfusion [101]. The Prospective Observational Prospective Multicentred Major Trauma Transfusion study (PROMMT) revealed that in the first 6 h, patients with ratios <1:2 were 3–4 times more likely to die than patients with ratios ≥1:1. Higher plasma and platelet ratios early in resuscitation were associated with decreased mortality in patients transfused at least three units of blood products during the first 24 h after admission. RBCs [11, 102–104]. The Pragmatic Randomized Optimal Plasma and Platelet Ratios (PROPPR) trial compared 1:1:1 (Plasma:Platelets:RBCs) to 1:1:2 (Plasma:Platelets:RBCs) in a multicentred trial including 680 severely injured trauma patients that met PROPPR criteria. The difference in 24 h and 30 day mortality were not statistically significant. Secondary outcome revealed that at the 2.9 h mark, high ratio resuscitation was significantly different. The study became unblinded once haemostasis was achieved and the administered blood products were revealed to the practitioners [5, 105, 106]. High ratio resuscitation has become the mainstay of practice within the United States.

The European guideline on management of major bleeding and coagulopathy following trauma: (fifth edition) recommends, for increased fibrinolytic activity (by viscoelastic monitoring) and a low fibrinogen concentration (< 1.5 Gm/L), early administration of TXA. Most trauma centres administer cryoprecipitate or fibrinogen concentrate to treat low fibrinogen levels. With a low intrinsic fibrinogen concentration, FFP administration will not rapidly increase fibrinogen levels in the bleeding trauma patient in isolation. There is also a lower incidence of TRALI (Transfusion Related Acute Lung Injury, a respiratory complication of blood product transfusion) with a decrease in the use of plasma as well as a decrease in haemodilution and decrease in haemoglobin concentration [88]. There exists a difference in transfusion practices between the USA, Europe and Canada. Perhaps there is a hybrid in philosophy that needs to be developed between the two methods of resuscitation.

Freeze dried lyophilized plasma has made a resurgence (FDP). The advantages of FDP are a long shelf life, stability at extremes of room temperature, easy and rapid reconstitution [107, 108]. The Israeli Defense Force (IDF) have reported successful administration of FDP (and TXA) at the point of injury [109].

Low titre fresh whole blood provides in vivo haemostatic properties, simplified logistics, lower transfusion volumes as well as less haemodilution. Also less anticoagulant that is used for component preservation and transport is introduced into the resuscitation process [110, 111]. Whole blood storage methods decrease the effects of storage lesions that are found in components of whole blood. Red blood cells and platelets undergo biochemical as well as morphologic changes as their shelf lives increase. As shelf life increases there is a release of microparticles, oxygen carrying capacity decreases, membrane ATP concentrations decrease and there is an increase inflammatory mediators. These changes have been noted as early as day 7 of shelf-life [112]. Logistics prove to be the main obstacle in the use of low titre leuko-reduced fresh whole blood in the civilian population. Most civilian blood banks do not keep low titre leuko-reduced blood on hand. Leukoreduction may prove to be a caveat depending on the type of leukoreduction filter used. Platelet sparing versus nonplatelet sparing filters must be used in order to maintain the quality and haemostatic properties of the fresh whole blood being transfused [113].

Conclusion

Trauma related death due to haemorrhage accounts for approximately 30 to 40% of the mortality in the civilian trauma population. Haemorrhage results from both coagulopathy as well as surgical bleeding. The rapid diagnosis and timely treatment of the patient with TIC determines the immediate and long term outcomes of these patients. The mechanisms and theories of TIC remain a hybrid between fibrinolysis, activated protein C, hypo-fibrinogenaemia and endothelial surface layer degradation. Rapid response from pre-hospital emergency medical personnel is key and transporting the patient to a trauma centre in a timely fashion is paramount. Prehospital administration of TXA, whole blood, fibrinogen concentrate, freeze dried plasma or component therapy have been shown to decrease the amount of blood product administration in hospital, decrease morbidity and improve outcomes. The availability and dosing of prehospital therapies varies between countries, civilian, military and local emergency medical services.

The key point from this review is that there needs to be a consensus for the care of the trauma patient from the point of injury to definitive treatment at the nearest trauma centre. There is an integral team approach from point of injury and delivery of the patient to definitive care. In instances of prolonged extrication or transport time patients in shock should be given TXA by emergency personnel pre-hospital. A hybrid of high ratio resuscitation, TXA and factor concentrates seems to be the ideal resuscitation method in order to provide the best haemostasis with limiting the complications of high volumes of resuscitation components. Research is ongoing and current trials may provide us with needed data to refine our global approach in the treatment of the patient with Trauma Induced Coagulopathy.

Questions

1. Which of the following ions are essential cofactors in clotting?
   (a) Potassium
   (b) Calcium
   (c) Phosphate
   (d) Chloride
   (e) Sodium
2. Tranexamic acid is effective in haemostasis by:
   (a) Decreasing clot formation time
   (b) Increasing platelet cross linking
   (c) Promoting generation of fibrinogen
   (d) Decreasing fibrin breakdown
   (e) Decreasing plasma levels of Protein C
3. Which of the following are scoring systems used in prediction of blood product requirements?
   (a) TASH score
   (b) ABC score
   (c) McLaughlin score
   (d) MARCH score
   (e) GCS
4. The presence of acute traumatic coagulopathy increases mortality by what degree:
   (a) 3 fold
   (b) 5 fold
   (c) 7 fold
   (d) 9 fold
   (e) 12 fold
5. Which clotting factor is the final common pathway between intrinsic and extrinsic systems in the classical model of coagulation?
   (a) VIIa
   (b) VIIIa
   (c) Xa
   (d) XII
   (e) XIII

Answers

1. b
2. d
3. a, b, c
4. d
5. c

References

1. Miniño AM. Death in the United States, 2010. NCHS Data Brief. 2012;99:8.
2. Alberdi F, García I, Atutxa L, Zabarte M. Epidemiology of severe trauma. Med Intensiva Engl Ed. 2014;38(9):580–8.
3. World Health Organization, Department for the Management of Noncommunicable Diseases D Violence and Injury Prevention. Injuries and violence: the facts 2014 [Internet]. 2014 [cited 2020 Jan 7]. Available from: http://apps.who.int/iris/bitstream/10665/149798/1/9789241508018_eng.pdf?ua=1
4. Vos T, Abajobir AA, Abate KH, Abbafati C, Abbas KM, Abd-Allah F, et al. Global, regional, and national incidence, prevalence, and years lived with disability for 328 diseases and injuries for 195 countries, 1990–2016: a systematic analysis for the Global Burden of Disease Study 2016. Lancet. 2017;390(10100):1211–59.
5. Holcomb JB, Tilley BC, Baraniuk S, Fox EE, Wade CE, Podbielski JM, et al. Transfusion of plasma, platelets, and red blood cells in a 1:1:1 vs a 1:1:2 ratio and mortality in patients with severe trauma: the PROPPR randomized clinical trial. JAMA. 2015;313(5):471.
6. Mitra B, Cameron PA, Mori A, Fitzgerald M. Acute coagulopathy and early deaths post major trauma. Injury. 2012;43(1):22–5.
7. DeMario VM, Sikorski RA, Efron DT, Serbanescu MA, Buchanan RM, Wang EJ, et al. Blood utilization and mortality in victims of gun violence: transfusion and mortality in gunshot victims. Transfusion (Paris). 2018;58(10):2326–34.
8. MacLeod JBA, Lynn M, McKenney MG, Cohn SM, Murtha M. Early coagulopathy predicts mortality in trauma. J Trauma. 2003;55(1):39–44.
9. Cohen MJ, Bir N, Rahn P, Dotson R, Brohi K, Chesebro BB, et al. Protein C depletion early after trauma increases the risk of ventilator-associated pneumonia. J Trauma Injury Infect Crit Care. 2009;67(6):1176–81.
10. Chang R, Cardenas JC, Wade CE, Holcomb JB. Advances in the understanding of trauma-induced coagulopathy. Blood. 2016;128(8):1043–9.

11. Holcomb JB, del Junco DJ, Fox EE, Wade CE, Cohen MJ, Schreiber MA, et al. The prospective, observational, multicenter, major trauma transfusion (PROMMTT) study: comparative effectiveness of a time-varying treatment with competing risks. JAMA Surg. 2013;148(2):127–36.
12. Wright IS. The nomenclature of blood clotting factors. Can Med Assoc J. 1962;86(8):373–4.
13. Hoffman M. Remodeling the blood coagulation cascade. J Thromb Thrombolysis. 2003;16(1/2):17–20.
14. Midwinter MJ, Woolley T. Resuscitation and coagulation in the severely injured trauma patient. Philos Trans R Soc B Biol Sci. 2011;366(1562):192–203.
15. Davenport RA, Brohi K. Cause of trauma-induced coagulopathy. Curr Opin Anaesthesiol. 2016;29(2):212–9.
16. Peng N, Su L. Progresses in understanding trauma-induced coagulopathy and the underlying mechanism. Chin J Traumatol. 2017;20(3):133–6.
17. Reynolds BR, Forsythe RM, Harbrecht BG, Cuschieri J, Minei JP, Maier RV, et al. Hypothermia in massive transfusion: have we been paying enough attention to it? J Trauma Acute Care Surg. 2012;73(2):486–91.
18. Holcomb JB, Wade CE. Defining present blood component transfusion practices in trauma patients: papers from the trauma outcomes group. J Trauma Injury Infect Crit Care. 2011;71:S315–7.
19. Duke MD, Guidry C, Guice J, Stuke L, Marr AB, Hunt JP, et al. Restrictive fluid resuscitation in combination with damage control resuscitation: time for adaptation. J Trauma Acute Care Surg. 2012;73(3):674–8.
20. Dobson GP, Letson HL, Sharma R, Sheppard FR, Cap AP. Mechanisms of early trauma-induced coagulopathy: the clot thickens or not? J Trauma Acute Care Surg. 2015;79(2):301–9.
21. Davenport R, Manson J, De'Ath H, Platton S, Coates A, Allard S, et al. Functional definition and characterization of acute traumatic coagulopathy. Crit Care Med. 2011;39(12):2652–8.
22. Tapia NM, Chang A, Norman M, Welsh F, Scott B, Wall MJ, et al. TEG-guided resuscitation is superior to standardized MTP resuscitation in massively transfused penetrating trauma patients. J Trauma Acute Care Surg. 2013;74(2):378–86.
23. Sankarankutty A, Nascimento B, Teodoro da Luz L, Rizoli S. TEG® and ROTEM® in trauma: similar test but different results? World J Emerg Surg. 2012;7(Suppl 1):S3.
24. Johansson PI, Sørensen A, Perner A, Welling K, Wanscher M, Larsen CF, et al. Disseminated intravascular coagulation or acute coagulopathy of trauma shock early after trauma? An observational study. Crit Care. 2011;15(6):R272.
25. Brohi K, Cohen MJ, Ganter MT, Schultz MJ, Levi M, Mackersie RC, et al. Acute coagulopathy of trauma: hypoperfusion induces systemic anticoagulation and hyperfibrinolysis. J Trauma Injury Infect Crit Care. 2008;64(5):1211–7.
26. Wada H, Matsumoto T, Yamashita Y. Diagnosis and treatment of disseminated intravascular coagulation (DIC) according to four DIC guidelines. J Intensive Care. 2014;2(1):15.
27. Rizoli S, Nascimento B, Key N, Tien HC, Muraca S, Pinto R, et al. Disseminated intravascular coagulopathy in the first 24 hours after trauma: the association between ISTH score and anatomopathologic evidence. J Trauma Injury Infect Crit Care. 2011;71:S441–7.
28. Gando S, Wada H, Thachil J. The Scientific and Standardization Committee on DIC of the International Society on Thrombosis and Haemostasis (ISTH). Differentiating disseminated intravascular coagulation (DIC) with the fibrinolytic phenotype from coagulopathy of trauma and acute coagulopathy of trauma-shock (COT/ACOTS). J Thromb Haemost. 2013;11(5):826–35.
29. Moore HB, Moore EE, Gonzalez E, Chapman MP, Chin TL, Silliman CC, et al. Hyperfibrinolysis, physiologic fibrinolysis, and fibrinolysis shutdown: the spectrum of postinjury fibrinolysis and relevance to antifibrinolytic therapy. J Trauma Acute Care Surg. 2014;77(6):811–7.
30. Madurska MJ, Sachse KA, Jansen JO, Rasmussen TE, Morrison JJ. Fibrinolysis in trauma: a review. Eur J Trauma Emerg Surg. 2018;44(1):35–44.
31. Davenport RA, Guerreiro M, Frith D, Rourke C, Platton S, Cohen M, et al. Activated protein C drives the hyperfibrinolysis of acute traumatic coagulopathy. Anesthesiology. 2017;126(1):115–27.
32. Ferreira CN, Sousa MO, Dusse LMS, Carvalho MG. A cell-based model of coagulation and its implications. Rev Bras Hematol E Hemoter. 2010;32(5):416–21.
33. Romney G, Glick M. An updated concept of coagulation with clinical implications. J Am Dent Assoc. 2009;140(5):567–74.
34. Brohi K, Cohen MJ, Ganter MT, Matthay MA, Mackersie RC, Pittet J-F. Acute Traumatic coagulopathy: initiated by hypoperfusion: modulated through the protein C pathway? Ann Surg. 2007;245(5):812–8.
35. Cohen MJ, Christie SA. Coagulopathy of trauma. Crit Care Clin. 2017;33(1):101–18.
36. Cohen MJ, Call M, Nelson M, Calfee CS, Esmon CT, Brohi K, et al. Critical role of activated protein C in early coagulopathy and later organ failure, infection and death in trauma patients. Ann Surg. 2012;255(2):379–85.
37. Feistritzer C, Schuepbach RA, Mosnier LO, Bush LA, Di Cera E, Griffin JH, et al. Protective signaling by activated protein C is mechanistically linked to protein C activation on endothelial cells. J Biol Chem. 2006;281(29):20077–84.
38. Levi M, Poll T. Coagulation in patients with severe sepsis. Semin Thromb Hemost. 2015;41(01):009–15.
39. Bir N, Lafargue M, Howard M, Goolaerts A, Roux J, Carles M, et al. Cytoprotective-selective activated protein C attenuates *Pseudomonas aeruginosa* –

induced lung injury in mice. Am J Respir Cell Mol Biol. 2011;45(3):632–41.
40. University of Texas Health Science Center, Wade CE. Pulmonary contusion on admission chest X-ray is associated with coagulopathy and mortality in trauma patients. Emerg Med Trauma Surg Care. 2015;2(3):1–5.
41. Lustenberger T, Talving P, Kobayashi L, Barmparas G, Inaba K, Lam L, et al. Early coagulopathy after isolated severe traumatic brain injury: relationship with hypoperfusion challenged. J Trauma Injury Infect Crit Care. 2010;69(6):1410–4.
42. Jansen JO, Scarpelini S, Pinto R, Tien HC, Callum J, Rizoli SB. Hypoperfusion in severely injured trauma patients is associated with reduced coagulation factor activity. J Trauma Injury Infect Crit Care. 2011;71:S435–40.
43. Burggraf M, Payas A, Kauther MD, Schoeneberg C, Lendemans S. Evaluation of clotting factor activities early after severe multiple trauma and their correlation with coagulation tests and clinical data. World J Emerg Surg. 2015;10(1):43.
44. Chapman MP, Moore EE, Moore HB, Gonzalez E, Gamboni F, Chandler JG, et al. Overwhelming tPA release, not PAI-1 degradation, is responsible for hyperfibrinolysis in severely injured trauma patients. J Trauma Acute Care Surg. 2016;80(1):16–25.
45. Campbell JE, Meledeo MA, Cap AP. Comparative response of platelet fV and Plasma fV to activated protein C and relevance to a model of acute traumatic coagulopathy. Lenting PJ, editor. PLoS ONE. 2014;9(6):e99181.
46. Rahbar E, Cardenas JC, Baimukanova G, Usadi B, Bruhn R, Pati S, et al. Endothelial glycocalyx shedding and vascular permeability in severely injured trauma patients. J Transl Med. 2015;13(1):117.
47. Uchimido R, Schmidt EP, Shapiro NI. The glycocalyx: a novel diagnostic and therapeutic target in sepsis. Crit Care. 2019;23(1):16.
48. Johansson PI, Stensballe J, Rasmussen LS, Ostrowski SR. A high admission syndecan-1 Level, A marker of endothelial glycocalyx degradation, is associated with inflammation, protein C depletion, fibrinolysis, and increased mortality in trauma patients. Ann Surg. 2011;254(2):194–200.
49. Johansson PI, Stensballe J, Rasmussen LS, Ostrowski SR. High circulating adrenaline levels at admission predict increased mortality after trauma. J Trauma Acute Care Surg. 2012;72(2):428–36.
50. Henriksen HH, McGarrity S, SigurÐardóttir RS, Nemkov T, D'Alessandro A, Palsson BO, et al. Metabolic Systems Analysis of Shock-Induced Endotheliopathy (SHINE) in Trauma: A New Research Paradigm. Ann Surg. 2019;1
51. Naumann DN, Hazeldine J, Midwinter MJ, Hutchings SD, Harrison P. Poor microcirculatory flow dynamics are associated with endothelial cell damage and glycocalyx shedding after traumatic hemorrhagic shock. J Trauma Acute Care Surg. 2018;84(1):81–8.
52. Haeger SM, Liu X, Han X, McNeil JB, Oshima K, McMurtry SA, et al. Epithelial heparan sulfate contributes to alveolar barrier function and is shed during lung injury. Am J Respir Cell Mol Biol. 2018;59(3):363–74.
53. Li J-P, Kusche-Gullberg M. Heparan sulfate: biosynthesis, structure, and function. In: International review of cell and molecular biology [Internet]. Elsevier; 2016 [cited 2020 Jan 7]: [215–73 pp.]. Available from: https://linkinghub.elsevier.com/retrieve/pii/S193764481630020X
54. Zhang L. Glycosaminoglycan (GAG) biosynthesis and GAG-binding proteins. In: Progress in molecular biology and translational science [Internet]. Elsevier; 2010 [cited 2020 Jan 7]: [1–17 pp.]. Available from: https://linkinghub.elsevier.com/retrieve/pii/S1877117310930019
55. Fries D, Martini WZ. Role of fibrinogen in trauma-induced coagulopathy. Br J Anaesth. 2010;105(2):116–21.
56. Peng HT, Nascimento B, Tien H, Callum J, Rizoli S, Rhind SG, et al. A comparative study of viscoelastic hemostatic assays and conventional coagulation tests in trauma patients receiving fibrinogen concentrate. Clin Chim Acta. 2019;495:253–62.
57. Hagemo JS, Stanworth S, Juffermans NP, Brohi K, Cohen M, Johansson PI, et al. Prevalence, predictors and outcome of hypofibrinogenaemia in trauma: a multicentre observational study. Crit Care. 2014;18(2):R52.
58. Cartwright BL, Kam P, Yang K. Efficacy of fibrinogen concentrate compared with cryoprecipitate for reversal of the antiplatelet effect of clopidogrel in an in vitro model, as assessed by multiple electrode platelet aggregometry, thromboelastometry, and modified thromboelastography. J Cardiothorac Vasc Anesth. 2015;29(3):694–702.
59. Mengoli C, Franchini M, Marano G, Pupella S, Vaglio S, Marietta M, et al. The use of fibrinogen concentrate for the management of trauma-related bleeding: a systematic review and meta-analysis. Blood Transfus [Internet]. 2017 [cited 2020 Jan 7]; Available from: https://doi.org/10.2450/2017.0094-17
60. Morrison JJ, Ross JD, Dubose JJ, Jansen JO, Midwinter MJ, Rasmussen TE. Association of cryoprecipitate and tranexamic acid with improved survival following wartime injury: findings from the MATTERs II study. JAMA Surg. 2013;148(3):218.
61. Morrison JJ. Military application of tranexamic acid in trauma emergency resuscitation (MATTERs) study. Arch Surg. 2012;147(2):113.
62. Roberts I, Shakur H, Afolabi A, The CRASH-2 Collaborators. The importance of early treatment with tranexamic acid in bleeding trauma patients: an exploratory analysis of the CRASH-2 randomised controlled trial. The Lancet. 2011;377(9771):1096–1101.e2.

63. Lopez E, Srivastava AK, Pati S, Holcomb JB, Wade CE. Platelet-derived microvesicles: a potential therapy for trauma-induced coagulopathy. Shock. 2018;49(3):243–8.
64. Midura EF, Kuethe JW, Rice TC, Veile R, England LG, Friend LA, et al. Impact of platelets and platelet-derived microparticles on hypercoagulability following burn injury. SHOCK. 2016;45(1):82–7.
65. Kornblith LZ, Kutcher ME, Redick BJ, Calfee CS, Vilardi RF, Cohen MJ. Fibrinogen and platelet contributions to clot formation: Implications for trauma resuscitation and thromboprophylaxis. J Trauma Acute Care Surg. 2014;76(2):255–63.
66. Verni CC, Davila A, Balian S, Sims CA, Diamond SL. Platelet dysfunction during trauma involves diverse signaling pathways and an inhibitory activity in patient-derived plasma. J Trauma Acute Care Surg. 2019;86(2):250–9.
67. Solomon C, Traintinger S, Ziegler B, Hanke A, Rahe-Meyer N, Voelckel W, et al. Platelet function following trauma: a multiple electrode aggregometry study. Thromb Haemost. 2011;106(08):322–30.
68. Stalker TJ, Traxler EA, Wu J, Wannemacher KM, Cermignano SL, Voronov R, et al. Hierarchical organization in the hemostatic response and its relationship to the platelet-signaling network. Blood. 2013;121(10):1875–85.
69. Moore HB, Moore EE, Chapman MP, Gonzalez E, Slaughter AL, Morton AP, et al. Viscoelastic measurements of platelet function, not fibrinogen function, predicts sensitivity to tissue-type plasminogen activator in trauma patients. J Thromb Haemost. 2015;13(10):1878–87.
70. Coleman JR, Moore EE, Kelher MR, Samuels JM, Cohen MJ, Sauaia A, et al. Female platelets have distinct functional activity compared with male platelets: implications in transfusion practice and treatment of trauma-induced coagulopathy. J Trauma Acute Care Surg. 2019;87(5):1052–60.
71. Nunez TC, Voskresensky IV, Dossett LA, Shinall R, Dutton WD, Cotton BA. Early Prediction of Massive Transfusion in Trauma: Simple as ABC (Assessment of Blood Consumption)? J Trauma Injury Infect Crit Care. 2009;66(2):346–52.
72. Cotton BA, Dossett LA, Haut ER, Shafi S, Nunez TC, Au BK, et al. Multicenter validation of a simplified score to predict massive transfusion in trauma: J Trauma Injury Infect Crit Care. 2010;69(Supplement):S33–9.
73. Schluter PJ. The trauma and injury severity score (TRISS) revised. Injury. 2011;42(1):90–6.
74. Brockamp T, Maegele M, Gaarder C, Goslings J, Cohen MJ, Lefering R, et al. Comparison of the predictive performance of the BIG, TRISS, and PS09 score in an adult trauma population derived from multiple international trauma registries. Crit Care. 2013;17(4):R134.
75. DeMuro JP, Simmons S, Jax J, Gianelli SM. Application of the shock index to the prediction of need for hemostasis intervention. Am J Emerg Med. 2013;31(8):1260–3.
76. Torabi M, Mirafzal A, Rastegari A, Sadeghkhani N. Association of triage time shock index, modified shock index, and age shock index with mortality in emergency severity index level 2 patients. Am J Emerg Med. 2016;34(1):63–8.
77. Torabi M, Moeinaddini S, Mirafzal A, Rastegari A, Sadeghkhani N. Shock index, modified shock index, and age shock index for prediction of mortality in Emergency Severity Index level 3. Am J Emerg Med. 2016;34(11):2079–83.
78. Schroll R, Swift D, Tatum D, Couch S, Heaney JB, Llado-Farrulla M, et al. Accuracy of shock index versus ABC score to predict need for massive transfusion in trauma patients. Injury. 2018;49(1):15–9.
79. Yazer MH, Spinella PC, Allard S, Roxby D, So-Osman C, Lozano M, et al. Vox Sanguinis International Forum on the use of prehospital blood products and pharmaceuticals in the treatment of patients with traumatic haemorrhage. Vox Sang. 2018;113(7):701–6.
80. El-Menyar A, Mekkodathil A, Abdelrahman H, Latifi R, Galwankar S, Al-Thani H, et al. Review of existing scoring systems for massive blood transfusion in trauma patients: where do we stand? Shock. 2019;52(3):288–99.
81. Pommerening MJ, Goodman MD, Holcomb JB, Wade CE, Fox EE, del Junco DJ, et al. Clinical gestalt and the prediction of massive transfusion after trauma. Injury. 2015;46(5):807–13.
82. Inaba K, Branco BC, Rhee P, Blackbourne LH, Holcomb JB, Teixeira PGR, et al. Impact of plasma transfusion in trauma patients who do not require massive transfusion. J Am Coll Surg. 2010;210(6):957–65.
83. Roberts I, Shakur H, Coats T, Hunt B, Balogun E, Barnetson L, et al. The CRASH-2 trial: a randomised controlled trial and economic evaluation of the effects of tranexamic acid on death, vascular occlusive events and transfusion requirement in bleeding trauma patients. Health Technol Assess [Internet]. 2013 Mar [cited 2019 May 7]: [17(10) p.]. Available from: https://www.journalslibrary.nihr.ac.uk/hta/hta17100/
84. Spinella P. Tranexamic acid mechanisms and pharmacokinetics in traumatic injury - full text view - ClinicalTrials.gov [Internet]. ClinicalTrials.gov. 2019 [cited 2020 Feb 27]. Available from: https://clinicaltrials.gov/ct2/show/NCT02535949?term=tranexamic+acid+trauma
85. Roberts I, Belli A, Brenner A, Chaudhri R, Fawole B, Harris T, et al. Tranexamic acid for significant traumatic brain injury (The CRASH-3 trial): Statistical analysis plan for an international, randomised, double-blind, placebo-controlled trial. Wellcome Open Res. 2018;3:86.
86. Committee on Trauma of the American College of Surgeons. ACS TQIP Massive Transfusion in Trauma Guidelines [Internet]. American College of Surgeons; 2014 [cited 2020 Feb 27]. Available from: https://www.facs.org/-/media/files/quality-programs/trauma/tqip/transfusion_guildelines.ashx

87. Rossaint R, Bouillon B, Cerny V, Coats TJ, Duranteau J, Fernández-Mondéjar E, et al. The European guideline on management of major bleeding and coagulopathy following trauma: fourth edition. Crit Care. 2016;20(1):100.
88. Spahn DR, Bouillon B, Cerny V, Duranteau J, Filipescu D, Hunt BJ, et al. The European guideline on management of major bleeding and coagulopathy following trauma: fifth edition. Crit Care. 2019;23(1):98.
89. NICE. Major trauma: assessment and initial management [Internet]. National Institute for Health and Clinical Excellence; 2016 [cited 2019 Sep 18]. Available from: https://www.nice.org.uk/guidance/ng39/evidence/full-guideline-2308122833
90. Chang R, Eastridge BJ, Holcomb JB. Remote damage control resuscitation in austere environments. Wilderness Environ Med. 2017;28(2S):S124–34.
91. Moore HB, Moore BA, Sauaia A, Moore EE. Clinical relevance and practical assessment of fibrinolysis shutdown. ANZ J Surg. 2020;90(4):413–4.
92. Moore HB, Moore EE, Huebner BR, Stettler GR, Nunns GR, Einersen PM, et al. Tranexamic acid is associated with increased mortality in patients with physiological fibrinolysis. J Surg Res. 2017;220:438–43.
93. Moore HB, Moore EE, Huebner BR, Dzieciatkowska M, Stettler GR, Nunns GR, et al. Fibrinolysis shutdown is associated with a fivefold increase in mortality in trauma patients lacking hypersensitivity to tissue plasminogen activator. J Trauma Acute Care Surg. 2017;83(6):1014–22.
94. Neeki MM, Dong F, Toy J, Vaezazizi R, Powell J, Wong D, et al. Tranexamic acid in civilian trauma care in the California prehospital antifibrinolytic therapy study. West J Emerg Med. 2018;19(6):977–86.
95. Wafaisade A, Lefering R, Bouillon B, Böhmer AB, Gäßler M, Ruppert M, et al. Prehospital administration of tranexamic acid in trauma patients. Crit Care. 2016;20(1):143.
96. El-Menyar A, Sathian B, Asim M, Latifi R, Al-Thani H. Efficacy of prehospital administration of tranexamic acid in trauma patients: a meta-analysis of the randomized controlled trials. Am J Emerg Med. 2018;36(6):1079–87.
97. Boudreau RM, Deshpande KK, Day GM, Hinckley WR, Harger N, Pritts TA, et al. Prehospital tranexamic acid administration during aeromedical transport after injury. J Surg Res. 2019;233:132–8.
98. Fleming A, Bishop M, Shoemaker W, Appel P, Sufficool W, Kuvhenguwha A, et al. Prospective trial of supranormal values as goals of resuscitation in severe trauma. Arch Surg Chic Ill 1960. 1992;127(10):1175–9; discussion 1179–1181.
99. Borgman MA, Spinella PC, Perkins JG, Grathwohl KW, Repine T, Beekley AC, et al. The ratio of blood products transfused affects mortality in patients receiving massive transfusions at a combat support hospital. J Trauma. 2007;63(4):805–13.
100. Holcomb JB, Wade CE, Michalek JE, Chisholm GB, Zarzabal LA, Schreiber MA, et al. Increased plasma and platelet to red blood cell ratios improves outcome in 466 massively transfused civilian trauma patients. Ann Surg. 2008;248(3):447–58.
101. Stinger HK, Spinella PC, Perkins JG, Grathwohl KW, Salinas J, Martini WZ, et al. The ratio of fibrinogen to red cells transfused affects survival in casualties receiving massive transfusions at an army combat support hospital. J Trauma Injury Infect Crit Care. 2008;64(Supplement):S79–85.
102. Holcomb JB, Fox EE, Wade CE. The prospective observational multicenter major trauma transfusion (PROMMTT) study. J Trauma Acute Care Surg. 2013;75:S1–2.
103. Robinson BR, Cotton BA, Pritts TA, Branson R, Holcomb JB, Muskat PC, et al. Application of the Berlin definition in PROMMTT patients: the impact of resuscitation on the incidence of hypoxemia. J Trauma Acute Care Surg. 2013;75(1 0 1):S61–7.
104. Holcomb JB, Fox EE, Zhang X, White N, Wade CE, Cotton BA, et al. Cryoprecipitate use in the PROMMTT study. J Trauma Acute Care Surg. 2013;75:S31–9.
105. Dzik W. Misunderstanding the PROPPR trial. Transfusion (Paris). 2017;57(8):2056.
106. Janelle GM, Shore-Lesserson L, Smith CE, Levy JH, Shander A. What is the PROPPR transfusion strategy in trauma resuscitation? Anesth Analg. 2016;122(4):1216–9.
107. Bux J, Dickhörner D, Scheel E. Quality of freeze-dried (lyophilized) quarantined single-donor plasma. Transfusion (Paris). 2013;53(12):3203–9.
108. Jost D, Lemoine S, Lemoine F, Lanoe V, Maurin O, Derkenne C, et al. French lyophilized plasma versus normal saline for post-traumatic coagulopathy prevention and correction: PREHO-PLYO protocol for a multicenter randomized controlled clinical trial. Trials. 2020;21(1):106.
109. Glassberg E, Nadler R, Gendler S, Abramovich A, Spinella PC, Gerhardt RT, et al. Freeze-dried plasma at the point of injury: from concept to doctrine. Shock Augusta Ga. 2013;40(6):444–50.
110. Repine TB, Perkins JG, Kauvar DS, Blackborne L. The use of fresh whole blood in massive transfusion. J Trauma Inj Infect Crit Care. 2006;60(Supplement):S59–69.
111. Manno CS, Hedberg KW, Kim HC, Bunin GR, Nicolson S, Jobes D, et al. Comparison of the hemostatic effects of fresh whole blood, stored whole blood, and components after open heart surgery in children. Blood. 1991;77(5):930–6.
112. Jones AR, Frazier SK. Consequences of transfusing blood components in patients with trauma: a conceptual model. Crit Care Nurse. 2017;37(2):18–30.
113. Haddaway K, Bloch EM, Tobian AAR, Frank SM, Sikorski R, Cho BC, et al. Hemostatic properties of cold-stored whole blood leukoreduced using a platelet-sparing versus a non-platelet-sparing filter. Transfusion (Paris). 2019;59(5):1809–17.

In Hospital REBOA for Major Trauma

16

Tim J. Stansfield

- Introduction: Concept, purpose, effect and use of REBOA within a MTC
- Definition
- Indications/contraindications
- Types of REBOA: level of balloon deployment, duration of balloon inflation, strategy of occlusion, environment of insertion access type, access location and type of balloon catheter
- Risk analysis for REBOA
- Practical considerations in the conduct of REBOA
- System optimisation for REBOA

Introduction

Resuscitative Endovascular Balloon Occlusion of the Aorta (REBOA) is a resuscitative adjunct used by trauma teams with the intent to benefit selected major trauma patients [1]. Colloquially sometimes termed "blowing a balloon up in the aorta", it is a conceptually attractive, technically straightforward intervention. It requires the trans-luminal passage of a catheter mounted compliant or semi-compliant balloon into a selected aorta segment and then inflation (distension) of the balloon with an appropriate liquid. This concept is demonstrated in Fig. 16.1. At higher volumes of inflation the balloon will form a circumferential seal with the aortic wall, sustained throughout each cardiac cycle. In the context of major trauma, the trauma team will decide whether they intend to use this capability, or whether they intend to inflate without full occlusion of an aortic segment. In either case, the aim of REBOA is to temporally obstruct aortic flow within the targeted aortic segment to improve the resuscitative management of the patient. The operator expectation is that such an improvement will be favourably reflected in the long-term outcome for the patient.

Assumptions

1. Unless otherwise implicitly stated, all reference to REBOA in this chapter will be in its' role as a resuscitative adjunct in selected major trauma patients. Strategies and effects of use in other contexts, for example post-partum major haemorrhage or aortic aneurysm rupture, are not directly considered.
2. Unless otherwise stated anatomical descriptions in this chapter refer to normal adult anatomy. Conventional REBOA catheters are designed for operation in adults; data and

T. J. Stansfield (✉)
The Leeds Vascular Institute, Leeds Teaching Hospitals NHS Trust, Leeds, UK

Royal Army Medical Corps, London, UK
e-mail: tim.stansfield@nhs.net

P. Lax (ed.), *Textbook of Acute Trauma Care*, https://doi.org/10.1007/978-3-030-83628-3_16

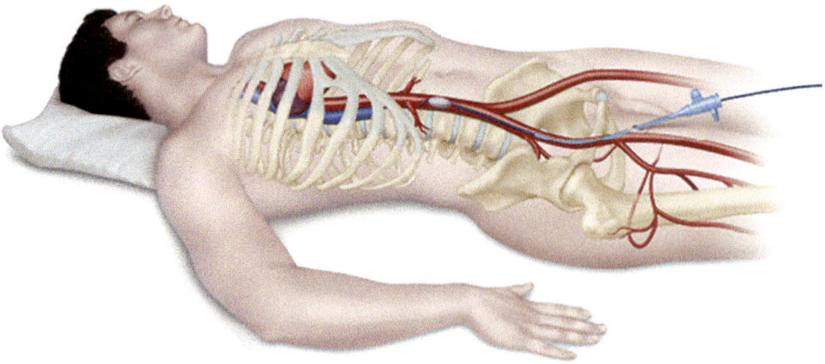

Fig. 16.1 Image courtesy of UK REBOA trial protocol. "blowing a balloon up in the aorta": A catheter mounted balloon device is inflated in the aorta, inserted via a right femoral access sheath

descriptions of use refer to the adult population.

3. Consent for REBOA is not discussed or implied as it is assumed that patients for REBOA will have such an injury and treatment profile as to not have capacity to consent. The procedure is performed in line with other lifesaving interventions—in the patient's best interests. Explanations, albeit brief in time critical situations, to the conscious patient is almost always appropriate regardless of lack of capacity. Clearly in the very unlikely event the patient has capacity then consent must be sought, albeit appropriately tailored such that gaining consent does not disproportionately threaten their life.

Purpose of REBOA

The similarities with open extraluminal aortic control are manifest. In humans, the benefits of REBOA are not fully defined by empirical human data, in part an extrapolation is made from other types of aortic control and animal data. With such formulation the potential benefits include:

1. Alteration of the aortic arch haemodynamics to the advantage of the coronary and cerebral circulation in the same way as open extraluminal aortic control.
2. Reduction of arterial blood flow and pressure distal to the inflated balloon and therefore:
   (a) Decreased blood loss, primarily from arterial bleeding. There may be a reduction in venous bleeding (for example, by reducing inflow into an organ or region, venous outflow may be proportionately reduced).
   (b) Improved visualisation of the operative field as it will be less continuously obfuscated by ongoing bleeding. For example, this may make damage control laparotomy (DCL) considerably more efficient.
   (c) Improved probability of clot formation in injured tissues.
3. Reduction in the associated morbidity of open aortic exposure and extraluminal aortic control, if that was to be the alternative strategy. For example, the wound generated by left lateral thoracotomy and the potential to cause intercostal avulsion on manoeuvring to clamp the descending thoracic aorta (DTA).

REBOA is not sustained or implanted, rather it is a temporary measure while an acceptable level of definitive haemorrhage control is achieved. For REBOA to be worthwhile, it is implicit that the potential benefits described above must come at an acceptable:

- *Risk*. For example: the physiological cost to the patient; principally in the ischaemic hit to the tissues oxygenated by flow distal to the balloon and the subsequent reperfusion hit.
- *Opportunity-cost*. This includes opportunity-cost to the:
  - Patient; whether an alternative strategy may be more efficient or effective and to
  - Healthcare resource; whether the benefit to the patient justifies any compromise to delivering healthcare to other patients. Decisions on healthcare resource cost clearly need to be pre-established by the

hospital system rather than by the responding trauma team. In large well-resourced medical facilities cost to healthcare resource is likely to be far less impactful compared to a facility with limited resources.

Probable Haemodynamic Effect of REBOA in Humans

REBOA increases cardiac afterload and proximal aortic pressure, and improves perfusion of the heart and brain [2, 3]. This is supported by basic science data in large animal models [4, 5] and is consistent with modelling of cardiac physiology such as the Frank-Starling law. In trauma, the mean increase in systolic blood pressure (SBP) from REBOA has recently been calculated from selected published literature as 78.9 mmHg [6]; the individual increase will clearly depend on the REBOA type (see below) and patient factors. In uninjured porcine models with total REBOA [7], reduced flow in the IVC, hepatic vein and portal vein with increased flow in the SVC has been noted.

Use of REBOA Within a MTC

REBOA is used in many Major Trauma Centres (MTCs) worldwide. The frequency of use in a trauma centre with REBOA capability probably depends on the population at risk presenting to the MTC (including the pre-hospital healthcare pathway), the trauma centre protocol and where the trauma team analyses the balance of risk to lie. In the UK, in-hospital REBOA as an adjunct for trauma resuscitation has effectively been initiated by the UK-REBOA trial. The vast majority of in-hospital REBOA use in the UK, outside the Royal London Hospital, is for patients who have been randomised to REBOA as part of this trial.

Key Points

Based on UK-REBOA trial protocol [8] and recruitment so far [9], UK major trauma centres in the future may on average select one patient every 2–3 months for the intervention.

This frequency is slightly less than that indicated by a TARN dataset gap analysis for exsanguinating sub-diaphragmatic bleeding [10]. With greater clarity on the trauma patient groups that are likely to clinically benefit from REBOA and with more familiarity of its' use, it is conceivable that it becomes a modestly more frequent intervention than highlighted. It may be there is a very rare role for UK Trauma Unit (TU) use of REBOA either as a transfer adjunct or for on-site DCL. However, it is very unlikely that a TU trauma team in the UK would be able to justify the opportunity cost in training to use REBOA compared to other priorities for training.

REBOA preparation, decision making, and conduct is within the context of the trauma team managing a major trauma patient with a potentially life-threatening injury. Such processes require integration into the in-hospital resuscitation pathway through the pre-arrival preparation phase, ED management phase, operating (conventional or hybrid theatre) or CT imaging phase, and then beyond. Trauma teams need to be able to conduct Damage Control Resuscitation (DCR) including blood product transfusion while maintaining a minimal and survivable duration of REBOA that meets the resuscitation strategy. This also requires concurrent interface with and transition through various hospital departments within a few hours from arrival in hospital. Therefore those seeking to optimise their REBOA processes should ensure familiarity with:

- Human factor considerations in complex processes, for example those described in the Human Factors and Decision Making in Damage Control Surgery chapters within this textbook.
- DCR imperatives
- Key decision points regarding definitive haemorrhage control, for example those described in the Decision Making in Damage Control Surgery chapter.
- REBOA specific considerations:
  (a) Probable haemodynamic effects of REBOA
  (b) Patient selection and strategy for REBOA
  (c) Practical technique of performing REBOA

- These REBOA specific considerations are described in this chapter.

Definition

REBOA is the action of inflation of a catheter mounted balloon device within a discrete aortic segment, for a discrete time interval, with the intent of facilitating resuscitative efforts for the patient.

Indications/Contraindications

The purpose of REBOA has been described above. Indications and contraindications of use are partly dependent on the type of REBOA and are considered in the patient and strategy selection section of this chapter. Identifying absolute contraindications for REBOA (Table 16.2) early will help avoid siting an unused and unnecessary larger access sheath.

Types of REBOA

REBOA is not one entity. There several variables in the conduct, which create different combinations and therefore "types of REBOA". In considering these variables, the analysis should be approached through a risk and benefit (risk reduction) assessment using slow cognitive decision-making in order to optimally select appropriate patients and REBOA conduct. Clearly, such an analysis requires an understanding of each variable. The variables are:

1. Level of balloon deployment
2. Strategy of occlusion
3. Duration of balloon inflation

} The crux combination of variables for the conduct of REBOA principally effecting the physiological benefit and burden

4. Environment of insertion
5. Access type
6. Access location
7. Type of balloon catheter

} These variables may confer different risks of complications and effects on the wider DCR pathway, such as time to proximal control. Without serious complication, they do not directly carry a material difference to the physiological benefit or burden.

Level of Balloon Deployment

The level of balloon deployment refers to the anatomical aortic segment targeted; these are divided into three zones.

- *Zone 1 REBOA*
  The balloon is contained entirely within the aortic segment between the left subclavian artery (SCA) and the coeliac axis. The principle patient group for the use of zone 1 REBOA is in those known or thought to have a sub-diaphragmatic visceral or torso vascular exsanguinating injury not amenable to more distal occlusion. For example, a patient with exsanguinating arterial bleeding from a liver laceration, as shown in Fig. 16.2(a). Primary survey identification of this patient group will be discussed later in this chapter. For the majority of adults, zone 1 is an approximately 20 cm length segment.
- *Zone 2 REBOA*
  The balloon is deployed across part or the full length of visceral aortic segment (the segment

that includes the coeliac axis to the lower renal artery). Currently, this is not considered a reasonable target for balloon deployment. This is because of:

- The real risk of dissection or thromboembolism into the arterial branch ostia caused by an abutting balloon. Such complications may cause organ infarction, multiorgan failure and death.
- The significant practical difficultly in accurately deploying a balloon in zone 2 without fluoroscopic or intravenous ultrasound (IVUS). Such an attempt would likely have significant opportunity cost in the time and effort required.

  In the majority of adults zone 2 is an approximately 3 cm length segment.

• *Zone 3 REBOA*

  The balloon is contained entirely within the infrarenal aortic segment. The key patient group for the use of zone 3 REBOA is in those patients known or thought to have exsanguinating bleeding from iliac arterial territory injury. For example, a patient with exsanguinating arterial bleeding from a pelvic fracture bleeding, as shown in Fig. 16.2(b). Primary survey identification of this patient group will be discussed later in this chapter. In the majority of adults zone 3 is an approximately 10 cm length segment.

Strategy of Occlusion

A strategy of occlusion refers to the targeting of an aortic pressure proximal to and/or distal to the balloon. There is no definition as to the level within the arterial tree that these pressure measurements are taken from. However, the proximal pressure measurement will usually be taken from a transducer connected to the lumen of an appropriate balloon mounted catheter or a radial arterial line, and the distal pressure measurement will usually be taken from the insertion sheath side port. In an alternative rare example, if the balloon mounted catheter has been inserted via an upper

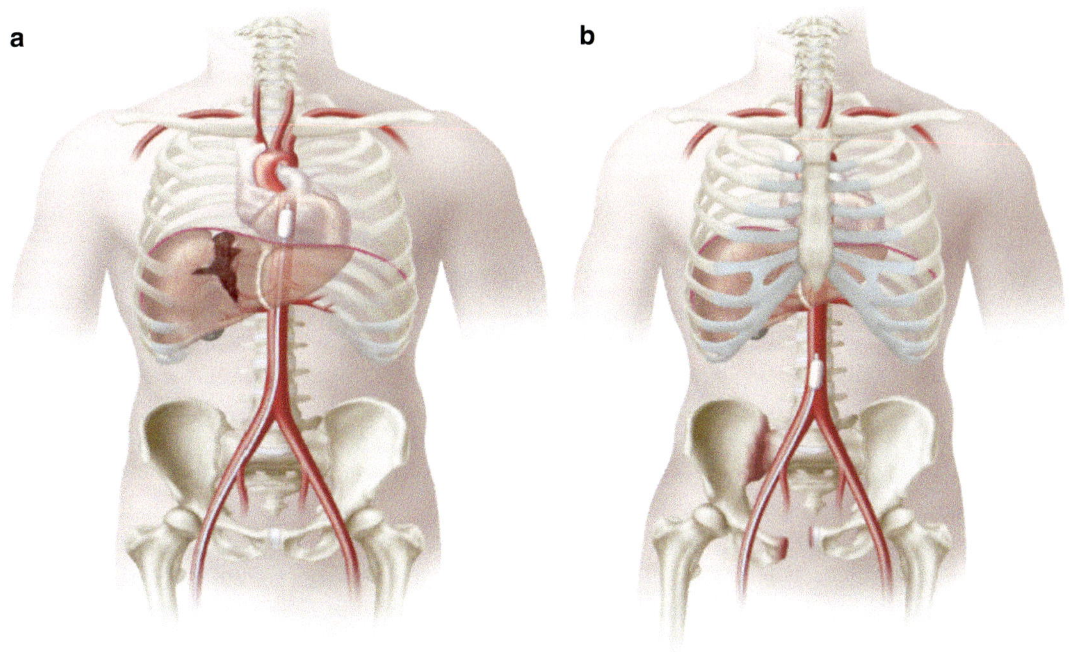

Fig. 16.2 Image courtesy of UK REBOA trial protocol. (**a**) Zone 1 balloon total occlusion for a liver laceration. (**b**) Zone 3 balloon total occlusion for pelvic fracture and associated significant vessel bleed

limb access site, then a transducer connected to the sheath side arm or radial arterial line will measure the proximal pressure, and a transducer connected to the balloon mounted catheter or a groin femoral access sheath will measure the distal pressure. It is not mandated to take invasive pressure measurements to use REBOA, however significant situational awareness is likely to be lost with regards to the ongoing resuscitation effort without such measurements. This cannot be recommended as usual practice in a hospital setting.

The quantity of fluid inflated into the balloon is not directly proportionate to the diameter of the balloon; the exact relationship is principally dependent on the construct of the occlusion balloon and the external forces acting on the balloon. The fluid volume inflated into the balloon not infrequently requires alteration as the resuscitation progresses to maintain the desired effect. The aorta is an elastic structure in healthy individuals and will distend, particularly in systole, as the patient is returned to euvolemia. The strategies described below may be combined together and do not have precise boundaries between one another. For example, on completion of total REBOA, gradually deflating the balloon before removal will retain a transient partial occlusive effect during deflation.

- *Total (aka complete or continuous)*
  A total REBOA strategy aims to achieve occlusion of an aortic segment. In other words the balloon forms a circumferential seal with an aortic wall segment, sustained throughout each cardiac cycle. This balloon strategy will provide, as an initial effect for an individual patient, the most reduced distal aortic flow and the greatest afterload increase of all the strategies. This is usually confirmed by loss of the biphasic arterial line signal distal to the balloon and a distal pressure drop to less than 15 mmHg. Note the pressure distal to total REBOA, in an active circulation state, is greater than 0 mmHg.
- *Partial*
  A partial REBOA strategy aims to deflate the balloon to ensure a degree of distal aortic flow to mitigate the ischemic and/or reperfusion hit, while not overtly compromising the benefit in reducing active bleeding. Based on blood pressure, this is clearly not an exact science. Furthermore, there is no consensus for precisely how this should be performed. Targeting a 5–10 mmHg increase from the total REBOA distal pressure may generate the optimal balance as suggested by the UK REBOA trial protocol [8]. There is evidence from the Japanese registry [11] that a median occlusion time of 58 min with partial REBOA was as well tolerated as a median occlusion time of 33 min for total REBOA.
- *Proximal target pressure only*
  Targeting a proximal pressure with REBOA without reference to the distal pressure potentially offers a similar effect to partial REBOA with the potential advantages of:
  - Maximising the distal flow at any given acceptable level of proximal perfusion
  - No mandated requirement to connect a second transducer to monitor the distal pressure.
- A systolic pressure just below the probable normal baseline systolic pressure is probably the optimal target, for example, 110 mmHg in a usually fit and well young adult. Therefore, as a successful resuscitation progresses, a greater distal flow may be achieved. This may or may not achieve a more optimal balance of blood loss against distal ischaemia/reperfusion.
- *Intermittent*
  The balloon is emptied entirely and re-inflated to a proximal or distal blood pressure target after a time interval. There is no consensus on the duration of the time interval. Intermittent REBOA aims to allow the maximum distal aortic flow at the risk of:
  - A critical perfusion loss to the carotid and coronary circulation as the proximal aortic pressure may significantly decrease on complete balloon deflation, depending on the resuscitative progress.
  - Clot disruption and blood loss from the distal arterial distribution at complete balloon deflation.

- Significant blood pressure variability between inflation and deflation; this may have a deleterious impact on organ function compared to a patient with the same average but more consistent blood pressure.

Intermittent REBOA may be performed intentionally. Alternatively, if total REBOA has been deflated after haemostasis is thought to have been achieved and there is a later sustained precipitous fall in blood pressure or additional distal bleeding requiring aortic control then the balloon may be reinflated thus mimicking an intermittent strategy.

Duration of Balloon Inflation

This refers to the length of time the balloon is inflated.

Consider with Level and Strategy of Occlusion

The triumvirate of duration of balloon inflation, level and strategy of occlusion are most informative when described together. Every minute of zone 1 complete occlusion is associated with a relatively significant incremental increase in morbidity and mortality, possibly in an exponential relationship. The UK REBOA trial [8, 9] currently recommends a target of less than 30 min of complete occlusion at zone 1, which is consistent with international consensus [12]. The UK REBOA trial also currently recommends a target of less than 90 min of complete occlusion at zone 3, whereas international consensus recommends targeting less than 60 min. Such targets are clearly not purporting to be "windows of safety" rather a reasonable balance of risk against giving enough time for adequate definitive control. A systematic review of the literature [13] in studies that recorded the occlusion time identified the average zone 1 time in 190 cases to be 58.5 min, and the average zone 3 time in 32 cases to be 68 min. The strategy of balloon occlusion was not recorded, nor was this data linked to outcome. Therefore, such mean duration times only provide an indication of published practice rather than guidance on conduct.

Environment of insertion

The environment of insertion refers to the physical space and surroundings that the REBOA catheter is inserted. This is most straightforwardly categorised into:

- *Pre-hospital REBOA*
  This is where REBOA is performed "in the field" rather than the hospital facility. London HEMS performed the world's first pre-hospital REBOA in 2014. Pre-hospital REBOA may be performed in very challenging environments and may confer a higher risk of access complications, prolonged ischaemic times and balloon dislodgement. Such interventions must balance the risk of prolonged scene times to complete the procedure (although noting that it is technically possible to perform REBOA at risk on a moving medical evacuation platform) against the benefits of shortening transfer times to hospital; where complications of REBOA may be fewer and a more comprehensive DCR package can be implemented. To ensure governance parity with the wider healthcare network, services employing pre-hospital REBOA must ensure that usage is subject to proper peer review, standardisation and morbidity and mortality analysis. The receiving trauma team should have specific training be able to manage an insitu REBOA in any network offering this as a prehospital intervention. A specific aide-memoire or checklist for trauma teams receiving a patient with REBOA in situ may reduce the risk of missed balloon dislodgment or catheter malposition.
- *In hospital REBOA*
  When performed in hospital, REBOA is probably most commonly initiated in the ED resuscitation trauma bay. However, the ongoing conduct of REBOA may then move to various locations in the hospital depending on resuscitation and definitive haemorrhage control imperatives. Outcomes and complication profiles from in hospital REBOA may be significantly different to pre-hospital REBOA within the same regional service. For example, (1)

pre-hospital REBOA may allow a sicker group of patients, who would have otherwise have died, reach hospital and (2) accessing the femoral artery may be more challenging in the pre-hospital space in terms of lighting, equipment specification and operator ergonomics.

Access Type

Endovascular balloon catheters are almost exclusively deployed via a sheath. It is possible to cut down onto an artery, gain proximal and distal control, perform an arteriotomy and direct the catheter into the artery without a sheath. Indeed, the first reported cases of REBOA in trauma by Hughes were performed by such a technique [14]. However, arterial access sheaths:

- Often have a haemostatic valve to the main lumen that will limit blood loss
- Provide atraumatic navigation for catheters and guidewires into the lumen (for example, avoiding traumatising the intima opposite the arteriotomy)
- Generally allow invasive pressure monitoring via the sheath side arm with a catheter and/or guidewire in situ. This is particularly useful in REBOA in providing more options and accuracy for the strategy of occlusion.

Arterial access for REBOA is broadly categorised into:

- *Percutaneous access*
  The sheath access (usually in the CFA segment) is inserted directly through the skin and soft tissues into the artery. This is probably most often done under ultrasound guidance to mitigate the risk of malposition or inadvertent vessel injury. A subsequent cut down for sheath removal with or without embolectomy may be required. In most circumstances, percutaneously inserted sheaths of 8 French (F) gauge or smaller do not routinely require a formal arteriotomy closure; either with a percutaneous closure device or cut down and surgical closure. Pressing on the sheath exit site for 3 min multiplied by the French gauge is usually sufficient. For example, approximately 20 min following removal of a 7F sheath, graduating from very firm pressure to lighter pressure during this time period. Failure to establish haemostasis in these circumstances will lead to a groin haematoma and possibly an arterial pseudoaneurysm. A patient with a significant trauma associated coagulopathy may need formal arteriotomy closure following a 7F or 8F sheath. Unless there are hostile access reasons in the groin (e.g. very significant subcutaneous fat, heavily calcified femoral artery), percutaneous access is likely to be the optimal and first line option.
- *Open Access*
  The sheath access is inserted under direct vision into the exposed artery; usually by a cut down onto the CFA segment. Exposing the CFA segment in the groin is not without risk of injury to the common femoral vein (rarely potentially life-threatening bleeding). Percutaneous access has significantly fewer wound complications than open access. Depending on the orientation of the arterial exposure wound it may be beneficial to insert the sheath through the skin, into the exposure wound and then into the arterial segment. Such an approach in selected patients will allow a more appropriate angle of approach to the artery (not confined by the wound edges) and provide more stability to the sheath.

A recent systematic review [13] of the published literature identified 310 percutaneous and 79 cut downs were performed in providing access for REBOA. Interestingly, some of the large matched cohort studies [15], while not recording proportions of access type, estimated a 50:50 split in usage.

Access Location

The arterial segment for sheath access is likely to be defined by the department SOP or protocol. All protocols are likely to use the Common Femoral Artery (CFA) segment as the first line.

If a trauma team is able to use upper body access locations then this gives more flexibility to the resuscitation effort. Different arterial segments have different complication profiles in terms of the region they perfuse. Access locations for REBOA can be broadly categorised to:

- *CFA*
  REBOA sheath access is almost exclusively sited into the CFA segment, thus providing retrograde access into the aorta via the external and common iliac artery. A systematic literature review [13] identified of all the published cases of REBOA used for trauma, where the access location was specified; 388 out of 390 were via the CFA.
- *Brachial Artery*
  Technically the brachial artery can be used for access. However, this will need to be done over a guidewire under fluoroscopy (to avoid aortic arch injury or catheter misdirection) and requires an expert, practiced endovascular skillset. These are significant limitations in time critical, unplanned, circumstances. The brachial artery segment is generally optimally accessed immediately above the biceps tendon. It's potential use is where the CFA segments do not provide suitable access, for example, if there is suspected or known discontinuity to both iliac vessels. However, in such circumstances it is very likely that an alternative strategy to REBOA will be more appropriate. It is worth noting that the average adult brachial artery is approximately 4–5 mm in diameter. In contrast, the average CFA is 7–8 mm in diameter—brachial access may therefore confer a higher risk of distal flow compromise especially from larger sheaths.
- *Other*
  Examples of other balloon catheter access points include intra laparotomy (iliac or aorta) and axillary. There is one recorded case of carotid access in the literature [13]. De-novo carotid access independently confers a higher risk of stroke and death. It is very unlikely that REBOA via carotid access can ever be justified.

Type of Balloon Catheter

There are many different types of balloon catheters that have been used to perform REBOA. Table 16.1 lists most currently used catheters with their principle advantages and disadvantages. This table:

- Aims to provide an insight into how balloon catheter selection may impact on the conduct of REBOA
- Is not a recommendation for an particular balloon catheter
- Cannot be relied on for reference values; operators should refer to the instructions for use (IFUs) issued with any particular device
- Does not contain all data on the catheters (for example: working length, catheter French guage, bending stiffness)

Risk Analysis for REBOA

With similarity to other resuscitative interventions, meaningful patient selection for REBOA will depend on an appraisal of the risk and benefit it confers against the alternative strategy or strategies considered by the trauma team. The alternative strategy is likely to be to proceed to damage control laparotomy without REBOA; where the options for open aortic control are weighted (see Decision Making in Damage Control Surgery chapter). It is worth noting that risk in these circumstances is inclusive of opportunity cost and that benefit is probably more easily considered as risk reduction.

Key Points
Risk analysis to insert a balloon catheter and inflate the balloon utilises slow (deliberate) thinking decision making in order to ensure an optimal decision based on the available information.

Table 16.1 Comparison of REBOA catheters

Balloon catheter	Manufacturer	Minimal sheath access[a]	Effective Catheter length	Maximum balloon diameter and compliance	Volume of inflation	Wire diameter mandated	Advantages	Disadvantages	Comment
ER-REBOA™ catheter	Prytime Medical™, Texas	7F	72 cm	32 mm Compliant	24 ml	N/A	• Positioned accurately by length of insertion from CFA sheath entry point (in both adult male or female torsos) and designed to not require zonal confirmation on imaging. • Length marks on one side catheter to guide insertion length. • Capability to measure pressure proximal to balloon via catheter lumen. • No guidewire needed which is one less step for REBOA. Has looped tip to aid atraumatic positioning. • Radiopaque marker bands to confirm balloon position with fluoroscopy.	• Not guidewire compatible: cannot use to position wire across aortic lesion already crossed. • Expensive.	• Straightforward to use, seemingly low catheter insertion complication profile and excellent training facilitation have made this the first choice of REBOA catheter for those trauma centres participating in the UK-REBOA trial. • 8Fr sheath access probably gives more reliable distal arterial signal.

ER-REBOA™ plus catheter	Prytime Medical™, Texas	7F	72 cm	32 mm Complaint	24 ml	N/A	• Advantages as per ER-REBOA™ catheter • Length marks on both sides of the catheter, with zonal markers, to guide insertion length. • No guidewire needed, however 0.025″ guidewire compatible to allow wire. This allows positioning of an aortic guidewire and subsequent endovascular manoeuvres. • Peel away sheath is pre-packaged over the balloon to reduce preparation time.	• Most expensive catheter.	• Next generation of the ER-REBOA™ catheter.
Coda® LP Balloon catheter	Cook® Medical, Ireland	12F	120 cm	32 mm Semi-compliant	40 ml	0.035″	• Very inexpensive. • Radiopaque marker bands to confirm balloon position with fluoroscopy.	• Requires positioning over a guidewire. This is: (1) More cumbersome as the protruding wire end needs to be retrievable throughout catheter insertion (2) An additional step. • Flexible catheter, therefore requires either long sheath or ridged wire to maintain position and prevent loop formation.	• The initial London HEMS pre-hospital REBOA programme used a Coda® catheter. The team managed to overcome the wire challenges in difficult environments.

(continued)

Table 16.1 (continued)

Balloon catheter	Manufacturer	Minimal sheath access[a]	Effective Catheter length	Maximum balloon diameter and compliance	Volume of inflation	Wire diameter mandated	Advantages	Disadvantages	Comment
Reliant™ Stent Graft Balloon catheter	Medtronic, Inc., California	12F	100 cm	46 mm compliant	60 ml	0.038″ or smaller	• Inexpensive. • Radiopaque marker bands to confirm balloon position with fluoroscopy.	• Requires positioning over a guidewire (see above for disadvantages). • Flexible catheter, therefore requires either long sheath or sufficiently ridged wire to maintain position and prevent loop formation.	
Rescue Balloon™ catheter	Tokai Medical Products, Japan	7F	80 cm	40 mm compliant	24 ml	0.025″	• Inexpensive. • Radiopaque tip and marker bands to confirm balloon position with fluoroscopy.	• Requires stiff stylet wire to be inserted after catheter insertion, before balloon inflation otherwise significant increased risk of balloon migration.	Has recently received (2020) CE approval for European use.
ResQ™ occlusion balloon catheter	QXMédical, Roseville, MN	11F	67 cm	38 mm compliant	30 ml	0.035″	• Inexpensive. • Radiopaque marker bands to confirm balloon position with fluoroscopy.	• Requires positioning over a guidewire (see above for disadvantages). However, given catheter length shorter a more manageable wire can be used.	

F = French. (F = times 3 the diameter of the catheter in mm; i.e., approximately the catheter outer circumfrence in mm. Therefore, 1F = 1/3 mm diameter catheter with approximately 1 mm circumference)

[a]For some catheters and sheath combinations, operators may find one French size greater than the minimum stated allows (1) a more reliable pressure transduction from side port and (2) an easier complete withdrawal of the balloon catheter when REBOA finished.

Importantly, such an analysis will be partly dependent on the readiness to deploy the balloon catheter, in other words the degree of further action required to perform REBOA.

Escalation of Readiness for REBOA

Full readiness to perform REBOA is at the end point of: suitable arterial access acquired, the REBOA plan is articulated and the balloon catheter system is prepared for insertion. Such readiness will:

1. Reduce the time between the definitive decision to use REBOA and the deployment of the balloon in the appropriate zone. Thus there is less opportunity cost of REBOA compared to an alternative strategy at the point of the definitive decision.
2. Have "sunk costs" of access risk. In other words, the risk from attempting access and the risk of failing to achieve access will not need to be considered in the decision to perform REBOA as access will already have been achieved.

Therefore, while not lessening the overall risk, a full or higher level of readiness will make the decision to perform REBOA less complex and more responsive to the dynamic situation. Escalation towards such readiness is conducted from the pre-alert of the patient's arrival though to the primary survey and resuscitation phase. It is thus integrated into the DCR process and can be achieved mostly by rapid thinking and minimal bandwidth expenditure, certainly in a well rehearsed team. Figure 16.3 schematically represents the rapid thinking readiness escalation process in the yellow boxes and the slow thinking risk analysis of whether to proceed with balloon catheter insertion and inflation in the blue box.

Readiness should be discontinued if REBOA is no longer a reasonable prospect due to:

- The current resuscitation efforts ending due to patient death, futility or the patient is sufficiently euvolemic without evidence of active bleeding, or
- The patient has been transferred to immediate definitive haemorrhage control; either surgical, endovascular or hybrid, or
- Aortic control has been achieved by extra luminal means

Table 16.2 explains the risk analysis process of readiness in more detail giving examples of where thresholds are met to perform the actions.

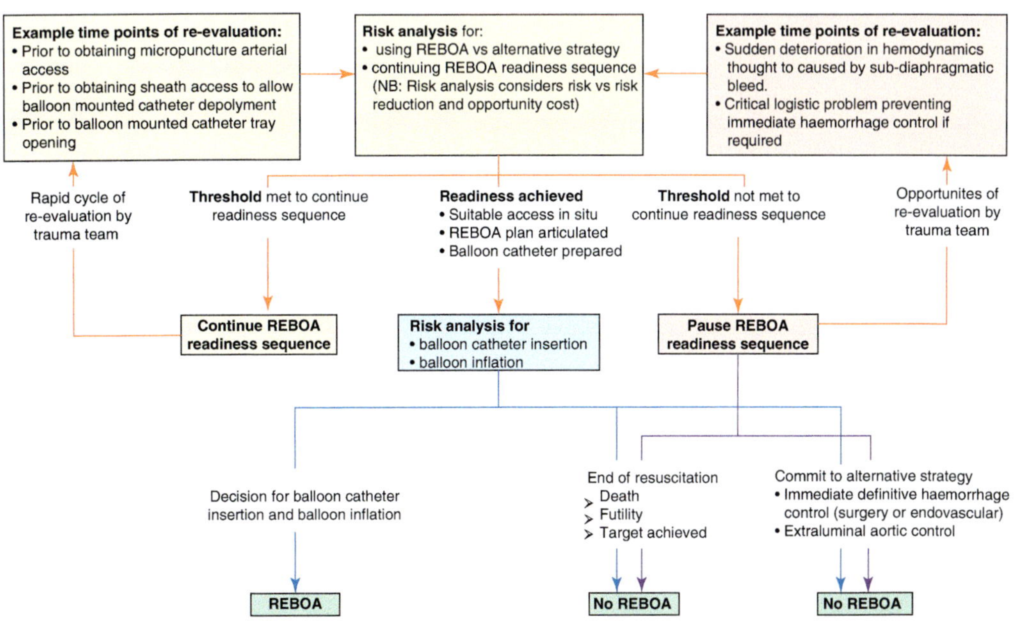

Fig. 16.3 REBOA readiness escalation process

Table 16.2 Example of risk analysis for escalation of readiness for REBOA

Phase	Actions	Risk and opportunity cost of action	Mitigation of risk	Benefit (risk reduction) of action	Example of threshold to make decision for action
Prepare	Ready Ultrasound (US) machine	• This preparation is likely to be part of the standard primary survey protocol for a major trauma patient and therefore should not carry additional risk or opportunity cost. • Most US machines carry the risk of a uncharged battery and therefore sudden loss of function at a critical stage.	Departmental daily functionality checks for US and ensure the battery has been appropriately charged prior to use.	Reduces the opportunity cost of spending time readying the US machine for: – eFAST – sheath access at a more critical phase of the resuscitation.	On pre-alert for major trauma patient.
	Ready mobile radiography (if trauma team intend to use)	• If this readiness is part of the standard primary survey protocol for such a major trauma patient then no additional risk or opportunity cost will be carried. • If radiography is not normally used as a primary survey adjunct then this rare event may carry small frictions in choreography and communication with the wider team.	Include logistics and choreography of radiographs in major trauma team training simulation.	Reduces the opportunity cost of spending time readying mobile radiology for: – The primary survey adjunct investigations (chest and pelvic radiographs) – For guidewire fluoroscopy.	On pre-alert for major trauma patient.
	Ensure all REBOA kit available, including: – local anaesthetic unless already appropriately analgised and/or unaware – trolley to set up kit	The individual allocated to do this will potentially lose situational awareness (SA) of the trauma team.	• If possible, ED should call forward the trauma team in advance of a code red patient; in sufficient time for all preparation and briefing (with a fudge factor for kit malfunction). This may need a call more than 10 min before the patient is due to arrive. • Allow the staff member conducting this step to regain SA on return, possibly through a pre-patient arrival brief.	If done prior to patient arrival reduces risk of: – Loss of SA – Opportunity cost of spending time setting up at a more critical phase of the resuscitation.	• On pre-alert for major trauma patient in haemodynamic shock or • On pre-alert for code red patient.

Table 16.2 (continued)

Phase	Actions	Risk and opportunity cost of action	Mitigation of risk	Benefit (risk reduction) of action	Example of threshold to make decision for action
	Ready arterial pressure transducers ×2	Opportunity cost: this action will need some additional preparation time and has a lower priority than, for example, preparation of airway management.		• If done prior to patient arrival reduces risk of: – Loss of SA – Opportunity cost of spending time setting upat a more critical phase of the active resuscitation. • There is a reasonable chance that at least one arterial pressure transducer may be used regardless of REBOA.	• On pre-alert for major trauma patient in haemodynamic shock or • On pre-alert for code red patient.
	Ready and open access kit onto suitable preparation trolley	• Need for space allocation; this could be outside or slightly away from the resuscitation bay • Need for about 5 min of time to set up which may cause a loss of SA by the staff member responsible for set up		• If done prior to patient arrival reduces risk of: – Loss of SA – Opportunity cost of spending time setting upat a more critical phase of the active resuscitation. • Laying out the access kit in an immediately accessible format probably: – Makes the technical aspect of procedure much easier – Gives higher chance of maintaining relative sterility in stressful circumstances.	<u>Any of:</u> • On pre-alert for code red patient if consistent with exsanguinating haemorrhage. • ATMIST handover and patient consistent with exsanguinating haemorrhage. • At primary survey if haemodynamically shocked and no obvious absolute contraindication for REBOA.

(continued)

Table 16.2 (continued)

Phase	Actions	Risk and opportunity cost of action	Mitigation of risk	Benefit (risk reduction) of action	Example of threshold to make decision for action
Access	Obtain micropuncture access (e.g. 4F sheath) if percutaneous access intended	• Arterial line access complications (see below). Although the purpose of micropuncture is to mitigate these risks, these access risks are still carried to a degree • Time spent gaining access by an appropriately trained healthcare provider; who could be otherwise performing a more essential task (opportunity cost) • Time spent gaining access that could otherwise be spent escalating the patient to definitive haemorrhage control	• Perform all percutaneous arterial access under US guidance where possible • Escalating readiness via micropuncture access probably reduces the arterial access risk as there is an additional assurance the sheath is in the lumen prior to attempted larger sheath entry.	• If trajectory looks likely for REBOA then early arterial access: – Negates the unknown quantity of access complications or inability to achieve access at a more complex DCR period – Negates the opportunity cost of trying to gain access while there is a window to escalate to definitive haemorrhage control.	Both of: • Patient deemed haemodynamically shocked on primary survey (this can rapidly be established if the performs horizontal resuscitation and assessment). • No contra indication for ipsilateral balloon mounted catheter.
	Upsize access (e.g. 4F to a 7F sheath) to allow deployment of balloon mounted catheter. OR Obtain de-novo access: – percutaneous sheath – open cut down and sheathin order to allow deployment of balloon mounted catheter.	Arterial access complications These are significantly affected by patient factors such as pre-existing arterial disease and subcutaneous tissue covering. The chief complications to consider are: • Venous injury/ arterial injury with haemorrhage that cannot be managed by direct pressure • Accidental venous cannulation • Limb ischaemia or infarction from: – Artery dissection(including proximal extension) and sequelae – Arterial spasm around sheath – Thromboembolism – Air embolism	• The first choice CFA access site should be contralateral to any significant lower limb injury. Lower limb injury is not an absolute contraindication to sheath insertion, however if required then: – Aim for sheath removal – as early as possible – Anticipate an additional ischaemic hit to the leg from CFA arterial spasm.	• Advantages of access independent to REBOA: – Provides an invasive arterial – Pressure measurement to guide resuscitation – If performed in CFA segment then this will likely give a more consistent pressure measurement than the usual alternative of radial artery access.	All of: 1. Met the requirements for micropuncture access (whether or not a microsheath in situ). 2. None of the following **absolute contraindication** for REBOA: – Cardiac tamponade – Known aortic injury that is likely to convert to a propagating aortic dissection or full thickness laceration – Life-threatening intra-thoracic bleeding. 3. On the balance of probabilities will receive REBOA unless circumstances improve significantly.

Table 16.2 (continued)

Phase	Actions	Risk and opportunity cost of action	Mitigation of risk	Benefit (risk reduction) of action	Example of threshold to make decision for action
		• Generating surgical needs, for example: – Infection requiring surgical intervention – Patch angioplasty – Arterial bypass – Amputation • Generally later presenting complications that may need surgery – Stenosis of artery – Pseudoaneurysm – AV fistula Note: The addition of a serious access complication may contribute to the patient's death	• Consider setting a time threshold and attempt number threshold for access (for example; the healthcare provider should discontinue further access attempts at a particular groin if more than 3 access attempts are unsuccessful or the time spent on trying to achieve access exceeds 5–10 min). This will hopefully reduce the risk of flailing with attempting access and causing arterial injury without benefit.		
		• Depending on sheath size and circumstance, the sheath access site may need: – A percutaneous vascular closure device – A subsequent open cut down onto the artery to remove the sheath and close the arteriotomy. Opportunity costs • Time spent gaining access by an appropriately trained health care provider; who could be otherwise performing a more essential task. • Time spent gaining access that could otherwise be spent escalating the patient to definitive haemorrhage control.			

(continued)

Table 16.2 (continued)

Phase	Actions	Risk and opportunity cost of action	Mitigation of risk	Benefit (risk reduction) of action	Example of threshold to make decision for action
		Concurrent injury exacerbation • In order to gain adequate views and space for access into the CFA an in situ pelvic binder (depending on its' construct) will probably need to – have a wedge cut from its fabric over the CFA region while maintaining the pelvic binder functionor – be removed with manual stabilisation of the pelvis in place This may compromise the pelvic stabilisation with result bleeding. • If there is a lower limb injury ischaemia associated with sheath insertion (eg arterial spasm) may convert a salvageable limb into an unsalvageable limb or other less favourable outcome.			

Table 16.2 (continued)

Phase	Actions	Risk and opportunity cost of action	Mitigation of risk	Benefit (risk reduction) of action	Example of threshold to make decision for action
Ready REBOA plan	Decide on: • initial zone for balloon (1 or 3) • initial balloon strategy	• Potential distraction from other decision making. • Additional bandwidth required. • Making decision too early may risk needing to rethink decision if there is a material change in the patients' circumstances prior to balloon inflation.	• Trauma team familiarity with the effect and rationale of aortic occlusion; trauma team simulation training likely to help with this.	By planning this decision, it probably allows the decision to be made in less stressful circumstances, with improved bandwidth reserve and situational awareness compared to making the decision at the point of balloon catheter insertion. This may therefore increase the probability of making a "better decision".	Following primary survey (including mechanism of injury analysis) and eFAST, where approximate anatomical level(s) of likely ongoing bleeding established.
	Exit strategy Once REBOA in situ the decision is usually between OT or CT (corresponding to first key decision point; KDP1 discussed in chapter 30_6.1)	This decision making is largely predicated by the zone and strategy of REBOA already identified in the preceding step. For example, a total zone 1 REBOA is probably less likely to survive a move to CT than to the OT. Therefore, the exit strategy is unlikely to confer much additional cognitive effort by the team and the risk and opportunity cost should be minimal. The exit strategy is effectively the output of KDP1.		A balloon inflation should not be seen as an end in itself. A temporarily lower aortic pressure may be the marginal gain required to trigger clot formation. However, the distal ischaemic/reperfusion sequelae clock starts at balloon inflation and this precious time should not be spent on decisions that could have been made pre-emptively.	As part of KDP1.

(continued)

Table 16.2 (continued)

Phase	Actions	Risk and opportunity cost of action	Mitigation of risk	Benefit (risk reduction) of action	Example of threshold to make decision for action
Ready REBOA catheter	Open balloon catheter tray	Cost of balloon catheter kit (may cost >£2000).	Ensure Trauma Team Leader confirms with the other trauma team members that the decision to proceed to REBOA is in accordance with plan.	• Allows immediate catheter use when a decision for REBOA is made • Note: The short time interval between readying the REBOA kit and deploying the balloon once the preceding readiness sequence steps have occurred means that there may be minimal advantage in doing this before a clear decision on REBOA has been taken.	Either: • At the decision to proceed to REBOA (requires risk analysis for balloon catheter insertion and inflation) Or • Concurrent to REBOA planning (above).
	• Prepare balloon mounted catheter for insertion (for example, if using ER-REBOA™ catheter: flush lumens and measure zone 1 and zone 3 distances, then standby to connect arterial pressure transducers). • Ready guidewire for insertion if required for balloon deployment.	• Time (balancing the opportunity cost) and an appropriately trained operator are required. • It is possible to damage a balloon prior to insertion if not handled with care. • Kit may desterilise if accidently falls or hangs off trolley.	• Ensure preparation trolley is sufficiently large to accommodate all kit. • A REBOA assistant can manage the kit trolley.		As soon as balloon catheter kit opened.

Within each phase the actions are considered in an escalatory order; although not all actions (for example, micropuncture access) are necessarily needed to reach the final step. The risk analysis of whether the patient has an injury profile amenable to aortic balloon inflation is clearly vital and concurrent
SA Situational Awareness, *US* Ultrasound, *OT* Operating Theatre

This process begins with the initiation of readiness on the pre-alert of a major trauma patient's arrival, such steps can be initiated en masse if the patient arrives in ED without warning. Although full readiness is achieved with catheter preparation, the financial cost of an opened and unused expensive balloon catheter is difficult to justify. Therefore, while it may be reasonable to move to full readiness with a lesser expensive balloon catheter, this readiness step may be better done in conjunction with a deliberate decision to perform REBOA if the team is using the more expensive balloon catheters. These risk analyses deliberately do not consider access type, access location, type of balloon catheter and environment of insertion. Such decisions are most likely to be pre-emptively made based on the resources available, the skill set of the operators and institutional protocol or experience.

Rationale to Gain Femoral Access with REBOA Decision Not Yet Made

Access for REBOA is not the exclusive reason to gain femoral arterial access. Monitoring the blood pressure in sick major trauma patients is best performed by invasive arterial lines. This is often via the radial artery, although there is evidence that radial arterial cannulation has a higher failure rate than femoral [16]. There is also evidence from non-trauma critically ill patients that there are significant differences in invasively monitored blood pressures between radial and femoral lines in the same patient [17–22]. This difference increases as the amount of vasoconstriction increases, and so the central arterial pressure of a hypotensive trauma patient may be higher than that displayed by an under-reading radial arterial line. Establishing femoral access for arterial pressure monitoring early in the patient's pathway is therefore a useful adjunct to resuscitation. To minimise the complication rate of such arterial access, a microsheath (e.g. 4F) should be used; a smaller gauge causes less of an injury to the artery and a femoral artery is less likely to circumferentially seal with the sheath, which would potentially cause limb ischaemia. If the patient subsequently requires further readiness for REBOA then the access may be straightforwardly upsized to a larger French gauge sheath by the following steps:

1. Insert an access guidewire (e.g. J tipped 0.035 inch).
2. Full withdrawal of the original access sheath with groin pressure onto the proximal CFA segment to minimise haematoma formation.
3. Enlarge the skin entry wound if required under local anaesthetic. This is particularly important if upsizing to a much larger French gauge.
4. Insert a larger sheath (mounted on obturator/introducer) that is compatible with the selected balloon catheter.
5. Remove access guidewire and obturator.
6. Aspirate and heparin-saline flush of the sheath side port.

Specific Injuries Affecting Access Considerations

When deciding on the site of access the trauma team must consider factors that may exacerbate concurrent injuries or make balloon catheter navigation difficult or impossible to achieve. These are:

- Ipsilateral limb injury.
  This is a relative contraindication to arterial access and will be dependent on the extent of the limb injury in the context of the overall injury burden. It is possible, for example, to place CFA access ipsilateral to a comminuted open knee fracture without appreciable adverse consequences. However, if access is sited ipsilateral to a significant downstream arterial injury or mangled limb and the same limb subsequently requires major amputation, it will probably not be possible to rule out that the access contributed to the amputation or a higher level of amputation than would otherwise have been needed. In such situations, the more straightforward method of risk analysis will be to assume access will precipitate limb sacrifice or a higher level amputation. Therefore sheath access for REBOA ipsilateral to a significant downstream arterial injury will only be justified if there is no reasonable alternative to save the patient's life. It should be noted that causing a lower limb infarction also presents a risk to life either through the ischaemic hit or subsequent additional surgical burden in an already very sick patient.
- Iliac arterial injury.
  This may be:
  - Presumed. For example, an pulseless groin with a penetrating ipsilateral iliac fossa injury.
  - Known. For example, through definitive identification on CTA imaging or intraoperative direct visualisation.

In either circumstance, siting ipsilateral access and/or attempting to navigate a guidewire or balloon catheter across an iliac injury carries very significant risk. Specifically, a quiescent, manageable, injury may be converted into active life-threatening bleeding or a viable lower limb may be converted into a life-threatening non-viable lower limb. In certain circumstances, such a risk may be sufficiently low as to be justifiable if performed by a highly experienced operator who first crosses the lesion using a guidewire under detailed fluoroscopy. Such an undertaking is not appropriate in a conventional ED resuscitation bay.

- Pelvic binder in situ
  Pelvic binders can save lives by reducing the pelvic volume through circumferential compression and therefore allowing pelvic clot stabilisation. A pelvic binder lies at the level of the greater trochanters, unfortunately significantly obstructing CFA access. In the vast majority of major trauma patients requiring REBOA attempting balloon catheter navigation from upper limb/ torso sites is impractical. Therefore, it is probably reasonable to remove the pelvic binder, maintain manual pelvic stabilisation and prioritise proximal control in the following circumstances:
  - Where life threatening pelvic bleeding appears active during primary survey despite initial resuscitative efforts including with a pelvic binder In situ as this is less likely to stop spontaneously.
  - Evidence of life threatening sub diaphragmatic abdominal bleeding regardless of pelvic injury

Once access is gained the pelvic binder can usually be reapplied. It is also occasionally possible to cut a wedge of material from some pelvic binder constructs without significantly compromising their effectiveness, while adequately exposing the CFA for access. Attempting CFA access with compromised views from an in situ pelvic binder should be avoided. There is a greater risk of flailing at a time critical phase and potentially compromising the skin entry point—displacing the operator to an accidental SFA or distal EIA access.

Risk Analysis for Conduct of REBOA

Decision making as to whether or not to use REBOA, optimally involves a focused risk analysis that considers:

1. Insertion of the balloon catheter via the accessed arterial system into the aorta, including guidewire insertion if required.
2. Inflation of the balloon in the aortic lumen.

Whether to proceed with these two actions is likely to be most efficiently decided by coupling their risk analysis (risk, risk reduction, opportunity cost) rather than considering them separately. This process is outlined at Table 16.3 and forms the basis for the deliberate decision making (slow thinking) for the use of REBOA. This decision making will likely be optimised by a brief team discussion. With familiarity of the process and using time during the initial DCR to beginning weighing the risks and merits, a decision may be made, discussed and shared within about 30 s. It is certainly not practical to use Table 16.3 as a step by step aide memoire in time critical circumstances.

There may be some circumstances where the trauma team decide to insert the balloon catheter without immediate balloon inflation, for example, reserving balloon inflation for progressive patient deterioration or for further trauma team re-assessment. However, catheter insertion via a femoral sheath is likely to be rapid whether or not a guidewire is required; the time benefit is very marginal. The patient circumstances are unlikely to have sufficiently changed during the time required for insertion to merit a re-assessment. Inserting a balloon catheter for it not to be used will have carried patient risk for no discernible benefit. Therefore the standard protocol should be to only insert a balloon catheter if there is the immediate intent to inflate the balloon. It is not clear whether it is possible to justify a rare exception to this rule in terms of mitigating the risk of transfer through the hospital of an actively bleeding patient using an in-situ uninflated aortic balloon catheter.

Table 16.3 Risk analysis for conduct of REBOA

Actions	Risk and opportunity cost of actions	Mitigations of risk	Benefit (risk reduction) of actions
Insert balloon catheter to correct zone	<u>Balloon catheter insertion complications</u> (Including use of guidewire): • Vessel dissection including causing stroke • Rupture of femoral/iliac/aortic vessel segments (or cava if miss-sited into venous system) • Catheter exit from vessel laceration • Cannulation of aorto/iliac/vessel side branch Consequences of these complications range from asymptomatic self-correcting, through to rapid irretrievable death. <u>Catheter at incorrect arterial aortic zone</u> Due to: • Insertion issue: fluoroscopic/ US misinterpretation (if used), mismeasurement to the correct zone, balloon migration, catheter coiling or a catheter insertion complication. • Catheter migration or slippage from the force of aortic pressure. • If the balloon catheter is secured (fixation is advised to avoid slippage and free an otherwise fixed hand) and a decision is made to alter the zone level, then time will be required to unfasten or otherwise unsecure the catheter and resecure it at the appropriate level.	<u>Balloon catheter insertion complications</u> • Ensure catheter not sited via potential injured vessel segment (for example, avoid siting via a left CFA access if there is a LIF penetrating wound). • Catheters can cross a dissected aortic segment without exacerbating an injury. However, if an aortic and/or iliac dissection is known (e.g. post CTA) or suspected then the trauma team will need to decide whether this risk is justifiable. There is no straightforward algorithm to make such a decision. <u>Catheter at incorrect arterial aortic zone</u> • Once catheter is at the correct zone, ensure it is fixed and either: – marked or – the insertion measurement recorded so that any slippage is recognised • The sheath and/ or guidewire insertion should also be monitored for slippage particularly if the balloon mounted catheter system relies on such structural support to maintain position.	Highest level of readiness prior to a decision for balloon distension. However, for reasons described in the main text, balloon distension should be immediate if sited correctly.

(continued)

Table 16.3 (continued)

Actions	Risk and opportunity cost of actions	Mitigations of risk	Benefit (risk reduction) of actions
Inflation of Balloon accounting for the following parameters: 1. Level • Zone 1 REBOA • Zone 3 REBOA 2. Duration "Clock on" time monitoring 3. Strategy of occlusion • Total • Partial • Proximal target pressure only • Intermittent	Incorrect arterial segment/aortic zone For reasons described in the row above. Inflation of the balloon in these circumstances may exacerbate the catheter insertion complications described above. For example, balloon catheter slippage is far more likely if unsecured. Aortic occlusion risks • An ischemic and subsequent reperfusion hit to the following distributions: – Zone 3: bilateral common iliac segment distribution +/-IMA and lower lumbar arteries. – Zone 1: Zone 3 distribution as above + the visceral aortic segment, gonadal, IMA and lumbar arteries. Every additional minute of zone 1 total occlusion is likely to materially affect the mortality and morbidity. Visceral organ perfusion compromise may cause: MOF AKI Liver dysfunction Bowel ischaemia or infarction requiring surgical intervention • Cardiac stroke volume reduction from increased afterload (in many circumstances this may not confer a risk). • ARDS • Paraplegia: permanent or temporary. For example from spinal cord ischaemia. The range of consequences from these complications are asymptomatic self resolving through to rapid irretrievable death. Balloon rupture This may be: • Recognised: The team will need to decide whether to: – insert a further balloon catheter (most likely course of action), this may take an additional minimal 2–3 min to source and prepare another catheter. – Pursue an alternative strategy, given the "sunk costs" into REBOA the trauma team are less likely to pursue this course of action. • Unrecognised: The risk this presents will be dependent on the burden of injury, the duration the ruptured balloon is unrecognised and/or the efficiency of ongoing DCR. Unintended consequences • Relating to increased bleeding from the arterial tree proximal to the balloon. This may range from a trivial affect through to triggering exsanguinating haemorrhage or worsening cardiac tamponade. Such risks may lead to death or the need for a resuscitative thoracotomy or other open thoracic or junctional surgical access procedure.	Incorrect arterial segment/ zone It is useful to keep a running record of the: – Catheter insertion length – Volume in balloon – Time balloon inflated As these parameters may help to risk stratify prognosis or risk of organ failure/ dysfunction. Aortic occlusion risks • The team should target the shortest time possible in any particular zone. • A shared mental model that every minute of aortic balloon inflation potential contributes to a compromise or potentially fatal ischaemic sequelae hit should be held. This probably helps drive sufficient urgency to establish adequate definitive haemorrhage control. • For zone 1 inflation, the team should target no more than 30 min of total occlusion. It may be possible to extended this to more than 60 min without fatal consequences if performed with a strategy that allows sufficient distal flow. • Concurrent efficient DCR including infusion of warmed blood products should be performed to ensure no exacerbation of hit due insufficient resuscitative effort. • The team should have a rationale (supported were required by eFAST or pelvic X-ray) for the zone of occlusion, to avoid an unnecessary zone 1 occlusion Balloon rupture Maintain an index of suspicion for balloon rupture; monitor the arterial pressure transducer connected above and below the balloon, if – unintendingly equivalent and – no resistance on balloon inflation then presume balloon rupture. Unintended consequences • As stated previously, do not perform REBOA with an absolute contraindication. Where there is a justifiable risk of initiating non-compressible exsanguinating bleeding from the proximal arterial system or cardiac tamponade from aortic balloon inflation then do not perform REBOA, unless this risk is deemed significantly mitigated by the capability to perform an immediate resuscitative thoracotomy.	Inflating the balloon will likely cause a reduction in blood loss in the distal distribution and reduce the associated sequelae of such blood loss. Part of the reduced blood loss may result from reduced distal pressure allowing clot formation—"the first clot is the best clot". In circumstances where the alternative strategy is open DTA or infra renal aortic occlusion then REBOA avoids the surgical exposure related risks these procedures carry (unless, for example, a resuscitative thoracotomy is subsequently needed). These avoided risks for open DTA occlusion via a thoracotomy include: • Cardiac laceration • Descending thoracic aortic injury or aortic branch injury • Oesophageal injury • Lung injury including a bronchopleural fistula • Later chest wall and pleural complications (that may require surgical intervention) such as empyema, sternal non-union, wound infection, rib fractures. For clarity, risks that are likely equivocal regardless of whether occlusion is external or intraluminal (REBOA) include: • Ischaemic and re-profusion hit downstream to the occlusion • Stroke.

DTA Descending Thoracic Aorta

Identifying the Highest Impact Group

By identifying the patient group that will receive most benefit from REBOA and differentiating these from the patient group that will receive little or no benefit, may give a more efficient framework for determining where REBOA risk is most justifiable. The literature on REBOA outcome in relation to patient cohort is discussed later in this chapter. On the balance of probabilities, those patients with exsanguinating sub diaphragmatic haemorrhage, that have not become physiologically irretrievable, are the major trauma group most likely to benefit from REBOA. London HEMS use the clinical "Hateful 8" signs to help differentiate the prehospital exsanguinating trauma casualty to those causalities that have a shock mimic (for example: vagal response from peritoneal irritation, spinal cord injury above the T6 root, impact brain apnoea, other major head injury, cardiac tamponade, tension pneumothorax). Better selection of patients with the most favourable risk/benefit profile for REBOA use may therefore involve identifying exsanguinating subdiaphragmatic haemorrhage through:

- Identifying the Hateful 8 signs or a similar system of signs.
- Ensuring the mechanism of injury is potentially consistent with exsanguination (accepting that pre-hospital information may be vague or incorrect).
- Primary survey, eFAST findings and/or pelvic radiograph findings consistent with proposed method of exsanguination.

Identifying Level of Bleeding

If REBOA is delayed until definitive bleeding point identification is made at DCL or CTA, then the cost to the patient in terms of hypoperfusion and blood loss may be substantial or life-threatening. The classic Stannard [1] algorithm for determining optimal balloon occlusion level based on primary survey findings suggested trauma patients who were non responders or transient responders with a systolic blood pressure of less than 90 mmHg with no evidence of mediastinum haematoma on CXR should be targeted with:

- Zone 1 REBOA for those with a (1) positive abdominal FAST (perihepatic, perisplennic or pelvic peritoneal fluid identified) in or (2) negative abdominal FAST and no evidence of pelvic fracture.
- Zone 3 REBOA for those with a negative abdominal FAST and pelvic fracture.

This chapter has proposed a less algorithmic method of determining REBOA catheter use. However, the Stannard algorithm appears to be a highly efficient way of identifying the initial target zone of occlusion without delaying a decision to definitive bleeding point identification. Rational adjustments to such an algorithm in terms of occlusion zone include:

- Initiate a zone 1 REBOA inflation if the patient is profoundly shocked, periarrest or in a low outflow state, for resuscitative purposes despite only meeting Stannard zone 3 criteria. The balloon occlusion should then be moved to zone 3 after aggressive resuscitation in order to continue to target bleeding control.
- If following a zone 3 REBOA inflation the patients' haemodynamic parameters worsen then this may be explained by a false negative FAST and exacerbation of abdominal bleeding. If there is no life threatening alterative identified (tension pneumothorax, cardiac tamponade, balloon malposition) then the balloon occlusion should be moved to zone 1.
- If a patient meeting zone 3 criteria has had significant external blood loss, e.g. from a traumatic amputation, it is conceivable the abdominal FAST may not become definitively positive until patient filling. Repeating the FAST in such circumstances following 1–2 units of volume resuscitation may then declare an abdominal bleed justifying a move to zone 1 REBOA.

Ensuring an Immediate Exit Strategy

As indicated in Table 16.2, identifying a intended pathway to balloon deflation (a REBOA exit strategy) prior to inserting a balloon catheter is a appropriate readiness step.

Key Points
The distal ischaemic and subsequent reperfusion sequelae clock starts ("clock on") at balloon inflation and this precious time should not be spent on decisions and logistic organisation that could have been made pre-emptively.

In the real world the operating suite, CT scan (with subsequent interventional endovascular intent) or hybrid suite may not be immediately available following balloon occlusion, and/or the patient's clinical situation may evolve to merit an alteration to the REBOA exit strategy. However, in order to minimise the associated risk, the trauma team should avoid, for example, calling the theatre coordination hub to arrange theatre space for DCL only once a zone 1 total REBOA occlusion is fully deployed.

Practical Considerations in the Conduct of REBOA

Equipment Readiness

The initial readiness step for REBOA is to prepare the equipment. There are many process similarities between preparing for REBOA and preparing for a resuscitative thoracotomy; both manoeuvres, although technically straightforward to execute, require equipment readiness and assistance for optimal efficiency. The cognitive aid shown in Table 16.4 for REBOA preparedness is intended to remove the burden on trauma team of bandwidth that can otherwise be expended for the resuscitative effort. Those well-rehearsed with REBOA equipment set up are unlikely to find this useful. Such preparedness, at first glance, appears if it will carry significant time-based opportunity costs (for example, alternatively spending this time on a direct path to achieving definitive haemorrhage control). In fact, a well organised equipment bag and rehearsed setup will compare favourably in efficiency to an alternative strategy, for example, resuscitative thoracotomy.

Figure 16.4 shows an organised REBOA equipment bag aiming to reduce bandwidth expenditure and accelerate readiness to perform REBOA. The exact details of the preparedness process will depend on the hospital facility, the access choices and the balloon mounted catheter device being used.

Technique of REBOA Catheter Use

Technique for REBOA catheter insertion is well described in other texts [23]. Clearly there are differences in technique between institutions and operators depending on personal experience, the available catheter mounted balloon, corresponding instructions for use (IFU), the ancillary and access kit used and method of balloon position confirmation. The following is a description of the core technique that will be broadly applicable to many but not all circumstances:

Sheath Access (in this Example: CFA and Percutaneous)

Note: It is quicker and more straightforward to work with a dedicated assistant, particularly for those that do not use similar equipment regularly.

1. Set up the equipment. It may be helpful to refer to a preparation checklist, for example Table 16.4. Include a vascular closure device if desired (e.g. Angio-Seal™ VIP vascular closure device).
2. Wash hands with soap and don sterile gloves.
3. Select groin for insertion. If this is equivocal then a right handed operator standing on the patients' right, aiming for a right CFA puncture with the US machine on the patients right to allow machine control adjustment (and vice versa for left handed operators) may be the most ergonomic configuration.
4. Disinfect skin (eg ChloraPrep BD 10.5 ml applicator; 2% chlorhexidine gluconate and 70% isopropyl alcohol w/v) in selected groin and upper thigh.
5. Cover lower limbs with sterile drape to allow sterile zone for sheath and ancillaries (can also use this for guidewire and balloon catheter if remains sterile between interval of sheath insertion and REBOA decision).
6. Advance obturator/introducer into sheath and ensure secured.

Table 16.4 Leeds MTC REBOA preparation checklist

Ser	Equipment	Readiness description	Confirm or tick when ready
(a)	(b)	(c)	(d)
1	REBOA bag	Move REBOA kit bag from hanging hook to selected resuscitation bay	
2	Ultrasound	US switched on and check basic function Cognitively rehearse switching tranducers between CFA access (linear array 5–10 MHz) and eFAST (curvilinear array 3.5–5 MHz +/− linear array +/− phased array 2–8 MHz) Power supply plan (for example: battery with plan for socket backup)	
3	Pressure transducers	Arterial pressure transducers ×2 ready to use with flushed lines and hung on drip stand.	
4	Trolley for access (kit opened)	Sterile trolley cover for working space Sterile Gloves: for operator and assistant Ultrasound ancillaries • Coupling medium (e.g.: sterile KY Gel) • Sterile sleeve cover and securing bands ChloraPrep™, BD 10.5 ml applicator Local anaesthetic • Lignocaine 1% 10 ml • 5 ml syringes ×2 Percutaneous micropunture access Kit (including e.g. 4F MAK™, Merit) Percutaneous Access Kit (e.g. 7F Avanti®+, Cordis, 18G access needle, 0.035 short guidewire) Scalpel size 11 20 ml 0.9% saline prefilled syringes ×2 Gauze swabs Temporary sharps holder	
5	Ready REBOA kit (unopened)	ER-REBOA™ Catheter, Prytime Medical™ Sterile fenestrated Drape 170 cm × 150 cm 10 ml 0.9% saline prefilled syringes ×2	
6	Ready securing kit (unopened)	Suture silk size 0 Large Tegaderm™, 3M™ dressings ×2 ER-REBOA™ Catheter clamp	

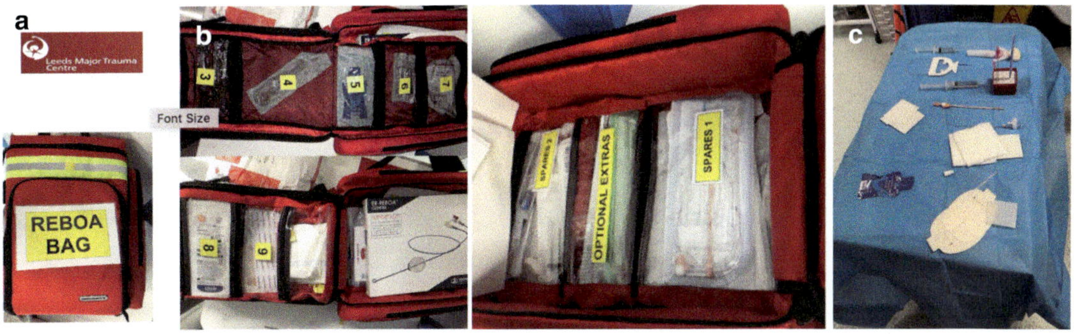

Fig. 16.4 REBOA equipment bag organisation at Leeds MTC. This bag was opened prior to a major trauma patient's arrival at Leeds MTC: (**a**) The REBOA bag unopened with a security seal tag to facilitate equipment replenishment process, (**b**) the bag opened displaying the contents of the main pouches within the bag, (**c**) access equipment from bag laid out and ready (micropuncture catheters were a later addition to the kit bag). In the event arterial access was not required and this opened kit on the trolley was ultimately discarded without use

7. Flush sheath via side port and introducer with sterile 0.9% saline.
8. Identify a suitable segment of CFA to puncture on US.
   (a) The artery can be identified as it is:
      – relatively noncompressible compared to vein. In a severely hypovolaemic patient this may not be so obvious.
      – obviously pulsatile unless low flow state or cardiac arrest. Pulsatility should be identified on B-mode in axial view and identification can be reinforced with colour or waveform mode.
      – lateral to the vein. Note that exceptions to this are so rare (e.g. some variants of persistent sciatic artery, previous extra anatomical bypass that alters the configuration) that they can be effectively discounted unless overwhelming evidence to the contrary.
   (b) Identify an entry point for the needle tip into the CFA. This point should allow for (1) compression on sheath removal if the intent is not to use a vascular closure device or open cut down and/or (2) subsequent cut down for sheath retrieval or complication straightforward and (3) being in a wide enough part of the artery to accommodate sheath. The CFA/ distal EIA may circumferentially spasm around the sheath at any point along its' length and attempting to enter the artery at the CFA bifurcation to offset this is probably futile. Therefore, while acknowledging the CFA may be of very short length with a high profunda femoris take off, the operator should ideally target:
      – the anterior wall of CFA
      – at least 1 cm below the inguinal ligament (compressing the distal EIA via the groin is often ineffective and fixing complications with a surgical approach is more straightforward at the CFA segment than the distal EIA segment)
      – at least 1 cm above the femoral bifurcation. It is less straightforward to repair complications and close arteriotomies directly at the bifurcation.
9. Infiltrate local anaesthetic into skin (eg lignocaine 1% about 3 ml) and overlying subcutaneous tissue.
10. Under US longitudinal and/or short axis visualisation insert the needle (for the sheath guidewire) at approximately 45 degrees to the groin skin plane in line with the long axis of the CFA. Longitudinal visualisation is preferred for insertion as the length of the needle can be visualised and the depth of the needle tip can be more consistently judged. Some US machines allow dual on screen short and longitudinal axis imagery.
11. Confirm the needle is in the arterial lumen with:
    (a) US visualisation
    (b) arterial back bleeding through the needle. Note that in low flow, hypoxic and/ or hypovolaemic states this may not spurt and /or may not appear to be obviously oxygenated blood.
12. Keep hold of the needle, place ultrasound probe on the sterile drape and insert the sheath guidewire (e.g. J tip 0.035 inch) through the needle. This should pass easily and the US should be used to confirm the wire is in the lumen. The guidewire should be advanced at least about 10–15 cm. If the wire does not pass easily then the needle and/ or guidewire are either:
    (a) Extra arterial
    (b) Within the arterial wall. This can potentially cause a problematic dissection, especially if the operator perseveres against resistance.
    (c) Within a side branch from the CFA/ distal EIA (this may not cause resistance)
    (d) Pushed against the posterior arterial wall preventing egress of the guidewire

    The former two situations require removal of the needle; with the exception of a needle that has passed "through – through the artery"—it is often possible to withdraw the needle into the lumen. The latter two situations may be salvaged by altering the position of the needle tip within the lumen and rotating the guidewire on advancing it into the artery. If the operator is in doubt the needle must be withdrawn.

13. Withdraw the needle over the guidewire and make a small incision in the skin (e.g: 3 mm for a 8F sheath). The operator must ensure this incision completely connects to the guidewire skin entry point, otherwise there will be effectively be no incision for the sheath insertion, potentially resulting in sheath kinking.
14. Insert the prepared sheath over the guidewire to its' hilt. Note the guidewire end must be visible at all times to prevent embolisation of the entire wire into the vessel. Troubleshoot as follows:
    (a) If the sheath fails to advance at the skin entry point and the skin is tight around the sheath and/or obturator then enlarge the incision.
    (b) If the sheath advances partly into the artery but not fully, then do not force. Given otherwise success of the preceding steps described above it is most likely the guidewire is in a side branch. Either attempt to reposition the guidewire under US visualisation or remove the sheath and the guidewire (provided the sheath size is appropriate to direct removal), compress the groin and consider other access locations for REBOA or an alternative strategy.
15. Remove the guidewire and obturator (aka introducer or dilator).
16. Use a 10 or 20 ml syringe three-quarters full with heparin-saline (10 IU/ml) to aspirate:
    (a) from sheath side or
    (b) directly from sheath lumen

    depending on the sheath design. The aspirate should be consistent with arterial blood with the caveats already described. Flush the aspirated lumen with 5–10 ml of heparin-saline; this should (1) flow easily and (2) be conducted with the syringe angled downwards to reduce the risk of an air embolism into the artery. If these steps are unsuccessful then the assumption must be that the sheath end is not in the arterial lumen.
17. Secure the sheath to the skin with at least one suture (e.g. 1-0 silk)

Balloon Catheter Insertion

Note: if the balloon catheter does not have a proximal pressure monitoring capability then a radial arterial line is likely to be the most straightforward option to measure proximal pressure following a femoral catheter insertion.

1. Ensure an appropriate size sheath, with regards to:
    (a) Diameter. The sheath must be able to accommodate the catheter French size, preferably including enough space to simultaneously transduce the fluid column in continuity with the sheath side arm with the catheter in situ; particularly if such a pressure measurement is part of the intended strategy.
    (b) Length. Long enough to support the inflated balloon to prevent balloon migration if required. A zone 3 REBOA is less likely to require such long sheath support as it can be "floated down" to the aortic bifurcation. The sheath must not be so long as to interfere with balloon inflation.

    If a smaller sheath is in situ, this can straightforwardly be exchanged for a larger sheath over an appropriate length guidewire. Enlarging the skin incision may be required at this stage depending on the size discrepancy.
2. Connect the pressure transducer to the sheath side arm.
3. If required, insert the balloon catheter guidewire (e.g.: Lunderquist or Amplatz guidewire) of appropriate length into sheath lumen. Note that the wire will usually be at least a 2 m length. This is optimally done under fluoroscopic visualisation.
4. Taking care not to desterilise the catheter mark the shaft distance from the sheath entry

point to zone 1 and to zone 3. For example, with an ER-REBOA™ Catheter this is from the sheath entry point, along the iliac aortic curvature, to where the apex of the pig tail aligns with the:
   (a) Suprasternal notch for zone 1
   (b) Xiphisternum for zone 3.
5. Insert the balloon catheter (over guidewire if required) and attach a pressure transducer to the appropriate catheter lumen if the catheter design allows.
6. Confirm deflated balloon position if required to do so based on personal and institute practice. For example, use of a plain film radiograph demonstrating integral radio-opaque markers are at the appropriate vertebral level or aortic balloon visualisation in relation to the heart or aortic bifurcation with US or IVUS.
7. Insert stylet into catheter if required (i.e. when using a Rescue Balloon catheter)
8. Inflate balloon in accordance with the balloon strategy to the desired pressure response. Note, the:
   (a) Balloon catheter must be held in position so that it doesn't migrate or slip.
   (b) Inflation fluid should be a sterile fluid (e.g. 0.9% saline). It may be mixed with IV contrast solution (e.g. Omnipaque 300) if fluoroscopic visualisation of the balloon during inflation or more precise position confirmation is required.
   (c) End point for balloon inflation will be guided by any or all of the:
      (i) device IFUs for a particular aortic zone
      (ii) blood pressure response and occlusion strategy
      (iii) loss of femoral pulse(s)
      (iv) tactile feedback on the syringe and catheter. Note resistance to inflation in less compliant balloons requires any additional inflation to be performed under fluoroscopy to mitigate the risk of aortic rupture.
9. The operator must ensure communication with the TTL, and hence the trauma team, to ensure appropriate situation awareness. The trauma team needs to record the zone, pressure strategy and duration. The use of a data capture capability, if available on the patient monitor (e.g.: Tempus Pro) may facilitate the record.
10. Either continue to hold the balloon catheter in situ (this will be awkward for transfers) or secure the balloon catheter to the skin using proprietary adhesive dressing and fastener or an alternative secure fix.

Adjusting Level of Aortic Balloon Occlusion

This is done in conjunction with the TTL and anaesthetist; acknowledging that this may be the same person if this step is intraoperative and resuscitative leadership has been passed to the anaesthetist. The technique will depend on the balloon catheter and an analysis of the balance of risk:

- Deflating the balloon completely will probably have highest risk of bleeding exacerbation and/or clot disruption
- Deflating the balloon to partial REBOA may mitigate such a bleeding risk, however, floating a partially inflated balloon across the visceral segment may cause or exacerbate aortic intimal injury (dissection). Aortic dissection can be unsalvageable and/or cause multiorgan failure.
- Retrograde movement of the balloon catheter though the aortic lumen is probably more likely to cause intimal injury or exacerbation of injury than antegrade movement.
- It is very likely that an aortic injury will not have been recognised or defined at this stage of the resuscitation.

On this basis deflating the balloon completely prior to moving aortic zone, regardless of direction, is likely to be the safest option. Therefore the optimal technique may be with two operators:

1. Release the catheter security dressing or suture as required.
2. Holding the sheath in place, advance or withdraw the balloon catheter to either the:

  (a) appropriate level pre-marked on the catheter or recorded distance on catheter cm markings
  (b) correct vertebral level under fluoroscopic guidance and visualisation of the radiopaque markers.
3. Reinflate the balloon in accordance with the desired balloon occlusion strategy.
4. Hold or re-secure the balloon catheter to the skin appropriately as described above.

In Conjunction with Definitive Haemorrhage Control

The "clock is on" once balloon occlusion is initiated and the patient should be moved to the operating theatre for DCL, the CT scan suite (with subsequent interventional endovascular intent) or the hybrid suite. In practice, a patient is unlikely to survive with zone 1 REBOA if taken to a CT scan suite and a lifesaving definitive abdominal haemorrhage control intervention is required. Balloon inflation to definitive haemorrhage control via a CT scan in most institutions may often exceed the survivable zone 1 REBOA time, particularly for total REBOA. If CT is performed then consideration should be given to moving to partial REBOA or complete balloon deflation for the duration of the scan. If a rapid protocol CT angiogram is used (e.g. Bastion) then such risk of clot disruption or additional bleeding is likely to be tolerable. The trauma team have the option of reinflating the balloon and accepting a suboptimal CT if this is not physiologically tolerated.

Key Points

The trauma team should anticipate an improvement in patient consciousness, possibly precipitating agitation, on balloon inflation.

This is particularly the case for zone 1 REBOA where carotid flow may be restored to within normal limits. Adjustments in analgesic and hypnotic drug dosage may be necessary in reaction to this.

Intraoperatively the surgeon or surgical assistant can directly control the balloon catheter, however, concurrent critical balloon manoeuvres and critical in cavity surgical manoeuvres will not be possible. A scrubbed REBOA operator, familiar with the device, who does not have concurrent duties at the operating table such as the scrub staff, surgeon or surgical assistant is probably therefore optimal. The surgical team will have access to the aorta and are able to corelate invasive pressure readings with presence or absence of aortic pulsation. Deflation of the balloon may be more optimally transitioned to manual external aortic compression. For example, particularly if a segment of infra renal aorta is sufficiently exposed. The principle rationale for such an approach is that currently available balloon technology has a sharp inflection point for release of occlusion, as described below.

The paradigm of DCL including a decision on four quadrant packing is extant with a clear priority for balloon deflation immediately after the most likely source(s) of exsanguinating bleeding have been identified and the relevant inflow artery selectively controlled (e.g. clamped). If the surgical plan is to remove an injured organ (e.g. splenectomy), there is no intrinsic need to do so prior to balloon deflation, unless it is required to provide access to another source of significant bleeding. If on balloon deflation a point of bleeding declares then the surgeon, in conjunction with the trauma team, should decide whether this requires balloon reinflation to address.

In moving total REBOA from total zone 1 to total zone 3 it is probably optimal to weight the risk of exacerbation of visceral segment distribution bleeding vs pre-emptive action. For example, a zone 2 retroperitoneal haematoma may convert to a life threatening bleed from transected renal artery clot blowout. Transitioning such a REBOA zonal move though a short period of partial zone 1 REBOA during which the supracolic and retroperitoneal structures are observed may be beneficial.

Balloon Deflation and Removal of Catheter

The REBOA operator and trauma team should be aware that with currently available balloon technology, deflation does not allow for the same degree of aortic flow control compared to carefully releasing aortic control at open surgery. This is likely to be due to:

- a "windsock" effect where the deflating balloon deforms via a pear shape to continue a circumferential seal with the aortic wall until an inflection point where a tiny volume change results in complete loss of this seal and very significant reduction in the obstruction to flow.
- elasticity of the aorta (particularly in the younger adult cohort) allowing blood to move past a partially inflated balloon in systole but not in diastole.

Balloon deflation, whether as part of intermittent REBOA, adjusting the occlusion strategy or with the intent of catheter removal, is clearly a critical step for the patient and requires careful coordination by the trauma team. The blood pressure drop and reperfusion sequalae should be anticipated by the anaesthetic team and an appropriate plan formulated, particularly for prolonged duration zone 1 Total REBOA. For example, if resuscitative and haemorrhage control goals have been achieved, then the anaesthetic team should aggressively trend the patient towards vasodilation and euvolemia so that the patient will more likely optimally respond to further volume filling and vasoconstrictive agents if required at balloon deflation. A workable technique for total balloon deflation that prioritises communication and controlled deflation is:

1. Agreement with the anaesthetic team/TTL for total balloon deflation.
2. Incremental deflation of the balloon with withdrawal of 0.5 ml volumes at time intervals that allow appropriate "blood pressure catch up", if required, by the anaesthetic team.
3. Alternatively, transition through sequential reperfusion:
   - Zone 1 total REBOA deflation transitions to partial REBOA (e.g. 5–10 mmHg increase in distal pressure) and resuscitation in accordance with response.
   - Zone 1 partial REBOA transitions to zone 3 REBOA and resuscitation in accordance with response.
   - Zone 3 REBOA transitions to selective iliac control if available. For example:
     - intraoperatively at DCL using external control
     - using a concurrent iliac occlusion balloon catheter in situ.

   This allows sequential reperfusion of the lower limbs and, to some extent, hemi pelvis with an appropriate resuscitation interval in between. Note: attempting to inflate an aortic balloon in the iliac segment in order to provide the same effect is technically possible, however, risks iliac rupture.
4. Remove the balloon catheter. It is important to confirm complete balloon deflation before attempting this in order to reduce the possibility of the balloon becoming stuck in the sheath. If a guidewire is in situ and there is no intent for endovascular intervention on the aortic segment or aortic branches then this should be removed simultaneously or immediately after catheter removal. If the deflated balloon catheter becomes stuck then:
   (a) If the operator is sure the balloon is contained entirely within the sheath then it can be removed as one entity in accordance with a sheath removal plan (see below).
   (b) If the balloon is stuck at the sheath end such that some folds of the balloon may be protruding into the arterial lumen then re-advance the catheter, ensure complete balloon deflation and then rotate the catheter while pulling it back through the sheath. Ultimately if the operator cannot withdraw the catheter completely into the sheath or is not sure that the balloon segment has been withdrawn fully into the sheath then an open cut down and retrieval should be performed. It is technically possible to withdraw a stuck, protruding, deflated balloon and low profile sheath through an artery wall without complication. However, this cannot be recommended as it may cause a significant laceration to the artery resulting in serious associated complications including pseudoaneurysm, major haemorrhage and/or vessel dissection that otherwise may be avoided.

5. Following removal of the balloon catheter, if it is still serviceable and the access is still in situ, then the operator may wish to reserve the ability to reinsert it in the immediate future. If practicable, the device can be reprepared and kept sterile for such a need until definitive haemorrhage control has been achieved.

Sheath Management Plan

The final step directly related to REBOA is for the trauma team, guided by the REBOA operator, to identify a sheath management plan. This is based on a risk analysis between keeping the sheath in situ with reassessment of the situation within the next few hours and sheath removal. When considering sheath removal the sheath side port (or sheath lumen if no side port) should be aspirated to assess for clot. It is important to note that the REBOA patient cohort has significant differences to an elective vasculopathic patient cohort and therefore the risk assessment has differences. Consider the:

- Risk to the limb.
  This requires an assessment of thrombosis risk, whether there is a distal limb injury, the general perfusion state of the limb and whether an access complication was recognised. It may be reasonably obvious that arterial intervention is required, for example:
- Presence of gross ipsilateral limb ischaemia
- Available imaging demonstrating thrombus
- Clot is removed from the side port of the sheath

In such circumstances open cut down with confirmation of inflow and appropriate outflow management (e.g. Fogarty balloon trawl) is very likely the safest overall option, rather than attempting an endovascular solution. "Monitoring" asymptomatic known thrombus in these circumstances carries a risk of limb loss. Ruling out a risk to the limb is not so straightforward. In trauma patients a pink foot does not necessarily correlate to a viable foot. In particular, those patients that have received a significant overall tissue injury from trauma and surgery, and have had a massive transfusion should be presumed to have prothrombotic characteristics. Individual institutions will usually decide where to set the threshold for open exploration of the arterial tree in those patients that do not have an obvious indication. This is likely to be based on their own experience; for example institutions that exclusively perform REBOA on obviously exsanguinating patients are likely to have a significantly higher yield from open thrombectomy than those institutions which have a lower threshold for REBOA use.

- Intent for definitive endovascular intervention.
  The sheath can be upsized as required and/or may provide convenient access for angioembolisation, covered stent deployment or other endovascular procedure. This may negate the risk of a further access attempt. However, if endovascular intervention is only a possibility rather than a definite immediate intent, then the rationale to keep in situ is significantly less strong.
- Type of access
  - *Open access*
    Open access will require a combination of sheath removal, arteriotomy closure and wound closure. This should be done as soon as possible; target a limit of 12 h from the index incision.
  - *Percutaneous access*
    Percutaneous access can potentially be left in situ with a slow heparin-saline infusion via the side port for 24–48 h. However, in a patient who is coagulopathic and/ or with a risk of rebleeding this may be undesirable. The size of the sheath, location of the sheath and coagulation status of the patient will inform on whether immediate direct pressure is a reasonable option for arteriotomy closure following sheath removal. If in doubt then the operator should choose between:

    a percutaneous vascular closure device (note there are device and access specific considerations to decide as to whether this is a reasonable option), or an open cut down, sheath removal, Fogarty balloon trawl and arteriotomy closure.

Key Points
In formulating a sheath management plan the trauma team including the REBOA operator will need to decide where their risk toleration lies; this will depend on the patient's profile, burden of injury and the logistics of the hospital facility.

Early sheath removal (target within 1 to 2 h of insertion) is likely to be the optimal balance of risk for the majority of patients. As a general rule, low profile sheaths (for example up to 7F or 8F) that:

- were inserted in-hospital without complication
- have no significant clot on sheath side arm aspiration
- are not upstream to an ischaemic limb
- have been in situ for less than 2 h, and
- are sited in patients that can be safety monitored and intervened on if signs of limb ischaemia develop

Can probably be removed directly at low risk. If these criteria are not met then the intervention as per *a risk to the limb,* described above, should be followed.

Lower Limb Fasciotomies

In order to manage the risk of compartment syndrome the trauma team should be aware that lower limb fasciotomies may be required. Patients at higher risk of lower limb compartment syndrome include those that have had:

- A prolonged REBOA inflation time (particularly total occlusion)
- An ischaemic complication to a lower limb.

In isolated ischaemic circumstances (i.e. in patients with no significant contributing ipsilateral limb fracture or direct soft tissue injury component), prioritising the anterio-lateral leg compartment is probably reasonable. Thigh and buttock fasciotomies are very rarely indicated.

Current Literature Perspective

Major trauma related literature review informs the risk analysis described in this chapter by quantifying some of the risk and benefit related to REBOA.

Comparison to Resuscitative Thoracotomy

Outcomes for resuscitative thoracotomy (RT) for subdiaphragmatic bleeding provide a potential extrapolation and/ or comparison group for REBOA. Both share a paradigm for decision making based on rapid risk analysis (for RT principally in terms of futility) in major trauma patients that usually results in aortic occlusion. However, characterising REBOA only as an endovascular alternative to an open DTA occlusion clamp in these circumstances is an oversimplification of the more nuanced risk-benefit analysis described in this chapter. The benefit of in-hospital open DTA occlusion prior to damage control laparotomy in patients with exsanguinating sub-diaphragmatic bleeding have been historically unclear [24–26]. Historical case series' (pre 2000) have suggested an overall survival rate of about 4.5% [27] in such patients with traumatic cardiac arrest and

1. penetrating abdominal injury with signs of life in the pre-hospital environment
2. blunt abdominal injury with signs of life on arrival to hospital.

who undergo open DTA occlusion; compared to a survival rate without occlusion of 0%. These may be two groups of patients where heuristics from RT decision familiarity and outcome can drive the REBOA risk-benefit analysis.

Extrapolating Epidemiological Data Is Problematic

Besides these potential groups are there others that may benefit from REBOA? Historical data has consistently attributed about 1 in 3 trauma deaths in the first 24 h to haemorrhage independent of head injury [28]. Trauma specialists have hypothesised that some of these deaths will be in patients who survived to hospital with non-compressible subdiaphragmatic haemorrhage who would have survived if they had sooner bleeding control [29]. Extrapolating data from quality trauma mortality studies needs to be done with caution.

- An analysis of a single Canadian trauma centre identified 1 in 3 in-hospital haemorrhagic deaths after blunt trauma as being preventable due to a delay to definitive haemorrhage control [30]. However, over 85% of these deaths were due to several hours of delay in obtaining angioembolisation for pelvic bleeding *after* initial damage control pelvic and abdominal surgery. REBOA may be able to help form an initial clot, however it cannot mitigate against such logistic challenges that many hospital systems may experience. This Canadian study makes a very reasonable case for a hospital hybrid suite; but their data should not be used as a strong case for REBOA.
- Variations in the definition of preventable deaths suggests that identifying these patients is not as objectively obvious as perhaps could be suggested, such variations are particularly prevalent in pre-hospital studies [31]. Therefore caution needs to be exercised in extrapolating the significant numbers of pre-hospital haemorrhage related deaths classified as potentially preventable as a case for in-hospital aortic control manoeuvres [32]. Perhaps a reasonable case for thinking creatively about the delivery of earlier high impact care, but again, not necessarily a strong case for REBOA.

REBOA Human Evidence Base

In order to more clearly identify potential patient groups that could benefit from REBOA, the current Oxford CEBM level 3 evidence base (observational studies) is summarised in Table 16.5. There is no current OCEBM level 1 or 2 evidence base regarding REBOA. Some of the data sources used by the studies overlap, such that the same patient cases appear in more than one study. The caveats regarding the interpretation of non-randomised trauma evidence described in chapter 30_6.1 apply to these studies. The findings of this evidence base can be summarised as:

1. It remains unclear as to the group of patients (categorised by physiological and/ or injury profile) where survivorship favours REBOA compared to an alternative strategy. There remains the possibility that such a group will not be clearly identified for the foreseeable future.
2. Partial REBOA is, on the balance of probabilities, more favourable than total REBOA in some patients (perhaps all patients, although this seems unlikely).
3. REBOA survivors, on the balance of probabilities, have a very low level of clinically significant balloon catheter complications.

These human data sets therefore do not provide an assured or comprehensive set of answers about how to conduct REBOA or who may benefit from REBOA (if anyone).

Future Availability of OCEBM Level 2 Evidence

The UK REBOA trial is the first randomised controlled trial (RCT) aiming to determine the clinical effectiveness of REBOA. It is a multicentre trial, recruiting non-pregnant trauma patients over the age of 16 (or thought to be so at the point of recruitment) from Major Trauma Centres (MTCs). Patients randomised are believed, by the trauma team, to have life threatening non-compressible torso haemorrhage amenable to REBOA in the context of a potentially survivable injury. The patients are randomised to either REBOA (with no mandated level, duration or strategy of occlusion) or to standard treatment. Between 2018 and October 2020 59 patients out of a target of 120 have been randomised. There

Table 16.5 Summary of human study evidence for REBOA

Study	Data source	OCEBM level	Dates conducted	Design	Population	Intervention group	Comparison group	Outcome	Study Limitations	Comment
Norri et al. [33]	Japan Trauma Data Bank (national registry)	3	2004 to 2011	• Retrospective, national registry, matched cohort study. • Propensity matched REBOA cases with non-REBOA cases on treatment likelihood. The authors used a logistic regression model for propensity score based on: age, sex, calendar year, RTS, mechanism of injury, maximum AIS for each of the nine body regions and treating facility.	• 1807 blunt trauma patients with survival data • >18 years old • Treated at trauma centres that use REBOA	• 351 REBOA • Precise criteria for REBOA use not clear	• 1456 non-REBOA • Propensity matched as described in design column	• REBOA conferred a lower chance of survival to leave hospital. OR = **0.30**, 95% CI = 0.23–0.40 • Subgroup analyses: – Isolated abdominal injury (OR for survival, **0.32**; 95% CI = 0.08–1.23) – Isolated serious pelvis/lower extremity injury (OR, **0.27**; 95% CI = 0.03–2.7)	• No record of vital signs at admission for improved injury stratification. • REBOA survivors vs non-survivors had a mean GCS, 11.6 vs. 7.2 (p = 0.0001). This implies that concurrent CNS injury contributed to worse survival. Some of the REBOA signal strength may have been lost by this effect. • There were no shock mimic data (for example, non-therapeutic laparotomy data not shown): Some of the REBOA use may not have been for the purpose of haemorrhage control. • No timing of intervention analysis available and therefore some patients may have been further down the line of irretrievability—some of the REBOA may have been "last ditch". However, note the 24% survival rate for REBOA patients is much better than the survival rate of RT and open DTA occlusion for blunt trauma; suggesting the REBOA cohort were not in as much extremis as a traumatic cardiac arrest cohort. • Complications were not recorded.	• Presumably analysed data also used by other Japan registry studies [34, 35]. • External validity to UK may be compromised: – There was an average of 3 h from point of injury to definitive intervention and 2 h to blood transfusion—this is a significantly different practice to Europe and US. – The mean age of the patients was 51.8 years (51.6 in the REBOA group).

Moore et al. [15]	US Trauma registry data from two level 1 trauma centres in Texas	3	Jan 2012 to June 2013	Retrospective, local registry, matched cohort study.	• 96 trauma patients • >= 16 years old • No intrathroacic haemorrhage (suspected or confirmed) • No penetrating chest trauma	• 24 REBOA • Criteria: – SBP < 90 and partial/ non-responder – Zone 1 (Z1) if FAST +ve or no pelvic fracture – Zone 3 (Z3) if FAST -ve and pelvic fracture • Z1 = 19, Z3 = 5 • Approx. 50% femoral cut down, 50% percutaneous	72 RT patients with standard care for exsanguinating haemorrhage from abdomen or pelvis	REBOA conferred higher trend of survival to leave hospital, however, OR was indeterminate: OR = **2.88**, 95% CI = 0.94–8.87	• Characteristics of the control and interventional group significantly differed biasing for a better REBOA outcome: – ISS = 75 in 6.3% of REBOA and 21.3% of RT groups. – 33% of the REBOA group were having CPR on arrival to ED compared to 63% of the RT patients. • There were no shock mimic data; the relevance of this is described in the row above. • No complication outcome data recorded.	• 87.5% REBOA and 14.3% RT deaths survived to ICU to die of head injury. Most deaths in the RT group were from haemorrhage in ED.
DuBose et al. [36]	The Prospective Observational Aortic Occlusion for Resuscitation in Trauma and Acute Care Surgery (AORTA) study: 8 participating level 1 trauma centres in the US (5 of which offered REBOA)	3	Nov 2013 to Feb 2015	Prospectively recorded registry data, matched cohort study.	• 114 trauma patients undergoing interventional aortic occlusion after injury for shock • >= 18 years old • Some patients had associated chest trauma: – 4.4% had cardiac repair – 3.5% had a non-anatomical lung resection	• 46 REBOA • Z1 = 36, Z3 = 10 • Approx. 50% open cut down, 50% percutaneous • Mean time from decision to REBOA was 6.6 min	• 68 open aortic occlusions (laparotomy or thoracotomy) • Mean time from decision to occlusion was 7.2 min	• REBOA conferred a higher trend of survival to leave hospital. However, OR was not clearly determinate: OR = **2.04**, 95% CI = 0.82 = 5.07 • REBOA complications: – 1/46 (2.2%) arterial pseudoaneurysm at the access site – 2/46 (4.3%) distal embolic events – No infection or need for amputation – 2/46 (4.3%) balloon migration after deployment	• Characteristics of the control and interventional group significantly differed potentially biasing for a better REBOA outcome: – Open aortic occlusion group more likely to have airway managed without pre-hospital intubation. – REBOA was performed by an attending in 93.5% of cases, whereas open aortic occlusion was performed by an attending in 57.3% of cases	• The mean age of the patients was 40.8 years old. • Presumably analysed data also used by Brenner et al. [37]. However, this study used a less precise comparison group.

(continued)

Table 16.5 (continued)

Study	Data source	OCEBM level	Dates conducted	Design	Population	Intervention group	Comparison group	Outcome	Study Limitations	Comment
								• Open aortic occlusion complications: – 1/68 (1.4%) retained haemothorax requiring operative evacuation – 2/68 (2.9%) local wound infections requiring additional surgical intervention. • Note AKI with dialysis required in 4/114 (3.5%) patients overall: – 2/46 (4.3%) in the REBOA group – 2/68 (2.9%) in the open aortic occlusion group ($p = 0.660$)	• Characteristics of the control and interventional group differed with an indeterminate effect on the outcome: – Open aortic occlusion group were more likely to suffer a penetrating injury (47.1% vs. 23.9%, $p = 0.013$)	

Brenner et al. [37]	The Prospective Observational Aortic Occlusion for Resuscitation in Trauma and Acute Care Surgery (AORTA) study: 11 participating level 1 trauma centres in the US and Canada (all of which offered REBOA)	3	Nov 13 to Jan 17	Prospectively recorded registry data, matched cohort study.	• 285 trauma patients undergoing interventional aortic occlusion after injury for shock • >=18 years old • No penetrating thoracic injury with an AIS>=2 • Complete survival data available • All aortic interventions were initiated in ED • Penetrating mechanism in 41.4% of patients	• 83 Z1 REBOA • Approx. 50% cut down and 50% percutaneous	202 RT patients with open DTA occlusion	• REBOA conferred a higher chance of survival to leave hospital, (total of 13/285 survivors) OR = **4.20**, 95% CI = 1.33–13.25. • Subgroup analysis, REBOA vs RT: – If CPR required before hospital then total of 5/172 (2.9%) survivors, OR = **2.05**, 95% CI = 0.33–12.69. – If CPR started in ED prior to aortic occlusion then total of 1/57 (1.8%) survivors – If no CPR prior to aortic occlusion then total of 7/56 (12.5%) survivors, OR = **8.00**, 95% CI = 0.89–17.58. • REBOA complications: – 2/83 (2.4%) requirement for patch angioplasty – 1/83 (1.2%) requirement for lower limb amputation – 4/83 (4.8%) distal embolism – 3/83 (3.6%) balloon migration	• There were very few overall survivors to calculate ORs; type 1 error may be more likely. • Characteristics of the control and interventional group significantly differed potentially biasing for a better REBOA outcome: – 75% of the open DTA occlusion group had CPR before hospital compared to 25% of the REBOA group. • Characteristics of the control and interventional group differed with an indeterminate effect on the outcome: – 16.9% REBOA vs 51.5% open DTA occlusion had penetrating mechanism ($p < 0.001$) – Duration of aortic occlusion, median: for REBOA was 31 min, and for open DTA occlusion was 19 min; however the strategy of occlusion was not recorded. – There was a transition to institutions preferring ER-REBOA balloon catheter use during the study.	Presumably analysed data also used by DuBose et al. [36]. However, this study used a more precise comparison group.

(continued)

Table 16.5 (continued)

Study	Data source	OCEBM level	Dates conducted	Design	Population	Intervention group	Comparison group	Outcome	Study Limitations	Comment
Joseph et al. [38]	American College of Surgeons Trauma QIP data set (740 participating hospitals)	3	2015 to 2016	• Retrospective, national registry, matched cohort study.	• 420 trauma patients alive on arrival • > = 18 years old • no RT • all physiological parameters recorded	• 140 REBOA • Precise criteria for REBOA use not clear	• 280 non- REBOA. • Propensity matched as described in design column	• REBOA conferred a lower chance of survival to leave hospital OR = **0.42**, 95% CI = 0.27–0.66. • Complications: – AKI: 10.7% REBOA group vs 3.2% non-REBOA group (p = 0.02) – Extremity amputation 3.6% REBOA group vs 0.7% non-REBOA group. – No difference in complications (all recorded as 0) for DVT, PE, stroke, MI, extremity compartment syndrome	• REBOA survivors vs non-survivors had a mean GCS, 11.6 vs. 7.2 (p = 0.0001). This implies that concurrent CNS injury contributing to worse survival. Some of the REBOA signal strength may have been lost by this effect. • There was no documentation as to the patient responsiveness to fluid resus; a useful determinate in rate of active bleeding and may sometimes indicate shock mimics.	• Presumably analysed data also used by other US registry studies [15, 37]. • The mean age of the patients was 44 years old.

	• Propensity matched REBOA cases with non-REBOA cases on treatment likelihood. The authors used a logistic regression model for propensity score based on: demographics, vital signs (pre-hospital and ED SBP, HR, and GCS score), mechanism of injury, ISS, each body region AIS, pelvic fractures (intact, incompletely disrupted, and completely disrupted pelvic ring), lower extremity vascular injuries and fractures, number and AIS for intraabdominal solid organ injuries (liver, spleen, and kidney injuries).		• REBOA may have conferred a quicker time to – Laparotomy: median 33 min (IQR = 26–62) in the REBOA group vs 45 min (IQR = 35–69) in the non-REBOA group – Angioembolisation: median 46 min (IQR = 31–69) in the REBOA group vs 59 min (IQR = 39–78) in the non-REBOA group	

(continued)

Table 16.5 (continued)

Study	Data source	OCEBM level	Dates conducted	Design	Population	Intervention group	Comparison group	Outcome	Study Limitations	Comment
Abe et al. [34]	Japan Trauma Data Bank (national registry): 234 participating hospitals	3	2004 to 2013	• Retrospective, national registry, matched cohort study. • Propensity matched REBOA cases with non-REBOA cases on treatment likelihood. The authors used a logistic regression model for propensity score based on: age, gender, mechanism of injury, transport type, pre-hospital treatment, vital signs at ED, ISS	• 304 trauma patients alive on arrival to hospital • >= 14 years old • complete data sets • No AIS = 6 for any one injury • Did not have both REBOA and aortic cross clamping	• 152 REBOA • Precise criteria for REBOA use not clear	152 open aortic occlusions (laparotomy or thoracotomy)	• REBOA conferred a higher chance of survival to leave hospital OR = **3.84**, 95% CI = 1.91–7.69.	• Characteristics of the control and interventional group significantly differed with an indeterminate effect on the outcome: The REBOA group had a lower AIS thorax score 3.8 vs 4.2 ($p < 0.001$), but the groups did not differ in ISS. • No record on how REBOA was conducted (e.g. zone, time, strategy) or time of open aortic occlusion. • No complication outcome data recorded.	• Presumably this study analysed data also used by other Japan registry studies [33, 35]. • The mean patient age was 53.7 years. • See comment on external validity for the Norii et al. [33] study.
Aso et al. [35]	Inpatient data extracted from the Japanese Diagnosis Procedure Combination database: 1000 participating hospitals	3	Jul 2010 to Mar 2014	• Retrospective, national registry, matched cohort study. • Propensity matched REBOA cases with non-REBOA cases on treatment likelihood. The authors used a logistic regression model for propensity score based on: age, sex, BMI, aetiology, Japan Coma Scale, presence of head injury, CPR on admission, severity of injury, hospital facility.	• 269 Trauma patients • >=15 years old • No penetrating thoracic injury	• 191 REBOA • Precise criteria for REBOA use not clear	68 RT	• Adjusted by propensity score, there was no significant difference between REBOA and RT in: – In Hospital mortality HR = **0.94**; 95% CI = 0.60–1.48 ($p = 0.79$) – Ventilator free days – ICU free days • Authors noted no lower limb amputations in either group • Comparing REBOA to non-adjusted RT conferred a higher chance of survival to leave hospital in favour of REBOA OR = **2.69**, 95% CI = 1.49–4.88	• Characteristics of the control and interventional group significantly differed potentially biasing for a better REBOA outcome: – *CPR*: 22% of REBOA group vs 62% of RT group ($p < 0.00001$) – *Receiving interventional radiology*: 40% of REBOA group vs 26.5% of RT group ($p < 0.05$) – *Receive exploratory laparotomy*: 9% of REBOA group vs 18% of RT group ($p < 0.05$) • No record regarding: – Pre-hospital transport time – How REBOA was conducted (e.g. zone, time, strategy) – Trauma Score or precise injury details that may have effected propensity scoring	• Presumably analysed data also used by other Japan registry studies [33, 35] • See comment on external validity for the Norii et al. [33] study.

Sadeghi et al. [39]	Aortic Balloon Occlusion Trauma Registry: 13 participating hospitals in Russia, Sweden, Israel, Finland, Japan, Italy	3	Nov 2011 to Sep 2016	Initially retrospective then prospectively recorded registry data, matched cohort study.	• 96 Trauma patients who all had a balloon inflated in aorta	• 50 Total REBOA • Precise criteria for REBOA use not clear • 46% <30 min occlusion time • 14% >60 min occlusion time	• 46 Partial or Intermittent REBOA • Precise criteria for REBOA use not clear • 29% <30 min occlusion time • 38% >60 min occlusion time	• Total REBOA conferred a lower trend of 30 day survival OR = **0.75**, 95% CI = 0.35–1.62 • No statistical difference between the complications: <u>Total REBOA:</u> – Extremity compartment syndrome 11% – Balloon migration 2% – Balloon rupture 2% – Embolisation signs 4% – MOF in survivors 33% <u>Partial or intermittent REBOA:</u> – Extremity compartment syndrome 0 – Balloon migration 7% – Balloon rupture 5% – Embolisation signs 2% – MOF in survivors 36%	• Incomplete outcome dataset • Possible significant differences in the conduct of DCR (including the prehospital phase) between centres participating with registry may have had significant impact on findings.	• 67% of cases were from Japan. See comment on external validity for the Norii et al. [33] study. • Presumably analysed data also used by the Japanese registry studies [33–35]. • 88% blunt trauma. • Mean age 52 years.

RT Resuscitative Thoracotomy, *CI* Confidence Interval, *OR* Odds Ratio

was a trial pause during part of the COVID pandemic, and last recruitment is now scheduled for 2023. The advantage of conducting this study in the UK was that, at incept, there was virtually no in-hospital REBOA conducted nationwide. Trauma team equipoise was probably therefore more guided by the evidence base and standardised REBOA training rather than by ad hoc enthusiastic, albeit competent, early adopters. Bayesian experimental design allows this seemingly small recruitment number to determine:

- The primary clinical outcome of 90-day mortality (defined as death within 90 days of injury, before or after discharge from hospital).
- The primary economic outcome of lifetime incremental cost per QALY gained, from a health and personal social services perspective.

There are a range of secondary outcome measures, including functional outcome at six months and complications. Knowing beyond reasonable doubt whether, in those patients that share the characteristics of the trial population group, REBOA is advantageous or not will greatly enhance the ability to conduct a risk-benefit analysis for a critically ill trauma patient presenting to ED.

System Optimisation for REBOA

There are several other considerations for institutions and hospitals offering REBOA that will, in principle, optimise delivery of this intervention.

Access to a Suitable Training Programme

The UK REBOA trial conducts standardised training to establish and sustain recruiting centres. There are also well-established courses in the US: ESTARS [40], modified ASSET [41] and BEST [42]. Many centres are likely to run their own in-house training programme instead of or in addition to such national courses. Collective training is probably helpful given the myriad of human factor considerations involved in delivering REBOA in a DCR context.

Audit and Clinical Governance

Given the risk profile of the REBOA intervention and the relative complexity of integrating REBOA decision making within the context of DCR, it is likely there will always be a benefit in ensuring there is a forum where areas of improvement can be identified.

REBOA Protocol or Guidance

This is likely to be mandated in most institutions. One approach is to construct a straightforward protocol for use such as the Stannard algorithm described in the *risk analysis for REBOA* section of this chapter. An alternative approach is to allow for a more nuanced risk analysis which may offer the team more options and adaptability to dynamic situations. The details of the protocol will therefore depend on the local trauma faculty view on how to best to manage the uncertainties regarding the use of REBOA.

Conclusion

- REBOA is an adjunct to DCR in severely injured trauma patients.
- The group of patients most likely to benefit from REBOA are almost certainly those with exsanguinating sub-diaphragmatic haemorrhage. Whether REBOA in this patient group is superior to an alternative strategy conducted by the trauma team is unclear based on the current literature.
- Understanding the risks, opportunity costs and risk reductions REBOA offers may help make a more optimal decision in its use.

Questions

1. In a conscious trauma patient, with isolated exsanguinating sub diaphragmatic torso bleeding, the most consistent haemodynamic consequence of a Zone 1 total REBOA is likely to be:
   (a) Increased IVC flow rate
   (b) Increased renal artery flow
   (c) Increased aortic arch intraluminal pressure
   (d) Decreased carotid artery intraluminal pressure
   (e) Exacerbation of subdiaphragmatic bleeding
2. Zone 1 partial REBOA:
   (a) Results in less distal flow than a Zone 1 total REBOA
   (b) Will not exacerbate subclavian artery bleeding
   (c) May reduce the overall re-perfusion insult compared to zone 1 total REBOA
   (d) Is usually determined by the mean arterial pressure
   (e) Mandates fluoroscopy to assure position
3. With regards readiness for REBOA:
   (a) Sheath access prior to a decision to perform REBOA is optimal
   (b) Sheath access following a decision to perform REBOA is optimal
   (c) An unassisted operator is usually more efficient
   (d) Microsheath use (e.g. 4F) has no role
   (e) Sheath access site is solely determined by operator ergonomics
4. If clot is removed from a percutaneously inserted 7F sheath side port then the management option likely to carry the lowest risk of limb threatening distal thromboembolism is:
   (a) Flush with side port with 10 IU/ml heparin, 0.9% saline mix
   (b) Systemic heparinisation targeting the APTTr between 2.0 and 3.0
   (c) Angiographic imaging and risk assessment for intervention
   (d) Open cut down and thromboembolectomy
   (e) Remove sheath immediately and provide external compression to prevent haematoma formation.
5. In a patient who has had 20 min of zone 3 total REBOA and then complete balloon deflation:
   (a) There is no risk of compartment syndrome
   (b) Severe arterial lacerations within the pelvis may be haemostatic
   (c) Mandatory lower limb fasciotomies are required
   (d) There is no risk of reperfusion injury
   (e) Sequential reperfusion of the common iliac arteries is mandated

Answers

1. c
2. c
3. a
4. d
5. b

References

1. Stannard A, Eliason JL, Rasmussen TE. Resuscitative endovascular balloon occlusion of the aorta (REBOA) as an adjunct for hemorrhagic shock. J Trauma. 2011;71(6):1869–72.
2. Dunn EL, Moore EE, Moore JB. Hemodynamic effects of aortic occlusion during hemorrhagic shock. Ann Emerg Med. 1982;11(5):238–41.
3. Spence PA, Lust RM, Chitwood WR, Iida H, Sun YS, Austin EH. Transfemoral balloon aortic occlusion during open cardiopulmonary resuscitation improves myocardial and cerebral blood flow. J Surg Res. 1990;49(3):217–21.
4. Markov NP, Percival TJ, Morrison JJ, Ross JD, Scott DJ, Spencer JR, et al. Physiologic tolerance of descending thoracic aortic balloon occlusion in a swine model of hemorrhagic shock. Surgery. 2013;153(6):848–56.
5. Biffl WL, Fox CJ, Moore EE. The role of REBOA in the control of exsanguinating torso hemorrhage. J Trauma Acute Care Surg. 2015;78(5):1054–8.
6. Borger van der Burg BLS, van Dongen TTCF, Morrison JJ, Hedeman Joosten PPA, DuBose JJ, Hörer TM, et al. A systematic review and meta-analysis of the use of resuscitative endovascular balloon occlusion of the aorta in the management of major exsanguination. Eur J Trauma Emerg Surg Off Publ Eur Trauma Soc. 2018;44(4):535–50.

7. Izawa Y, Hishikawa S, Matsumura Y, Nakamura H, Sugimoto H, Mato T. Blood flow of the venous system during resuscitative endovascular balloon occlusion of the aorta: Noninvasive evaluation using phase contrast magnetic resonance imaging. J Trauma Acute Care Surg. 2020;88(2):305–9.
8. Jansen J. UK REBOA Trial Protocol - Version 3 [Internet]. 2017 [cited 2020 Oct 31]. Available from: https://w3.abdn.ac.uk/hsru/REBOA/Public/download.aspx
9. UK-REBOA [Internet]. [cited 2020 Oct 31]. Available from: https://w3.abdn.ac.uk/hsru/reboa/public/public/index.cshtml
10. Barnard EBG, Morrison JJ, Madureira RM, Lendrum R, Fragoso-Iñiguez M, Edwards A, et al. Resuscitative endovascular balloon occlusion of the aorta (REBOA): a population based gap analysis of trauma patients in England and Wales. Emerg Med J. 2015;32(12):926–32.
11. Matsumura Y, Matsumoto J, Kondo H, Idoguchi K, Ishida T, Kon Y, et al. Fewer REBOA complications with smaller devices and partial occlusion: evidence from a multicentre registry in Japan. Emerg Med J. 2017;34(12):793–9.
12. Borger van der Burg BLS, Kessel B, DuBose JJ, Hörer TM, Hoencamp R. Consensus on resuscitative endovascular balloon occlusion of the Aorta: a first consensus paper using a Delphi method. Injury. 2019;50(6):1186–91.
13. Borger van der Burg BLS, van Dongen TTCF, Morrison JJ, Hedeman Joosten PPA, DuBose JJ, Hörer TM, et al. A systematic review and meta-analysis of the use of resuscitative endovascular balloon occlusion of the aorta in the management of major exsanguination. Eur J Trauma Emerg Surg Off Publ Eur Trauma Soc. 2018;44(4):535–50.
14. Hughes CW. Use of an intra-aortic balloon catheter tamponade for controlling intra-abdominal hemorrhage in man. Surgery. 1954;36(1):65–8.
15. Moore LJ, Brenner M, Kozar RA, Pasley J, Wade CE, Baraniuk MS, et al. Implementation of resuscitative endovascular balloon occlusion of the aorta as an alternative to resuscitative thoracotomy for noncompressible truncal hemorrhage. J Trauma Acute Care Surg. 2015;79(4):523–32.
16. Greer MR, Carney S, McPheeters RA, Aguiniga P, Rubio S, Lee J. Radial arterial lines have a higher failure rate than femoral. West J Emerg Med. 2018;19(2):364–71.
17. Arnal D, Garutti I, Perez-Peña J, Olmedilla L, Tzenkov IG. Radial to femoral arterial blood pressure differences during liver transplantation. Anaesthesia. 2005;60(8):766–71.
18. Dorman T, Breslow MJ, Lipsett PA, Rosenberg JM, Balser JR, Almog Y, et al. Radial artery pressure monitoring underestimates central arterial pressure during vasopressor therapy in critically ill surgical patients. Crit Care Med. 1998;26(10):1646–9.
19. Mignini MA, Piacentini E, Dubin A. Peripheral arterial blood pressure monitoring adequately tracks central arterial blood pressure in critically ill patients: an observational study. Crit Care Lond Engl. 2006;10(2):R43.
20. Compton FD, Zukunft B, Hoffmann C, Zidek W, Schaefer J-H. Performance of a minimally invasive uncalibrated cardiac output monitoring system (Flotrac/Vigileo) in haemodynamically unstable patients. Br J Anaesth. 2008;100(4):451–6.
21. Galluccio ST, Chapman MJ, Finnis ME. Femoral-radial arterial pressure gradients in critically ill patients. Crit Care Resusc J Australas Acad Crit Care Med. 2009;11(1):34–8.
22. Kim WY, Jun JH, Huh JW, Hong SB, Lim C-M, Koh Y. Radial to femoral arterial blood pressure differences in septic shock patients receiving high-dose norepinephrine therapy. Shock Augusta Ga. 2013;40(6):527–31.
23. Morrison J, Reva V, Lonn L, Matsumoto J, Matsumara Y, Holcomb J, et al. REBOA. In: Top Stent [Internet]. 1st ed. The Journal of Endovascular Resuscitation and Trauma Management; 2017 [cited 2020 Oct 31]. Available from: https://jevtm.com/top-stent/
24. Ledgerwood AM, Kazmers M, Lucas CE. The role of thoracic aortic occlusion for massive hemoperitoneum. J Trauma Inj Infect Crit Care. 1976;16(8):610–5.
25. Millikan JS, Moore EE. Outcome of resuscitative thoracotomy and descending aortic occlusion performed in the operating room. J Trauma Injury Infect Crit Care. 1984;24(5):387–92.
26. Wiencek RG, Wilson RF. Injuries to the abdominal vascular system: how much does aggressive resuscitation and prelaparotomy thoracotomy really help? Surgery. 1987;102(4):731–6.
27. Rhee PM, Acosta J, Bridgeman A, Wang D, Jordan M, Rich N. Survival after emergency department thoracotomy: review of published data from the past 25 years. J Am Coll Surg. 2000;190(3):11.
28. Kauvar DS, Lefering R, Wade CE. Impact of hemorrhage on trauma outcome: an overview of epidemiology, clinical presentations, and therapeutic considerations. J Trauma. 2006;60(6 Suppl):S3–11.
29. Morrison JJ, Rasmussen TE. Noncompressible torso hemorrhage: a review with contemporary definitions and management strategies. Surg Clin North Am. 2012;92(4):843–58.
30. Tien HC, Spencer F, Tremblay LN, Rizoli SB, Brenneman FD. Preventable deaths from hemorrhage at a level I Canadian trauma center. J Trauma. 2007;62(1):142–6.
31. Oliver GJ, Walter DP. A call for consensus on methodology and terminology to improve comparability in the study of preventable prehospital trauma deaths: a systematic literature review. Acad Emerg Med Off J Soc Acad Emerg Med. 2016;23(4):503–10.
32. Davis JS, Satahoo SS, Butler FK, Dermer H, Naranjo D, Julien K, et al. An analysis of prehospital deaths: who can we save? J Trauma Acute Care Surg. 2014;77(2):213–8.
33. Norii T, Crandall C, Terasaka Y. Survival of severe blunt trauma patients treated with resuscitative endo-

vascular balloon occlusion of the aorta compared with propensity score-adjusted untreated patients. J Trauma Acute Care Surg. 2015;78(4):721–8.
34. Abe T, Uchida M, Nagata I, Saitoh D, Tamiya N. Resuscitative endovascular balloon occlusion of the aorta versus aortic cross clamping among patients with critical trauma: a nationwide cohort study in Japan. Crit Care. 2016;20(1):400.
35. Aso S, Matsui H, Fushimi K, Yasunaga H. Resuscitative endovascular balloon occlusion of the aorta or resuscitative thoracotomy with aortic clamping for noncompressible torso hemorrhage: a retrospective nationwide study. J Trauma Acute Care Surg. 2017;82(5):910–4.
36. DuBose JJ, Scalea TM, Brenner M, Skiada D, Inaba K, Cannon J, et al. The AAST prospective aortic occlusion for resuscitation in trauma and acute care surgery (AORTA) registry: data on contemporary utilization and outcomes of aortic occlusion and resuscitative balloon occlusion of the aorta (REBOA). J Trauma Acute Care Surg. 2016;81(3):409–19.
37. Brenner M, Inaba K, Aiolfi A, DuBose J, Fabian T, Bee T, et al. Resuscitative endovascular balloon occlusion of the aorta and resuscitative thoracotomy in select patients with hemorrhagic shock: early results from the american association for the surgery of trauma's aortic occlusion in resuscitation for trauma and acute care surgery registry. J Am Coll Surg. 2018;226(5):730–40.
38. Joseph B, Zeeshan M, Sakran JV, Hamidi M, Kulvatunyou N, Khan M, et al. Nationwide analysis of resuscitative endovascular balloon occlusion of the aorta in civilian trauma. JAMA Surg. 2019;154(6):500–8.
39. Sadeghi M, Nilsson KF, Larzon T, Pirouzram A, Toivola A, Skoog P, et al. The use of aortic balloon occlusion in traumatic shock: first report from the ABO trauma registry. Eur J Trauma Emerg Surg Off Publ Eur Trauma Soc. 2018;44(4):491–501.
40. Villamaria CY, Eliason JL, Napolitano LM, Stansfield RB, Spencer JR, Rasmussen TE. Endovascular skills for trauma and resuscitative surgery (ESTARS) course: curriculum development, content validation, and program assessment. J Trauma Acute Care Surg. 2014;76(4):929–36.
41. Kuhls DA, Risucci DA, Bowyer MW, Luchette FA. Advanced surgical skills for exposure in trauma: a new surgical skills cadaver course for surgery residents and fellows. J Trauma Acute Care Surg. 2013;74(2):664–70.
42. Brenner M, Hoehn M, Pasley J, Dubose J, Stein D, Scalea T. Basic endovascular skills for trauma course: Bridging the gap between endovascular techniques and the acute care surgeon. J Trauma Acute Care Surg. 2014;77(2):286–91.

Anticoagulants in Trauma

17

Robert Greig

Introduction

Death due to haemorrhage remains the primary cause in 2.3 million trauma deaths per annum worldwide. As described in the haemostasis and coagulopathy chapter, trauma induced coagulopathy (TIC) develops in about 10 to 25% of trauma patients. The presence of acute traumatic coagulopathy (ATC), a component of TIC, increases mortality almost nine-fold, and is unrelated to transfusion practice.

Patients with ATC have a higher incidence of multi-system organ failure, prolonged hospital and intensive care stay as well as increased blood product utilisation. Death from exsanguination occurs within 2 to 3 h (median time) after presentation, accounting for nearly 50% of trauma deaths. Early recognition and treatment of TIC, along with massive transfusion guidelines, represent an opportunity to improve outcomes in trauma resuscitation.

But what if the patient was already anticoagulated prior to the trauma?

Millions of people worldwide are anticoagulated and they are anticoagulated for various indications. The multitude of indications also reflects a variety of ages that are anticoagulated. With increased age ("silver trauma" for example) there is increased likelihood of anticoagulation reflecting the pathologies of old age e.g. NVAF, Stroke prevention, DVT.

In the past there were few alternatives to warfarin. Today in 2021 while warfarin is still the predominant anticoagulant used worldwide, there is a growing population of patients anticoagulated with a newer breed of anticoagulants (Direct oral anticoagulants (DOAC)) that the trauma team need to be aware of and prepared to manage. In the UK, as in many other countries, DOACs are now used first line in anticoagulation for non-valvular AF and VTE treatment & prevention.

This chapter aims to provide a background knowledge to anticoagulants and how to reverse their properties rapidly in the trauma setting—it does not describe FFP to packed red blood cell resuscitation ratios which are considered elsewhere. The basis of this chapter is to take a pharmacologically anticoagulated patient and put them on a "normal coagulation footing" for which they will then need typical blood product resuscitation as per any "non anticoagulated" trauma patient.

R. Greig (✉)
Emergency Medicine, Jersey, Channel Islands, UK

P. Lax (ed.), *Textbook of Acute Trauma Care*, https://doi.org/10.1007/978-3-030-83628-3_17

Anticoagulants: Types and Assessing Anticoagulant Effect

This section aims to cover most anticoagulants and can also be applied to non-traumatic anticoagulated haemorrhage e.g. gastrointestinal and intracranial bleeds. One often assumes that trauma happens outside of the care environment but falls also happen in medical facilities and not every patient is on warfarin or a DOAC; many patients will be on injectable anticoagulants such as low molecular weight heparins. Figure 17.1 outlines the sites of action of the anticoagulant agents that are considered individually below.

Vitamin K Antagonists (VKA) Also Called Coumarins: Warfarin (Coumadin), Dicumarol (Dicoumarol), Acenocoumarol (Sinthrome), Phenindione

Pharmacology The most commonly used VKA is warfarin and its effects on coagulation are complex. Taken orally, VKA inhibits the Vitamin K conversion cycle affecting both the prothrombotic factors II, VII, IX, X, and also the antithrombotic Proteins C & S.

When first initiated warfarin exerts a procoagulant effect with the onset of anticoagulant action typically developing from 24 to 72 h. Warfarin metabolites are excreted 92% renally.

Monitoring Anticoagulant Effect INR (International Normalised Ratio) or PT (Prothrombin Time) are both increased with warfarin. INR is the standard test to assess VKA/Warfarin anticoagulation. Once steady state has been achieved, the APTT will also be prolonged due to Factor IX depletion, and this may be a guide as to whether the patient is in a pro-or anticoagulant phase of the warfarin effect.

Direct Oral Anticoagulants (DOACs: Formerly Called NOACs (Novel Oral Anti Coagulants))

These fall into two groups:

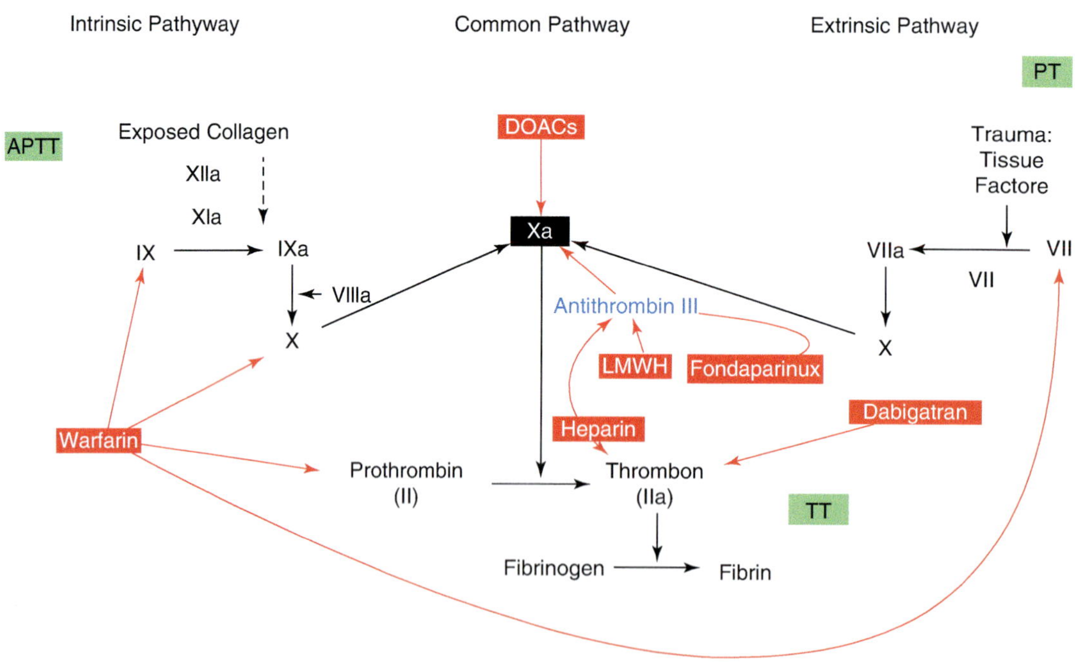

Fig. 17.1 Effect Sites of Anticoagulants on the Normal Clotting Pathway

Direct Thrombin Inhibitors: Dabigatran (Pradaxa)

Pharmacology Dabigatran is a competitive reversible direct inhibitor of the active site of thrombin (Factor IIa). Dabigatran inhibits thrombin, preventing the conversion of fibrinogen into fibrin, the final point of the clotting cascade. The onset of anticoagulant action peaks at 1.5 h and a steady state of anticoagulation is achieved after 3 days of continuous dosing.

Dabigatran's half-life (T 1/2) ranges from 12 to 14 h after continuous dosing. The half-life is increased to >24 h in patients with a creatinine clearance of <30 mL/min and with severe renal impairment dabigatran may be detected up to a week after the last dose.

Dabigatran is mostly subject to renal excretion and excreted unchanged, hence the anticoagulant effect will increase as renal function declines. In overdose, its effects can be reduced with haemodialysis, but this is exceptionally rare.

Factor Xa Inhibitors: Apixaban (Eliquis), Edoxaban (Lixiana) and Rivaroxaban (Xarelto)

Pharmacology These agents act by reversible direct inhibition of free and clot-bound Factor Xa. Inhibiting Xa prevents formation of thrombin, hence the "-xa-" in the names of these agents.

Maximum effect varies between 1 and 4 h post dosing and the half-life also varies from 5 to 9 h with rivaroxaban, 9–14 h with apixaban and 10–14 h with edoxaban. Edoxaban has a much larger volume of distribution. Apixaban and rivaroxaban are currently more commonly prescribed as edoxaban is a newcomer to the market, though recent cost reductions in edoxaban have meant patients who are newly diagnosed with atrial fibrillation are preferentially started on edoxaban in the UK. Many patients who take apixaban and rivaroxaban may be transitioned over to edoxaban if there is no clinical contraindication.

Approximately one third of the excretion of Factor Xa inhibitors is via the renal route. Edoxaban also has three metabolites that act as anticoagulants in laboratory tests, but are produced in a small amount which are highly protein bound, so that they are not felt to clinically contribute to the anticoagulant effects of edoxaban [1].

Factor Xa inhibitors have similar clinical indications to warfarin, with the exception of prosthetic heart valve prophylaxis or valvular AF. Some (particularly rivaroxaban) have other rapidly growing indications, e.g. rivaroxaban with aspirin in peripheral arterial or coronary artery disease, but usually at lower doses [2–5].

Monitoring Anticoagulant Effect of Both Groups DOACs were intended to be anticoagulants that don't require monitoring—i.e. "anticoagulation that you can turn your back on". Xa-inhibitors prolong PT (Prothrombin Time) and APTT (Activated Partial Thromboplastin Time) to a varying degree. The APTT cannot be used for evaluation of FXa inhibitory effects because of the weak correlation and variability of assays [6].

PT prolongation is related linearly and dose-dependently to the Factor Xa-inhibitor concentration. The effect on the PT depends both on the *assay* and the *FXa inhibitor*. Anti-FXa assays are commercially available yet there is currently no data that associate a coagulation parameter or a drug concentration with bleeding risk [7]. That being said, 30 ng/ml of DOAC is considered to be the *cut-off of safety* for emergency surgery or consideration for thrombolysis based on expert opinion [8, 9]. Warfarin provides continuous anticoagulation which can be measured, however DOACs operate on peaks and troughs which decline to very low levels with 24-hour dosing, or low levels with 12-hour dosing. Measuring PT/APTT or DOAC level is therefore time dependent—some centres can (and will) measure DOAC levels pre- and 2–3 h post dose where there is a particular issue e.g., absorption or other potential drug interactions. There is a lot of variation between laboratories in the effects of DOAC on PT/APTT due to different thromboplastin reagents; with some reagents apixaban will give normal PT/APTT at peak levels for example. A very long PT/APTT may be a clue to a higher level of DOAC but it is not reliable (something like a lupus anticoagulant or dietary vit k deficiency may also prolong PT/APTT).

> *In essence, the standard coagulation result can be normal or abnormal and it does not reflect the degree of anticoagulation or bleeding risk.*

Dabigatran concentrations may be measured either directly, or by using surrogates such as coagulation tests. However, when the use of the most common tests such as the standard coagulation screen or global screen have been considered APTT, PT, and INR have been found to be clumsy in regard to the anticoagulation effect of dabigatran [10, 11]. Hawes et al. found 29% of patients had normal PT and 29% had normal APTT whilst taking Dabigatran 150 mg BD [12]. Standard coagulation tests are affected to varying degrees by dabigatran. The sensitivity of PT and APTT varies considerably based on the assays used - APTT shows a curvilinear dose-response with a steep increase at low concentrations whilst PT is relatively insensitive. However Thrombin Time (TT) is a sensitive measure which could be used for assessing low concentrations of dabigatran [13]. Most clinicians do not have access to liquid chromatography-mass spectrometry assays to determine plasma dabigatran concentrations and questions still arise as to the clinical validity of the result.

Therefore, instead of measuring dabigatran concentrations directly, the TT could be used as a surrogate to determine dabigatran concentrations and its clinical effect. TT is a test that is more widely available and familiar to some clinicians. However Brett et al. [11] concluded that the TT is not a perfect surrogate for dabigatran concentrations as it is associated with false positive results (i.e. the TT was prolonged not only in patients who had clinically relevant dabigatran levels, but was also prolonged in some patients who did not have significant levels of dabigatran). This finding was the same as in the CORIDA study [14]; while a normal TT 100% predictive of having a low dabigatran concentration that is safe for surgery, a high TT may be due to the presence of dabigatran or another factor.

In a study by Ebner et al. [13], 481 samples from 96 DOAC-treated patients were tested using PT, APTT, TT, DOAC-specific assays (anti-Xa activity, diluted TT), and liquid chromatography-tandem mass spectrometry (the latter being the gold standard for DOAC quantification). Sensitivity and specificity of test results to identify DOAC concentrations <30 ng/ml were calculated.

The study addressed can '*test x*' identify if '*patient y*' has *negligible* DOAC levels. Sensitivity (the ability of a test to rule out anticoagulation in this study) represented the percentage of samples correctly identifying DOAC levels <30 ng/ml i.e. excluding anticoagulation. Specificity (the ability of a test to rule in anticoagulation in this study) represented the percentage of samples identified as DOAC >30 ng/ml ruling in anticoagulation.

Ebner et al. found that normal PT and APTT provide insufficient specificity to safely identify DOAC concentrations <30 ng/mL (rivaroxaban PT: specificity 77% & sensitivity 94%; apixaban PT: specificity 13% & sensitivity 94%. Dabigatran aPTT: specificity 49% & sensitivity 91%). A substantial proportion of cases with DOAC levels *above* an accepted safe treatment threshold of 30 ng/ml would have normal global results for PT/APTT, and (with the exception of dabigatran as mentioned above) a normal TT.

Ebner et al. conclude that with regard to DOAC treated patients, abnormal APTT/PT/TT results may reflect a presence (but not the degree) of anticoagulation and that *normal results are clinically meaningless* [13]. However, if the TT is near normal there is very little dabigatran left on board—this may be useful in certain circumstances, e.g. the last dose was taken a couple of days ago and the patient has minor renal impairment.

In summary, normal test results of global coagulation assays are simply not suited for emergency coagulation (or anticoagulation) assessment in DOAC treated patients [10, 13, 15]. A calibrated quantitative anti-FXa assay may help to inform clinical decisions in exceptional situations about use of apixaban, edoxaban or rivaroxaban, for example in overdose and emergency surgery, although this is not available in most centres. However, use of anti-FXa assays should not be used to measure the effectiveness of andexanet alfa (the *antidote* to rivaroxaban and apixaban, see later) as the results may not be reliable. Treatment monitoring should be based mainly on clinical parameters indicative of appropriate response (achievement of haemostasis) and lack of efficacy (re-bleeding) [15].

Francart et al.[16] found of patients taking Rivaroxaban, 32% had a normal PT.

There is no acute reliable measure of DOAC anticoagulation and no coagulation test can be applied to decide whether a reversal agent is required or not.

If a patient is on a DOAC or has had a dose in the preceding 24 hours one must assume the patient is anticoagulated and must be reversed if clinically significant bleeding is proven or suspected [13]

Low Molecular Weight Heparin (LMWH), Heparin (Unfractionated Heparin, UFH) and Fondaparinux

Pharmacology *Low molecular weight heparins (LMWH)* activate antithrombin III, which in turn binds to and inhibits Xa. Lack of Xa prevents activation or conversion of prothrombin to thrombin stopping the common clotting pathway or reducing its efficacy.

Unfractionated Heparin (UFH) not only deactivates Xa by activating Antithrombin III but the molecular chain is longer (higher molecular weight), allowing UFH to bind and block Thrombin, preventing conversion of Fibrinogen to Fibrin. Binding of both Antithrombin III and Thrombin is termed "the bridging effect". This is achieved by the longer, larger molecular size. LMWHs are too small to have this effect.

There is also a secondary effect: UFH not only prevents fibrin formation but also prevents thrombin-induced activation of platelets and of factors V and VIII [17].

Fondaparinux works in a similar way to LMWHs but its anti-Xa activity is seven-fold that of other LMWHs. It is a synthetic analogue of the Antithrombin III binding pentasaccharide sequence found in UFH and LMWH. Its molecular weight is much lower than that of the LMWHs at 1728 compared to the average of 5000 for LMWHs. The pentasaccharide sequence is chemically modified to increase the affinity (by a factor of approximately 300) for Antithrombin III compared to UFH and LMWH.

Fondaparinux is an *indirect* Xa inhibitor (compared with direct Xa inhibition of DOACs). Its anticoagulant effect makes no change to PT/INR/APTT results whilst being 100% renally excreted unchanged [18].

Fondaparinux has pure Xa activity compared to LMWHs which have some effect on Factors II, IX, XI, and XII. The half-life of Fondaparinux is much longer at 21 h compared to a mean of 4 h for LMWHs, however this rises to 72 h when creatinine clearance is <30 ml/min. Usage of fondaparinux is low in an era of DOACs.

Monitoring Anticoagulant Effect *UFH anticoagulation* may be reflected in the prolongation of APTT or the APTT ratio or Anti FXa levels. Monitoring these parameters allows titration of the intravenous infusion rate. In truth, APTT is poor at measuring the anticoagulation effect of heparin [19], but it is the best test available immediately. Most institutions in the United States utilise anti-FXa or APTT to monitor UFH therapy [20].

During the COVID pandemic, Anti-FXa and APTT were found to be prone to monitoring inaccuracies and lead to under dosing of UFH in the severely ill. Medication, e.g. propofol, or Antiphospholipid antibodies (raised in critically ill COVID cases) have been found to falsely increase anti-FXa levels. APTT levels are also affected by COVID via raised fibrinogen levels found in the critically ill COVID cases. [20–23]

The same cannot be applied to LMWH or Fondaparinux. These medicines (like DOACs) were designed not to be routinely monitored.

LMWHs do affect the APTT but results are considered suboptimal for monitoring. APTT displays a linear dose response to LMWH but is less strongly correlated with anti-Xa activity. There is variation between APTT assays and types of LMWH [24]. Alternatively, Anti-Xa assays are performed using chromogenic mass spectrometry with the result given in international units per millilitre (iu/ml): LMWH therapeutic range is 0.5–1.2 iu/ml and the prophylactic range is 0.1–0.4 iu/ml. The Anti-Xa test is not a method of global coagulation and cannot predict bleeding risk. It is an expensive time-consuming test with no current role in the trauma patient as it is not readily available in most places and difficult to perform.

Fondaparinux does not cause any change in PT/APTT/INR tests. The standard assay for Anti-Xa activity does not reflect on Fondaparinux because of the vast affinity difference between Fondaparinux and LMWH for Xa, although bespoke assays for fondaparinux are possible to create [25].

APTT is insensitive to both LMWH and Fondaparinux.

Antidotes for Anticoagulants

For Warfarin

Vitamin K

Can be given IV or PO, with reversal effects within 12–24 h. In acute trauma Vitamin K has no role in the acute management of coagulation reversal, *however* vitamin K is the only true antidote to warfarin which will allow manufacture of replacement clotting factors. It can be given as follow up to urgent reversal with Prothrombin Complex Concentrate (PCC) as Vitamin K begins to take effect after 6 h to assist synthesis of new clotting factors [26]. PCC will give a time-limited window of "normal" clotting of 6–12 h, but without additional Vitamin K then anticoagulation may reoccur without additional medication given.

4 Factor Prothrombin Complex Concentrate (PCC). Beriplex or Octaplex

Beriplex (manufacturer CSL Behring UK LTD) 4 factor dried human complex of clotting factors. Contains Factors II, VII, IX, X coupled with Protein C & S. Administered IV: *Each loaded syringe of prepared Beriplex will be 20 ml in volume and should be administered as a slow push = 8 ml per minute or over 2.5 min.*

The dose is 30–50 iu/kg (note: max 100 kg body weight). Alternatively, 3000 iu for most VKA anticoagulated adults is adequate if working off approximate weights in traumatic haemorrhage including neuroaxial bleeds (Brain-Spine-Eye bleeds). Often clinicians cannot wait for the INR to return from the lab or they may be working in the pre-hospital environment.

Haemostasis should be achieved 30 minutes after injection and a coagulation screen should be repeated at that point. Repeated administration of Beriplex taking the total dose beyond 5000 iu is not advised.

Octaplex (manufacturer Octapharma) is also a 4 factor PCC. It is also administered IV but it must be given more slowly than Beriplex initially: 1 ml per minute for the first 5 min then increasing by 1 ml per minute over subsequent 3 min to maximum rate of 8 ml/min. In this author's opinion, this seems impractical compared to *Beriplex* administration. A "standard" dose of 30 iu/ml for all patients regardless of INR. If the patient's weight is unknown: 2000 iu for majority of female patients and 2500 iu for a majority of male patients.

The maximum dose is 3000 iu and haemostasis is reported at 60 min, compared with 30 min for *Beriplex*. Octaplex is cheaper than Beriplex, so some hospitals have locally agreed protocols which have pre-specified doses of 1000–3000 iu dependent on patient weight and INR (if known) and over a shorter period.

There is some controversy regarding the use of four factor PCC to reverse DOACS [27–30]. If andexanet alfa is not available, the author advises 50 iu/kg of Beriplex.

For Dabigatran

Idarucizumab (*Praxbind*, Boehringer Ingelheim)

This is a specific reversal agent (humanised monoclonal antibody fragment) for dabigatran

(*Pradaxa*) indicated for when rapid anticoagulation reversal is necessary. The affinity of Praxbind for dabigatran is 300-fold more potent than the affinity of dabigatran for thrombin. Praxbind removes dabigatran from thrombin, forming a stable complex that results in neutralisation of dabigatran's anticoagulant effect.

The dose is 5 g via intravenous infusion and administered as two consecutive infusions over 5 to 10 min each or as a bolus injection. Idarucizumab binds specifically to dabigatran reversing its direct thrombin inhibition. Idarucizumab has no effect on any other anticoagulants [31] and has an immediate effect; once in circulation the dabigatran is neutralised.

Both dabigatran and idarucizumab are excreted by the kidneys, *either separately or as a complex*. In porcine trauma models, animals with blunt liver injury developed low urinary volumes presumably due to haemorrhagic shock. *Clinicians must bear this in mind* when dealing with dabigatran enhanced haemorrhagic shock, if renal perfusion pressure is not restored, dabigatran anticoagulation will return, irrespective of dosing with idarucizumab. A further treatment of 10 g may be required within 24 h if further bleeding is evident. In the same trauma models, administration of idarucizumab resulted in termination of bleeding and restored kidney perfusion [32].

If idarucizumab is not available, do not consider PCCs as they will not work and theoretically may have an increased risk of thromboembolic events based on laboratory data [33–35]. However, dabigatran is excreted in the urine (80% renally excreted with a T1/2 of approximately 13 h with a glomerular filtration rate (GFR) of >80 ml/min, and 18 h with a GFR of 30–50 ml/min) so it's vital that renal perfusion pressure is maintained. Clinicians could consider haemodialysis, as dabigatran is not protein bound (unlike direct Xa inhibitors) although this is highly unlikely to occur in the resuscitation room!

For Direct Factor Xa Inhibitors:
(Apixaban, Edoxaban and Rivaroxaban)

Andexanet Alfa (Ondexxya or Andexxa Manufactured by Alexion)

Andexanet alfa is a high affinity decoy molecule for Factor Xa inhibitors. It sequesters apixaban and rivaroxaban, inhibiting them from binding to endogenous Xa. Thus, Xa function returns and so does thrombin formation. Andexanet alfa is administered as a bolus over 15 min ("low dose" regimen) or 30 min ("high dose" regimen) followed by an infusion over 120 min (Fig. 17.2).

It works rapidly (within 2–10 min); in healthy volunteers on apixaban (Annexa-A study) 100% thrombin generation is restored to above lower limit of normal range, and in the case of rivaroxaban (Annexa-R study) it is restored to 96% after bolus administration [36, 37]. It is currently very expensive (approximately £25,000 per course), so its use may increase in future and may have to be authorised by a consultant haematologist depending on local arrangements.

There are two Andexanet alfa regimens depending on three elements:

Fig. 17.2 Reversal regimens for Factor Xa inhibitors from Summary of Product Characteristics

FXa inhibitor	Dose	Time since last dose		
		<8 hours	≥8 hours	Unknown
Apixaban	≤5mg	Low	Low	Low
	>5mg	High	Low	High
	Unknown	High	Low	High
Rivaroxaban	≤10mg	Low	Low	Low
	>10mg	High	Low	High
	Unknown	High	Low	High

(A) Which DOAC was taken? (apixaban or rivaroxaban) (there is currently *no licence for edoxaban reversal*)
(B) The DOSE of DOAC taken
(C) TIME since last dose

The above three elements will decide which of the two regimens will be used: "**High dose**" or "**Low dose**":

Often in trauma, it is unlikely that the clinician will be able to ascertain the time since last DOAC dose and the actual dose. Advised practice is to follow the HIGH DOSE Regimen for trauma with exsanguination or neuroaxial bleeding enhanced by DOAC anticoagulation.

The reversal effect will last for up to 14 hours, although peak normalisation is 4 hours from start of the drug administration

Edoxaban and Andexanet Alfa At time of writing there was insufficient data to grant andexanet alfa a licence in the reversal of edoxaban - partly because the numbers of patients on this drug are currently low making recruitment difficult. Annexa-4 enrolment is ongoing to specifically recruit further patients on edoxaban to address this. The initial Annexa-4 [38] analysis of 352 subjects attempted to look at andexanet and edoxaban reversal but the numbers were just too small.

A phase II pharmacokinetic and pharmacodynamic study [39] assessed andexanet alfa compared with placebo when administered to healthy volunteers on a steady dose of 60 mg edoxaban. In an andexanet dosing regimen of 600 or 800 mg bolus (which finished 3 and 5 h after the last dose of edoxaban respectively) and a bolus plus infusion regimen of 800 mg followed by 1 h of 8 mg/min infusion (which is half the time of the licensed high dose regimen), Xa activity returned to baseline within 2 min for the edoxaban groups where the largest reduction was observed for the bolus plus infusion (800/8 mg) cohort. In the edoxaban group, Xa activity was sustained for 1.5 h *after* the infusion *completed.* The duration of anti-Xa inhibition was half that observed in a parallel rivaroxaban cohort. The duration of the andexanet for edoxaban infusion was only 60 min compared to 120 min (i.e. *half* the licensed rivaroxaban and apixaban regimens) most likely because the volume of distribution is twice that of rivaroxaban. Thrombin generation lasted 2 h after the completion of the bolus plus infusion in both edoxaban and rivaroxaban cohorts.

The study authors acknowledge that 'reversal' was based on anti-FXa activity and thrombin generation levels rather than bleeding outcomes. However, correlation of these bleeding outcome surrogate markers has been shown to reflect anticoagulant bleeding correction in animal studies [40, 41].

The author would recommend following local guidance as use of andexanet alfa would be *off label* for the reversal of edoxaban but would advise that the "High Dose" regimen should be used in the face of traumatic life threatening edoxaban enhanced haemorrhage (where the dose and timing of the last dose is unknown): 800 mg bolus over 30 min followed by 8 mg/min over subsequent 120 min. *Readers are advised to further contact the manufacturer for further medical information regarding dosing and administration.*

4 Factor Prothrombin Complex Concentrate & DOAC Reversal

There is some controversy regarding the use of 4 factor PCC to reverse DOACs. If andexanet alfa is not available, the author advises 50 iu/kg of Beriplex [35, 42–46]. Figure 17.3 is a suggested decision tree for consideration of PCC vs andexanet in DOAC reversal.

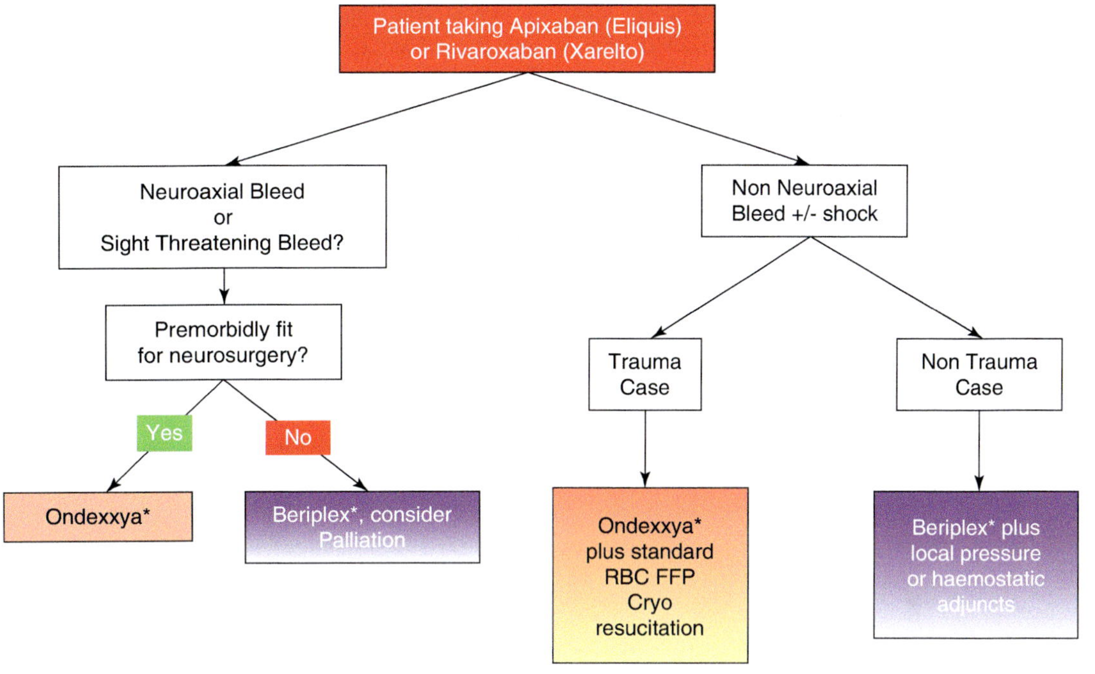

Fig. 17.3 Decision making in reversal of apixaban or rivaroxaban. *Do not co-administer other blood products within same IV line

For Unfractionated Heparin (UFH)/ Heparin

Protamine

Protamine is a drug that should not be used lightly and is rarely used outside of cardiopulmonary bypass surgery. It's also an ingredient in certain subcutaneous insulin preparations (protamine-zinc-insulin) and patients on these insulins are at an increased risk of allergic reactions to protamine reversal.

Side effects include pulmonary artery hypertension, histamine release, systemic hypotension, anaphylaxis, pulmonary oedema and paradoxical bleeding. Thus the author recommends a "low and slow" approach to protamine use [47, 48].

Protamine is given by peripheral intravenous infusion rather than centrally. Peripherally appears to be associated with less histamine release compared with central administration.

UFH is an anionic molecule that when exposed to the cationic protamine molecule forms a salt. This salt is inactive and has no anticoagulant properties.

The anti-heparin effect is rapid in onset, within 5 min, and the unbound half life is short at 10 min. Little is known about the metabolism of the UFH-Protamine salt. Studies suggest it is either subject to hepatic or renal metabolism.

Care is needed at all stages of protamine use, especially in terms of traumatic haemorrhage because excessive doses of protamine paradoxically cause impairment of platelet function, so may clinically cause bleeding.

Note: Protamine has no effect on Fondaparinux induced anticoagulation.

The dosing of protamine to reverse UFH and LWMH is controversial and varies in the medical literature. What is accepted is that 1 mg of Protamine reverses 1 mg (100 iu) of UFH/Heparin/LMWH [49].

The author advises clinicians in the United Kingdom (UK) to refer to either Toxbase or the

British Society of Haematology or their local haematologist for heparin/UFH/LMWH reversal.

Toxbase Guidance

In the UK clinicians will be familiar with and have 24 h access to www.toxbase.org, an online up to date database on poisons treatment. This guidance is taken from their database.

Protamine reversal for Heparin/UFH:

- Give a loading dose of 20–25 mg IV Protamine at a rate (not exceeding) 5 mg per minute.
- Repeat APTT after 4 h.

British Society for Haematology Guidance (BSH)

From the BSH guidance titled "Management of Bleeding in Patients on Antithrombotic Agents" [47] (dated 1st November 2012 with an addendum made in February 2019):

- Calculate the amount of Heparin given intravenously in the preceding 2-hour period.
- Assume that 1 mg of protamine reverses 100 iu of heparin: e.g. an infusion rate of 1250 iu/h. requires a reversal dose of 25 mg. Given slowly at a rate not exceeding 5 mg/min via intravenous infusion.
- Bleeding soon after 5000 iu loading bolus needs 50 mg.
- The reversal affect can be measured using APTT.

The BSH also states that a maximum dose of 50 mg is sufficient to reverse heparin/UFH in most settings.

Further information regarding Protamine: as mentioned at the start of this section, protamine is not a drug to be used lightly given the potential severity of its side effects. It is a proven valuable reversal agent for heparin induced anticoagulation.

Clinicians should be prepared for the side effects: have ready access to cardiovascular rescue drugs during administration including vasopressors and inotropes coupled with intramuscular adrenaline if anaphylaxis develops.

IV steroids and H1 & H2 antagonists should also be at hand to calm any histamine based allergic response. If a mild allergic response occurs and an infusion is required consideration should be given to either slowing the rate of infusion to over 16 h with prophylactic administration of steroids with H1 & H2 antagonists or considering an alternative medication. Certainly, if anaphylaxis develops protamine should be discontinued and andexanet alfa (as an off-licence, second line agent as described above) considered if life threatening or neuroaxial bleeding cannot be stopped.

Excess dosing of protamine negatively impacts on platelet function and the coagulation cascade thus paradoxically causing anticoagulation. Excess protamine can stimulate clot breakdown by decreasing thrombin concentration (in theory).

Andexanet alfa could be used as an alternative if anaphylaxis develops but bleeding continues [50]. *The author advises that andexanet use would be off label. Readers are advised to contact the manufacturer for further medical information regarding dosing and administration or their local haematologist.*

For Low Molecular Weight Heparin (LMWH)

Protamine

Protamine reverses approximately 60% of LMWH based on data from animal studies. Anti-Xa levels post protamine infusion do not correlate its likelihood of persistent bleeding. As with Heparin/UFH 1 mg of protamine reverses 100 iu or 1 mg of LMWH [48, 49].

Please see advisory guidance in the Heparin/UFH section regarding the clinical risk with protamine use.

Protamine Reversal for LMWH: Courtesy of Toxbase

- Administer a loading dose of 20 mg IV Protamine over 4 min.
- Then an infusion is required over the subsequent 8 h: the total dose of protamine (loading

and infusion) should match 1 mg of Protamine for every 1 mg or 100 iu of Enoxaparin, Tinzaparin or Dalteparin. e.g. if 100 mg Enoxaparin taken, 100 mg of protamine will be required: 20 mg as *loading* IV dose and 80 mg as IV *infusion* over 8 h.

- Note: it is unnecessary to monitor the APTT.

Andexanet Alfa

At the time of writing there were human and animal studies [38, 51] examining the validity and safety of using andexanet alfa to reverse the anticoagulant effects of LMWH in the face of life threatening haemorrhage. There still are insufficient studies to give FDA/EMA approval for LMWH reversal by andexanet.

The author advises that andexanet use would be off label but andexanet should be used as ***second line after protamine***. Readers are advised to contact the manufacturer for further medical information regarding dosing and administration.

For Fondaparinux

At the time of writing there were no identified antidotes to Fondaparinux induced anticoagulation.

Studies suggest that rFVIIa (*NovoSeven* manufactured by Novo Nordisk) affords some correction of global coagulation assays [47, 52, 53]. A placebo controlled study in healthy volunteers treated with therapeutic doses of fondaparinux and 90 μg/kg rFVIIa demonstrated correction of prolonged coagulation times and partial restoration of thrombin generation [54]. Currently the British Committee for Standards in Haematology advise use of rFVIIa [47].

***NovoSeven* rFVIIa** dose 90 mcg/kg IV [54] as a *slow push* over 5 min.

Readers are advised to contact the manufacturer for further medical information regarding dosing and administration or their local haematologist.

Theoretically andexanet alpha could also be used given that it's a decoy molecule for Xa inhibitors [55] but the data is still very limited.

Anti-Platelet Agents

Finally, a brief mention should be made regarding all anti-platelet agents in the trauma setting and consideration for platelet transfusion. This is a controversial area. The data is mixed and currently there is no evidence to suggest any mortality benefit from platelet transfusion in patients with traumatic intracranial haemorrhage taking anti-platelet agents nor significant reduction in haemorrhage progression or neurosurgical intervention [56, 57]. In one meta-analysis regarding traumatic intracranial haemorrhage, platelet transfusion shows a trend towards *decreased survival* [57]. Platelet transfusion theoretically increases the risk of arterial thrombosis. In patients taking anti-platelet medication, if there is significant bleeding or concern then the anti-platelet medication should be stopped. Patients will start to produce functional platelets themselves within 24 hours of stopping the medication.

Summary

Dealing with haemorrhagic trauma is complex enough, this can be compounded by the presence of medications—the worst being anticoagulants. It is vital that the clinical team has a working knowledge of the antidotes to reverse the plethora of anticoagulants now available.

- If a patient has taken any oral DOAC in the preceding 24 h, assume they are fully anticoagulated. However, patients who have taken rivaroxaban or edoxaban 24 h prior may have near normal bleeding times.
- There is no acute rapidly accessible test to determine the level of anticoagulation from a

DOAC, the PT & APTT could be normal yet the patient anticoagulated

- Often clinicians cannot ascertain the time or dose of last DOAC consumption (often because clinicians are unable or forget to ask or check medical records!).
- Reversal agents aren't true reversal agents: they buy you a period of normal coagulation, the effects of some anticoagulants can return.
- Coagulation screens produce clinically meaningless results in this setting. Do not be guided by them (unless the patient is anticoagulated with either VKA or UFH) in the decision-making process regarding anticoagulant reversal. Remember standard blood tests have a lag time before the results are available, but an expert local haematologist may be able to give some interpretation.
- Resuscitation rooms should have standard operating procedures (SOPs) for reversal agent use including pictorial instructions on drug reconstitution because often reversal agents are either rarely used or very expensive and therefore not stocked in large volumes—mistakes can be costly in more ways than one, and antidotes should be rapidly available when needed.
- *Do not use FFP to reverse anticoagulants as* there is a risk of volume overload in some patients due to the large amount of FFP needed to have sufficient effect to reverse anticoagulants, regardless of other considerations. *Use blood products to resuscitate whilst removing the anticoagulant from the equation with antidotes.*
- **Trauma units should stock reversal agents within the resuscitation room, not in remote departments.**

Multiple Choice Questions

1. Which of the following are Factor Xa Inhibitor Anticoagulants?
   (a) Apixaban
   (b) Edoxaban
   (c) Dabigatran
   (d) Fondaparinux
   (e) Warfarin

   Answer: Correct = A & B are Factor Xa Inhibitors.

   Incorrect = C is a Direct thrombin Inhibitor; D is an Indirect FXa Inhibitor via Antithrombin III; E inhibits the formation of Factor X.

2. In regard to Factor Xa Inhibitor Anticoagulants: which of the following is true…
   (a) The effect on PT depends on either the assay or the Xa Inhibitor
   (b) They act by forming an irreversible blockade of both free and clot bound FXa thus preventing Thrombin from being formed
   (c) The degree of anticoagulation or bleed risk cannot be reliably ascertained by standard laboratory testing.
   (d) There is no acute reliable measure of DOAC anticoagulation

   Answer:

   A, False: it depends on both.

   B, False: the effect is reversible.

   C, True: Its consensus opinion that a plasma level of DOAC below 30 ng/ml is considered the cut off of safety for emergency surgery, but this is far from a standard laboratory test (currently).

   D, True: Mass spectrometry may exclude DOAC levels, but this isn't a rapid test in the acute haemorrhagic situation.

3. Regarding dabigatran anticoagulation: which of the following is false…
   (a) Clinicians must be aware that the idarucizumab-dabigatran complex is renally excreted and therefore optimum urinary output must be maintained
   (b) Idarucizumab is a monoclonal antibody, which forms a complex with dabigatran, with an affinity for dabigatran 300 times more than that of dabigatran to thrombin.
   (c) If idarucizumab is not available, then dialysis may be an option as it is not protein bound
   (d) If idarucizumab is not available, then 4 factor PCC is a reversal option

(e) A normal TT is indicative of a subject suitable for emergency surgery.

Answer: D is the false answer, the rest are true.

4. Reversal of heparin anticoagulation with protamine: true or false
   (a) Protamine is a low-risk drug
   (b) Protamine is best administered peripherally
   (c) UFH and Protamine combine to form a salt
   (d) Fondaparinux is reversed by protamine

   Answer:

   A, False: It has multiple side effects including paradoxical bleeding, systemic hypotension and anaphylaxis. Clinicians should be prepared for the side effects including having IM adrenaline nearby.

   B, True: Its associated with less histamine release given peripherally IV.

   C, True: This salt is subject to renal or hepatic metabolism. The exact pathway has yet to be described.

   D, False: There is no antidote to Fondaparinux anticoagulation. Although NovoSeven can be tried.

5. True or False: Regarding Andexanet alfa… before deciding on the dosing regimen (High dose or Low Dose) you need to ascertain
   (a) the DOAC taken
   (b) the TIME of last dose
   (c) the DOSE taken
   (d) the PT & APTT

   Answer: A: True, as andexanet alfa doesn't currently have a license to reverse edoxaban, however early indications suggest that you would follow the High Dose regimen in an emergency.

   B, True.

   C, True.

   D, False: No measurements are required only proof of haemorrhage.

References

1. Parasrampuria DA, Truitt KE. Pharmacokinetics and pharmacodynamics of edoxaban, a non-vitamin K antagonist Oral anticoagulant that inhibits clotting factor Xa. Clin Pharmacokinet. 2016;55:641–55.
2. Anand SS, Bosch J, Eikelboom JW, Connolly SJ, Diaz R, Widimsky P, et al. Rivaroxaban with or without aspirin in patients with stable peripheral or carotid artery disease: an international, randomised, double-blind, placebo-controlled trial. Lancet. 2018 Jan;391(10117):219–29.
3. McClure GR, Kaplovitch E, Narula S, Bhagirath VC, Anand SS. Rivaroxaban and aspirin in peripheral vascular disease: a review of implementation strategies and management of common clinical scenarios. Curr Cardiol Rep. 2019 Oct;21(10):115.
4. Combining rivaroxaban with aspirin in stable atherosclerotic vascular disease: clinical evidence from the COMPASS study. Br J Cardiol [Internet]. 2020 [cited 2020 Sep 4]; Available from: https://bjcardio.co.uk/2020/03/combining-rivaroxaban-with-aspirin-in-stable-atherosclerotic-vascular-disease-clinical-evidence-from-the-compass-study/
5. Bonaca MP, Bauersachs RM, Anand SS, Debus ES, Nehler MR, Patel MR, et al. Rivaroxaban in peripheral artery disease after revascularization. N Engl J Med. 2020 May 21;382(21):1994–2004.
6. Samuelson BT, Cuker A, Siegal DM, Crowther M, Garcia DA. Laboratory assessment of the anticoagulant activity of direct Oral anticoagulants. Chest. 2017 Jan;151(1):127–38.
7. Demir M. Coagulation testing for new Oral anticoagulants. J Atr Fibrillation. 2015 Nov;8(3):1089.
8. Drouet L, Bal dit Sollier C, Steiner T, Purrucker J. Measuring non-vitamin K antagonist oral anticoagulant levels: when is it appropriate and which methods should be used? Int J Stroke. 2016 Oct;11(7):748–58.
9. Ahmed N, Steiner T, Caso V, Wahlgren N. For the ESO-KSU session participants. Recommendations from the ESO-Karolinska stroke update conference, Stockholm 13–15 November 2016. Eur Stroke J. 2017 Jun;2(2):95–102.
10. Cuker A, Siegal DM, Crowther MA, Garcia DA. Laboratory measurement of the anticoagulant activity of the non–vitamin K Oral anticoagulants. J Am Coll Cardiol. 2014 Sep;64(11):1128–39.
11. Brett OF, Brett CN, Chin PK. The effect of routine preoperative interruption of dabigatran therapy on coagulation parameters and dabigatran plasma levels in a mixed surgical population. Anaesth Intensive Care. 2019 Mar;47(2):183–8.
12. Hawes EM, Deal AM, Funk-Adcock D, Gosselin R, Jeanneret C, Cook AM, et al. Performance of coagulation tests in patients on therapeutic doses of dabigatran: a cross-sectional pharmacodynamic study based on peak and trough plasma levels. J Thromb Haemost. 2013 Aug;11(8):1493–502.

13. Ebner M, Birschmann I, Peter A, Härtig F, Spencer C, Kuhn J, et al. Emergency coagulation assessment during treatment with direct Oral anticoagulants: limitations and solutions. Stroke. 2017 Sep;48(9):2457–63.
14. Godier A, Dincq A-S, Martin A-C, Radu A, Leblanc I, Antona M, et al. Predictors of pre-procedural concentrations of direct oral anticoagulants: a prospective multicentre study. Eur Heart J. 2017 Aug 14;38(31):2431–9.
15. Medicines and Healthcare products Regulatory Agency, UK Government, Drug Safety Update. Direct-acting oral anticoagulants (DOACs): reminder of bleeding risk, including availability of reversal agents [Internet]. GOV.UK. [cited 2020 Jul 16]. Available from: https://www.gov.uk/drug-safety-update/direct-acting-oral-anticoagulants-doacs-reminder-of-bleeding-risk-including-availability-of-reversal-agents
16. Francart SJ, Hawes EM, Deal AM, Adcock DM, Gosselin R, Jeanneret C, et al. Performance of coagulation tests in patients on therapeutic doses of rivaroxaban: a cross-sectional pharmacodynamic study based on peak and trough plasma levels. Thromb Haemost. 2014;111(06):1133–40.
17. Hirsh J, Anand SS, Halperin JL, Fuster V. Mechanism of action and pharmacology of unfractionated heparin. Arterioscler Thromb Vasc Biol. 2001 Jul;21(7):1094–6.
18. Weitz JI, Middeldorp S, Geerts W, Heit JA. Thrombophilia and new anticoagulant drugs. Hematology. 2004 Jan 1;2004(1):424–38.
19. Kitchen S. Problems in laboratory monitoring of heparin dosage. Br J Haematol. 2000;111(2):397–406.
20. Adie SK, Farina N. Impact of COVID-19 on monitoring of therapeutic unfractionated heparin. J Thromb Thrombolysis. 2020 Aug;19:1–3.
21. Bowles L, Platton S, Yartey N, Dave M, Lee K, Hart DP, et al. Lupus anticoagulant and abnormal coagulation tests in patients with Covid-19. N Engl J Med. 2020 Jul 16;383(3):288–90.
22. Vlot EA, Van den Dool EJ, Hackeng CM, Sohne M, Noordzij PG, Van Dongen EPA. Anti Xa activity after high dose LMWH thrombosis prophylaxis in covid 19 patients at the intensive care unit. Thromb Res. 2020 Dec;196:1–3.
23. White D, MacDonald S, Bull T, Hayman M, de Monteverde-Robb R, Sapsford D, et al. Heparin resistance in COVID-19 patients in the intensive care unit. J Thromb Thrombolysis. 2020 May;22:1–5.
24. Thomas O, Lybeck E, Strandberg K, Tynngård N, Schött U. Monitoring low molecular weight heparins at therapeutic levels: dose-responses of, and correlations and differences between aPTT, anti-factor Xa and thrombin generation assays. PLoS One. 2015;10(1):e0116835.
25. Johnson PN, Benefield EC, Bui P-YN, Gausman JN, Marlar RA, Gessouroun MR. Fondaparinux monitoring: need for a local Fondaparinux-calibrated anti–factor Xa assay. J Pediatr Pharmacol Ther JPPT. 2013;18(4):318–9.
26. Hanley JP. Warfarin reversal. J Clin Pathol. 2004 Nov;57(11):1132–9.
27. Tellor KB, Barasch NS, Lee BM. Clinical experience reversing factor Xa inhibitors with four-factor prothrombin complex concentrate in a community hospital. Blood Transfus. 2018 Jul;16(4):382–6.
28. Zada I, Wang S, Akerman M, Hanna A. Four-factor prothrombin complex concentrate for the reversal of direct Oral anticoagulants. J Intensive Care Med. 2019 Nov;20:885066619882909.
29. Müller M, Eastline J, Nagler M, Exadaktylos AK, Sauter TC. Application of prothrombin complex concentrate for reversal of direct oral anticoagulants in clinical practice: indications, patient characteristics and clinical outcomes compared to reversal of vitamin K antagonists. Scand J Trauma Resusc Emerg Med [Internet]. 2019 Apr 23 [cited 2020 July 16];27. Available from: https://www.ncbi.nlm.nih.gov/pmc/articles/PMC6480883/
30. Grottke O, Schulman S. Four-factor prothrombin complex concentrate for the management of patients receiving direct oral activated factor X inhibitors. Anesthesiol J Am Soc Anesthesiol. 2019 Nov 1;131(5):1153–65.
31. Pollack CV, Reilly PA, Eikelboom J, Glund S, Verhamme P, Bernstein RA, et al. Idarucizumab for dabigatran reversal. N Engl J Med. 2015 Aug 6;373(6):511–20.
32. Glund S, Gan G, Moschetti V, Reilly P, Honickel M, Grottke O, et al. The renal elimination pathways of the dabigatran reversal agent Idarucizumab and its impact on dabigatran elimination. Clin Appl Thromb Off J Int Acad Clin Appl Thromb. 2018 Jul;24(5):724–33.
33. Grottke O, Aisenberg J, Bernstein R, Goldstein P, Huisman MV, Jamieson DG, et al. Efficacy of prothrombin complex concentrates for the emergency reversal of dabigatran-induced anticoagulation. Crit Care [Internet]. 2016 [cited 2020 July 16];20. Available from: https://www.ncbi.nlm.nih.gov/pmc/articles/PMC4850655/
34. Shaw JR, Siegal DM. Pharmacological reversal of the direct oral anticoagulants—a comprehensive review of the literature. Res Pract Thromb Haemost. 2018 Mar 26;2(2):251–65.
35. Eerenberg ES, Kamphuisen PW, Sijpkens MK, Meijers JC, Buller HR, Levi M. Reversal of rivaroxaban and dabigatran by prothrombin complex concentrate: a randomized, placebo-controlled, crossover study in healthy subjects. Circulation. 2011 Oct 4;124(14):1573–9.
36. Siegal DM, Curnutte JT, Connolly SJ, Lu G, Conley PB, Wiens BL, et al. Andexanet alfa for the reversal of factor Xa inhibitor activity. N Engl J Med. 2015 Dec 17;373(25):2413–24.
37. The ANNEXA-A and ANNEXA-R Trials | NEJM [Internet]. [cited 2020 Jul 16]. Available from: https://www.nejm.org/do/10.1056/NEJMdo005043/full/
38. Connolly SJ, Crowther M, Eikelboom JW, Gibson CM, Curnutte JT, Lawrence JH, et al. Full study report of Andexanet alfa for bleeding associated

with factor Xa inhibitors. N Engl J Med. 2019 Apr 4;380(14):1326–35.
39. Lu G, Conley PB, Leeds JM, Karbarz MJ, Levy GG, Mathur VS, et al. A phase 2 PK/PD study of Andexanet alfa for reversal of rivaroxaban and edoxaban anticoagulation in healthy volunteers. Blood Adv. 2020 Feb 25;4(4):728–39.
40. Lu G, Pine P, Leeds JM, DeGuzman F, Pratikhya P, Lin J, et al. Andexanet alfa effectively reverses edoxaban anticoagulation effects and associated bleeding in a rabbit acute hemorrhage model. PLoS ONE [Internet]. 2018 Mar 28 [cited 2020 July 16];13(3). Available from: https://www.ncbi.nlm.nih.gov/pmc/articles/PMC5874076/
41. Grottke O, Braunschweig T, Rossaint R, Akman N, Leeds JM, Conley PB, et al. Transient or extended reversal of apixaban anticoagulation by andexanet alfa is equally effective in a porcine polytrauma model. Br J Anaesth. 2019 Aug;123(2):186–95.
42. Arachchillage DRJ, Alavian S, Griffin J, Gurung K, Szydlo R, Karawitage N, et al. Efficacy and safety of prothrombin complex concentrate in patients treated with rivaroxaban or apixaban compared to warfarin presenting with major bleeding. Br J Haematol. 2019 Mar;184(5):808–16.
43. Grandhi R, Newman WC, Zhang X, Harrison G, Moran C, Okonkwo DO, et al. Administration of 4-factor prothrombin complex concentrate as an antidote for intracranial bleeding in patients taking direct factor Xa inhibitors. World Neurosurg. 2015 Dec;84(6):1956–61.
44. Durie R, Kohute M, Fernandez C, Knight M. Prothrombin complex concentrate for the management of severe traumatic bleeding in a patient anticoagulated with apixaban. J Clin Pharm Ther. 2016 Feb;41(1):92–3.
45. Zahir H, Brown KS, Vandell AG, Desai M, Maa J-F, Dishy V, et al. Edoxaban effects on bleeding following punch biopsy and reversal by a 4-factor prothrombin complex concentrate. Circulation. 2015 Jan 6;131(1):82–90.
46. Pahs L, Beavers C, Schuler P. The real-world treatment of hemorrhages associated with dabigatran and rivaroxaban: a Multicenter evaluation. Crit Pathw Cardiol. 2015 Jun;14(2):53–61.
47. Makris M, Van Veen JJ, Tait CR, Mumford AD, Laffan M. The British Committee for Standards in haematology. Guideline on the management of bleeding in patients on antithrombotic agents. Br J Haematol. 2013 Jan;160(1):35–46.
48. Applefield D, Krishnan S. Protamine. In: StatPearls [Internet]. Treasure Island (FL): StatPearls Publishing; 2020 [cited 2020 July 16]. Available from: http://www.ncbi.nlm.nih.gov/books/NBK547753/
49. Cuenca JS, Diz PG, Sampedro FG, Zincke JMG, Acuña HR, Fontanillo MMF. Method to calculate the protamine dose necessary for reversal of heparin as a function of activated clotting time in patients undergoing cardiac surgery. J Extra Corpor Technol. 2013 Dec;45(4):235–41.
50. Siddiqui F, Tafur AJ, Hoppensteadt D, Walenga J, Jeske W, Bontekoe E, et al. Andexanet alpha differentially neutralizes the anticoagulant, Antiprotease and thrombin generation inhibitory effects of unfractionated heparin, enoxaparin and Fondaparinux. Blood. 2019 Nov 13;134(Supplement_1):1158.
51. Pine P, Lu G, Canivel D, Pratikhya P, DeGuzman F, Karbarz M, et al. Andexanet alfa reverses anticoagulation effects of enoxaparin and associated bleeding in a rabbit acute hemorrhage model. Blood. 2016 Dec 2;128(22):1445.
52. Gatt A, van Veen JJ, Woolley AM, Kitchen S, Cooper P, Makris M. Thrombin generation assays are superior to traditional tests in assessing anticoagulation reversal in vitro. Thromb Haemost. 2008;100(08):350–5.
53. Desmurs-Clavel H, Huchon C, Chatard B, Negrier C, Dargaud Y. Reversal of the inhibitory effect of Fondaparinux on thrombin generation by rFVIIa, aCCP and PCC. Thromb Res. 2009 Mar;123(5):796–8.
54. Bijsterveld NR, Moons AH, Boekholdt SM, van Aken BE, Fennema H, Peters RJG, et al. Ability of recombinant factor VIIa to reverse the anticoagulant effect of the Pentasaccharide Fondaparinux in healthy volunteers. Circulation. 2002 Nov 12;106(20):2550–4.
55. Siddiqui F, Tafur A, Bontekoe E, Iqbal O, Jeske W, Mehrotra S, et al. Assay-based differentiation in the neutralization profile of unfractionated heparin, enoxaparin, and Fondaparinux by Andexanet alfa. Clin Appl Thromb. 2020 Jan 1;26:107602961989512.
56. Alvikas J, Myers SP, Wessel CB, Okonkwo DO, Joseph B, Pelaez C, et al. A systematic review and meta-analysis of traumatic intracranial hemorrhage in patients taking prehospital antiplatelet therapy: is there a role for platelet transfusions? J Trauma Acute Care Surg. 2020 Jun;88(6):847–54.
57. Batchelor JS, Grayson A. A meta-analysis to determine the effect on survival of platelet transfusions in patients with either spontaneous or traumatic antiplatelet medication-associated intracranial haemorrhage. BMJ Open. 2012;2(2):e000588.

Part IV

Pre-hospital Aspects of Trauma Care

History of Pre-Hospital Medicine in the UK

18

Matthew Beardmore

Abbreviations

ALS	Advanced Life Support
BASICS	British Association of Immediate Care Schemes https://www.basics.org.uk/
BMJ	British Medical Journal https://www.bmj.com/
CCP	Critical Care Paramedic
CPD	Continuing Professional Development
CPR	Cardiopulmonary resuscitation
ECG	Electrocardiogram
ECMO	Extracorporeal Membrane Oxygenation
ED	Emergency Department
EMS	Emergency Medical Services
FPHC	Faculty of Pre-Hospital Care https://fphc.rcsed.ac.uk/
HCPC	Health and Care Professions Council https://www.hcpc-uk.org/
ICU	Intensive Care Unit
IV	Intravenous
JESIP	Joint Emergency Services Interoperability Principles https://www.jesip.org.uk/home
JRCALC	Joint Royal Colleges Ambulance Liaison Committee https://www.jrcalc.org.uk/
MICU	Mobile intensive Care Unit
NCEPOD	National Confidential Enquiry into Patient Outcome and Death www.ncepod.org.uk/
NICE	National Institute of Health and Clinical Excellence https://www.nice.org.uk/
PAD	Public Access Defibrillator
PHEA	Pre-hospital emergency anaesthesia (current terminology for 'pre-hospital RSI')
PHEM	Pre-hospital Emergency Medicine (implicit in this, physician-led)
RAF	Royal Air Force
REBOA	Resuscitative Endovascular Balloon Occlusion of the Aorta
RSI	Rapid Sequence Induction (of Anaesthesia)
SAMU	Service d'Aide Médicale d'Urgence = MICU Network & Dispatch
SMUR	Service mobile d'urgences et réanimation = MICU
TARN	Trauma Audit Research Network https://www.tarn.ac.uk/

M. Beardmore (✉)
Department of Anaesthesia, Royal Cornwall Hospitals NHS Trust, Cornwall, Truro, UK

Devon Air Ambulance Trust, Exeter, Devon, UK
e-mail: matthew.beardmore1@nhs.net

P. Lax (ed.), *Textbook of Acute Trauma Care*, https://doi.org/10.1007/978-3-030-83628-3_18

- Early examples of pre-hospital care largely centre around the battlefields of antiquity and the middle ages. Provision of medical care at the point of injury and the rapid transport of casualties to field hospitals were to form the modern concept of an 'ambulance'.
- Significant advances in casualty care developed during the American Civil War were rapidly transferred to the large U.S. cities and European capitals such as Vienna and Paris in the mid-to late 1800s. Similar progress in the UK would take many more decades and be pioneered by city police and fire services.
- Ambulances used during World War I were redeployed onto the UK mainland post-war, forming the Home Ambulance Service. This rapidly expanded in both size and scope, with the gradual acknowledgement that first aid training of attendants was crucial.
- Following World War II, the epidemics of polio, trauma and cardiovascular disease would drive rapid change in medical science and pre-hospital systems. Training of ambulance personnel in these advanced skills heralded the era of the professional ALS paramedic. Opportunities for further specialism within the profession were to follow soon after.
- Doctors' involvement in on-scene pre-hospital civilian care would progress from ad hoc volunteering with BASICS and 'flying squads' to the formation of a sub-specialty training programme in 2012.
- Helicopter emergency medical services spread through the UK in the late 1980s and 1990s. In parallel, the Faculty of Pre-hospital Care was formed and professional examinations in the domain were developed. The range of pre-hospital personnel and interventions has expanded rapidly in the twenty-first century.

The story of how UK emergency medical services (EMS) developed into their modern form spans more than 150 years. Local developments, international experiences and geographical barriers have all influenced their development. The medical literature gives intermittent glimpses and insights into this fascinating tale of innovators, early adopters and individuals determined to change the system for the better. As such the story rarely forms a 'joined-up' narrative and no text can hope to credit every notable step of progress nor address every controversy in this field. Indeed, many lessons have been learned for a frustratingly long time and are often re-learned. Those frustrations are more than balanced by the truly inspirational figures on whose shoulders our professions now stand: Sir William Knott-Bower; Dr. Frank Pantridge; Dr. Douglas Chamberlain; Dr. Ken Easton to name but a few. What follows is a brief history of the EMS system with a focus on the development of UK pre-hospital emergency medicine. The very earliest examples of pre-hospital care as well as relevant international influences are included to put the story of progress on these small islands into perspective.

Antiquity to Early Modern

Hippocrates (460–370 BC) provides one of the first entries in the medical literature to recognise the importance of providing care at the optimal moment [1]:

> there are proper moments during diseases, … One must sometimes act quickly… These favourable moments will pass by quickly… Death will ensue if one defers [treatment]… One must grasp the opportunity

Military campaigns have often been the catalyst for improvements in immediate care. Early examples [2] include the surgeons accompanying Philip II of Macedon's army units in the mid-300 s BC. Stretcher bearers would be encouraged to bring in the wounded from the battlefield. Specially tasked horse units with modified saddles provided more rapid evacuation of casualties from battle in the armies of sixth century AD Byzantium. Horse drawn carriages were later utilised to transport wounded crusaders from battles to hospital in Jerusalem—the precursor to the chivalrous order of the Knights of St John. The latter would be recognised in the name of the well-recognised international first aid organisation formed in 1877 and still active today.

The invention of firearms would transform immediate care, starting on the battlefields of France. Undoubtedly influenced by the royal surgeon Abroise Paré, King Henry II of France ordered the provision of mobile hospitals to treat the ill and injured in 1550 [1]. Paré was a pioneer in many regards – an early battlefield surgeon credited with refinements in amputation technique, the invention of new surgical instruments and designing prostheses amongst many others. Later, Larrey (1766–1842) would quickly realise the implications of the newly developed and highly mobile artillery on battlefield care. Ambulances would require similar levels of mobility [1]. Leaving the wounded until after combat and then ponderously transporting to hospitals more than a league (2.42 miles) behind the lines meant a transit time of more than 24 h from injury. Many arrived dead or beyond help. Horse-drawn "flying ambulances" were to provide urgent treatment on the battlefield before rapidly transporting to field hospitals. Napoleon credited these as one of the greatest inventions of the 1700s and Larrey is recognised as the father of the modern concept of an ambulance [2].

Other remarkable examples of early pre-hospital care include [1]: a description of mouth-to-mouth artificial ventilation in 1761 by Dr. Samuel-Auguste Tissot; public access drowning first aid boxes in 1774 in Paris by Philippe-Nicolas Pia; and possibly the first successful use of defibrillation in 1775 by Danish veterinary surgeon Abildgaard. He describes the experimental delivery of an electric shock to a variety of animals; having shocked a domestic cockerel it appeared "completely dead" but thankfully "briskly flew off" after a subsequent shock "in the chest" [3].

Key Points

- The importance of timely treatment of critical illness has long been acknowledged in medical publications.
- For many centuries casualties were slowly evacuated to distant field hospitals, with relatively few examples of rapid on-scene treatment and transport.

Late Modern: 1860–1945

The service one would receive in the case of illness or injury in London in the 1860s would depend on one's wealth. Those with the means could call on a cab [2], otherwise ad hoc arrangements with carts, stretchers or other 'unsuitable conveyances' would need to be made. It was recognised that rough, inexpert handling of casualties caused harm. The British Medical Journal (BMJ) would explain why the famous surgeon Percival Pott, having fractured his leg in the street, fought off assistance from bystanders with his cane [4]:

> well he knew the danger which a man has suffered an accident is liable to undergo at the hands of those who undertake his conveyance to a surgeon

The limb- and life-threatening consequences of rough handling rendering a closed fracture open in the pre-antibiotic era were a major concern of the day. Recommendations for effective pre-hospital care in the same article of 1860 seem very prescient [4], especially when one considers how much longer it would take to establish an ambulance service in London:

1. Surgeons in suitable localities, possessed of a stock of splints, bandages, pillows, etc., whose duty it is to obey every call to succour the injured.
2. Printed instructions put into circulation by the authorities, with regard to what persons ought to do who are near to or who are witnesses of any serious accident.
3. Ambulances, held in readiness for the immediate transit of persons who have met with severe injuries-the slings in common use, and other modes of conveyance, being more or less inconvenient or objectionable.

Across the Atlantic, the American Civil War (1861–1865) was raging. William Green Morton, credited with the first public demonstration of surgical anaesthesia with ether in 1846, was treating soldiers of the Northern United States. Witnesses state [1] he would regularly anaesthetise more than 100 men per day and demand to be conveyed to the front to visit hospitals. The delivery of anaesthesia on the battlefield lead to the then Surgeon General William Alexander Hammond to announce the end of the "medical Middle Age" [1]. At the end of the conflict, the experience gained in casualty management was transferred promptly into civilian life in US cities. Horse-drawn ambulances with surgeon-ambulance men and medical equipment appeared in Cincinnati in 1865 and New York in 1869 at Bellevue Hospital. The latter had an impressive telephony service resulting in rapid casualty location and conveyance to the wards. Their system of "holding of coroner's inquests ..., by which grand opportunities for studying forensic medicine are afforded" [5] exceed many UK pre-hospital services' current routine follow-up practise.

These experiences were brought across to Europe and slowly adopted. Henri Nachtel is credited with importing them to France, where he eventually gained the support of Victor Hugo to initiate one of Europe's first pre-hospital physician-based municipal ambulance services in 1887. Saint Louis hospital housed on-call facilities (a stable!) for an intern, a coach driver, a telephone operator and the horses [1]. Vienna however gains the credit for Europe's first organised EMS system with the founding of Vienna's voluntary society for rescue in 1881 in the wake of a large theatre fire [6].

Back in London, comparatively little progress had been made during the two decades outlined above. The 'St John Ambulance litter' or 'Furley stretcher' was developed for civilian practise and introduced around 1880 in London [7]. Police, fire-fighters, and taxi-drivers would variably convey patients on these wheeled stretchers to hospitals and surgeries. Around this time horse-drawn ambulance carriages for the transport of patients with infectious diseases, and shortly afterwards for all patients, were introduced by the London Metropolitan Asylums Board [2]—these would remain in service until 1912. The Asylums Board had 6 ambulance stations, meaning the whole of London was within a 3-mile radius of a station [8].

The bicycle and the electric vehicle are both making come backs within UK practise more than a century after their debuts. The bicycle was first utilised in Leicester in 1892, securing a stretcher between two bicycles, and a later development in Birmingham using tandems in a similar arrangement [2]. It would be the year 2000 before these would again feature, this time in London [8]. Easily a century ahead of its time, however, was the electrically powered ambulance introduced in 1907 by the City of London Police [9]. That the police would invest such in an ambulance demonstrates the marked EMS system differences compared to today. At the turn of the century, police in Manchester and Liverpool had developed more advanced services than the capital [10].

This had not gone unnoticed by Sir William Knott-Bower, commissioner of the City of London police. He recognised that his officers would often be the first to attend most cases and thus a policy of first aid training for every policeman was implemented. Determined to bring London's ambulance provisions up to speed, he attempted in a 1904 report to persuade the Police Committee to invest in a combined mounted police patrol and ambulance system:

> to meet the requirements of the City of London such as has been available for many years in Liverpool, Manchester, and many of the large towns in the provinces, in Paris and Vienna, and in nearly all the great cities of America [9]

His criticisms of the ambulance provisions to the population of London echo Hippocrates' earlier quote and the recommendations of the BMJ article published 43 years earlier:

> [the hand litter] has the disadvantages of length of time necessarily taken in bringing it to the scene, and in removing the patient, want of prompt first-aid on the spot, lifting and carrying of the patient by unskilled persons...Thus, even where the hand-litter is available, a simple fracture may often become compound before arrival at the hospital, a patient may sink from exhaustion or haemorrhage whom earlier skilled aid might have saved [9].

Knott-Bower's vision was to place two senior St Bartholomew medical students to act as 'surgical dressers'; his request was however declined on the grounds of cost [9]. The parallels with the Paris-based system implemented in 1887 are no coincidence—Dr. Nachtel is credited by the Commissioner as being the "first [to bring] the question of Horse Ambulances to the notice of the Court of Common Council" [9]. He oversaw the installation of 52 electric street call boxes, so effectively used in New York 40 years previous, that could be used by any police constable to summon an ambulance [10]. The system was impressive in its efficiency: ambulance response times averaging 4 min; delivery of the patient to the accident ward (including rendering of first aid on the spot) averaging 9.5 min.

Political pressure and frustrated calls for a dedicated municipal ambulance service rapidly mounted in the medical literature in the first decades of the twentieth century. This is notable in correspondence to the Lancet in 1910, lamenting "ancient and out-of-date … stretchers", lack of any "organisation… for dealing with cases of accident" [in suburban London] and patients being conveyed by "obsolete wheeled litters, a passing growler, or a greengrocer's van" [10]. Street and road accidents were already resulting in large numbers of casualties, and the problem was growing rapidly. 1907 saw 17,055 injuries with 283 fatal in such incidents; this compares to 10,540 and 155 respectively in 1905 [10]. Clearly the increasingly busy and mechanised post-industrial streets of the city were giving an early insight into the looming pandemic of trauma to follow later in the century.

Once again, war would drive progress in the civilian ambulance services. The vast numbers of casualties in World War I and huge progress made in casualty 'flow' from the front lines to rehab would positively influence pre-hospital care in the UK [2]. The Red Cross ambulances themselves, jointly with the Order of St John, would be redeployed onto the UK mainland to form the 'Motor Ambulance Service for England, Ireland and Wales' [11], or the 'Home Ambulance Service'. The review of its first year, published in 1920, details its 256 operational ambulances having carried over 7000 cases in return for a small fee, "remitted in necessitous cases" [11]. Progress was rapid, by 1925 some 1500 cases were transported per week, and the need for first aid skills amongst its staff was gaining recognition with yet more evidence of the rising death toll on our roads [12]:

> the increasing demand on the service to deal with road accidents has emphasised the need for skill in first aid on the part of the attendants serving with the ambulances… In road accidents, involving perhaps several persons, it often falls to the lot of the attendants to handle difficult case without professional supervision [of doctors or nurses]. A good deal of harm may be done by unskilful handling.

Rather remarkably the service also provided an "x-ray car" "for private patients and cottage hospitals within a reasonable radius of London" allowing radiographs to be taken in patient's bedrooms [12].

The Local Government Act resulted in responsibility for ambulance provision in London being transferred to London County Council in 1930 [8], the earliest recognisable version of today's London Ambulance Service. This re-structuring was applied to the rest of the country post-war, forming county ambulance services. It is important to note that the Home Ambulance Service worked alongside rather than replace numerous other pre-existing voluntary, police- and fire-led ambulance services, some of which continued to function until 1948 [2].

The next sentinel moments in the development of UK pre-hospital practise were seen in the mid-1930s. Orkney County Council awarded the first contract for an air ambulance covering the northern Scottish Isles to Highland Airways in 1934 [13]. Following a fire on Wimpole Street, London, which resulted in jammed operator telephone lines and a delayed response, the world's first universal emergency number was introduced [14]. 999 went live in 1936, fully 32 years before its equivalent in the USA.

The outbreak of World War II led to the formation of the London Auxiliary Ambulance Service to work alongside the London County Council Ambulances during the Blitz. This was not a knee-jerk response to the declaration of war in

September 1939, rather the culmination of years of preparation for mass casualty events, re-organisation of the hospital network and the creation of extra bed capacity [15]. Initially staffed by 5000 volunteers, 50% of whom were women, the service swelled to 10,000 staff at its peak and was disbanded in 1945 [2].

Key Points

- As early as 1860, the importance of high quality, basic on-scene care by trained individuals and careful handling of casualties was well recognised.
- Major US cities, Vienna and Paris developed advanced, medicalised pre-hospital systems decades before the UK. The police and fire services of UK cities formed the very earliest versions of an ambulance service.
- The Home Ambulance Service was formed following World War I, supplementing the services provided by the fire and police. These endured until the end of World War II.

Contemporary: 1945—Present

Medical progress following World War II proceeded at a high pace, driven simultaneously by polio epidemics, ever-increasing civilian trauma deaths and developments in the cardiovascular sciences.

The polio epidemic far surpassed the capabilities of medical services to provide artificial ventilation. Iron-lung external negative pressure ventilators were first utilised clinically in 1928 in Boston, with invasive positive pressure ventilation coming into use in Denmark in 1952 [1]. Expertise was however centred in a few hospitals nationwide with, for example, only two centres in the whole of France. Patients would often die in transit from the provinces to these hospitals. Recognising this situation, Maurice Cara would create physician-staffed ambulances with portable ventilators (of both types) in 1956. In-transit mortality rates for high-risk patients fell rapidly from 50% to 1% [1].

World Health Day 1961 focussed on civilian trauma deaths—"Accidents Need Not Happen"—already the world's third cause of early mortality [16]. Remaining in the political spotlight, the seminal 1966 report by the National Academy of Sciences in the USA published "Accidental Death and Disability: The Neglected Disease of Modern Society" would result in marked improvements to trauma care. The report was particularly damning of the current situation [17]:

> expert consultants returning from both Korea and Vietnam have publicly asserted that, if seriously wounded, their chances of survival would be better in the zone of combat than on the average city street

> Approximately 50 per cent of the country's ambulance services are provided by 12,000 morticians, mainly because their vehicles can accommodate transportation on litters

> Although it is possible to converse with astronauts in outer space, communication is seldom possible between an ambulance and the emergency department that it is approaching

> In contrast to the days when an intern accompanied every ambulance on an emergency call, the pendulum may have swung too far toward total dependence on ambulance personnel

The recommendations of this report would lay the foundations for modern pre-hospital trauma systems: data collection; research; public access first aid materials; instruction manuals for healthcare professionals; co-ordination of ambulance provision; multi-disciplinary radio channels resembling today's multiagency working principles (e.g. JESIP); and a single, universal public emergency number.

On the other side of the Atlantic, exciting developments in pre-hospital cardiac care were in motion in Belfast. The post-war years had witnessed the first successful treatment of ventricular fibrillation in humans – during open chest surgery in 1947 [18] and by the external application of current to a closed chest in 1956 [19]. Coronary thrombosis was another feared early killer and it often did so quickly. Epidemiologists Bainton and Peterson demonstrated that 63% of patients dying from acute coronary thrombosis did so within the first hour of their presentation [20]. The average age of their 1963 patient cohort was just 45 years.

Further evidence would demonstrate that 10% of this patient group died in an ambulance on their way to hospital [21]. If such rhythm disturbances occurred on a cardiac ICU survival rates of approximately 50% were described [22].

Dr. Frank Pantridge recognised that it "seemed silly to keep the ICU in the hospital and that the thing to do was take both the equipment and expertise to the patient" [21]. Defibrillators of that era however were exclusively mains powered. In the winter of 1965, assisted by technician Alfred Mawhinney and his Senior House Officer John Geddes, he converted a mains defibrillator to function from two 12 V 63-amp car batteries in series with a static inverter [21]. The first 'portable' defibrillator weighed 70 kg! Placed in an ambulance with a junior doctor and a nurse, the mobile intensive care unit (MICU) went live on first January 1966. General practitioners would make priority calls to the hospital switchboard who then alerted the duty doctor and ambulance control. Response times were less than 15 min for 78% of calls [23].

Early results of this innovation were published in 1967 to a remarkably mixed response. Of the 312 patients attended over 15 months, no patients died in transit. This compares to a pre-MICU study of coronary deaths showing 102 of 414 patients arriving dead at hospital. Ventricular fibrillation had been successfully treated in 10 patients outside of hospital, 4 of whom were in-transit; 5 of these patients survived to discharge from hospital [24]. Dr. Pantridge describes his perceptions of the UK medical establishment's response to this seminal development thus [21]: "we were voices in the wilderness"; "we were disbelieved and indeed, to some extent, ridiculed". The response in the USA was far more positive. 'Time' magazine featured this work just a month after it appeared in the Lancet [24] and it is reported that Air Force One was fitted with a defibrillator given President Johnson's cardiac history [21]. St Vincent's hospital in New York imitated this physician staffed MICU in 1968 [24]. Miami pioneered ECG telemetry to the hospital which would act as a "Trojan horse" for the delegation of physician-level interventions at distance [24]. Subsequent iterations in 1969 in six different US states utilised 'paramedics' drawn from fire departments to provide early care for victims of myocardial infarcts and for primary cardiac arrests [24]. Amongst these, the Seattle programme is highly regarded for [24]:

- Its implementation of a 'tiered' emergency response—CPR trained firemen initially, followed by defibrillation-trained paramedics.
- Physician supervision during the unit's first 10 months allowed for the teaching of endotracheal intubation, ECG interpretation and administration of IV cardioactive medications; these paramedics would then work solo with physician advice available by radio.
- Large-scale citizen CPR training—100,000 Seattle residents were trained within a few years of the programme's inception.

The year 1970 saw the inception of the pioneer 'Advanced Life Support' (ALS) paramedics. The UK ambulance service was undergoing major changes during these years. Pre-1966 all that was required to work on an ambulance was a driving license and the promise that one would attend a first aid course in service [25], the time-frame for which was not defined. It was possible to work for some time without any healthcare training at all. Dr. E L M Millar would chair a committee reporting to the Minister for Health on ambulance service equipment and training. His 1966 reports proposed an 8-week basic training programme and civil defence training with a heavy practical element [26, 27]. After 12 months' experience on the roads a variety of tests would follow before the award of the 'Ambulance Services Proficiency Certificate', or colloquially a 'Millar certificate' [25]. The ambitions of these reports are clear [28]:

> the working party would like to see advanced courses for those seeking promotion, special courses for instructors and control room operators, and refresher courses of 1 week every 3 years

> stresses the need for practical training under the conditions simulating the actual work of an ambulance service

> During his first year he should spend at least a week in the casualty department of an approved hospital
>
> …ambulance services council should be set up, with representatives of the Royal Colleges… it might well have a standing committee for training…

This could be considered an early call for the Joint Royal Colleges Ambulance Liaison Committee (JRCALC) which would not convene for the first time until 1989.

Lessons had been learnt during the Blitz in appropriately training ambulance crews with "enough background knowledge to make sensible decisions and behave calmly in critical situations"; the old teaching of "rush the casualty to the nearest hospital" was fast becoming outdated [28]. The curriculum outlined by Millar is 'broadly similar' to today's ambulance technician qualification, indeed the programme evolved into the Institute of Health and Care Development technician programme [25]. It would be another 19 years before 'extended trained ambulance staff', or ALS paramedics, would be similarly established at a national level in the UK [29].

The latter half of the 1960s saw the rapid expansion of volunteer immediate care doctor schemes [30] and more frequent descriptions of 'flying squads' [31].These aimed to fill the "therapeutic vacuum" [32] affecting those trapped and critically injured in road and industrial incidents between scene of accident and meaningful intervention at hospital. Dr. Ken Easton founded the UK's first general practitioner immediate scheme with 34 of his colleagues covering 1000 square miles in the North Riding of Yorkshire [30]. An ex-RAF doctor, he worked at a practise in Catterick near the A1 corridor, a road notorious for its high accident rate. He worked alongside Mr. Ron Exelby, who having inherited a haulage firm upon leaving the RAF recognised the need for a vehicle rescue and recovery business in the area [33]. By 1973 there were 28 such schemes around the UK, ranging in membership from 1 to 100 [30]. Dr. RAA Johnson recounts his experiences of visiting 9 of these [30]:

> the potential of radio-telephones is becoming tremendous with new, more sophisticated equipment the natural reluctance shown by some ambulance services… and the fear that the ambulance men will become drivers and porters if doctors attend incidents… almost without exception, these fears have been allayed

His description outlines the equipment, tasking, governance arrangements and the beginning of multidisciplinary training with police, fire, and ambulance personnel at staged incidents. Most of these schemes were funded by charitable donations from the public; indeed, the only scheme at that time receiving hospital funding was the Northern Region Hospitals Board of Scotland [30].

Dr. Easton went on to be the first chair of the British Association of Immediate Care Schemes (BASICS) at its inception in 1977, inspiring the next generation of immediate care doctors, though gaining government support proved far more challenging [33].

An early description of an 'Accident Flying Squad' based at the Derbyshire Royal Infirmary in 1966 recounts a dynamic and prescient prehospital team [31]. With "no available standards for guidance" they equipped themselves with a portable ventilator (requiring a portable power supply), medications, surgical instruments and even plasma [31]. Their first ever call was a delayed primary response to a multiply injured patient at a cottage hospital, assisted by the Derby Borough Police. Another case recounts a rendezvous with an ambulance to provide timely resuscitation of the victim. The squad actively prepared for major incidents, encouraged multi-agency working and were to install the UK's first hospital radio-transmitter to allow two-way communication with local ambulances.

Similar such arrangements were in place in both France and Germany from 1957 [1, 6]. The critical difference on the Continent was the rapid recognition of their value. The French government made physician-staffed mobile intensive care units (SMUR) a national service in 1965 and created a national specialist dispatch service (SAMU) in 1968 [1]. That same year the German anaesthetist Frey started trials of helicopter EMS; they would become a national service just 3 years later [6].

Another innovator of UK pre-hospital medicine was working to make Brighton "the Seattle of the UK" [34]. Dr. Douglas Chamberlain was reportedly motivated to improve the ambulance response having witnessed the 999 response to a patient suffering a sudden cardiac arrest in front of him in 1970 [34]:

> ...the ambulance which arrived after a protracted time with a defibrillator that took two men to lift. When it was turned on it exploded and caught fire. I thought we ought to be able to do better...

A pioneer in many regards, his work to establish the 'extended skills' (defibrillation, endotracheal intubation) of UK 'paramedics', jointly establish the Joint Royal Colleges Ambulance Liaison Committee (See Figure 18.1—'What is JRCALC?') and advocate for the first public access defibrillators (PAD) are perhaps some of his finest achievements. PADs were distributed far and wide [34]: Brighton and Hove Football ground in 1977 [35]; Victoria station, London; and British Caledonian Airlines aircraft. Not to mention the huge mark left on the academic world of resuscitation: training the first Resuscitation Officer; key member of the Resuscitation Council UK, European Resuscitation Council, and International Liaison Committee on Resuscitation; and Editor-in-Chief of *Resuscitation* journal from 1990.

Figure 1: A Brief Outline of JRCALC

What is JRCALC?

Joint Royal Colleges Ambulance Liaison Committee first convened in 1989, bringing a multidisciplinary approach to training, education, and standards to the UK ambulance service [68]. It publishes frequently updated clinical guidelines for pre-hospital care, the first version of which was published in the year 2000. Guideline development sub-groups bring multidisciplinary experts with pre-hospital experience together to produce these [68]. The 'JRCALC guidelines' form the basis for paramedic practise in the UK. One of its original roles was to provide oversight to the ambulance services, though this has become less prominent now that all Ambulance Trusts have a medical director [68].

With continued political pressure from the likes of Pantridge, Chamberlain and their peers, local versions of the Brighton "experimental" [29] 'paramedic' training schemes slowly spread and evolved during the 1980s to other parts of the UK [36]. This was formalised in 1985 with the Department of Health introducing a national training scheme for such 'extended trained ambulance staff' [29]. The goal was to train enough paramedics to ensure their presence on each emergency ambulance by 1996. This target was achieved by most services; the UK finally had an ALS-based ambulance service [36].

By now the UK's first air ambulances were appearing and trauma was back on the medico-political agenda. Long since used to transport critically injured patients in Europe, it was acknowledged that we needed to "catch up experts and systems in other countries" [37]. Starting in Cornwall in 1987 they spread quickly, numbering 10 by 1999 [38]. London's helicopter flew its first mission in 1989 and the iconic helipad on the roof of the Royal London was built in 1990 [39]. Initially the helicopter system was instituted solely for the treatment of trauma [40].

The Surgical Colleges take much of the credit for bringing trauma back onto the political agenda from 1988. A review of 1000 trauma deaths showed that up to one third of trauma deaths were potentially preventable and that UK trauma management "still leaves much to be desired" [41]. The average age of this patient cohort was 41 years—many life-years were being lost. Of grave concern was that many of the deaths judged to have been preventable were due to failure to stem haemorrhage, prevent hypoxia and delays to (or absence of) surgical treatment [41]. The "Report on the Management of Patients with Major Injuries" recommended enhanced training for ambulance staff, more sophisticated methods of transport and improved communication between ambulances and receiving hospitals [42]. The British Orthopaedic Association made increasingly strong calls for centralisation of trauma services and US-style trauma networks in their reports of 1989, 1992 and 1997 [43–45].

The North Americans were simultaneously developing trauma management; the changes implemented either side of the Atlantic differed [46]. While the United States focused on pre-hospital triage based on physiology and mechanism of injury, the UK focused on in-hospital trauma expertise and seniority [46]. UK consultant trauma involvement almost doubled between 1989 and 1997, while the severity adjusted odds of trauma death reduced by 60% in long-standing Trauma Audit Research Network (TARN) participant hospitals [46]. Most of these gains had been made by 1994, with stagnation the key message between 1994 and 2000 [46]. The question became: Should we be addressing the pre-hospital phase of treatment?

More frequent and urgent calls for reform of UK pre-hospital care would follow from the mid-90s. The British Medical Association Board of Science and Education recognised BASICS as a valuable national resource in 1993, recommending central funding [47]. The value doctors could offer pre-hospital beyond the competencies of a 'Level 2' paramedic was formally acknowledged. Cooke highlights some of the deficiencies of immediate care schemes, citing the part-time nature and "variability of the service", variable geographical cover where "audit…is sparse" [48]. His call for recognition of "the practitioner in immediate care…as a specialist" requiring a training program and examinations would remain unmet until pre-hospital emergency medicine (PHEM) was approved by the General Medical Council as a medical sub-specialty in 2011.

The Royal College of Surgeons of Edinburgh were characteristically early to adapt to developments in urgent care, having already introduced the Specialty Fellowship in Accident & Emergency Medicine in the 1970s [49]. The Faculty of Pre-hospital Care (FPHC) was formed within the College in 1996 with the primary aim of setting and maintaining standards in pre-hospital care [49]. This further strengthened the calls for change. It was becoming increasingly unacceptable that "the pre-hospital phase is the only part of the health service in which management of the individual patient is not the responsibility of a senior clinician" (a hospital specialist or a General Practitioner) [38]. Noting that the average ambulance service paramedic would see only one severely injured patient per year, there was a strong argument to use helicopters to deliver an expert trauma team to the scene of severe injuries [38]. Training was in short supply for doctors however, with only one pre-hospital 'training scheme' for registrars and a total of 2 NHS appointed consultants in the specialty in 1999 [38].

However, training and career development opportunities were fast expanding for paramedics in the early part of the twenty-first century. State registration of paramedics with the Council for Professions Supplementary to Medicine came in 2000 along with publication of the first iteration of JRCALC guidelines [29]. A year later the term 'paramedic' becoming a protected title and the first UK BSc (Hons) Paramedic Sciences degrees would produce graduates [29]. A more flexible paramedic workforce was proposed to meet efficiency and resource targets. Emergency Care Practitioners would be educated to degree level, work across professional and organisational barriers in Emergency Departments (ED), hospital and primary care settings [50]. The "confusing variation" [51] and the "number of different terminologies" [52] around this role that ensued required clarification for other healthcare professionals and patients alike. The more standardised term 'specialist paramedic' was recommended by the College of Paramedics in 2014 [52], mandating a minimum of post-graduate diploma level education for such roles. These changes coincided with the formal end of the Millar certificate era [50]. Paramedics are now regulated by the Health and Care Professions Council (HCPC) and their college publishes a professional journal and CPD resources for their 10,000+ members.

The debate on 'pre-hospital and retrieval medicine' continued formally in print in 2005. It began: "the provision of on scene medical support to ambulance services in the UK is fragmented, disorganised, and largely unregulated" [32]. The need for a medically regulated and specifically trained workforce to provide immediate care was once again stressed by Dr. R Mackenzie. It was accompanied by a detailed outline of potential accreditation pathways and, in retrospect, a highly accurate framework of today's PHEM subspecialty training pathway [32]. The reactions from learned societies and Royal

Colleges were largely positive. Calls to ensure this new specialty was multidisciplinary were multiple and many feared alienating or discouraging long-standing immediate care doctors [32].

Enough momentum had been gained and progress was rapid. The NCEPOD 2007 report 'Trauma: Who Cares' commented on the potential need for personnel capable of delivering pre-hospital anaesthesia and considered the current structure of pre-hospital management insufficient for those with severe injuries [53]. Such specialist resources were available in *some* areas, *some* of the time, depending who was on-call; the issue became that of inequality of access. This "geographical lottery" of emergency care seen in so many counties [54] was, the Royal College of Surgeons would inform parliament, resulting in preventable deaths in the UK [55]. The scale of this inequality was starkly presented in a wide-ranging 2009 survey of ambulance services, air ambulances, BASICS schemes and emergency departments [56]. Accounting for incomplete data collection, it was estimated that volunteer doctors made almost 10,000 scene attendances per year. None of these schemes had a guaranteed 24 h service. 45% of their doctors reported having the capability to provide rapid sequence induction of anaesthesia (RSI), latterly known as pre-hospital emergency anaesthesia (PHEA). The hospital 'flying squad' was largely obsolete with only 2% of EDs being able to provide an 'RSI-capable' team. Air ambulances operations were largely restricted to daytime taskings with only 29% operating with a doctor 7 days per week.

The Intercollegiate Board for Training in PHEM was formed in 2009. The aim of the training scheme was to produce specialists equivalent to independently practising consultants. As such, an expansive medical curriculum with associated knowledge, skills and behavioural elements was devised [57]. The FPHC exams would be core to demonstrating this high standard: The Diploma in Immediate Medical Care (dating from 1988); and the Fellowship in Immediate Medical Care (dating from 2000) [49]. Graduates of the scheme would be expert providers of pre-hospital critical care, transfer and retrieval medicine. Predictions estimated that their "high level on-scene and in-transit medical support" would benefit approximately 0.5–1% of emergency calls, acknowledging that 99% of pre-hospital care demand was met "to a high standard" by paramedics [58]. The first PHEM registrar began training in the East of England in 2012; more than 50 trainees have now completed this training programme [58]. In response the early concerns, provisions for experienced immediate care doctors to accredit as consultants and multi-disciplinary access to the national summative PHEM assessments were made.

Calls for major improvements in pre-hospital governance would continue in 2011 despite this progress. The lack of national standards for provider competencies, training and revalidation, the absence of a central governing body and increasing interest of the Care Quality Commission in the sector remained high on the agenda [59]. The rapid expansion of the UK pre-hospital world came with some complications:

- Even with guidance on nomenclature relating to 'specialist' paramedic roles [52], large variations exist in the regional training and competencies of critical care paramedics (CCP) around the UK [60].
- The medical workforce expanded, with a wider range of backgrounds and experience. Many assume that staff on air ambulances would have critical care capabilities but "many employ[ed] doctors that do not have these skills" [56].
- Combinations of the above working within very different pre-hospital organisations with different 'sign-off' expectations for solo practise of sedation and/or anaesthesia.

The net effect of this being that there could be considerable uncertainty about the skill set of an air ambulance or 'critical care' resource arriving at a tasking; and marked differences in services both in and between regions. The FPHC Practitioner levels clarify this to some extent (see Table 18.1 'Levels' and Skill sets of UK Pre-hospital practitioners—A brief guide), but some carefully targeted questions may still be needed to establish this on-scene.

Table 18.1 'Levels' and Skill sets of UK Pre-hospital practitioners—A brief guide. As outlined in the main text, role nomenclature in UK pre-hospital practise is confusing and in an almost constant state of flux. The below table outlines current conventional role 'boundaries' and skill sets to help clarify this [57, 60, 61]. There will undoubtedly be examples of different local practises and individuals who perhaps do not fit neatly into this; please accept my apologies for any oversights or oversimplifications

FPHC descriptor	FPHC definition	Practitioner 'Level'	Example role title	Example skill set
F	Non-registered healthcare practitioner	3	Senior healthcare assistant/ technician	– Basic resuscitation skills (BLS, airway, 02, defibrillation) – Trauma skills (spinal immobilisation, fracture Mx, haemorrhage control, wound management) – Measurement of vital signs and 12-lead ECG – Entonox analgesia – Limited range of emergency drugs for ACS, asthma anaphylaxis and hypoglycaemia.
		4	Associate ambulance practitioner	
G	Registered pre-hospital care 'Practitioner'	5	Paramedic	All the above, plus: – Tracheal intubation (N.B. variation between ambulance trusts) – Needle thoracocentesis – Needle cricothyroidotomy – IV cannulation & analgesia – Oral/IM/IV drug administration of a wide JRCALC pharmacopoeia
		6	Critical care paramedic Also: Nurse, Physician's assistant, Some medical staff	Large variations in scope of practise and local arrangements, including: – Procedural and post-ROSC sedation – Administration of muscle relaxant – Ultrasound/ECHO competencies – Thoracostomy – Surgical airway – Amputation – Non-invasive ventilation – Arterial and central venous access – Chest drain insertion In current practise, doctor-only: – Rapid sequence induction of anaesthesia – Thoracotomy – REBOA – ECMO
H	Registered pre-hospital care 'Advanced Practitioner'	7	Post-DIMC experienced Dr., CCP or nurse	
		8	Post-FIMC Dr., CCP or nurse	
–		9	Senior pre-hospital management	

There is much to celebrate in the advances that have been made in the UK EMS system. A new generation of pre-hospital professionals are beginning their careers with many exciting developments and challenges afoot. Both the Association of Anaesthetists of Great Britain and Ireland and NICE have set quality standards for pre-hospital RSI and FPHC guidelines are being published with a high frequency [62–64]. Our trauma systems are world-renowned, with a 2015 paper highlighting regular emergency thoracotomies in London having good neurological outcomes in 15%, versus just one successful such procedure in the whole of the USA [65]. A Masters degree in pre-hospital care has recently opened at the Institute of Pre-hospital Care in London [66] and the development of extended roles for paramedics leads both the USA and

Australia [50]. There are a number of potentially 'meaningful interventions' that we may choose to expand in the short term: point-of-care blood tests; telemedicine; various imaging modalities; REBOA; and ECMO. Funding of specialist pre-hospital teams will likely remain challenging. Many PHEM trainees and critical care paramedics learn their trade entirely within charitable organisations. The government recently allocated a "one-off" £10 million to 9 different air ambulances to improve their equipment and facilities [67]; a small minority of services are centrally commissioned. For parting thoughts, what lessons will we continue to re-learn in the modern era? Upon what unmet needs and neglected patient groups will the next generation reflect?

Key Points

- The 25 years following World War II saw the development of invasive ventilation, external cardiac defibrillation and their rapid adoption in the pre-hospital setting. The world's first ALS paramedics were trained to deliver these interventions in the USA.
- Prior to 1966, all that was required to work on a UK ambulance was a driving license and to agree to sign up to a first aid course. The Millar Report of that year was to formalise the training of ambulance personnel.
- It would take another 20 years before a national UK training programme for 'ALS paramedics' was instituted. Professional registration, post-graduate opportunities and diversification of paramedic roles followed relatively quickly.
- Meanwhile, numerous volunteer immediate care doctor schemes and flying squads were to fill the "therapeutic vacuum" facing critically injured, trapped trauma victims on-scene.
- Pre- and in-hospital trauma management has featured prominently in the medico-political agenda since the mid-1980s. In parallel, UK Helicopter emergency medical services have rapidly expanded. Key development since then include: the development of standards; more equitable geographical provision; and professionalisation of training for these services.

Conclusion

This history of UK pre-hospital care charts the progression from basic first aid and stretcher conveyance of casualties to advanced helicopter-based critical care interventions over the course of a few centuries. Taking the time to understand this journey, sometimes tortuous and slow, is critical to understanding the current system and potential future developments. To those of you who will shape the future of this specialty, I hope that you find the accounts and anecdotes of the pioneers included in the text both instructive and inspiring. Notably, these pioneers are not limited to medical inventors and visionaries, but also to those who tirelessly published and lobbied to raise the profile of the neglected diseases of their times. Despite the apparent complexity of modern EMS systems, the astute reader will have noted the basic lessons of pre-hospital care being relearned through each generation covered by the text. Let us not forget these as we look forward to an exciting future in this specialty.

Acknowledgements I would like to thank Professor Myles Gibson for his correspondence, Dr. David Hume for his review of this manuscript and Dr. Peter Lax for his advice and guidance.

Questions

1. Regarding historical developments in emergency medicine, the following were first reported prior to 1900:
   (a) successful external cardiac defibrillation of a human being
   (b) 'iron lung' ventilation
   (c) successful external cardiac defibrillation of a chicken
   (d) mouth-to-mouth ventilation
   (e) an electric-powered ambulance

   Answers: FFTTF

2. Communication between pre-hospital teams and the destination hospital is crucial. Which of these statements are true:
   (a) the universal emergency number, 999, was introduced in the UK in 1936

(b) by the 1980s, communication between UK ambulances and receiving hospitals was advanced
(c) telephone links between incident scenes and Bellevue hospital, NYC, were in place by 1869
(d) horse-drawn flying ambulances were proposed to be one of the greatest inventions of the 1800s
(e) telemetric transfer of ECGs from scene to local hospital was pioneered in Miami in the late 1960s

Answers: TFTFT

3. Pre-hospital pioneers and 'firsts'. Which of these statements are true?
   (a) the first portable defibrillators used in the UK weighed 70kg
   (b) the 'Millar certificate' marked a significant step towards professional, highly trained paramedics
   (c) physician-staffed mobile intensive care units became a national standard in France in 1965
   (d) Helicopter emergency medical services (HEMS) were widely established in Germany in 1971
   (e) the UK's first HEMS unit was established by 1981

   Answers: TTTTF

4. Service provision and nomenclature within UK pre-hospital practice. Which of the following are true?
   (a) Specialist clinical roles have a limited range of tightly regulated, clearly defined terms
   (b) Provision and availability of physician-led pre-hospital critical care is uniform throughout the UK
   (c) IBTPHEM is the organisation responsible for GMC-approved pre-hospital doctor training
   (d) the NMC is the professional body that represents UK paramedics
   (e) only doctors are eligible to sit the FPHC exams (DipIMC/FIMC)

   Answers: FFTFF

5. Which of the following correctly quote seminal reviews, commentary and reports into pre-hospital care?
   (a) *Although it is possible to converse with astronauts in outer space, communication is seldom possible between an ambulance and the emergency department that it is approaching [1966]*
   (b) *...the fear that the ambulance men will become drivers and porters if doctors attend incidents... almost without exception, these fears have been allayed... [1974]*
   (c) the provision of on scene medical support to ambulance services in the UK is consistent, well-organised, and highly regulated [2005]
   (d) *very little harm may be done by unskilful handling [1925]*
   (e) it seemed silly to keep the ICU in the hospital and that the thing to do was take both the equipment and expertise to the patient [1965]

   Answers: TTFFT

References

1. Club de l'histoire de l'anesthésie et de la réanimation, France. Anesthésie, analgésie, réanimation, Samu: notre histoire, de 1945 aux années 2000. Tome III, Paris: Éditions Glyphe; 2016.
2. Pollock A. Ambulance services in London and Great Britain from 1860 until today: a glimpse of history gleaned mainly from the pages of contemporary journals. Emerg Med J. 2013;30(3):218–22.
3. Abildgaard P. Societatis Medicae Havniensis Collectanea [Internet]. Joann Gottlob Rothe; 1775. 334 p. (Societatis Medicae Havniensis Collectanea). Available from: https://books.google.co.uk/books?id=ZtJcAAAAcAAJ
4. British Medical Journal. BMJ. 1860;s4-1(207):980–2.
5. Mapother ED. An address on American medicine. Br Med J. 1870;2(514):477–9.

6. Roessler M, Zuzan O. EMS systems in Germany. Resuscitation. 2006;68(1):45–9.
7. Sir John Furley and St John Ambulance [Internet]. Museum of the Order of St John. 2019 [cited 2020 May 3]. Available from: http://museumstjohn.org.uk/sir-john-furley-and-st-john-ambulance/
8. Our History [Internet]. London Ambulance Service NHS Trust. [cited 2020 May 3]. Available from: https://www.londonambulance.nhs.uk/about-us/who-we-are/a-brief-history/
9. Police ambulances | City of London Police [Internet]. [cited 2020 May 3]. Available from: https://colp.mpw.cds.co.uk/police-forces/city-of-london-police/areas/city-of-london/about-us/about-us/police-ambulances/
10. Hardy HN. An ambulance Service for London. Lancet. 1910;176(4533):195–7.
11. British Medical Journal. Br Med J. 1920;1(3099):713–7.
12. British Medical Journal. Br Med J. 1925;2(3374):388–92.
13. Bloice L, Baxter G, Gray D. Report on the social and cultural importance.pdf [Internet]. 2017 Feb [cited 2020 Mar 3]:[42 p.]. (SPARA Project). Report No.: Deliverable 7.1. Available from: https://rgu-repository.worktribe.com/output/246807/report-on-the-social-and-cultural-importance-of-remote-and-peripheral-airports
14. Why 999 for an emergency? 2010 May 13 [cited 2020 May 3]; Available from: http://news.bbc.co.uk/local/london/hi/people_and_places/history/newsid_8675000/8675199.stm
15. Denham M. As we once were the wartime emergency medical service and the future NHS | British Geriatrics Society [Internet]. British Geriatric Society. 2015 [cited 2020 May 3]. Available from: https://www.bgs.org.uk/resources/as-we-once-were-the-wartime-emergency-medical-service-and-the-future-nhs-2
16. Cardiology: Immediate Counterattack. Time [Internet]. 1967 Sep 1 [cited 2020 May 3]; Available from: http://content.time.com/time/magazine/article/0,9171,837241,00.html
17. National Academy of Sciences (US) and National Research Council (US) Committee on Trauma, National Academy of Sciences (US) and National Research Council (US) Committee on Shock. Accidental Death and Disability: The Neglected Disease of Modern Society [Internet]. Washington (DC): National Academies Press (US); 1966 [cited 2020 May 3]. Available from: http://www.ncbi.nlm.nih.gov/books/NBK222962/
18. Beck CS. Ventricular fibrillation of long duration abolished by electric shock. JAMA. 1947;135(15):985.
19. Zoll PM, Linenthal AJ, Gibson W, Paul MH, Norman LR. Termination of ventricular fibrillation in man by externally applied electric countershock. N Engl J Med. 1956;254(16):727–32.
20. Bainton CR, Peterson DR. Deaths from coronary heart disease in persons fifty years of age and younger: a community-wide study. N Engl J Med. 1963;268(11):569–75.
21. Pantridge JF. An unquiet life: memoirs of a physician and cardiologist. Place of publication not identified: publisher not identified; 1995.
22. Pantridge JF, Geddes JS. Cardiac arrest after myocardial infarction. Lancet. 1966;287(7441):807–8.
23. Pantridge JF, Geddes JS. A Mobile intensive-care unit in the management of myocardial infarction. Lancet. 1967;290(7510):271–3.
24. Eisenberg MS, Pantridge JF, Cobb LA, Geddes JS. The revolution and evolution of prehospital cardiac care. Arch Intern Med. 1996;156(15):1611–9.
25. Kilner T. Educating the ambulance technician, paramedic, and clinical supervisor: using factor analysis to inform the curriculum. Emerg Med J. 2004;21(3):379–85.
26. Millar ELM. Ambulance training and equipment. Part 1. Training [Internet]. Great Britain: Ministry of Health; 1966 [cited 2020 May 3]. Available from: http://archive.org/details/op1269011-1001
27. Millar ELM. Ambulance training and equipment. Part 2. Equipment and vehicles [Internet]. Great Britain: HMSO; 1967 [cited 2020 May 3]:[55 p.]. Available from: https://archive.org/details/op1269012-1001/page/n53/mode/2up
28. Training the ambulance man. Lancet. 1966;287(7438):649.
29. The Journey of the College | About Us [Internet]. 2019 [cited 2020 May 3]. Available from: https://web.archive.org/web/20190418131938/https://www.collegeofparamedics.co.uk/about_us/the-journey-of-the-college
30. Johnson RA. Immediate care schemes. J R Coll Gen Pract. 1974;24(149):847–50.
31. Collins J. Organization and function of an accident flying squad. BMJ. 1966;2(5513):578–80.
32. Mackenzie R, Bevan D. For Debate...: A license to practise pre-hospital and retrieval medicine. Emerg Med J. 2005;22(4):286–93.
33. A Brief History of BASICS [Internet]. British Association for Immediate Care. [cited 2020 May 3]. Available from: https://www.basics.org.uk/brief-history-basics/
34. Baskett P. Douglas Chamberlain CBE DSc (hon) FRCP FRCA FACC FESC—A man for all decades of his time. Resuscitation. 2007;72(3):344–9.
35. Jaggarao NSV, Sless H, Grainger R, Vincent R, Chamberlain DA. Defibrillation at a football stadium: an experiment with Brighton and Hove Albion. BMJ. 1982;284(6327):1451–3.
36. Carney CJ. Prehospital care - a UK perspective. Br Med Bull. 1999;55(4):757–66.
37. Earlam R. Trauma Helicopter [Internet]. [cited 2020 May 3]. Available from: http://www.richardearlam.com/trauma-helicopter/
38. Coats T, Goode A. Opportunity to improve pre-hospital care in the UK. Lancet. 1999;353(9161):1292.
39. Our History | London's Air Ambulance [Internet]. [cited 2020 May 3]. Available from: https://www.londonsairambulance.org.uk/about-us/history

40. Kirk CJC, Earlam RJ, Wilson AW, Watkins ES. Helicopter emergency medical service operating from the Royal London Hospital: the first year. Br J Surg. 1993;80(2):218–21.
41. Anderson ID, Woodford M, de Dombal FT, Irving M. Retrospective study of 1000 deaths from injury in England and Wales. BMJ. 1988;296(6632):1305–8.
42. Saleh M. Commission on the provision of surgical services. The management of patients with major injuries. Ann R Coll Surg Engl. 1989;71(4 Suppl):58.
43. The British Orthopaedic Association. The Management of Trauma in Great Britain. London; 1989.
44. British Orthopaedic Association. The Management of Skeletal Trauma in the United Kingdom. London: British Orthopaedic Association; 1992.
45. British Orthopaedic Association. The Care of Severely Injured Patients in the United Kingdom. London: British Orthopaedic Association; 1997.
46. Lecky FE. Lack of change in trauma care in England and Wales since 1994. Emerg Med J. 2002;19(6):520–3.
47. British Medical Association Board of Science and Education. Immediate care schemes. London: BMA; 1993.
48. Cooke MW. Immediate care: specialty or pastime? Injury. 1994;25(6):347–8.
49. Gibson M. Letter to author. 2020.
50. Brooks IA, Cooke M, Spencer C, Archer F. A review of key national reports to describe the development of paramedic education in England (1966–2014). Emerg Med J. 2016;33(12):876–81.
51. Jashapara A. Critical care paramedics - Delivering enhanced pre-hospital trauma and resuscitation care: A cost-effective approach [Internet]. NHS Confederation; 2011 [cited 2020 May 3]:[16 p.]. Available from: https://pure.royalholloway.ac.uk/portal/en/publications/critical-care-paramedics%2D%2Ddelivering-enhanced-prehospital-trauma-and-resuscitation-care-a-costeffective-approach(c7d9148f-9d24-4be2-95f8-94a77cc47081)/export.html.
52. College of Paramedics. Paramedic Curriculum Guidance [Internet]. College of Paramedics; 2014 [cited 2020 May 3]. Available from: https://collegeofparamedics.co.uk/COP/ProfessionalDevelopment/Paramedic_Curriculum_Guidance.aspx
53. Findlay G, Martin IC, Carter S, Smith N, Weyman D, Mason M. A report of the National Confidential Enquiry into Patient Outcome and Death 2007. p. 151.
54. Lockey D. International EMS systems: geographical lottery and diversity but many common challenges. Resuscitation. 2009;80(7):722.
55. House of Commons Hansard Debates for 11 Jun 2008 (pt 0001) [Internet]. Hansard. 2008 [cited 2020 May 3]. Available from: https://publications.parliament.uk/pa/cm200708/cmhansrd/cm080611/halltext/80611h0001.htm
56. Hyde P, Mackenzie R, Ng G, Reid C, Pearson G. Availability and utilisation of physician-based pre-hospital critical care support to the NHS ambulance service in England, Wales and Northern Ireland. Emerg Med J. 2012;29(3):177–81.
57. Curriculum - The Intercollegiate Board for Training in Pre-Hospital Emergency Medicine | IBTPHEM [Internet]. The Intercollegiate Board for Training in Pre-Hospital Emergency Medicine; 2015 [cited 2020 May 3]. Available from: http://www.ibtphem.org.uk/curriculum/
58. Mackenzie R. Brief history of pre-hospital emergency medicine. Emerg Med J. 2018;35(3):146–8.
59. Nutbeam T. Clinical governance and prehospital care in the UK. Emerg Med J. 2011;28(2):91–2.
60. von Vopelius-Feldt J, Benger J. Critical care paramedics in England: a national survey of ambulance services. Eur J Emerg Med. 2014;21(4):301–4.
61. Black JJM, Davies GD. International EMS systems: United Kingdom. Resuscitation. 2005;64(1):21–9.
62. Lockey DJ, Crewdson K, Davies G, Jenkins B, Klein J, Laird C, et al. AAGBI: safer pre-hospital anaesthesia 2017: association of anaesthetists of Great Britain and Ireland. Anaesthesia. 2017;72(3):379–90.
63. Consensus Statements - The Faculty of Pre-Hospital Care [Internet]. [cited 2020 May 3]. Available from: https://fphc.rcsed.ac.uk/my-fphc/resources/consensus-statements
64. NICE. NICE Quality Standard 166: Trauma [Internet]. National Institute for Health and Clinical Excellence; 2018 [cited 2020 Jan 12]. Available from: https://www.nice.org.uk/guidance/qs166/resources/trauma-pdf-75545603800261
65. Wilson MH, Habig K, Wright C, Hughes A, Davies G, Imray CHE. Pre-hospital emergency medicine. Lancet. 2015;386(10012):2526–34.
66. The Institute – IoPHC.co.uk [Internet]. [cited 2020 May 3]. Available from: http://iophc.co.uk/about-us/the-institute
67. £10 million awarded to 9 air ambulance charities [Internet]. GOV.UK. 2019 [cited 2020 May 3]. Available from: https://www.gov.uk/government/news/10-million-awarded-to-9-air-ambulance-charities
68. About | [Internet]. [cited 2020 May 3]. Available from: https://www.jrcalc.org.uk/about/

19 Aviation Considerations in PHEM

Joe Moore and Peter Lax

- Differences between HEMS and Air Ambulance taskings
- UK Aviation legislation and exemptions
- Specific sites of interest
- Carriage of patients and escorts
- Tasking and radio procedures
- Navigation and lookout
- Weather and flight safety
- Landing sites
- Specific flight zones and limitations

The use of helicopters in aeromedical evacuation and emergency medical response can be traced back to World War II. In Burma in January 1945, a Sikorsky YR-4 helicopter was used to extricate a 21-year-old soldier who had accidentally shot himself through his hand from the Naga Hills back to Myitkyina [1]. Modern helicopters are more technologically advanced, and the legal considerations of operating a helicopter around built-up areas are not insubstantial. Pilots must have good knowledge of both technical and legal aspects of the relevant issues surrounding helicopter emergency medical services (HEMS) duties before being selected as a HEMS pilot. While HEMS have been used in the military (most notably the UK MERT in Afghanistan [2, 3]), taskings and training are more specific to the theatre of operations for the deployment depending on the perceived threats. Many basic principles are the same in military and civilian operations, but this chapter will focus specifically on UK civilian practice and regulations. The general considerations for HEMS aviation in the UK are outlined, and the Agusta Westland AW109 helicopter is used as an example. However, at the time of writing, seven different models of helicopters are operated in the UK in the HEMS role by various charities. Each operator will have different policies and standard operating procedures. Where specific details are given below, they are related to operations at The Air Ambulance Service in the UK and Sloane Helicopters as the operator.

While each airframe will have specific operating characteristics and limitations, the principles below are applicable for all airframes within their operating flight envelope. The AW109 helicopter is a twin-engine, single pilot helicopter. It is the fastest helicopter in use by any UK HEMS organisation, typically cruising at 150–180 mph. In the HEMS role, it is a legal requirement for the aircraft to be crewed by a HEMS pilot and a HEMS TCM (Technical Crew Member) or two HEMS pilots. These are supplemented with a doctor or

J. Moore
Sloane Helicopters, Sywell, Northampton, UK

The Air Ambulance Service (TAAS), Rugby, Warwickshire, UK

P. Lax (✉)
Tactical Medical Wing, Royal Air Force, Brize Norton, Oxfordshire, UK

The Air Ambulance Service (TAAS), Rugby, Warwickshire, UK
e-mail: p.lax@NHS.net

P. Lax (ed.), *Textbook of Acute Trauma Care*, https://doi.org/10.1007/978-3-030-83628-3_19

second paramedic. There is typically the ability to carry one further person in addition to the patient, and this capacity is used for crew training, observing or, occasionally, to bring an escort for a patient (e.g. parent of an injured child). It consumes around 240 kg of fuel per hour (4 kg per min, approximately 5 L/min).

HEMS vs Air Ambulance

Helicopter Emergency Medical Services (HEMS) and Air Ambulances are two separate entities, though they are often grouped together when discussing the use of helicopters in pre-hospital and transfer medicine. The most significant distinction between a HEMS operation and an Air Ambulance is that HEMS aircraft are allowed to land on previously unsurveyed sites to treat patients and then transfer them to a hospital. In contrast, Air Ambulances can only land in locations that have been pre-surveyed and fly to another pre-surveyed site. Simply put, Air Ambulances most commonly transport patients between hospitals, but HEMS aircraft will fly from a base to the scene of an accident and then on to a hospital. In the UK, the RAF survey landing sites (and occasionally a secondary site) for every hospital to allow for Air Ambulance flights. These landing sites may not be on the hospital site but located a short distance away, depending on the layout and location of the hospital.

Where there are helicopter landing pads on-site, the approaches are assessed to ensure they are free of obstructions such as wires, high trees or other hazards to the aircraft. In hospitals without helipads, the nominated site may be a large sports field in the hospital's vicinity, which will require a land ambulance transfer to or from the landing zone (LZ), known as a secondary transfer. In the case of hospitals that require a secondary transfer to get from the LZ to the hospital itself, ambulance availability and distance may play a part in the selection of destination hospitals for patients. To avoid unnecessary delays, it is always prudent to request a ground ambulance from control when loading a patient onto a helicopter before taking off from the scene if it will be needed on arrival at the LZ!

Aviation Legalities

Helicopter operators hold an Air Operators Certificate (AOC) that entitles them to complete Commercial Air Transport (CAT). This is the same base certification that is needed for any fee-paying flight service. In addition, selected operators hold some additional permissions that allow them to operate a Helicopter Emergency Service (HEMS). To maintain this, the UK aviation regulatory body (the Civil Aviation Authority—CAA) audits each operator and completes a flight with each service at least once a year.

To be a legally authorised HEMS flight and operate with HEMS exemptions, the aircraft must:

- Be tasked by Ambulance Control
- Have either a HEMS pilot and HEMS TCM, or two HEMS qualified pilots on board.
- Have a landing site larger than twice the diameter of the main rotor blades (otherwise known as a 2D site, 26 metres in the AW-109).
- Be operating within the Class 1 helicopter performance envelope when arriving at a hospital. This refers to the performance in the event of one engine failing during a critical phase of flight, such as landing or takeoff. Factors such as patient/escort weight and current fuel level need to be dynamically calculated on each tasking as they will change on scene, as opposed to fixed weights that will be static throughout the shift such as equipment and crew.

Those four factors are the minimum mandated hard limits. However, there are many other factors to consider.

Permissions and Exemptions

SERA (Standardised European Rules of the Air) is where the basis for UK Aviation Rules are laid down. Exemptions to some of these rules can only be issued by the CAA, subject to certain conditions being met. The authoritative regulations are found in Part-SPA, Subpart J—HEMS [4], but below is a brief overview of some of the exemptions in use for HEMS in the UK.

Minimum Heights SERA3105

For all civilian aircraft, Visual Flight Rules state that unless taking off or landing any aircraft should fly at least 500 ft. above the highest person, vehicle or structure within a 150-metre radius of the aircraft in non-congested areas (i.e. over the countryside). In congested areas (i.e. metropolitan areas), the minimum altitude is at least 1000 ft. above the highest person, vehicle or structure within a 600-metre radius of the aircraft. The CAA has issued an exemption from the 1000 ft. rule in the UK for HEMS flight, but HEMS are not exempt from flying within 500 ft. of any person, vessel, vehicle or structure.

Prisons

There are several prisons with a no-fly zone around them, as depicted on standard aviation maps. While HEMS are exempt from these exclusions, and prison no-fly zones (NFZ) are typically marked up on HEMS aviation maps manually (e.g. with a coloured sticker) to show this. Still, it is good practice to avoid the NFZ unless critical.

Nuclear Facilities

All nuclear facilities have a no-fly zone around them, as depicted on aviation maps. HEMS are permitted into these areas (as stated in the CAA exemption), but each NFZ has specific restrictions. On the rare occasion HEMS may be tasked into one of these areas, the pilot should be given a few minutes of extra planning time to check the individual NFZ requirements before entering.

Landing and Taking off Near Open-Air Assemblies

Under the Rules of the Air regulations 5 (1)(b) [5], a helicopter shall not land in a congested area or near an open-air assembly without the permission of the CAA. HEMS are exempt from this as long as they are acting as an 'Emergency Services Helicopter'.

Pilot Duty Period and Discretion

Pilots are usually scheduled to work a 10- or 12-hour day depending on the operator, including time at the start and end of shift to prepare the aircraft and paperwork. They are permitted to extend their working day past 10 h at their discretion, i.e. if they are happy to do so. Potentially this may lead to a delayed start to the next days' shift if the pilot has to reclaim any of the additional hours worked. The maximum duty periods are also limited by how many consecutive days are worked and (theoretically) by how much flying has been done [6]. While the mission profile of most HEMS services is one of multiple short flights, there are maximum limits of how many flying hours can be accrued over specific periods (Fig. 19.1). HEMS pilots are unlikely to come close to these limits, as most flights are under 20–30 min. Turnaround and standby times (as well as time on scene) mean that even on busy days it is improbable that a pilot would come close to violating the 9-hour flight rule [7].

Crews cannot work more than seven consecutive days and must have a 2-day rest period if they work seven consecutive days. There are additional restrictions on 14-day working and an absolute limit on flight hours in any 3-day period (18 h), 28-day period (90 h) or 12 month period (800 h). Again, the mission profile of most HEMS units means that pilots would rarely come close to these limits.

Carriage of Patients

One utility of HEMS is to bring medical capability closer towards the point of injury and decrease the time from injury to assessment by advanced medical teams. A second implied use is to transport patients from the point of injury to a hospital, though not all patients are suitable for air transportation. The following scenarios merit some considerations:

Patient Height Certain helicopters may struggle to fit an over extended scoop stretcher; if the patient needs to be laid completely flat. Another

20.8 Maximum flying hours

The Maximum number of Flying Hours which a pilot may be permitted to undertake are:

Single day	Table E
Any 3 consecutive days	18 hours
Any 7 consective days	30 hours
Any 3 consecutive 28 day periods	240 hours

Table E - FDP- Helicopters

Local time of start	Single Pilot		Two pilots	
	Length of FDP in hours	Max. flying time in hours	Length of FDP in hours	Max. flying time in hours
0600-0659	9	6	10	7
0700-0759	10	7	11	8
0800-1359	10	7	12	8
1400-2159	9	6	10	7
2200-0559	8	5	9	6

Fig. 19.1 Taken from Overseas Territories Aviation Circular 121 [8]

consideration that should be made is if there is a Kendrick or other traction splint in place, as this will usually extend beyond the end of the scoop. Alterations can be made to the seating in the helicopter for patient loading/unloading in extreme circumstances, but this is the exception rather than the rule as it may take time to reconfigure the aircraft. If this is longer than the time it would take to move the patient to the hospital by road with an available ambulance, consideration should be given to moving the clinical crew to the land ambulance to escort the patient instead of flying them.

Weight Patient weight is a consideration in both fuel calculations for flight and for landing performance (Class 1 weight as described above).

Circumference All patients and their escorts need to be secured in the aircraft, typically with four-point harnesses on the stretcher. Largely obese patients may prove challenging and can only be carried if the sliding door immediately next to the stretcher can be safely closed with the patient secured. The patient must also be able to lay flat, and their body habitus may preclude this.

Contaminated/Off-Gassing A small amount of contaminant inside the small volume of the helicopter cabin can make it very unpleasant for the crew and potentially incapacitate the pilot, causing a serious risk to flight safety. Patients who have been involved in incidents with chemicals that could impair safe flight would not be flown. This includes specific incapacitants such as tear gas, common agents such as petrol or diesel fuel, patients involved in industrial chemical agents or infectious diseases.

Suicidal Patients Patients who have attempted suicide or are psychiatrically unwell are not carried (unless they have been given a general anaesthetic) as they could pose a risk to flight safety if they make a further attempt.

Near Term Pregnancy Typically, carrying heavily pregnant patients should be avoided as delivering a baby in a helicopter is not ideal. Still, this may have to be done in extreme cases after an individual risk/benefit analysis. Depending on the reason for transport and necessity to lay the patient supine, it also may not be possible to provide manual displacement of the uterus or lateral tilt in flight to relieve aortocaval compression.

Unstable Patients Patients with severe cardiorespiratory instability pose a challenging dilemma as they may benefit the most from rapid transfer to hospital. However, the cramped environment of the helicopter and use of safety restraints for both clinical crew and passengers limit the interventions which can be performed. Very unstable patients are usually best transported by land, but if there is no other option or the transfer time is significantly longer, they can be transported by air. There are no absolute rules in this situation, but each patient should be considered on a case by case basis. It also needs to be established that the benefit of transferring a patient by air outweighs the risk, however small that risk may be. If a patient has a non-time-critical minor injury and can be transported by land without causing a deterioration in their condition, they should not be flown.

Carriage of Escorts

There are occasions when it is appropriate to carry an escort, the most obvious being a parent when transporting a child. Before offering the escort a seat, clinicians should consult the pilot. The pilots' primary consideration is the additional weight and its effect on aircraft performance, but other factors exist too:

- Has the escort flown in a helicopter before?—If they are scared, how will they react?
- How stable is the patient?—How will the escort react if the patient deteriorates?
- Was the escort involved in what happened to the patient? Are there any other reasons that they should not be transferred with the patient from a forensic or safeguarding perspective?
- Is the rear seat medical crewmember happy that the escort will not distract them from the patient's care? For the majority of incidents where HEMS are tasked, the police may be able to transport relatives or escorts on blue lights to the hospital if required.

The rear seat crew member can indicate to the pilot if they feel that the escort may not be appropriate to fly, and crews should discuss this scenario at morning briefings before it occurs.

Call Taking and Tasking

Generally, the TCM or doctor will answer the base emergency phone and take details of the tasking from ambulance control. The most crucial information to obtain is the location (grid ref., town, etc.) so that it can be plotted on the overview map to allow for flight route planning by the pilot. Several factors come into play. Amongst these are the current and predicted weather, NOTAMS (Notice to Airmen—temporary warnings or restrictions in some areas), ATZs (air traffic zones), danger areas, likely destination hospitals, fuel considerations (current fuel load, projected usage and ability to be under class 1 weight when arriving at hospital, timings (last landing and FTLs—flight time limitations), additional kit and route for departing the airfield.

Once a plan has formed, the pilot will start the helicopter while the crew continue to take further details such as type of incident, injuries, number and age of patients, other assets travelling etc.

Radio Procedures

Radio communication can be complicated as two separate radio systems are used in flight.

The first deals with the aviation side of HEMS, typically speaking to air traffic control towers, radar services and occasionally talking to other aircraft when needed. These are the pilot's responsibility, and specific radio licenses and qualifications are required by the CAA (Civil Aviation Authority) before being authorised to use these systems. The second is the radio communication system used by the ambulance service for taskings, updates, and "flight following"- both systems may be overheard by all crew for situational awareness. While this may be useful, it occasionally can be distracting as people operating exclusively on the aviation system cannot hear when the ambulance system is broadcasting and vice versa and may "cross-talk". Transmissions and messages on the aviation system always take priority as they may be transmitting instructions that could pose an immediate threat to life if not heard (e.g. aircraft vectoring instructions for collision avoidance). There is also an intercom system so that the crew can communicate within the helicopter over the noise of engines and wind rush.

The busy times on the radios are takeoffs and landings, departing the airport, updating control on the estimated time of arrival on scene, passing through other ATZ's and coming back into the base, so conversation on the intercom is kept to a minimum during these times. Especially important is the concept of a "sterile cockpit" when descending through 300 ft. into a scene. This is the idea that everyone should be silent. There should be no transmissions unless there is a safety-critical issue that has been spotted to allow the pilot to concentrate on the landing—this includes answering routine radio messages.

Comms Panel in the Aircraft

The comms units in each aircraft will vary, so new crewmembers should take local guidance. However, there are a couple of universal principles to note. There are always at least three settings that can be modified on the comms box of each aircraft, and it is not always obvious what they do. These settings are:

Vox—This changes how sensitive a microphone is. Turned fully anti-clockwise, the microphone is 'live' the whole time, meaning that all incidental aircraft noise will be picked up. Conversely, if it is turned fully clockwise, the crew member would have to shout very loudly to get the microphone to pick up! This setting should be adjusted so that the microphone will pick up when the crew member speaks at a comfortable volume but doesn't pick up breathing noise.

ICS—This stands for Intercom System and is the volume that conversations from crewmates are heard.

RX—This is the volume for ALL radios, so it will vary how loudly all the radio transmissions that come into the helicopter are heard (both ambulance and aviation).

Maps and Charts

Pilots use specific aviation charts for navigating, which detail ATZs, airspace etc. The two carried as standard are the 1:250000 (quarter mil) used for most taskings, and the 1:500,000 (half mil) used if there is a significant distance to fly and show less detail due to the scale. Ordnance Survey (OS) maps and street A-Z maps are carried to fine-tune navigation the aircraft gets closer to the scene (Fig. 19.2).

The UK Grid Reference System

The British Isles are split into a series of 100 km × 100 km squares on a 1:50,000 scale map, and a 6 figure grid reference is used to plot a point, e.g. "SP 123456". This reference will be accurate to within 100 m of an incident which is good enough for HEMS purposes. Each square is given a two-letter code. The Northern ones have the prefix 'N' (NA, NB, NC......), the Southern ones have the prefix 'S', and the Eastern ones have the prefix 'T'. This is where the alphabetical component comes from in the example (Fig. 19.3).

The numerical component is split into 2 × 3 figures (i.e. in the example above, it is "123" and

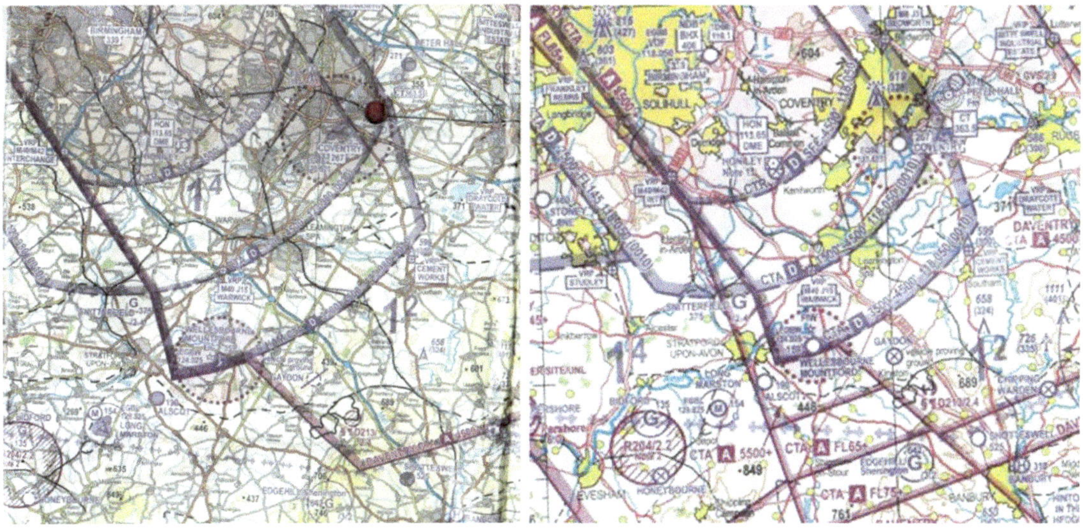

Fig. 19.2 Quarter (top) and half mil aviation maps (reproduced with the permission of NATS)

			HO	HP		
			HT	HU		
	HW	HX	HY	HZ		
NA	NB	NC	ND	NE		
NF	NG	NH	NJ	NK		
NL	NM	NN	NO	NP		
	NR	NS	NT	NU		
	NW	NX	NY	NZ	OV	
		SC	SD	SE	TA	
		SH	SJ	SK	TF	TG
	SM	SN	SO	SP	TL	TM
	SR	SS	ST	SU	TQ	TR
SV	SW	SX	SY	SZ	TV	

Fig. 19.3 UK OS Map grids (Produced with kind permission of Ordnance Survey)

"456"). Each of the squares within the map segment designated by the alphabetical code (e.g. SP, SK) is split into 1 km^2. Therefore, each two-letter square represents 100 km × 100 km. Specific points within these two-letter squares are referenced by how many Easterly (left to right) and then Northerly (bottom to top) subdivisions are used. The order of sequences is often remembered as "along the corridor then up the stairs". The first two numbers of each sequence give the number of **full** squares that are moved (e.g. in the example, 12 along and 45 up within the SP square). The final number of each three-digit set comes from splitting the designated square into tenths to give a location within a 100-metre radius.

In Fig. 19.4, the grid reference for the centre of the highlighted square would be TL625335 (i.e. the large map square is TL, the specific square to localise it is 62 across and 33 up). Within that box, it is 5/10th across and 5/10th up. If the location desired was in the top left corner of the same highlighted box, the reference would be TL621339, i.e. the same box but 1/10th across and 9/10th up.

In the example above of SP123456, think of the coordinates as being in the SP square and then moving along to the East 12.3 squares, finally going up 45.6 squares. The key for reading an OS Map is printed on every map.

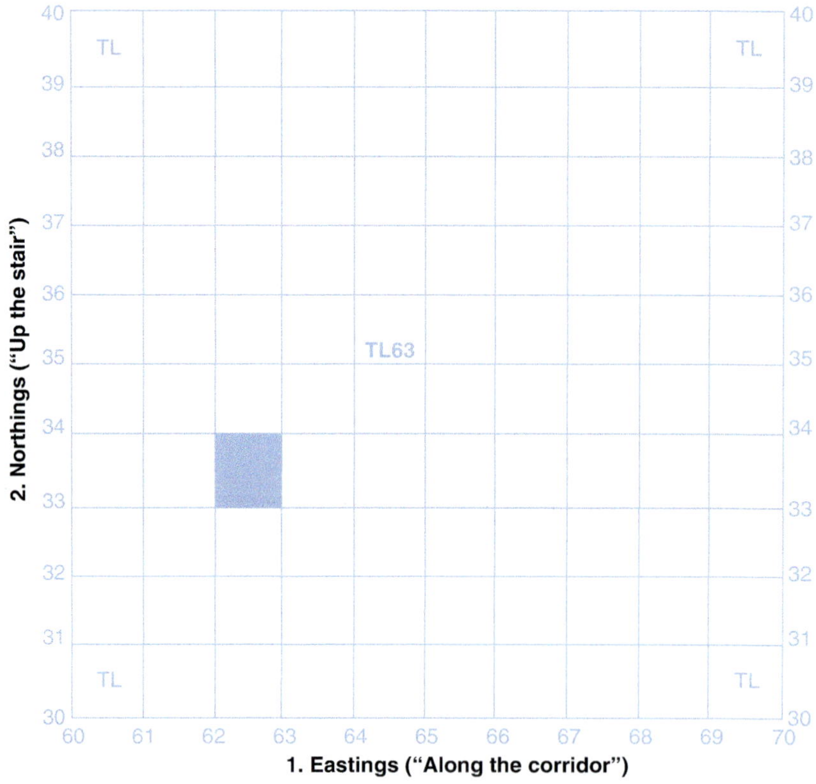

Fig. 19.4 Calculating a specific grid reference (Produced with kind permission of Ordnance Survey)

A-Z Maps or Street Mapping

Precise street mapping is completed using iPads or similar devices and is usefl when landing in conurbations and an incident is on a particular road. Hard copy A-Z maps can be carried as a backup option (Fig. 19.5). The crew can either look for the road name in the index at the back of the book for the relevant county or plot the grid from the grid reference. In this example, the previous SP123456 location will be used. The Ordnance Survey website (https://gridreferencefinder.com/) can be used to display the grid used in this example.

Find out roughly from the OS map where it is; the example is just east of Evesham in the County of Worcestershire.

Look on the back cover of the AZ, find Evesham and look up the page number required—for this example, it is page 164/165.

On that page, look across the bottom and up the left-hand side. The grid reference numbers are visible, and 123,456 has been plotted in the below picture. One thing to note on A-Z maps is that they are twice the magnification of OS maps, so the Eastings and Northings are spread across two squares in the book compared to one square on a folding map.

In-Flight Navigation

On the way to an incident, the TCM will provide a route brief to the pilot at an appropriate time using an aviation chart, generally after exiting the base's controlled air space. This brief should include a gross error check (e.g. 'We will pass Rugby on our left'), any pertinent aviation hazards or NOTAMS en-route, including any tall obstacles if the cloud base is low.

The medical passenger should be looking out for other traffic or aviation hazards. The TCM will continuously be updating the location on the map in case the weather closes in, or there is a diversion to another incident and the need to plan a new route. The TCM should also point

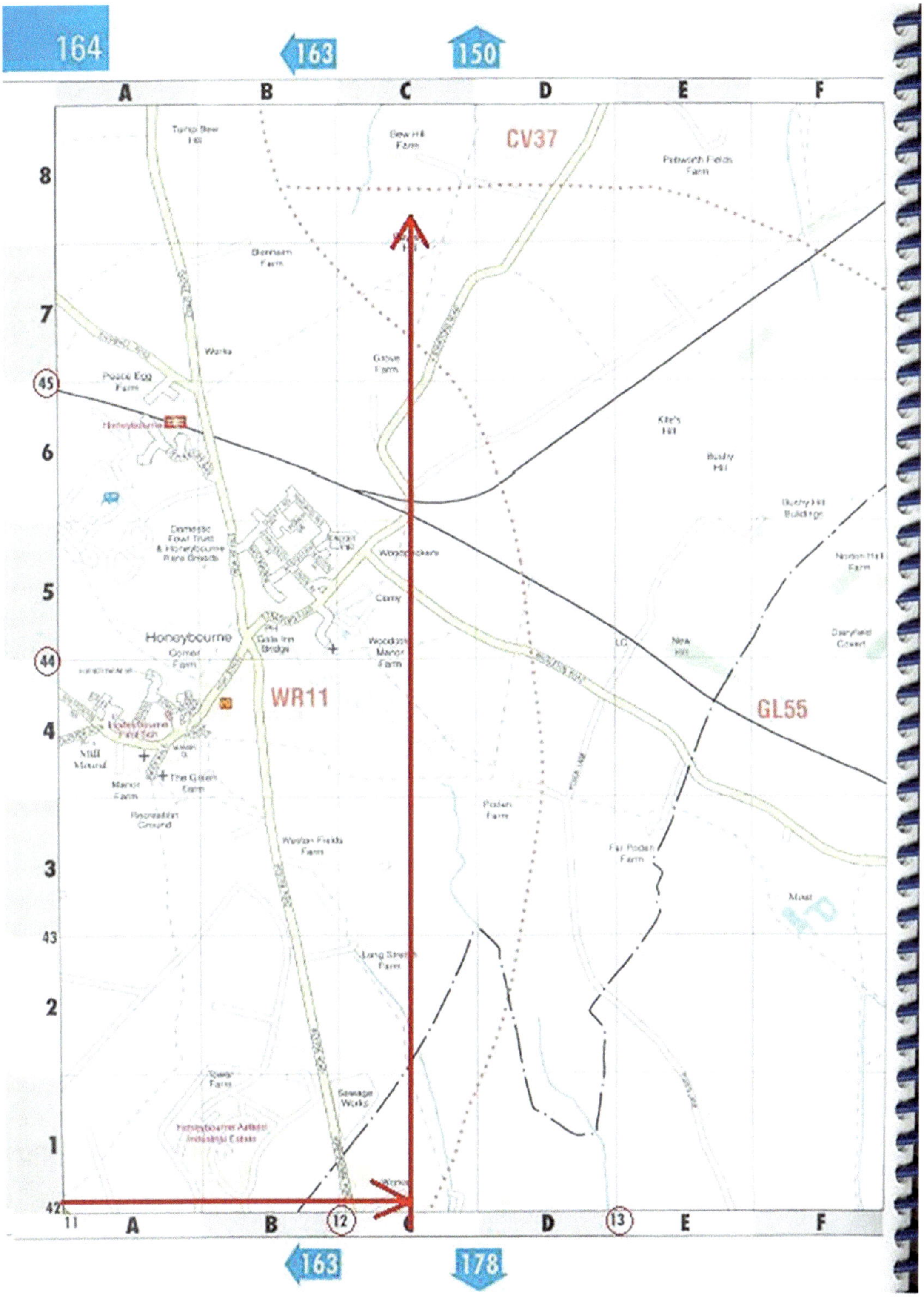

Fig. 19.5 A-Z map used for short-distance navigation

out any relevant target headings, e.g. 'That village with the spire is the one we're heading for' and any additional briefings required on the location of the incident. This template for briefing and navigation will be repeated for all flights for the TCM, i.e. flights to hospital and back to base.

Lookout and the Clock Code

Airspace in the UK is mainly uncontrolled (i.e. it is up to individual pilots to see other aircraft and avoid collisions); therefore, a good lookout is essential. This is particularly true when leaving or re-entering controlled airspace around airports or when looking for a landing site when all eyes are drawn to the scene. To communicate that a crew member has seen another aircraft, the clock code is to identify where it is relative to the helicopter (Fig. 19.6). 12 o'clock is straight ahead of the aircraft, 6 o'clock is directly behind, 3 o'clock is 90° to the right, and 9 o'clock is 90° to the left.

If an aircraft is seen, it is also referred to as being above ("high") at the same height ("level") or below ("low") as the helicopter, e.g. "Plane at 2 o'clock, high". This system can also be used for describing ground-based obstructions, e.g. "Wind turbines, 3 o'clock".

The pilot is responsible for overall lookout and flight safety, but the diagram below shows areas of responsibility during high workloads; ORANGE for pilot, YELLOW for TCM & GREEN for rear-seat crew members (Fig. 19.7).

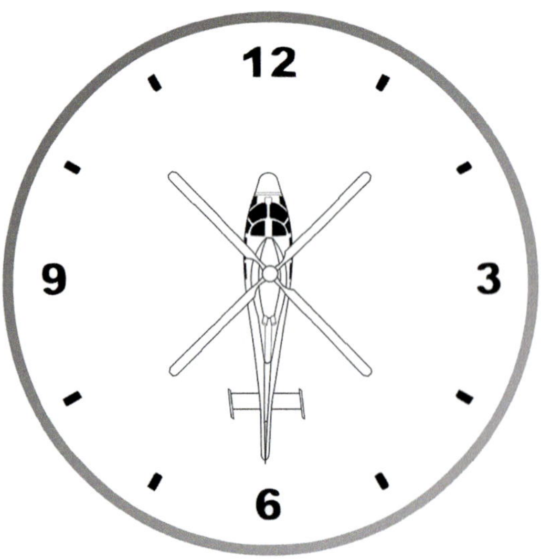

Fig. 19.6 The clock code is used to describe relative positions to the aircraft

Weather Limitations

Most small aircraft (both helicopters and aeroplanes) operate to Visual Flight Rules (VFR). This means that they need to see where they are going, maintain visual contact with the ground, and keep away from clouds. Larger aircraft and airliners operate to Instrument Flight Rules (IFR); this means they can navigate by sole reference to their instruments, radio beacon or GPS rated navigation and use instrument landing systems (ILS) at airports where they are equipped.

Figure 19.8 shows the difference between weather limits for Air Ambulance and HEMS and also the difference that carrying a TCM makes as a comparison. Despite being allowed to fly at 300 ft. under CAA exemptions, HEMS aircraft do not have an exemption to the 500 ft. minimum cloud base restriction. Usually, a HEMS aircraft will not accept a tasking on safety grounds unless there is a 500 ft. cloud base and 1.5 km of visibility.

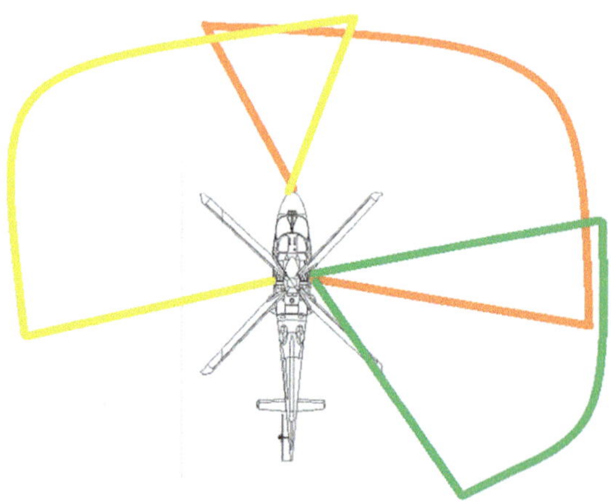

Fig. 19.7 lookout zones on aircraft and arcs of responsibility

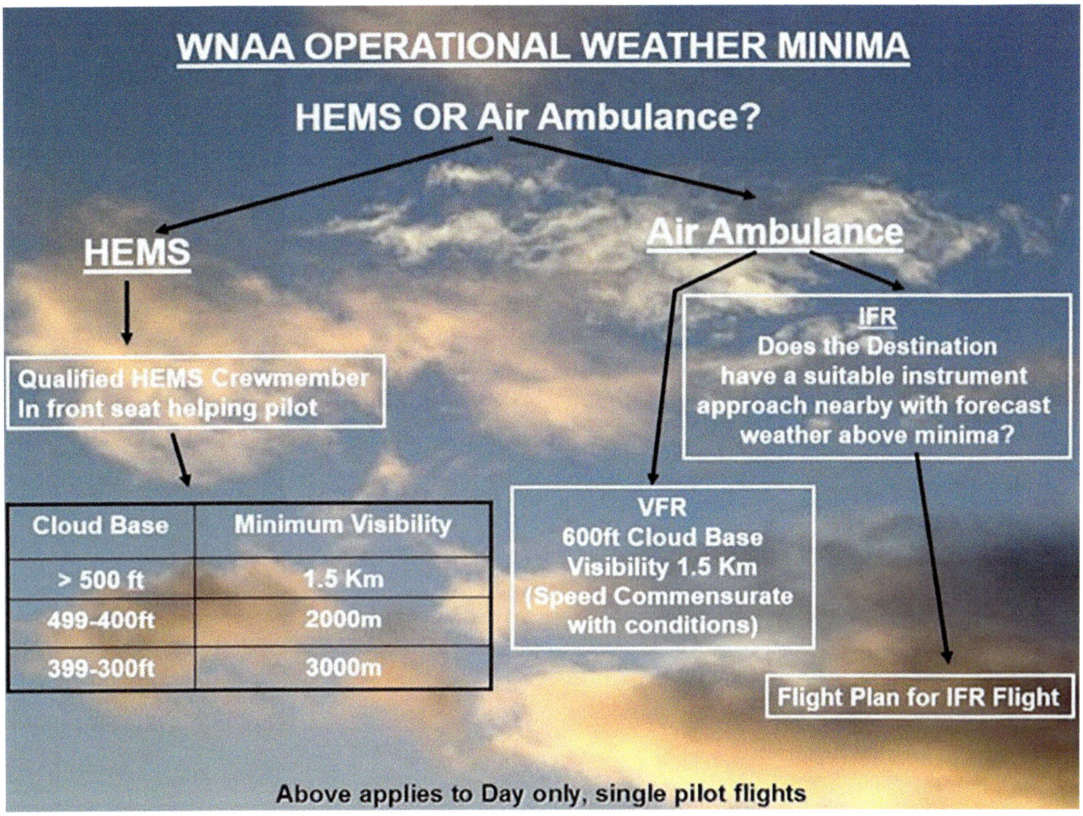

Fig. 19.8 Visibility minimum standards for operations

Sometimes HEMS aircraft will depart on a tasking within these limits, but if the weather worsens en route they may not be able to complete the tasking. One UK-based example of this would be a tasking in the Peak District where low cloud cover or fog obscures the ground and removes the ability to land or operate safely. There is the option to convert to IFR flight and recover back to a suitably equipped airfield in these instances. IFR flight will allow appropriately equipped aircraft with specifically trained and current crews to navigate between set points at set altitudes in poor visibility. Still, it will not allow them to land anywhere. Landing in poor visibility requires ILS (Instrument Landing System) equipment, a related but separate capability. This is only possible in large airports with the appropriate equipment, not on scene or in hospital helipads. Regardless of equipment and currency, HEMS aircraft cannot fly in fog, thunderstorms or icing conditions for safety reasons.

Disc Safety

Main Rotor

This is inclined forwards on the AW109 and so is low at the front of the helicopter (Fig. 19.9), therefore, disc discipline is paramount! The most significant danger periods are during startup or shutdown when the disc's rotational speed is below that which will provide sufficient lift to stop the disc from dropping.

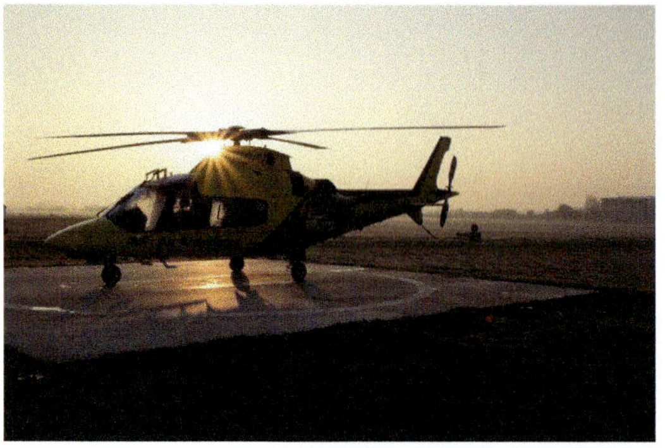

Fig. 19.9 AW109 helicopter. Note the main rotor disk is tilted forwards and so is lower at the nose

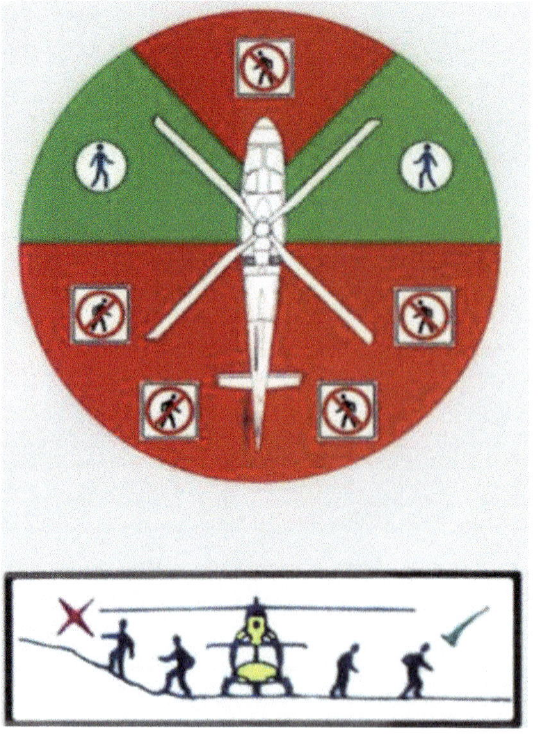

Fig. 19.10 Safe zones of entering and leaving the disc

Tail Rotor

The tail rotor counterbalances the rotational force generated by the engines, and the rotor itself can change orientation to allow rotation of the body of the aircraft. It is hard geared to the main rotor so that they will rotate at a fixed ratio to each other. In the event of the loss of tail rotor effectiveness, the helicopter cannot be controlled and will spin uncontrollably. The tail rotor is positioned low, and a 'stinger' under the tail rotor provides a visual reminder of its presence, and safety around this area is also paramount. One solution to decrease risk from the tail rotor initially developed by the Hughes Aircraft Company is the use of a NOTAR (NO TAil Rotor) system [9]. This uses the Coanda effect to generate a jet of air which can be directed to provide counter-torque in the place of a tail rotor. While it avoids the physical presence of a blade, is quieter than tail-rotor systems, reduces aircraft vibration, and there are no significant differences in flying characteristics, there are downsides. These are principally decreased fuel efficiency, reduced manoeuvrability at high forward airspeeds and greater complexity due to the increased number of parts in the system. Subsequently, NOTAR systems have only been employed by MD helicopters. A halfway compromise between these two systems is the Fenestron system [10, 11]. This houses a fan in place of the tail rotor and is principally used by Eurocopter/Airbus Helicopters. The fan is housed in the body of the tail and has between eight and eighteen blades which can be placed at different angles to minimise noise. Housing the fan inside the tail assembly also decreases the risk of rotor strike on either the ground or people with poor disc discipline.

Disc Discipline

Entry under the disc (whether it is already running or about to start up) is only allowed if a crewman is wearing their helmet with the visor down and they have received a "thumbs up" acknowledgement from the pilot. The pilot will only let personnel under the disc if it is stopped or at ground idle speed, as in between the disc can be unstable and move in the wind. The crew member responds with a thumb up to show they have acknowledged the clearance and they must only walk in the green areas indicated in Fig. 19.10 (between 9 and 11 o'clock or between 2 and 3 o'clock). Sloping ground also presents a hazard as this can reduce the clearance between personnel and the disc.

Disc Protection on Landing and Take off

When landing on scene, it is imperative that all the crew remain in communication and maintain a good lookout for people running towards the aircraft until the rotors have stopped; particular attention is paid to the tail rotor area. After landing, the pilot will opt for one of three levels of disc protection from the crew. Generally, a medium threat level is assumed whenever the public is nearby, but even members of other emergency services may approach the disc without thinking!

Minimum Threat Clear to open doors, stand outside of the aircraft and under the disc if the crew wishes to. This is used when the risk of people approaching is low (e.g. isolated location with no one in the immediate vicinity of the LZ). The crew is still to look out and be ready to react if required.

Medium Threat Clear to open doors; crew mandated to stand outside of the aircraft and under the disc. The crew remain plugged into the aircraft communication system but stand outside next to the helicopter, so they are a visible deterrent and can react quickly if someone approaches. Should a threat appear, the rest of the crew should be informed, and the crew member who has seen the danger should put their hand out in front of them to signal the approaching person to stop. The crew should be aware of the disc while putting their hand out directly ahead of them rather than above their head to avoid injury. If the crewmember believes the approaching person will not stop, then they should ask the pilot for permission to come off comms and exit the disc to intercept them. As mentioned previously, the crew should bear the risk posed by upsloping ground in mind.

Maximum Threat Clear to open doors and cleared to stand outside of the disc area if required. This level is used when the crew believes that a person will not stop from coming under the disc. The crew member should tell the pilot what they are doing until they come off comms. The crew member must remember to disconnect their headset, or they will be pulled back towards the aircraft when they run out of cable! They can then exit the disc, bearing in mind the hazard posed by upsloping ground.

Depending upon the scene, these three levels can also be used on takeoff as people can be unpredictable at this stage too. Usually, HEMS crews will try to recruit Police, Ambulance staff, (or within reason) responsible members of the public to help them keep the crowd back to a safe distance during takeoff.

Takeoff and Landing Checks

The very nature of HEMS means that time is a valuable commodity, and efficiency should be embraced wherever possible. However, this needs to be balanced against the potentially catastrophic results of making mistakes in aviation. To minimise the risk of forgetting something important, 'read and response' checklists are used before every takeoff and landing to address the biggest threats to the aircraft. Some aircraft may have additional items, but these are the minimum necessary checks. When the pilot is ready, he will ask for the checks, they are:

<u>Pre Take Off</u>

- Both engines............At flight
- Fuel Pumps and cocks............on
- Captions and lights............On, as required
- Limiter............On
- Instruments and radios............Set
- Secure in the front............Check
- Secure in the back............Check

<u>Pre Landing</u>

- Site Survey............Discussed
- Gear Down............Three Greens
- Secure in the front............Secure
- Secure in the back............Secure

Note. 'Secure in the front' means helmets secure (pilot and TCM are to check each other's straps), seatbelts are worn and correctly secured, the doors are latched (pins into holes), and there are no loose objects in the cockpit. 'Secure in the back' means helmets and seatbelts are secure for all persons, including patients and escorts, the doors are latched, and all equipment is stowed and secured.

Landing Site Selection

Usually, the aim is to land as close to the patient as possible to minimise the distance carrying equipment from the landing site to the patient, or the patient back to the aircraft. Sometimes the closest site isn't always the quickest, e.g. if the landing site is a tight space or has blockages to exits. The crew should consider this during the landing recce (Fig. 19.11). Although HEMS aircraft can land in areas as small as '2D' (twice the dimension of the largest diameter of the disc, 26 metres in an AW109), it has to be agreed by the crew that the landing site is appropriate for the tasking they believe they are going to. The 5 S's of a safe landing site - size, shape, surroundings, surface, and slope- should be considered when assessing potential landing areas.

- **Size.** Is it big enough? The minimal diameter required, as previously mentioned, is 2D or twice the largest rota diameter.
- **Shape.** Does its shape lend itself to an approach or departure in a specific direction?
- **Surroundings.** Obstacles—trees, fences or wires.
- **Surface.** A surface composition such as dust/sand or snow can cause problems with visibility when in the final phases of landing. Mud can also cause problems if the surface is waterlogged or not firm enough to support the helicopter's weight after it has landed. FOD (or Foreign Object Debris) is any substance, object or debris which could cause damage to the aircraft or personnel or property in the immediate vicinity. The downwash created by the rotor blades can be severe enough to knock people over. It can cause anything not secured to the ground to be moved which could cause injury to people or animals under trees, or be sucked into an engine or rotor and cause damage to the helicopter.
- **Slope**. Is there an excessive slope that will cause the aircraft to be unstable or put the crew or public at risk of rotor strike?

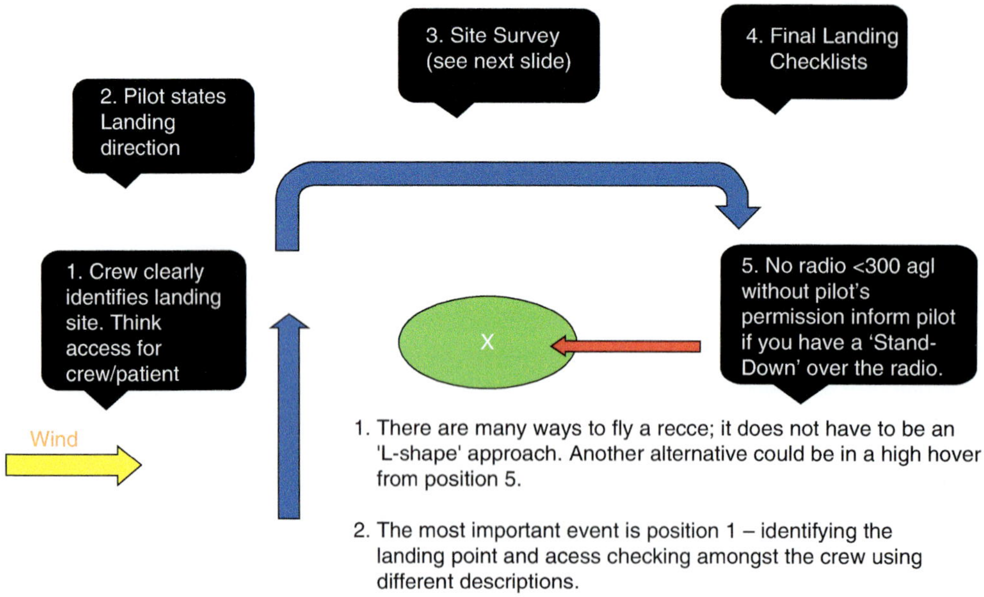

Fig. 19.11 Landing site selection procedure

The height of objects near the landing site is also a consideration. For exampole, an Operators guidance might be that nothing can be higher than 3 feet within 1D on any landing site (i.e. under the disc itself). Between 1-2D, nothing can be over 5 ft. The tail rota must be clear of all objects.

Access and egress from the landing site to the patient should be considered. It may be time-critical to get a doctor or paramedic to a patient immediately after landing, so landing somewhere which involves climbing over a wall to get out may be necessary. However, access to the site or repositioning of the helicopter may subsequently be required to ensure the patient can be loaded into the aircraft if needed for onward transport.

Landing Site Recce: Arrival and Approach

- **Cabin security**. Before the rear crew member can open the door, all loose objects must be secured—this includes jackets, paperwork, maps etc.
- **Personal security.** Double-check seat belts are fastened and visors lowered to prevent dust from blowing into eyes.
- **Briefing.** Ensure that all crew know where they are aiming to land in the site.

Ensure the crew know how their seat rotates/tracks and that they can close the door if required.

The pilot will then state "clear for doors"; the response is "door opening", and the rear crew member then ensures the door is fully open and locked in position. They may also rotate their seat to better view the tail area and down to the landing site. They will then state one of three options:

1. Good to continue down as briefed.
2. The site is unsuitable—"Up, Up, Up" are the words to be used.
3. Stop—there are things to be aware of before proceeding. The door operator will point out hazards currently stopping the aircraft from landing, and the pilot will see if they can manoeuvre the helicopter to mitigate these. If they can safely reduce the risk, the aircraft will land; if not, the pilot will abort the landing, and the aircraft will be flown away and a new landing site selected. Before the helicopter flies away, the door is closed, and the pilot informed that the door is securely shut.

Wheels and Stinger Check

Once landed on scene, the pilot may ask for a wheel and stinger check if the ground is exceptionally soft or if there is uneven ground around the tail rotor. Once the wheels are on the ground, the rear door operator will rotate their seat and lean out, and the front door operator will lean out to look at how far the wheels have sunk in the mud. This then can be communicated to the pilot in terms of simple fractions, e.g. "halfway up the wheels". The maximum amount of sinkage that is allowed is approximately half the diameter of the main landing gear. The rear door operator may also have to look through the gap between the open door and the helicopter to get a good view and check that the stinger is not touching the floor. If the stinger is getting close, the rear crew-member must communicate this to the pilot to prevent a tail rotor strike.

If for any reason the landing site is unsuitable, then the helicopter may have to be repositioned. All doors must be closed and the pilot informed that the door is securely shut before the helicopter is repositioned.

Specific Landing Site Considerations

Railways

In the event of a HEMS helicopter being deployed to a rail incident, under no circumstances will the helicopter land on or near any part of the track, nor will any part of the helicopter protrude within three meters of the railway track. There is also the risk of overhead wires to consider near the incident.

Reservoirs

There are two types of reservoirs that merit consideration:

Underground Reservoirs These generally are large open areas with a grass cover on them (and from the air can look a very enticing landing spot!). As well as the potential risk of damage to the structure or helicopter, another concern is that a helicopter weighing over three tons landing on it might disturb the internal structure that covers the reservoir and lead to bits of rust flaking off and contaminating the water. This would require divers to inspect the tank or for it to be drained with subsequent disturbance of the water supply to a large geographic area, so it is best to avoid landing on these sites.

Open Lakes During the summer when the water gets low, the land around open lake reservoirs looks good to land on, but there have been problems where the undercarriage has gone through the crust and started to sink. Therefore these sites should be avoided.

Beaches

When landing on beaches, it is advisable to pick a landing site above the high water mark in case the tide starts coming in and the engines cannot be restarted! If that is not possible, consider a rotors-running drop-off or even keeping the engines running, bearing in mind the risk from sand to the helicopter and personnel on the ground.

Prisons

Many operators have a policy that they will not land in prisons. It may be that Ambulance Control informs HEMS units that the Governor of the prison has given his permission to land inside its grounds, but even in this instance operators still may choose to not land within their perimeter. The reason is that if the inmates discover what triggers a helicopter being sent, they potentially could stage an incident and use a helicopter as an escape plan or worse. Even overflying high-security prisons is prohibited for most aircraft, as the area above them is considered permanently restricted airspace.

Industrial Incidents

When travelling to an industrial incident, the nature of any substances that may be involved will play a part in HEMS activity. The crew should consider the direction of the prevailing wind. The landing site should be upwind from the incident to avoid contaminating the aircraft or exposing the pilot and crew to any risk of incapacitation. When moving patients from these incidents, it may not be possible to fly them if they have been contaminated by certain chemicals that pose a flight risk if they were to "off-gas" and incapacitate the pilot. Similar consideration must be given to patients exposed to CS gas or pepper spray in police or military incidents—if they are at risk of off-gassing, they cannot be flown and must be transported by land.

Airport Landings

IFR Recoveries

If the weather turns poor and IFR conditions are encountered, the aircraft will need to descend through the cloud at an airfield with a suitable Instrument Landing System (ILS), Performance Based Navigation (PBN) approach or use a Non-Directional Beacon (NDB) approach. All types of approach require pilots to navigate by the details supplied on

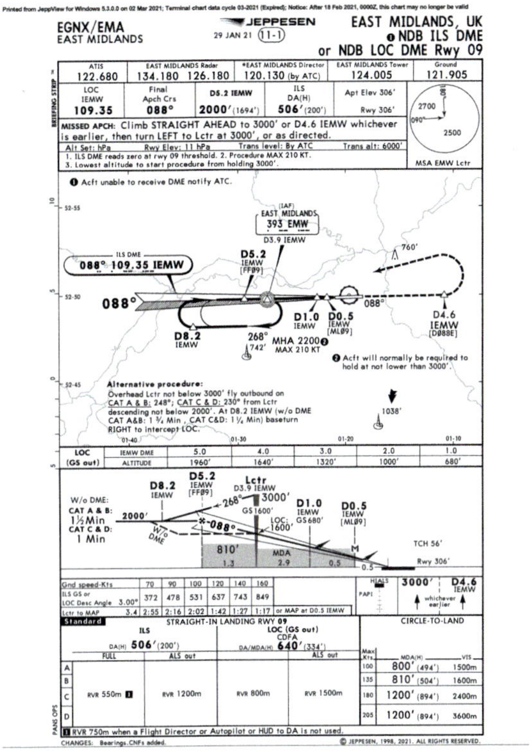

Fig. 19.12 IFR Chart for landing at East Midlands Airport

'the plate' (Fig. 19.12). This is a navigational document for each aircraft that details a flight path in these conditions. Below is an example with the crucial details listed:

- Airfield, Runway & Approach details
- ILS Frequency (detailed ×2)
- NDB frequency
- Inbound heading
- Inbound height
- Top of drop
- Check heights
- Decision Altitude & vis
- Go Around details

Night Flying

To ensure safe operating, pilots must undertake additional training and have currencies with additional equipment such as night-vision goggles. This is before considering the need for more planning time before taking off and (depending on aircraft type) the potential need for an additional pilot. As the risk and associated costs are higher and the response times are increased because of extra planning time, in most areas operating in night conditions does not offer the same advantages as HEMS during daylight. This is especially true in metropolitan areas which are supplied with good traffic systems and motorways. However, there are some areas of the country where night HEMS may still be a valuable and viable option. What must be considered by all HEMS personnel is the impact of a prolonged tasking close to night hours. This leads to two scenarios that must be planned for:

- Once landed on scene it becomes official night, and a night departure procedure is undertaken.
- Having left scene for either hospital or base, it becomes official night while flying.

Factors to be aware of include weather limits (when planning, the weather suitability for taking off or flying VFR at night the cloud base and visibility should be greater than 1500 ft. and 5 km), hospital landing site facilities and transfer times. Not all hospitals are approved for night landings or takeoffs. If the hospital is not suitably equipped, then the aircraft must have left the hospital landing site before official night. If the aircraft has landed and is on an unequipped pad and night falls before departure, then it must be left in situ until the following day.

Procedures for Departure from a HEMS Site at Night

Size The site has to be at least 100 m × 60 m with no obstacles higher than 40 ft. in the backup area for a helipad departure. The crew must deploy portable landing site lights per Fig. 19.13.

Marshalling Signals

If it becomes necessary for the pilot to reposition the helicopter at the scene of an incident, the TCM or medical passenger may be asked to assist the pilot by watching the approach and giving suitable hand signals to guide them in safely. There are several marshalling signals, as shown in Fig. 19.14.

Aircraft Emergency Procedures

A full explanation of in-flight emergencies is beyond the scope of this text, and the exact procedures will differ between aircraft and operators. In the unlikely event of an in-flight aviation emergency, the pilot will take any immediate actions, but then the TCM will use the appropriate Emergency Checklist. Most emergencies will require the defective system to be shut down. A decision is then made about whether the mission can continue as planned, if a diversion is necessary, or if a landing is a better option and how quickly this needs to happen.

For emergencies that require a forced landing (e.g. double engine failure), the TCM will activate the Emergency Locator Transmitter (ELT)

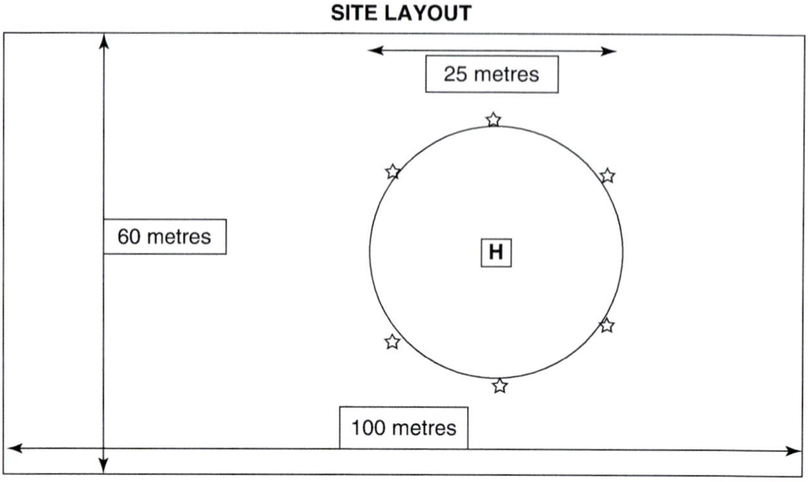

Fig. 19.13 Night light setup for departure after dark from a HEMS landing site

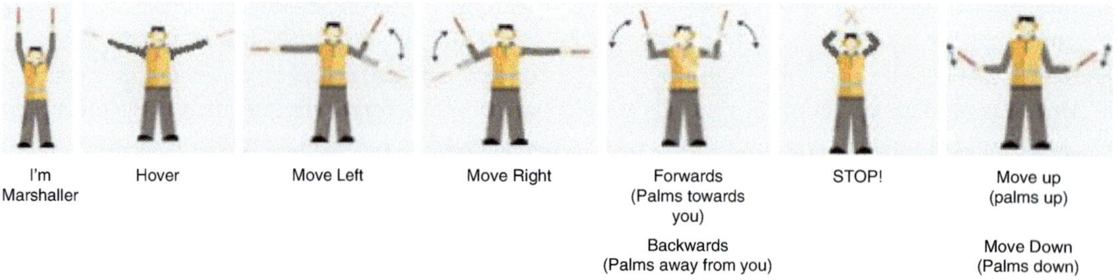

Fig. 19.14 Common marshalling signals

and, if time allows, update control on their location and intention. The rear seat passenger will ensure their seat is in the rearward facing position and turn the oxygen supply off to minimise the risk of fire on landing. All loose objects should be secured and the brace position adopted.

Batteries

Many items are carried on board that contain batteries. Two central problems with this need to be considered:

- Lithium batteries, if damaged, can cause very intense fires.
- The cargo compartment of the aircraft may not have any smoke or fire detection systems.

A battery fire in the cabin would be bad, but the crew would know about it. However, if the fire was in the cargo compartment near where many of the aircraft's electronic systems are located, it could be catastrophic.

Therefore any kit that contains batteries must be checked to ensure there is no damage to the battery or the equipment before it is put on board the aircraft.

Conclusions

HEMS operations in the UK are fully funded by distinct and dedicated charities, with no centralised Government funding. While they are expensive to operate, they bring multiple advantages to the care of critically injured patients, either by decreasing the time taken to get to definitive care or by bringing clinical teams who can provide advanced levels of care to the point of injury. Safety is the priority at all times; due to this, there has only been one fatal helicopter crash in UK HEMS operation since 1987 [12] despite over 270,000 flights. This model is safe; however, the tasking, training and governance requirements around HEMS operations are necessarily strict about maintaining this standard, and meet or exceed the same essential standards for other commercial aircraft operators.

Questions

1. The limitations on air ambulances are the same as HEMS aircraft.
   (a) True
   (b) False
2. Helicopters were first used as medical evacuation platforms in the Vietnam war.
   (a) True
   (b) False
3. The zone of safety when entering a running rotor disk is either at the three or nine o'clock position.
   (a) True
   (b) False
4. Patients who have been in an industrial chemical accident should not be transported by air.
   (a) True
   (b) False
5. The minimum size of a HEMS landing site is twice the maximum size of the rotor disc
   (a) True
   (b) False

Answers

1. b
2. b
3. b
4. a
5. a

References

1. Martin T. Aeromedical transportation: a clinical guide. 2nd ed. CRC Press; 2006.
2. Woolley T, Round JA, Ingram M. Global lessons: developing military trauma care and lessons for civilian practice. Br J Anaesth. 2017;119(Suppl_1):i135–42.
3. Clarke JE, Davis PR. Medical evacuation and triage of combat casualties in Helmand Province, Afghanistan: October 2010–April 2011. Mil Med. 2012;177(11):1261–6.
4. European Aviation Safety Agency. Acceptable Means of Compliance (AMC) and Guidance Material (GM) to Annex V Specific approvals [Part-SPA] of Commission Regulation (EU) 965/2012 on air operations [Internet]. Mar, 2017. Available from: https://www.easa.europa.eu/regulations
5. UK Government. The Rules of the Air Regulations 2015 [Internet]. 840 2015. Available from: https://www.legislation.gov.uk/uksi/2015/840/contents/made

6. Air Safety Support International. Overseas Territories Aviation Circular: Fatigue Management - Commercial Air Transport Operations [Internet]. 2013 [cited 2019 Dec 26]. Available from: https://www.airsafety.aero/getattachment/13c7713a-0abd-44df-b6e9-2e5682481322/Fatigue-Management-—-Commercial-Air-Transport-Operations-Printable-Version.aspx
7. Great Britain, Civil Aviation Authority. The avoidance of fatigue in aircrews: guide to requirements. London: Civil Aviation Authority; 2004.
8. Air Safety Support International. OTACs | OTAR Part 121 - Commercial Air Transport Operations - Large Aeroplanes | Fatigue Management – Commercial Air Transport Operations | Section B - The Scheme [Internet]. [cited 2020 Jun 8]. Available from: https://www.airsafety.aero/Requirements-and-Policy/OTACs/OTAR-Part-121-Commercial-Air-Transport-Operation/Fatigue-Management-%E2%80%93-Commercial-Air-Transport-Ope/Section-B-The-Scheme.aspx
9. NOTAR: More than What it Appears to Be [Internet]. Rotor & Wing International. 2012 [cited 2020 June 8]. Available from: https://www.rotorandwing.com/2012/09/01/notar-more-than-what-it-appears-to-be/
10. Scott J. Aerospaceweb.org | Ask Us - Fenestron Tail Rotor [Internet]. 2005 [cited 2020 June 8]. Available from: http://www.aerospaceweb.org/question/helicopters/q0212a.shtml
11. McAdams T. Fantails | [Internet]. 2012 [cited 2020 June 8]. Available from: https://blog.aopa.org/aopa/2012/06/04/fantails/
12. Chesters A, Grieve PH, Hodgetts TJ. A 26-year comparative review of United Kingdom helicopter emergency medical services crashes and serious incidents. J Trauma Acute Care Surg. 2014;76(4):1055–60.

Scene Safety

20

Jenny Mealey and Peter Lax

- Environment
- Traffic
- Kit Management
- Being prepared and escalating concerns
- PPE
- Training, SOP'S and sign off
- Equipment checks
- Driving
- Multiagency working
- Dynamic risk assessment
- Manual handling
- IP&C
- Police & evidence
- Fire & rescue
- Communication
- Team debrief

Introduction

Working in the pre-hospital environment is vastly different from working in a well-resourced, warm and well-lit hospital. Performing even simple tasks can become more complicated, and the environment itself can cause or compound medical issues (e.g. hypothermia as a primary pathology or worsening coagulopathy in trauma patients). The majority of health care professionals work in an indoor environment and may not fully understand the challenges or limitations that working outdoors poses. Placing a cannula in a comfortable ward environment differs from performing the same task in the dark and rain in a ditch. Some of the challenges and mitigations that can be put in place are as follows.

Environment

Temperature and Weather

Both hot and cold weather can present challenges for patients and practitioners. For example, patients involved in road traffic collisions may be unable to move due to either physical entrapment, pain or injuries that require coordinated and specialist extrication, and the environment can compound this. Patients cannot be left enclosed in vehicles in extreme heat or cold for any length of time without potentially suffering complications. The effects of the environment must be consid-

J. Mealey (✉)
The Air Ambulance Service (TAAS), Rugby, Warwickshire, UK
e-mail: jenny.mealey@theairambulanceservice.org.uk

P. Lax
Tactical Medical Wing, Royal Air Force, Brize Norton, Oxfordshire, UK

The Air Ambulance Service (TAAS), Rugby, Warwickshire, UK
e-mail: p.lax@NHS.net

P. Lax (ed.), *Textbook of Acute Trauma Care*, https://doi.org/10.1007/978-3-030-83628-3_20

ered when performing interventions such as exposure for examination. Exposure needs to be adequate for assessment, but also avoid unnecessary heat loss. While ensuring timely and safe medical care is a paramount consideration, a degree of compromise may be needed to account for the effects of the environment. As General Patton famously said, "A good plan violently executed now is better than a perfect plan next week". Working in safety equipment in the heat is physically demanding (as is working in multiple layers of clothing in the cold weather), especially where a degree of dexterity is required.

The weather will affect all aspects of scene management. In cold and wet weather, a quicker extrication strategy may be the preferred option due to the risk of thermal injury to the patient during a prolonged extrication. Modifications of standard operating procedures may also need to be considered in light of the effects of weather. For example, a Rapid Sequence Induction is typically performed with 360° access in optimised space on scene [1]. In the rain, the location may need to be changed to make the procedure safer for the patient and technically easier for the operator. One example would be to perform an RSI in the centre of the ambulance with the side door opened to create space rather than outside. This may decrease heat loss, provide more light and improve the chances of first-pass success in a critical intervention. Bright sunlight can also hinder videolaryngoscopy by causing glare artefacts on the screen [2, 3], and practitioners should consider this during the set up for the procedure. The operating temperature of individual pieces of equipment may also be exceeded in the pre-hospital environment; they may cease to function or require changes to their use. While this is less likely in temperate climates, practitioners who work in extremes of cold or heat may be more familiar with this issue.

Traffic

It is very easy to become task-focused and lose situational awareness. This is true not just on roads but railway lines, industrial areas and anywhere where the location cannot be fully closed down to allow for a "sterile" work area. Do not be tempted to rush in, even if there are already resources on scene. Take a few seconds to look around the environment; fully appreciate the risks and hazards, look for them, listen for them and don't forget the sense of smell. Scenes always have four dimensions—front and back, left and right, top and bottom and time. Hazards can emerge from any direction at any point, and while a scene may be safe at the initial time of assessment, there is no guarantee it will stay that way. Scene safety is an individual and team responsibility that cannot be devolved—each practitioner is as responsible for their teams' safety as they are their own. Often, other agencies such as police or fire departments may already be on scene and have made initial safety checks, but this is not always the case [4]. Team and patient safety always take precedence over clinical treatment. A useful starting point is to clarify with other agencies what has been done to make the scene safe—do not assume anything has been done. For example, a railway line may have been made safe in one direction, but the parallel line may still be live (meaning trains passing very close or electrical current still passing through it). If in doubt, check—it is far better to make two phone calls to the Rail Operator than none at all, and scene safety should be one of the first and most frequently enforced lessons for new practitioners working in pre-hospital care. Motorways are very dangerous; drivers passing the scene are distracted and can easily cause further collisions by "rubbernecking". Try and allow at least one clear lane for a safety margin on an active tasking, or move to a safer location as soon as possible. While shutting a busy motorway may not be an ideal course of action, in certain circumstances (e.g. landing an air ambulance), it may be mandatory to close one or both directions of traffic flow temporarily. In the event of a fatal incident, the road will be closed by Police to preserve the scene and collect forensic evidence for the ensuing investigation.

Kit Management

Have a kit dump which is close to hand but not so close that it is being stepped on or covered in oil (or worse, other responders helping themselves to your equipment!). The Fire Service will designate an area where all hydraulic tools are located if they are not being immediately used. Tools are returned to this area once they have been used and thus avoid cluttering up space around the patient. Medical equipment should be managed similarly with an emphasis on safety. For example, if a cannula needs to be placed, ensure a sharps box is to hand, the needle is made safe, and all equipment is removed from the area around the patient after cannulation. Pre-hospital clinicians are there to enhance the capabilities of existing teams, not to create more work or hazards for them. Personal kit should also be appropriately managed, but what is carried will vary from person to person depending on role and experience. A basic cannulation kit, trauma shears, gloves and a head torch are a good starting point, as well as a mobile phone or radio in the event of needing to summon help in an emergency. Preparation of kit may also decrease scene times and time to intervention as well as reducing cognitive loads on pre-hospital teams, so training and standardisation in equipment preparation can have a direct patient benefit [5, 6].

Being Prepared and Escalating Concerns

When working in the pre-hospital environment as part of an enhanced care team, practitioners should expect to be sent to the sickest, most injured patients and the most complex of taskings and should prepare accordingly. Arriving at a scene without essential safety equipment is unacceptable and will make the team appear amateurish. Team and scene safety is paramount; if something looks unsafe then speak up. This does not need to be in an aggressive manner in the first instance, but can be escalated as required. There will always be a level of risk in all emergencies - the key is to look for them, mitigate risk where possible and verbalise the subsequent plan to others. If the threat has not been acknowledged, the verbal escalation can increase from "I am concerned..." to "This is unsafe..." and finally "STOP, this is dangerous." The mnemonic CUS can be used to remember this schema. For example, "I'm concerned that beam could cause a safety hazard, has it been secured?". If no action has been taken it can escalate to "Team I've noticed this beam above us looks very unsafe, can anyone confirm it has been secured?". If there is still no acknowledgement or feedback, this is then followed finally by "Everyone stop! That beam is unsafe, move now!".

Personal Protective Equipment (PPE)

Under UK law, employers should provide employees with the appropriate clothing and safety equipment required under the Personal Protective Equipment at Work Regulations (1992) and Section 9 of the Health and Safety at Work Act (1974). A helmet (for example, to be used at RTCs and on building sites) is essential. Ensure that if these are for communal use, they are checked for cleanliness, serviceability and fitted correctly at the start of a shift. High visibility jackets should be readily available; again, ensure there is one in an appropriate size for each team member. Working in a jacket that is too big or small will make tasks more difficult and appear amateurish.

Boots are essential equipment, and many people choose to purchase a preferred style or brand. Ensure that they are fit for purpose with good non-slip soles and reinforced toe caps. Diesel and other fuels are extraordinarily slippery, and falling over not only can cause injury but can be embarrassing on a busy scene! Gloves are also essential workwear. Both latex or nitrile examination gloves and a set of heavy-duty industrial gloves for use at RTC's are crucial. Practitioners may wear examination gloves underneath RTC gloves to save time, but for assisting with the patient's extrication, a good set of RTC gloves will minimise the risk of any minor cuts from glass or sharp surfaces. Goggles or safety glasses can be used to prevent contamination from blood and body fluids and as eye protection when glass or vehicles are being cut. They may not be used as frequently as other PPE but should be easily to hand. Knee pads should be purchased if the employer's clothing does not have built-in knee protection - this is a worthwhile investment as they will save a lot of bruising and discomfort.

Training SOP's and Sign Off

All institutions and schemes should have a period of training and sign off before authorising solo practice. Even practitioners with significant prior experience can make the most of this time by watching how others operate in the pre-hospital environment, debriefing even simple jobs to understand the decision-making process and scene etiquette. This is especially true for personnel who have lots of hospital experience but limited exposure to working in the pre-hospital environment; clinical medical skills are not necessarily the essential part of each case. Standard operating procedures (SOP's) should be agreed on at an organisational level, with dissemination amongst all clinical staff and regular audit to ensure compliance or identify areas for improvement. There should also be appropriate senior support available for each shift, and personnel should never doubt who to call if they find themselves in a difficult or complicated situation. Simulation training is an excellent way to learn in a safe and supportive environment. Staff should be honest about their weaknesses and ask peers and mentors to develop scenarios that will help strengthen skills in these areas. For example, staff who do not regularly deal with children in their daily practice may benefit from paediatric simulations. Try and ensure the simulations are as real as possible—if there is a check sheet for kit or procedures, then use it in the simulation; if a kit dump is required, then set one up. Particular emphasis should be placed on adequate kit familiarity and preparation. All staff should rehearse the set up for an RSI and know how to set up the ventilator. The first time this is done should not be on scene where stress levels will be high, and something could easily be missed. The more uncommon procedures such as thoracotomy and resuscitative hysterotomy should be practised using simulation where possible and thoroughly discussed. Many schemes have an "Emergency of the day" for the team to discuss, or perhaps an SOP of the week so that these are frequently reviewed, and any amendments required can be actioned promptly.

Organisational learning is also essential, and each individual should also ensure they are familiar with the adverse incident reporting procedures within the organisation. There may be several levels of reporting, from discussing a case at a morbidity and mortality meeting to immediate actions should equipment fail.

Beginning of Shift Checks and Procedures

Daily briefings should be an established part of any enhanced care team. These should include any kit or equipment issues, hospital issues, weather, crew issues and confirmation of senior on-call arrangements as necessary. This is in addition to legally mandated checks such as stock checking/signing out of controlled or scheduled drugs.

There should be a communications check to ensure at least two forms of communication within the team (e.g. radio and mobile phone). This is an opportunity to check or confirm familiarity with any issues that may arise with equipment. Is the on-call senior listed as "on-call", "Dr X", or "Dave" on the phone? Is there a passcode on the phone? Do all team members know how to use the radio effectively? Can they unlock it, adjust the volume and change the channel? Proper voice protocols and procedures are essential for effective working in pre-hospital care and will improve with practice and experience. Messages should be short, unambiguous and to the point; rehearse the message before transmitting it to develop this skill, and consider if it could be refined before pressing the send button. Be confident in using the radio, think before speaking, be clear and don't waffle! If team members lack confidence in radio communications, then incorporate it into simulation practice. Practice giving a situation report, requesting further resources or handing over a patient to a hospital via radio communications.

Driving

There may be a requirement to be appropriately trained and practised in emergency response ("blue light") driving. While this is often considered an exciting part of the job, it is also challenging. There are minimum standards to be met and rules to be adhered to, and most organisations will have an appropriate course to undertake before being allowed to drive on blue lights. The individual should always drive within their limitations. Ensure that any vehicle used for emergency response driving is well maintained and has had basic oil, water and tyre checks regularly. If a responder is a passenger and a colleague is driving, it is the passenger's responsibility to co-drive. Co-driving involves navigation, safety checks when approaching junctions, being alert to dangers and communication with the tasking service and other responders as necessary. Some response schemes utilise a "sterile cockpit" ethos and prohibit talking while driving unless highlighting a safety issue or updating the driver on mission-critical information. This has to be balanced against the need to create a shared mental model of what should happen on arrival if a high-stakes intervention needs to occur rapidly (e.g. who is doing which part of a maternal resuscitation/resuscitative hysterotomy). Ensure that the vehicle is as safe on the inside as possible. If something has to be taken in the ambulance, ensure it is strapped in as a ventilator flying through the air at 40 mph will cause damage to whomever or whatever it hits! Communication extends into the car; if any individual is unhappy with the speed or style of driving, they should be able to raise this, e.g. "I'm not comfortable doing this speed in the rain. Can we slow down please?"

Multiagency Working

It is rare to attend a scene as part of an enhanced care team and not find other agencies there. The most important thing to do is to approach every scene and try and establish clear communication. This can be as simple as approaching the team who are present and saying, "Hello, I'm......., this is Jenny, what can we do to help?". This immediately shows an intention to work as a team and not take over or push people out of the way. Life is much easier if first respond agencies don't feel threatened or marginalised by other practitioners! CRM is an important skill, and using personnel to the best of their abilities should be encouraged.

Conversely, if a responder is becoming overwhelmed or given a task that they do not feel confident undertaking, provide them with a job they feel happy with rather than exclude them from patient care. For example, "Could you run through a bag of fluids please?" or "Can you get the scoop and cut those trousers?". This approach will help the responder to feel they participated and were useful, despite feeling overwhelmed. It may also help improve working relationships between services. Enhanced care teams can be exposed to major trauma regularly. However, in the UK, most ambulance crews will attend perhaps one major trauma incident a year [7]. Emphasise what the team needs to do, make sure everyone has a job that they can perform even if its something simple.

Dynamic Risk Assessment

In practical terms, this is the process of assessing risk and monitoring that risk. This involves every part of a scene—the patient, the geography, the weather, other agencies, relatives etc. No incident will be risk-free, but having an appreciation of the risk with active mitigation can make the scene safer. This process is continuous; for example, the arrival of friends or relatives who are being held back by the Police can cause conflict and risk. This can generally be managed by going and speaking to them if possible. Friends and relatives are understandably worried, and straightforward communication and information can be enough to defuse the situation to the point that they may be able to see the patient calmly. For example, "Hello, I'm Laura, one of the doctors.

Ben has suffered the following injuries, we are currently treating him, and we will take him to University Hospital". This will not always work or be possible (especially if there are drink or drugs involved), but the fear of a friend or relative dying is behind most aggression when bystanders try to get to the patient.

It is prudent to learn some basic de-escalation strategies. Be mindful of (and learn and emulate) the tone and body language that experienced individuals use. Be polite and respectful; if the situation is volatile, then leave until Police can gain control. Getting into a shouting match is pointless, unprofessional and does nothing to add to patient care. It can be challenging to reason with someone who has consumed drugs, alcohol or both; if this person is the patient, then an element of chemical control may be required [8–10]. Any benefits gained from drug administration have to be balanced against the risks of the procedure. In some cases, assistance from the Police (either by talking the patient down or other limited forms of restraint) can prevent the need for pharmacological intervention.

Practitioners should always be aware of their surroundings and avoid letting their exit routes be blocked. As part of their daily briefing (or before operational sign off), they should also know how to operate the radio's emergency button. Once the button has been pressed, they should also know what happens and how they can help get information across to control or the Police. Something as simple as saying, "come on, put the knife down and let's get out of the kitchen", gives colleagues vital information about the incident, weapon and location on scene.

Chemical suicide has become more prevalent in recent years [11, 12]. The methods vary from mixing chemicals that will create a toxic gas to ingesting chemicals. If the patient appears deceased in an enclosed space such as a car, take a moment to look for evidence of chemicals. Are the windows taped, is there a sign in the window? If chemical suicide is a potential mechanism, and toxic compounds may still be in the environment, do not enter. Request the Fire Service and HART (Hazardous Area Response Team) to attend. They can enter in the necessary§ PPE and assess the threat and the casualty. For ingested chemicals (e.g. sodium nitrate), consulting Toxbase will tell inform the practitioner of the risks of off-gassing into the environment. This may impact transport options, as individual patients may not be able to be emplaned onto a helicopter if they pose a risk to flight safety (see aviation chapter for more details).

Confined area working is not an uncommon occurrence. Examples of recent cases in confined spaces include building collapse, RTCs and incidents in tunnels, mines or lift shafts. Medical teams should only enter these areas when deemed safe, generally by the fire brigade. These can be challenging environments as access to equipment will be restricted, movement will be minimised, and it is easy to become anxious and unable to operate. If small spaces are a source of anxiety for individuals, it may be worth adding these into simulated practice or asking a colleague to go into the space instead. Multiagency working with partner agencies (e.g. Fire service or Mountain Rescue services) who have access to specialist training areas and equipment is excellent for overcoming fear, developing strategies and building relationships before working with each other on scene. The balance of extrication versus in-situ training can be a difficult one. Occasionally the most crucial intervention on scene will be extrication rather than anything medical, and the environment may preclude any meaningful interventions with the patient in their current location. Good communication and a flat hierarchy between agencies should aid in effective decision making and optimise patient care.

Manual Handling

There are many adjuncts available to assist with moving patients, and where possible, these should be utilised to minimise risk to responders. If they cannot be used, then try to have as many people as possible to distribute the weight and effort required to move the patient. Even in a snatch rescue, there is time to get multiple rescuers to grab part of the patient and move to a safer location rather than one individual. A responder who injures themselves moving a patient may be unable to treat them once they have been relocated, but a team member who stands back while everyone else lifts is not one who will be remembered kindly!

Infection Control

A danger added to any scene by medical responders is sharps and the additional risk of injury - this appears to be an international phenomenon [13–15]. Ensure if a needle or scalpel is used (preferably a "sharp-safe" model) that it is immediately put in a sharps bin. Ideally, all sharps should be used once and safely discarded. However, if a scalpel is required to be used again on the same patient (e.g. at two different stages in an amputation), then it should be retained by the individual practitioner, not on the floor or anywhere else it could accidentally harm anyone or pose an infection risk to the patient.

Eye protection should be worn where there is a risk of splashing body fluids. Although the risk is higher at some times than others (e.g. when performing invasive procedures), it is ever-present. There are reports of colleagues who have had blood flicked in their eyes by the elastic of an oxygen mask being removed.

Gloves should always be worn. If there is likely to be a lot of contamination with body fluids, consider double gloving. This method not only provides extra protection, but the top soiled pair can be removed when a cleaner pair is required. Always double glove for a thoracotomy or thoracostomy where rib fractures are suspected.

Police and Evidence

In the UK, the Police are the lead agency on scene in overall command and control, unless they cede this authority to the Fire Service to deal with specific safety concerns. The Police require only a few pieces of information in the initial phase of any incident. The most important of these being the potential for life-threatening or life-changing injuries (e.g. paralysis, significant head injury or loss of a limb). This information allows them to escalate or de-escalate their response to the scene quickly. Responses range from calling in collision investigation and forensic teams and closing the road for hours or merely marking locations and taking photographs. They will also require the patient details, as they often have to deliver the news of a severely injured or deceased patient to the next of kin—a job none of us would like.

If pronouncing death at a scene (which will obviously require extensive police investigation), it would be highly advisable to remove any kit or equipment from the patient's immediate vicinity before confirming the death. At some point, every pre-hospital scheme has had vital equipment impounded as part of the crime scene by an over-zealous police officer! Discretely move the bags, monitor and other equipment back toward the vehicle or the ambulance (although these too can be impounded) before stopping resuscitation and confirming death. If someone has already pronounced death or followed the local recognition of life extinct (ROLE) protocol, then do not approach the scene as this may disturb or destroy evidence. The more people that contaminate a scene, the harder it is for the Police to preserve evidence an establish a solid case for their investigation. Other forensic considerations are outlined in the forensic chapter, and while lifesaving interventions should take priority over the preservation of a scene, needlessly destroying evidence helps no-one. For example, when cutting a stab victim's clothes to expose injuries, cut away from the tears made by the weapon where possible. Another example would be in major incident care; if a body needs to be moved to gain access to a live casualty, move it but take a picture of the position the body was found in before relocating it. This will help with criminal and coronial investigations following the incident.

Fire and Rescue Services

The fire service will monitor the scene safety and discuss with the medical teams the options for extrication and agree on the best extrication plan. Firefighters have authority over medical teams on safety matters, though they will largely go out of their way to accommodate medical teams and interventions. Basic principles of extrication are described below. However, specific vehicle extrication methods are beyond the scope of this textbook, and dedicated texts on extrication methodology are available. Ask the fire crews via the Officer in Charge (OIC) what they can do, let the OIC know if the patient can or cannot be moved in specific ways, come up with a plan together, and then let the crew carry it out. Try not to stop them frequently to check the patient and avoid leaving unnecessary equipment in the middle of an active scene. Monitors such as small finger pulse oximeters are useful as they can be placed on a patient without trailing wires and getting in the way of firefighters who may be using hydraulic cutting equipment. Establish a position where the patient can be observed for deterioration or the need for intervention without obstructing firefighters. The number of procedures that can be carried out on an entrapped patient is minimal; the severely injured patient will often benefit more from an emergency or rapid extrication than they will a "heroic" or misguided procedure. Stories of performing RSI's while hanging through a sunroof are (more often than not) tales of systems failing rather than succeeding. If a procedure increases time to extrication and makes the management or movement of a deteriorating, critically ill patient more complex, the balance is rarely in favour of performing it.

The JESIP principles [16–18] offer sound practical advice about setting up command points next to each other for ease of communication and additional mutual support. There are courses nationally, and attendance is highly recommended. The individuals in overall charge of their team should be identifiable, and this may be by using a tabard or a different coloured helmet—if unsure of who to speak to, ask.

Everyone at the scene of an incident is working toward the same goal of getting the patients out in the best possible condition. Communication between the agencies is critical; discuss what needs to happen and be realistic about what can be done. A truly trapped patient cannot be released in 5 min no matter how sick they are or who is shouting loudest! A helpful tool is to liaise between medical and fire leadership regularly on scene, setting time periods to review extrication plans and patient condition as the scene evolves.

Communication

Good or poor communication is usually the most consistent feedback point raised from all serious or multiagency incidents. It is a recurring theme, and lessons are not learned as well as they should be, even in high profile cases. For example, the 1987 King's Cross fire highlighted the limitations and issues around communicating above and below ground with radios causing poor dissemination of information and impacting situational awareness and decision making [19, 20]. This issue was highlighted again in 2005 with the 7/7 bombings, with official reports into the incident stating that communication difficulties had not been dealt with adequately despite recommendations from the King's Cross fire report [21, 22]. Communication difficulties on scene have also been highlighted as causing problems as recently as the Grenfell Tower Inquiry [23, 24]. Effective communication within and between agencies, as well as to patients and bystanders, will expedite most incidents. There should be an ethos of equality within any team and an ingrained understanding of the primacy of safety. Any team member should be to be able to speak up if they see something they are not sure about or have any concern about on scene. Any such concern should be taken seriously, discussed on an even gradient. It does not matter who is the most medically qualified person on scene; safety is everyone's concern. It is very often the most qualified clinician who becomes fixated on a medical issue and becomes unable to see the broader picture. The idea of "Doctor knows best" in pre-hospital care is rightfully being replaced with "What is the team consensus".

Verbal and Non-Verbal Communication

The moment a team arrives on scene, people are watching to see their demeanour and reaction. The first responding team may have been unsure whether to ask for additional resources, or they may not have asked for any at all and be surprised by others arrival! While walking to the scene, take it in. Walk with purpose and do not allow body language to convey apathy, boredom or arrogance. For some patients, this is the worst day of their lives, and while a practitioner may forget individual incidents, someone will remember the team who looked after them and their attitude. The team should introduce themselves and use their first names. This is an excellent human factors technique and will help reduce any perceived authority gradient with other agencies and make them feel comfortable raising concerns. "Lucy, I'm concerned about this patient's leg." "Ok, Paul. I'll come and have another look, thanks." is far less formal than "Dr Smith I'm concerned about this patients leg". When discussing the plan of action, involve the wider team; experienced teams use this approach and should be suitably experienced that the plan will be no surprise to them. Ask the wider group, "can anyone think of a better way to do this? Does anyone think there is something else we can do?". It may be that there isn't, but the team has been asked and the opportunity to offer an opinion given. Humility on scene and acknowledgement that there is a large amount of experience both within and outside of the team will improve communication, and ultimately, patient care. An arrogant individual who believes they have all of the answers and do not need to listen to anyone else has no place working in pre-hospital care.

If a traumatic procedure is to be performed, tell people what to expect and give them the option to leave—especially non-medical colleagues. For example, before a thoracotomy warn personnel that the internal organs will be visible, and they may see steam come from the chest. Not everyone will be able to cope with this, so use them to go and complete another practical task (e.g. "could you get the scoop stretcher and the bed, please?"). Soft skills are essential in getting the best out of teams—if a responder is made to feel like a failure because they can't cope with seeing an intervention, they may shut down and refuse to work on scene, both now and in future taskings. If they are given a task where they are made to feel useful and contribute to patient care without seeing something distressing, they are still available to help with work and scene management. If responders are required to hold a tarpaulin, ask them to face away and tell them when it is safe to look back. Do not underestimate how much these things can traumatise onlookers, both professionals and bystanders.

Team Debriefing

Hot debriefings should be conducted where possible, and managers should undertake formal welfare checks after any distressing incident. Wherever possible, a "cold" team debrief should be held, inviting all services involved. Responders should have an opportunity to ask questions and debrief honestly; if something went wrong, say so. Offer a phone number or email address as a point of contact for the pre-hospital organisation or clinical manager. This gives all services a chance to understand decision-making processes and the interventions carried out. Having this opportunity and information can help people process what may have been the worst job they have ever attended.

Key Points

- Exposure needs to be adequate for assessment, but also avoid unnecessary heat loss
- Perform an RSI in the centre of the ambulance with the side door opened to create space rather than outside. This may decrease heat loss, provide more light and improve the chances of first-pass success in a critical intervention.
- Take a few seconds to look around the environment; fully appreciate the risks and hazards, look for them, listen for them and don't forget the sense of smell. Scenes always have four dimensions—front and back, left and

right, top and bottom and time. Hazards can emerge from any direction at any point.

- Medical equipment should be managed similarly with an emphasis on safety. For example, if a cannula needs to be placed, ensure a sharps box is to hand, the needle is made safe, and all equipment is removed from the area around the patient after cannulation.
- Arriving at a scene without essential safety equipment is unacceptable and will make the team appear amateurish. Team and scene safety is paramount; if something looks unsafe then speak up. This does not need to be done aggressively in the first instance but can be escalated as required.
- All institutions and schemes should have a period of training and sign off before authorising solo practice. Even practitioners with significant prior experience can make the most of this time by watching how others operate in the pre-hospital environment, debriefing even simple jobs to understand the decision-making process and scene etiquette.
- There should be a communications check to ensure at least two forms of communication within the team (e.g. radio and mobile phone).
- If a responder is a passenger and a colleague is driving, it is the passenger's responsibility to co-drive. Co-driving involves navigation, safety checks when approaching junctions, being alert to dangers and communications.
- Life is much easier if first respond agencies don't feel threatened or marginalised by other practitioners!
- The arrival of friends or relatives who are being held back by the Police can cause conflict and risk. This can generally be managed by effective communication where possible.
- Practitioners should always be aware of their surroundings and avoid letting their exit routes be blocked. Knowledge of the emergency operation of radios is essential.
- Multiagency working with partner agencies (e.g. Fire service or Mountain Rescue services) who have access to specialist training areas and equipment is excellent for overcoming fear, developing strategies and building relationships before working with each other on scene.
- A responder who injures themselves moving a patient may be unable to treat them once they have been relocated, but a team member who stands back while everyone else lifts is not one who will be remembered kindly!
- The Police require only a few pieces of information, such as the potential for life-threatening or life-altering injuries in the initial phase of any incident. This allows them to determine their response and should take no more than 10 s.
- Try not to stop fire crews frequently to check the patient, and avoid leaving unnecessary equipment in the middle of an active scene. Monitors such as small pulse oximeters are useful as they can be placed on a patient without trailing wires and getting in the way of firefighters who may be using hydraulic cutting equipment.
- A truly trapped patient cannot be released in 5 min no matter how sick they are or who is shouting loudest!
- The moment a team arrives on scene, people are watching to see their demeanour and reaction.
- While walking to the scene, take it in, walk with purpose and do not allow body language to convey apathy, boredom or arrogance.
- If a traumatic procedure is to be performed, tell people what to expect and give them the option to leave—especially non-medical colleagues. For example, before a thoracotomy warn personnel that the internal organs will be visible, and they may see steam come from the chest. Not everyone will be able to cope with this, so use them to go and complete another practical task (e.g. "could you get the scoop stretcher and the bed, please?").
- Hot debriefings should be conducted where possible, and managers should undertake formal welfare checks after any distressing incident.

Conclusion

Working in the pre-hospital environment poses more challenges than in-hospital practice. Clinical medicine is only one facet that needs to be considered, and the environment can both cause and worsen clinical presentations. As well as the risk to patients, the environment can be hazardous to unwary or inexperienced practitioners. Effective teamwork is even more essential to ensure safety and optimise patient outcomes than in a well-lit, warm, well-resourced hospital. This chapter is not an exhaustive list of the factors and hazards associated with the environment for individuals who currently or wish to work in the pre-hospital environment. For those staff who receive patients in emergency departments, it is hopefully an insight into some of the issues that have faced crews that present neatly packaged patients from frequently chaotic incidents. It is also an illustration of why everything may not have been completed in a hospital textbook standard manner.

Questions

1. The term sterile cockpit refers to
   (a) Infection control issues during procedures
   (b) Decontamination of the aircraft between jobs due to covid-19
   (c) Maintaining silence during critical phases of flight or response driving (except in an emergency)
2. When should a hot debrief be conducted
   (a) Only when requested by the fire & rescue team
   (b) After every job
   (c) After jobs where unusual or uncommon procedures have taken place
3. When arriving on scene, the most critical priority is
   (a) Getting to the patient
   (b) Personal safety
   (c) Establishing a cordon
   (d) Finding the officer in charge
   (e) Deciding which hospital to go to
4. When arriving at a rail incident
   (a) You can walk on the lines as they'll have been turned off
   (b) You can walk down the side of the track wearing a hi-vis as all the train drivers will see you
   (c) The ambulance service will turn off the electricity
   (d) Only go on the tracks when advised by network rail that it is safe
5. On arriving at an RTC, you find a patient trapped under a car and a bystander who is a first aider, also under the car comforting the patient. Should you
   (a) Ask the bystander to come out from under the car
   (b) Leave them as they're first aid trained
   (c) Wait till the fire service arrive
   (d) Ask the first aider to start treatment, such as o2 application.

Answers

1. c
2. c
3. b
4. d
5. a

References

1. Crewdson K, Lockey D, Voelckel W, Temesvari P, Lossius HM, EHAC Medical Working Group. Best practice advice on pre-hospital emergency anaesthesia & advanced airway management. Scand J Trauma Resusc Emerg Med. 2019;27(1):6.
2. Savino PB, Reichelderfer S, Mercer MP, Wang RC, Sporer KA. Direct versus video laryngoscopy for prehospital intubation: a systematic review and meta-analysis. Acad Emerg Med. 2017;24(8):1018–26.
3. Pieters BM, van Zundert AA. Videolaryngoscopes differ substantially in illumination of the oral cavity: a manikin study. Indian J Anaesth. 2016;60(5):325–9.
4. McQueen C, Bexon K, Wyse M. A safe scene? Emerg Med J. 2013;30(8):687.
5. Schyma BM, Wood AE, Sothisrihari S, Swinton P. Optimising remote site airway management kit dump using the SCRAM bag—a randomised controlled trial. Perioper Med. 2020;9(1):11.

6. Swinton P, Corfield AR, Moultrie C, Percival D, Proctor J, Sinclair N, et al. Impact of drug and equipment preparation on pre-hospital emergency Anaesthesia (PHEA) procedural time, error rate and cognitive load. Scand J Trauma Resusc Emerg Med [Internet]. 2018 Sep 21 [cited 2020 July 8]:[26 p.]. Available from: https://www.ncbi.nlm.nih.gov/pmc/articles/PMC6150998/
7. Findlay G, Martin IC, Carter S, Smith N, Weyman D, Mason M. A report of the National Confidential Enquiry into Patient Outcome and Death. London: National Confidential Enquiry into Patient Outcome and Death; 2007. p. 151.
8. Gillings M, Grundlingh J, Aw-Yong M. Guidelines for management of acute behavioural disturbance (May 2016).pdf [Internet]. The Royal College of Emergency Medicine; 2016 [cited 2020 July 8]. Available from: https://www.rcem.ac.uk/docs/College%20Guidelines/5p.%20RCEM%20guidelines%20for%20management%20of%20Acute%20Behavioural%20Disturbance%20(May%202016).pdf
9. Scheppke KA, Braghiroli J, Shalaby M, Chait R. Prehospital use of IM ketamine for sedation of violent and agitated patients. West J Emerg Med. 2014;15(7):736–41.
10. Isenberg DL, Jacobs D. Prehospital agitation and sedation trial (PhAST): a randomized control trial of intramuscular haloperidol versus intramuscular midazolam for the sedation of the agitated or violent patient in the prehospital environment. Prehospital Disaster Med. 2015;30(5):491–5.
11. Anderson AR. Characterisation of chemical suicides in the United States and its adverse impact on responders and bystanders. West J Emerg Med. 2016;17(6):680–3.
12. Reedy SJD, Schwartz MD, Morgan BW. Suicide fads: frequency and characteristics of hydrogen Sulfide suicides in the United States. West J Emerg Med. 2011;12(3):300–4.
13. Elder A, Paterson C. Sharps injuries in UK health care: a review of injury rates, viral transmission and potential efficacy of safety devices. Occup Med. 2006;56(8):566–74.
14. Shaban RZ, Creedy DK, Clark MJ. Management of sharps in ambulance care: a state-wide survey of paramedic knowledge and reported practice. Aust Infect Control. 2004;9(4):120–5.
15. Alhazmi RA, Parker RD, Wen S. Needlestick injuries among emergency medical services providers in urban and rural areas. J Community Health. 2018;43(3):518–23.
16. Pollock DK. Local interoperability in UK emergency management: a research. Report. 2017;53
17. Flanagan J. Joint emergency services interoperability programme: working together saving lives. J Paramed Pract. 2014;6(6):284–7.
18. JESIP - Working together, Saving Lives [Internet]. [cited 2020 July 8]. Available from: https://www.jesip.org.uk/principles
19. Allinson RE. Saving human lives: lessons in management ethics. Dordrecht: Springer; 2005. p. 354. (Issues in business ethics)
20. Fennell D. Investigation into the King's cross underground fire: presented to parliament by the secretary of state for transport by command of her majesty, November 1988. London: HMSO; 1988. p. 247.
21. Great Britain, Intelligence and Security Committee, Murphy P. Report into the London terrorist attacks on 7th July 2005. London: Stationery Office; 2006.
22. London Assembly, Greater London Authority, editors. Report of the 7 July Review Committee. London: Greater London Authority; 2006. 3 p.
23. Galea E. Interim Phase 1 Recommendations for the Grenfell Inquiry from Prof ED Galea [Internet]. 2019 [cited 2020 July 8]. Available from: https://www.grenfelltowerinquiry.org.uk/evidence/professor-ed-galeas-report-interim-recommendations
24. Inquiry TGT. Grenfell Tower Inquiry: Phase 1 Report Overview [Internet]. London: Her Majesty's Stationary Office; 2017 [cited 2020 July 8]:[32 p.]. Available from: https://www.grenfelltowerinquiry.org.uk/phase-1-report

Mechanism of Injury

21

Thomas G. D. Woolley, Steve Dick, and Darren Reid

- Understanding the physical forces involved
- Classification of injury mechanisms
- Road traffic collisions: Cars
- Road traffic collisions: Pedestrians
- Road traffic collisions: Bicycles and Motorcycles
- Falls from height
- Equestrian accidents

T. G. D. Woolley (✉)
Royal Army Medical Corps, Department of Anaesthesia, Nottingham University Teaching Hospitals NHS Trust, Nottingham, UK

The Air Ambulance Service (TAAS), Rugby, Warwickshire, UK
e-mail: thomas.woolley@nhs.net

S. Dick
East Midlands Ambulance Service NHS Trust, Nottingham, UK

The Air Ambulance Service (TAAS), Rugby, Warwickshire, UK
e-mail: Steve.Dick@emas.nhs.uk

D. Reid
Royal Centre for Defence Medicine, Birmingham, UK

The Air Ambulance Service (TAAS), Rugby, Warwickshire, UK
e-mail: Steve.Dick@emas.nhs.uk

Introduction

The term 'mechanism of injury' (MOI) is used to describe a process of considering the forces involved in an injury-causing event. In a patient with traumatic injuries, this process is used to suggest possible patterns of injuries and thus guide assessment and treatment. It is important to note that the physical forces involved in an individual incident will include a vast array of variables. As such, the MOI can only provide a guide to potential injuries rather than a prescriptive list.

The MOI assessment considers the application of mechanics to understand the movement of objects, the forces applied to the structures of the human body, knowledge of the underlying anatomy and how this is affected by these forces. Understanding these interactions is also merged with scientific data relating to common injury patterns to provide clinicians with guidance on the likelihood of specific injuries and injury patterns [1].

Certain MOIs can be used to decide on the level of clinician response dispatched to the scene alongside patient symptoms via the MPDS (Medical Priority Dispatch System) criteria utilized by most ambulance services in the UK [2–6]. However, most major trauma triage tools utilize the MOI to identify "high-risk" patients to transfer to major trauma centres, though the validity of this approach has recently been challenged [7, 8]. Commonly included mechanisms that may trigger admission to a major trauma centre include traumatic death of occupant in the

P. Lax (ed.), *Textbook of Acute Trauma Care*, https://doi.org/10.1007/978-3-030-83628-3_21

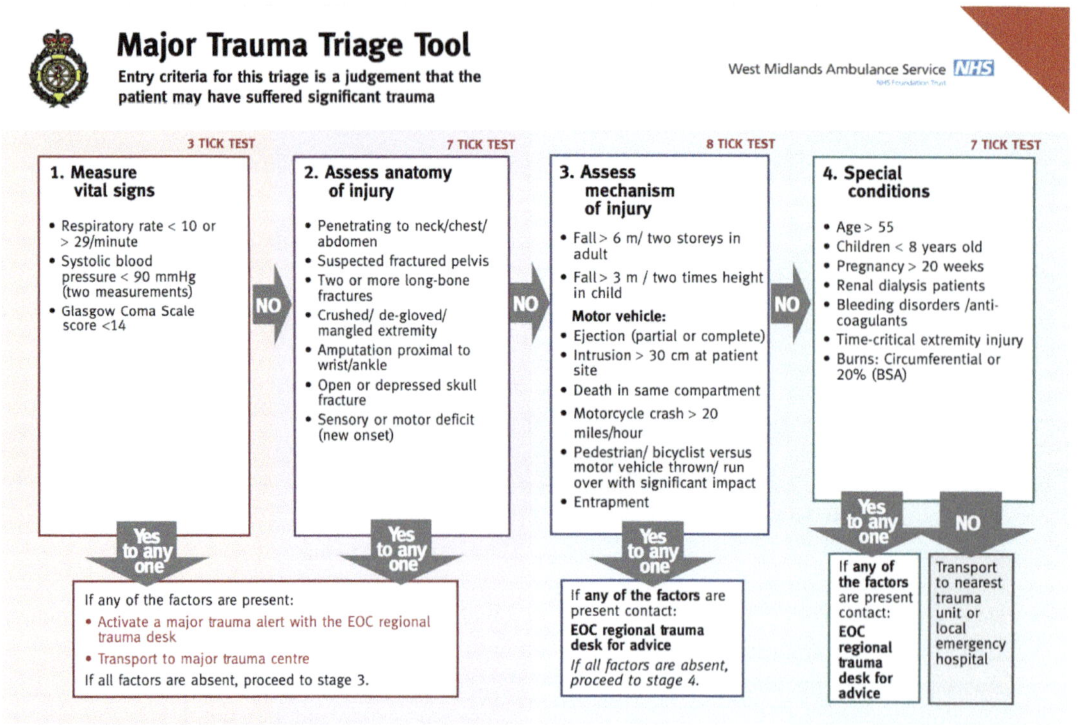

Fig. 21.1 2015 West Midlands Ambulance Triage Tool (incorporating mechanism of injury)

same passenger compartment, ejection from the vehicle, significant intrusion into the passenger compartment, falls from >20 ft, and motorcycle crash >20 mph (Figs. 21.1 and 21.2).

It should be noted that while the MOI is often used in high speed, high force accidents, such as a head-on collision between two cars, it can be equally helpful in predicting injury patterns in low force incidents.

By way of an example, consider an elderly patient falling from standing. While the forces involved are lower, clinicians must consider the nature of the fall, the material the patient fell onto and the relative vulnerability to injury caused by the ageing process or frailty.

Understanding the Physical Forces Involved

To effectively utilize MOI assessments, it is essential to understand how the forces involved in an injury-causing event are generated and dissipated. This requires a basic understanding of several underlying physical principles.

Firstly, consider Newton's laws of motion [9]:

- A body in motion or at rest will remain in that state until acted upon by an outside force.
- The sum of forces applied to an object is equal to the mass of that object multiplied by its acceleration.
- When a body exerts a force on a second body, the second body will simultaneously exert a force of equal magnitude and in the opposite direction to the first body.

To apply these concepts to traumatic injury, one must look at their effect on a patient. Picture the rider of a bicycle thrown from the saddle when travelling at a speed of 25 mph who falls to the floor. If we crudely estimate that the rider strikes the floor and stops immediately, we can understand the force applied by the ground to the rider. We must also be aware that while the rider may stop almost instantaneously, their internal

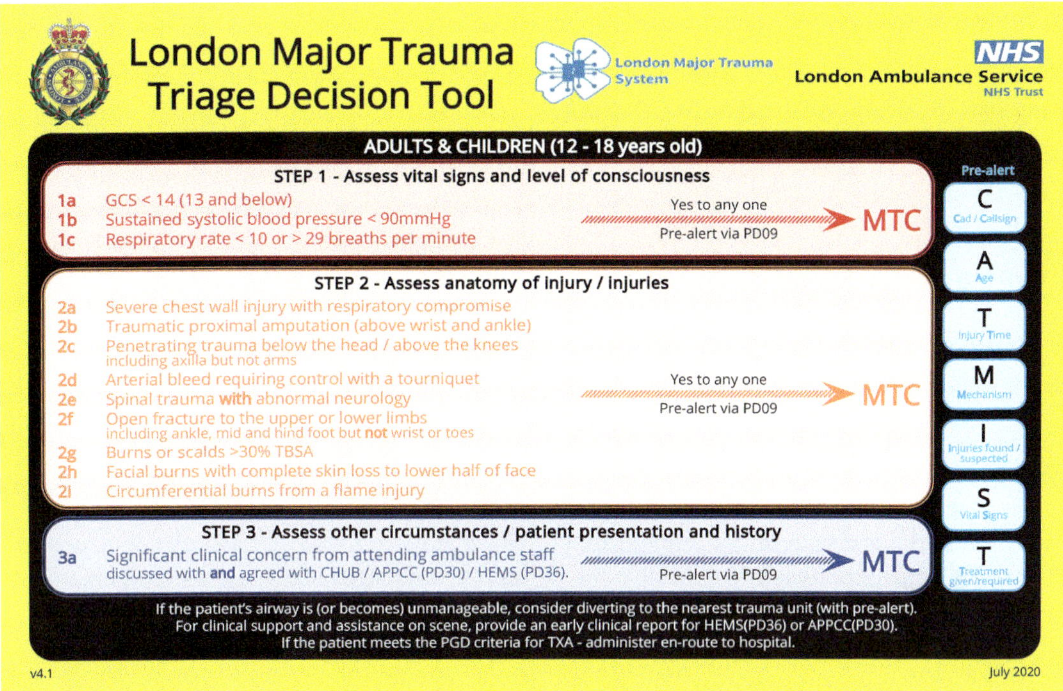

Fig. 21.2 2020 London Ambulance Service Major Trauma Triage decision tool (note mechanism of injury has been removed favouring anatomical and physiological data)

organs are still travelling at 25 mph and will continue to move and collide with other internal structures, generating sheering and other forces.

The second consideration is the amount of energy liberated at the moment of impact. The kinetic energy of a moving object can be found from [2]:

$$\text{Kinetic Energy} = 1/2\,\text{mass} \times \text{velocity}$$

When we apply this formula to the cyclist from our previous example, we can see that velocity, or speed, is the most significant driver of kinetic energy. An identical cyclist falling from his bicycle at 5 mph would generate significantly less kinetic energy.

Conversely, even a slight increase in the cyclist's speed would substantially affect the kinetic energy produced.

An increase in mass has a far more negligible effect on the total kinetic energy released on impact; a slow-moving lorry will potentially cause less damage than a car travelling at high speed.

Impulse momentum theory describes the relative rate of change in the momentum of an object. It demonstrates that the relative changes in momentum (ΔP) and the time over which these changes occur (ΔT) determine the level of force applied to an object.

$$F = \frac{\Delta P}{\Delta T}$$

To better understand this concept, visualize a person undertaking a bungee jump. If they were to jump when attached to an ordinary rope, their fall would be arrested once the entire length of line had been used. Their change in momentum would be significant and near-instantaneous, resulting in a massive transmission of force through their harness and likely causing substantial injuries. Now consider the use of the elasticated rope seen during bungee jumps. The momentum change is identical when compared to jumping with a static line. However, the gradual reduction in speed increases the time over which momentum is changed, reducing the force transmitted to the harness and the jumper.

This concept has driven several design changes to improve safety [10–14] and aid in reconstructing incidents for investigation [15]. Increasing the time over which momentum is changed can be relatively straightforward—for example, placing padding around hard objects and fitting vehicles with seatbelts and airbags. More complicated engineering innovations which perform the same function have been seen, such as the development of vehicle crumple zones and seatbelt pre-tensioners.

Grouping of Injury Types

It is important to note that certain types of injury are specific to particular injury mechanisms. These mechanisms can be broadly divided into four groups; blunt trauma, penetrating trauma, ballistic trauma, and acceleration/deceleration trauma. The effect of these four mechanism groups on the human body differs significantly and warrant further discussion.

Blunt Trauma

The term 'blunt trauma' is used to define mechanisms of injury in which the initial force applied to the patient is limited to contact with the outer surface of the body and where there is no penetration into a cavity. Blunt trauma may cause body cavities to become open, such as the evisceration of bowel or the creation of an open skull fracture. Still, these injuries differ from true penetrating injuries in that the open cavity is a result of the force dissipating through the body. Typically, blunt trauma mechanisms involve a relatively high ratio of contact area to force, whereas the opposite is true for penetrating injuries. Mechanisms of injury leading to blunt trauma can range from a simple fall from standing to being struck by a falling object or a person being struck by a vehicle.

Penetrating Trauma

Penetrating trauma is used to group all injuries in which a foreign body penetrates a body cavity. The most obvious example of this is a stab wound caused by a sharp object, but further examples include impalement, industrial accidents and falling debris. While gunshot wounds are a form of penetrating trauma, ballistic injuries cause different injury patterns and are discussed below.

Penetrating trauma involves the transmission of force through an object with a relatively small surface area, transmitting the energy to a small area of the body. Generally, this results in a predictable injury pattern based upon the estimated route the object took through the body cavity and the tissues it encountered during its journey. Unlike ballistic trauma, there is generally little force transmitted outside of this path.

A common pitfall in making a diagnosis of injures based on the assessment of the entry wound in penetrating trauma is not to appreciate the actual depth and direction that the penetrating object may have travelled. For example, depending on the length and force of the penetration, wounds to the buttocks and groin may be associated with injuries to the abdominal and even thoracic viscera.

Ballistic Trauma

Ballistic injuries generally involve projectiles travelling at extremely high velocity that cause significant damage beyond the path they take through a cavity. The MOI relating to ballistic injuries is covered in detail within the ballistics chapter. Therefore, it will not be covered here other than highlighting that these injuries have additional management considerations compared to more conventional penetrating injuries.

Acceleration and Deceleration Trauma

Newton's second law of motion describes the relationship between the forces acting upon a body, its mass and acceleration or deceleration and gives us the formula: Force = mass × acceleration.

For a body with a fixed mass, the rate of acceleration or deceleration is, therefore, the primary determinant of the amount of force transmitted.

For example, a faster deceleration during a head-on motor vehicle collision will lead to a more forceful impact of the driver's torso against the steering wheel or their head onto the windscreen.

Acceleration and deceleration are also commonly the cause of compression and shearing injuries to thoracic and abdominal viscera and vascular structures.

Shearing injuries such as damage to the aortic arch occur as a direct result of deceleration forces. Additionally, these forces can cause internal organs such as the heart and liver to pull away from their ligamentous attachments leading to significant internal haemorrhage.

Road Traffic Collisions

Road Traffic Collisions (RTCs) are among the most common causes of trauma death and injury in the UK, with 1870 deaths and 25,950 serious injuries from July 2018 to June 2019 [16].

By understanding the forces involved in collisions, it is possible to relate these to associated injury patterns.

Road traffic collisions involving vehicles can be broadly categorized into frontal or head-on collisions, lateral impact collisions and rear-end collisions. They can also be further subdivided depending on the type of vehicles or road user involved.

Frontal/Head-on

A head-on motor vehicle collision is the mechanism of collision that accounts for the majority of both driver (58%) and front seat passenger (53%) deaths [14].

This mechanism results in rapid deceleration of the vehicle as it impacts, with direct transmission of large forces to the vehicle and, consequently, the occupants.

Front-seat occupants will continue to move forward after the vehicle has impacted.

If unrestrained, they may either collide with the vehicle dashboard, steering wheel, roof, windscreen or "submarine" under the steering wheel and into the footwell, depending on how well restrained they are and what impact technology is in the car.

This can result in lower limb and pelvic injuries due to the impact of the knees against the dashboard, chest and abdominal injuries from impact with the steering wheel and head and facial injuries from impact with the windscreen, as well as physical entrapment from a variety of causes.

There is also a high chance of ejection from the vehicle through the windscreen with additional injuries from impact with the ground.

Unrestrained rear seat occupants may also collide with the front seats, causing injury to themselves as well as further injury to front-seat occupants.

As previously mentioned, the presence of safety devices such as airbags, seat belts, and the crumple zone in modern vehicles have helped dissipate some of the force projected onto the patient and reduce some of the effects of blunt impact trauma. However, the vehicle occupants can still suffer significant injuries despite these.

Seat belts can cause abrasions and lacerations across the neck, torso and abdomen, and contusions and perforations of the abdominal viscera.

Summary of Injury Patterns

- Various degrees of traumatic brain injury
- Scalp injuries
- Facial injuries
- Flexion and extension injuries to the cervical spine
- Seatbelt injuries
- Rib fractures, flail chest, sternal fractures, pulmonary/cardiac contusions
- Abdominal visceral injuries, ruptured diaphragm
- Upper limb injuries
- Pelvis and acetabular injuries, fracture/dislocation of femur and patella

Impact with airbags can cause facial injuries. The talcum powder, which is used to lubricate the airbags as they deploy, is dispersed and can cause respiratory irritation or breathing problems. Patients may experience temporary deafness from the explosion of an airbag in a confined space.

Scene Findings Associated with Significant Injury
- Intrusion into the passenger compartment
- Deformity of lower door sills
- Damage to "A" post caused by pedestrian
- Movement of passenger seats within a compartment
- Damage to dashboard around steering wheel (indicating knee strike)
- Separation of the engine from the vehicle
- Report of secondary collision (e.g. Car vs Car, then into a wall)

Rear Impacts

Rear-end collisions are commonly associated with whiplash injuries of the cervical spine and injuries to the lower back. On the whole, serious rear-end collisions are less frequent than frontal impact collisions.

Absent or poorly adjusted headrests may exacerbate neck injuries, and a rear-end shunt at high speed may cause a subsequent frontal collision with associated injuries.

Summary of Injury Patterns
- Hyperextension of the lumbar spine
- Hyperextension and hyperflexion of the neck
- Shear injuries to kidneys, liver and spleen

Side on/"T-Bone" Collision

Despite the increase in strength in modern vehicles, their sides are still less well designed to tolerate impacts than the front or rear. The narrower diameter of the vehicle wall and smaller distance between the outside and passenger compartment compared to the vehicle's longitudinal axis cannot accommodate a sufficient crumple zone. This means that impacts along the lateral axis are unable to dissipate the force of impact in the same way as the longitudinal axis of the vehicle.

The proximity of the shell of the vehicle to the occupant means that they are much more likely to suffer injuries as a result of intrusion into the passenger compartment.

Indicators of high risk in these cases include significant damage to the B post and damage or lateral movement of the occupant's seat. Another factor to consider is that the human body has a different tolerance to G-forces depending on the axis, duration, duration and location of their application [17, 18]. This is depicted in Fig. 21.3.

Summary of Injury Patterns
- Head injury through impact with the side of the car (then possibly with adjacent occupant)
- Shear injuries to kidneys, liver and spleen
- Pelvic and long bone injuries
- Pulmonary contusion and diaphragmatic injury
- Lateral hyperextension of the neck
- Arm and leg injuries

Rollover

A rollover is defined as a crash in which the vehicle is overturned by at least a quarter turn, and therefore resting on its side, but may also include those that end up on their roof or even back on their wheels. Rollovers may occur due to rapid directional change at high speeds or following a

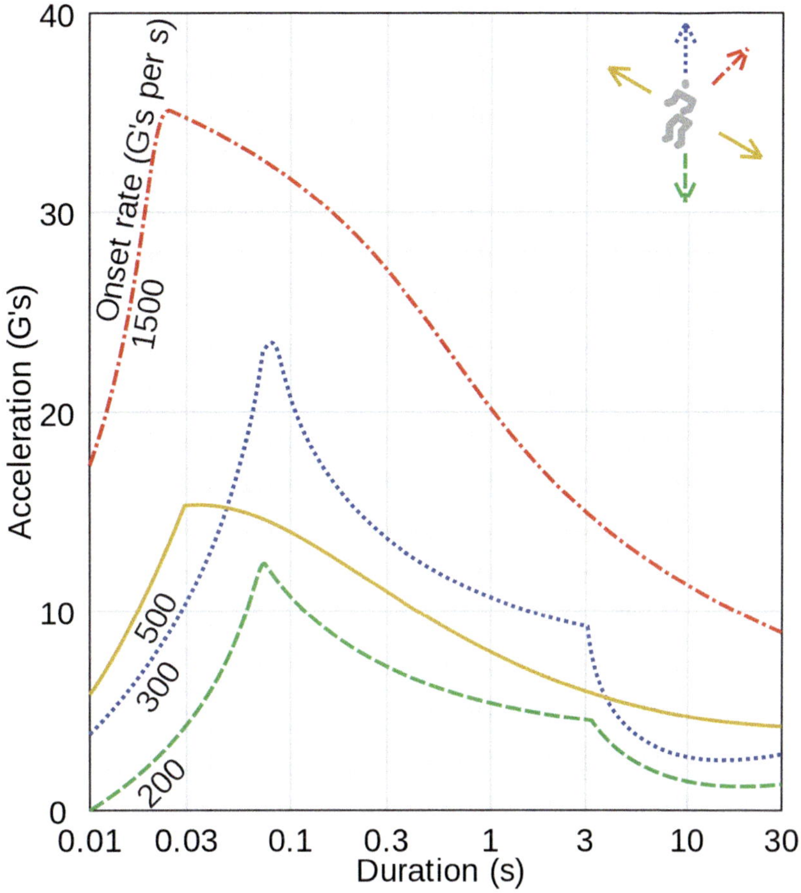

Fig. 21.3 Differential tolerance of G-forces depending on loading direction (Cmglee via Wikimedia, based on data from Brulle [18])

collision with road furniture or other vehicles. Vehicles may overturn on their side (short axis) or end over end (long axis).

Motor vehicle rollovers represent a small but significant proportion of crashes. Despite occurring in only 2.5% of all vehicle crashes, they account for over a third of motor vehicle accident-related occupant deaths [19]. They are also associated with increased injury severity compared to non-rollover collisions with specific injury types, including severe spinal cord injuries and significant injuries to the torso and spleen.

Restrained passengers will typically remain in their seat but will be struck by unrestrained objects or other occupants in the vehicle. Head injuries and spinal injuries due to impact with the sides and roof of the car are common. If casualties are unrestrained, they may be ejected from the vehicle leading to a higher mortality rate.

Factors associated with increased injury severity include roof crush (a notably weak part of many vehicles), entrapment, ejection and intrusion of the B-post into the passenger compartment.

Look for deformation of the roof, multiple body panels and damage to the environment. Due to the nature of rollover incidents, almost any injury is possible, and occupants require a high index of suspicion.

Pedestrian

The most common mechanism is a frontal collision of a pedestrian with a car, which accounts for over 80% of pedestrian road traffic collisions. Accidents involving larger vehicles such as buses and lorries are less common but usually occur due to significant blind spots in these vehicles. They are also more likely to have fatal outcomes as a result of the significant forces involved.

A vehicle's impact will typically result in a significant transfer of force to the pedestrian with little impact on the vehicle. This means that while there may often be little visible damage to the vehicle, the pedestrian may still have suffered significant injuries. Visible damage to more robust parts of the car such as bumper, windscreen and A-post should lead to a very high index of suspicion of significant pedestrian injury (Fig. 21.4.).

Pedestrian impact with vehicles is usually thought of as three separate collisions; the initial impact with the front of the vehicle, the secondary impact with the bonnet, windscreen and roof and finally, the impact with the ground.

The height of the pedestrian shows some correlation with the patterns of injury.

In adults, the point of impact will usually be between the front bumper or bonnet edge and the pedestrian's lower limbs. This often causes the pedestrian to be thrown upwards and onto the bonnet and roof of the car. Therefore, the most frequent combination of injuries is lower limb and pelvis injuries with a traumatic head injury (Fig. 21.5).

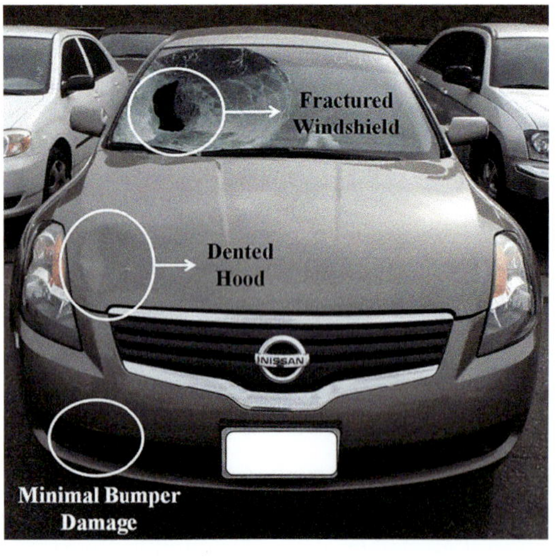

Fig. 21.4 Damage profile to a vehicle that has hit a pedestrian

Shorter patients and children will take the impact of the vehicle across the centre of their body, and as a result, will be thrown forwards of the vehicle. The transmission of forces is more significant in this case due to its being a direct blow to the centre of mass instead of an off-centre impact.

Associated injuries in these cases are therefore more likely to include pelvic, abdominal and thoracic trauma.

Summary of Typical Pedestrian Injury Patterns

- Sheer injuries to kidneys, liver and spleen
- Lower limb injuries
- Hyperextension/hyperflexion injuries to the neck
- Head Injuries
- Chest injuries
- Pelvic fractures

Cyclists and Motorcyclists

Road traffic accidents involving cyclists and motorcyclists may include falls, collisions with other vehicles and collisions with stationary objects.

Cyclists will be propelled forwards, hitting either the vehicle or object they have collided with or impacting directly with the ground. This will commonly cause injuries to the head and neck as well as thoracic and upper limb injuries.

Falls onto outstretched arms are common and associated with wrist fractures and shoulder injuries such as dislocation and clavicle fractures. High velocity falls may also cause fractures to the scapula.

This mechanism of fall is also associated with a high risk of head-first impact, with the ground causing hyperextension or hyperflexion injuries of the cervical spine and associated vertebral fractures, with the potential of a high spinal cord injury as a result.

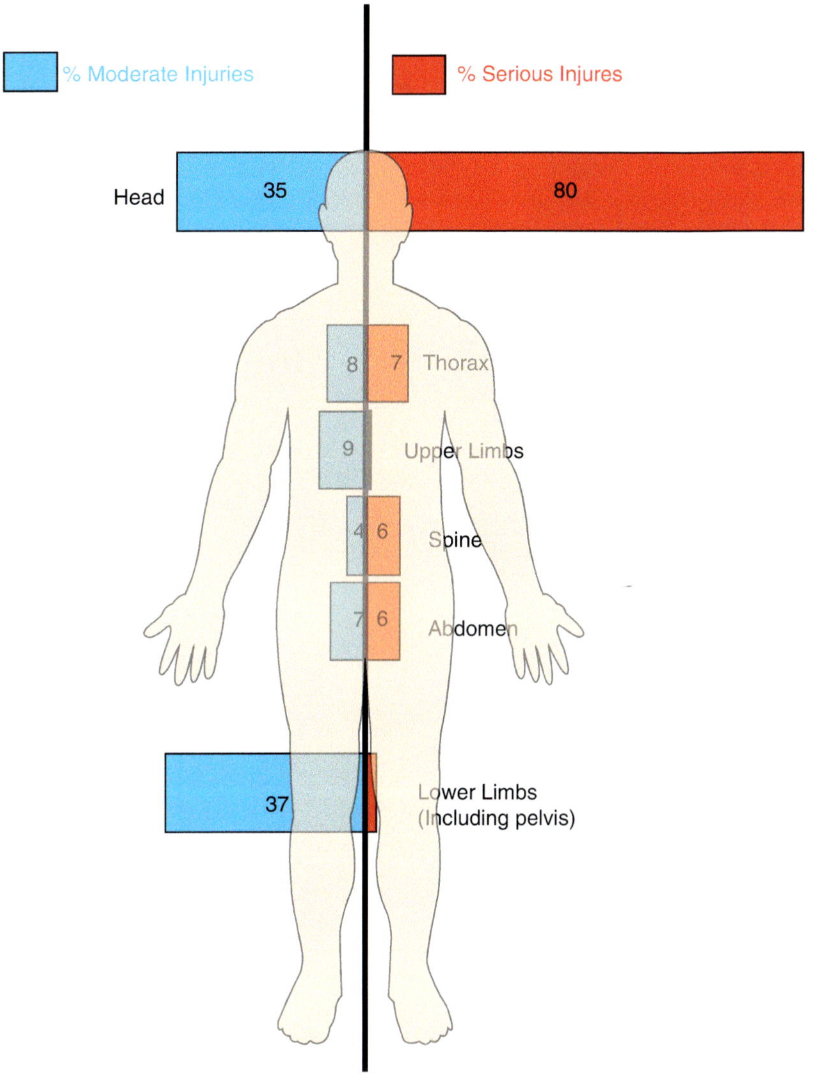

Fig. 21.5 Patterns of moderate or severe injuries in pedestrian vs car collisions (based on data from Jain [20])

Motorcyclists may be thrown forward and upwards on frontal impact, causing them to sustain pelvic and femoral fractures as they collide with first the fuel tank and then the handlebars [21, 22].

Depending on the nature of the accident, some of the force of impact may be dissipated by the rider rolling or sliding down the road. This may even be sufficient for the rider to avoid any serious injury. Furthermore, protective clothing worn may help motorcyclists may also prevent significant abrasions and cuts. Modern motorcycle helmet and protective clothing design have reduced the risk of traumatic brain injury and cervical spine injury, but a high degree of suspicion should remain.

A motorcyclist who falls from a bike due to lateral forces is said to have “high-sided” or “low-sided” [23]. A high-siding motorcyclist effectively travels up and over the motorbike, generating forces associated with a fall from a height, an impact at speed with the ground and a significant rotational force. A low-siding motorcyclist will fall from the bike's low side, often sliding away from or underneath the bike. This can generate injuries associated with crushing between the bike and the road but is generally associated with less significant injuries (Fig. 21.6).

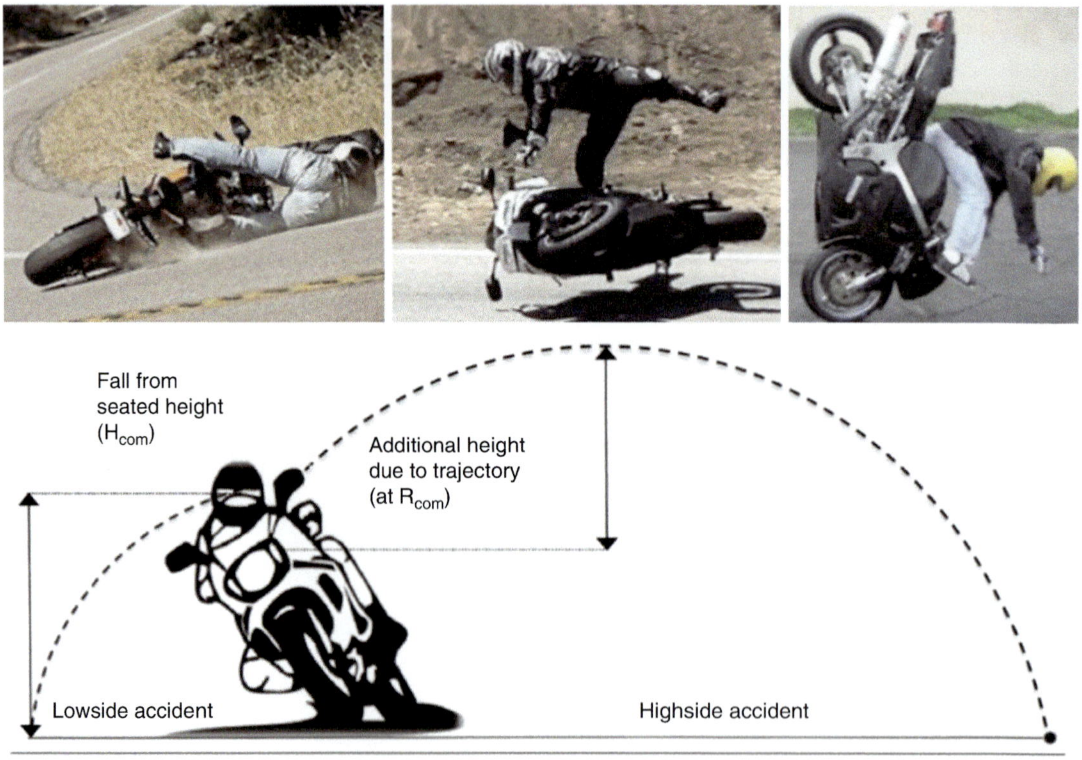

Fig. 21.6 High side vs low side ejection (from Lloyd [23])

Falls

Falls from a height are a common cause of blunt trauma and are associated with a high rate of injury and mortality.

The most important factor influencing the severity of the injury is the height fallen. Falls from >20 ft for adults or >10 ft for children will generally trigger a major trauma centre admission. However, other aspects that will also determine the severity of the fall include the impact surface, the rate of deceleration and the parts of the body striking the ground [24].

Injuries associated with a fall from height onto feet typically include calcaneal fractures, lumbar spine blowout fractures and possibly unstable vertical shear pelvic injuries. Head-first falls are associated with often severe head injuries, and hyperflexion or hyperextension injuries of the cervical spine.

Falls from standing in the elderly will often produce injuries such as a neck of femur fracture and wrist fractures as a result of their lower bone density.

Equestrian Accidents

As large and powerful animals, it should not be surprising that incidents involving horses often result in significant injuries. Approximately 20% of all horse riders will suffer an injury requiring hospitalization or other medical treatment in their riding career, with a fatality rate of 1 in 10,000 riders, usually from head injury [25]. While an emphasis has traditionally been placed on the size of the horse involved, it is more important to consider the speed, relative positioning of rider and horse, the trajectory of any fall and any contact made between the horse and rider after they separate. Where an injury occurs before a rider is mounted, for example, a kick or trampling incident, the duration of any contact or number of kicks is important [26].

Kicks

Horses generate and transfer massive forces when kicking, and these forces are transmitted through a relatively small contact area around the hoof. When applied to the human body, this force, which has been reported to be up to 10,000 Newtons, can cause significant injuries. Kick injuries from horses to the patient's head are associated with a high incidence of skull fracture and high-grade Le Fort fractures. Kicks to the thorax and abdomen can cause significant damage to underlying organs, including reported cases of aortic rupture. This is particularly important to consider in the later management of patients as contusions, and more subtle injury may not be immediately apparent on the first CT images.

Falls from a Horse

Falls from horses are associated with a high incident of head and pelvic injuries. Factors influencing the severity of injury include the use of protective equipment (helmets and automatically inflating air jackets), whether the rider remained connected to the horse in any way (instinctively keeping hold of the reins or a foot getting trapped in a stirrup) and contact between the horse and rider after the fall.

"Rotational" falls are a specific mechanism which are recognized as extremely dangerous and have been associated with numerous fatalities. A rotational fall typically occurs when a horse and rider attempt to navigate a jump over a fixed obstruction rather than a collapsible obstacle such as a typical jump found at riding schools. In a rotational fall, the horse typically strikes its chest or forelegs on the object, causing a pivoting motion of the horse and resulting in a somersault-like rotation over the object. Consequently, the rider is either catapulted from the horse at significant speed or, more troublingly, rotates through the initial impact in combination with the horse. This results in an impact with the floor or jump, followed by the horse landing on top of the rider. The range of injuries that can be sustained in a rotational fall from a horse is vast. As such, any rider reported to have suffered a rotational fall ought to be very thoroughly examined, imaged and observed.

Summary

Mechanism of injury allows us to understand the magnitude of forces involved in an incident, the direction they occur in and knowledge of the underlying anatomy to deduce the potential injuries that a patient may suffer.

Once the mechanism and mode of injury are known, injuries can be broadly split into four distinct types: blunt, penetrating, ballistic, and acceleration/deceleration.

Key points to remember are:

- Pedestrians are at high risk of serious injury if struck by moving vehicles and should be considered to have such injuries until proved otherwise, even if there is no visible damage to the vehicle.
- Patients ejected from their vehicle or involved in a rollover are at increased risk of death.
- Falls from height carry a risk of significant injury, especially from above 6 m.
- The external wounds sustained by victims of stabbings may not reflect the internal damage.
- Rapid deceleration and acceleration may damage internal organs through shearing forces without visible external signs of injury.

Questions

1. Mechanisms of injury are commonly categorized in all of the following terms EXCEPT:
   (a) Penetrating
   (b) Ballistic
   (c) Blunt
   (d) Invasive
2. Which mechanism of motor vehicle collision is most commonly associated with driver and front seat passenger death.
   (a) Frontal Impact
   (b) Side on/T-bone Impact

   (c) Rear Impact
   (d) Rollover
3. Which of the following suggests the highest likelihood of injury to the driver of a vehicle in a side-on or t-bone vehicle collision:
   (a) Lateral movement or damage to the driver's seat
   (b) Lateral movement or damage to the front passenger seat.
   (c) Damage to the side panels without intrusion into the passenger compartment
   (d) Significant damage to the rear of the car without intrusion into the passenger compartment.
4. A high-side ejection from a motorbike is when:
   (a) There is a collision that impacts the side of the bike.
   (b) The rider slides away from or underneath the bike
   (c) The rider travels up and over the bike during the fall.
   (d) The rider is ejected over the handlebars of the bike.
5. The most important factor influencing the severity of injury in a fall from height is:
   (a) The weight of the person falling
   (b) The height fallen
   (c) The speed of the fall
   (d) The impact surface

Answers

1. d
2. a
3. a
4. c
5. b

References

1. Mackay M. Mechanisms of injury and biomechanics: vehicle design and crash performance. World J Surg. 1992 May;16(3):420–7.
2. Clawson JJ, Dernocoeur KB, Murray C. Principles of emergency medical dispatch. 5th ed. Salt Lake City, UT: Priority Press; 2014.
3. Deakin CD, Sherwood DM, Smith A, Cassidy M. Does telephone triage of emergency (999) calls using advanced medical priority dispatch (AMPDS) with Department of Health (DH) call prioritization effectively identify patients with an acute coronary syndrome? An audit of 4, 657 emergency calls to Hampshire Ambulance Service NHS Trust. Emerg Med J. 23(3):232–5.
4. Hardeland C, Olasweegen T, Lawrence R, et al. Comparison of medical priority dispatch (MPD) and criteria based dispatch (CBD) relating to cardiac arrest calls. Resuscitation. 2014;85(5):612–6.
5. Bohm K, Kurland L. The accuracy of medical dispatch - a systematic review. Scand J Trauma Resusc Emerg Med. 2018 Nov 9;26(1):94.
6. Cameron PA, Gabbe BJ, Smith K, Mitra B. Triaging the right patient to the right place in the shortest time. BJA Br J Anaesth. 2014 Aug 1;113(2):226–33.
7. Staudenmayer K, Wang NE, Weiser TG, Maggio P, Mackersie RC, Spain D, et al. The triage of injured patients: mechanism of injury, regardless of injury severity, determines hospital destination. Am Surg. 2016 Apr;82(4):356–61.
8. Ryan JL, Pracht E, Langland-Orban B, Crandall M. Association of mechanism of injury with overtriage of injured youth patients as trauma alerts. Trauma Surg Acute Care Open [Internet]. 2019 Dec 29 [cited 2020 Sep 5];4(1). Available from: https://www.ncbi.nlm.nih.gov/pmc/articles/PMC6937421/
9. Kieser J, Taylor M, Carr DD. Forensic biomechanics. Chichester, West Sussex: Wiley-Blackwell; 2012. p. 164. (Essentials of forensic science)
10. Xu F, Wan X, Chen Y. Design optimization of thin-walled circular tubular structures with graded thickness under later impact loading. Int J Automot Technol. 2017 June 1;18(3):439–49.
11. Xu J, Li YB, Chen X, Ge DY, Liu BH, Zhu MY, et al. Automotive windshield — pedestrian head impact: energy absorption capability of interlayer material. Int J Automot Technol. 2011 Aug 19;12(5):687.
12. Choi HY, Shin J, Oh CJ, Bae JH. Occupant injury risk analysis at NASS/CDS database. Int J Automot Technol. 2017 Oct 1;18(5):851–60.
13. Lee YH, Joo YJ, Park JS, Kim YS, Yim HJ. Robust design optimization of frontal structures for minimizing injury risks of flex pedestrian legform impactor. Int J Automot Technol. 2014 Aug 1;15(5):757–64.
14. Frampton R, Page M, Thomas P. Factors related to fatal injury in frontal crashes involving European cars. Annu Proc Assoc Adv Automot Med. 2006;50:35–56.
15. Han I. Impulse-momentum based analysis of vehicle collision accidents using Monte Carlo simulation methods. Int J Automot Technol. 2015 Apr 1;16(2):253–70.
16. Department for Transport. Reported road casualties in Great Britain: provisional estimates year ending June 2019 [Internet]. Stationery Office; 2019 [cited 2020 Sep 6]. Available from: https://www.gov.uk/government/statistics/reported-road-casualties-great-britain-provisional-results-2019

17. Bibel GD. Beyond the black box: the forensics of airplane crashes. Baltimore: Johns Hopkins University Press; 2008. p. 393.
18. Brulle RV. Engineering the space age: a rocket scientist remembers. Maxwell Air Force Base, Ala: Air University Press; 2008. 268 p.
19. Champion HR, Lombardo LV, Shair EK. The importance of vehicle rollover as a field triage criterion. J Trauma. 2009;67(2):8.
20. Jain SSL. 'Dangerous instrumentality': the bystander as subject in automobility. Cult Anthropol. 2004 Feb;19(1):61–94.
21. Meredith L, Baldock M, Fitzharris M, Duflou J, Dal Nevo R, Griffiths M, et al. Motorcycle fuel tanks and pelvic fractures: a motorcycle fuel tank syndrome. Traffic Inj Prev. 2016 Aug 17;17(6):644–9.
22. Hurson C, Collins D, McElwain JP. Crotch rocket pelvic fractures. Injury Extra. 2004 Feb 1;35(2):17–9.
23. Lloyd JD. Biomechanics of solo motorcycle accidents. Forensic Biomech. 2016 Jan;7(1):6.
24. Alizo G, Sciarretta JD, Gibson S, Muertos K, Romano A, Davis J, et al. Fall from heights: does height really matter? Eur J Trauma Emerg Surg. 2018 Jun;44(3):411–6.
25. Havlik HS. Equestrian sport-related injuries: a review of current literature. Curr Sports Med Rep. 2010 Oct;9(5):299–302.
26. McCrory P, Turner M. Equestrian injuries. Epidemiol Pediatr Sports Injury. 2005;48:8–17.

22 Mass Casualty Incidents

Alexander G. Porthouse, Hannah M. Clancy, and Andrew Thurgood

- Definition of a major incident and mass casualty event
- Types of major incidents including CBRN incidents
- How to prepare for major incidents at an organisational and personal level
- CSCATTT as a useful approach to major incidents
- Use of the communication tool METHANE
- Triage sieve and sort for casualties
- Importance of debriefing, human factors and CRM

Introduction

Unfortunately, those working in healthcare, particularly the field of trauma, may be involved in a major incident or mass casualty event. This may be as a first responder, or in hospital as a clinician working in a receiving emergency department for victims of the incident. It is therefore essential for healthcare professionals to have an understanding of how to approach and work with teams involved in these incidents.

In the UK, the Major Incident Medical Management and Support (MIMMS) system is the most commonly used approach to exploring and dealing with major incidents. This chapter broadly follows the MIMMS approach [1].

A mass casualty event involves a large number of presenting casualties but usually within the capacity of responding services. A major incident is one which requires abnormal responses and measures.

An understanding of major incidents is vital for all levels of those involved; from the police and ambulance services responding on the ground through to hospital management ensuring bed space for post-surgery patients. Even members of the public including victims and bystanders may need a basic understanding of how to act in these events, particularly in the initial phases of an incident. This will further extend to those working in local authorities who will need to ensure travel and logistical infrastructure remains intact.

Types and Scope of Major Incidents

There are several ways to describe and think about major incidents. These can be related to their cause and origin and also consequential

A. G. Porthouse (✉)
Royal Army Medical Corps, Catterick Garrison, UK
e-mail: alexander.porthouse@nhs.net

H. M. Clancy
Royal Army Medical Corps, Leuchars, UK

A. Thurgood
Mercia Accident Rescue Service, Hereford, UK
e-mail: a.thurgood@citizenaid.org

P. Lax (ed.), *Textbook of Acute Trauma Care*, https://doi.org/10.1007/978-3-030-83628-3_22

effects of the incident. An initial categorisation of these incidents is to look at the cause to determine if it is **natural** or **human-made.** An example of a natural major incident could be an earthquake, such as in Nepal in 2015 [2], or wildfire, such as the 2019–2020 Australian bushfires [3, 4]. Human-made incidents can be just as varied and include train crashes, large traffic collisions and even accidents involving nuclear power plants such as the 2011 Fukushima nuclear power plant accident [5].

Incidents can be further categorised as **compensated** vs **uncompensated**. A compensated incident is one in which the requirements are matched by the resources available, whereas in an uncompensated incident demand outstrips locally available resources and requires external assistance. Either of these types of incident may also involve responding services and infrastructure (e.g. hospitals or major roads become unusable), thereby making it a **compound** incident.

The size and scope of an incident should also be considered as part of the above classification. However, these do not exist in a linear relationship, i.e. a "large-scale" incident does not always provide a guide to the severity and resources required. A large train derailing at low speed may appear as a large incident, but the carriages could well be empty; conversely, a small amount of explosive detonated in a bus full of passengers could be catastrophic. The usual amount of resource available may also determine the tipping point for declaring a major incident. A four-car RTC may just be an everyday tasking for a major metropolitan ambulance service with hundreds of vehicles; however, the same incident on an isolated small island may completely overwhelm the local health system.

The time frames involved should also be considered in planning for and dealing with major incidents as they may involve additional services beyond those normally expected to be involved. Local authorities may be required to coordinate relief efforts such as organising food deliveries and shelter to those affected whilst businesses such as supermarkets may need to implement special measures and deliveries as part of relief efforts. Local and regional infrastructure may be required to support aid efforts ensuring transport methods are available (road, rail) and power supplies are reliably maintained or rapidly restored.

There is much crossover between the terms mass casualty incident, major incident and disaster. A disaster tends to suggest a larger scale of incident. The International Foundation of the Red Cross defines a disaster as one in which "a sudden and calamitous event disrupts a community or society and the hazard impacts on vulnerable people" [6]. Whilst a major incident can be managed by emergency services, albeit with special measures put in place, a disaster usually involves the victims as actors and participants in relief efforts. This suggests that any capacity for response by typical infrastructure and services has been completely overwhelmed. Historically, major incidents can generally be managed by a nation's intrinsic resources and services, whilst disasters typically require an international effort.

The most recent example of a disaster is the August 2020 Beirut explosion [7]. In a system which was already under considerable economic strain and was due to go into lockdown for increasing COVID transmission, a large explosion of 2700 tons of ammonium nitrate occurred in the city docks. This was thought to be secondary to a fireworks storage facility catching alight and spreading to the neighbouring warehouse where the chemical was stored. The city was largely shielded from the blast by a grain silo (the main food reserve in the country which was also destroyed). Still, the pressure wave blew out windows and caused glass injuries kilometres away from the epicentre. Three hospitals have been rendered non-functional and two others damaged, with the majority of the imported medical supplies in the dock to combat the spread of COVID destroyed. Using the above classification, this is a human-made, uncompensated, compound incident. As one doctor put it, "My first instinct was to just put on my white coat and just go to try to see what happened… initially, I thought the hospital was safe. People are going to need us there. The biggest shock was to actually see that there was no hospital left" [8].

CBRNE3T

Major incidents may sometimes involve chemicals, nuclear threats, biological agents (natural or human-made) or explosions (Fig. 22.1 shows symbols related to these). These can be thought of within the umbrella "CBRNE3T" structure used to describe military incidents and hazards and will require specialist personnel and equipment to deal with—Table 22.1 provides a breakdown of these.

If an incident is expected to involve any of the above, then specialist advice and services may be required, such as involvement of ambulance Hazardous Area Response Teams (HART). Those responding will need to ensure they wear correct Personal Protective Equipment (PPE) and liaise with those in control of the scene such as Armed Response Police in an explosives incident.

Preparation

Those working in healthcare should be well aware of the importance of advanced preparation and planning. This is all the more pertinent in major incidents which can quickly overwhelm organisations and individuals.

Organisational Preparedness

Organisations that could be involved in a major incident should have pre-made plans which consider all hazards that may occur. These plans could be for an organisation that may be susceptible or at risk of a major incident, such as a predetermined attendance for a chemical factory fire by emergency services. Those that would be involved in the incident should have regular training and familiarisation with major incident plans.

Building on planning and training, tabletop exercises and simulations can further enhance preparedness at all levels. They may be conducted by individual organisations, or at a higher level involving multiple responding services with high fidelity simulation of a theoretical incident—for example, exercises mimicking a terror attack on a large shopping centre have been conducted in the UK [11]. This also allows for major incident plans to be tested to "breaking point" which will expose potential flaws and hitches in responses.

Other actions to ensure organisational preparedness could involve regular kit and equipment checks, confirming those within the organisation know where they can access basic first aid equipment and major incident packs. Adequate supplies of PPE should be maintained.

The NHS has drawn up Major Incident and Mass Casualty Clinical Guidelines (Fig. 22.2) to assist in preparedness which can be accessed via the Emergency Preparedness, Resilience and Response area of the NHS England website [13]. This stresses the importance of preparedness in receiving hospitals alongside providing quick references for various injuries and types of attack (e.g. CBRN).

Individual Preparedness

Whilst an organisation can go some way to preparing individuals, those involved in response to major incidents also bear a personal responsibil-

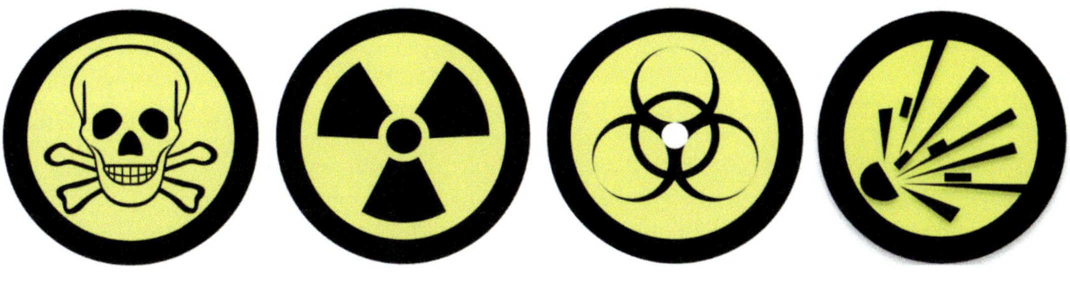

Fig. 22.1 Common symbols that may be related to CBRN incidents

Table 22.1 Description of CBRNE3T incidents

Type	What is it?	Example
Chemical	An incident involving intentional or accidental release of chemicals. Could result in contamination of the scene and workers and poisoning of casualties.	Novichok nerve agent poisoning in March 2018 in Salisbury [9]. This required extensive contact tracing, isolation and clean up. Fortunately, doctors were used to seeing the symptoms of organophosphate poisoning from the local agriculture industry, so quickly realised the Skripals were suffering from a similar toxidrome. This required a large-scale combined approach including specialists from the Defence Science and Technology Laboratory in Porton Down. This incident also highlights the importance of scene decontamination as there was a second round of exposure resulting in a fatality.
Biological	Similar to a chemical incident, this can involve the intentional or accidental release of biological agents, or these could be due to naturally spreading infection.	The 2001 Anthrax letter attacks in the United States could be considered a biological major incident. The incident resulted in a large-scale tracing and decontamination effort.
Radiological	An emission of radioactive material or radiation. This can cause widespread contamination.	2011 Fukushima nuclear power plant accident which led to a massive release of radiation and radioactive materials into the environment.
Nuclear	An incident involving a nuclear detonation or out of control reaction. There will be direct consequences of the release of large amounts of energy from the initial incident accompanied by the possibility of exposure to radiation and the spreading of radioactive materials.	1986 explosion at the Chernobyl nuclear power plant. The energy from the blast caused considerable damage to the reactor building allowing the release of large amounts of radioactive material. The two nuclear weapons used in Hiroshima and Nagasaki during the second world war demonstrate the devastation that the energy released from a nuclear explosion can cause.
Explosive/ Ballistic	All the effects of explosive activity on the human body including gunshot wounds, indirect fire, improvised explosive devices and bombs. With IEDs or bombs: Risk of primary trauma of the blast wave on gas containing structures, secondary trauma from the impact of airborne debris and tertiary injury following being thrown by the blast and sudden deceleration.	London Bombings 7 July 2005 [10]. The deliberate detonation of homemade explosives on public transport. These explosions occurred over multiple sites, some of which were difficult to access, such as an underground passenger train.
Environmental	Environmental conditions likely to cause harm, e.g. heat, cold and altitude.	The wildfires that burnt through Australia during 2019 and 2020 were a large scale environmental incident resulting in over 30 deaths and large amounts of damage [3, 4].
Endemic	Infectious diseases that pose a hazard to health but that are not deliberately released.	2014 Ebola outbreak in West Africa is an example of a large scale, long-running incident involving an infectious disease. More recently, COVID19 has been present on a global level.
Trauma	Traumatic injuries that are distinct to those caused by the above factors.	There are various examples of major incidents that can lead to traumatic injuries. Examples of events which these injuries could arise from include road traffic collisions or building collapses.

ity to make sure they are up to date with training and new techniques. In the UK, there are several courses catered to preparing individuals to deal with major incidents, MIMMS being one of the best known with derivatives for the military and hospital-specific major incidents.

Vehicles used for responding should be regularly serviced and well maintained, and personnel

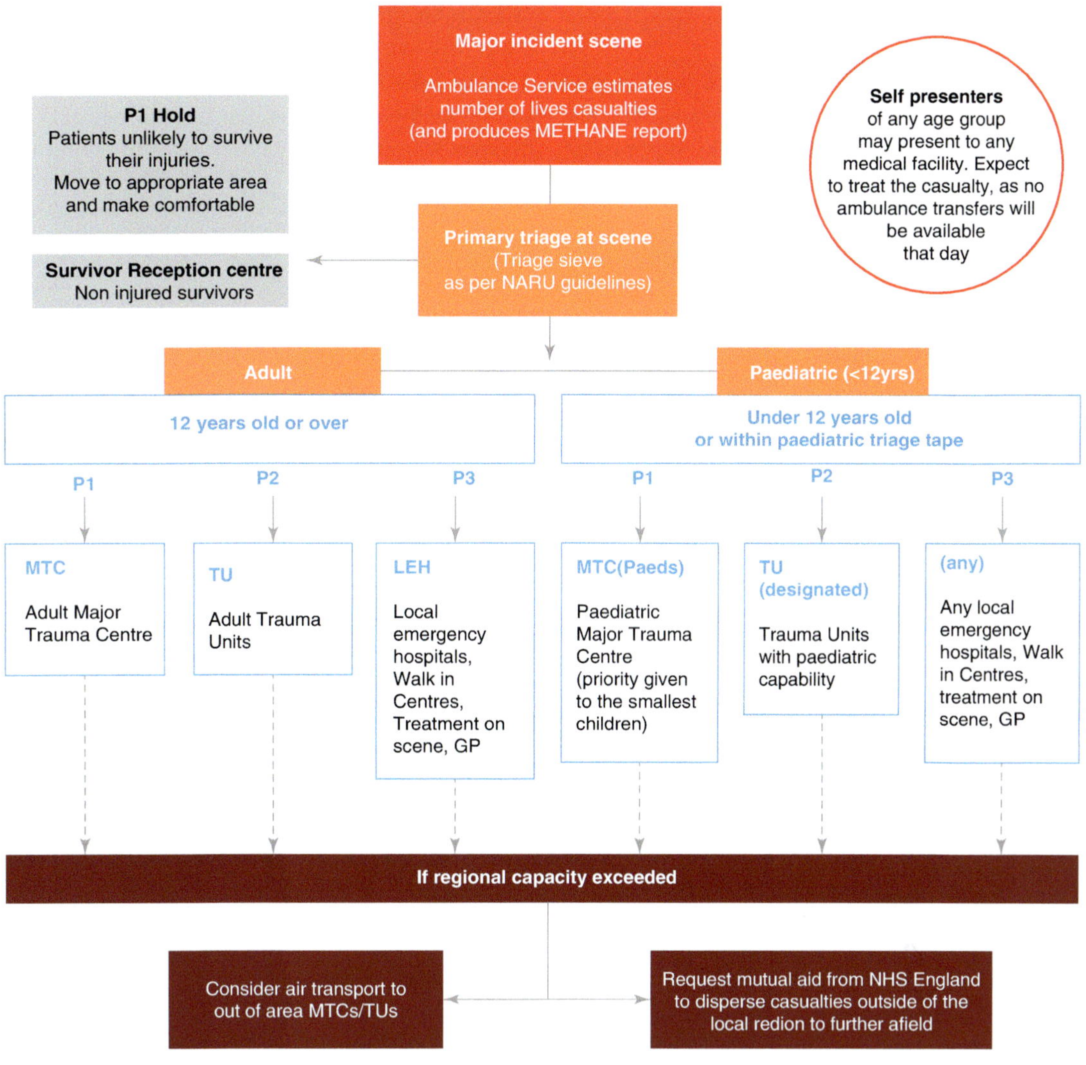

Fig. 22.2 From NHS clinical guidelines for major incidents [12]

that may be required to drive at speed to an incident should receive appropriate training.

Individuals responding in the pre-hospital phase of a major incident should be familiar with the PPE that they are expected to use. At a minimum, a correctly fitted helmet, eye protection, hearing protection, protective suit with high visibility markings and appropriate gloves (offering cut and heat protection) and footwear (with steel toe caps) should be worn by individuals. This can then be further added to or changed depending on the hazards present. Individuals should also ensure they have adequate warm kit and waterproof layers.

In hospital staff have similar responsibilities—at a minimum, each staff member should know where to report to if they are called in to work as part of a major incident response. Of the published data in the UK, approximately 50% of staff have not read their hospital's major incident plan or do not know what their role is in a major incident [14]—this is simply not acceptable. A potential solution would be credit-card-size action cards for each staff group, with the first steps of where to go, who to report to and relevant contact details given out at hospital induction and carried until needed.

Public Involvement

Events over recent years in Europe have seen a surge of deliberate attacks that have cumulatively resulted in hundreds of deaths and thousands of injuries. Unfortunately, the tempo of incidents is not slowing. Against this background of violence, the statutory emergency services have worked hard to firm up their resilience by adjusting tactics, revising their equipment and enhancing their communication capabilities. Much work has been done on system preparedness and multi-agency working by exercising scenarios that have chilling similarities to what has played out in real life.

During a firearm or knife attack, police firearms units will mobilise swiftly. Their priority will be to contain, and if necessary, neutralise the threat. Other services, and specifically medical and fire rescue services, will also be mobilised but will be held off until it is safe to move forward. This means that there will be no professional help immediately available: it is a deliberately staged response underpinned by the need to remain safe. Similar staging arrangements may be made in the event of non-terror related incidents if there are safety concerns. The fire and rescue services have overall control of safety issues on site and may refuse to let other agencies enter if safety concerns remain (e.g. fire or chemical contamination).

During terror incidents, the public may be more exposed and vulnerable in the immediate aftermath than in a conventional situation, simply put, they will be on their own until it is safe for others to arrive.

During this initial managerial and therapeutic vacuum, the injured will be reliant upon themselves or each other to survive; within the military this is called "self-aid" or "buddy-aid". Casualties with major haemorrhage will die if simple and effective treatment is not applied. The use of an improvised tourniquet is advocated if bleeding cannot be stopped by direct pressure and elevation of the limb. In the context of an amputated limb, a tourniquet is mandated.

The citizenAID team recognised the similarity between the members of the public in a mass casualty incident and the situation a soldier must cope with when dealing with combat casualties. A wounded soldier will not receive an immediate formal medical response, but instead will rely on his own actions or those of friends around him to render life-saving first aid. Only when the "fire-fight" has been won is it safe to evacuate the casualty. A member of the public caught up in a terrorist event is effectively isolated on a "battlefield", albeit on the streets of a city in a developed country.

The wounding pattern is exactly that seen from bullets, bombs, knives and vehicle accidents that are seen in conflict. The hard-won clinical lessons from the recent military conflicts have demonstrated extraordinary and unprecedented survival of severely injured service members. This, in part, is due to the immediate and timely interventions at the point of injury. These battlefield medical skills have been contextualised for the civilian environment within citizenAID.

The citizenAID program focuses on key principles that are proven to be effective and save lives [15, 16]. These are scene control, inward and outward communication and the treatment of the injured. Each element is then applied to the shooter, knife attacker or bombing incident. Information is also given on what to do when a suspect bomb is found. citizenAID takes any non-medically trained member of the public and enables them to save lives in the unlikely but not impossible chance of a terrorist attack. An important aspect of citizenAID is the development of a school program that aims to drive the key messages of citizenAID into both primary and middle schools. Cartoons have been designed and through allegory, inform children of what to do in these rare but not impossible situations.

In many countries around the world exposed to the risks of natural disaster, it is common to see government-led educational initiatives in schools preparing society for a disaster such as a tsunami or an earthquake. As much as we do not know when the next earthquake will occur, we will not be able to predict when the next terrorist assault will be. Still, by embracing citizenAID within society we can be better prepared, ultimately less scared, and equipped with basic skills to save lives in these rare events.

The UK National Counter Terrorism Security Office has warned hospitals and general practices that they may be targets for terrorist attacks, in updated guidance on protecting crowded places from a terrorist attack issued in June 2017 [17]. The document, which advises on ramping up the security of all crowded settings, has a specific section dedicated to healthcare. It tells health professionals, "It is possible that your hospital or surgery could be the target of a terrorist incident". This reinforces the importance of major incident plans, and organisational and personal preparedness, as previously discussed.

CSCATTT

The CSCATTT paradigm is a system initially developed as part of MIMMS which has since been adapted and used by multiple organisations such as the National Ambulance Resilience Unit (NARU) and the Joint Emergency Services Interoperability Programme (JESIP). Following this system allows prioritisation and greater unification between attending services and provides a common language and approach. It should be followed sequentially and applies across all echelons of response—from those first on scene all the way through to incident commanders at a strategic level.

Key Points

C—Command & Control
S—Safety
C—Communications
A—Assessment
T—Triage
T—Treatment
T—Transport

It uses a stepwise and straightforward approach to establish control and safety of an incident first before addressing other priorities such as triage, and finally, medical treatment. Effective communication and following this system allows good situational awareness to be maintained both at the incident and at distant sites where coordination of other resources may be occurring. This will also hopefully prevent the responder from merely rushing to the nearest casualty without appreciating the overall situation.

Command, Control and Coordination of an Incident

The various agencies involved in an incident will have individual command chains within their organisations. Alongside this, an incident will require an overall commander. Command is usually thought of as a vertical process (associated with hierarchy and formal rank structure) whereas control occurs as a horizontal process. NARU describes the action of command as exercising authority which is associated with a rank or role, and control as the application of the authority and management of resources [18].

Initially, command of an incident will fall to the most suitable person present until a full response is mounted. This may simply be the first ambulance on scene acting as a control point. The command and control process will begin with the declaration of a major incident; then as the incident and response evolves, each responding organisation will appoint their own commanders at up to three levels; Bronze, Silver and Gold. These have also been referred to as Tactical, Operational and Strategic tiers. While there can be multiple Tactical/Bronze commanders within one area, they will report to a single Operational/Silver commander who has oversight of that area.

In a disaster or very significant major incident, there may be multiple areas (each with a Silver commander) who will report to the Strategic/Gold commander who will be coordinating national resources. There is only ever one Gold commander. The use of Gold command is infrequent, but a theoretical example of how Bronze/Silver command can be used is a train crash with multiple casualties. Each carriage may have its own Bronze commander who is overseeing numerous paramedics and medical teams, and each Bronze commander would report to the

Silver commander who has overall control of the incident. There would be no need for Gold command in this scenario. However, if 15 trains crashed in different areas as part of a coordinated terror attack, then Gold command may be used to coordinate the response.

A major incident usually requires a response from multiple emergency services. Each service will have an individual command structure as discussed; however, one service will take primacy of responsibility for a scene and hence "control" the incident. The command tiers of Bronze, Silver and Gold can also relate to different cordons or "zones" (also may be called Cold, Warm and Hot) which assist with identification of threat level, scene access and egress, and control.

Training and tabletop planning can lead to predetermined attendance procedures within each service, with the immediate dispatch of specific numbers and types of vehicles, equipment and personnel in response to a major incident being called.

The Ambulance Commander and the Medical Commander lead the medical element of a response to a major incident. They should be easily identifiable and be closely linked to the Fire and Police service commanders. Ideally, all three should be co-located as the incident evolves and talk regularly to share mental models and priorities. The appointment of these personnel may be predetermined but is initially likely to be fluid, with the first crew on scene assuming this role and acting as a rendezvous point until a more senior officer arrives. Those operating in a command role should not be engaged in patient treatment as it limits situational awareness, constrains the ability to communicate with other services and act as a conduit to higher echelons.

Primacy at Scene

Fire and rescue will usually hold primacy at the scene of a major incident if there are safety concerns; otherwise the police will be in charge, especially if firearms or weapons are involved or there is suspicion that a crime may have occurred. The police are usually the last to leave the scene of a major incident as evidence preservation, collection and investigation falls to them. They are also important for closing off roads and controlling access points. When clinicians are working with the police at a crime scene, they should understand the importance of evidence preservation. However, clinical need may take priority at times (see forensic considerations chapter for further details). The medical response rarely has primacy, though most other organisations will be incredibly accommodating to ensure patients are treated as best possible. Medical teams do not have the ability to overrule either fire or police, but the corollary is not true!

Safety

Safety precautions should start long before arrival at the scene of a major incident—prevention beats any intervention. Prevention can be done at an individual level (for example, individuals ensuring their car is roadworthy before setting off on a journey) or at a population or organisational level such as implementing changes following root cause analysis of major incidents.

Those responding should consider donning PPE before setting off to the scene as hazards may be immediately present or offer little time to do this on scene. This is especially important in incidents involving hostile actors such as a firearms incident.

Key Points

There is a risk that those arriving at an incident (whether as assistance, members of the public, or the media) become part of the incident itself. An attempt to minimise this risk is through the enforcement of cordons. Safety of those responding to an incident is commonly referred to as "Safety 1-2-3":

1. Self
2. Scene
3. Survivors

If approaching an incident with an unknown hazard, then responders should follow STEP 1-2-3:

1. Step 1: one casualty—approach as normal
2. Step 2: two casualties—approach with caution
3. Step 3: three or more casualties—do not approach, evacuate the scene and seek further help

A responder who is unsafe, be it through incorrect PPE, neglecting an ongoing unmitigated threat, or through inadequate training, will be putting themselves and the casualties at increased risk rather than assisting. Teams such as HART (Hazardous area response team) or SORT (Special Operations Response Team) may be required to assist with treatment if there is an immediate or suspected CBRN threat.

Communication

Communication failures are frequently cited as a significant contributor to failings or poor outcomes in response to a major incident [19–24]. Major incident plans should be in place in every emergency service and hospital that may receive patients in response to these events, however, recognition and declaration of a major incident and initiation of these plans is a common limiting factor.

Various communication methods can be utilised at an incident but should be standardised, tested and well-practised by responding organisations before a major incident is declared. Communication can take place locally, such as between a group of Fire and Rescue personnel stabilising a car, or across a distance when an ambulance may need to update a control centre of its location.

Radios are commonplace amongst responding organisations in the UK. They typically have good reliability in open areas, but operators should be trained in their use and familiar with voice procedure and the phonetic alphabet (see Table 22.2). Mobile telephones may initially be useful in reporting an incident and establishing some coordination. Still, users should be aware that cellular networks could become swamped by calls or suffer disruption of supporting infrastructure, which will impair reliability [25].

Table 22.2 The NATO Phonetic Alphabet

Alpha, Bravo, Charlie, Delta, Echo, Foxtrot, Golf, Hotel, India, Juliet, Kilo, Lima, Mike, November, Oscar, Papa, Quebec, Romeo, Sierra, Tango, Uniform, Victor, Whiskey, X-ray, Yankee, Zulu
—The NATO Phonetic Alphabet

Methods of communication that can be used locally can include hand signals, loudspeakers and runners with written notes to ensure messages are passed accurately. Ideally, all critical communication should be conducted as part of a "closed-loop" where those communicating acknowledge receipt of the information and actions required.

Different organisations will use varying communication formats. The mnemonic METHANE (adopted by the Joint Emergency Services Interoperability Principles—JESIP) provides a structured way to make an initial report or update on an ongoing incident.

Key Points

M—Major incident declared/standby & My Callsign
E—Exact location: grid reference, landmarks, junction numbers
T—Type of incident
H—Hazards
A—Access and egress routes available or blocked
N—Number of casualties
E—Emergency services and equipment present and required

Using METHANE also allows the responder to think about the management of the scene in an organised way, prompting them to identify entry and exit routes to the scene and begin planning for which resources may be required in a logical order.

Another example of a useful communication tool for pre-alerting patients into a hospital during major incidents is the ATMIST system (Table 22.3). This mnemonic allows individual casualties to be quickly handed over with all the relevant information that healthcare providers downstream will require and can even be physically attached to the patient using slate cards.

Communication between medical, ambulance, police and fire commanders is vital in the coordination of an incident response. These command nodes should be clearly identified to each other and to all other members of the response through clearly labelled tabards, PPE and signposts and vehicle markings where appropriate.

Table 22.3 ATMIST Handover system

A	Age
T	Time of wounding
M	Mechanism of injury
I	Injuries sustained
S	Signs and symptoms (including patients obs in an ABCD format)
T	Treatments given

Assessment

An assessment of the scene needs to be made by those responding early in the incident to determine what other emergency resources are required. Initially, this may be completed by an inexperienced provider and the assessment can be built up throughout the implementation of CSCATTT. As discussed, METHANE is a powerful tool in that it encourages the user to start to assess and think about key areas of incident control.

Assessment of the scene is a continuum and is required at all levels as an incident develops. As the scene evolves and levels of command are established, accurate assessment allows optimisation of resource allocation. This will exist across a spectrum, from deciding what equipment and capabilities are required at the scene of the incident through to which receiving hospitals are the most appropriate for individual patients and if these hospitals need to start clearing space for casualties.

Incident assessment requires liaison across all responding services per JESIP (see Fig. 22.3) and will continue after the incident is wound up as part of the debrief process.

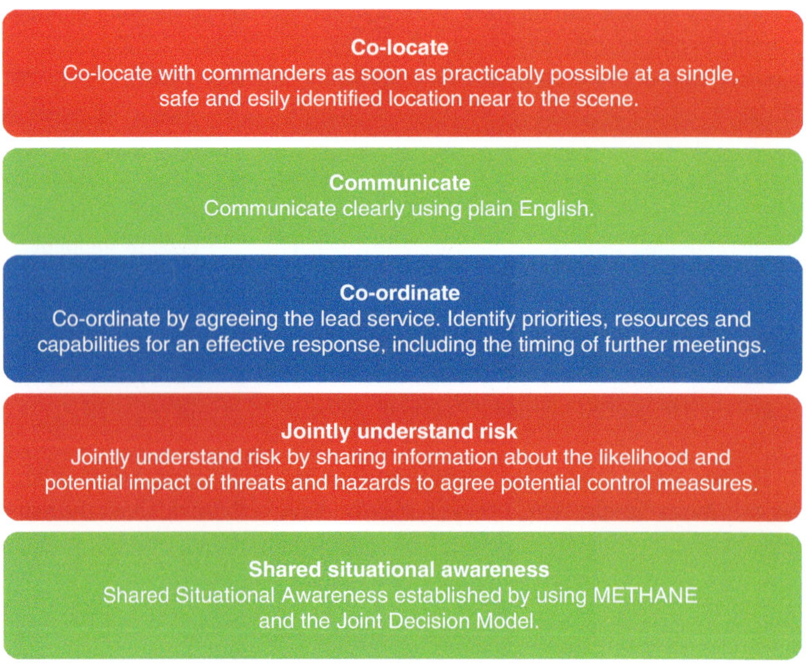

Fig. 22.3 Principles for joint working (From JESIP [26])

Triage

Triage is the process of sorting casualties into priority categories, usually based on physiological parameters, to guide urgency of treatment and evacuation and optimise treatment delivery in a system with finite resources. A casualty's triage category should be reassessed as an incident progresses.

Sorting patients by severity has roots deep within the warfare environment. The idea of "sorting" and "sieving" patients by injury and physiological reaction to that injury was brought to the fore by one of Napoleon's doctors in the early 1800s [27]. Initially focussed around returning those that could still fight to the frontline and separating those requiring surgery, triage has evolved into a complex discipline with a vast academic background and several widely adopted solutions.

The typical triage system used by UK responders is a sieve—sort system. It allows a rapid, reproducible and safe categorisation of patients at the point of wounding, and a more nuanced but reproducible sorting of patients further down the line. The ultimate aim is to deliver the correct patient to the correct care at the correct time. An example of good triage in action may be a police medic identifying an abdominal gunshot wound with uncontrolled bleeding and ensuring they are taken to a hospital with surgical capability quickly (well within the hour) and allowing another casualty with a dislocated shoulder to be further assessed on scene by experienced medical practitioners and directed to the most appropriate healthcare facility with appropriate use of resources.

In the UK, the vast majority of pre-hospital and emergency care providers use a similar triage system for the initial sieve. This focusses on easily measurable physiological parameters including level of consciousness, presence or absence of breathing abnormalities and whether cardiovascular compromise (manifested in heart rate abnormalities) is present. This can all be quickly and accurately measured in a chaotic situation. A note should be taken of numbers and categories of casualties for communication up-stream. Casualties and their classification can also be individually identified by physical makers such as wrist "snap-bands" or cruciform triage cards. Liaison with other locally responding units such as ambulance services and fire and rescue should be sought to ensure a commonly used and understood system of marking and communication.

An example of a commonly used triage sieve system is shown in Fig. 22.4. The practitioner performing triage would begin in the top left of the algorithm and follow the prompts to assign a category. It should be noted that if a casualty has had a tourniquet applied due to catastrophic haemorrhage, then they are triaged as a P1. Following the algorithm assesses the other physiological parameters as described above with prompts for limited interventions.

Key Points

The triage categories, as described by MIMMS [1] and similar systems, are:

- P1 (sometimes referred to as T1)—Those requiring immediate care. These are the sickest patients who cannot wait for life-saving interventions
- P2 (sometimes referred to as T2)—Those requiring urgent care. These are unwell casualties who require interventions within the next 2–4 h
- P3 (sometimes referred to as T3)—Those patients whose treatment can be delayed beyond 4 h (but they will still require assessment and further triage)

The triage tool demonstrated in Fig. 22.4 requires some training and healthcare-specific skills to use. Figure 22.5 illustrates a triage sieve that can be used by the public, or those without medical training, in a major incident as developed by citizenAID. It relies on easily measurable parameters, for example whether a casualty is talking, to assign a triage category and also contains prompts for simple interventions.

Triage is a prescriptive process which relies on adherence to a strict protocol and categorisation. The most appropriate person to perform the initial triage sieve may be the most junior clini-

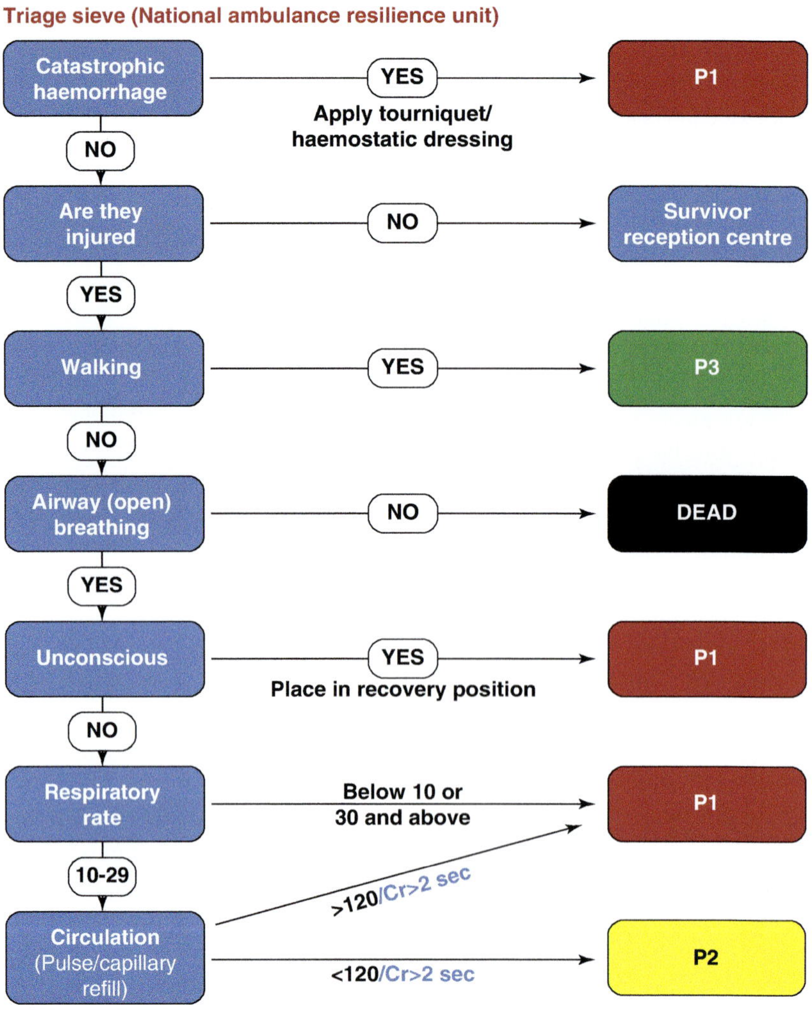

Fig. 22.4 Triage sieve as used by NARU [28]

cian (or non-clinical team member) who will follow the selected algorithm and allow more senior clinicians to gain an overview and start planning. There is evidence that senior clinicians performing triage results in less over-triage of patients (i.e. a reduction in patients inappropriately being sent to major trauma centres) [29]. There is also evidence that higher levels of over-triage paradoxically increases population mortality In major incidents [30], so there is a definite balance that must be struck between gaining situational awareness for senior clinicians and ensuring correct disposition arrangements. While every patient *may* benefit at an individual level from being sent to a major trauma centre, this benefit is not realised at a population level. There is a definite opportunity cost for less- or moderately-injured patients who are sent to a major trauma centre when they could be adequately managed at a trauma unit or smaller hospital.

As patients pass through the echelons of care, there may be more time and resources to assess the patient. In this case, it could be desirable to perform a triage sort on a patient allowing more accurate assignment to care in an appropriate time frame. An example of a triage sort system based on the Triage Revised Trauma Score (TRTS) is included above (Table 22.4).

Triage serves as a guide and suggestion to care that should be offered. It is best used when the clinical demands of a situation outstrip time and resources. Whilst there are robust systems for tri-

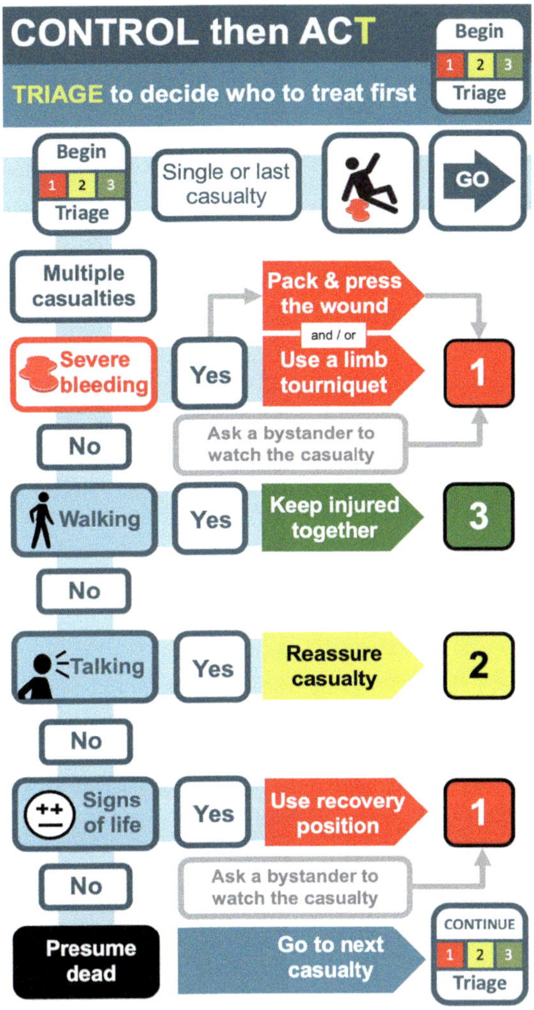

Fig. 22.5 Triage sieve as used by the public (citizenAID)

age, they should be used by trained practitioners and applied sensibly and appropriately. The practitioner should recognise that in some situations, clinical judgement and experience may trump algorithm based triage tools as alluded to above. The benefit of triage systems is that they "fail-safe" on an individual patient level, and provide a degree of medicolegal protection if they are followed. Triage systems can also be subject to under or over triage. Under triaging may result in an unwell patient being classified as less sick than they actually are as opposed to over triage which may cause patients to be classified as more unwell than they actually are. The underlying principle of triage is to "do the most, for the most", and by basing decisions on easily measurable physiological criteria, this approach follows egalitarian principles.

Triage tools currently in use in the UK are robust and can serve most of the population. If adult triage criteria are applied to the paediatric population, they fail-safe and will over triage children to higher levels of care than they would otherwise need [31, 32]. Again, while this is advantageous at an individual level, it may prove deleterious overall from a systemic perspective.

Unfortunately, children may be involved in major incidents, such as the 2017 Manchester Arena bombing, and normal physiological parameters vary with age. In this case, alternative triage tools (e.g. paediatric triage tape) are available to give responders a rough guide to the child's condition when they may not always

Table 22.4 Example of physiological triage sort based on MIMMS model [1]

Systolic Blood Pressure	Respiratory Rate	GCS	Score
>89	10-29	13-15	**4**
76-89	>29	9-12	**3**
50-75	6-9	6-8	**2**
1-49	1-5	4-5	**1**
0	0	3	**0**

Individual scores added together to give overall triage sort score and priority

Priority	Score
T1	1-10
T2	11
T3	12
Dead	0

know exact ages. These systems have recently come under some criticism as they appear to perform poorly in terms of explicitly identifying children who require life-saving interventions, and the data they are based on may be methodologically flawed [33].

It is worth remembering that all the difficulties of working in a major incident will apply during triage. Dark and noisy working conditions may obscure injuries, patients may be in an anxious or heightened state from previous activity, and PPE may lead to difficulty in measuring observations such as respiratory rate.

MPTT-24: A New Triage Tool

The Modified Physiological Triage Tool (MPTT) (Fig. 22.6) is a sieve derived from military data which has been shown to outperform previous triage methods in military and civilian scenarios [35]. It has been further refined into the MPTT-24; the name resulting from decreasing the upper limit of the Respiratory Rate bracket to 24 breaths per minute. Alongside the alteration to respiratory rate, the triage tool uses the AVPU scale (patient responding to voice) instead of the GCS scale, increasing performance and rapidity of use [34].

Treatment

Performing interventions takes time, and in the initial response to a major incident the objective is to achieve "the most for the most". To this end, limited treatment takes place and is usually governed by the skill of the responder, the equipment available, the injuries sustained and the total number of casualties. The triage sieves which were presented earlier in the chapter include some limited interventions such as application of tourniquets and placing casualties in the recovery position. The UK Defence Medical Services military triage sieve also includes airway positioning if the casualty is not breathing. Interventions are limited to allow all casualties to be fairly triaged in a short time frame.

Depending on the circumstances, it may be appropriate and desirable to ask survivors and

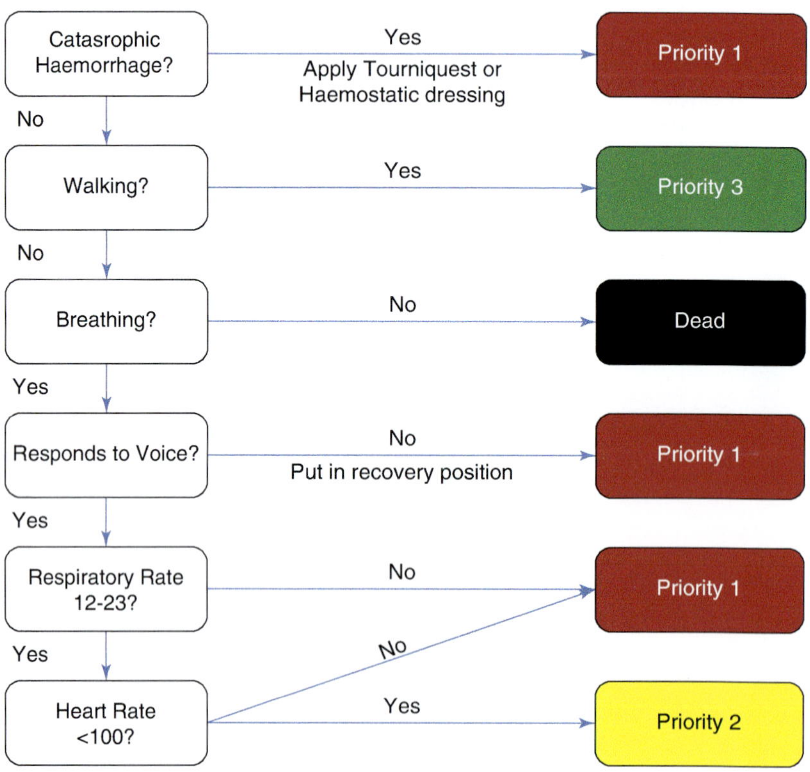

Fig. 22.6 The MPTT-24 triage tool [34]

walking wounded to self-clear from the area and attend a designated survivor reception centre or casualty clearing station for secondary triage. More unwell casualties may need assistance with extrication and evacuation. The casualty clearing station should be set up in an easy to access area where security can be guaranteed. It is here that casualties from all triage categories will go for secondary triage (sort systems as described above), resuscitation, treatments and onwards. At this stage, treatment should follow the MABCD approach.

In incidents involving firearms or terrorism, medical help may be delayed in getting to the casualties [36]. In these circumstances, bystanders and even casualties may need to apply basic first aid and interventions as described above.

Transport

While people traditionally think of injured personnel arriving at hospitals in a designated ambulance, in major incidents these resources are likely to be overwhelmed. This means there is a requirement for carefully considered use of available resources, matching a patient's clinical needs to the capabilities and equipment of a transportation platform.

The utilisation of improvised evacuation platforms, with consideration of the most appropriate destination, helps manage on scene and downstream patient flow and outcome. An awareness of local receiving centres and their capabilities can be drilled during tabletop exercises, and an overview of capacity can be maintained through Gold Command.

Airframes such as helicopters may be necessary for long-distance transfers if a patient requires specialist input (such as a burns centre). Still, they are limited in capacity of casualties they can carry and space for interventions once en route. Survivors and even walking wounded could travel in improvised platforms such as a coach with medical escort freeing up more clinically capable platforms such as ambulances to deal with priority 1 and 2 casualties.

At times, those in charge of arranging transport may have to take a nuanced approach when it comes to platform and destination selection. In an incident with large numbers of casualties, available ambulance vehicles may be at a premium resulting in a balance of risk vs benefit of travel time to certain facilities against a shorter journey time (with further secondary transfer) allowing an ambulance asset to be returned to the incident scene ready for a new tasking.

Some platforms may be unsuitable for a particular patient due to restrictions or requirements. Contaminated patients may not travel in an airframe due to the risk of contaminants (such as toxic agents) affecting the pilot and other aircrew. In the event of CBRN incident, specialist input from services such as HART should be sought, and subsequently, they may be able to utilise transport platforms best. Injuries and casualty type may also dictate which transport may be suitable; casualties that need to lie flat will not be able to travel via Patient Transport Service vehicle or bus for example. These considerations may ultimately mean that lower priority patients (P2/3) begin to leave the scene quicker than P1 patients depending on the availability of the platform.

What also needs to be considered is patients who will make their own way to the hospital without going through a sieve/sort system and can overwhelm capacity in short order. A recent example of this is the 7/7 bombings, where four bus drivers used their initiative to load patients onto double-deckers and arrived at the Royal London Hospital (the MTC) and overwhelmed it with walking wounded patients [10].

Crew Resource Management & Human Factors

Major incidents will require a large number of people to be involved at all levels and potentially in multiple locations (on scene, in a control room, at receiving hospitals). Those in charge should ensure that workforces are rotated to allow them to rest and that there is access to food, water and ablutions if the incident and subsequent recovery period are going to be prolonged. The usual amount of emergency work will continue during the incident—people elsewhere will still have heart attacks and strokes which need treating. Hence, the capacity for these patients in the system needs to be considered additionally. While elective and some urgent (e.g. cancer) services may temporarily be put on hold, this is only an ultra-short-term strategy as these patients will have worse outcomes if left for long periods and are then often uncounted victims of these incidents [37].

A well-rested workforce will go some way towards mitigating against errors due to human factors. Regular communication with all levels of personnel as to plan updates, expected timelines and perceived problems will also aid in this mitigation as well as a standardised and well-rehearsed major incident management system such as the MIMMS approach.

Debrief

Following the event, debriefing should occur at all levels. Those directly involved with hands-on work at the scene will require feedback on performance and a chance to raise their concerns. At higher levels, reports and investigations into the cause and management of the incident will help prevent similar incidents occurring and also improve outcomes. This highlights the need for accurate record-keeping throughout.

A debrief is not just a chance for learning but also to aid the mental resilience of those involved in the event. These incidents can often expose people to traumatic experiences, and staff welfare should be considered during and after the event (see Fig. 22.7).

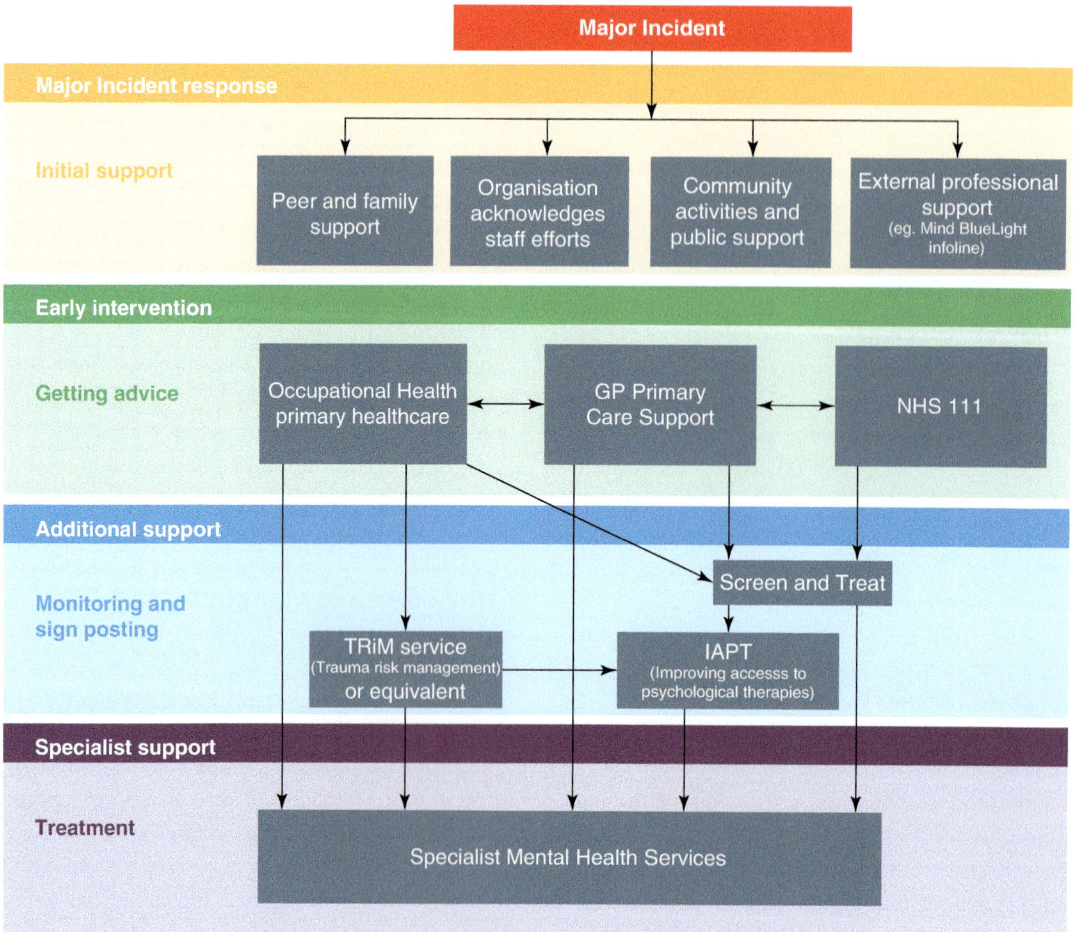

Fig. 22.7 NHS Clinical Guidelines for major incidents—Psychosocial support for staff [13]

Summary

It is essential to follow a structured and shared system, such as CSCATTT, when managing a major incident. Alongside a structured approach preparation will improve the response to an incident. This not only includes individual preparation but organisational readiness which can be further enhanced through exercises, either large scale and high fidelity or tabletop. Preparedness will also aid in generating resilience, although staff welfare and debriefing are essential as well.

Questions

1. Command and control differ in that:
   (a) Commander refers to a higher ranked individual than a controller
   (b) Command is a horizontal process and control a vertical one
   (c) Command involves exercising authority whereas control is the application of this and use of resources
   (d) Command is the application of authority and use of resources whereas control involves exercising authority
2. You are asked to lead the triage of casualties at a scene involving a train derailment. You have been assigned an area with three casualties. Casualty A is a 24-year-old male lying against a doorway with some blood slowly oozing around a leg wound, is talking but clearly distressed by what has happened to him and is confused. He has a respiratory rate of 27 with a heart rate of 112. Casualty B is not responding to you. She appears to be in her 30s and has an obvious head wound with no ongoing bleeding, a respiratory rate of 8 and a heart rate of 100. As you approach, casualty C walks over to you holding his wrist complaining of severe pain. At first glance he appears to be breathing quickly and is panicking about what has just happened. You have been told to use a standard triage sieve like that used by NARU. What is the correct triage category for the patients:
   (a) Casualty A is P1, Casualty B is P1, Casualty C is P2
   (b) Casualty A is P2, Casualty B is P1, Casualty C is P3
   (c) Casualty A is P2, Casualty B is Dead, Casualty C is P2
   (d) Casualty A is P1, Casualty B is P1, Casualty C is P1
3. In the METHANE mnemonic T stands for:
   (a) Triage categories of patients - to be reported to help facilitate the evacuation of patients to correct facilities
   (b) Total number of patients – to allow appropriate allocation of suitable vehicles for evacuation of patients
   (c) Telecommunications – to establish efficient and reliable communications between bronze level and silver / gold levels of command
   (d) Type of incident – to support the correct allocation of specialist resources and ensure use of correct PPE
4. Which of the following is correct at the scene of a major incident:
   (a) The police will have primacy at all incidents
   (b) If an incident leads to severe casualties in large numbers then the medical services will have primacy
   (c) The police are typically last to leave the scene
   (d) Evidence preservation may prevent some required medical interventions
5. When approaching a new scene with three or more unconscious casualties you should:
   (a) Approach with caution and ask for specialist equipment to be bought you in meantime
   (b) Do not approach at all until specialist equipment or services is on scene
   (c) Approach to within 2 m and call out to casualties to ascertain level of consciousness
   (d) Complete appropriate lifesaving treatments then safely withdraw from scene and await further helps

Answers

1. c
2. b
3. d
4. c
5. b

References

1. Mackway-Jones K, editor. Major incident medical management and support: the practical approach to pre-hospital incident command. 3rd ed. Chichester, West Sussex: Wiley-Blackwell; 2012. 181 p.
2. Giri S, Risnes K, Uleberg O, Rogne T, Shrestha SK, Nygaard ØP, et al. Impact of 2015 earthquakes on a local hospital in Nepal: a prospective hospital-based study. PLoS One. 2018;13(2):e0192076.
3. Filkov AI, Ngo T, Matthews S, Telfer S, Penman TD. Impact of Australia's catastrophic 2019/20 bushfire season on communities and environment. Retrospective analysis and current trends. J Saf Sci Resil. 2020;1(1):44–56.
4. Yu P, Xu R, Abramson MJ, Li S, Guo Y. Bushfires in Australia: a serious health emergency under climate change. Lancet Planet Health. 2020;4(1):e7–8.
5. Anzai K, Ban N, Ozawa T, Tokonami S. Fukushima Daiichi nuclear power plant accident: facts, environmental contamination, possible biological effects, and countermeasures. J Clin Biochem Nutr. 2012;50(1):2–8.
6. International Federation of Red Cross and Red Crescent Societies. What is a disaster? - IFRC [Internet]. 2020 [cited 2020 Sep 6]. Available from: https://www.ifrc.org/en/what-we-do/disaster-management/about-disasters/what-is-a-disaster/
7. Devi S. Lebanon faces humanitarian emergency after blast. Lancet. 2020;396(10249):456.
8. Dyer O. Beirut's battered hospitals struggle in aftermath of explosion. BMJ. 2020;m3171.
9. Hulse EJ, Haslam JD, Emmett SR, Woolley T. Organophosphorus nerve agent poisoning: managing the poisoned patient. Br J Anaesth. 2019;123(4):457–63.
10. Assembly L. Greater London authority, editors. Report of the 7 July review committee. London: Greater London Authority; 2006. 3 p.
11. Rucki A. If you hear loud noises coming from Manchester Arndale tonight don't be alarmed. Manchester Evening News [Internet]. Online. 2020 Feb 13 [cited 2020 Sep 7]; Available from: https://www.manchestereveningnews.co.uk/news/greater-manchester-news/manchester-arndale-emergency-services-training-17742721
12. NHS England. Clinical guidelines for major incidents and mass casualty events. NHS England; 2018.
13. NHS England. Clinical guidelines for major incidents [Internet]. NHS England. 2018 [cited 2020 Sep 6]. Available from: https://www.england.nhs.uk/ourwork/eprr/major-incidents/
14. Wong K, Turner PS, Boppana A, Nugent Z, Coltman T, Cosker TDA, et al. Preparation for the next major incident: are we ready? Emerg Med J. 2006;23(9):709–12.
15. Herron J, Hay-David A, Hodgetts TJ. citizenAID®: A life saving principle [Internet]. Worldwide Military Medicine. 2019 [cited 2020 Sep 6]. Available from: https://military-medicine.com/article/3774-citizenaid-a-life-saving-principle.html
16. Hodgetts TJ, Porter KM, Mahoney PF, Thurgood A, McKinnie C. Enhancing national resilience: The citizenAID initiative: Trauma [Internet]. 2017 Apr 1 [cited 2020 Sep 6]; Available from: https://journals.sagepub.com/doi/10.1177/1460408617694217
17. National Counter Terrorism Security Office. Crowded Places Guidance 2017 [Internet]. National Counter Terrorism Security Office; 2017 [cited 2020 Sep 7]. Available from: https://www.gov.uk/government/publications/crowded-places-guidance
18. National Ambulance Resillience Unit. National Ambulance Service Command and Control Guidance Version 3.0 [Internet]. National Ambulance Resillience Unit; 2019 [cited 2020 Sep 6]. Available from: https://naru.org.uk/wp-content/uploads/2019/06/NARU-COMMAND-AND-CONTROL-GUIDE-V3.0-03.2019-WEB-210619.pdf
19. Inquiry TGT. Grenfell Tower Inquiry: Phase 1 Report Overview [Internet]. London: Her Majesty's Stationary Office; 2017 [cited 2020 July 8]:[32 p.]. Available from: https://www.grenfelltowerinquiry.org.uk/phase-1-report
20. Fennell D. Investigation into the King's Cross Underground fire: presented to Parliament by the Secretary of State for Transport by command of Her Majesty, 1988. London: HMSO; 1988. p. 247.
21. Craigie RJ, Farrelly PJ, Santos R, Smith SR, Pollard JS, Jones DJ. Manchester Arena bombing: lessons learnt from a mass casualty incident. BMJ Military Health. 2020;166(2):72–5.
22. Burroughs JE. Three factors leading to the failure of communications in emergency situations [Internet] [PhD Thesis]. Walden University; 2017 [cited 2020 Sep 6]. Available from: https://scholarworks.waldenu.edu/cgi/viewcontent.cgi?article=4765&context=dissertations
23. Kerslake B. The Kerslake Report: An independent review into the preparedness for, and emergency response to, the Manchester Arena attack on 22nd May 2017 [Internet]. 2018 Mar [cited 2020 Sep 6] p. 226. Available from: http://www.kerslakearenareview.co.uk/documents/
24. Tovey O, Tolson J, Vinand A. Communication in a crisis in UK ambulance services: what is needed to improve incident communication? J Bus Contin Emerg Plan. 2018;11(4):309–16.
25. Ofcom. Connected Nations Report 2015 [Internet]. OfCOM; 2015 Dec [cited 2020 Sep 6]. Available from: https://www.ofcom.org.uk/__data/assets/pdf_file/0034/59479/resilient_comms.pdf
26. JESIP. Joint doctrine: The interoperability framework. Edition 2. [Internet]. JESIP; 2016 [cited 2020 Aug 5]. Available from: https://www.jesip.org.uk/joint-doctrine
27. Horne ST, Vassallo J. Triage in the defence medical services. J R Army Med Corps. 2015;161(2):90–3.
28. Lax P, Prior K. Major incident pre-hospital care. Surg Oxf. 2018;36(8):402–8.

29. Aylwin CJ, König TC, Brennan NW, Shirley PJ, Davies G, Walsh MS, et al. Reduction in critical mortality in urban mass casualty incidents: analysis of triage, surge, and resource use after the London bombings on July 7, 2005. Lancet. 2006;368:7.
30. Frykberg ER, Tepas JJ. Terrorist bombings: lessons learned from Belfast to Beirut. Ann Surg. 1988;208(5):569–76.
31. Wallis LA, Carley S. Validation of the paediatric triage tape. Emerg Med J. 2006;23(1):47–50.
32. Wallis LA, Carley S. Comparison of paediatric major incident primary triage tools. Emerg Med J. 2006;23(6):475–8.
33. Follows A, Vassallo J. Paediatric major incident triage tools for identifying those in need of life-saving interventions. Trauma. 2020;22(3):237–45.
34. Vassallo J, Smith JE, Wallis LA. Major incident triage and the implementation of a new triage tool, the MPTT-24. BMJ Military Health. 2018;164(2):103–6.
35. Smith JE, Vassallo J. Major incident triage: the civilian validation of the modified physiological triage tool. Emerg Med J. 2016;33(12):908.
36. Turner CDA, Lockey DJ, Rehn M. Pre-hospital management of mass casualty civilian shootings: a systematic literature review. Crit Care. 2016;20(1):362.
37. Maringe C, Spicer J, Morris M, Purushotham A, Nolte E, Sullivan R, et al. The impact of the COVID-19 pandemic on cancer deaths due to delays in diagnosis in England, UK: a national, population-based, modelling study. Lancet Oncol. 2020;21(8):1023–34.

23 Tactical Trauma Care

Hannah M. Clancy and Alexander G. Porthouse

- Describe the scope of tactical medicine and trauma care.
- Learn the key considerations for working practice and safety within the tactical environment.
- Review the MABCD management paradigm and the considerations that the tactical environment requires.
- Gain an understanding of the appropriate interventions at different phases of an incident and levels of care provision.

Introduction

Tactical medicine is a unique and specialised area of healthcare. While people frequently think of military medics applying tourniquets in foreign warzones, it is vital to stress that tactical care also occurs in domestic settings and when working with non-governmental organisations (NGOs) and civilian agencies. Tactical field care occurs when the threat is not necessarily neutralised in a semi-permissive or non-permissive environment.

Recent years have seen an increase in terror attacks both within the UK and abroad. Traditional sequential management by the emergency services to control or eliminate the threat is recognised to delay treatment to victims. To this end, emergency services are adapting their practices to allow lifesaving care to be delivered closer to the immediate incident wearing specialist personal protective equipment (PPE) [1, 2]. This falls in line with police armed response units adopting more aggressive military tactics to subdue better armed, equipped and trained threats. Indeed, police armed response teams will typically receive trauma training on their D13 course of a similar standard to that of a British Army Combat Medical Technician [3].

As states destabilise and fail, a power vacuum leaves parties vying for supremacy with internal as well as international conflict. Healthcare professionals may find themselves included in the response to this, working for global charities and NGOs and dealing with traumatic injuries. In non-conventional warfare and through domestic threats, it may be challenging to distinguish hostile persons and combatants from the civilian population. An appreciation of care within the tactical environment allows healthcare providers to better protect themselves and deliver an appropriate and safe level of care to their patients.

Many practices described within this chapter are based around those of the British Armed Forces. However, many of these principles are valid worldwide and are employed with other pub-

H. M. Clancy (✉)
Royal Army Medical Corps, Leuchars, UK
e-mail: hmclancy@doctors.org.uk

A. G. Porthouse
Royal Army Medical Corps, Catterick Garrison, UK
e-mail: alexander@porthouse.co.uk

P. Lax (ed.), *Textbook of Acute Trauma Care*, https://doi.org/10.1007/978-3-030-83628-3_23

lic, charitable and private organisations. Within the armed forces, many western countries follow very similar practices when delivering trauma care to ensure interoperability in multinational operations with organisations such as NATO. Some of these training methodologies have been passed on to other (non-military) organisations which operate in similar environments. This chapter explores some of the lessons learned from previous conflicts and how these fundamental principles can be applied in the civilian setting.

War Wounds on Home Soil

In recent years the world has seen an increasing number of marauding firearms terrorist attacks (MTFA) and roving terror attacks (RTA) [4]. These attacks, either by "lone-wolf" solo actors or planned groups of terrorists, are typically characterised by indiscriminate targeting of civilians. They occur in many forms, increasingly involving shooting or stabbing and bludgeoning. They may also involve explosives (either improvised or military-grade), starting fires, vehicular attacks, hostage-taking or sieges. Examples include Anders Breivik planning and executing a "lone-wolf" attack in Norway in 2011, killing 77 and injuring 319 [5], and the Islamic State attack in November 2015 by a group of nine terrorists in Paris, resulting in 137 deaths and 413 casualties [6]. While security services intercept many such attacks in the planning phase, some will still slip through the net. This is an international phenomenon, as shown in Table 23.1.

Those treating casualties will encounter wounding patterns similar to those sustained in combat, including gunshot wounds (GSW), stabbings and blast injuries, requiring tactical field care unless the threat has been eliminated. Injuries may affect multiple regions of the body (discussed later in the **Anatomy and Wounding** section) and may be complicated further by incidental environmental or intentional pathogenic contamination [7–9]. The civilian emergency response services are increasingly exposed to what may previously have been considered a military threat, and the public and personal safety and equipment considerations to mitigate for this are discussed later in this chapter.

Table 23.1 Recent terrorist attacks and casualty figures

Atrocity	Year	Dead	Injured
Madrid train bombings	2004	192	2000+
London bombings	2007	55	700+
Mumbai attacks	2008	174	300+
Norway (Brevik) attacks	2011	77	320
Boston Marathon bombing	2013	3	264
Kenya mall shooting	2013	67	200+
China Kunming knife attacks	2014	29	140
Tunisia resort shootings	2015	38	39
Paris Islamic state attack	2015	130	440
Brussels bombings	2016	32	300+
Nice bastille day vehicular attack	2016	86	458
Berlin Xmas market attack	2016	12	56
Westminster car/knife attack	2017	4	50
Manchester arena bombing	2017	23	500+
London bridge attack	2017	8	48
Barcelona las Ramblas attack	2017	14	120
Las Vegas concert shooting	2017	59	527
Average per attack		30	251+

Phases of Care

Working outside of a hospital in any environment poses unique challenges at the best of times, with some of these outlined in the Scene Safety chapter. When these issues are compounded by an ongoing threat to responders and their casualties, decision making and treatment options become even more pressurised and context-dependent. Working within the tactical environment exposes the practitioner to unique risks such as hostile personnel and potential CBRNE3 threats (see CBRN chapter for further details) and an ever-changing environment in addition to the "usual" constraints of pre-hospital practice.

As a NATO member, the UK armed forces separate an incident into "zones" or phases, guiding what can and cannot be achieved when delivering care within the tactical sphere and how the practitioner should view and respond to their environment. These are standardised between NATO members to enable interoperability (see Fig. 23.1) [10]. This is increasingly mirrored across civilian response services with uniformity of terminology and training to improve coordination between different emergency services and regions [11]. The point of these phases is not to restrict care, but is born from the necessity to pro-

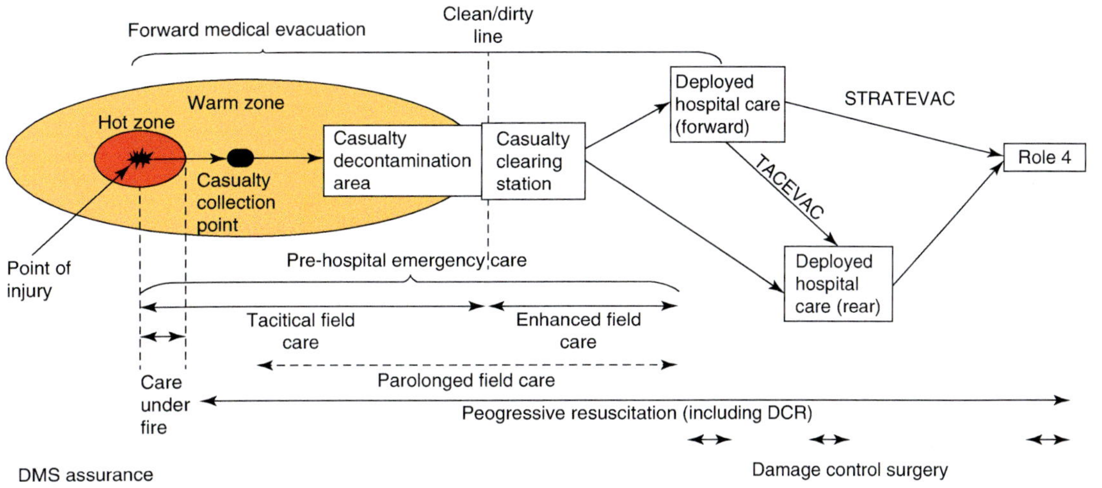

Fig. 23.1 The Operational Care Pathway (From JSP 950) [10]

tect the practitioner and casualty, enable safe and effective care and "do the most for the most". The priorities within each "zone" are based on those interventions that optimise resource, personnel and time allocation given the ongoing threat level. At times the phase of care will intuitively match the current zone of operation; in other words, "**care under fire**" will take place in the "hot zone" and "**tactical field care**" in the "warm zone". However, this will not always be the case, as the phase of care is determined by the threat level, not the patient location. This level can fluctuate with time and other factors determining the evolution of an ongoing incident. The appropriate level of care to provide should be under constant evaluation. The complexity of possible and appropriate interventions can be increased as the threat to those providing care is reduced.

Care Under Fire/Non-Permissive Environment

Care taking place in the hot "non-permissive" zone is commonly termed "care under fire". Here there is an ongoing imminent threat to both responders and the general population. The priority remains to contain or neutralise the threat rather than provide "gold standard" medical interventions. If the casualty is inaccessible to the responder and alert, they should be encouraged to perform self-aid, extricate, and/or seek cover until help can get to them. There is an increasing drive for public education in these matters through first aid schemes and initiatives such as the "CitizenAid" application [12, 13] in the UK and the "Stop the Bleed" campaign in the USA [14, 15].

All members of the British Armed Forces are trained to deliver basic first aid under these circumstances to themselves or others, termed 'self-aid' and 'buddy-aid'. This is similar to practice in other agencies worldwide who work in this environment (e.g. US law enforcement 'SWAT' teams). Only those immediately life-threatening injuries are addressed: tourniquets for massive haemorrhage and maintenance of an airway by positioning (recovery/three-quarter prone) alone. Within military practice, on operations where a high number of casualties are anticipated, a greater proportion of a unit's members may be upskilled to national equivalents of Team Medic, or potentially a Combat Medical Technician included in the task force (see Box 23.1) [16].

Tactical emergency medical services (TEMS) is an evolving civilian field. There is a recognition of the dangers present even on carefully planned tactical police operations and the potential need for increased medical support. Much of this is modelled around a military approach. There is debate about the utility of health care

Box 23.1 Levels of Care in the British Army—UK Armed Forces [16]

Battlefield Casualty Drills: All soldiers in the British Army have annual training in first aid, basic life support and basic principles of major trauma care, including the use of tourniquets. This includes delivery of care under fire by 'self-aid' and 'buddy-aid'.

Team Medic: A soldier from within the operational unit who has additional medical training primarily focussed on traumatic injuries and who carries minimal additional specialist medical equipment.

Combat Medical Technician: A medically trained soldier able to deliver protocol based primary health care, care under fire, resuscitation and stabilisation and in-transit monitoring for evacuation. They are regulated by the British Army Scope of Practice and Code of Conduct and will always work under supervision, even if this is remote.

Role 1: Led by Medical Officer (Doctor) or military nurse practitioner with BATLS (Battlefield Advanced Trauma Life Support) training. Capable of field resuscitation and early stabilisation. They usually belong to a larger unit (Regiment or Ship). Provides tactical and prolonged field care.

MERT (Medical Emergency Response Team): Senior physician-led (Emergency medicine/Anaesthetics/GP with advanced airway and resuscitation skills) and a team of variable size and skill mix. Can provide resuscitation with blood products, pre-hospital emergency anaesthesia and advanced decision making. May have a role in tactical field care and may bypass some treatment areas to allow a shorter time from the point of injury to damage control or definitive surgery.

Role 2: A Role 2 Medical Treatment Facility provides an initial surgical response capability and is characterised by its ability to perform surgical interventions and perform reception/triage of casualties. It can perform resuscitation and treatment of shock to a higher level than Role 1 facilities. In practical terms, this means the provision of damage control surgery (life, limb and function saving), basic laboratory and imaging services, limited intensive care capacity and a limited holding capacity for prolonged care of severely injured service personnel in austere and hostile environments. It is unlikely to operate in the tactical environment unless small teams are deployed within specialist environments.

providers in the hot and warm zones when organic team members can be trained in the initial lifesaving measures of haemorrhage control and airway management. The benefits of rapid access to a vocational provider's more advanced skill set have been questioned [17, 18]. Current practice in the USA does not generally support health care providers (physicians or mid-level providers) being placed in the hot or warm zone. The only situation this may be beneficial is if there is a mass casualty, where specially trained physicians may provide direct medical oversight of both initial triage and treatment areas which could be near the warm zone. There is a requirement for both those responding tactically and those responding in a medical capacity to appreciate each other's roles and capabilities, the tactics employed and pertinent legal elements of these situations [19]. There is a need to upskill those responding tactically so that they can assist their "buddies" in addition to assisting civilian casualties and wounded suspects. Physicians play a crucial role in the training of these advanced tactical team medics and should deploy with them whenever possible to be on scene in the "cold zone" as medical oversight for casualties. They should also be immediately available once the victim is extricated to the more permissive safe zone before transport. As a minimum, the medical responder should be aware that they will need to optimise cover from view and fire in this environment, and allow the armed response element to lead the event. In this scenario, medical elements are force enablers that support the overall mission rather than being the lead.

At this point, the priority is to win the firefight and preserve life before evacuation rather than providing definitive care. Only minimal and crucial interventions should be performed whilst the threat remains active. This can be at odds with a healthcare provider's instincts and may result in a hefty psychological burden following the event. Evacuation of a casualty to a more permissive environment and a higher level of care must be balanced with the safety to move without causing further casualties.

For the responder delivering care in this environment, it is essential that they wear correct personal protective equipment (PPE) for the threat encountered. This may include a ballistic helmet, goggles, body armour, chemical resistant suits and respirators. In some circumstances, camouflage (both visible and infrared) and identifying markers are necessary to allow other units and friendly actors in the area to identify the healthcare provider quickly. Personal equipment may also include a weapon issued to the individual for defence of themselves or their casualty. This should be maintained and familiar to the user as with the rest of their PPE.

Due to PPE requirements and the often physically demanding task of operating within the tactical environment, casualties and responders may be at risk of heat injury. This can manifest in the disturbance of physiological parameters even without injury. Raised temperature, respiratory rate and heart rate should alert the responder to the potential for heat injury. The risk of heat injury may be increased by working in already austere conditions and dehydration due to climate or lack of resources [20–22]. While PPE is essential in this environment, it is uncomfortable to wear for long periods and can degrade the performance of both tactical and medical tasks [23–26]. It can also decrease mobility and dexterity to perform interventions. The decision to remove a patient's PPE to examine and treat them depends on the prevailing scene dynamics and risk/benefit balance.

When all these issues are considered together, whole unit training (including medical contingency plans) should be undertaken in full PPE so that any limitations can be identified and solutions put in place before any live operations are undertaken. While challenging to seek real-life experience in these scenarios, it is essential to simulate and train as realistically as possible for these events. Training should include large-scale high-fidelity exercises and tabletop planning exercises, with specially trained physicians involved in the medical planning and logistics of the planned event.

Tactical Field Care/Semi-Permissive Environment

Once the threat is eliminated or a casualty is extracted from immediate danger to a semi-permissive environment, "tactical field care" commences. However, there continues to be a secondary threat of indirect fire or CBRNE3T (see later section). An example would be the cessation of enemy fire in a military firefight or a wounded police officer being removed from an area where there is still an ongoing siege with terrorists. Those working in this environment should always be aware of the potential for regression to a non-permissive environment. It is therefore important to continue with PPE, maintaining good tactical discipline and communication. Assessment of the casualty and access for treatment may be at the expense of removing their ballistic protection. Working under limited lighting in order to maintain security can make interventions challenging.

In the tactical field care phase, a full MABCD survey should be done (see later), interventions from the hot zone should be reviewed, and the patient should be stabilised for medical evacuation (MEDEVAC). There may be a greater availability or selection of kit and equipment at this stage. However, it should be stressed that actions taken in this phase should be swift but accurate, and again, only those actions appropriate to the level of threat should be performed.

All interventions up to this point fall under the umbrella of pre-hospital care; non-medically trained personnel can be given specific and targeted training in these techniques and have employed them effectively on operations [18]. In the military, this level of care is most likely delivered by a combat medical technician if they are attached to the operating force element. In situations where MEDEVAC can be based on a platform that is safe to take forward, advanced care providers can collect patients, and advanced interventions can begin in the tactical environment, effectively "bringing the hospital to the patient". The gold standard for this was the Medical Emergency Response Team (MERT) in Afghanistan, where a CH-47 Chinook permitted 360-degree access to the patient in flight. This capability also allowed patients more rapid evacuation to deployed hospital care.

Information passage between each of these levels of care is limited but vital and can be effectively achieved using the ATMIST tool (see Box 23.2), although others do exist.

It is always good practice to maintain kit discipline in the pre-hospital environment, but this is even more applicable in a tactical context. This not only includes maintenance and regular functions checks, but when using kit and equipment, only having the safe minimum requirement unpacked at any time for the survey or intervention. This allows a quick response to a change in the threat level or the arrival of an evacuation platform. There will likely be no clinical "white-space" available. Part of this care may be delivered in less than ideal environments that could be noisy, dirty or cold with limited ability to assess casualties. Depending on the tactical situation, the use of light and communications equipment may also be strictly controlled as this could alert hostile forces.

Box 23.2 ATMIST Report

A—Age & sex.

T—Time of wounding.

M—Mechanism of injury.

I—Injuries sustained.

S—Signs & symptoms.

T—Treatments given.

"I have an ATMIST report - 33-year-old male, time of wounding approx. 1940 hrs with a mechanism of stabbing during a possible terror attack. Injuries sustained are one stab wound to the chest and one to the abdomen. I suspect some internal abdominal bleeding. He has bruising around his abdomen but is currently alert with a resp rate of 26, heart rate of 120 and a palpable radial pulse. I have given him oxygen, applied a chest seal and abdo dressing and given him 5 mg of Morphine."

Resuscitation and Advanced Care/ Permissive Environment

This phase can occur when all nearby threats have been neutralised or the casualty and healthcare provider have been extracted to a safe area. Use of PPE and tactical discipline should still be adhered to as directed by those in charge of scene safety, but this phase should allow more conventional treatment to begin—essentially more akin to standard trauma care. It may be possible to run horizontal resuscitation with a well-staffed and equipped team and a manageable number of casualties.

The Physiology and Anatomy of Tactical Trauma Care

Physiology

The severity of a casualty is typically judged based on physiological parameters; heart rate, blood pressure, respiratory rate, oxygen saturation and temperature. Those that serve in the tactical environment are generally younger and fitter than the general population. This manifests as an ability to compensate for physiological insults until very unwell, when there is a rapid decompensation.

The nature of a warzone, site of a terror attack or disaster zone means that confusion and chaos often reign supreme. Casualties, whether bystanders or responders, will likely already have raised heart and respiratory rates if they have been running or fighting, which can lead to confusion during triage or treatment. However, even taking this into account, a casualty should be assumed to be at their worst triage category rather than mislabelled as "well but distressed" to avoid missing those that are injured. This approach does lead to an element of over-triage initially, but it is safer than under-triage.

Anatomy and Wounding

For those who frequently operate in the tactical environment, such as military personnel and specialist police officers, PPE is designed to mitigate risk. Combat body armour and helmets are the items most frequently seen, primarily protecting the head and thorax with some protection to the abdominal organs. As mentioned previously, body armour can be a double-edged sword in that it provides protection but limits mobility and can cause fatigue and so potentiate injury.

Data from terror attacks and recent conflicts demonstrate injury patterns commonly affecting the head, neck, chest, abdomen and junctional areas and commonly involving multiple areas [27]. Casualties may suffer penetrating injury from gunshot wounds, stabbing or shrapnel or blunt force trauma from direct impact or explosions. Alongside the obvious external wounding caused by explosives, there may be internal injuries such as blast lung or internal haemorrhage, and therefore adherence to a thorough format of assessment is crucial.

Unique Challenges of Tactical Trauma Care

While deaths from trauma have historically been described as trimodal (immediate from unsurvivable injuries, early primarily from haemorrhage or airway compromise and late from infection and SIRS response), there is an increasing shift away from this theory in an era of pre-hospital care, trauma networks, early resuscitation and critical care [28–30]. While outcome from trauma may, in the controlled environment, be linked to timelines to accessing care and at the level of care and expertise available, extended distances and accessibility of the casualty, either physically or due to ongoing threat, are significant contributors in the tactical environment.

CBRNE3T

The term "CBRNE3T" is an expansion of the widely recognised CBRN (chemical, biological, radiological and nuclear), acknowledging disease-non battle injury (DNBI) as the leading cause of casualties on operations (see Box 23.3) [31–36]. Defence describes its service personnel as operating in an "all-hazards environment", but this is increasingly becoming a factor that must be considered in all pre-hospital and major incident settings. Operational environments may have a known CBRNE3T threat that a chain of command can take steps to mitigate against, including donning of PPE in line with the perceived threat state and have a well-rehearsed response. Casualties and responders in the civilian environment are unlikely to have the benefit of this "pre-alert".

Box 23.3 CBRNE3T

Chemical—Threats from chemical agents or industrial chemicals and crowd control agents.

Biological—Weaponisation of live organisms, toxins and biological hazards.

Radiological—Release of ionising or non-ionising radiation.

Nuclear—Harnessing of nuclear fission/fusion reactions.

Explosive (ballistic)—Results of gunshot wounds, indirect fire, improvised explosive devices, shells and bombs and their collateral damage.

Environmental—Hazards emerging from heat, cold and altitude.

Endemic—Infectious diseases pose a risk even when not deliberately released.

Trauma—Not all trauma is a result of explosive activity.

Tactical field care is often delivered in austere environments where local flora and fauna, climate, terrain and disease may have a concurrent impact alongside operational threats. Patients in this setting may have been exposed to (and may continue to need protection from) any of these threats even once evacuated from the immediate incident. A high level of suspicion of should remain when responding to these incidents.

From the responder's perspective, a "Safety 1-2-3" approach towards an unwitnessed or suspicious incident where there may be a CBRNE3T element in play [37, 38]:

1. **One person incapacitated with no apparent cause**:
   approach using standard protocols
2. **Two people incapacitated with no apparent cause**:
   approach with caution, update control
3. **Three or more people incapacitated with no apparent cause:**
   use caution:
   - Evacuate those not involved from the scene
   - Communicate and advise that help is on the way
   - Disrobe patients in the immediate area—to minimise contamination
   - Decontaminate patients before they leave the "hot zone", dry decontamination

While the vocational medical responder's utility in the hot zone is debated, recognised roles, particularly in the CBRN environment, include:

Medical Reconnaissance—observation of signs and symptoms with the aim to identify a toxidrome and potential causative agent.

Triage—described in the "Major Incidents" chapter. May be undertaken by non-medical personnel but require adaptation in the presence of CBRN agents.

Trauma care—those withing the CBRN environment may still have other injuries that require treatment.

Antidote administration

Decontamination will then take place in the warm zone (see Fig. 23.2) [39].

The MABCD Approach in the Tactical Environment

Care in the non-permissive and semi-permissive environment is limited due to safety to the rescuer and efficacy of interventions in this setting. Here the suggested interventions are explored and broken down into each stage. The approach detailed here is similar to that used by the UK armed forces and most NATO forces. It is essential that practitioners receive training in tactical trauma care and that teams are familiar with one another's systems. The UK armed forces train their medical personnel in Battlefield Advanced Trauma Life Support (BATLS), an adapted version of the original Advanced Trauma Life Support (ATLS) course.

Care Under Fire

Care under fire occurs at the point of wounding, in a non-permissive environment where the priority remains to "win the firefight". Minimal interventions are performed at this stage and are usually provided by self-aid or buddy aid, not a specially trained responder. Soldiers and armed response officers should be trained in basic first aid, including control of massive haemorrhage, have annual refresher training, and carry equipment such as emergency care bandages and tourniquets. As public education on response to these events is developed, there is a push to provide this equipment in public areas or teach improvised techniques for bystanders to perform care under fire.

The SAFE approach to Care Under Fire

- **S**—Shout/send signal for help

  In the military setting, this involves shouting "man down" to inform members of the immediate subunit if tactically appropriate. From here, a member of the unit will be responsible for communicating this "contact report" to a higher echelon to give a location, time of enemy contact, number of enemies and their disposition and the commander's intent, usually via radio communications. In addition to this, when the

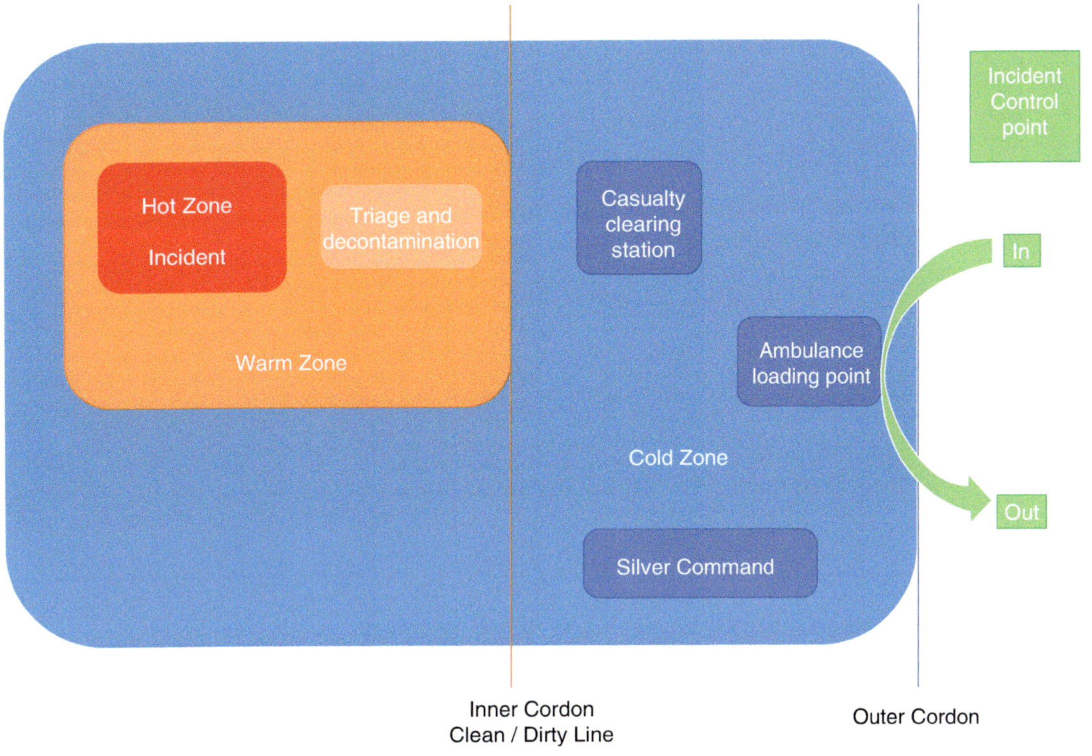

Fig. 23.2 Response to CBRN incidents and cordon control (based on Byers et al. [39])

tactical situation allows, a "nine-liner" report is made to request medical evacuation if needed. This is given in a specific format to save time and allow accurate transcription by personnel receiving the message in the event of communication difficulty (see Fig. 23.3). Casualties, if able, should make others around them aware of their injuries. Those responding to the scene should identify the likely need for assistance and request this early.

- **A**—Assess for danger: to self, patient and scene

  At this point, the priority is responding to the threat. This may involve neutralising the assailant. A safe approach route must be established, clear of secondary devices, considering the ongoing risk of indirect fire. As discussed previously, the Safety 1-2-3 approach is used in an instance with multiple casualties to consider the possibility of a CBRN threat. The structural integrity of any infrastructure must also be considered, both at the current time and with anticipation of how the firefight may evolve in the next few minutes.

- **F**—Find and free casualties

  Not all casualties are immediately identifiable, particularly those ejected from vehicles or thrown by a blast wave. All possible casualties need to be identified and accounted for. Casualties may be physically or functionally entrapped and need to be freed to permit treatment and evacuation. In a civilian setting this can involve multiple agencies, including the Fire Services and the Hazardous Areas Response Team. Speed of extrication is usually governed by the patient's condition. Control of c-spine and appropriate interventions will likely be dictated by the level of ongoing threat and the likelihood of injury. Of note, patients with penetrating ballistic neck injuries should not routinely have cervical spine collars applied as this worsens outcomes in patients who have potentially survivable injuries by causing airway compromise or hiding other life-threatening pathology. Patients

9 Liner Request		Date:			Time:		
1	Callsign						
2	Location of HLS						
3	Number of patients / priority	P1		P2		P3	
4	Specialist equipment required						
5	Pt type	Stretcher	Walking		Escort		Other
6	Security of HLS						
7	HLS Marking Method						
8	Number of Patients by nationality						
9	HLS Terrain / Obstacles						

Fig. 23.3 9 Liner template

with penetrating ballistic neck injuries and unstable spinal pathology die of their wounds very quickly [40]. If patients with these injuries are attended by medical teams, they should not have a cervical collar applied.

- E—Evaluate

  Assessing the casualty and their injuries. In this environment, only immediately life-threatening conditions are addressed.

Interventions appropriate during **care under fire**:

- **<M>—Massive Haemorrhage**

  Tourniquet applied by self-application or buddy aid. This is the primary method of haemostasis in the non-permissive environment. Improvised tourniquets may be used.
- **A—Airway**

  Turning the patient onto their front to allow postural drainage.

Tactical Field Care

Tactical field care takes place in a semi-permissive environment. Here there is an ongoing threat to consider danger from CBRNE3T, but a more thorough assessment and treatment can be provided. The interventions in each stage of the MABCD approach have been outlined in previous chapters. However, a brief list of appropriate interventions in the warm zone for each stage is laid out below.

- **M—Massive Haemorrhage**

  The ideal haemorrhage control follows a stepwise approach (see Fig. 23.4) [41]. The threshold for tourniquet application in the tactical environment is low in the non-permissive environment. The clinical requirement can be reassessed in the semi permissive environment and assessed for haemostasis [41, 42].

  If a tourniquet has been applied too proximally, an additional tourniquet should be applied as close to the wound as is viable. Once this is in place, the original tourniquet can be loosened slowly but left in place to assess for adequate haemostasis. If it is felt that a bleed can be adequately controlled by other means, then again, the tourniquet should be loosened slowly but not removed, with monitoring of adequate haemostasis. Equally, if ongoing bleeding despite a tourniquet, a second tourniquet more proximal than the first may be applied (See Fig. 23.5) [43].

Topical haemostatics include agents such as Celox. They are not indicated before a semi permissive environment is reached because of the time taken to apply correctly. Application of celox is ideally a two-person technique (see Fig. 23.6) [43].

- In those with penetrating trauma, a roll to identify any further injuries and exit wounds should be performed early to avoid missing other sources of haemorrhage. In those with blunt trauma should be minimal.
- **A—Airway**

  Inspection and clearing of the airway. Hand operated suction.

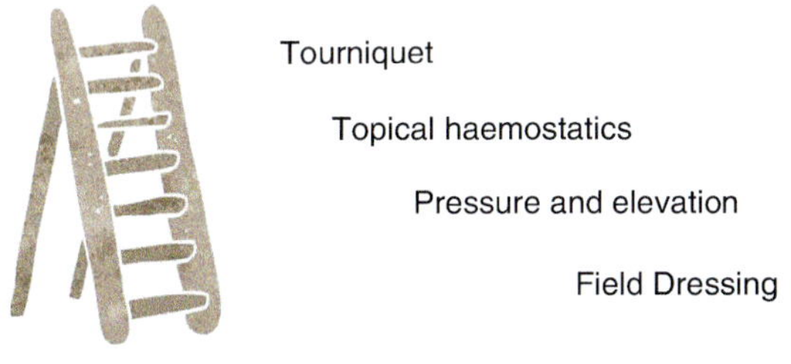

Fig. 23.4 Haemorrhage control ladder (Adapted from Moorehouse et al. [41])

  OPA/NPA sizing and insertion.

  Oxygen if available.

  Surgical airway if required and appropriately trained provider present.

- **c—Cervical Spine Control**

  Manual immobilisation.

  Care of a potential C-Spine injury must be balanced with the impact of an immobilised casualty on manoeuvrability out of an area of ongoing threat.

- **B—Breathing**

  A thorough assessment of the chest should be made using whatever means the responder is most familiar with (for example, see Box 23.4) [42]. Interventions performed in this environment include applying oxygen if available, analgesia, needle thoracentesis, thoracostomy, chest seal application and early recognition of the need to expedite evacuation.

- **C—Circulation**

  Intravenous or intraosseous access gained and fluids administered to restore a radial pulse.

  Administration of Tranexamic Acid, fluids or blood products if available.

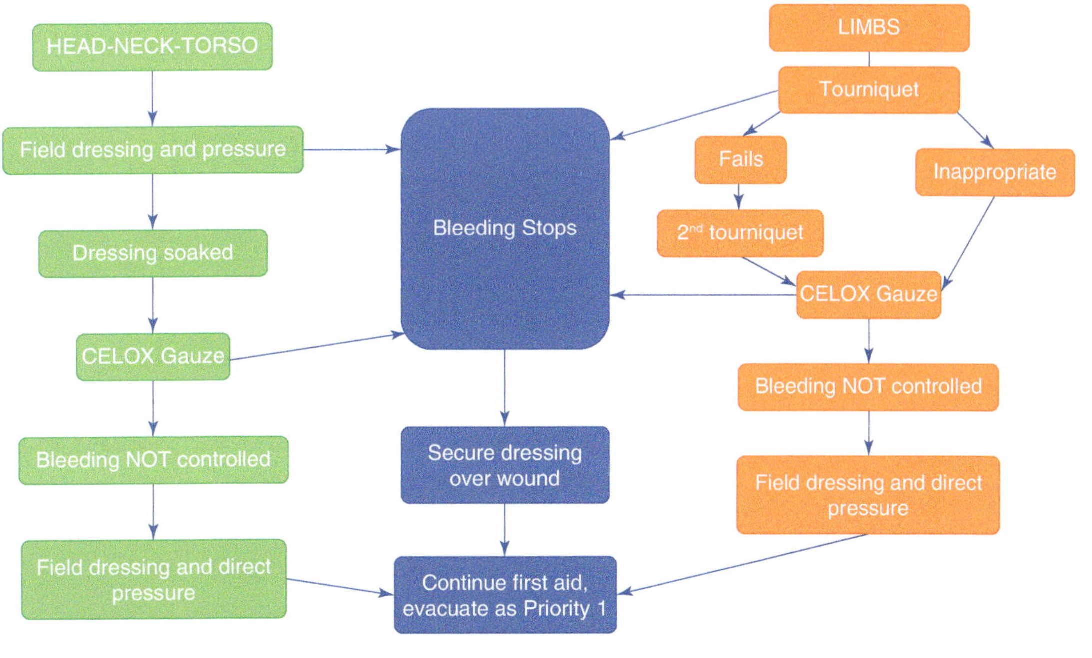

Fig. 23.5 Achieving haemostasis (based on BATLS Aide Memoire, 3rd Edition) [43]

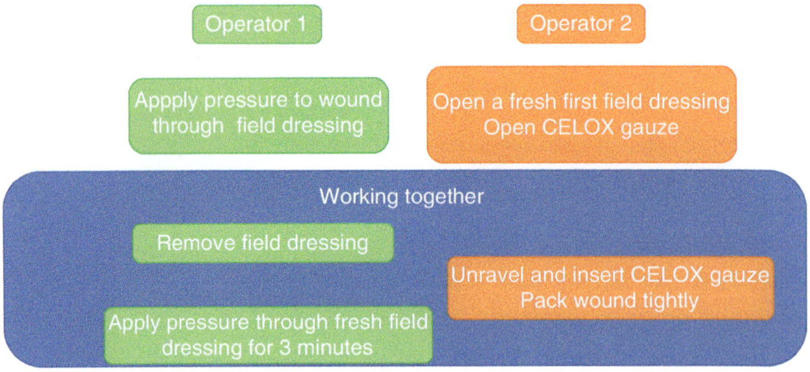

Fig. 23.6 Celox Application (based on BATLS Aide Memoire 3rd edition) [43]

- **D—Disability**

  Level of consciousness is generally assessed using one of two scales. The AVPU scale, or the Glasgow Coma Scale.

  AVPU stands for:

> **Box 23.4 BATLS Approach to Respiratory Assessment (Based on BATLS Aide Memoire, 3rd Edition) [43]**
>
> Currently, BATLS teaches a "RISE N FALL" assessment of the chest. This is designed to be a thorough assessment of the respiratory system in a uniformed format that all providers are familiar with.
>
> **R**—Respiratory Rate
> **I**—Injuries to chest and axillae
> **S**—Symmetry of chest wall
> **E**—Effort of breathing
> **N**—Neck assessment
> **T**—Trachea
> **W**—Wounds
> **E**—Emphysema
> **L**—Larynx
> **V**—Veins
> **E**—Complete neck assessment every time before applying a cervical collar
> **F**—Feel: for tender areas and bony crepitus
> **A**—Assess resonance (percussion)
> **L**—Listen to chest (auscultation)
> **L**—Look at the back

- **A**—Alert.
- **V**—Responds to verbal stimuli.
- **P**—Responds to painful stimuli.
- **U**—Unresponsive.

  AVPU is a quicker and simpler score to assess than the GCS but can still be used to identify deterioration.

- **E—Exposure/Environment**

  Patients should be packaged carefully for transport with minimal patient handling. All interventions should be checked and protected from dislodgement. Consider whether the patient has been offered sufficient analgesia prior to movement and whether antibiotic cover is indicated if they are available. The casualty will need protection from the environment to avoid hypothermia and hyperthermia and exposure to other CBRNE3T threats. Adequate documentation about the patient's injury and treatments will need to accompany the patient through the chain of care. Regular reassessments should be made while awaiting evacuation.

Challenges of International and Austere Working

The majority of medical care worldwide in mature healthcare systems is delivered in an environment that is safe, clean, well lit, protected from the elements and has almost immediate availability of senior support. Virtually all of these elements are missing in the tactical and austere environments. Security in the tactical setting is not guaranteed. This is particularly true for those working furthest forwards, embedded within front line fighting units or working with tactical emergency response units, providing the immediate interventions to save lives and prevent further injury. Even for those in comparatively safe rear echelons, there is a need to be concealed from the enemy and an ever-present risk of harm from rogue actors infiltrating accompanying organisations [44, 45], indirect fire (artillery and mortars) or long-range attacks such as airstrikes.

Displaying the red cross, crescent, or crystal should guarantee protection to the wearer, vehicle or building displaying it under the Geneva Conventions [46]. However, this is often not adhered to in non-conventional conflict [47–49]. Disruption of logistic and support chains is a potent method to render a fighting force ineffective. Healthcare facilities may even be seen as desirable targets by those wishing to create terror and psychological harm to a population. While remaining concealed from the enemy, aid posts need to be easily identified by the population they are there to serve.

The kit and equipment available are often limited to that which can be carried by the practitioner, or accommodated by the transportation platform. There are restrictions in terms of cold-chain supplies (items that require transport and storage in refrigerators), such as various drugs and blood products. There is a need to estimate the number and type of casualties in order to take an appropriate kit selection, often relying on improvisation or adaptation of existing equipment to perform multiple roles. Sourcing of kit and equipment can be difficult when dislocated from a supply chain, as some countries do not allow transit through or importation of certain medications. Monitoring equipment usually connected to a continuous power supply is now limited by battery life, and spare batteries can be bulky and heavy. Communications equipment presents yet another challenge; they require sufficient battery power and capacity to run reliably but may create electromagnetic signals or "splash" alerting hostile forces to their location. They may also require specific criteria to be met to send and receive signals, such as a direct line of sight or good prevailing atmospheric conditions depending on the type of communication bearer being used. These can all be limited in the austere environment or when working "at reach". Consideration should be given to capacity on the communication network for the passage of information. Those using radio equipment should be trained in its use and familiar with basic voice procedures and protocols [50].

The evacuation chain involved in the care of a patient injured in these circumstances is often complicated if it formally exists at all. While military operations will have a specific medical evacuation (MEDEVAC) plan as part of the medical planning aspect, charities and aid agencies may not have the luxury of being able to evacuate patients from or to hospitals outside of the region.

MEDEVAC typically relies on the coordination of several different organisations, potentially of different nationalities, who have not necessarily cooperated before. Each organisation will have their Standard Operating Procedures (SOPs), and there is no guaranteed congruency in these. Again, communications can be an issue here in terms of interoperability of systems or even common language.

Increasingly there is a need to provide "prolonged field care", not solely the immediate resuscitation. This comes with inherent challenges for kit requirements, monitoring, transport and ability to maintain functionality. Alongside this is the breadth of presentations to these aid posts. Everything from trauma to primary health care must be catered for, including the presentation of obstetric and paediatric patients. In tactical trauma care, there is often an element of scene appraisal and "reading the wreckage" in predicting injury patterns and the management of personnel who may not initially appear injured and, potentially, a need to triage patients to prioritise "the most for the most".

The natural and man-made challenges ordinarily faced in the pre-hospital environment are compounded by tactical requirements, such as minimal noise permitted and no white light as previously mentioned. The scope of tactical care is likely to increase as non-blood oxygen-carrying fluids, clotting products and medications that are more stable across different climatic conditions are developed.

Conclusion

Working in tactical and austere environments provides a unique and exciting challenge to medical practitioners. While the medical principles remain unchanged at their core, there are many considerations on top of these (such as safety, protective equipment and tactical discipline) that the care provider needs to take into account. Training and simulation can go a long way towards preparing someone to work in this setting.

An understanding of delivering care in the tactical environment is not just applicable to those practising in the military. Civilian responders could find themselves attending a major incident such as a terror attack or violent crime and may be tasked to work alongside specialist police units. If ever in doubt about what actions to take at this sort of incident, always consider responder safety and liaise with those in charge of the scene.

Questions

1. Which of the following is correct in the care under fire environment:
   (a) Responders should remove a casualty's PPE to get better access to them
   (b) Lifesaving interventions can be delivered by non-trained personnel
   (c) Catastrophic haemorrhage should be managed using the haemorrhage control ladder
   (d) Obstructed airways should be managed using a surgical airway
2. The "M" in ATMIST stands for:
   (a) "Mechanism of Injury."
   (b) "Management"
   (c) "My call sign."
   (d) "Major Incident declared"
3. Which of the following is incorrect regarding the semi-permissive environment?
   (a) A full MABCD assessment should be made
   (b) There remains an ongoing threat to the casualty and responder
   (c) C-spine immobilisation should be applied in all blast victims
   (d) A tourniquet applied during "care under fire" should never be removed
4. Which of these is a challenge to working in the austere environment?
   (a) Communications
   (b) Extremes of temperature and their effect on equipment and medications
   (c) Availability of resupply
   (d) All of the above
5. Which is incorrect regarding the "all-hazards environment"?
   (a) Care delivered may be limited by PPE
   (b) Casualties should be decontaminated at the outer cordon
   (c) ≥3 casualties presenting with similar symptoms should raise suspicion of a CBRN threat
   (d) Normal physiological parameters for triage can be used

Answers

1. b
2. a
3. c
4. d
5. b

References

1. Butler FK. TCCC updates: two decades of saving lives on the battlefield: tactical combat casualty care turns 20. J Spec Oper Med. 2017;17(2):166–72.
2. Callaway DW. Translating tactical combat casualty care lessons learned to the high-threat civilian setting: tactical emergency casualty care and the Hartford consensus. Wilderness Environ Med. 2017;28(2):S140–5.
3. Hartley F, Howells A, Thurgood A, Hall F, Porter K. Medical training for police officers in specialist role (D13): a retrospective review of patient report forms from 2010–2015. Trauma. 2018;20(1):20–4.
4. Graham D. Marauding terrorist firearms' attacks: a Practitioner's view of the UK's emergency service initial response arrangements to Deal with an active shooter. RUSI J. 2018;163(2):42–50.

5. Ranstorp M. 'Lone Wolf Terrorism'. The Case of Anders Breivik. S+F. 2013;31(2):87–92.
6. Service Médical du RAID. Tactical emergency medicine: lessons from Paris marauding terrorist attack. Crit Care. 2016;20(1):37.
7. Frickmann H, Sturm D, Finke E-J. Risks of Infection as a Result of Foreign Tissue Implantation Injuries and Sexual Violence in Asymmetric Conflicts [Internet]. military-medicine.com. 2019 [cited 2020 Aug 5]. Available from: https://military-medicine.com/article/3675-risks-of-infection-as-a-result-of-foreign-tissue-implantation-injuries-sexual-violence-in-asymmetric-conflicts.html
8. Kao RL, McAlister VC. Care of victims of suicide bombing. Can J Surg. 2018;61(6):S184–7.
9. Eshkol Z, Katz K. Injuries from biologic material of suicide bombers. Injury. 2005;36(2):271–4.
10. Defence Medical Services. Joint Service Publication 950 [Internet]. Ministry of Defence; 2016. Available from: https://www.gov.uk/government/publications/operational-patient-care-pathway
11. JESIP. Joint doctrine: The interoperability framework. Edition 2. [Internet]. JESIP; 2016 [cited 2020 Aug 5]. Available from: https://www.jesip.org.uk/joint-doctrine
12. Khorram-Manesh A, Plegas P, Högstedt Å, Peyravi M, Carlström E. Immediate response to major incidents: defining an immediate responder! Eur J Trauma Emerg Surg [Internet]. 2019 Apr 5 [cited 2020 Aug 5]; Available from: http://link.springer.com/10.1007/s00068-019-01133-1
13. Hodgetts TJ, Thurgood A, Porter K, Mahoney PF. CitizenAID [Internet]. citizenAID. [cited 2020 Aug 5]. Available from: https://www.citizenaid.org/citizenaid
14. Stop The Bleed [Internet]. Stop The Bleeding Coalition. [cited 2019 Aug 26]. Available from: https://stopthebleedingcoalition.org/
15. Zwislewski A, Nanassy AD, Meyer LK, Scantling D, Jankowski MA, Blinstrub G, et al. Practice makes perfect: the impact of stop the bleed training on hemorrhage control knowledge, wound packing, and tourniquet application in the workplace. Injury. 2019;50(4):864–8.
16. British Army. Health Service Support to Land Operations Handbook. Version 1, Edition 1. Ministry of Defence; 2019.
17. Metzger JC, Eastman AL, Benitez FL, Pepe PE. The lifesaving potential of specialized on-scene medical support for Urban tactical operations. Prehosp Emerg Care. 2009 Jan;13(4):528–31.
18. Kyle T, le Clerc S, Thomas A, Greaves I, Whittaker V, Smith JE. The success of battlefield surgical airway insertion in severely injured military patients: a UK perspective. J R Army Med Corps. 2016;162(6):460–4.
19. Schwartz R, Lerner B, Llwewllyn C, Pennardt A, Wedmore I, Callaway D, et al. Development of a national consensus for tactical emergency medical support (TEMS) training programs--operators and medical providers. J Spec Oper Med. 2014;14(2):122–38.
20. Cadarette B, Blanchard L, Staab J, Kolka M, Sawka M. Heat stress when wearing body armour. US Army Research Institute of Environmental Medicine; 2001. p. 20.
21. Lehmacher EJ, Jansing P, Kupper T. Thermo-physiological responses caused by ballistic bulletproof vests. Ann Occup Hyg. 2007;51(1):91–6.
22. Adams JD, McDermott BP, Ridings CB, Mainer LL, Ganio MS, Kavouras SA. Effect of air-filled vest on exercise-heat strain when wearing ballistic protection. Ann Occup Hyg. 2014;58(8):1057–64.
23. Tomes C, Orr RM, Pope R. The impact of body armor on physical performance of law enforcement personnel: a systematic review. Ann Occup Environ Med [Internet]. 2017 16 [cited 2020 June 3]:[29 p.]. Available from: https://www.ncbi.nlm.nih.gov/pmc/articles/PMC5434519/
24. Larsen B, Netto K, Aisbett B. The effect of body armor on performance, thermal stress, and exertion: a critical review. Mil Med. 2011;176(11):1265–73.
25. Dempsey PC, Handcock PJ, Rehrer NJ. Impact of police body Armour and equipment on mobility. Appl Ergon. 2013 Nov;44(6):957–61.
26. Kollock RO, Hale D, Vogelpohl R, Kremer L, Horner J, Cox C, et al. The influence of body armor on balance and movement quality. Int J Exerc Sci. 2018;11(1):648–56.
27. Arnold JL, Halpern P, Tsai M-C, Smithline H. Mass casualty terrorist bombings: a comparison of outcomes by bombing type. Ann Emerg Med. 2004;43(2):263–73.
28. de Knegt C, Meylaerts SAG, Leenen LPH. Applicability of the trimodal distribution of trauma deaths in a level I trauma Centre in the Netherlands with a population of mainly blunt trauma. Injury. 2008;39(9):993–1000.
29. Bardes JM, Inaba K, Schellenberg M, Grabo D, Strumwasser A, Matsushima K, et al. The contemporary timing of trauma deaths. J Trauma Acute Care Surg. 2018;84(6):893–9.
30. Gunst M, Ghaemmaghami V, Gruszecki A, Urban J, Frankel H, Shafi S. Changing epidemiology of trauma deaths leads to a bimodal distribution. Proc (Bayl Univ Med Cent). 2010;23(4):349–54.
31. Belmont PJ, Goodman GP, Waterman B, DeZee K, Burks R, Owens BD. Disease and nonbattle injuries sustained by a US Army brigade combat team during operation Iraqi freedom. Mil Med. 2010;175(7):469–76.
32. Agency I of M (US) MF-U, Joellenbeck LM, Russell PK, Guze SB. Risks to Deployed Forces [Internet]. Strategies to Protect the Health of Deployed US Forces: Medical Surveillance, Record Keeping, and Risk Reduction. National Academies Press (US); 1999 [cited 2020 Aug 5]. Available from: https://www.ncbi.nlm.nih.gov/books/NBK225082/
33. Le TD, Gurney JM, Nnamani NS, Gross KR, Chung KK, Stockinger ZT, et al. A 12-year analy-

sis of nonbattle injury among US Service members deployed to Iraq and Afghanistan. JAMA Surg. 2018;153(9):800–7.
34. Sanchez JL, Craig SC, Kohlhase K, Polyak C, Ludwig SL, Rumm PD. Health assessment of US military personnel deployed to Bosnia-Herzegovina for operation joint endeavor. Mil Med. 2001;166(6):470–4.
35. Defence Statistics (Branch). Types of Injuries Sustained by UK Service Personnel on Op HERRICK in Afghanistan, 1 April 2006 to 30 November 2014 [Internet]. London: Ministry of Defence; 2016 Feb [cited 2020 Aug 5]: [12 p.]. Available from: https://www.google.com/url?sa=t&rct=j&q=&esrc=s&source=web&cd=&ved=2ahUKEwj_5oHj9IPrAhWGYMAKHU8QDRwQFjAFegQIBxAB&url=https%3A%2F%2Fassets.publishing.service.gov.uk%2Fgovernment%2Fuploads%2Fsystem%2Fuploads%2Fattachment_data%2Ffile%2F502888%2F20160223_Afghanistan_Types_of_Injuries_Official_Statistic_Final_OS.pdf&usg=AOvVaw0hAqTF_sY-aF6ADq7eMtrb
36. McKee KT, Kortepeter MG, Ljaamo SK. Disease and nonbattle injury among United States soldiers deployed in Bosnia-Herzegovina during 1997: summary primary care statistics for operation joint guard. Mil Med. 1998;163(11):733–42.
37. Chilcott RP, Larner J, Matar H. UK's initial operational response and specialist operational response to CBRN and HazMat incidents: a primer on decontamination protocols for healthcare professionals. Emerg Med J. 2019;36(2):117–23.
38. Home Office. Initial Operational Response to a CBRN Incident [Internet]. Home Office; 2015 [cited 2020 June 3]. Available from: https://www.jesip.org.uk/uploads/media/pdf/CBRN%20JOPs/IOR_Guidance_V2_July_2015.pdf
39. Byers M, Russell M, Lockey DJ. Clinical care in the 'hot zone'. Emerg Med J. 2008;25(2):108–12.
40. Ramasamy A, Midwinter M, Mahoney P, Clasper J. Learning the lessons from conflict: pre-hospital cervical spine stabilisation following ballistic neck trauma. Injury. 2009;40(12):1342–5.
41. Moorhouse I, Thurgood A, Thurgood A, Walker N, Cooper B, Mahoney PF, et al. A realistic model for catastrophic external haemorrhage training. BMJ Military Health. 2007;153(2):99–101.
42. Lee C, Porter KM. Tourniquet use in the civilian prehospital setting. Emerg Med J. 2007 Aug;24(8):584–7.
43. Battlefield Advanced Trauma Life Support Course Manual. Department of Distributed Training, Defence School of Healthcare, Defence Medical Academy. Crown Copyright 2021.
44. Green-on-Blue Attacks in Afghanistan: The Data | RealClearDefense [Internet]. [cited 2020 June 2]. Available from: http://www.realcleardefense.com/articles/2017/03/21/green-on-blue_attacks_in_afghanistan_the_data_111015.html
45. Corera G. What lies behind Afghanistan's insider attacks? BBC News [Internet]. 2013 Mar 11 [cited 2020 June 2]; Available from: https://www.bbc.com/news/world-asia-19633418
46. International Committee of the Red Cross (ICRC). Geneva Convention Relative to the Protection of Civillian Persons in Time of War (Fourth Geneva Convention) [Internet]. International Committee of the Red Cross (ICRC); 1949 [cited 2020 June 2]. Available from: https://www.refworld.org/docid/3ae6b36d2.html
47. Red Cross: Health, Aid Workers Face Unabated Attacks | Voice of America - English [Internet]. VOA News. 2019 [cited 2020 June 3]. Available from: https://www.voanews.com/middle-east/red-cross-health-aid-workers-face-unabated-attacks
48. Izade E. Red Cross volunteers attacked in Guinea while trying to bury an Ebola victim. Washington Post [Internet]. 2104 Sep 24 [cited 2020 June 3]; Available from: https://www.washingtonpost.com/news/to-your-health/wp/2014/09/24/red-cross-volunteers-attacked-in-guinea-while-trying-to-bury-an-ebola-victim/
49. Farmer B. Taliban 'will no longer protect Red Cross staff in Afghanistan'. The Telegraph [Internet]. 2019 Jun 12 [cited 2020 June 3]; Available from: https://www.telegraph.co.uk/global-health/terror-and-security/taliban-will-no-longer-protect-red-cross-staff-afghanistan-amid/
50. Bricknell MC, Hanhart N. Stability operations and the implications for military health services support. J R Army Med Corps. 2007;153(1):18–21.

Trauma Retrieval

24

Holly A. Chambers, Graham M. Percival, and Robin D. Berry

- Understand the complexity of the transfer environment and the associated risks to the patient and 'crew'
- Recognise the requirement for trained, skilled staff
- Describe those factors required to deliver an adaptable, consistently safe and well-governed transfer service
- Promote the Defence Systems Approach to Training
- The multi-modal roles of simulation training
- The importance of Standard Operating Procedures
- Communication in all its forms as central to a "safety culture"

H. A. Chambers · R. D. Berry (✉)
Department of Anaesthesia and Critical Care Medicine, Derriford Hospital, Plymouth, UK

Tactical Medical Wing, Royal Air Force, Brize Norton, Oxfordshire, UK
e-mail: holly.chambers2@nhs.net; robin.berry@nhs.net

G. M. Percival
Emergency Medical Retrieval Service, Paisley, Scotland

Tactical Medical Wing, Royal Air Force, Brize Norton, Oxfordshire, UK

Introduction

Trauma transfer teams were initially developed by enthusiastic volunteers who recognised a local requirement and developed staffing and operational models to meet demand. More recently, lessons learned from conflict and the concentration of expertise into Major Trauma Centres (MTC's) has resulted in an increase in the number of trauma transfers and the complexity of interventions made before and during transit. This has seen the establishment of guidelines and minimum standards from governmental organisations and professional societies dealing with ICU transport and specific patient cohorts [1–3]. Today's transfers require motivated, highly trained individuals who have the pragmatism to function in a remote and austere environment, in addition to the mental agility and clinical skills necessary to deliver best practice care en route.

Whilst the medical management of injured persons is described elsewhere in this book, the purpose of this chapter is to consider those factors required to deliver an adaptable, consistently safe and well-governed transfer service.

Training

The transfer environment can be an overwhelming and unforgiving place for both patient and staff, with a wide variance in the published incidence of adverse events during intra-hospital

P. Lax (ed.), *Textbook of Acute Trauma Care*, https://doi.org/10.1007/978-3-030-83628-3_24

transfer [4–7]. It is a mistake to assume that a clinician who is clinically competent in the hospital setting will effectively function in the transfer role. Procedural skills alone do not prepare a practitioner to safely conduct trauma transfers without further training and exposure. Novices should not learn through trial and error but should have an introductory equipment course followed by closely supervised practice [8]. Transfers within a hospital do not guarantee immediate senior assistance, especially when remote locations are involved. Furthermore, there is now published evidence that specifically trained transfer teams have a lower incidence of complications [9, 10] than ad hoc crews. Consequently, hyperacute transfers of unstable patients (e.g. to Major Trauma Centres from Trauma Units) should be performed by the most experienced staff.

Many transfer services will choose to deliver the bulk of their training in-house with access to external courses when appropriate. Unfortunately, the cost of external training can become prohibitive for any except permanent staff members, and therefore a robust in-house system is essential for trainees.

The transfer setting deserves respect, and the delivery of a robust induction and training package demonstrates a commitment to preparing novices for working in a challenging environment. A significant component of transfer training is generic, but additional bespoke elements will be needed to address local transfer pathways, logistics and platforms. It is crucial that this initial instruction is planned in both time and content and not left to chance. Front loading with programmed lessons will ensure the novice is equipped with sufficient knowledge and skills to function safely in the early days whilst experience is gained. Exposure to "on the job" situations is valuable when supervised, but unsupported 'learning by mistakes,' should never be acceptable.

To reduce the potential for individual variation in training, all delivery should be based around objectives and learning outcomes. This can involve a significant amount of work in analysing exactly what a novice needs to know about a piece of equipment, for example, and then defining how that training will be delivered. Relying on "word of mouth" cascade training will undoubtedly lead to gradual dilution of information accuracy and relevance. The Defence Systems Approach to Training (DSAT) is a well-governed method of analysing, preparing and delivering training that is reproducible, auditable and educationally robust [11]. The DSAT step-wise process deconstructs a skill and takes training development from Training Needs Analysis right through to Key Learning Points and Lesson Plans. Any service wishing to demonstrate sound educational governance would be recommended in using such a systematic approach to its training planning and delivery. Failure to provide adequate training in the use of medical devices, in general, should be considered a significant clinical risk with subsequent litigation likelihood.

It is out of the scope of this chapter to define the content of induction and refresher training, but a variety of methods and resources should be available.

1. Hands-on instruction and training
2. Case-based discussions
3. Simulation/scenarios
4. Journal Club
5. Morbidity and Mortality review

Key Points in Transfer Medicine

The mountaineer Edward Whymper eloquently describes the mindset required; "Climb if you will, but remember that courage and strength are nought without *prudence*, and that a momentary negligence may destroy the happiness of a lifetime. Do nothing in haste; look well to each step, and from the beginning think what may be the end [12]."

Furthermore, these key points should be borne in mind:

1. *Transfer is not a treatment* and may expose the patient to significant risks as the patient does not settle into a steady state during the journey. Therefore, the risk-benefit assess-

ment must be clearly in favour of transfer before considering the task further. In the pre-hospital setting, the decision to transport the patient to ED is usually simple, but the timing and necessity for secondary transfers often require more thought. Similarly, whilst the hazards of inter-hospital transfer may be obvious, intra-hospital moves to facilitate imaging and damage control resuscitation deserve equal respect. One prospective study demonstrated that approximately 80% of intra-hospital transfers experienced some form of adverse event, with 33% of transfers being complicated by a critical incident [4], and the frequency of these adverse events increased with the complexity of the patient.

2. *Leave nothing to chance.* Transfer teams are frequently required to expedite patient moves, and to do this safely they need to create and share accurate mental models of the task and any anticipated problems [13, 14]. This skill is developed from effective training, familiarity with kit and operating platforms, along with local knowledge of patient care pathways.
3. *The transfer environment is hazardous—the casualty, all personnel and equipment must be safely secured* to ensure the safety of the patient, the transfer team, their escorts and the vehicle in which they are travelling.
4. The transfer of critically ill patients is a 'team sport'. Where possible, training should be conducted as a squad with both medical and allied health professional staff included.

Trauma Retrievals

The goal is to deliver injured persons to the point of definitive care as quickly as possible and in the best physiological state [15].

Trauma retrievals can be divided into three categories:

1. Primary retrieval (from the scene to the most appropriate receiving facility). This will be determined by time, the patient's physiology and the nature of their injuries. In this context, providers need to be competent and practised in primary survey and interventions such as rapid sequence induction (RSI), thoracostomy, intravenous and intra-osseous access, titrated fluid resuscitation and the use of sedation. Any procedures undertaken should be focused on those which are immediately life-saving or intended to prevent secondary brain injury. Currently, the transfer platforms used in civilian practice lack the size or physical access to allow many procedures to occur in transit. Consequently, experienced practitioners are needed to ensure the correct balance between 'scoop and run' or 'stay and play'.
2. Modified Primary Retrieval, the mission is undertaken as a primary retrieval but with the patient being collected from a small, local medical facility such as a GP Surgery or Community Hospital. This type of transfer may be "sold" as a secondary mission but represents all the clinical challenges usually associated with outdoor pre-hospital work, including limited access due to room size.
3. Secondary retrievals are performed after primary survey, imaging and damage control resuscitation in a trauma unit when the patient requires the tertiary services provided by an MTC. This transfer may be time-critical (for example, traumatic brain injury), but other injuries may allow for an extended timeline.

The risks of an extended journey to an MTC versus a pit stop in a closer trauma unit [30], potentially necessitating a subsequent secondary transfer, must be carefully but quickly evaluated. Stopping for limited interventions or diagnostic imaging is attractive to primary transfer teams, but it is difficult to maintain momentum once a hospital team becomes engaged. Unfortunately, the clinicians' natural desire to diagnose and treat can lead to delays in definitive care, which may significantly impact morbidity. Therefore, pit stops should only focus on life, limb and sight-saving interventions. This requires an understanding within trauma networks regarding the priorities of care, with trauma units being supported and prompted by the MTC trauma team leader.

Secondary transfer teams take critically ill patients from a relative place of safety and put them in a potentially hostile environment. Consequently, effective governance systems must be in place to control or minimise these hazards.

The patient should be conveyed without suffering harm or deterioration due to the transfer. This mandates that providers understand the physiology and evolution of trauma and the potential physiological effects of transfer [16, 17]. An effective transfer is not simply about the carriage of an individual but also about their ongoing management and optimisation within the confines of the operational space.

Human Factors

Human factors are those elements of behaviour and performance that can act as precursors to accidents and incidents. The number of factors is legion, but 12 common and inter-related elements have been identified in aviation and recur in accident investigation; the so-called, dirty dozen (Table 24.1). Whilst recognising and understanding these factors is crucial to creating, maintaining and developing a safe and efficient transfer service, it must be acknowledged that even the best drilled individuals and teams will make mistakes, occasionally leading to harm. The psychological safety of the team is vital to creating a culture that will allow accurate reporting, debriefing and sharing of lessons without fear of redress or humiliation. Similarly, support mechanisms must be in place for team members who need reassurance after witnessing or being party to an adverse event.

Table 24.1 The dirty dozen [18]

Lack of teamwork	Lack of assertiveness	Norms
Lack of awareness	Distraction	Fatigue
Lack of knowledge	Pressure	Complacency
Lack of communication	Stress	Lack of resources

Situational Awareness

Largely acquired through experience, this crucial skill demonstrates why novices should not be sent unaccompanied, and that provision should be made for trainees to learn alongside more experienced staff. At different stages of a patient move, individual team members will become relatively task-focused, emphasising that situational awareness must be a collective responsibility. In particular, the aeromedical world presents hazards related to noise and moving parts. In turn, aircraft are at risk from FOD (foreign object damage) and dangerous air cargo; therefore, patient packaging must be meticulous. It is mandatory that practitioners are familiar with the transport equipment and recognise the features of normal operation and any weaknesses in functionality. This enables full participation and troubleshooting as required.

Key Points

Zero-point surveys are used in resuscitation scenarios and can be readily adapted to promote the safe transfer of casualties [13]. At any point in the patient's journey where a change in location or position occurs, lines, tubes and monitoring are at potential risk of becoming dislodged. Zero-point surveys before each stage of transfer are helpful to confirm readiness to perform and conclude an activity.

S Self:—physical readiness, am I prepared, am I safe?

T Team:—who is leading, do others know their roles, deliver brief

E Environment:—hazards, space, light, noise, crowd control, temperature, shelter from the elements. It may not be possible to control the environment, such as aircraft noise and rotor downwash, therefore stop and check when out of those immediate environs.

P Patient:—MABCD assessment/check

U Update:—share mental model of patient status

P Priorities:—identify team goals, set mission trajectory

Team Structure and Function

When proposing a retrieval formation, it is important to be clear how staffing requirements have been calculated. The involvement of an experienced Human Resources practitioner when building and costing an establishment may reduce future management challenges, particularly when sessional staff are drawn from other employers.

Although there is considerable overlap in the team profile required to deliver primary and secondary retrievals, the pre-hospital environment has traditionally been seen as the realm of Emergency Medicine specialists, whilst critical care transfers are the domain of Anaesthetists and Intensivists. These divisions have related to the practical skill sets achieved during speciality training and the different experiences of providing organ support. With transfer training now codified into the training syllabi as part of a specialist trainee pathway for a variety of clinical specialities and sub specialities, these boundaries have faded. This has further been supported by the development of formal qualifications such as the Diploma in Retrieval and Transfer medicine from the Royal College of Surgeons of Edinburgh [19]. We are now seeing the evolution of practitioners with generic skill sets, who can provide best-practice care, whether at the incident scene or during primary or secondary transfer.

The most reliable and consistent performance will come from established transfer teams, with their size and composition determined by the service provider, patient population and the available means of transport. The military usually operates with four-person teams, but in the civilian setting, the size constraints of the transfer platform often serve to limit the medical squad to two. Typically, one will be a doctor, whilst the other could be a nurse, operating department practitioner or paramedic. Qualification in a particular field of practice should not confer automatic inclusion or exclusion to an individual. It is recognised that each profession brings its own skills, knowledge and perspective. The Emergency Medical Retrieval Service in Scotland has successfully created a generic Retrieval Practitioner role with recruitment from a Nursing (EM or ICU) or Paramedic background, acknowledging that nurses can be trained to do pre-hospital tasks and paramedics can be instructed in critical care transfers. These practitioners work in a variety of transport platforms, including rotary and fixed-wing aircraft. Successful teams function to a level greater than the sum of their parts, representing an amalgamation of skills, training and personality. Most teams exist in a state of flux, seeing changes of kit, personnel and vehicles with learning coming from collective experience, exposure, training and debriefing. Whilst every team must have a clear leader, any authority gradient must allow all team members to contribute. At different phases of the transfer, the skill set and practitioner required to execute an activity may change.

Standardisation and Processes

There are many aspects of the transfer process that can be controlled and made predictable by applying Standard Operating Procedures. These should aim to reduce individual variability without stifling clinical judgement. There should be standardisation of equipment, regular maintenance and function tests, regular re-qualification examinations, and hands-on simulation scenarios to facilitate this.

The precise configuration of the kit and ancillaries is to a certain extent dependent on the expected mode of transport and the reliance on this for operational capability. A service that can operate independently of a vehicles power and oxygen supply has the greatest flexibility, but often requires a greater payload to support this versatility.

Equipment must be compliant with extant legislation making it suitable for use in medical transport such as land and air ambulances. This extends to how equipment is secured in vehicles, and whenever available, specialist patient transfer trolleys with securing brackets should be used. CEN 1789 (European Committee on Standardisation) [20] and British Standards compliant electromed will have been tested to withstand the rigours of the transfer environment and have inbuilt dampening technology to prevent erroneous observations.

Checklists and Establishing the Appropriate Norms

Norms refer to the 'way we do things', with workplace practices developing over time, influenced by local experience and culture. Without scrutiny, actions can be both good and bad, safe and unsafe, with rogue elements deviating from best practice. Since norms are enforced through peer pressure and habit, it is essential to develop psychologically safe, well-governed services that follow best practice guidelines.

Medical teams are increasingly using checklists in their field of practice. They are of proven benefit in transfer medicine when packaging kit and drugs, or when performing interventions on the move [21]. Like any item of kit, they should have a specific location within the transfer bags and be readily accessible to the team.

Various process links have been made between medicine and aviation, particularly in the areas of communication, checklists and emergency action cards. The aviation industry accepted that it was unrealistic for aircrew to commit everything to memory and precisely recall information as required, especially in an emergency situation [22–25]. Checklists are not intended to replace team members expertise and knowledge, but removing the cognitive burden of simple tasks allows their timely progression and is evidenced based in support of safe procedures.

Key Points

In order to be effective, a checklist should have a number of features:

1. Purpose—To assist in a high-risk procedure or complex logistics pathway
2. Structured and logical
3. Have an endpoint that leads to an action/intervention, e.g. RSI checklist
4. Involve at least two people—the challenger and the responder
5. Each challenge should require a response, e.g. confirming that equipment is present or provide specific information.
6. Presented in a way that makes it legible (font size, text/background contrast), use of colour, borders and sections to ensure lines are not accidentally missed and provide an intermediate point to return to if the checklist is interrupted for some reason.
7. Mandated use by all team members in a predictable and consistent way.

An extension of the checklist is the Emergency Action Card (EAC) which is a method of confirming that the required actions in response to an event have been carried out correctly. Most actions in response to an emergency will be carried out immediately and from memory, with the EAC being used to confirm actions. If the situation remains unresolved, the EAC may be used to facilitate troubleshooting. This is especially useful in an environment where normal cues such as equipment alarms may go unnoticed due to excessive noise or poor lighting.

Examples of EAC topics:

- Accidental extubation
- Sudden fall in SpO_2
- Sudden rise in Peak Airway Pressure
- Falling $EtCO_2$

Simulation Training

Transfer medicine is well suited to simulation training. Every opportunity should be taken to rehearse a team before they go live wearing the necessary clothing and PPE to ensure safety and comfort. It is vital to thoroughly debrief these practice sessions and address any lessons learned—this is best facilitated by using a 'faculty' to run the scenario. The debrief should also form part of the wash-up after completing a patient move, and this should include all those directly involved. Inward looking debriefs rarely identify subtle problems and do not lead to sustained service development. These sessions can also be a valuable testbed for new procedures or checklists and can further identify potential hazards to staff or patients without placing either group in danger.

Drilling teams in common or emergency tasks using standardised equipment and procedures builds memory, creates more resilient individuals and permits the promulgation of lessons learned to the wider transfer network. Establishing a robust learning and audit culture is essential to developing a progressive transfer team that can communicate and implement lessons learned. However, implementing changes in practice will only be effective if they have been disseminated to the wider group. This can be a challenge when large numbers of part-time sessional staff are involved. Regular briefing communications should be distributed amongst all team members to encourage engagement with service development projects and learning from the experience of others. A robust governance system goes hand in hand with this learning culture, and team members should feel comfortable and have easy access to an event reporting system. This system needs to have a positive output and be seen as benefitting the service and individual development and safety.

Command and Control

Ideally, there should be a 'tasking authority' who receive transfer requests and deploy the appropriate medical assets. Acting as a focal point, they reduce the medical team's administrative burden, allowing them to focus on the mission. Transfer teams are purely present to deliver clinical care, not to facilitate timetables or crew duty hours. The control centre should act to manage these expectations whilst enabling conference calls between interested parties.

The control centre acts as the communication, transport and logistic hub for the transfer team. They will facilitate access to resources that are not routinely used on all missions, such as anti-malarials for international flights, blood products or specialist drugs. The control centre must have an empathetic relationship with the transfer team by ensuring missions run as seamlessly as possible, and personnel are recovered back to the home base with the minimum of delay, assuming that the next mission is always just about to hit the controllers screen. Good examples of established command and control hubs are The Royal Air Force Aeromedical Evacuation Control Centre (AECC) and the Scottish Ambulance Service (SAS) Specialist Services Desk (SSD).

Preparation

To reduce the risks to the patient, crew and vehicle, significant patient interventions should be performed before leaving a fixed location. Whilst road ambulances have the ability to stop quickly and provide a stable platform, that option is less readily available when air assets are used. Therefore, it is essential to confirm that all lines and tubes are well secured, and that staff have good access to intravenous ports. A general rule of thumb is to secure the lines and tubes to the patient, the patient to the stretcher and the stretcher to the transport. Any infusions should be changed at the point of departure, with prefilled replacements easily to hand.

Similarly, batteries should be fully charged and sufficient oxygen carried for twice the expected transit time. Preparing the patient with access and orientation guided by the transport platform can significantly reduce the amount of line and tube husbandry required once the patient is loaded. If the standard road ambulance has a stretcher position that makes access to one side of the patient more difficult, consider this when siting and securing IV cannulae or invasive pressure transducers. Equipment accessibility is an essential consideration during transport, particularly in small air platforms where bags may need to be stowed out of reach for safety and security. During road transport, bags are generally accessible but should be secured to avoid them becoming potential hazards should the vehicle turn or brake suddenly.

For longer transports, aspects of nursing care that are not often considered in shorter, primary transfers need to be contemplated. For example, patients should be rolled where possible to inspect and alleviate the impacts of pressure damage from lying in one position for prolonged periods. When packaging patients, consideration should be given to using devices such as vacuum mattresses to distribute pressure on "at risk" areas to mitigate against long periods of immobility, especially when anaesthetised [26, 27]. Prolonged contact with moist areas from leaking dressings or other bodily fluids can also contribute to skin damage, so inspection of wounds, monitoring of vacuum dressing systems or re-dressing saturated bandages need to be possible. Packaging also needs to take into account the ambient temperature, as patients can very easily become hypothermic following anaesthesia or trauma [28]; however, they can also become hyperthermic if packaged incorrectly.

During transfer, the aim should be to remain seated and secure whilst monitoring the patient and any ongoing therapies (Fig. 24.1). There should be no routine requirement for personnel to move around the back of an ambulance whilst travelling, as this exposes the whole team and patient to increased risk. Accessibility to equipment also includes items such as syringe pumps, the monitor and ventilator, which should be visible and within arm's reach of at least one of the team to enable changes to be made from the security of their seat.

Requesting the vehicle to pull over and stop, or in extremis asking a helicopter to land should always be a briefed option. However, this choice is not readily available to colleagues using fixed-wing assets.

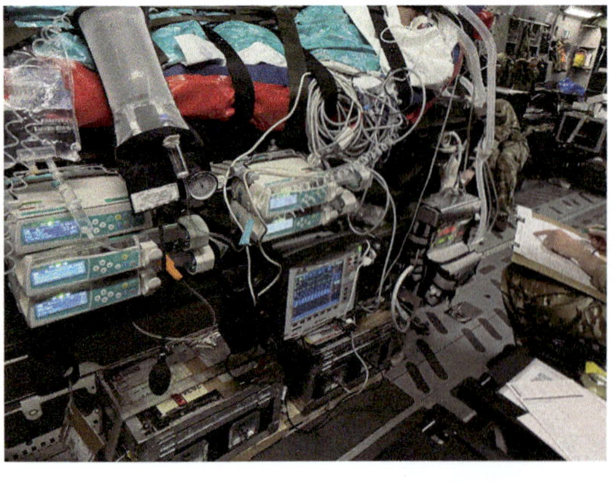

Fig. 24.1 An RAF CCAST repatriation. Note the equipment and monitoring is set up so that the accompanying team can remain seated during landing and takeoff and still have access to all monitoring and infusions

Loading Plan

Loading and unloading is a particularly challenging part of the transfer process when the chance of tube and line displacement is highest. There are several decisions to be made during this phase, and they should all be made well in advance of moving the patient:

- How will the patient be positioned?
- What access to the patient is possible?
- How does that fit with existing tubes and lines?
- Do any interventions need to occur?
- How will the patient, equipment, bags and transfer team be secured?

In most instances, the transport platforms available to individual teams will be limited, and teams must rehearse loading with the relevant crews.

Spatial constraints usually dictate the location of kit during the move, and this needs to be a consideration when packing bags.

Equipment Packaging and Carriage

To manage the patient's expected physiological path and to mitigate against potential untoward events, transfer teams should have considerable redundancy in the equipment, drugs, and consumables carried. Bags should be packed in accordance with a checklist so that the location of specific items is never in doubt or subject to individual variation. Consideration must be given to the manual handling implications of transfer bags and the weight consequences for the transport platform. Transfer teams working in the pre-hospital environment may have to access awkward locations and do not want to be impeded by heavy or bulky bags. An individual transfer bag should not exceed 20 kg as this becomes a manual handling issue. The stowage of bags in transit needs to allow for heavy braking, landing, or vehicular accidents and a suitably attached carabiner and webbing sling provides a simple but effective solution.

Visual and loud audible alarms within specific patient limits should be set on electromedical equipment to enable team awareness of changes to the patients' condition. A designated team member must have 'eyes on' the monitor at all times during the transfer, and they should be provided with effective means of gaining the attention of the rest of the team should the patient deteriorate.

Feeling Included

Within established teams and irrespective of rank or role, the use of first names is commonplace and demonstrates trust and bonding within the group. Frequently however, teams will rely on other allied health professionals (e.g. ambulance crews) to complete their missions. Asking for first names can promote inclusivity and reduce barriers to effective communication.

Communication within the Team

Effective communication maintains team situational awareness and shares the team leaders "mental model". All team members must feel empowered and have the confidence to converse with the wider group. In most circumstances, communication will be through normal conversation or via a headset, but predetermined hand signals can be used. In noisy, low lit environments, the use of headsets dramatically improves communication and reduces the fatigue experienced by otherwise hypervigilant staff. Established transfer teams with individual familiarity, strong SOP structure and a system of daily and pre-mission briefs will experience fewer communication problems in difficult environments. The team will share a common mental model where complex or urgent communication will be the exception to the norm, reducing the likelihood of misheard or misunderstood messages.

The military "SMEAAC" model of briefing can have some value when seeking a reproducible communication structure:

- Situation: What is happening at the moment?
- Mission: What do we plan to do?
- Execution: How are we going to achieve the plan?
- Actions on: What will we do if things go wrong?

Any questions?: An opportunity for the team to raise concerns or clarify any unclear points.

- Confirm understanding: Check team understanding.

Whilst the level of ambient environmental noise determines the method of communication and hearing protection required, it does not guarantee perfect and unambiguous message transfer in all circumstances. Effective use of aircraft intercom systems requires practice to become accustomed to voice distortion and lack of non-verbal cues.

Intercom systems should have the capability to "isolate" the transfer team to allow medical discussions without distracting the aircrew. However, these periods should be kept to a minimum to ensure that medical crew remain situationally aware of the aircraft state and overall mission progress.

Mission Communication

Good communication is paramount in trauma retrieval to eliminate unnecessary delays. Transfer teams need to know where they are going, how they are getting there, who will meet them and how long it will take. During the journey, it is desirable that tasking agencies and receiving facilities can be contacted in the event of delay, diversion or deterioration. Access to a reliable form of 2-way communication is essential, whether via mobile or Airwave system. For secondary transfers, a tripartite conversation between referring unit, receiving centre and transfer team ensures a common understanding of the patient condition and plans before departure. This significantly reduces the potential for misinterpretation of clinical information and facilitates an efficient handover on completion of the journey. A long narrative is not required, but the information provided as an ATMIST should assist the receiving team in planning for the patients' arrival and determining whether a Trauma Team or Code Red activation is required. There is no excuse for a critically injured patient to arrive unannounced at a receiving facility.

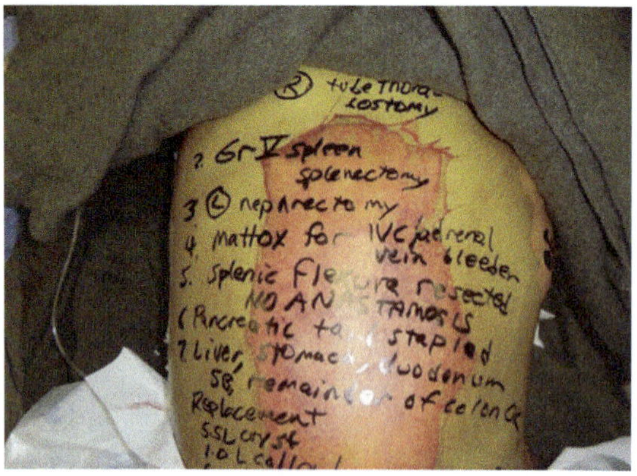

Fig. 24.2 Patient post damage control laparotomy who may be transferred for definitive care. The operative information may be passed on via a variety of means! [29]

Clinical Information

Where teams are working on regular referral pathways or within networks, documentation should be agreed upon and standardised to ensure effective communication and data collection for both clinical and audit purposes. For continuity of care and avoidance of significant omissions, it is imperative that the transfer team hand over and leave copies of all clinical information before they disperse. In its simplest form, handover includes patient details and an ATMIST/ AMPLE brief, but following DCR is likely to comprise operation notes and findings, imaging and reports, resuscitative fluids, drugs given, next of kin details and agreed ceiling of treatment/resuscitation status (Fig. 24.2). Wherever possible, trauma networks should enable image sharing between receiving hospitals and the MTC to limit the requirement for re-imaging and further exposure to ionising radiation. This is especially important in the paediatric population, where they are at greater risk of radiation-induced malignancy or infertility.

Team Welfare

The overall welfare of the team is the responsibility of the team leader but requires the attention of all team members. Fatigue is a natural physiological response to prolonged physical and or mental stress. It reduces concentration, impairs memory and degrades decision making as the individual becomes easily distracted and loses situational awareness. They may exhibit mood changes, becoming withdrawn or aggressive, but unfortunately transfers do not follow shift patterns or sleep cycles. Individuals may be stressed through hypervigilance and/or the effects of noise, vibration and travel sickness. Cumulative fatigue is a safety risk for the whole team, and it is the responsibility of all team members to recognise fatigue in themselves and others, particularly during overnight missions.

Daily routines should allow for meal breaks, although a team "welfare pack" with snacks, drinks and cash should be prepared for short notice moves. This pack should also include a small stock of team medications for minor but debilitating ailments such as headaches and motion sickness.

Infection Control

The team and gaining unit must be made aware if the patient is subject to source or protective isolation, applying to both active infections and colonisation. Provision of appropriate PPE, including eye and respiratory protection is vital. Alcohol-based hand rubs, sharps receptacles and decontamination materials must be available and easily secured for transport. Hand hygiene can be difficult in transit; larger platforms such as fixed-wing aircraft may offer toilets with sinks. While soap and water are preferable, hand wash wipes and alcohol-based hand rubs are acceptable substitutes. Enhanced cleans of vehicles are time consuming and impact on the availability of vehicles and equipment. This should be a consideration when planning multiple, sequential patient transfers.

Insertion of biomedical devices such as cannulas and the drawing up medications in a hospital setting will save time, effort and allow for the appropriate level of asepsis. Any devices placed in transit under 'suboptimal' conditions must be documented and handed over accordingly. Aseptic Non-Touch Technique (ANTT) can be maintained even in the transfer environment and should form a part of any training serials.

Recovery Phase

After a transfer, hardware needs to be decontaminated, consumables and drugs replaced, and electrical equipment placed on charge. Depending on the transfer service structure and the distances and time travelled, there may be a relief crew and a second set of equipment that is checked and ready to use. A team with a high mission rate may not always have time to restock before their next job, so there should be a degree of resilience in the capability. Local experience and circumstances will determine the amount of reserve equipment required, and for those teams involved in major incident response, this resilience becomes crucial. Depending on the time of day and duration of the mission, thought should be given to delaying critical replenishment tasks or delegating them to a 'reserve' team. This is because the effect of fatigue leading to mistakes or omissions in restocking bags is significant. Kit and equipment that cannot be replenished because of supply or servicing issues should be quarantined until returned to full complement.

Contemporary Transfer Medicine

Transfer Medicine is an emerging speciality and represents all the complexities of moving a critically injured patient safely. The significance of a Post Graduate Diploma in Retrieval and Transfer Medicine facilitated by the RCS in Edinburgh highlights the speciality's growing maturity and importance. The days of using the most junior or least missed members of a department to move a patient should be long gone, as the casualty requires skilled, senior involvement at all stages of their clinical journey. These rules should be applied to all transfers, whether within a hospital's confines or when moving a patient to definitive care.

Conclusion

Trauma transfers are potentially hazardous for both the patient and their escorts. They should only be undertaken by individuals trained for the task, familiar with the kit and the working environment. Classroom lessons and simulation exercises should be completed before supervised practice is allowed. Good communication strategies and the use of standard operating procedures with checklists will provide team members with a shared mental model allowing safe carriage of complex casualties.

Questions

1. Which of these is not one of the human factors dirty dozen?
   (a) Assertiveness
   (b) Distraction
   (c) Pressure
   (d) Stress
2. Which are the truly key points in transfer medicine?
   (a) Most patients settle into a steady state during transfer.
   (b) Patient escorts do not require seat belts as they need rapid access to their patient.
   (c) Leave nothing to chance.
   (d) Intra hospital moves can be safely conducted by junior staff under distant supervision.

3. Regarding Zero-point surveys
   (a) They are conducted as part of a wash-up debrief.
   (b) Include an assessment of 'self'.
   (c) Are patient focussed.
   (d) Are optional for individual team members.
4. Which of the following is not a feature of checklists
   (a) They are intended for high-risk procedures.
   (b) They are structured and logical.
   (c) They have an endpoint leading to an action.
   (d) No response is required to a challenge.
5. Which is not part of the SMEAC model of briefing
   (a) Situation: what is happening at the moment?
   (b) Mission: what do we plan to do?
   (c) Execution: how are we going to achieve the plan?
   (d) Actions on: what are the timings for the mission?

Answers

1. a
2. c
3. b
4. d
5. d

References

1. Faculty of Intensive Care Medicine, Intensive Care Society. Guidance On: The Transfer of the Critically Ill Adult [Internet]. 2019. Available from: https://www.ficm.ac.uk/sites/default/files/transfer_critically_ill_adult_2019.pdf
2. National Institute for Health and Care Excellence (Great Britain). Emergency and acute medical care in over 16s: service delivery and organisation. Chapter 34: [Internet]. Manchester: National Institute for Health and Care Excellence (NICE); 2018 [cited 2020 Oct 13]. Available from: https://www.nice.org.uk/guidance/ng94/evidence/34.standardised-systems-of-care-for-intra-and-interhospital-transfers-pdf-172397464673
3. AAGBI. Interhospital transfer [Internet]. The Association of Anaesthetists of Great Britain and Ireland; 2009 [cited 2020 June 19]. Available from: https://anaesthetists.org/Home/Resources-publications/Guidelines/Interhospital-transfer-AAGBI-safety-guideline
4. Jia L, Wang H, Gao Y, Liu H, Yu K. High incidence of adverse events during intra-hospital transport of critically ill patients and new related risk factors: a prospective, multicenter study in China. Crit Care [Internet]. 2016 Jan 18 [cited 2020 Oct 10]: [20 p.]. Available from: https://www.ncbi.nlm.nih.gov/pmc/articles/PMC4717618/
5. Parmentier-Decrucq E, Poissy J, Favory R, Nseir S, Onimus T, Guerry M-J, et al. Adverse events during intrahospital transport of critically ill patients: incidence and risk factors. Ann Intensive Care. 2013;3(1):10.
6. Knight PH, Maheshwari N, Hussain J, Scholl M, Hughes M, Papadimos TJ, et al. Complications during intrahospital transport of critically ill patients: focus on risk identification and prevention. Int J Crit Illn Inj Sci. 2015;5(4):256–64.
7. Lahner D, Nikolic A, Marhofer P, Koinig H, Germann P, Weinstabl C, et al. Incidence of complications in intrahospital transport of critically ill patients--experience in an Austrian university hospital. Wien Klin Wochenschr. 2007;119(13–14):412–6.
8. Paton L, Stenhouse J, Ruddy J, Howie N. Still preparing to fail by failing to prepare? A survey of trainees' experience of and training in interhospital transfers. J Intensive Care Soc. 2014;15(1):43–7.
9. Wiegersma JS, Droogh JM, Zijlstra JG, Fokkema J, Ligtenberg JJM. Quality of interhospital transport of the critically ill: impact of a mobile intensive care unit with a specialized retrieval team. Crit Care Lond Engl. 2011;15(1):R75.
10. Bellingan G, Olivier T, Batson S, Webb A. Comparison of a specialist retrieval team with current United Kingdom practice for the transport of critically ill patients. Intensive Care Med. 2000;26(6):740–4.
11. Macmillan A, Bricknell M. A view of future issues for defence medical training. RUSI J. 2004;149(6):48–54.
12. Whymper E. Scrambles amongst the Alps: in the years 1860–1869. Berkeley, CA: Ten Speed Press; 1981. 164 p.
13. Reid C, Brindley P, Hicks C, Carley S, Richmond C, Lauria M, et al. Zero point survey: a multidisciplinary idea to STEP UP resuscitation effectiveness. Clin Exp Emerg Med. 2018;5(3):139–43.
14. Hearns S. Peak performance under pressure [Internet]. 2019 [cited 2020 Oct 13]. Available from: http://www.vlebooks.com/vleweb/product/openreader?id=none&isbn=9781859598597
15. Davies G, Chesters A. Transport of the trauma patient. Br J Anaesth. 2015;115(1):33–7.
16. Beard L, Lax P, Tindall M. Physiological effects of transfer for critically ill patients. Anaesth Tutor Week. 2016;330:7.
17. Hale JJ, Hall DP, Dunn MJG. Physiology of patient transfer by land and air. Anaesth Intensive Care Med. 2019;20(10):595–9.

18. Dupont G. Human performance factors for elementary work and servicing [Internet]. Transport Canada; 2003 [cited 2020 Oct 7]. Available from: http://www.skybrary.aero/bookshelf/books/2038.pdf
19. DiplomainRetrievalandTransferMedicine-TheFaculty of Pre-Hospital Care [Internet]. [cited 2020 Oct 10]. Available from: https://fphc.rcsed.ac.uk/examinations/diploma-in-retrieval-and-transfer-medicine
20. CEN - Technical Bodies - CEN/TC 239 [Internet]. [cited 2020 Oct 13]. Available from: https://standards.cen.eu/dyn/www/f?p=204:32:0::::FSP_ORG_ID,FSP_LANG_ID:6220,25&cs=1B1D012F382EE77C2A7F801C99ADA007A
21. Chaparro A, Keebler JR, Lazzara EH, Diamond A. Checklists: a review of their origins, benefits, and current uses as a cognitive aid in medicine. Ergon Des. 2019;27(2):21–6.
22. Ross P. Human factors issues of the aircraft checklist. J Aviat/Aerosp Educ Res. 2004;13(2):7.
23. Clay-Williams R, Colligan L. Back to basics: checklists in aviation and healthcare. BMJ Qual Saf. 2015;24(7):428–31.
24. Barshi I, Mauro R, Degani A, Loukopoulou L. Designing Flightdeck Procedures - NASA Technical Memorandum 2016–219421 [Internet]. NASA; 2016 [cited 2020 Oct 13]. Available from: http://www.sti.nasa.gov
25. Degani A, Wiener EL. Cockpit checklists: concepts, design, and use. Hum Factors J Hum Factors Ergon Soc. 1993;35(2):345–59.
26. Sheerin F, de Frein R. The occipital and sacral pressures experienced by healthy volunteers under spinal immobilization: a trial of three surfaces. J Emerg Nurs. 2007;33(5):447–50.
27. Chan D, Goldberg RM, Mason J, Chan L. Backboard versus mattress splint immobilization: a comparison of symptoms generated. J Emerg Med. 1996;14(3):293–8.
28. Langhelle A, Lockey D, Harris T, Davies G. Body temperature of trauma patients on admission to hospital: a comparison of anaesthetised and non-anaesthetised patients. Emerg Med J. 2012;29(3):239–42.
29. Galante JM, Gordon WT, Martin MJ, Rodriguez CJ. Managing dismounted complex blast injuries in military & civilian settings: guidelines and principles. 1st ed. Cham: Springer; 2018: Imprint: Springer; 2018. 1 p
30. Nirula R, Maier R, Moore E, Sperry J, Gentilello L. Scoop and run to the trauma center or stay and play at the local hospital: hospital transfer's effect on mortality. J Trauma. 2010;69(3):595–9. discussion 599–601

Sedation and Field Amputation

25

Caroline Leech and Jonathan Veitch

- An introduction to sedation for painful procedures.
- Sedation for field amputation
- Indications for prehospital amputation and consideration of the potential risks of the procedure.
- Preparation of equipment and checklists for actions: including for use before decision to perform, immediately before procedure, and post emergency amputation (immediate and delayed actions).
- The surgical technique for emergency limb amputation in the field: including standard guillotine technique and novel methods in extreme circumstances.
- An overview of the pharmacology, doses and side effects of drugs commonly used for procedural sedation

C. Leech (✉)
Emergency Department, University Hospitals Coventry and Warwickshire NHS Trust, Coventry, UK

The Air Ambulance Service (TAAS), Rugby, Warwickshire, UK
e-mail: Caroline.Leech@uhcw.nhs.uk

J. Veitch
Department of Anaesthesia, Nottingham University Teaching Hospitals NHS Trus, Nottingham, UK

212 Field Hospital (Reserves), Sheffield, UK
e-mail: jveitch@doctors.org.uk

Introduction

Emergency limb amputation is a very rare procedure that may be necessary in the pre-hospital setting to save a life. Amputation may be required due to entrapment in the wreckage of a road traffic collision, building collapse, or industrial and agricultural machinery. There is limited literature on pre-hospital amputation [1], with the exception of heterogenous case reports which are prone to publication bias [2]. While most of these publications have focussed on the mechanics and technical conduct of surgical amputation, often little consideration is given to the strategy of sedation to facilitate the procedure. There is morbidity and mortality associated with sedation, which can be increased in isolated environments and with sicker patients [3, 4]. This chapter aims to outline some considerations around the use of sedation for painful procedures, both in- and pre-hospital with specific reference to the performance of emergency amputation. There is also an overview of some of the common sedative agents and considerations of which agents may be most appropriate in specific circumstances.

Sedation

Appropriate and safe use of sedation has the potential to reduce pain and anxiety, decrease Post Traumatic Stress Disorder (PTSD) [5, 6] and increase the ease of transportation of injured

P. Lax (ed.), *Textbook of Acute Trauma Care*, https://doi.org/10.1007/978-3-030-83628-3_25

patients. It can facilitate life or limb-saving therapeutic procedures to be undertaken outside of the theatre environment in a humane way. The requirement to reduce fractures and dislocations, in order to treat neurovascular compromise, can be function- or even limb-saving.

The ideal sedating agent would allow titration, be cardiovascularly stable, provide maintenance of respiratory drive and airway reflexes, along with a rapid reversal if required. Currently no such agent fulfils these requirements completely so the choice of agent (or agents) rests on the end point required. The "classic triad" of anaesthesia that should be considered is analgesia, amnesia and paralysis. All three elements may not be required in each instance and the degree and depth of each element that is required also changes.

Gaining experience with sedation is vital and initial training should be done in a fully monitored hospital environment with an experienced supervisor. There must be consideration of individual patient variation in pharmacodynamics and pharmacokinetics (especially in those who are cardiovascularly compromised). Even experienced anaesthetists and procedural sedationists are caught out occasionally; the important thing is to be able to deal with any potential complications. There are multiple guidelines for safe sedation practices in various settings and across different populations [7], but the common theme is that there are minimum standards of training and monitoring that are required, and that continual audit and standardisation of procedures should be undertaken to ensure safety [8].

Sedation in Practice

The art of sedation is based around achieving a blend of hypnosis, anxiolysis and analgesia appropriate for the clinical situation. No one drug provides all these in an easily titratable way, therefore a combination of agents is commonly used. However, the number of agents used should be kept as low as possible as many drugs will act synergistically and may lead to over-sedation. Complex regimes are more prone to failure or complications than simple ones, and increasing depth of sedation is associated with a higher risk of complications [9]. The following are examples of sedation regimes in commonly occurring situations: they are by no means the only combination that will work, nor the best in every individual patient or in each setting (pre-hospital vs ED vs operating theatre). Experience will shape the choice of agent and help avoid common pitfalls. Institutional or organisational guidelines should be developed in conjunction with all parties who may be involved in sedation, and with reference to established national guidelines where relevant [7, 8, 10]. Regular audit and feedback should be employed to continually improve local practice.

When performing procedural sedation, it is important to ensure an appropriate level of monitoring (including end-tidal CO_2 levels) and to plan for all potential complications. Common factors to consider should be over- or under-sedation, loss of the airway and subsequent desaturation, dysphoria (if using ketamine) and vomiting. A pre-sedation brief (ideally supported by a checklist, such as Fig. 25.1) should be completed and all members of staff involved should

Procedural Sedation Checklist

Indication?	Agreed
Assessment of potential problems?	Discussed
Oxygen (+1 spare cylinder)	Check
IV access (check patency)	Check
Monitoring (ECG / NIBP / Sats / ETCO2)	Check
Rescue equipment (Suction / BVM / Airway kit)	Check
Action plan & equipment	Check
Roles allocated	Check

Fig. 25.1 Pre-sedation checklist (reproduced with permission of The Air Ambulance Service)

know the plan in each of these scenarios and have equipment to hand to effectively manage them. Ideally, two points of patent IV or IO access should be achieved in case one point becomes dislodged or fails mid-procedure, and further sedation or emergency drugs need to be given quickly.

Sedation for Painful Procedures

There are many procedures in trauma care that require short periods of sedation, either in- or pre-hospital. These include application of traction splints or insertion of chest drains in patients with haemothoraces or pneumothoraces. The pain of traumatic dislocation and/or fracture of a joint can be significantly relieved by early relocation of the joint or reduction of the fracture. Many of the methods described below would be appropriate for these procedures or circumstances, with the exception of inhaled agents in patients with chest trauma.

The aims of sedation for fracture manipulation or joint relocation are short lived analgesia and relaxation of muscles. Analgesia may be sufficient for fracture manipulation, and occasionally can be achieved with just a short acting opiate, entonox or methoxyflurane in isolation. Both gases have analgesic onset in around 6–8 breaths and as an example, alfentanil will have onset within 60 s. On cessation of inspiration of the gas or after the last bolus of alfentanil, the duration of analgesia will only be a few minutes. Occasionally, some muscle relaxation may be needed to aid the procedure, especially in cases of prosthetic hip dislocation or prolonged time before attempted relocation. This muscle relaxation may be achieved with midazolam, which may also cause some amnesia of the events and anxiolysis [11]. Commonly a dose of 1–2 mg will suffice if another agent is being used (and is insufficient on its own—e.g. propofol), without leading to excessive sedation after successful relocation. Further longer acting analgesia should be considered once the procedure has been completed and the patient is more awake. The pitfall to avoid is the administration of long acting analgesics before joint relocation, as once the painful stimulus has decreased then over-sedation purely from analgesics is a distinct possibility. In terms of agent choice, propofol in isolation is associated with a faster recovery time than midazolam in isolation due to its pharmacological profile (3 min with propofol vs 45 min with midazolam in one recent study) [12]. The use of propofol target controlled infusions (TCI) is ideal in these cases as the majority of propofol offset is from redistribution rather than metabolism, and TCI pumps will alter their infusion rates automatically to maintain a fixed (and titratable) concentration set by the sedationist. These pumps are commonly used in operating theatres and require training, so may not be practical in other settings by non-anaesthetic staff, though current evidence suggests a lower rate of complications, lower overall drug dose but the same depth and desired duration of sedation [13].

Sedation for Amputation

Emergency amputation in the pre-hospital environment is uncommon but may be required due to entrapment with deterioration necessitating rapid extrication to allow life threatening injuries to be treated immediately (Fig. 25.2). The techniques and equipment required are discussed later in this chapter. In the awake, or semi-conscious patient, this will require a high degree of sedation and analgesia. In an ideal situation, general anaesthetic with a protected airway would be provided, to allow judicious analgesia and guarantee amnesia. However, in cases of entrapment access to the airway may be significantly compromised and intravenous access difficult.

In these complex scenarios, the intraosseous route or intramuscular route may still be achievable. All intravenous agents can be given in the same dose through the intraosseous route with similar onset times, but intramuscular dosing requires an increase dose to allow for reduced absorption and has a longer onset. In the cardiovascularly unstable patient, poor peripheral perfusion can significantly reduce the intramuscular absorption of drugs further, rendering the blood concentration subtherapeutic and with a more prolonged onset time. For these reasons, IM sedation is an option of last resort. Every effort should be made to gain intravenous or intraosseous access, especially before initiating sedation. In combative patients, IM administration of sedation may allow the patient to be sedated enough to achieve IV or IO access before proceeding with any other necessary intervention [14, 15].

Emergency amputation is a life saving procedure but this does not diminish the requirement for anaesthesia, analgesia and amnesia. Ideally the patient should have full monitoring attached and full access to the airway; this is due to the level of sedation required for an amputation being much deeper than the other procedures so far discussed.

Given the difficulties in this situation, ketamine seems the obvious choice. It provides excellent analgesia, a dissociative anaesthesia and has the greatest chance of maintaining respiratory drive along with airway reflexes. There is also the benefit in the haemodynamically compromised patient where other anaesthetic agents typically reduce cardiac output. Gaining experience with ketamine is essential before using it in these demanding situations. It can be difficult to assess adequate depth of sedation with ketamine for novice users, as vocalisations from the patient are common [16] and can be misinterpreted as them being inadequately sedated and in pain.

Emergency limb amputation in the prehospital setting is demanding and will require one dedicated practitioner to manage the sedation of the patient and a second to perform the amputation—one person cannot do both safely.

Indications for Pre-Hospital Amputation

1. An immediate and real risk to the patient's life due to a scene safety emergency e.g. fire, drowning.
2. A deteriorating patient physically trapped by a limb when they will almost certainly die during the time taken to secure extrication.
3. The patient is dead and their limbs are blocking access to potentially live casualties in the case of a multi-casualty major incident. Before moving bodies or amputating limbs, a picture should be taken of the body in place for the purposes of further forensic examination [1].

Figure 25.2 illustrates a scenario where the patient may be physically trapped by the lower limbs but will not survive to await mechanical extrication by the fire service.

Amputation may be considered for a completely mutilated non-survivable limb retaining minimal attachment, which is delaying extrication and evacuation from the scene in a non-immediate life-threatening situation. However, where possible this should be avoided, as it is very difficult to assess the likelihood of limb salvage in this setting. There have been cases where amputation was

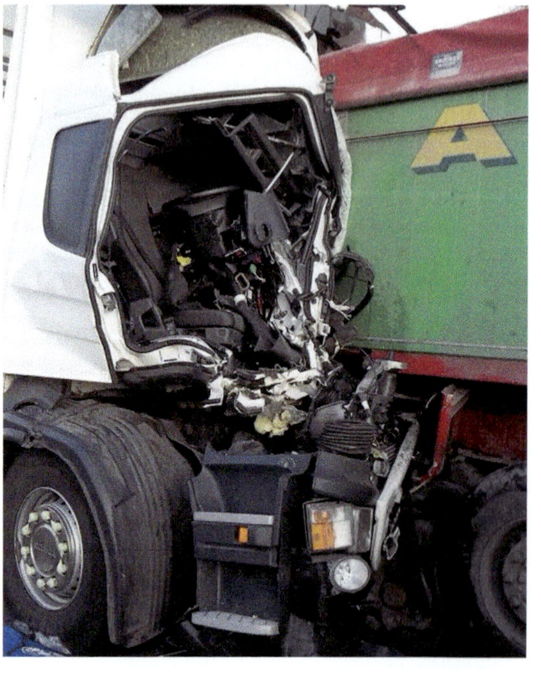

Fig. 25.2 Amputation may be required for the deteriorating patient physically trapped by a limb when they will almost certainly die during the time taken to secure extrication. Entrapment in the cab of an articulated lorry represents a situation where conventional rapid extrication may not be possible with a deteriorating patient

considered but the patient rescued, and subsequently the patient recovered with a functioning limb.

Equipment for Pre-Hospital Amputation

The following equipment is required for the surgical pre-hospital guillotine amputation:

- Commercial tourniquet (for prophylactic haemorrhage control × 2)
- Scalpel size 23 (for cutting skin and muscle)
- Gigli saw handles and wire (for cutting bone—more than one wire will be necessary in case of breakage)
- Spencer Wells Forceps (for passing and protecting wire)
- Paramedic shears (for cutting muscle)
- Artery forceps (for clamping of large vessels)
- Haemostatic gauze and emergency bandage (for pressure dressing of the stump)
- Sharps box (for safe disposal of sharps)

Consideration should be made to use alternative equipment to cut through the bone if the Gigli saw should fail e.g. using a hacksaw which is normally carried on fire service vehicles.

Main Risks of the Procedure

- Emergency amputation carries risks of sharps injuries from the equipment or fractured bone, and the risk of communicable diseases from blood exposure.
- Due to the entrapment, practitioners may be working in a confined space or an area with environmental risks.
- If the tourniquet fails to be used effectively, there is a risk of catastrophic haemorrhage.
- There is a risk of psychological trauma to emergency service workers and bystanders who have witnessed the case. This should be considered before the event to minimize unnecessary exposure, and after the event for psychological support.

Pre-Procedure Checks

Prior to proceeding with sedation and amputation, the pre-hospital practitioner should make the following checks:

1. Is there any other option for extrication? A discussion should take place between the Emergency Medical and the Fire Service personnel to ensure that all other options have been exhausted. There should be a shared mental model of the plan with all key individuals on scene. All equipment should be prepared for the procedure in a kit dump.
2. It is recommended that where possible, practitioners call their 'top cover' senior or peers for medical advice in their organisation to quickly discuss the case. This may provide additional ideas for rescue in a high-pressured environment and will ensure that support is available to the team immediately after.
3. A photograph of the scene and the entrapment should be taken to inform future debrief and investigation of the case.
4. Roles should be allocated for the emergency services team so that there is no time-lag when the patient is freed. This includes staff to manually handle the patient from the wreckage, a designated person to provide immediate haemorrhage control and dressing of the stump, and another to lead on primary survey and resuscitation of the patient after extrication. There is a risk that following the amputation, the practitioner who has performed the surgical procedure will have exceeded their bandwidth. Where there are multiple members of advanced critical care staff on scene, it is useful for one to concentrate only on the surgical procedure and another to only focus on the resuscitation when the patient is freed. An individual should be designated to look after sharps safety.
5. A pit stop area should be identified and laid out close to the entrapment for the patient to be received into immediately after the extrication. This is for immediate haemorrhage control and ABC life-saving interventions before moving on to more comprehensive care.

6. Tranexamic acid should be given, and a proximal haemorrhage control tourniquet should be applied and fully tightened with the time of application recorded.
7. The ambulance (and crew) which will be used to transport the patient to hospital should be identified and prepared. The vehicle should be orientated so that it can leave scene immediately without delay, the driver appropriately briefed, and internal heaters turned on to minimise heat loss from the patient and optimise conditions during transfer. If possible, a pre-alert phone call made to the receiving hospital informing them of the patient's status and current plan for amputation may be beneficial if there is a short transfer time to hospital.

Immediately Before the Procedure

The reaction of the patient to the pain of the tourniquet will indicate the level of sedation required to safely facilitate the procedure. In some cases, the patient will be moribund and no sedation will be required. In others, a carefully titrated sedative will be necessary. This should be titrated according to current blood pressure, conscious level, and the patient's level of pain.

Adequate Personal Protective Equipment (PPE) must be used, including eye protection.

The limb should be quickly inspected to identify the site of amputation and to ensure that the tourniquet has been applied with sufficient space to maintain compression on the stump after the limb has been removed. If the distance between amputation and tourniquet is too small, the tourniquet may fall off. If there is an obvious fracture site in the limb at the appropriate level, this should be chosen for the incision to facilitate a very quick amputation.

Immediately before starting the procedure, all members of staff on scene should be made aware so they can be focused on the procedure and their imminent tasks.

The Surgical Procedure

Once adequate analgesia/dissociative anaesthesia has been established and the tourniquet verified, the limb should be amputated as distally as possible to retain as much tissue and functional limb as possible. It is likely that the stump will need to be revised subsequently and the remaining limb length will be further shortened, so starting with as much tissue as possible is beneficial.

A scalpel is used to divide the skin circumferentially, cut through the subcutaneous tissues and open the fascia of the underlying muscle groups, and can continue to cut through the muscles. If this is difficult due to sharp safety, paramedic or "trauma" shears may be used to cut through muscle tissue. At this point, no attempt should be made to identify and clamp individual vessels, as this may prolong the time taken to complete the procedure. Limited access to the patient will impair identification of vessels, combined with the retraction of the vessels being cut. Prior correct placement and application of the tourniquet is the mainstay of haemostasis in this procedure.

After the soft tissues have been circumferentially incised, the Gigli wire is passed under the bone of the limb by picking up one end of the wire with the Spencer Wells forceps and passing it to the other side (Fig. 25.3). The handles should

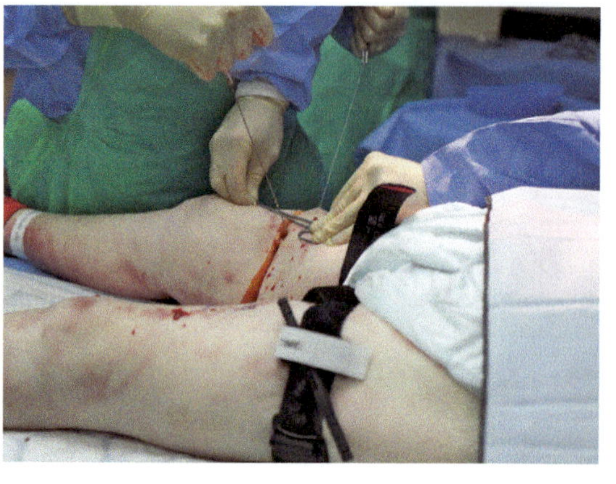

Fig. 25.3 Demonstration of guillotine amputation on a cadaveric lower limb (note Spencer Wells forceps ready to avoid injury from the Gigli wire after bone separation)

be applied at both ends of the wire and a back-and-forth action used to cut through the bone. An assistant should hold the Spencer Wells forceps over the gap to avoid the wire coming up into the practitioners face when the bone has been separated. Posterior soft tissue and skin may then need to be incised with scalpel or paramedic shears to complete the amputation if they are still attached.

Immediate Actions Post Procedure

The patient should be immediately extricated and moved to the pit-stop area for haemorrhage control and life-saving ABC management.

Haemorrhage control should include checking the stump for any bleeding. If there is active bleeding, the tourniquet should be tightened until bleeding stops. If this remains ineffective a second tourniquet can be applied more proximal to the first and fully tightened. Any obvious vessels at this point can now be clamped using artery forceps. A pressure bandage (+/− haemostatic gauze) should be applied with compression to the stump. Given the degree of anaesthesia needed (and for humanitarian reasons), performance of a rapid sequence intubation may be considered for airway protection. This should be discussed before starting the procedure and prepared for in advance, whilst weighing up the risks of further deterioration in a hypovolaemic patient.

Ongoing assessment and resuscitation of the patient should proceed, with evacuation to a Major Trauma Centre and definitive care as soon as possible. There is a real risk of slowing down at this point; momentum should be maintained to avoid unnecessarily long scene times.

If a prophylactic tourniquet has been applied to other limbs during entrapment (as the distal limb could not be inspected for haemorrhage in the trapped state) these should be reassessed and considered for removal if upon direct inspection there is no active bleeding.

The fire crew should be asked to continue to attempt to extricate the trapped body part where feasible and it should be transported to hospital as the skin may be used for surgical reconstruction later. However, this may not be safe or achievable.

Intravenous prophylactic antibiotics should be administered on route to hospital.

Delayed Actions After Procedure

The procedural crew should ensure that an appropriate hot debrief of the case is undertaken with the rest of the emergency services team. It is likely that many staff will never have seen this procedure before, and the experience may be psychologically challenging. Staff may have questions about the indications for the procedure and how this fit into the patients life-saving management.

The team who conducted the amputation should ensure that they contact the seniors in their own organisation to inform them that the procedure has taken place and to obtain support. Comprehensive documentation of the clinical decision-making for amputation and the patient management should be made on the patient report form and the organisational database. The patient should be followed up for outcome, and the case should be routinely discussed in a mortality and morbidity meeting. Any learning points from rare cases such as these should be fed back into the organisational governance process. A full check list for pre-hospital amputation can be found in Fig. 25.4.

Novel Techniques for Surgical Amputation

Human cadaveric studies have identified that fire service equipment may be effectively used for amputation in cases of complex limb entrapment [17]. If the Gigli wire used for bone cutting snaps and is no longer available for use, then a suitable alternative is the simple handheld hacksaw which is normally provided on a fire service vehicle.

Studies have assessed the reciprocating saw and the Holmatro dedicated cutter ('jaws of life') and found them to be rapid and effective at cutting through a limb direct to skin. The reciprocat-

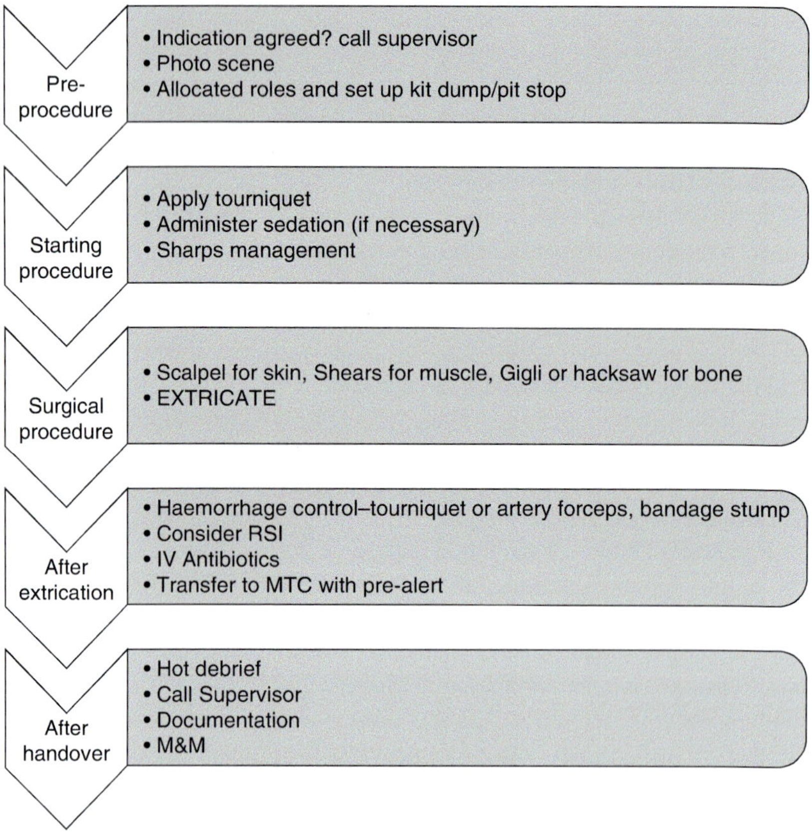

Fig. 25.4 Suggested checklist for amputation

ing saw carries significant risks of aerosolation of blood with splatter and infection control risks, as well as concerns around use in a confined space with limited visibility where other viable body parts may be injured by the uncontrolled saw blade. The dedicated cutter can be used under water but is difficult to insert circumferentially in a confined space and there is a time lag waiting for the "dead-mans handle" to open again after the first cut. Novel devices should only be used where the standard surgical methods are not possible due to a scene safety emergency or failure of standard equipment.

Training for the Procedure

All pre-hospital practitioners who may be expected to perform pre-hospital amputation should be adequately trained and operate within the governance and standard operating procedures for their organisation. Training should focus on the human factors elements of a potential entrapment as well as the surgical practical skills. This may include a combination of cadaveric skills practice, as well as scenario training. When training is being undertaken, staff should consider that they are likely to be working with limited access and poor visibility. An 'amputation checklist' may be useful as these procedures are rare.

Overview of Drugs Commonly Used in Procedural Sedation

Midazolam

Midazolam is a water-soluble imidazobenzodiazepine and is available as a clear solution in a variety of concentrations. It can be administered intravenously, intramuscularly or orally. The bioavailability of the latter routes are 80–100% and

15–27% respectively [18]. This means that the doses given will vary by route in fit and well patients, and their effects may have a high variability in patients who are critically unwell.

Midazolam has a variety of effects centred around activation of GABA receptors: hypnosis, sedation, anxiolysis, amnesia and anticonvulsant activity. If administered intravenously the onset of effects is within 60 s. The extent of these effects is dose dependant, with interpatient variability. Sedation is achieved with 0.07–0.1 mg/kg, titrated to effect, and the end point should be drowsiness but following commands. In most patients, respiratory drive and cardiovascular stability is maintained, however apnoea will occur in 10–77% if higher doses are administered [19, 20]. Emergency reversal is possible using flumazenil though this should not be routine practice as flumazenil decreases seizure threshold and may precipitate malignant arrhythmias such as ventricular tachycardia. Flumazenil should not be used in cases of mixed overdose, and especially not in cases of patients who have developed long term benzodiazepine tolerance [21].

Ketamine

Ketamine is a phencyclidine derivative and is available as a colourless solution is a variety of concentrations (10/50/100 mg/ml), so care is needed to check the dose and concentration prior to administration [22].

Ketamine provides analgesia and dissociative anaesthesia by non-competitive antagonism of the NDMA receptor. It can be administered intravenously, intranasally, intramuscularly or orally. The oral bioavailability is 20%. The analgesic effects of ketamine begin at approximately 0.1 mg/kg, with sedative effects starting at 0.5 mg/kg. Anaesthesia is obtained with intravenous doses of 1–2 mg/kg and the onset is within 30 s. Intramuscular dose for anaesthesia is 10 mg/kg, which can limit the usefulness of this mode of delivery due to the volume required. Maintenance of anaesthesia can be delivered with an infusion of 0.05 mg/kg/min.

Ketamine is cardiovascularly stable, causing a tachycardia, increase in cardiac output and blood pressure by an increase in sympathetic tone via endogenous catecholamine release. Whilst this is advantageous in most circumstances, in patients who have mounted a sustained catecholamine response (e.g. prolonged sepsis), induction of anaesthesia with ketamine may cause hypotension if the patient's endogenous adrenaline reserves have been depleted. This is because ketamine is intrinsically a myocardial depressant, however the stimulant effects of catecholamine release offset this [23]. Caution is needed in patients with a history of ischaemic heart disease who may not tolerate tachycardia. There is noted increase in respiratory rate with preservation of airway reflexes. Cerebral blood flow is increased along with cerebral metabolism. This does not preclude the use of ketamine as an induction agent in intracranial trauma as the improved cardiovascular profile reduces the chances of hypotension and subsequent secondary brain injury. Historically, ketamine was thought to increase intracranial pressure (ICP) and be contraindicated in head injury. However this was largely based on poor quality, small observational studies which made no effort to control other confounding variables which contributed to increasing ICP, (chiefly CO_2) in patients with pre-existing impairment of CSF drainage [24, 25]. More recent studies and reviews have shown ketamine does not increase ICP, and may be neuroprotective in terms of preserving or increasing cerebral perfusion pressure and decreasing neuronal cell death [23, 26–28].

Propofol

Propofol is a phenol derivative and the most commonly used anaesthetic induction agent in the United Kingdom, given in over 90% of anaesthetic inductions in hospital [29]. It is a white oil-in-water emulsion, either in a 1% or 2% concentration. It has no analgesic properties and is solely a hypnotic agent through its potentiation of the GABA receptor in the cerebral cortex. Propofol is only used intravenously and has no effect orally due to very high first pass metabolism. Induction doses of 1.5–2.5 mg/kg result in anaesthesia within one arm-brain circulation, commonly 30 s. Infusion rates of 4–12 mg/kg/h maintain anaesthesia or 2–6mg/ml blood concentration is aimed for using a Target Controlled Infusion (TCI) device. There is a wide variety of effective sedative doses in propofol, but some effects can be seen with 0.5 mg/kg doses, especially in older patients or those who have taken other depressant drugs.

The cardiovascular effects of propofol can be significant in elective patients, and exacerbated even further in an already compromised patient. Vascular resistance falls without a compensatory rise in heart rate. This causes a reduction in cardiac output. There is obtundation of the laryngeal reflexes which assists in providing optimal intubating conditions, although apnoea is very common. Metabolism is primarily in the liver and results in a rapid wake up after bolus or cessation of infusion. Propofol is of limited use for induction of anaesthesia in trauma due to its unfavourable pharmacodynamic profile in hypovolaemic patients. It is of some use for maintenance of anaesthesia or procedural sedation when it is given in lower doses over a longer period of time. Multiple methods have been described ranging from intermittent boluses [12], use in a target controlled infusion device [13] or in combination with other drugs such as ketamine ("ketofol") [30–32], but dose reductions are needed in comparison to "normal" induction of anaesthesia. Propofol must be given with an analgesic agent when used for procedural sedation due to the previously mentioned lack of intrinsic analgesic effect.

Methoxyflurane

Methoxyflurane is a volatile anaesthetic agent which was previously withdrawn from clinical use over safety concerns, as in concentrations required to maintain surgical anaesthesia it was found to cause renal failure [33]. It is unusual amongst inhaled anaesthetic agents in that it provides analgesia in addition to hypnosis, and for this reason it has been re-marketed as an inhalational analgesic under the brand name Penthrox [34]. It has been used extensively in Australia and is now being introduced to the UK as a competitor to nitrous oxide. It has several logistical advantages over nitrous oxide in that it is not a compressed gas, does not require pressure regulators and cannot give a hypoxic mixture, unlike Entonox which will separate out into its constituent gasses below −6 °C. It is licenced for the relief of moderate to severe pain in trauma. Each inhaler contains 3 ml of agent, with a maximum allowable dose of 6 ml per 24 h. period. Patients are advised to intermittently inhale through the device and analgesia should begin within 6–10 breaths. With continuous use, the inhalers provide analgesia for 20–30 min and with intermittent use this can be significantly extended. Caution should be used in those with cardiovascular or respiratory compromise and its use in head injuries or chest injuries is contraindicated. Use of methoxyflurane in an enclosed space has the potential to produce effects on clinicians or other staff in proximity: therefore it should not be used in patients who are being transported or will be transported by helicopter in case it incapacitates the pilot. There is some data supporting safety for ground ambulance staff [35].

Morphine

Morphine is an opioid and a phenanthrene derivative. It is available in a variety of concentrations of clear, colourless liquids, or in oral formats in a variety of doses. The effects occur by agonist activity of the mu- and kappa- opioid receptors. Intravenous dose is 0.05–0.1 mg/kg but peak effect may not occur for 20 min due to hepatic transformation to the more active morphine-6-glucuronide metabolite [18]. Morphine, like most opioids, causes respiratory depression with a decreased ventilatory response to hypoxia and hypercarbia. It may also cause release of histamine, leading to bronchoconstriction and a decrease in systemic vascular resistance. The gastrointestinal effects are most commonly nausea and decreased gastric motility.

Morphine is most commonly used in intermittent bolus for analgesia, but may also be used as an infusion along with a hypnotic agent for sedation. Rates of infusion are 0.05–0.1 mg/kg/h. depending on the level of sedation and analgesia required [36]. The effects of morphine can be completely reversed with naloxone, with the exception of intrathecal or epidural administration, in which circumstance the analgesic and sedative effects remain.

Fentanyl

Fentanyl is a potent synthetic opioid and derivative of phenylpiperidine, it is a highly selective mu-receptor agonist. It is available as a clear, colourless liquid in 50 mcg/ml concentration that can be administered intravenously, intramuscularly, intranasal, intrathecally or epidurally. By the intravenous route, analgesic doses are initially in the range of 1–3 mcg/kg, but doses of up to 100 mcg/kg can be used to induce anaesthesia for cardiothoracic cases, with peak effect for both indications in 2–5 min. Smaller doses have a duration of action of between 30 and 60 min but higher doses may be effective of 4–6 h. Fentanyl may be used for analgesia in moderate to severe pain or as a co-induction agent in anaesthesia. It obtunds the sympathetic response to laryngoscopy and intubation, reducing the hypertensive response and associated tachycardia. Fentanyl is a potent depressor of respiratory drive by reducing the response to hypoxia and hypercapnia.

Alfentanil

Alfentanil is a synthetic opioid derived from anilinopiperidine. It is available in two concentrations, 0.5 mg/ml and 5 mg/ml, both used only intravenously. Like fentanyl, it is a highly selective mu-receptor agonist with the same analgesia, cardiovascular and respiratory effects. Intravenous boluses are 10–50 mcg/kg with peak effect in 90 s. The duration of action is shorter than fentanyl at 5–10 min.

The fast onset and significant sympathetic obtundation make it a useful co-induction agent when hypertension is to be avoided, such as in intracranial haemorrhage. Alfentanil has a relatively short context sensitive half-life which makes it suitable for continuous infusion for sedation during transfer or on intensive care. Infusion rates are 0.5–1 mcg/kg/min.

Entonox

Entonox™ is a 50/50 mixture of oxygen and nitrous oxide delivered as a vapour in pressurised cylinders. It is most commonly used via a patient demand valve which regulates pressure from the cylinder and allows spontaneous respiration. Entonox produces analgesia and central nervous system depression in a dose dependent fashion. Slight depression of the respiratory drive and a small decrease in myocardial contractility is noted. Nausea is also a common side effect in approximately 15% of patients [20].

The delivery of Entonox is patient controlled which confers some degree of safety. It can provide reasonable analgesia for the relocation of joints or the reduction of fractures. Caution should be observed in head, abdominal and chest injuries as the diffusion of nitrous oxide expands any gas filled spaces, thus increased intracranial pressure, abdominal pressure respectively, with a risk of causing expansion of a pneumothorax due to the low solubility of nitrous oxide in the blood. For this reason, Entonox should not be used in cases where there is chest trauma where there is a risk of any form of pneumothorax. In normal operating temperatures the concentration of oxygen delivered remains around 50%, however, if the cylinders are kept below −6 °C, then separation of the nitrous oxide and the oxygen can occur. This leads to an initially higher inspired concentration of N_2O and possibly a hypoxic mixture. Nitrous oxide in itself can be used to augment anaesthesia and has been used as an analgesic or anaesthetic since 1800, though repeated or prolonged use of nitrous has been found to interfere with folate metabolism and can cause bone marrow suppression and megaloblastic anaemia [37].

Conclusion

Sedation is a critical skill to acquire for both pre- and in-hospital emergency staff. There are multiple, equally valid ways of performing sedation with a variety of drugs, and a one-size-fits-all approach is not appropriate. Each situation has to take into account patient, logistical and organisational factors, but which ever method is used should have patient safety at its core. This should be underpinned by organisational commitment to peer review and standardisation of training and implementation as much as is practicable. Performing sedation in the pre-hospital environment can be demanding, as too can performing an amputation. One practitioner doing both of these things well is not an achievable target, as the cognitive bandwidth required for both interventions is substantial. While these procedures are thankfully rare, training and regular simulation will mitigate some of the anxiety surrounding performing these procedures when necessary.

Questions

1. Which of the following would be an appropriate indication for amputation?
   (a) patient is trapped by leg in rising flood water with loss of consciousness
   (b) patient is trapped in vehicle by the steering wheel on their torso
   (c) patient is trapped by arm in machinery with no obvious method of extrication
   (d) patient is trapped by arm in machinery with distal catastrophic haemorrhage
   (e) patient has been released but there is a 1 cm wide section of bridging tissue connecting the mangled pulseless limb
2. Which of the following is essential before performing an emergency lower limb amputation on a peri-arrest patient?
   (a) intravenous access
   (b) application of a tourniquet
   (c) administration of analgesia
   (d) loss of central pulses
   (e) failure of extrication within 15 min of arrival
3. Following amputation and extrication of the patient, which of the following actions must be performed before leaving scene?
   (a) photo the scene
   (b) administer IV antibiotics
   (c) anaesthetize and intubate the patient
   (d) check the stump for bleeding and provide haemorrhage control
   (e) extricate the amputated part
4. Which sedative drug would be most appropriate for emergency amputation (assuming all were available)?
   (a) Midazolam IV
   (b) Propofol IV
   (c) Ketamine IV
   (d) Ketamine IM
   (e) Entonox INH
5. Ketamine should be administered at which of the following starting doses?
   (a) 0.5 mg/kg IV for analgesia
   (b) 1.0 mg/kg IV for analgesia
   (c) 0.5 mg/kg IV for sedation
   (d) 1 mg/kg IV for sedation
   (e) 1 mg/kg IM for sedation

Answers

1 a
2 b
3 d
4 c
5 c

References

1. Porter KM. Prehospital amputation. Emerg Med J. 2010;27(12):940–2.
2. Gander B. Prehospital amputation: a scoping review. J Paramed Pract. 2020;12(1):6–13.
3. Sheahan CG, Mathews DM. Monitoring and delivery of sedation. Br J Anaesth. 2014;113(Suppl_2):ii37–47.
4. Hughes CG, McGrane S, Pandharipande PP. Sedation in the intensive care setting. Clin Pharmacol Adv Appl. 2012;4:53–63.
5. Hughes CG, McGrane S, Pandharipande PP. Sedation in the intensive care setting. Clin Pharmacol Adv Appl. 2012;4:53–63.
6. Galarza Vallejo A, Kroes MCW, Rey E, Acedo MV, Moratti S, Fernández G, et al. Propofol-induced deep sedation reduces emotional episodic memory reconsolidation in humans. Sci Adv [Internet]. 2019 Mar 20 [cited 2020 July 8]: 5(3). Available from: https://www.ncbi.nlm.nih.gov/pmc/articles/PMC6426467/
7. National Institute for Health and Care Excellence. NICE Evidence Search - Sedation Guidelines [Internet]. NICE Evidence Search. 2020 [cited 2020 Jan 10]. Available from: http://tiny.cc/NICEsedation
8. Academy of Medical Royal Colleges Safe Sedation Practice Working Group. Safe Sedation Practice for Healthcare Procedures [Internet]. London: Academy of Medical Royal Colleges; 2013 Oct [cited 2020 May 24]: [37 p.]. Available from: https://www.aomrc.org.uk/reports-guidance/safe-sedation-practice-1213/
9. Jacques KG, Dewar A, Gray A, Kerslake D, Leal A, Lees F. Procedural sedation and analgesia in a large UK emergency department: factors associated with complications. Emerg Med J. 2011;28(12):1036–40.
10. Royal College of Anaesthetists, Royal College of Emergency Medicine. Safe Sedation of Adults in the Emergency Department - Report and Recommendations.pdf [Internet]. 2012 [cited 2020 Jan 10]. Available from: https://www.rcem.ac.uk/docs/Col-

lege%20Guidelines/5z7.%20Safe%20Sedation%20in%20the%20Emergency%20Department%20-%20Report%20and%20Recommendations.pdf
11. Tomita S, Matsuura N, Ichinohe T. The combined effects of midazolam and propofol sedation on muscle power. Anaesthesia. 2013;68(5):478–83.
12. Dunn T, Mossop D, Newton A, Gammon A. Propofol for procedural sedation in the emergency department. Emerg Med J. 2007;24(7):459–61.
13. Fyntanidou B, Papadopoulos I, Nikolaidis C, Nasro H, Lazaridou A. Conscious sedation with TCI-propofol versus manual propofol for patients undergoing vertical infraclavicular blockade: A-510. Eur J Anaesthesiol. 2006;23:132–3.
14. Gillings M, Grundlingh J, Aw-Yong M. Guidelines for management of Acute Behavioural Disturbance (May 2016).pdf [Internet]. The Royal College of Emergency Medicine; 2016 [cited 2020 July 8]. Available from: https://www.rcem.ac.uk/docs/College%20Guidelines/5p.%20RCEM%20guidelines%20for%20management%20of%20Acute%20Behavioural%20Disturbance%20(May%202016).pdf
15. Scheppke KA, Braghiroli J, Shalaby M, Chait R. Prehospital use of IM ketamine for sedation of violent and agitated patients. West J Emerg Med. 2014;15(7):736–41.
16. Rowland LM. Subanesthetic ketamine: how it alters physiology and behavior in humans. Aviat Space Environ Med. 2005;76(7):8.
17. Leech C, Porter K. Man or machine? An experimental study of prehospital emergency amputation. Emerg Med J. 2016;33(9):641–4.
18. Payne K, Mattheyse FJ, Liebenberg D, Dawes T. The pharmacokinetics of midazolam in paediatric patients. Eur J Clin Pharmacol. 1989;37(3):267–72.
19. Luck H, Morgan P. Prehospital emergency anaesthesia: considerations, pitfalls, and controversies. Intensive care Med. 2019;8
20. Scarth E, Smith S. Drugs in Anaesthesia and Intensive Care. 5th ed. Oxford University Press; 2016. (Oxford Medical Publications; vol. 1)
21. An H, Godwin J. Flumazenil in benzodiazepine overdose. Can Med Assoc J. 2016;188(17–18):E537.
22. Warner LL, Smischney N. Special K with no license to kill: accidental ketamine overdose on induction of general Anesthesia. Am J Case Rep. 2018;19:10–2.
23. Pai A, Heining M. Ketamine. Contin Educ Anaesth Crit Care Pain. 2007;7(2):59–63.
24. Albanese J, Arnaud S, Rey M, Thomachot L, Alliez B, Martin C. Ketamine decreases intracranial pressure and electroencephalographic activity in traumatic brain injury patients during Propofol sedation. Anesthesiol J Am Soc Anesthesiol. 1997;87(6):1328–34.
25. Filanovsky Y, Miller P, Kao J. Myth: ketamine should not be used as an induction agent for intubation in patients with head injury. CJEM. 2010;12(02):154–7.
26. Chang LC, Raty SR, Ortiz J, Bailard NS, Mathew SJ. The emerging use of ketamine for Anesthesia and sedation in traumatic brain injuries. CNS Neurosci Ther. 2013;19(6):390–5.
27. Zeiler FA, Teitelbaum J, West M, Gillman LM. The ketamine effect on ICP in traumatic brain injury. Neurocrit Care. 2014;21(1):163–73.
28. Bar-Joseph G, Guilburd Y, Tamir A, Guilburd JN. Effectiveness of ketamine in decreasing intracranial pressure in children with intracranial hypertension. J Neurosurg Pediatr. 2009;4(1):40–6.
29. Anaesthesia, Surgery and Life-Threatening Allergic Reactions. Report and findings of the Royal College of Anaesthetists' 6th National Audit Project: Perioperative Anaphylaxis [Internet]. NIAA Health Services Research Centre; London; 2018 May [cited 2020 June 18] [234 p.]. Report No.: 6. Available from: https://www.niaa.org.uk/NAP6Report
30. Ferguson I, Bell A, Treston G, New L, Ding M, Holdgate A. Propofol or ketofol for procedural sedation and analgesia in emergency medicine—the POKER study: a randomized double-blind clinical trial. Ann Emerg Med. 2016;68(5):574–582.e1.
31. Daniel J. Pallin MD. Propofol vs. Ketofol for Procedural Sedation in the ED. NEJM J Watch [Internet]. 2016 July 29 [cited 2020 May 24];2016. Available from: https://www.jwatch.org/NA41955/2016/07/29/propofol-vs-ketofol-procedural-sedation-ed
32. Arora S. Combining ketamine and Propofol ("Ketofol") for emergency department procedural sedation and analgesia: a review. West J Emerg Med. 2008;9(1):20–3.
33. Jephcott C, Grummet J, Nguyen N, Spruyt O. A review of the safety and efficacy of inhaled methoxyflurane as an analgesic for outpatient procedures. Br J Anaesth. 2018;120(5):1040–8.
34. PENTHROX 3mL inhalation vapour, liquid - Summary of Product Characteristics (SmPC) - (emc) [Internet]. [cited 2020 May 22]. Available from: https://www.medicines.org.uk/emc/product/1939/smpc
35. Frangos J, Mikkonen A, Down C. Derivation of an occupational exposure limit for an inhalation analgesic methoxyflurane (Penthrox®). Regul Toxicol Pharmacol. 2016;80:210–25.
36. Narayanan M, Venkataraju A, Jennings J. Analgesia in intensive care: part 1. BJA Educ. 2016;16(2):72–8.
37. Banks A, Hardman JG. Nitrous oxide. Contin Educ Anaesth Crit Care Pain. 2005;5(5):145–8.

Part V

Radiology in Trauma

Point of Care Ultrasound (POCUS) 26

Jake Turner and Justin Squires

- The physics of ultrasound: Waveforms, mechanics, resolution, artefacts & Doppler
- A system based approach to pre-hospital point of care ultrasound
  - Airway: Difficult airway assessment
  - Breathing: Chest trauma
  - Circulation: Differentiating shock states
  - Disability: Intracranial pressure monitoring
  - Exposure: Musculoskeletal injury
- The role for ultrasound in cardiac arrest
- Limitations of pre-hospital ultrasound
- Ultrasound governance

Introduction

Point of care ultrasound (POCUS) has increased in popularity and allows real-time imaging of body systems to aid diagnosis, facilitate triage and guide interventions. The use of pre-hospital POCUS must be balanced against the challenges of the environment and time to definitive care for time-critical patients. Considerations include distance to transfer, scene time, operator experience, training and local governance. POCUS is a well established investigation in hospital based critical care to assess for fluid status, cardiac performance and presence of time-critical pathology such as pneumothorax or cardiac tamponade [1–3].

This chapter describes the basics of ultrasound physics, settings on commonly used hand-held devices, a system based approach to POCUS, the role of POCUS in cardiac arrest and limitation/governance considerations. Competency in POCUS is attained through courses, hands on experience, peer review and certification by approved trainers.

The original version of this chapter was revised. The correction to this chapter can be found at https://doi.org/10.1007/978-3-030-83628-3_45

The authors composed, revised and approved this manuscript. The work is original. There are no conflicts or relevant disclosures.

J. Turner (✉)
Department of Anaesthesia, Nottingham University Teaching Hospitals NHS Trust, Nottinghamshire, UK

The Air Ambulance Service (TAAS), Rugby, Warwickshire, UK

Midland's Air Ambulance (MAA), West Midlands Ambulance Service, West Midlands, UK
e-mail: jake.turner3@nhs.net

J. Squires
The Air Ambulance Service (TAAS), Rugby, Warwickshire, UK

Emergency Medicine Department, Sheffield Teaching Hospitals, Sheffield, UK
e-mail: justin.squires1@nhs.net

P. Lax (ed.), *Textbook of Acute Trauma Care*, https://doi.org/10.1007/978-3-030-83628-3_26

Physics

Ultrasound

Ultrasound is a high-frequency sound wave outside the range of human hearing (>20 KHz) with medical ultrasound being in the frequency range of 1–13 MHz. The higher the frequency of ultrasound the better the resolution of the image, but the shallower the depth of penetration. Superficial vessels and nerves are imaged with 6–13 MHz probes whereas imaging of the heart and abdominal viscera is with 1–5 MHz probes.

Ultrasound is created by the passage of an alternating current across piezoelectric crystals, causing them to vibrate in the ultrasound frequency range and generate sound waves. These piezoelectric crystals have a unique property where they can 'receive' reflected sound waves causing them to vibrate and generate an electrical output; this is the principle of ultrasound detection and subsequent image generation. Evolving technology, using semiconductors to generate and receive the ultrasound waves rather than piezoelectric crystals, offers the possibility for smaller, cheaper and more versatile units.

Waveform

Ultrasound waves have a sinusoidal pattern and consist of both positive and negative oscillations around an axis (Fig. 26.1). The wavelength is the distance between two sound waves with the intensity of the sound wave proportional to the amplitude (volume). The frequency is defined as the numbers of waves per second (Hertz), and in the audible sound range is identified as the pitch.

Sound waves travel through air and body tissues at different velocities (Table 26.1). This change in velocity creates a reflection of the ultrasound wave at tissue interfaces and therefore, visualisation of the tissues by the ultrasound transducer. Noting the significant difference in speed between air and human tissues generally explains why there is such a strong reflection at any boundary with air that is difficult to image through. The gel used between the probe and the patient eliminates air at the probe/skin interface to avoid this problem.

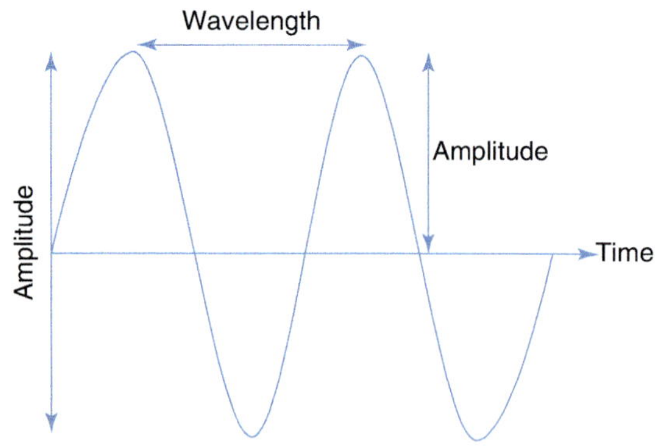

Fig. 26.1 Sound Waveform

Table 26.1 Speed of sound through air & human tissues [4]

Soft tissue (m/s)	Speed of sound (m/s)
Air	330
Fat	1450
Liver	1550
Blood	1570
Muscle	1585
Bone	4080

The speed of sound (c) is a product of the wavelength (λ) and frequency (f), $c = \lambda f$. As the sound wave velocity changes on transition across different tissues, the wavelength must then also change to accommodate this, as the frequency is constant.

Key Points

- Medical ultrasound is in the frequency range of 1–13 MHz
- The higher the frequency of ultrasound, the better the resolution
- The lower the frequency of ultrasound, the deeper the penetration
- Sound waves travel through air and body tissues at different velocities
- Sound wave reflection occurs at tissue interfaces, and is the principle behind image acquisition

Mechanics

For image acquisition, the ultrasound waves transmitted through the body must be reflected and then detected at the transducer. The intensity of reflected waves detected, and the time delay for detection will influence the echogenicity and depth of the image formed respectively. However, as sound waves travel through the body, they weaken in intensity through a variety of mechanisms affecting image quality (Fig. 26.2):

- **Refraction:** Sound waves vectors are altered as they pass through soft tissue interfaces. This may result in waves that are reflected by deeper structures being unable to return to the transducer for detection
- **Transmission:** Sound waves continue through the soft tissue without reflection and therefore are not detected by the transducer
- **Scatter:** Sound waves are reflected in multiple vectors, with only those in plane with the transducer being detected
- **Attenuation:** Sound wave amplitude attenuates as the waves move away from their point of origin and through soft tissue

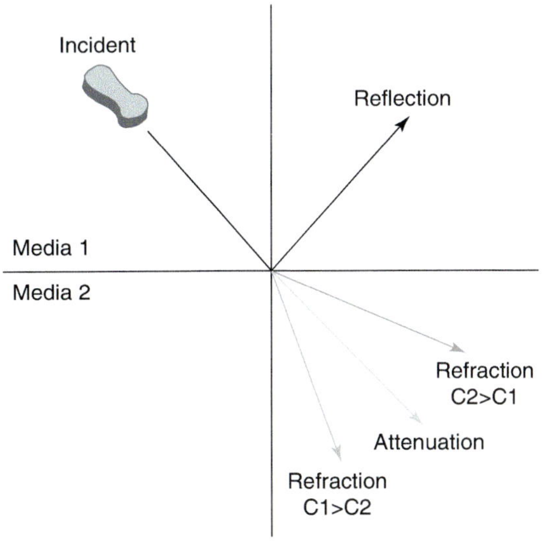

Fig. 26.2 Sound Wave Mechanics (from Shin and Jeong) [5]

The echogenicity (brightness) of a structure is directly proportional to the number of ultrasound waves that are reflected as the sound waves transition through the tissue interface. Fluid-filled structures are anechoic (black), soft tissues are grey and dense tissues are echogenic (bright white) with dropout artefact behind them (absence of transmitted ultrasound). Anisotropic structures are structures which have a variable image quality depending on the angle the ultrasound waves interact with it, such as nerves, tendons and muscle fibres where probe orientation is paramount for image quality (Figs. 26.2 and 26.3).

Air-filled structures scatter the sound waves at the soft tissue interface giving an echogenic line with artefact behind this, in the gas-filled structure. For example, the aerated lung has a bright white pleural interface with A-line artefacts transitioning across the lung field with the same spacing as the distance from the probe to the pleural interface. They demonstrate the presence of air below the pleural interface and are therefore present in healthy aerated lung (Fig. 26.4).

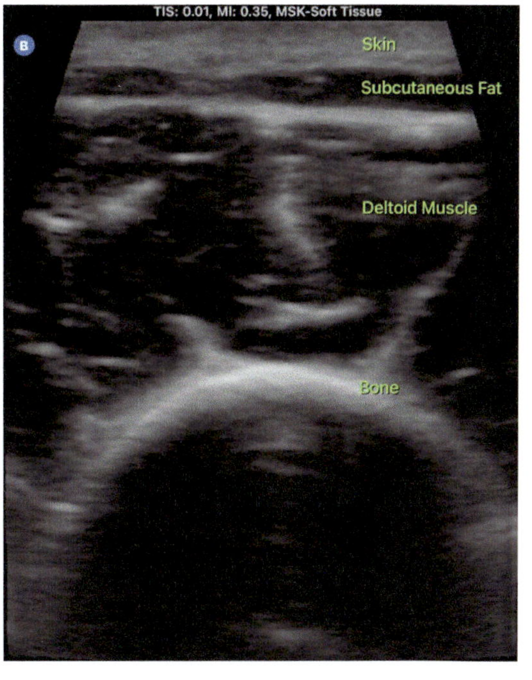

Fig. 26.3 Soft Tissue Interfaces of the shoulder (courtesy Dr. J Squires)

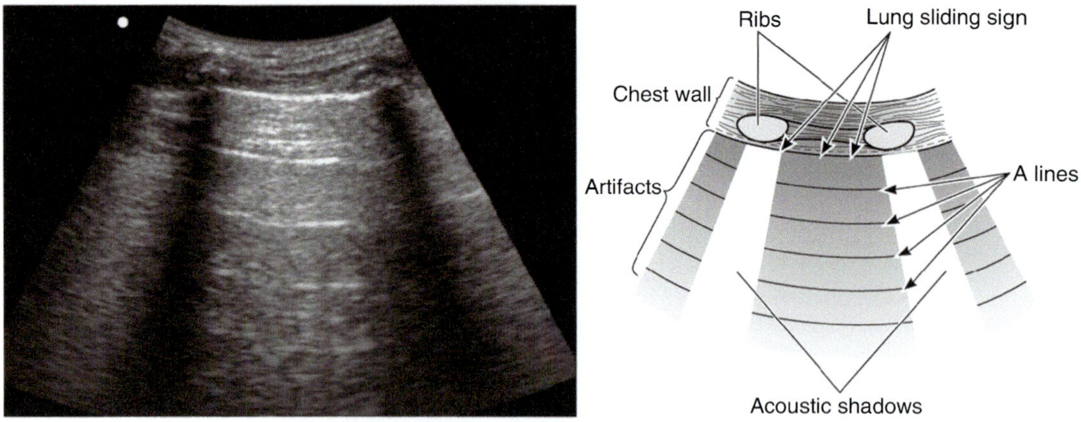

Fig. 26.4 Pleural Interface (from Ma and Mateer [6])

Resolution

Resolution is defined as the ability to distinguish echoes in terms of space, time or strength, and is therefore essential in image quality:

- **Contrast Resolution**: Differentiation between tissues with differing characteristics (e.g. nerves appear different to surrounding muscles as they reflect ultrasound differently)
- **Temporal Resolution:** Changes in anatomy that occur over time can be used to demonstrate or quantify pathology (e.g. presence of lung sliding, or degree of contractility in echocardiography)
- **Spatial Resolution:** Structures that are close together can be delineated and displayed separately, in both axial and lateral planes (Fig. 26.5)
  - Axial resolution (depth of scan) is improved by higher frequency sound waves. This can be achieved by shorter wavelengths/pulse, manipulating gain settings (though higher gain decreases resolution) and decreasing the field of view (a smaller field improves resolution).
  - Lateral resolution is improved by narrowing the focal zone so neighbouring objects can be interrogated separately and moving the zone of interest into the central axis of the beam

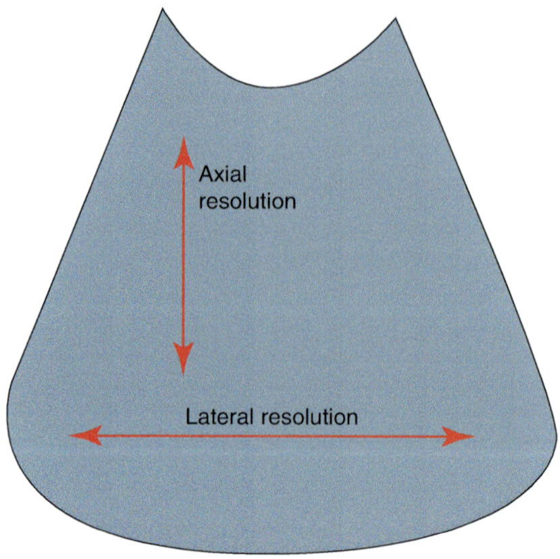

Fig. 26.5 Spatial Resolution

Key Points Echogenicity and depth of images are determined by sound wave reflection intensity and delay

- Refraction, attenuation and scatter of sound waves are responsible for ultrasound image degradation
- Resolution is the ability to distinguish between echoes of sound, in terms of space, time or strength

Artefacts

Artefacts can be both helpful (e.g. pleural interface disruption, gallstone identification) or unhelpful, by obscuring details and mimicking pathologies (Fig. 26.3). Acoustic shadowing occurs when very dense objects cast acoustic shadows as the ultrasound waves are absorbed or reflected (e.g. bones or gallstones). This causes a void or dark area behind the dense structure and means that deeper tissues cannot be visualised. Acoustic enhancement occurs when ultrasound passes through a structure which conducts ultrasound without reflecting it, principally fluid-filled structures such as a full bladder or cyst. As a result, structures behind the fluid-filled structure appear to be brighter as time gain compensation (see below) overcompensates and makes these posterior structures appear more echogenic.

Edge shadowing occurs when velocity differentials of sound waves across rounded structures cause the edges to lose resolution/appear blurred. Reverberation is caused by ultrasound pulses bouncing off parallel reflecting surfaces which are almost perpendicular to the direction of the beam before returning to the probe. Some of the pulse becomes caught between the two surfaces and has a delayed return to the probe after being reflected multiple times. This results in a series of "ghost" images deep to the original image and depends on how much of the pulse is dissipated, the size of the surfaces and how far apart they are. An example of this is a comet tail artifact, when multiple calcific or crystalline structures are imaged (such as bile duct stones or renal calculi) and appear to emit a tail further away from the probe.

Mirror images occur where there is a highly reflective structure directly in the path of the beam (e.g. diaphragm), which reflects the beam back. Rather than the beam going directly to the probe, it encounters another reflective structure on its return and is turned back towards the first reflective surface in a "Z" shaped manoeuvre, which subsequently returns the pulse to the probe. These surfaces reflect sound so perfectly that on screen two images can form a perfect mirror image.

Doppler

As sound waves are reflected from moving objects, the speed of the moving structure influences the frequency of the reflected sound waves, called the Doppler effect. This explains the commonly heard change in pitch of a vehicle or a siren as it passes by the observer. The Doppler effect can be utilised to measure the velocity of a moving target (blood), and the vector of its movement can be shown in colour with reference to the position of the probe (Fig. 26.6).

Using Doppler to measure the velocity of flow relies on the vector of the ultrasound wave to be in alignment with blood flow, any discrepancy will introduce error into the Doppler equation and subsequent velocity calculation. Also, there are a variety of Doppler modes with varying limitations, and in the pre-hospital environment may have impaired reliability.

Key Points

- Artefacts such as acoustic shadowing, edge shadowing and mirror images can be helpful, or impede image interpretation
- The Doppler effect occurs when sound waves are reflected from moving objects, influencing the frequency of the reflected sound waves
- The Doppler effect can be utilised to measure the velocity of a moving target, and the vector of its movement

Hardware

Probes

There are three main types of ultrasound probes used for medical ultrasound (Fig. 26.7):

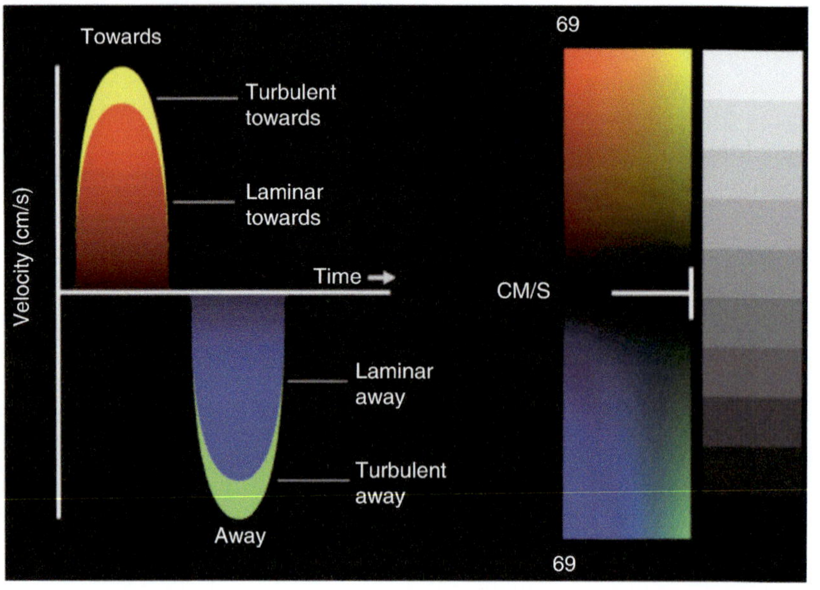

Fig. 26.6 The Doppler effect (Image reproduced with permission from http://pie.med.utoronto.ca/tee)

- **Linear Array** = Rectangular footprint with high-frequency ultrasound (5–10 MHz) ideal for high resolution but with poor penetration. Used for imaging the pleural surface, identifying veins for cannulation or nerves for regional anaesthesia
- **Curvilinear** = Curved footprint with lower frequency ultrasound (2–5 MHz) ideal for deep penetration in abdominal imaging
- **Phased Array** = Small footprint with lower frequency ultrasound (2–5 MHz) ideal for imaging between rib spaces in echocardiography

Probe orientation is critical, and there is a marker on the ultrasound screen that will correlate to a mark on the ultrasound probe. Most ultrasound machines also have programmed presets (cardiac, chest, vascular, nerve, abdominal) that can be used to optimise contrast, frequency and focal zone.

Image Optimisation

Once the correct machine pre-sets have been selected, image quality can be further optimised by considering depth, focus and gain of the machine. The depth of the image should be just beyond the area of interest to optimise both image quality and size. The focal zone can be adjusted on some machines so that the area of highest resolution can be targeted to the area of interest. Most small machines, however, cannot be adjusted and the depth controls, therefore, control the focal zone. This is usually two-thirds of the depth selected for the scan.

Time gain constant adjustments can be made to attempt to counter the reduction in reflections from objects further away from the probe by increasing the gain of signals reflected. Overall gain can be controlled on most machines and works by increasing the amplitude of the detected returning ultrasound. Adjusting the gain will increase the brightness of the image, which can help to ameliorate issues with attenuation, but this will also increase the strength of detected 'noise'.

Modes

There are three main modes available in medical ultrasound; 2-Dimensional (2D), Motion-mode (M-mode) and Doppler. With 2D, this is the visual imaging of structures below the probe.

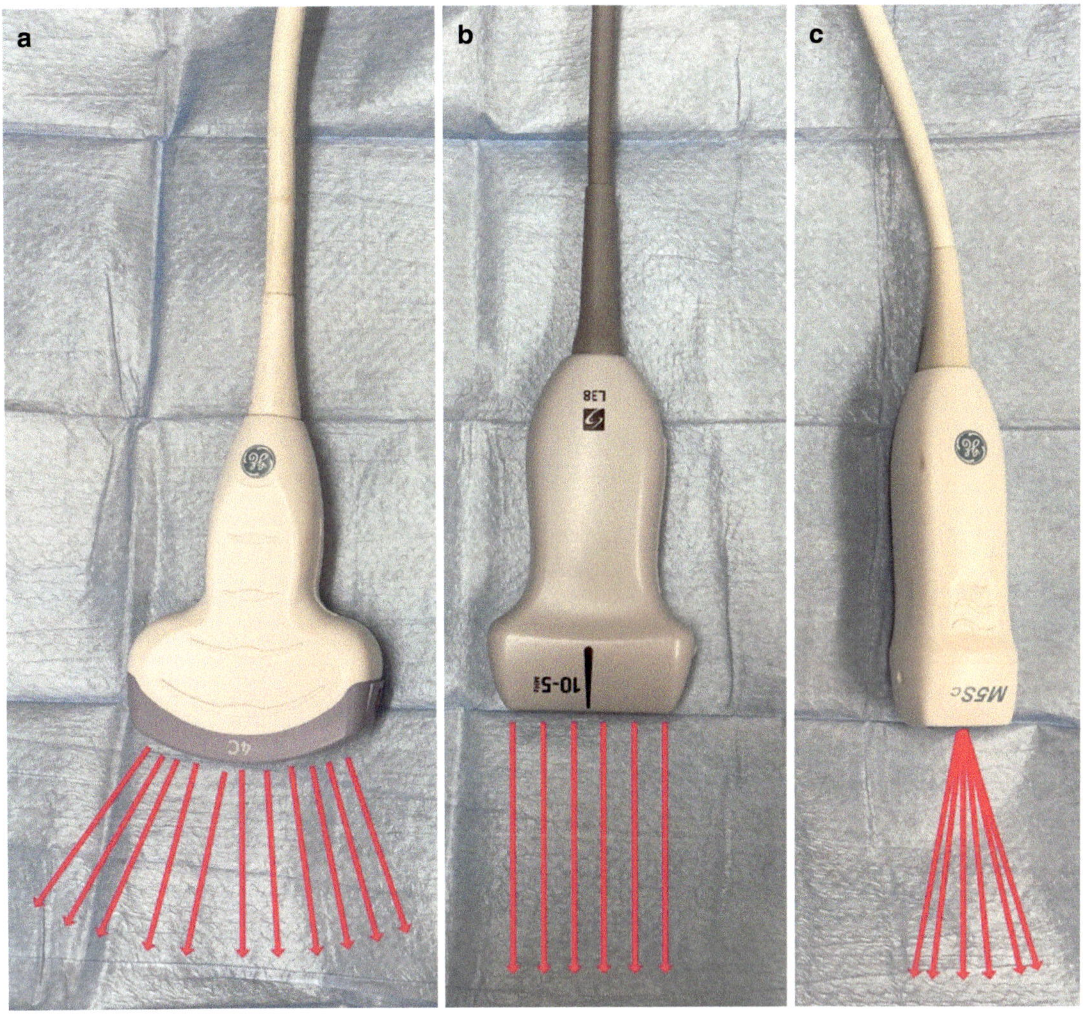

Fig. 26.7 Ultrasound Probes—A: Curved array probe, B: Linear array probe, C: Phased array probe

Doppler, as described above, will allow the velocity and vector of a moving structure to be measured. M-mode is a time-motion display along a chosen ultrasound line and provides a single-dimensional display of movement along that chosen line (Fig. 26.8).

2D is the commonest mode used for image acquisition, Doppler mode is useful for measuring flow when calculating cardiac output or differentiation between non-pulsatile/pulsatile structures, and M-mode is useful for identifying a normal pleural interface/excluding a pneumothorax.

Probe Handling

There are several co-ordinated techniques for handling an ultrasound probe that must be mastered to optimise image quality and reliability. The first principle is to avoid holding a probe with an unsupported hand; always try to rest the hypothenar eminence of the hand against the patients' body to stabilise the image. Following this, several probe handling techniques can be utilised to optimise image acquisition (Fig. 26.9);

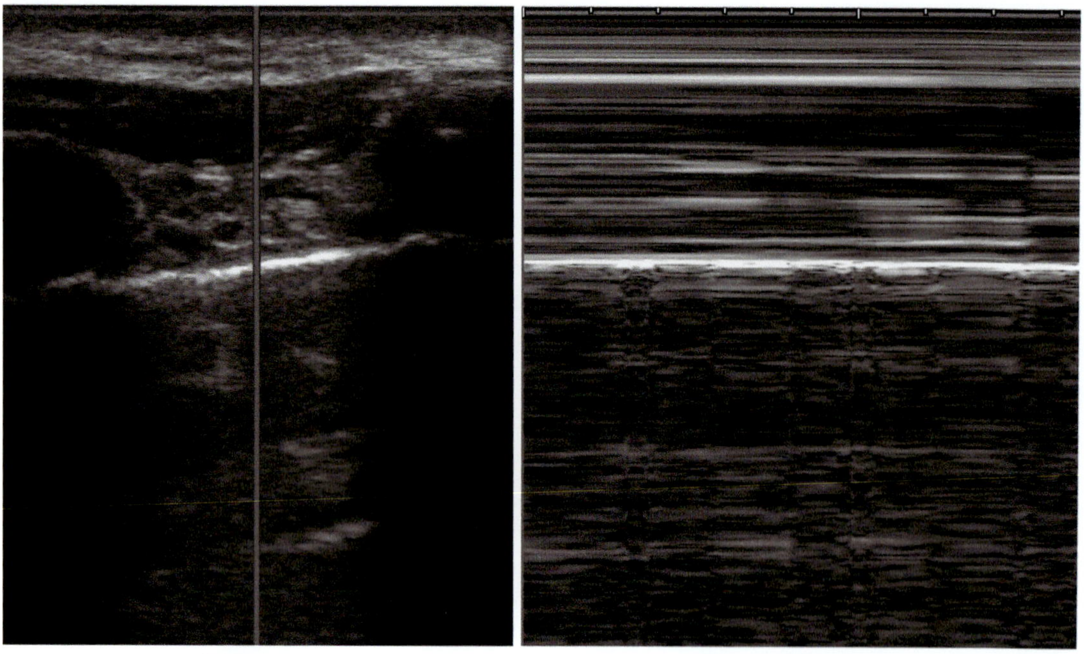

Fig. 26.8 2D and M-Modes of pleural interface

- Pressure—Applying/Releasing pressure
- Alignment—Translating the probe in the horizontal plane
- Rotation—Rotating the probe in the horizontal plane
- Tilting—Tilting the probe in the vertical plane.

It is useful to make one alteration at a time and see the effect on the image quality rather than simultaneously combining manoeuvres.

Key Points

- There are three main types of probes, all with different ultrasound frequency ranges and imaging profiles: phased array, linear array and curvilinear
- Image optimisation is a complex task, requiring consideration of pre-sets, depth, focus and gain
- There are different modes of operation, each with specific functions: M-mode, 2D-mode and Doppler
- Probe handling techniques are complex, and require practice to optimise image quality: pressure, alignment, rotation and tilt

Video Resources

There are an abundance of good learning resources which will demonstrate pathological findings on ultrasound. The Society of Point of Care Ultrasound website (https://spocus.org/resources-programs/foamed/) is useful for visualising the pathological signs that are explained in the following sections and for further reading, and the reader is advised to make use of them alongside this text:

Systems

Airway

Front of neck access for "can't intubate, can't oxygenate" scenarios is an essential skill for clinicians managing airways in trauma. Ultrasonographic identification of the cricothyroid membrane is becoming an expectation of care in the assessment of patients with potentially difficult airways for in-hospital practice (Fig. 26.10).

Breathing

Pneumothorax

Chest ultrasound has a sensitivity that exceeds that of X-ray and approaches that of computerised tomography (CT) in ruling out a pneumothorax via demonstration of an intact pleural interface with the following features [8]:

- Presence of pleural sliding
- Presence of B-lines
- Seashore M-mode (Fig. 26.11)

M-mode records the movement of points on the scan line over time. Points which are not moving (like the relatively fixed tissues of the chest wall) will be recorded as a horizontal line (like waves crashing on the seashore). This can be compared with a pleural interface that expands and contracts with respiration and thus shows a motion effect. The "sand" of the lungs is clearly different from the "waves" of the pleura and subcutaneous tissue above. If there is reduced/no motion where the lung should be

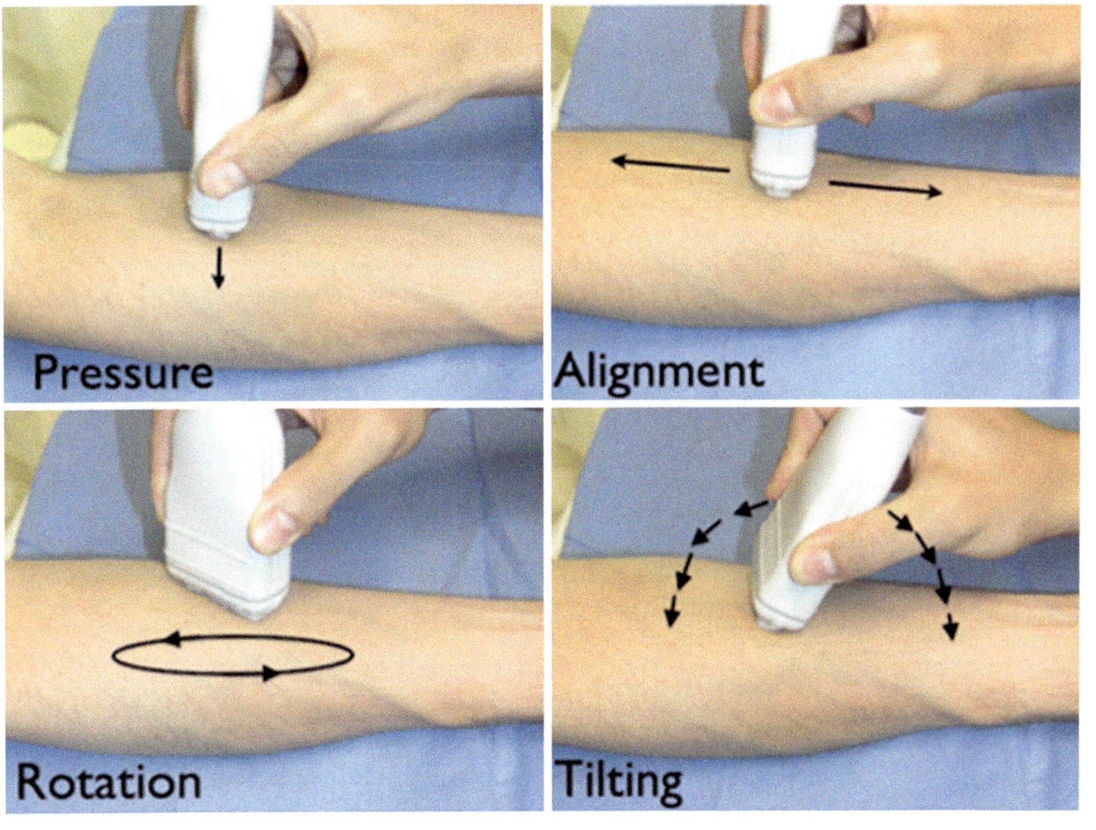

Fig. 26.9 Probe Handling Techniques

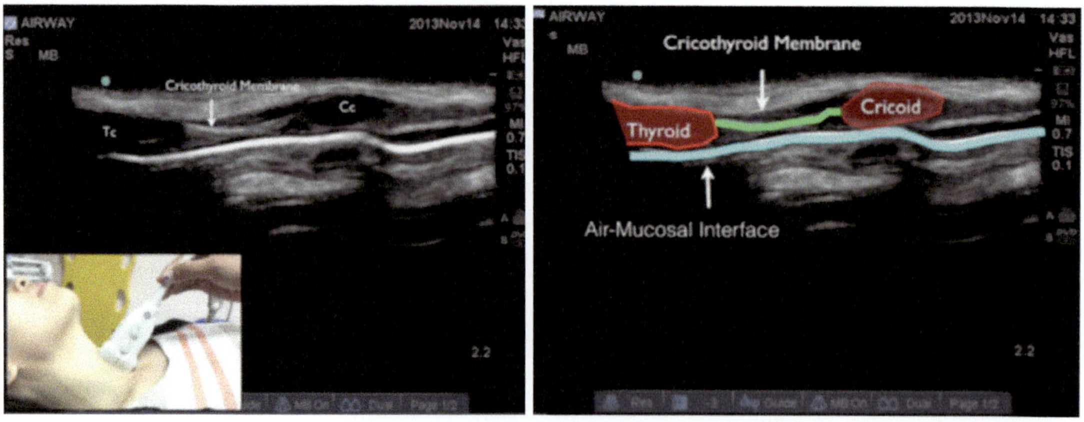

Fig. 26.10 Front of neck ultrasound (from Osman and Sum [7])

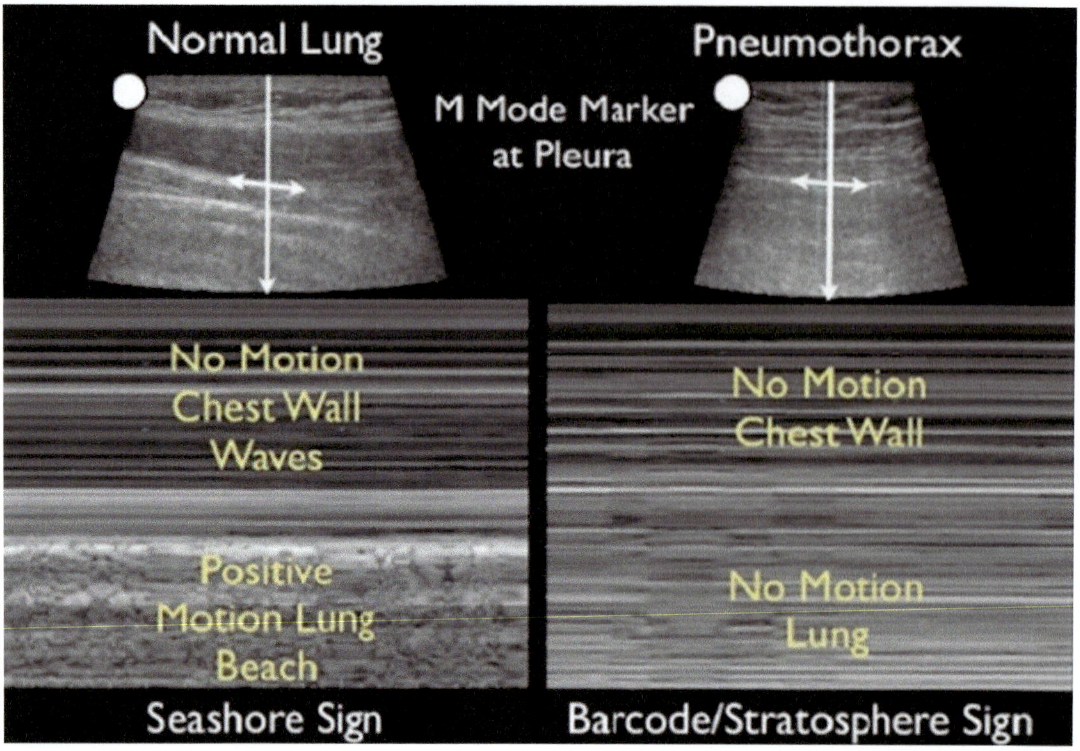

Fig. 26.11 M-Mode in normal lung vs pneumothorax (from Seif et al., https://doi.org/10.1155/2012/503254)

(due to a pneumothorax), then the horizontal lines of the "waves" are seen throughout the entire image. The presence of a lung point (transition point from a normal to an abnormal pleural interface) is pathognomonic of pneumothorax and can reliably rule in its presence if seen.

Chest ultrasound has a sensitivity and specificity that exceeds X-Ray and approaches that of CT in diagnosing a haemothorax through visualisation of pleural fluid [9]. Ultrasound can be used to guide the placement of intercostal drains or as a tool to identify the focus of bleeding for surgical intervention in the shocked trauma patient (see FAST).

Intra-Alveolar Fluid

Chest ultrasound can identify consolidatory changes in lung tissue which can be a result of fluid, infection or blood/contusions. Ultrasound can differentiate between pulmonary contusions and pneumothorax as the cause for hypoxia, guide initial management and stabilisation of patients prior to full-body CT.

Key Points

- Ultrasound can be used to identify the cricothyroid membrane in patients with difficult airway anatomy, to facilitate surgical cricothyroidotomy
- Chest ultrasound has a sensitivity that exceeds that of X-ray and approaches that of computerised tomography (CT) in ruling out a pneumothorax
- Chest ultrasound has a sensitivity and specificity that exceeds X-Ray and approaches that of CT in diagnosing a haemothorax
- Chest ultrasound can identify consolidatory changes in lung tissue which can be a result of fluid, infection or blood/contusion

Circulation

Cardiac

Focused echocardiography can be used to assess the heart for filling, contractility, dilatation, hypertrophy and presence of cardiac tamponade. How to undertake this skill is beyond the scope of this book. However, the The Society of Point of Care Ultrasound website (https://spocus.org/resources-programs/foamed/) highlight the usefulness of such scans in the assessment of a shocked patient. The information gathered from a focused echocardiogram can be used to assess and guide treatment of both the shocked trauma patient and those in cardiac arrest.

Abdominal

Focused assessment with sonography in trauma (FAST) is a well-established skill in the ED and has excellent specificity for ruling in a haemoperitoneum [10, 11]. Extended FAST (e-FAST) includes these four views as well as the lung/pleura (see earlier for chest ultrasound):

- Hepatorenal space (Morrison's pouch)
- Splenorenal space
- Retro-vesicular space (Pouch of Douglas in women)
- Pericardial space

In modern day trauma care, spiral CT and proximity of scanners to the emergency department make whole body CT (WBCT) a favourable imaging modality. Notwithstanding, the REACT-2 trial failed to demonstrate a statistically significant mortality benefit with WBCT compared to conventional imaging and selective CT in blunt trauma [12]. FAST scanning however, may have a role in those patients in extremis for whom an ultrasound scan can guide resuscitation and operative intervention prior to a delayed CT.

Abdominal ultrasound can also demonstrate occult retroperitoneal haemorrhage from a ruptured abdominal aneurysm with varying specificity and sensitivity [13].

Vascular Access

Ultrasound can help place intravenous cannulae or central vascular access in patients with difficult vascular access. Retrograde endovascular balloon occlusion of the aorta (REBOA) is an emerging concept in pre-hopsital emergency medicine (PHEM), requiring ultrasound-guided femoral arterial guide wire placement.

Disability

Raised intracranial pressure (ICP) is challenging to exclude on clinical examination alone, and the instigation of neuroprotective measures reduce morbidity and mortality. Early studies have shown that ultrasound may be a sensitive tool for ruling out raised ICP via the assessment of the optic nerve sheath diameter at the optic disc [14] (Fig. 26.12).

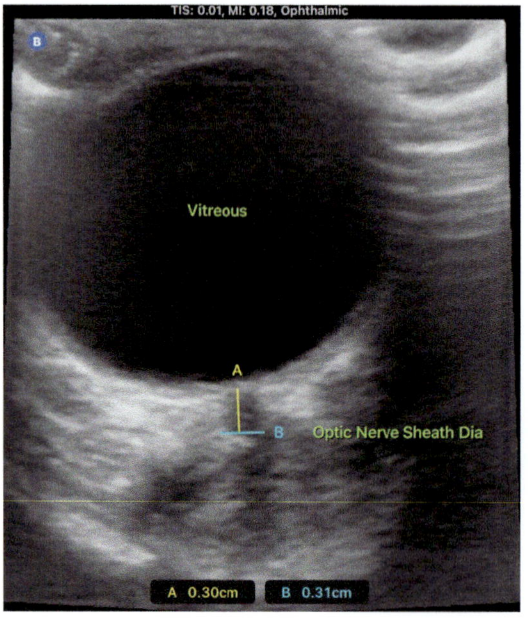

Fig. 26.12 Optic Nerve Sheath Diameter measurement. The optic nerve sheath is a linear hypoechoic structure posterior to the globe. Measurement A identifies the location for measurement of sheath diameter (3 mm behind the retina). Measurement B is the measurement of the optic nerve sheath diameter (3.1 mm). Image courtesy of Dr. J Squires

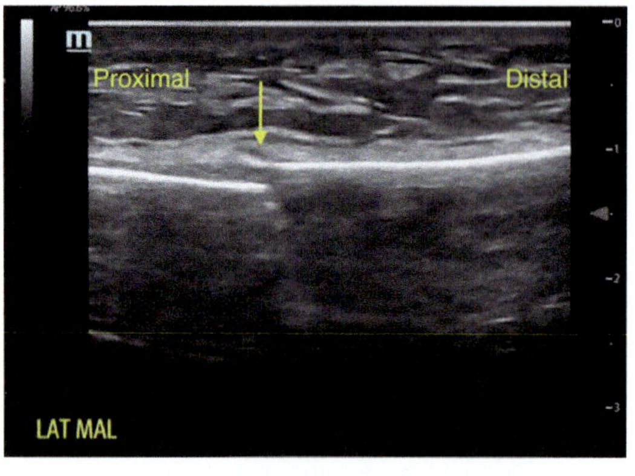

Fig. 26.13 Cortical step indicating bony fracture (from Crombach et al [15])

Exposure

Ultrasound can be used to identify cortical steps in fractured bones and help to guide the pre-hospital management of injuries (Fig. 26.13) in resource-limited environments. Ultrasound-guided nerve blocks for the pre-hospital management of distal injuries and limb entrapments are a developing concept, whereas ultrasound-guided nerve blocks are well established in hospital practice.

Cardiac Arrest

A focused echocardiogram can be used in cardiac arrest to identify aetiology, guide treatment and facilitate decision-making. Ultrasound can be used to identify the following pathologies; Pseudo-pulseless electrical activity (PEA), Hypovolaemia, Contractility, Massive PE and Cardiac Tamponade.

Pseudo PEA (occasionally referred to as a "low-flow" state as opposed to a "no-flow" state) is a severe shock state, distinct from true electromechanical dissociation. If cardiac activity is seen on ultrasonography (e.g. in severe hypovolaemia or cardiac tamponade) then treatment is directed at the aetiology of the shock rather than CPR and standard ALS algorithms. True PEA is where there is electromechanical dissociation, no evidence of cardiac pulsation on echocardiography, and treatment is guided by ALS algorithms.

The role of pre-hospital ultrasound remains contentious [16–19] with the uptake variable across HEMS providers. However, the value of ultrasound in the demonstration of irreversible pathology and the benefit of this when making decisions to cease resuscitation should also be taken into consideration.

Key Points

- Focused echocardiography can be used to assess the heart for filling, contractility, dilatation, hypertrophy and presence of cardiac tamponade
- Focused assessment with sonography in trauma (FAST) has excellent specificity for ruling in a haemoperitoneum
- Ultrasound may be a sensitive tool for ruling out raised ICP via the assessment of the optic nerve sheath diameter

- Ultrasound can be used to identify cortical steps in fractured bones and help to guide the pre-hospital management of said injuries
- A focused echocardiogram can be used in cardiac arrest to identify aetiology, guide treatment and facilitate decision-making

Limitations & Governance

The in-hospital use of POCUS is well established, and several courses are available through the Royal College of Emergency Medicine and affiliated organisations (RCEM and ICS) that allow clinicians to train in the use of POCUS, maintain currency and continued professional development. In the pre-hospital environment, there needs to be a consideration of whether the additional information gained by ultrasound will change patient management without delaying scene times.

Many UK HEMS staffing models include pre-hospital physicians who may be trained in POCUS from their base hospital speciality. The Air Ambulance Association (AAA) guidance on POCUS advises that all services undertaking pre-hospital POCUS should have appropriate training, governance and standards of imaging as would be expected in hospital practice [20]. POCUS is not currently part of the IBTPHEM sub-speciality curriculum, and training should be aligned to neighbouring institutions and adapted to PHEM. An RCEM approved level 1 course would be a good starting point.

There are numerous practical limitations with performing pre-hospital ultrasound that must be considered so that they can be anticipated and mitigated; sunlight, vibration and movement during land or air transport can impact on image quality. POCUS must not delay scene times for time-critical patients. Patients are not prepared as they would be in an outpatient setting so full stomachs and empty bladders impacting on image quality. Screen size may impact on image quality and interpretation.

Usual hospital-based practice, supported by the AAA guidance on POCUS, also suggest that the following clinical governance issues must be considered when introducing ultrasound to pre-hospital care teams:

1. An ultrasound lead with appropriate experience and training should be appointed
2. All physicians undertaking pre-hospital POCUS should have the required training to do so with a logbook supporting continued professional development and currency
3. Regular training and updates should be provided by the service to all clinicians involved in pre-hospital POCUS
4. Documentation of POCUS use in the diagnosis and management of patients must be kept, and images stored digitally in a central database for audit, review/examination and training

Key Points

- The in-hospital use of POCUS is well established, and several courses are available to facilitate training and maintain currency
- The Air Ambulance Association (AAA) advises all services should have appropriate training, governance and standards as would be expected in hospital practice
- There are numerous practical limitations with performing pre-hospital ultrasound, nor should it delay scene times for time-critical patients

Conclusion

POCUS is a useful skill that has several uses in care of the trauma patient. In the pre-hospital environment it may give information which would otherwise not be available without CT scanning, and in-hospital in select groups it may lead to the avoidance of ionising radiation or logistically difficult transfers to CT scanners. While there is an acknowledged degree of inter-operator variability in the interpretation of scans [21–23], by picking gross sonographic end points rather than relying on fine details, this should be largely mitigated against. Ultrasonography should be subject to established governance and training requirements whether used in- or pre-hospital, and its use will likely increase in the next few years as scanners become cheaper, smaller and more durable.

Questions

1. What is the frequency range of medical ultrasound?
   (a) >20 Hz
   (b) >20 KHz
   (c) 1–5 MHz
   (d) 6–13 MHz
   (e) 1–13 MHz
2. Sound waves can weaken in intensity as they travel through the body by a variety of different mechanisms. Which of the following mechanism definitions is correct?
   (a) Refraction: Sound waves vectors are altered as they pass through soft tissue interfaces. This may result in waves that are reflected by deeper structures being unable to return to the transducer for detection
   (b) Transmission: Sound wave amplitude attenuates as the waves move away from their point of origin and through soft tissue
   (c) Scatter: Sound waves continue through the soft tissue without reflection and therefore are not detected by the transducer
   (d) Attenuation: Sound waves are reflected in multiple vectors, with only those in plane with the transducer being detected
3. Resolution is the ability to distinguish between two echos/objects in terms of space, time or strength. Which of the following resolution definitions is correct?
   (a) Contrast Resolution: Changes in anatomy that occur over time can be used to demonstrate or quantify pathology
   (b) Temporal Resolution: Differentiation between tissues with differing echo characteristics
   (c) Spatial Resolution: Structures that are close together can be delineated and displayed separately, in both an axial and lateral plane
4. Chest ultrasound can rule out a pneumothorax via demonstration of an intact pleural interface with the following features:
   (a) Presence of pleural sliding
   (b) Absence of B-lines
   (c) Presence of D-lines
   (d) Presence of C-lines
   (e) Barcode/Stratosphere M-mode
5. the AAA guidance on POCUS suggest that the following clinical governance issues must be considered when introducing ultrasound to pre-hospital care teams:
   (a) An ultrasound lead with appropriate experience and training should be considered
   (b) All physicians undertaking pre-hospital POCUS should have the required training to do so with a logbook supporting continued professional development and currency
   (c) Regular training and updates should be provided by the clinicians parent hospital
   (d) Documentation of POCUS use in the diagnosis and management of patients must be kept, written examination summaries stored digitally in a central database

Answers

1. e
2. a
3. c
4. a
5. b

References

1. Pontet J, Yic C, Díaz-Gómez JL, Rodriguez P, Sviridenko I, Méndez D, et al. Impact of an ultrasound-driven diagnostic protocol at early intensive-care stay: a randomized-controlled trial. Ultrasound J. 2019;11(1):24.
2. Wilson S, Mackay A. Ultrasound in critical care. Contin Educ Anaesth Crit Care Pain. 2012;12(4):190–4.
3. Hall DP, Jordan H, Alam S, Gillies MA. The impact of focused echocardiography using the focused intensive care echo protocol on the management of critically ill patients, and comparison with full echocardiographic

studies by BSE-accredited sonographers. J Intensive Care Soc. 2017;18(3):206–11.
4. Reid C. Sonography training oriented to retrieval medicine manual [Internet]. Greater Sydney Area HEMS; 2016 [cited 2019 June 20]: [88 p.]. Available from: https://nswhems.files.wordpress.com/2016/06/sonography-training-oriented-to-retrieval-medicine-manualsm.pdf
5. Shin S-J, Jeong B-J. Principle and comprehension of ultrasound imaging. J Korean Orthop Assoc. 2013;48(5):325–33.
6. Ma OJ, editor. Ma and Mateer's emergency ultrasound. 3rd ed. New York: McGraw-Hill; 2013.
7. Osman A, Sum KM. Role of upper airway ultrasound in airway management. J Intensive Care. 2016;4(1):52.
8. Chen L, Zhang Z. Bedside ultrasonography for diagnosis of pneumothorax. Quant Imaging Med Surg. 2015;5(4):618–23.
9. Brooks A, Davies B, Smethhurst M, Connolly J. Emergency ultrasound in the acute assessment of haemothorax. Emerg Med J. 2004;21(1):44–6.
10. Farahmand N, Sirlin CB, Brown MA, Shragg GP, Fortlage D, Hoyt DB, et al. Hypotensive patients with blunt abdominal trauma: performance of screening US. Radiology. 2005;235(2):436–43.
11. Sirlin CB, Brown MA, Andrade-Barreto OA, Deutsch R, Fortlage DA, Hoyt DB, et al. Blunt abdominal trauma: clinical value of negative screening US scans. Radiology. 2004;230(3):661–8.
12. Sierink JC, Treskes K, Edwards MJR, Beuker BJA, den Hartog D, Hohmann J, et al. Immediate total-body CT scanning versus conventional imaging and selective CT scanning in patients with severe trauma (REACT-2): a randomised controlled trial. Lancet Lond Engl. 2016;388(10045):673–83.
13. Hwang J, Harbison Kimberly H, Liteplo A, Sajed D. Ultrasound for abdominal aortic aneurysm [Internet]. EBMedicine.net. 2011 [cited 2019 June 20]. Available from: https://www.ebmedicine.net/topics.php?paction=showTopicSeg&topic_id=252&seg_id=4863
14. Blaivas M, Theodoro D, Sierzenski PR. Elevated intracranial pressure detected by bedside emergency ultrasonography of the optic nerve sheath. Acad Emerg Med Off J Soc Acad Emerg Med. 2003;10(4):376–81.
15. Crombach A, Azizi N, Lameijer H, El Moumni M, ter Maaten JC. Point-of-care bedside ultrasound examination for the exclusion of clinically significant ankle and fifth metatarsal bone fractures; a single blinded prospective diagnostic cohort study. J Foot Ankle Res. 2020;13(1):19.
16. El Zahran T, El Sayed MJ. Prehospital ultrasound in trauma: a review of current and potential future clinical applications. J Emerg Trauma Shock. 2018;11(1):4–9.
17. Bøtker MT, Jacobsen L, Rudolph SS, Knudsen L. The role of point of care ultrasound in prehospital critical care: a systematic review. Scand J Trauma Resusc Emerg Med. 2018;26(1):51.
18. Ketelaars R, Reijnders G, van Geffen G-J, Scheffer GJ, Hoogerwerf N. ABCDE of prehospital ultrasonography: a narrative review. Crit Ultrasound J. 2018;10(1):17.
19. El Sayed MJ, Zaghrini E. Prehospital emergency ultrasound: a review of current clinical applications, challenges, and future implications. Emerg Med Int. 2013;2013:1–6.
20. Masud S. Use of Ultrasound in Pre-Hospital Emergency Medicine [Internet]. Association of Air Ambulances; 2016 [cited 2020 Aug 9]. Available from: https://associationofairambulances.co.uk/wp-content/uploads/2017/11/AAA-C09-Ultrasound-BPGDi.docx.pdf
21. Rippey JCR, Royse AG. Ultrasound in trauma. Best Pract Res Clin Anaesthesiol. 2009;23(3):343–62.
22. Vázquez Martínez JL, Quiñones Coneo KL, Villegas TV, Sánchez Porras M, Macarrón CP-C, Pérez AC, et al. Applicability of a modified EFAST protocol (r-EFAST) to evaluate hemodynamically unstable patients after percutaneous cardiac intervention. Crit Ultrasound J [Internet]. 2017 June 12 [cited 2020 Aug 10]: [9 p.]. Available from: https://www.ncbi.nlm.nih.gov/pmc/articles/PMC5468180/
23. Greatrex F, Montefiori E, Grupp T, Kozak J, Mazzà C. Reliability of an integrated ultrasound and stereophotogrammetric system for lower limb anatomical characterisation. Appl Bionics Biomech. 2017;2017:1–8.

Recommended Further Reading

Sonography Training Orientated to Retrieval Medicine Manual, Justin Bowra
Emergency Ultrasound Course Manual, Justin Bowra
Focused Intensive Care Echocardiography, Intensive Care Society
Ultrasound in Emergency Medicine Level 1, Royal College of Emergency Medicine
ABC in Pre-Hospital Emergency Medicine, Nutbeam & Boylan
Manual of Emergency and Critical Care Ultrasound, Noble & Nelson

Diagnostic Radiology in Trauma

27

Haripriya Ramotar and Constantinos Tingerides

- Introduction and importance of trauma imaging
- Trauma imaging modalities: Digital radiography, ultrasonography, computed tomography, magnetic resonance imaging, fluoroscopy, catheter angiography
- Injury patterns in major trauma based on anatomical regions
- Special considerations: Children, pregnancy, elderly
- Adverse events associated with administration of intravenous contrast

Introduction

On 8 November 1896, German physicist Wilhelm Roentgen produced an image of his wife's hand using electromagnetic radiation in a wavelength range he called X-rays [1]. Within weeks this new technology was used to image skeletal trauma; the following year, it was used near the battlefield during the Greco-Turkish War [2]. Since then, several breakthroughs in imaging technology have yielded new modalities. Fluoroscopy, Catheter angiography, Computed Tomography (CT), Ultrasonography, Magnetic Resonance Imaging (MRI) and Nuclear Medicine techniques all have a role in the investigation and treatment of trauma patients.

Trauma can affect a single area or it can be multifocal. It also ranges in severity from trivial to life-threatening. Imaging techniques are associated with a cost, can take up valuable time and even have the capacity to harm the patient, for example, through ionising radiation or the use of potentially nephrotoxic intravenous contrast agents. The fundamental principle of trauma imaging is to obtain accurate and sufficient information in a timely fashion with minimum risk to the patient. To achieve this, front line services work closely with radiology departments to produce and continuously review patient pathways, guidelines and protocols. All trauma team members must have a sufficient understanding of contemporary imaging strategies as suboptimal utilisation may lead to suboptimal results. This chapter primarily deals with imaging strategies in major trauma, i.e. patients suspected to have injuries that can result in death or severe disability, defined as an ISS score of >15.

Trauma Imaging Modalities

The Royal College of Radiologists has published guidelines for radiology in major trauma [3]. This document outlines the role of different modalities in this field. Digital radiography and

H. Ramotar (✉)
Department of Clinical Radiology, Whittington Health, London, UK
e-mail: haripriya.ramotar@nhs.net

C. Tingerides
Radiology Department, Leeds General Infirmary, Leeds, UK

P. Lax (ed.), *Textbook of Acute Trauma Care*, https://doi.org/10.1007/978-3-030-83628-3_27

ultrasonography can be performed at the bedside, while CT and MRI examinations require transferring the patient. Catheter angiography is often used in major trauma in an interventional radiology or hybrid suite, principally with a view to performing embolisation.

Digital Radiography

Digital radiography must be available in the emergency room. It is a workhorse in the initial assessment of many forms of trauma. It is invaluable in assessing chest trauma as it is a fast way of detecting pneumothorax and haemothorax. Such complications of chest trauma may require urgent intervention. Digital radiography has also traditionally been used in the assessment of the c-spine and the pelvis and is widely used in suspected limb fractures after excluding life-threatening injuries.

From combined meta-analyses, chest radiography has a pooled high specificity of 0.99 in detecting pneumothoraces (1.00 for tension pneumothoraces only). Still, it lacks sensitivity compared to other modalities, which may be due to many factors such as the pneumothorax size, location of air, projection used, and interpreter level of skill. Haemothoraces are detected with high specificity (1.00) and variable sensitivity (0.20–0.63) [4].

The use of cervical spine radiographs is decreasing as they are technically challenging to perform and have poor sensitivity compared to CT [5]. Similarly, many units have abandoned the routine use of pelvic radiographs, opting for a lower threshold of assessment with CT. In other units, pelvic radiographs remain a useful screening tool to rapidly determine the need for immediate interventions [6]. The effective dose for an AP pelvic x-ray is 0.7 mSv and 2.9–3.9 mSv for a pelvic CT, but fundamentally the use of plain film is in transition for trauma in most well-resourced areas. Hospitals have protocols in place guiding how the information gained from each modality (plain film vs straight to CT) guides patient management in their centre [7]. Digital radiography is not helpful in assessing abdominal trauma because of its low sensitivity and specificity in this area.

Ultrasonography

Ultrasound examinations can be performed at the bedside by appropriately trained operators. They have a role in the assessment of blunt or penetrating injury to the thorax and abdomen. Particular protocols termed Focused Assessment with Sonography for Trauma (FAST) or 'extended-to-thorax' extended—FAST (eFAST) have been developed. These can be used in the pre-hospital environment or immediately on arrival to hospital for suspected haemoperitoneum, haemopericardium, haemopneumothorax and inferior vena cava/aortic assessment [8]. A 3–5 MHz sector probe or curved linear array probe for the abdomen is often used. If eFAST is used, a sector scanner probe to visualise between the ribs can be helpful—see the POCUS chapter for a further discussion on scanning techniques.

FAST for haemoperitoneum has a median sensitivity of 0.64 and specificity of 1.0 with a lower sensitivity of 0.63 for any solid organ injury. Not all solid organ injury is associated with haemoperitoneum in the acute setting. Therefore, a negative FAST scan does not rule out significant intraabdominal or pelvic traumatic pathology [4]. Consequently, the use of FAST in major trauma as a sole imaging technique may result in a substantial underestimation of the presence and severity of solid organ injury.

eFAST for detecting pneumothoraces has a variable sensitivity of 0.40 and specificity of 1.00 for detecting tension pneumothoraces, and pooled sensitivity of 0.84 and specificity of 0.98 for pneumothoraces. Overall this diagnostic yield is higher than that for plain chest radiography [4]. Technically, a higher frequency (and possibly a sector scanner) probe is the most useful [8].

Computed Tomography

CT scans can be performed quickly and offer higher sensitivity and specificity than bedside tests for a variety of skeletal and soft tissue injuries. They are instrumental in detecting haemorrhage and guiding management to achieve haemostasis as fast as possible. They also have disadvantages. Transfer of the patient to the scanning room is needed, which may be hazardous in haemodynamically unstable patients. CT scanning uses ionising radiation, and most protocols require the administration of an intravenous contrast agent that may be nephrotoxic or cause an allergic reaction. Therefore the use of CT scanning must be justified for each patient.

In general, CT scans are indicated when:

- There is haemodynamic instability (the scan is performed after or during resuscitation).
- There is an obvious severe injury on clinical assessment.
- Bedside imaging has suggested significant injuries such as pneumothorax on chest radiographs or intra-abdominal fluid on FAST assessment.
- The mechanism of injury suggests that there may be severe occult injuries. Such mechanisms include high-speed vehicle collision and fall from height.

After a decision to perform a CT scan is taken, the team must decide which areas need to be scanned. Generally speaking, there are two strategies for performing a CT scan in major trauma. One approach is to use CT to scan the areas where an injury is clinically suspected, guided by bedside tests including digital radiography. The second is to scan the entire body (termed whole-body CT—WBCT). The advantage of the first strategy is that reducing the scan volume reduces the radiation to the patient. The disadvantage is that clinically excluding injury in one area when there is a significant or distracting injury elsewhere is often difficult; inaccurate assessment may lead to delayed diagnosis and extra trips to the scanner. WBCT provides a comprehensive evaluation of life-threatening traumatic injuries, reduces trips to the CT scanner, and mitigates the necessity for other imaging modalities such as radiography and ultrasound.

Several studies have shown benefits to WBCT, claiming increased probability of survival and decreased time in the emergency department. However, these studies have been retrospective and are plagued with selection bias. The REACT-2 Trial is the first randomised controlled trial to compare these two strategies [9]. The authors concluded that WBCT does not reduce in-hospital mortality compared with the standard radiological workup. Future research may help identify subgroups of patients that benefit from WBCT.

Using intravenous contrast agents in trauma CT allows the reporting radiologist to detect bleeding and improves the assessment of solid organ and other injuries. The timing of image acquisition in relation to the administration of contrast determines the phase of the scan. For example, in an arterial phase abdominal scan, images are acquired around 20 s after injecting intravenous contrast. This allows accurate assessment of the arteries and improves the sensitivity of detecting arterial abnormalities. If images are acquired again a few seconds later, the contrast will be more concentrated in the parenchyma of the solid organs and venous structures (portal-venous phase). In a split bolus scan, two variably sized contrast boluses are given at different times to enhance the abdominal arterial and venous systems simultaneously. Again, there are several possible combinations of phases, and the radiologist must tailor each scan according to the clinical information.

In 2005 Nguyen et al. first published the use of a biphasic contrast protocol in a combined study between centres in Baltimore, US and Geneva, Switzerland [10]. This 'top-to-toe' approach starts with an unenhanced CT of the head +/− the neck to assess for haemorrhage. Then contrast is administered in two different volume boluses at different rates (the exact volumes of which can vary slightly from centre to centre) and a single acquisition from either the base of skull or lung apices to the ischial tuberosities. A 5 min delayed acquisition was then performed through the region of a suspected injury to further assess for bleeding. This protocol is commonly referred to as the Bastion Protocol in the UK as military radiologists adopted it in Camp Bastion in Afghanistan.

In many centres, a dedicated CT scanner is situated next to (and in some cases within) the emergency department to make the transfer of patients less hazardous. Bedside imaging examinations should not delay transfer to CT for imaging. One possible exception is the chest radiograph in an unstable patient, as chest drain insertion may help in the efforts to render the patient haemodynamically stable for transfer to CT. However, as described in the breathing and chest injury chapter, tension pneumothorax is rare in spontaneously breathing patients and should primarily be a clinical diagnosis in ventilated patients.

Magnetic Resonance Imaging

There are instances where magnetic resonance imaging (MRI) is indicated in the context of neurological trauma, and it must be available at all times in a major trauma centre. MRI can be considered if there is strong clinical suspicion of spinal injury, even if no abnormality is seen on radiographs. There may be some subtle, indirect markers that raise the suspicion of a ligamentous neck injury on a trauma CT (e.g. anterior vertebral soft tissue swelling), but pure ligamentous injuries are best detected with MRI. Sequences that highlight tissue oedema, such as inversion recovery, are particularly useful. Compressive soft tissue lesions such as extradural haematomas of the spinal canal may cause spinal cord injury. Penetrating neurological trauma with non-magnetic materials (such as wood) can be assessed with MRI, where additional information on associated contusions, haematomas and/or intraventricular blood may provide further prognostic information [11].

Fluoroscopy

There are instances where fluoroscopic procedures may be indicated to aid care in severely injured patients. Fluoroscopy is a technique where real-time screening x-rays are used to monitor the movement of radio-opaque structures such as bones. Contrast can also be used to monitor the flow of liquids and check the integrity of fluid containing structures, such as the urinary system. One such use is when there is suspected urethral injury in an uncatheterised patient. The presence of blood at the urethral meatus, particularly in males, should raise the suspicion of a renal collecting system, bladder or urethral injury. A retrograde urethrogram can be done to assess the integrity of the urethra [12]. This should be done in a dedicated suite or theatre with the ability to obtain real-time fluoroscopic images.

If there is a suspicion of a bladder injury in a catheterised patient, retrograde cystography can be performed. This involves instilling contrast until the bladder is full and obtaining images with fluoroscopy. A retrograde cystogram can also be performed during the initial CT assessment by performing another CT after the bladder is filled.

Catheter Angiography

Interventional Radiologists perform catheter angiography, often to achieve haemostasis through embolisation or the use of stent grafts. This technique is the basis of many interventional radiology procedures, which are discussed in the interventional radiology chapter.

Injury Patterns in Major Trauma

Head and Neurological Trauma Imaging

Image findings in significant cranial trauma include fractures of the skull, parenchymal contusion, intracranial bleeding and sequelae of raised intracranial pressure. Such injuries are often associated with maxillofacial fractures. Data are acquired with a single pass of the patient through the CT gantry. The data are used to create several sets of images designed to optimise the detection of different types of injuries. The sets of images vary in the orientation, windowing (degree of post-acquisition adjustments made to highlight certain tissue types, e.g. bone or lung) and slice thickness.

Calvarial fractures can range from overt displaced deformities (Fig. 27.1) to subtle non-displaced fractures requiring review of multiplanar reformats for identification (Fig. 27.2). Base of skull fractures may already be evident clinically with the classic Battle's sign or Panda eyes. However, radiologically they can be very complicated as they require an assessment of several important base-of-skull features and vascular structures (Fig. 27.3). Bone injuries can be identified on an unenhanced study with specific bone reconstructions.

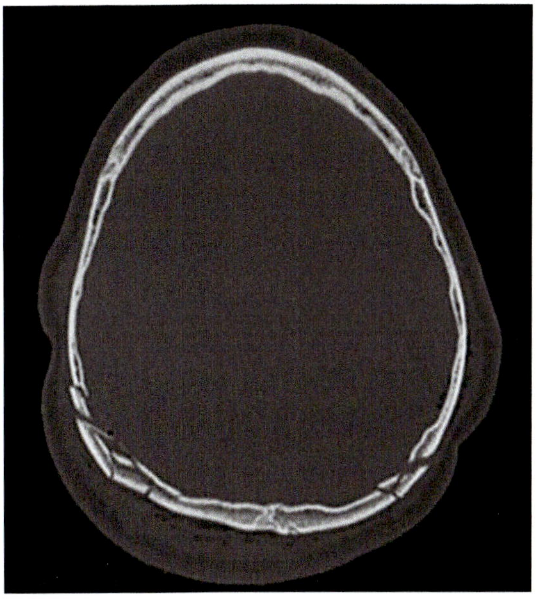

Fig. 27.1 Axial CT with bone reformatting to reveal extensive calvarial fractures of the parieto-occipital region

Brain injury in the setting of trauma can occur with or without calvarial or base of skull fractures. Injury patterns include contusional injuries, extradural/subdural/subarachnoid haemorrhage and hypoxic brain injury (Figs. 27.4, 27.5 and 27.6). All of these injuries can be potentially identified in an unenhanced study. Intravenous contrast is very rarely needed, with the only benefit found in the enhancement of small intra-axial contusional injury that is not high density at the time of scanning. The addition of intravenous contrast is thought to introduce added perfusional stress to neural tissue because of disturbance of the blood-brain barrier [13]. Intracranial bleeding can cause raised intracranial pressure (Fig. 27.7). Disruption in the equilibrium between blood, brain tissue and CSF fluid in a fixed space can result in brain herniation with catastrophic consequences.

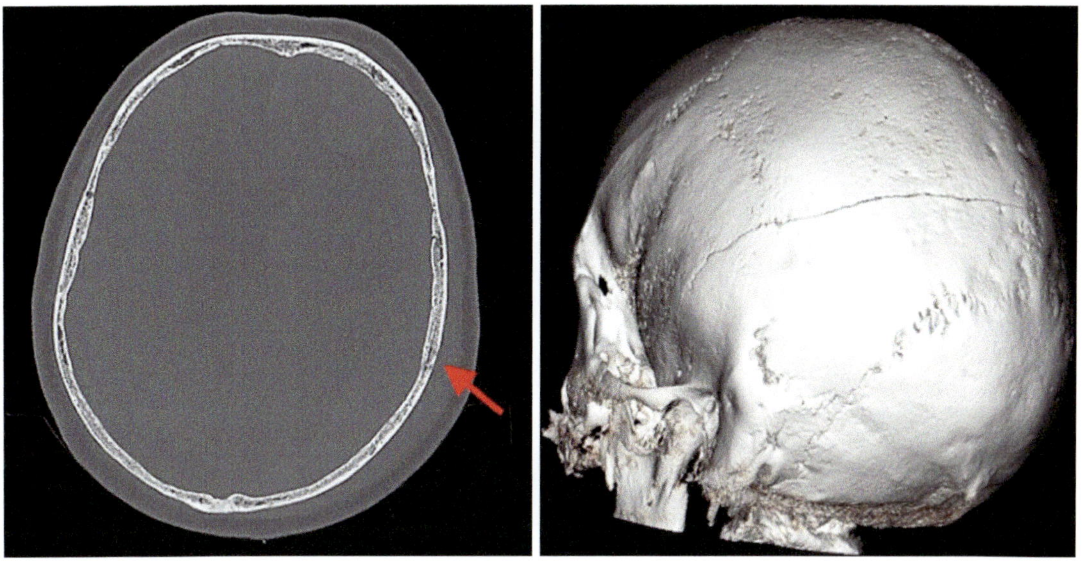

Fig. 27.2 Comparison of axial CT of the head with bone reformats and 3D reconstructions demonstrating a subtle left parietal bone fracture that is better visualised on 3D reconstructions

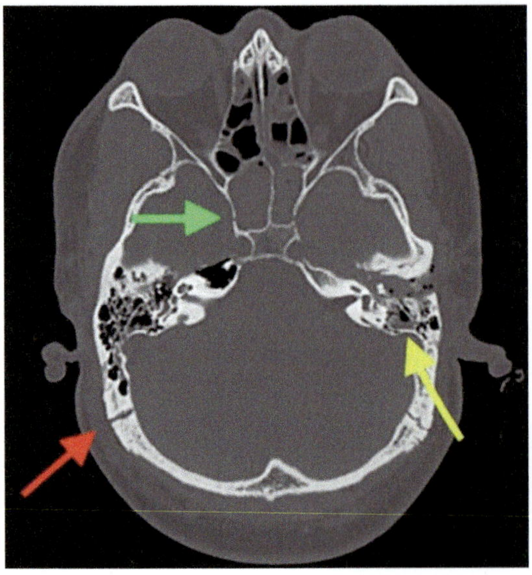

Fig. 27.3 Base of skull fractures with diastasis of the right lambdoid suture (red arrow). There are further fractures through the sphenoid sinuses (green arrow) and the left mastoid air cells (yellow arrow)

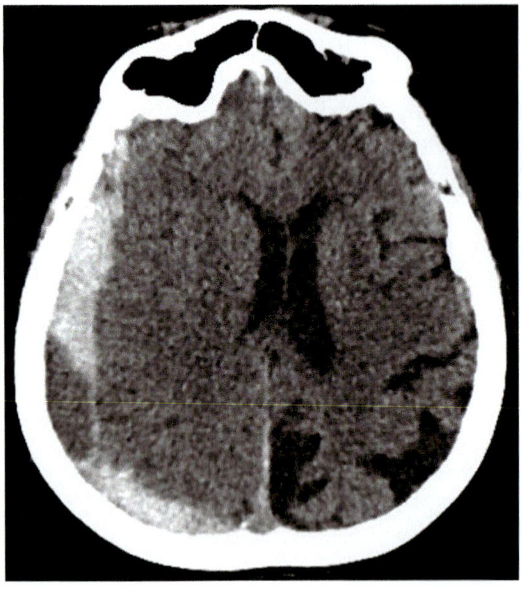

Fig. 27.4 A large right sided cresentic high density subdural haematoma is visualised. Low density areas within it represent flow artefact from ongoing brisk bleeding

Blunt cervical vascular injury (BCVI) is a term used for injuries to the carotid and vertebral arteries secondary to non-penetrating trauma. Although BCVI is rare, it can lead to devastating outcomes, including stroke and death. Current

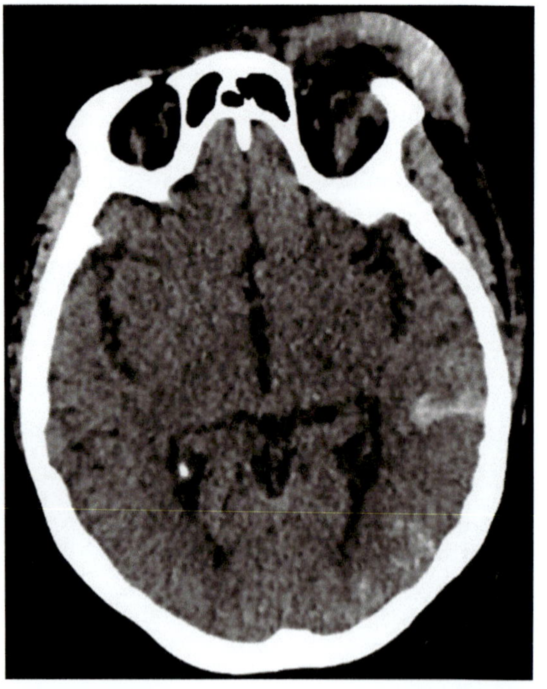

Fig. 27.5 High density outlining the sulci of the left parietal lobe represents subarachnoid haemorrhage. A concurrent left periorbital haematoma is the point of impact of injury

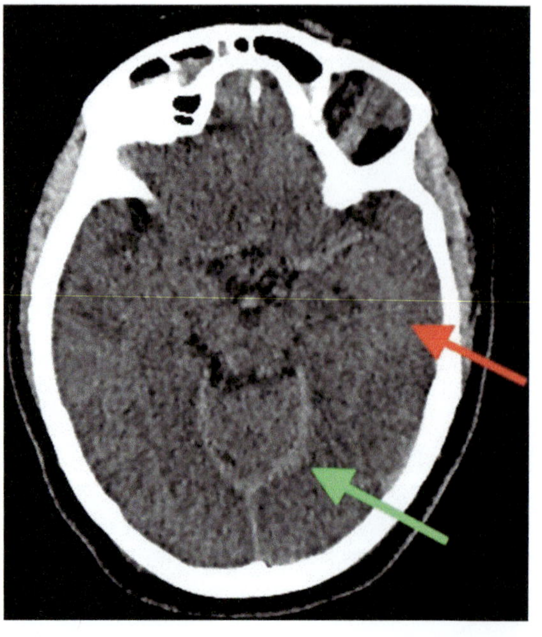

Fig. 27.6 Axial CT image demonstrating global hypoxic injury with a reversal of gray-white matter density (red arrow). As a result the posterior falx cerebri and tentorium cerebelli are relatively dense, creating the 'pseudosubarachnoid' sign (green arrow)

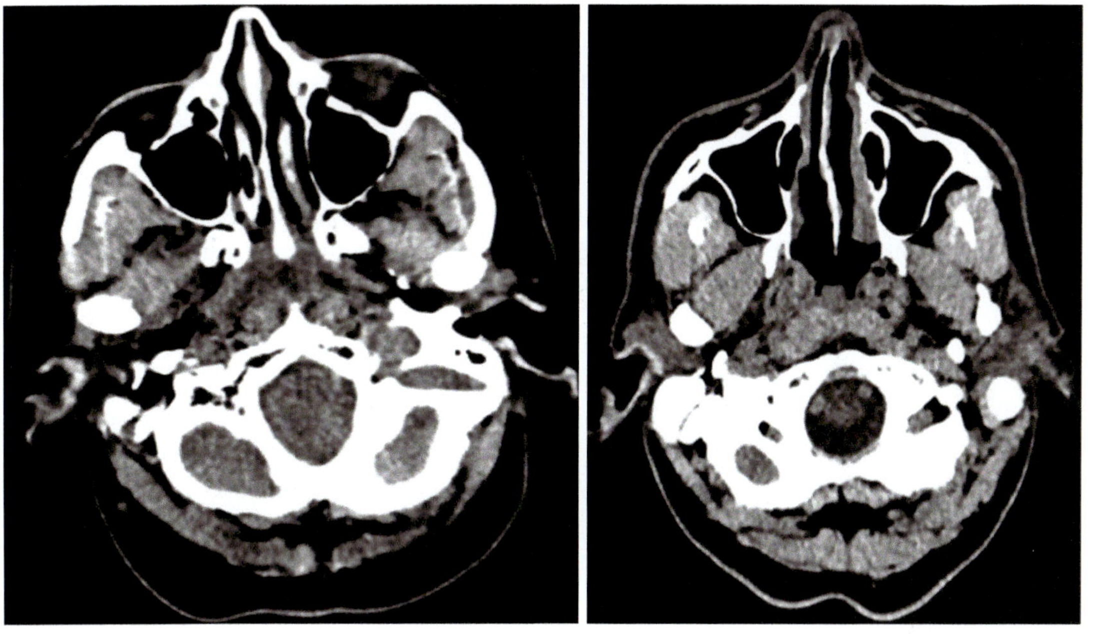

Fig. 27.7 Two axial plane CT scans demonstrating fullness of the foramen magnum (left) and a normal foramen magnum with visible CSF (right). The former is a result of descent of the cerebellar tonsils due to raised intracranial pressure

treatment strategies for BCVI range from antiplatelet and anticoagulation therapy to endovascular stents and mechanical thrombectomy. When there is clinical suspicion of BCVI, a CT angiogram of the neck can be used to diagnose the injury in the first instance. In some cases however, BCVI is asymptomatic, or it occurs in patients with other neurological trauma. Such injuries can present with delayed onset of neurologic injury that may have been avoided if BCVI was recognised and treated. Screening for BCVI in high-risk patients may improve outcomes, and therefore screening criteria have been developed and are in use in trauma centres [14, 15].

Injuries of the spine require careful clinical and radiological assessment. In the setting of isolated cervical spine injury, the National Emergency X-Radiography Utilization Study (NEXUS) provides a set of validated criteria for patients <65 years old to determine which patients require imaging. If the patient is alert and stable, there is no focal neurology, no altered level of consciousness, no intoxication, no midline spinal tenderness or distracting injuries, then there is a sensitivity of 99.6% for ruling out cervical spine injury [16]. Over the age of 65, these criteria are less reliable, and a clinical decision regarding imaging is needed. The Canadian C-Spine Rule (CCR) also provides an algorithm for use to decide which patients require at least radiography of the cervical spine. CT with sagittal and coronal reconstructions is the primary imaging tool in Major Trauma Centres (Fig. 27.8). Otherwise, if this facility is not available, plain film radiographs from the occiput to T1 with lateral, AP, and odontoid views (Fig. 27.9) should be done if the patient fits the criteria for imaging [17].

In the context of the Severely Injured Patient, the spine is assessed as a part of WBCT with axial, sagittal and coronal bone reconstructions of the whole spine. CT imaging can identify bony injuries, which may need concomitant treatment consideration, but it does not assess the cord itself unless there is catastrophic disruption. If there is clinical or radiological suspicion of spinal cord injury, an urgent MRI is recommended once the patient is stable and the imaging resources are available. MRI can be used to identify prognostic features such as spinal cord swelling, oedema or contusion. As previously mentioned, MRI is also better at detecting purely ligamentous injuries which may require treatment.

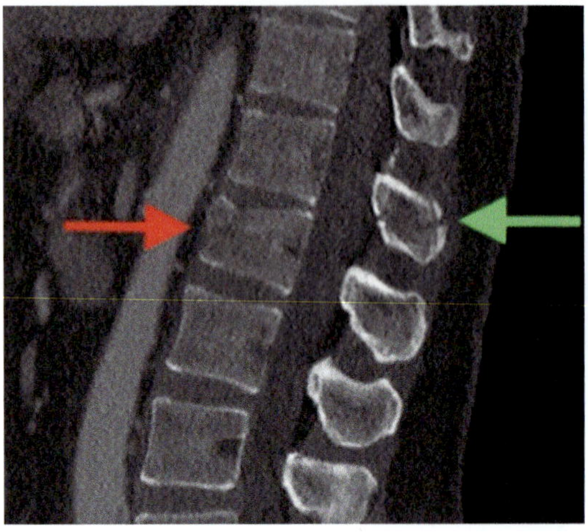

Fig. 27.8 A selected image from a sagittal view of the spine with bone reformats demonstrating a Chance fracture. A horizontal fracture through a vertebral body (red arrow) extends into the spinous process (green arrow)

Chest Trauma Imaging

Injuries can occur anywhere from the extrathoracic tissues to the heart. The most concerning injuries are those that cause significant injury of the aorta or directly to the heart. Lung injury in the form of pulmonary contusions or lacerations may also be the source of significant morbidity and mortality. The chest portion of trauma CT is usually performed in the arterial or split-bolus phase with contrast opacifying the systemic (i.e. non-pulmonary) arteries to outline traumatic abnormalities and points of haemorrhage.

Injuries that involve the pleural space include pneumothoraces (particularly in penetrating injuries) and haemothoraces (Fig. 27.10). Air can be introduced in the pleural space secondary to alveolar rupture from sudden increased intrathoracic pressure (blunt trauma) or from the external environment (penetrating injury (Fig. 27.11). Particularly worrying is a tension pneumothorax (Fig. 27.12) with penetrating injury when a valve system in the chest wall is created that allows air to be continually drawn in but not released. The result is a rise in intrathoracic pressure above that

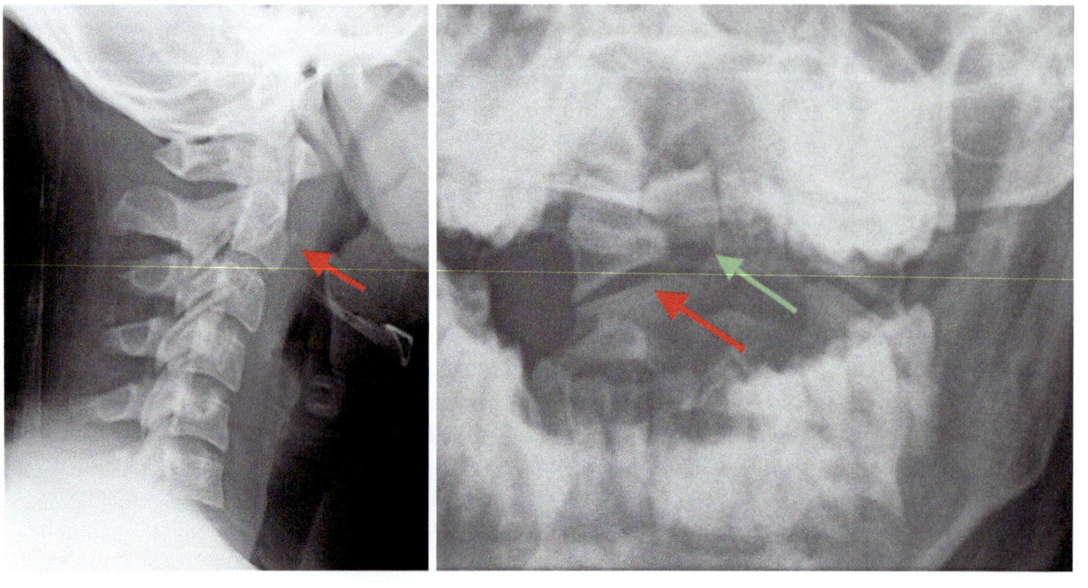

Fig. 27.9 These images are not from the same injury. On the left a sagittal cervical spine view shows a small avulsion fracture of the anterior C2 body. On the left an open-mouth peg view demonstrates asymmetry between the C1 right lateral mass and the C2 body (red arrow) and widening at the atlantodental interval (green arrow)

of the atmosphere that can compromise venous return to the heart and cardiac function, and cause contralateral lung collapse worsening the patient's cardiorespiratory status. A tension pneumothorax is a clinical diagnosis at the initial assessment stage and should be treated before any imaging is carried out. Imaging a pneumothorax with plain radiography can prove difficult as air accumulates medially and anteriorly in the supine position, and apically in the erect position. As most trauma x-rays are performed with the patient lying supine on a bed, anterior pneumothoraces can be quite large before showing the typical loss of vascular markings or a "lung edge" at the periphery. Pneumothoraces demonstrated on CT but not on plain film are called 'occult' pneumothoraces. These are particularly important if a patient is to be ventilated—a small pneumothorax can increase in size under ventilation and become clinically significant. The term haemothorax refers to blood in the pleural space and can be caused by bleeding from several sources such as mediastinal vascular structures, the lungs or intercostal vessels. Emergency chest drain insertion may be necessary to improve ventilation.

Pulmonary contusion is a common injury in blunt chest trauma. It is caused by injury to the alveoli with associated alveolar haemorrhage. As such, the usual appearances are of patches of ill-defined airspace consolidation at the location of impact, with sometimes an opposing contra-coup contusion. It is reasonably short-lived, with reso-

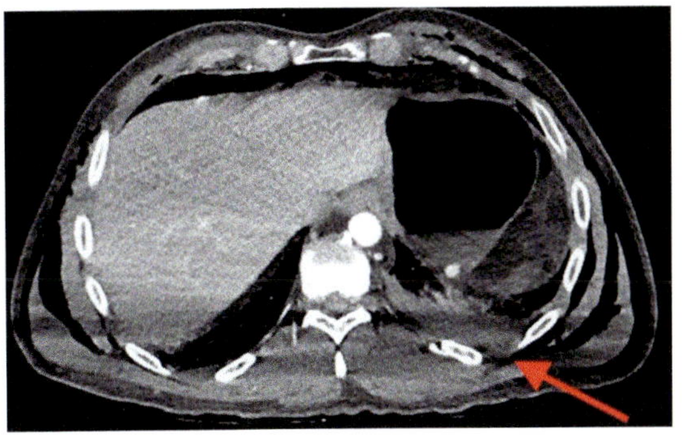

Fig. 27.10 Axial plane CT image of a high density left sided haemothorax (red arrow)

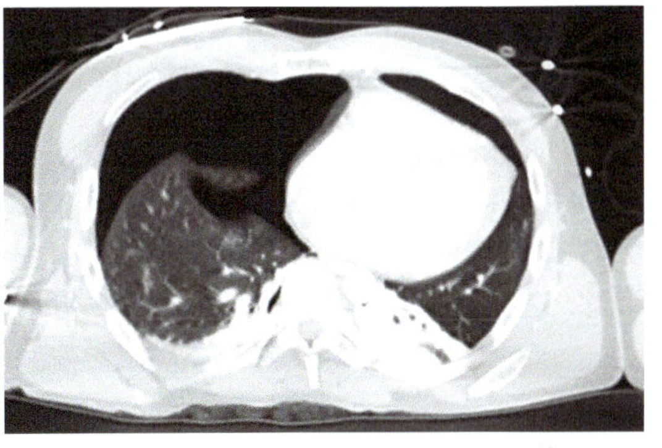

Fig. 27.12 A large right-sided tension pneumothorax displaces the mediastinum to the left. There is also a small volume left-sided pneumothorax present

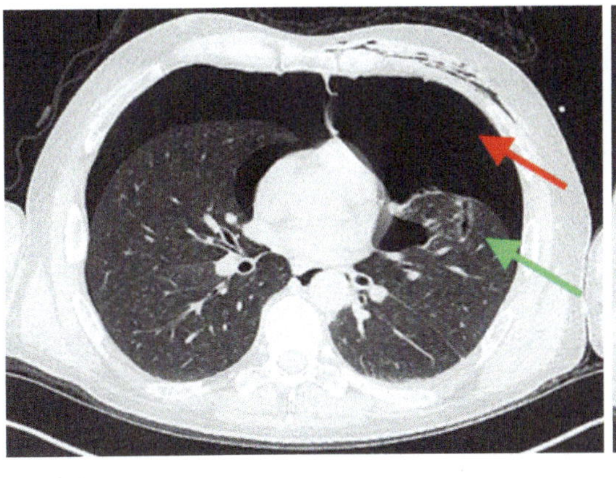

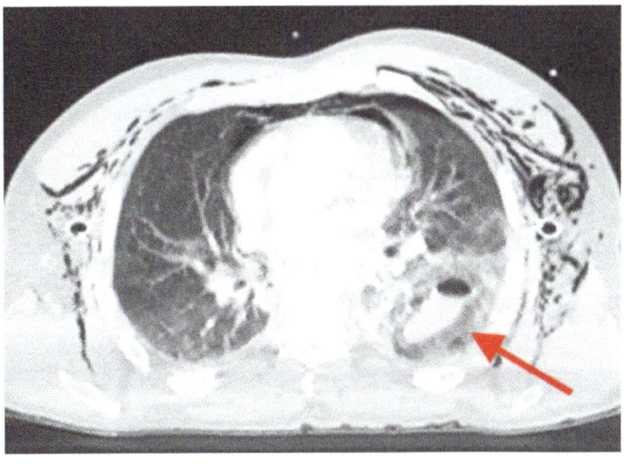

Fig. 27.11 On the left bilateral pneumothoraces (red arrow) with a linear left-sided pulmonary laceration (green arrow) from a penetrating chest injury are visible. On the right there is a posterior left pulmonary laceration with cavitation and a concurrent haematocoele. (red arrow)

lution beginning within 24–48 h after the injury. However, extensive pulmonary contusions (or moderate-sized ones in patients with pre-existing lung disease) can cause a significant respiratory compromise in this period [18].

Pulmonary lacerations from penetrating or blunt injuries (shearing or rib fractures) present as oval or rounded cavities along the tract of the laceration rather than as a linear defect like those seen in solid visceral lacerations. This is due to the elastic recoil of the lung tissues that cause the lung parenchyma to move away from the laceration. They can be filled with air, blood or both [18].

Injury to the heart and thoracic aorta can be direct due to penetrating injury that breaches the myocardium or aortic wall at the point the penetrating object enters, or indirect in the case of deceleration injury. Common locations of aortic injury are the proximal descending aorta, aortic arch, aortic root, distal descending aorta and the aortic hiatus where there are aortic attachments. Periaortic haematoma is often present and can be an indirect sign of vascular injury (Fig. 27.13). Further changes such as intramural haematoma, pseudoaneurysm, an intimal flap and thrombus are best visualised on CT [18]. Imaging of aortic injury is also discussed in the interventional radiology chapter.

Bronchial and tracheal lacerations are rare. Patients with these injuries often die before arriving at a hospital due to respiratory arrest, pneumothorax, haemorrhage or associated injuries related to high energy trauma. Deceleration injury can compress the upper airway between the thoracic spine and the sternum, shear the airway at fixed points or cause rupture when the intrathoracic pressure is raised against a closed glottis [19]. Complete transection of the bronchi results in a 'dropped lung' appearance. Bronchoscopy to confirm the diagnosis is often recommended if a tracheobronchial injury is demonstrated or suggested on CT. Complications include pneumonia, empyema, bronchiectasis and airway obstructions to name a few, and therefore treatment in a specialist unit is needed.

Chest wall injuries range from simple broken ribs to flail segments, scapular fractures and significant chest wall soft tissue injuries. In a flail segment, the fractured portion moves paradoxically on respiration and poses a problem with ventilation. Flail segment is a clinical diagnosis, but it should be raised in a CT report when there are three or more consecutive ribs with fractures in two or more places [20].

Abdominal and Pelvic Trauma Imaging

Deceleration, external compression and crush injuries make up the majority of blunt injury forces causing vascular and solid visceral injury. Points of fixation such as vascular pedicles and

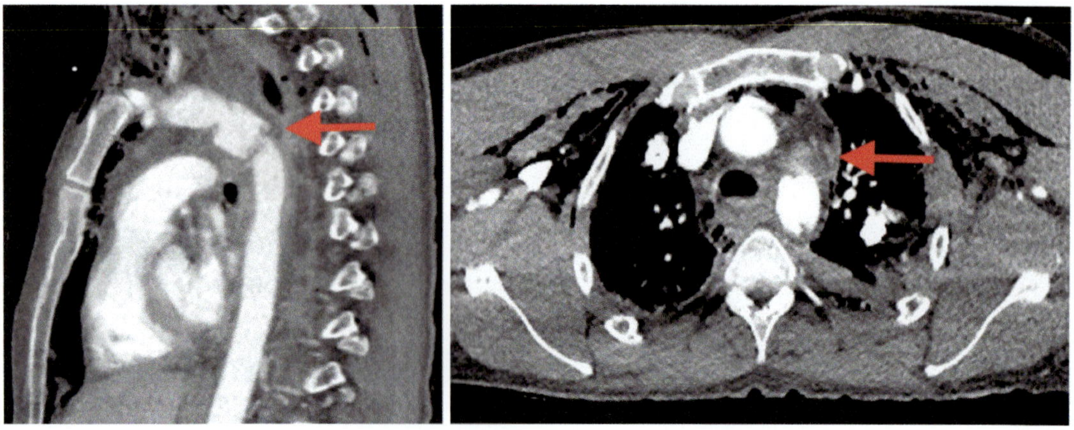

Fig. 27.13 Sagittal and axial contrast enhanced CT images showing a proximal descending thoracic aortic incomplete transection (left) with a resultant mediastinal haematoma (right)

mesenteric attachments are placed under considerable shear forces and can tear in deceleration injury, causing bleeding (Fig. 27.14). Hollow visceral structures and the diaphragm may rupture when external compression forces create a sudden rise in intraabdominal pressure. Crushing forces compress the solid organs between the abdominal wall and spine. This may cause tears, and consequently bleeding may occur from damaged arterial or venous structures. Performing a delayed phase study of the abdomen and pelvis can assess pooling of any extravasated contrast if a blush was identified on the survey of the initial study by the radiologist with the patient on the CT table. Sometimes even if there is no point of bleeding demonstrated, high-density free fluid in the abdomen and pelvis can serve as indirect evidence of bleeding and indicate the need for early operative intervention. Low energy penetrating traumas cause lacerations along the path of object entry (Fig. 27.15). High-energy penetrating traumas such as gunshot wounds cause regional soft tissue injury and cavitation along the tract [21].

The spleen, liver, kidneys and small bowel are the solid organs that are most commonly injured [22], with linear lacerations being the most common injury (Fig. 27.16). At the scene or on arrival to the emergency department, a FAST scan can assess for the presence of free fluid that may suggest a more severe injury if the patient is haemodynamically unstable and may require emergency surgical intervention. CT scanning is the gold

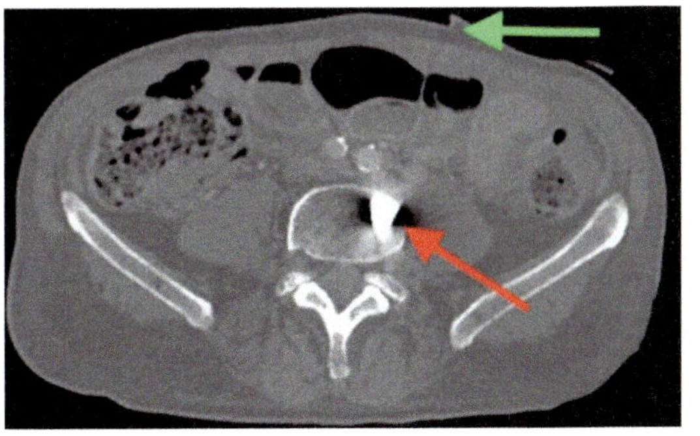

Fig. 27.15 Axial CT with bone reformats through the abdomen demonstrates a very high density triangular object in the vertebral body (red arrow), which represents the broken off tip of a knife blade responsible for a penetrating abdominal injury wedged in the bone. A skin defect at the entry site in the anterior left abdominal wall is visible (green arrow)

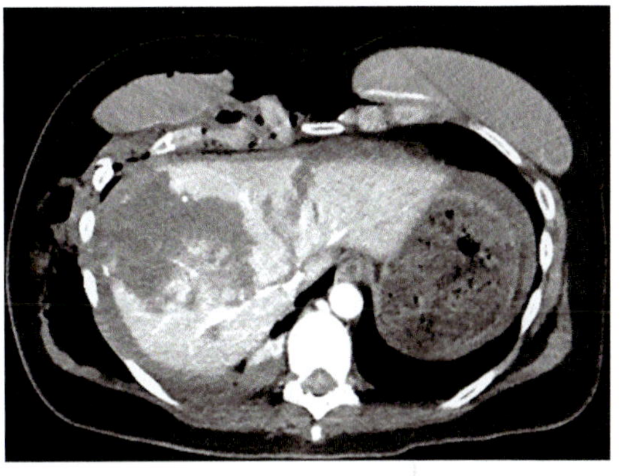

Fig. 27.16 Multiple low density linear lacerations of the liver extend to the hilum. Surrounding fluid likely represents haematoma

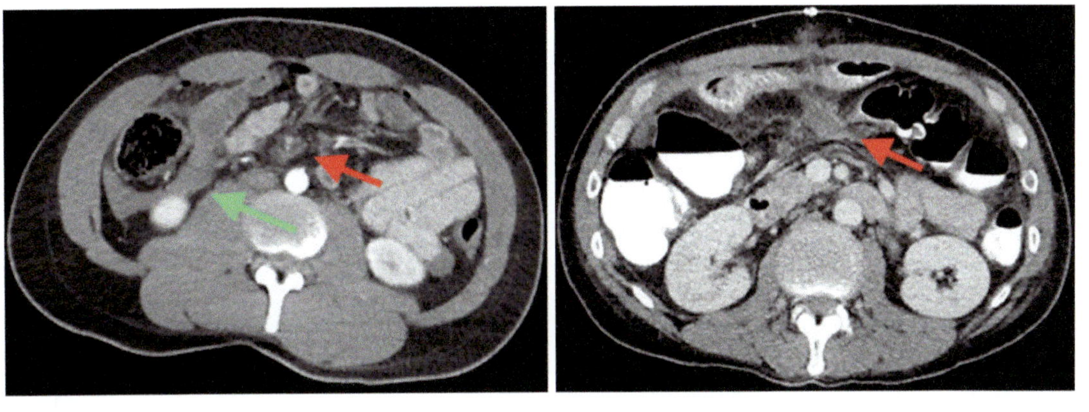

Fig. 27.14 On the left an axial contrast enhanced CT image shows discontinuity of the superior mesenteric artery (red arrow). Concurrent lack of enhancement of right-sided small bowel (green arrow) compared with enhancing left-sided bowel represents resultant small bowel hypoperfusion and possibly ischaemia. On the right image, a dense mesenteric haematoma (red arrow) indicates significant mesenteric injury

standard, and those patients who are more severely injured have the most to gain from WBCT per a recent multi-centre, retrospective analysis [23]. While FAST is a useful technique if positive in haemodynamically unstable patients who need emergency treatment and cannot be taken for a CT scan, a negative FAST does not rule out significant intra-abdominal bleeding [24]. Paradoxically, the false-negative rate increases with more severely injured blunt trauma patients (i.e. those with an ISS of >25) [25]. The anatomical locations assessed are the hepatorenal fossa, left subphrenic space, both paracolic gutters and the pouch of Douglas. Free fluid in the pelvis of young women of reproductive age can be equivocal in significance and be related to their menstrual cycle. However, free fluid in men is more strongly indicative of solid visceral injury. Ultimately if the mechanism of injury is significant enough and the patient is objectively symptomatic with external signs of injury, transfer to CT should not be delayed. Diagnostic peritoneal lavage is not commonly performed and does not feature in the NICE guidelines for assessing bleeding in abdominal trauma.

Injuries to the mid-upper abdomen (e.g. from a steering wheel or handlebars) can result in pancreatic and/or duodenal injury with a 70–95% specificity of CT in detecting these injuries [26]. In the first 12 h post injury, the pancreas may appear normal with a small volume of peripancreatic fluid, fluid around the splenic vein and thickening of the fascia. If there is delayed onset of abdominal pain, a repeat study can be done in 24–48 h [19]. Lacerations can extend through the neck and body to variable degrees, but ultimately injury to the main pancreatic duct is associated with high morbidity and mortality [27]. Isolated duodenal injuries are rare. Isolated subserosal haematomas can present gastric outflow obstruction.

Injury to the stomach, bowel and mesentery are uncommon but delaying the diagnosis of this injury for even 8–12 h can lead to the development of peritonitis and sepsis, increasing morbidity and mortality [28]. Indicators of hollow viscous injury are pneumoperitoneum, pneumoretroperitoneum, focal discontinuity in the bowel wall, transection, or more indirectly, bowel wall thickening or poor enhancement [19]. Diffuse foci of mesenteric haemorrhage or extravasation of intravenous contrast from small mesenteric vessels can also be seen and is often an indication for urgent laparotomy.

The kidneys and ureters are vulnerable to injury in road traffic accidents, with frank haematuria being a reliable indicator of such an injury. In a study by Erlich and Kitrey, 84–95% of renal trauma was managed conservatively [29]. Vascular injury or injury to the intra- or extrarenal collecting systems require surgical assessment. If perirenal free fluid is visualised on the CT, renal collecting system injury with a urinoma should be suspected (Fig. 27.17). A delayed phase CT would be needed to opacify the renal collecting system to identify the point of injury. This can be done at the initial trauma CT or later once the patient is stable. The vascular pedicle of the kidney can be avulsed in a deceleration injury. A differential lack of enhancement of the kidney may indicate such an injury [19]. Renal cortical lacerations are visualised as linear areas of low attenuation that may extend anywhere from the capsule to the renal pelvis with associated haematoma, subcapsular haematoma or renal parenchymal contusion according to the American Association for the Surgery of Trauma (AAST) renal injury scale [30]. A delayed phase study

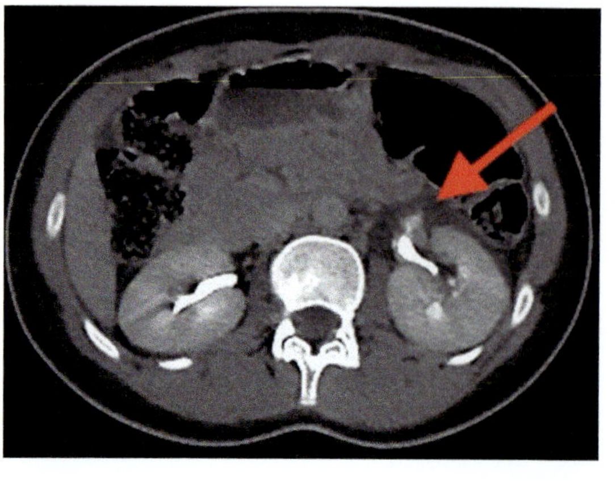

Fig. 27.17 This contrast-enhanced delayed-phase axial CT of the abdomen shows a blush of contrast around the left renal pelvis (red arrow) indicating rupture of the left renal collecting system

may highlight pooling of extravasated contrast to confirm a point of bleeding if there is a suspicion of it on the arterial or split bolus phase.

Urinary bladder injury or rupture is often due to a combination of a full bladder and compressive forces to the pelvis that may result in a pelvic fracture. Frank haematuria in the presence of a pelvic fracture warrants a cystogram, again either at the time of the injury if the patient has a functioning urinary catheter in situ, or at a later time once the patient has been catheterised. Cystograms involve injecting contrast agent via a catheter to distend the bladder. Then imaging is performed by CT or by fluoroscopy. Bladder ruptures can be intraperitoneal (Fig. 27.18) or, more commonly, extraperitoneal (80–90%) [31]. In the former, contrast that escapes the bladder can be seen outlining intraabdominal structures such as the bowel and collecting along peritoneal reflections. In the latter contrast outlines extraperitoneal structures and spaces.

The pelvis is a bony ring with very rigid fibrous joints. A fracture of this ring at a single point cannot be presumed to be isolated, and careful evaluation of the trauma CT is needed to look for other injuries. Compression forces may be in the AP plane, laterally, vertically shearing or a combination. Haemorrhage and pelvic visceral injury are common serious sequelae of pelvic fractures (Fig. 27.19). The elderly, frail patients or those at

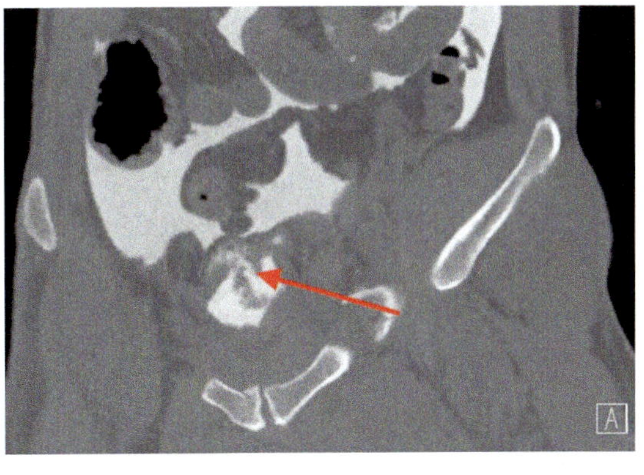

Fig. 27.18 Coronal CT of the pelvis after injection of contrast agent into the urinary bladder via a urethral catheter. A large defect in the superior aspect of the bladder (red arrow) represents an intraperitoneal rupture of the bladder with contrast outlining the bowel and mesentery

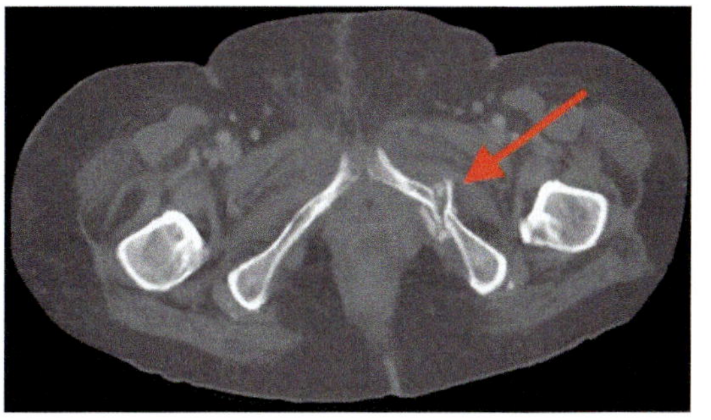

Fig. 27.19 Axial CT through the lower pelvis with bone reformats shows a fracture of the left interior pubic ramus (red arrow) with a surrounding high density haematoma

risk of bleeding (e.g. anticoagulation or hypocoagulable conditions) may bleed significantly due to minor lateral compression injury. A pelvic binder is often applied if there is a suspected pelvic fracture in the context of hypotension. This binder can temporarily reduce unstable fractures and halt venous bleeding. If no pelvic fracture is demonstrated on WBCT, a radiograph is required after removal of binder.

Special Considerations

Children

Generally, the use of adult trauma imaging protocols is seen as inappropriate in the paediatric trauma population. Developing tissues are more radiosensitive with a cumulative radiation risk over a lifetime. Children have a longer projected lifetime in which the effects of these cumulative doses can manifest. It is predicted that cancers later in life will occur in 1 in 1000 patients who have a CT as a child [32]. Specific lower dose paediatric protocols and assessment by paediatric surgeons can help avoid unnecessary radiation exposure.

Pregnancy

The physiological and anatomical changes of pregnancy add to the complexity of trauma management. Moreover, in addition to the life of the pregnant patient, the life and wellbeing of the fetus is at risk. Fetal loss rates approach 40–50% in life-threatening trauma [33]. The priority in caring for the pregnant trauma patient is to stabilise the mother, as maternal demise will almost always lead to foetal demise. As already discussed, some of the best imaging techniques in trauma involve ionising radiation. It is thought that fetal radiation doses of less than 50 mGy are not associated with increased fetal anomalies or fetal loss throughout pregnancy. The radiation dose of WBCT is well below this threshold, and therefore it should not be withheld if clinically indicated [34]. WBCT is associated with higher radiation than strategies that do not involve CT. The approximate whole-body CT effective dose can be around 30 mSV, which is more than that of any combination of plain film equivalents. However, in the case of trauma in pregnancy, plain films do not play a large diagnostic role. Information yield, especially with respect to potential bleeding and visceral injury, is higher with WBCT. As the dose is below that implicated in fetal abnormalities, WBCT is the investigation of choice [35]. Every effort should be made to use as low a radiation dose as achievable. This can be done by adjusting technical parameters on the CT protocol and by avoiding overlapping imaged areas that include the uterus and fetus.

There are several pregnancy-specific injuries such as placental abruption, uterine rupture, premature rupture of the membranes and spontaneous abortion. Identification of such injuries may require imaging by more than one modality [34]. The contribution of the obstetrics team is invaluable in the management of the Seriously Injured pregnant patient, and early involvement is highly recommended.

Elderly

Declining physiological reserve and pre-existing conditions have been shown to influence patient outcomes after trauma adversely. The overall effect of even low energy trauma on an ageing patient (>65 years old) or a frail person can be devastating. In a study by Kirshenbom et al., coronary artery disease, renal failure, dementia and warfarin use were associated with a higher mortality rate during the patient's hospital admission after trauma [36]. A lower threshold for performing WBCT may be justified in this population.

Adverse Events Associated with Administration of Intravenous Contrast

The use of intravenous contrast agents is generally considered safe but not without risk. Adverse events vary from minor physiological reactions to life-threatening events. The risk can be reduced through screening and patient selection strategies. Teams should screen for predisposing factors that may contraindicate the use of contrast agents or increase the risk of reactions. In some cases, premedication or pre-hydration are also used to reduce risk: steroids are used to prevent allergic reactions, and pre-hydration is used to reduce the risk of contrast-induced nephropathy. The team must be able to promptly recognise and treat reactions when they do occur to reduce harm.

Adverse reactions can be classified as allergic-like or physiologic. Allergic-like reactions involve the release of histamine and other biologic mediators. They can range from limited urticaria to life-threatening laryngeal oedema, bronchospasm and cardiac arrest. Physiological reactions are associated with the molecular toxicity of each agent as well as physical and chemical characteristics such as osmolality and viscosity. Physiologic reactions range from a warm feeling to cardiovascular collapse. Distinguishing allergic-like reactions from physiologic reactions is vital as they require different treatments. Moreover, physiologic reactions do not require pre-medication with steroids in the future.

Contrast-induced nephrotoxicity (CIN) is a term used to describe a sudden deterioration in renal function following the administration of intravenous contrast agents. The validity of this condition has been questioned in the literature. This is because confounding medical conditions may also explain any observed reduction in renal function. The link between contrast agent administration and nephrotoxicity has not yet been fully clarified. Nevertheless, several local, national and international bodies have guidelines that outline steps to reduce the risk.

The risk of CIN is considered low in patients with stable renal function. A risk/benefit analysis should be performed in patients known or suspected of having reduced renal function. Indicated examinations should be tailored to allow the clinical questions to be answered with the lowest possible dose of contrast medium. When the patient's condition allows, pre-hydration should be performed as it is thought to reduce the risk of CIN. In the Severely Injured Patient with a high pre-test probability of haemorrhage, contrast-enhanced studies are performed regardless of renal function status [37].

Key Points

- All trauma team members must have a sufficient understanding of contemporary imaging strategies as suboptimal utilisation may lead to suboptimal results.
- Particular protocols termed Focused Assessment with Sonography for Trauma (FAST) or 'extended-to-thorax' extended—FAST (eFAST) have been developed and can be used in the pre-hospital environment or immediately on arrival to hospital for suspected haemoperitoneum, haemopericardium, haemopneumothorax and inferior vena cava/aortic assessment.
- Generally speaking, there are two strategies for performing a CT scan in major trauma. One strategy is to use CT to scan the areas where an injury is clinically suspected guided by bedside tests, including digital radiography. The second is to scan the entire body (termed whole-body CT—WBCT).
- The timing of image acquisition in relation to the administration of contrast determines the phase of the scan.
- There are instances where magnetic resonance imaging (MRI) is indicated in the context of neurological trauma, and it must be available at all times in a major trauma centre.
- The presence of blood at the urethral meatus, particularly in males, should raise the suspicion of a renal collecting system, bladder or urethral injury. A retrograde urethrogram can be done to assess the integrity of the urethra.
- Blunt cervical vascular injury (BCVI) is a term used for injuries to the carotid and vertebral arteries secondary to non-penetrating trauma. Although BCVI is rare, it can lead to devastating outcomes, including stroke and death. Current treatment strategies for BCVI range from antiplatelet and anticoagulation therapy to endovascular stents and mechanical thrombectomy.
- If there is clinical or radiological suspicion of spinal cord injury, an urgent MRI is recommended once the patient is stable and the imaging resources are available. MR can be used to identify prognostic features such as spinal cord swelling, oedema or contusion.
- Flail segment is a clinical diagnosis, but it should be raised in a CT report when there are three or more consecutive ribs with fractures in two or more places.
- While FAST is a useful technique if positive in haemodynamically unstable patients who need emergency treatment and cannot be taken for a CT scan, a negative FAST does not rule out significant intra-abdominal bleeding.
- It is predicted that cancers later in life will occur in 1 in 1000 patients who have a CT as a child. Specific lower dose paediatric protocols and assessment by paediatric surgeons can help avoid unnecessary radiation exposure.
- There are several pregnancy-specific injuries such as placental abruption, uterine rupture, premature rupture of the membranes and spontaneous abortion. Identification of such injuries may require imaging by more than one modality.
- The risk of CIN is considered low in patients with stable renal function. A risk/benefit analysis should be performed in patients known or suspected of having reduced renal function. Indicated examinations should be tailored to allow the clinical questions to be answered with the lowest possible dose of contrast medium.

Conclusion

Advances in technology have given imaging a pivotal role in managing the Severely Injured Patient following Major Trauma. The effective use of imaging techniques requires a high level of expertise and teamwork, and early collaboration with radiologists and radiographers who can recommend the most useful imaging strategy. Imaging is associated with risk which stems from the need to move a haemodynamically unstable patient, the use of ionising radiation and the use of intravenous contrast agents. Risk can be reduced by performing risk/benefit analysis on every case and tailoring techniques to each patient.

Questions

1. What is the most appropriate first line imaging investigation for suspected brain injury?
   (a) Intracranial catheter angiography
   (b) Contrast enhanced CT head and cervical spine
   (c) MRI head
   (d) Unenhanced CT head and cervical spine
   (e) skull radiograph
2. What is the most appropriate investigation for a suspected urethral injury
   (a) Urethral ultrasound
   (b) Pelvic CT
   (c) Pelvic MRI
   (d) Retrograde urethrogram
   (e) Cystoscopy
3. Which of the following statements about Focused Assessment with Sonography for Trauma (FAST) is false
   (a) FAST scan can exclude an aortic injury
   (b) It can be used to detect haemoperitoneum
   (c) It has replaced diagnostic peritoneal lavage in many centres
   (d) It can be used to detect haemopericardium
   (e) It can be performed by an appropriately trained emergency physician
4. Which of the following areas is NOT included in the FAST scan protocol
   (a) Perisplenic space
   (b) Hepatorenal recess
   (c) Perihepatic space
   (d) Pericardium
   (e) Peripancreatic space
5. Which of the following statements about bladder injury is false:
   (a) Bladder injuries are associated with pelvic fractures
   (b) Bladder ruptures are most commonly intraperitoneal
   (c) Fluoroscopic studies can have a role in the assessment of bladder injury
   (d) A bladder injury is often due to a combination of a full bladder and compressive forces to the pelvis
   (e) A retrograde CT cystogram is performed after injecting contrast directly into the bladder via a urinary catheter

Answer Key

1. d
2. d
3. a
4. e
5. b

References

1. Brodsky A, Kathren RL. Historical development of radiation safety practices in radiology. Radiographics. 1989;9(6):1267–75.
2. Graham RNJ. Battlefield radiology. Br J Radiol. 2012;85(1020):1556–65.
3. Radiologists TRCO. Standards of Practice and Guidance for Trauma Radiology in Severely Injured Patients [Internet]. Royal College of Radiologists; 2011 [cited 2020 Feb 28]. 24 p. Available from: https://www.rcr.ac.uk/system/files/publication/field_publication_files/bfcr155_traumaradiol.pdf
4. NICE. Major trauma: assessment and initial management [Internet]. National Institute for Health and Clinical Excellence; 2016 [cited 2019 Sep 18]. Available from: https://www.nice.org.uk/guidance/ng39/evidence/full-guideline-2308122833
5. Holmes JF, Akkinepalli R. Computed tomography versus plain radiography to screen for cervical spine injury: a meta-analysis. J Trauma. 2005;58(5):902–5.
6. Verbeek DO, Burgess AR. Importance of pelvic radiography for initial trauma assessment: an orthopedic perspective. J Emerg Med. 2016;50(6):852–8.
7. Ward R, Carroll WD, Cunningham P, Ho S-A, Jones M, Lenney W, et al. Radiation dose from common radiological investigations and cumulative exposure in children with cystic fibrosis: an observa-

tional study from a single UK centre. BMJ Open. 2017;7(8):e017548.
8. Richards JR, McGahan JP. Focused assessment with sonography in trauma (FAST) in 2017: what radiologists can learn. Radiology. 2017;283(1):30–48.
9. Sierink JC, Treskes K, Edwards MJR, Beuker BJA, den Hartog D, Hohmann J, et al. Immediate total-body CT scanning versus conventional imaging and selective CT scanning in patients with severe trauma (REACT-2): a randomised controlled trial. Lancet. 2016;388(10045):673–83.
10. Nguyen D, Platon A, Shanmuganathan K, Mirvis SE, Becker CD, Poletti P-A. Evaluation of a single-pass continuous whole-body 16-MDCT protocol for patients with polytrauma. AJR Am J Roentgenol. 2009;192(1):3–10.
11. Kazim SF, Shamim MS, Tahir MZ, Enam SA, Waheed S. Management of penetrating brain injury. J Emerg Trauma Shock. 2011;4(3):395–402.
12. Ingram MD, Watson SG, Skippage PL, Patel U. Urethral injuries after pelvic trauma: evaluation with urethrography. Radiographics. 2008;28(6):1631–43.
13. Mauser HW, van Nieuwenhuizen O, Veiga-Pires JA. Is contrast-enhanced CT indicated in acute head injury? Neuroradiology. 1984;26(1):31–2.
14. Bensch FV, Varjonen EA, Pyhältö TT, Koskinen SK. Augmenting Denver criteria yields increased BCVI detection, with screening showing markedly increased risk for subsequent ischemic stroke. Emerg Radiol. 2019;26(4):365–72.
15. Nagpal P, Policeni BA, Bathla G, Khandelwal A, Derdeyn C, Skeete D. Blunt cerebrovascular injuries: advances in screening, imaging, and management trends. AJNR Am J Neuroradiol. 2018;39(3):406–14.
16. Hoffman JR, Wolfson AB, Todd K, Mower WR. Selective cervical spine radiography in blunt trauma: methodology of the national emergency X-radiography utilization study (NEXUS). Ann Emerg Med. 1998;32(4):461–9.
17. Stiell IG, Wells GA, Vandemheen KL, Clement CM, Lesiuk H, De Maio VJ, et al. The Canadian C-spine rule for radiography in alert and stable trauma patients. JAMA. 2001;286(15):1841–8.
18. Kaewlai R, Avery LL, Asrani AV, Novelline RA. Multidetector CT of blunt thoracic trauma. Radiographics. 2008;28(6):1555–70.
19. Soto JA, Anderson SW. Multidetector CT of blunt abdominal trauma. Radiology. 2012;265(3):678–93.
20. Sangster GP, González-Beicos A, Carbo AI, Heldmann MG, Ibrahim H, Carrascosa P, et al. Blunt traumatic injuries of the lung parenchyma, pleura, thoracic wall, and intrathoracic airways: multidetector computer tomography imaging findings. Emerg Radiol. 2007;14(5):297–310.
21. Rhee PM, Moore EE, Joseph B, Tang A, Pandit V, Vercruysse G. Gunshot wounds: a review of ballistics, bullets, weapons, and myths. J Trauma Acute Care Surg. 2016;80(6):853–67.
22. Arumugam S, Al-Hassani A, El-Menyar A, Abdelrahman H, Parchani A, Peralta R, et al. Frequency, causes and pattern of abdominal trauma: a 4-year descriptive analysis. J Emerg Trauma Shock. 2015;8(4):193–8.
23. Huber-Wagner S, Biberthaler P, Häberle S, Wierer M, Dobritz M, Rummeny E, et al. Whole-Body CT in haemodynamically unstable severely injured patients – a retrospective, multicentre study. PLoS One [Internet]. 2013;8(7). [cited 2019 Aug 26] Available from: https://www.ncbi.nlm.nih.gov/pmc/articles/PMC3722202/
24. Savatmongkorngul S, Wongwaisayawan S, Kaewlai R. Focused assessment with sonography for trauma: current perspectives. Open Access Emerg Med. 2017;9:57–62.
25. Becker A, Lin G, McKenney MG, Marttos A, Schulman CI. Is the FAST exam reliable in severely injured patients? Injury. 2010;41(5):479–83.
26. Velmahos GC, Tabbara M, Gross R, Willette P, Hirsch E, Burke P, et al. Blunt pancreatoduodenal injury: a multicenter study of the research consortium of New England Centers for trauma (ReCONECT). Arch Surg. 2009;144(5):413–9. discussion 419–420
27. Wong YC, Wang LJ, Lin BC, Chen CJ, Lim KE, Chen RJ. CT grading of blunt pancreatic injuries: prediction of ductal disruption and surgical correlation. J Comput Assist Tomogr. 1997;21(2):246–50.
28. Killeen KL, Shanmuganathan K, Poletti PA, Cooper C, Mirvis SE. Helical computed tomography of bowel and mesenteric injuries. J Trauma. 2001;51(1):26–36.
29. Erlich T, Kitrey ND. Renal trauma: the current best practice. Ther Adv Urol. 2018;10(10):295–303.
30. Kozar RA, Crandall M, Shanmuganathan K, Zarzaur BL, Coburn M, Cribari C, et al. Organ injury scaling 2018 update: spleen, liver, and kidney. J Trauma Acute Care Surg. 2018;85(6):1119–22.
31. Gross JS, Rotenberg S, Horrow MM. Resident and fellow education feature bladder injury: types, mechanisms, and diagnostic imaging. Radiographics. 2014;34(3):802–3.
32. Kharbanda AB, Flood A, Blumberg K, Kreykes NS. Analysis of radiation exposure among pediatric trauma patients at national trauma centers. J Trauma Acute Care Surg. 2013;74(3):907–11.
33. Mattox KL, Goetzl L. Trauma in pregnancy. Crit Care Med. 2005;33(10 Suppl):S385–9.
34. Raptis CA, Mellnick VM, Raptis DA, Kitchin D, Fowler KJ, Lubner M, et al. Imaging of trauma in the pregnant patient. Radiographics. 2014;34(3):748–63.
35. Hui CM, MacGregor JH, Tien HC, Kortbeek JB. Radiation dose from initial trauma assessment and resuscitation: review of the literature. Can J Surg. 2009;52(2):147–52.
36. Kirshenbom D, Ben-Zaken Z, Albilya N, Niyibizi E, Bala M. Older age, comorbid illnesses, and injury severity affect immediate outcome in elderly trauma patients. J Emerg Trauma Shock. 2017;10(3):146–50.
37. Beckett KR, Moriarity AK, Langer JM. Safe Use of Contrast Media: What the Radiologist Needs to Know. Radiographics. 2015;35(6):1738–50. x

Interventional Radiology in Trauma

28

Chris Miller and Constantinos Tingerides

- Introduction to the development and growing role of interventional radiology in trauma.
- Endovascular equipment and embolic agents used in trauma.
- Resuscitative endovascular balloon occlusion of the aorta (REBOA).
- Common traumatic injuries amenable to endovascular intervention.
- Aftercare following endovascular procedures.

Introduction

Since its origin in 1964 with the first peripheral angioplasty procedure and subsequently the first endovascular embolisation for gastrointestinal haemorrhage in 1971 [1], interventional radiology has grown and evolved into a speciality that now performs a wide range of procedures diagnosing and treating a spectrum of pathologies. The integration of the interventional radiologist into the trauma team has been propagated by growing expertise honed in embolisation techniques in the non-acute setting combined with the technological advances in endovascular devices and imaging equipment. The almost ubiquitous availability of multi-slice whole body computed tomography now allows a rapid assessment and a targeted, minimally invasive intervention strategy to be employed where historically open surgery may have been performed [2].

Initially, endovascular management of trauma was reserved for patients who were haemodynamically stable falling into a non-operative management category. More recently, new devices and procedures are being utilised in the unstable patient and in initial resuscitation [3]. Endovascular techniques can be used as the primary therapy for haemostasis or following damage control trauma surgery when there is ongoing haemorrhage. It is generally accepted that avoiding open surgery where possible is beneficial, potentially reducing blood loss, procedure time and the requirement for a general anaesthetic [4].

The primary aim of the Interventional Radiologist in the management of traumatic injuries is to gain endovascular control of hemorrhage through either endovascular occlusion or re-lining of a damaged vessel with as little tissue damage as possible. This chapter reviews the indications, equipment and different techniques that are frequently used.

C. Miller (✉) · C. Tingerides
Radiology Department, Leeds General Infirmary, Leeds, UK
e-mail: christopher.miller6@nhs.net

P. Lax (ed.), *Textbook of Acute Trauma Care*, https://doi.org/10.1007/978-3-030-83628-3_28

Equipment and Devices

Basics

Access to the arterial system is usually through the common femoral artery. Although radial access is a safe alternative route, it is not yet widely used in trauma [5]. For the majority of embolisation procedures a 4Fr or 5Fr vascular access sheath can be used keeping the arteriotomy size to a minimum. If a large vessel stent graft is to be deployed then sheath diameters of up to 24Fr are needed. The artery can be punctured using ultrasound guidance or palpation and anatomical landmarks, although in shocked patients the femoral pulse may be difficult to palpate.

Subsequently the target vessel (usually identified on computed tomography in advance) is accessed using a combination of angiographic catheters and wires (Fig. 28.1) with a variety of properties based on their intrinsic design [6]. A microcatheter through the parent catheter and vascular access sheath (tri-axial system) permits cannulation of bleeding small branch vessels and "superselective" embolisation. Real time fluoroscopy is used when guiding to a specific location in the body, whilst digital subtraction angiography, often with high flow rates of contrast, is essential to detect an abnormal or bleeding vessel.

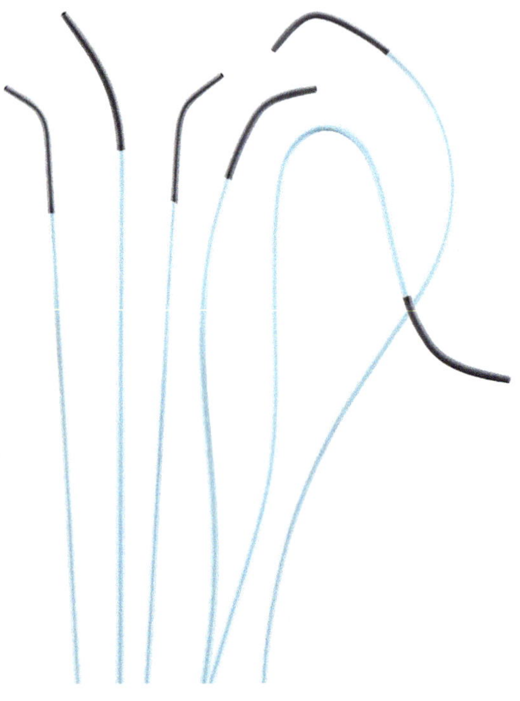

Fig. 28.1 Diagnostic angiographic catheters. The different shapes are used to access vessels throughout the body

Embolic Agents

There are a variety of embolic agents available which have different characteristics useful for specific scenarios. These can be classified by mechanism of action and by whether they produce a temporary or permanent effect. All work to cause vessel occlusion or decrease blood flow [7]. One of the priorities of any interventional radiologist performing embolisation procedures is to reduce blood flow in or occlude only the intended target vessel and minimise embolisation of healthy tissue (commonly known as non-target embolisation). It is therefore essential to understand and be familiar with the different embolic agents available and how they behave in vivo.

Coils are one of the most common types of devices used in trauma embolization (Fig. 28.2). These exert a mechanical embolic effect by physically blocking the vessel in addition to providing a thrombogenic surface and causing vascular endothelial damage and release of clotting factors. Coils are made of stainless steel or platinum and can have a fibre coating that increases thrombogenicity [8]. Coils are available in sizes varying from 1 mm up to several centimetres. They can be used in the smallest diameter arterial branches up to major trunk vessels, with the latter often requiring several coils to achieve full embolisation. Standard coils are designed for delivery through 4Fr angiographic catheters. Microcoils are designed to be delivered through microcatheters which can be advanced through small, tortuous vessels permitting embolisation of peripheral target vessels. Some coils include a retrievable mechanism and so can be repositioned if initially deployed in an unsuitable position. Coils are easily visible on angiography and, with

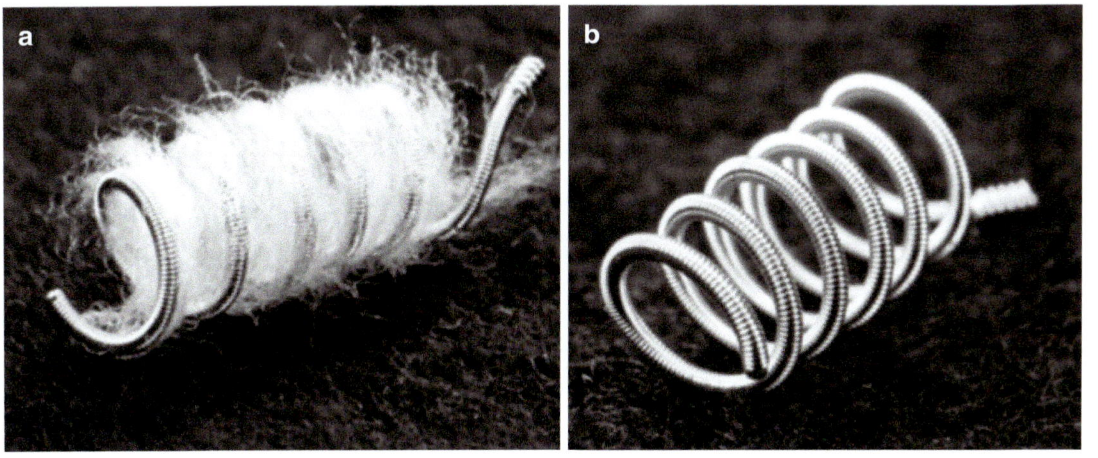

Fig. 28.2 Embolization coils made from platinum with (**a**) and without (**b**) nylon fibres, the fibres promote thrombosis

experience, can be accurately placed minimising the risk of non-target embolisation.

Vascular plugs are similar to coils in that they rely on a mechanical effect and induced thrombosis to cause vessel occlusion. They can be repositioned for accurate placement and are quick to deploy. Their main disadvantage over coils is that they are difficult to advance through tortuous anatomy. Also depending on size they require a larger size delivery catheter and so are more suited to larger, proximal vessels [9].

As already discussed, both coils and vascular plugs rely on the ability of the body to form thrombus in addition to their mechanical occlusion properties. In severe trauma that results in deranged clotting, the time to vessel occlusion following embolisation may be prolonged and ideally correction of underlying coagulopathy is undertaken prior to and alongside the interventional procedure [8].

Liquid embolic agents used in trauma include glue (Cyanoacrylate—Histoacryl, B Braun, Italy) and Onyx—an ethylene-vinyl alcohol copolymer (Onyx, Micro Therapeutics Inc., Ca, USA). A main advantage is that these agents do not require the patient to a have a normal coagulation to achieve a successful embolisation. Liquid embolics have complex in vivo properties and can have undesirable effects if used inappropriately by inexperienced operators [10]. Onyx co-polymerizes on contact with blood creating a lava substance controlled by gradual injection, this solidifies into a cast of the vessel over several minutes resulting in a permanent mechanical occlusion [11]. Cyanoacrylate is mixed with lipiodol before being injected to allow it to become radio-opaque and delay polymerization. The ratio of dilution influences viscosity. It solidifies quicker than Onyx and in addition to its mechanical effect causes an inflammatory response on the vessel wall. It can be more difficult to control as locules are carried distally by flow in the vessel [11].

Particulate embolic agents including polyvinyl acryl particles (PVA) and polymer spheres are less commonly used in trauma. Particles embolise distally occluding the distal vascular and capillary bed of the target vessel/organ resulting in a permanent occlusion and so could be used where distal haemorrhage control has not been successfully gained with another agent [12].

Another common agent used in trauma is Gelfoam (Pfizer, New York). This is purified porcine skin gelatin which is engineered into a porous sponge [13]. The sponge induces the clotting cascade thought to be due to platelet damage on contact with the intricate sponge lattice and also acts as a mechanical support to thrombus formation resulting in vessel occlusion [14]. One of the theoretical advantages of Gelfoam in trauma over other embolic agents is that it produces only a temporary effect as over time the agent is completely absorbed and target vessel is often recanalized [15]. Whilst this may seem counter-intuitive, the purpose of embolisation in trauma is to resolve haemorrhage whilst limiting end-organ ischaemia which can be achieved with temporary occlusion. Gelfoam is usually prepared as either a pledglet with the intention of creating a plug in a vessel or it can be cut into small pieces and mixed with contrast and saline to form a slurry which is injected resulting in embolisation distal to the catheter tip [16].

Stent-Grafts

Often injury occurs to larger vessels that cannot be sacrificed with embolisation. In such cases, endovascular repair of the vessel can be undertaken with a stent graft as an alternate to open surgical techniques (Fig. 28.3). Primarily designed for aneurysmal and peripheral vascular disease, stent-grafts were pioneered in the 1980s [17, 18]. In the last three decades their use has increased dramatically as endovascular repair has been associated with the healthcare ideal of lower perioperative mortality and reducing the length of stay in hospital following the procedure; the long term outcomes of endovascular treatments compared to surgical repair are however still contentious.

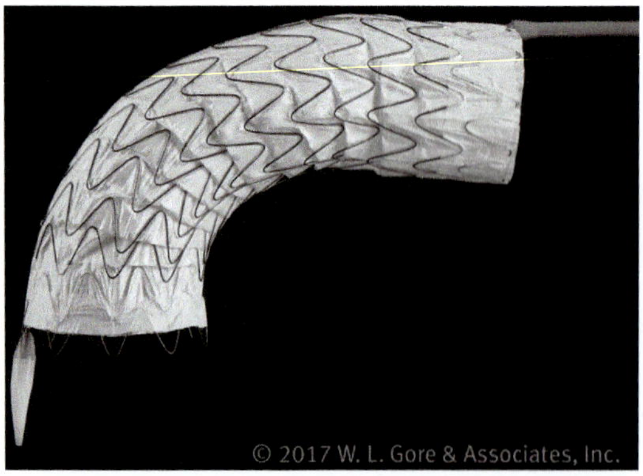

Fig. 28.3 Thoracic aortic stent graft. This model has metallic Nitinol (Nickel-Titanium alloy) stents supporting an ePTFE (expanded polytetrafluoroethylene) polymer graft

A range of stent-grafts are commercially available, the fundamental design being a metal-compound stent scaffold with a material cover such as polyester or polytetrafluoroethylene (PTFE). The grafts are either self-expanding relying on an intrinsic outward radial force to fix them to the vessel wall or are mounted on a balloon which is inflated in the artery until the stent is opposed to the wall. When deployed the stent-graft relines the vessel wall sealing the defect/injured segment and achieving haemostasis while maintaining vessel patency [10].

Closure Devices

On completion of the procedure, haemostasis must be achieved at the percutaneous arteriotomy access site. Very rarely the arterial sheath is left in situ to be used for arterial blood pressure monitoring or for access if a second endovascular procedure is considered very likely. If left in situ the sheath should be sutured and attached to a pressurised saline flush to prevent thrombus formation in the lumen.

Haemostasis is traditionally achieved by manual digital compression of the arteriotomy site and is often considered the gold standard. However, this can be time consuming, especially in the context of trauma where coagulopathy may be deranged. It also requires a period of flat bed rest recovery which might not be practical in patients with multiple injuries. Vascular closure devices were first introduced in the 1990s with the aim of achieving haemostasis rapidly and allowing earlier mobilization [19]. A range of closure devices are now available with different mechanisms of action. This includes those where the artery is approximated by deployment of a permanent suture or metal clip (Proglide, Starclose SE; Abbott Vascular), or where an absorbable sealant/plug is deployed over the arteriotomy site (Angio-Seal, St Jude Medical; Mynx-Grip, Cordis Cardinal Health).

Haemostasis can now be achieved in even the largest percutaneous arteriotomies and success rates of closure devices are high. The operator needs to be aware of and be able to manage complications that can arise. These include haematoma, pseudoaneurysm formation, acute ipsilateral leg ischaemia and failure to achieve haemostasis [20].

Targets for Endovascular Therapy

REBOA

Resuscitative endovascular balloon occlusion of the aorta (REBOA) is a minimally invasive technique utilised in patients in extremis from uncontrollable torso or lower limb haemorrhage. Traditionally resuscitative thoracotomy and aortic cross clamping is used to occlude the aorta and rapidly gain control in these cases. Whilst first described in two patients in the Korean war [21] the concept of balloon occlusion has only become more enthusiastically adopted in the twenty-first century largely driven by the wars in Iraq and Afghanistan where endovascular techniques were implemented in combat [22].

The principle of aortic balloon occlusion is similar to that of cross clamping—blood flow distal to the inflated balloon is halted or significantly reduced preventing further hemorrhage whilst proximally, coronary and carotid flow improve with a raised mean arterial pressure [23]. The technique for inserting the balloon is familiar to an experienced endovascular interventionist. First access is gained via the common femoral artery and a vascular sheath inserted. Through this the balloon is inserted to the desired level in the aorta—either zone 1 (between the left subclavian artery and the coeliac axis) for suspected abdominal visceral haemorrhage or zone 3 (below the renal arteries and above the aortic bifurcation) when the bleeding is suspected from the pelvis with pelvic fractures. Zone 2 is the visceral segment where balloon inflation should be avoided to prevent damage to the major abdominal branches [24]. External landmarks are used to estimate how far the balloon should be inserted without image guidance. The balloon is then inflated. Arterial pressure measurements can be taken from both the balloon catheter tip and arterial sheath, which should improve and diminish respectively.

Rapid progression of management following balloon insertion is of paramount importance. The time of inflation should be recorded and the length of time the aorta is occluded kept to a minimum so normal circulation can be restored promptly preventing ischaemic injury distal to the occlusion. This necessitates a rapid multidisciplinary decision on further definitive management which will either be an emergency laparotomy or endovascular embolisation to control the haemorrhage. Following deflation and removal of the balloon the common femoral arteriotomy will have to be closed in the groin using a closure device or surgery. Lower extremity perfusion should be assessed and any loss of peripheral pulses (or other evidence of ischaemia) should trigger immediate investigation.

Head and Neck Vascular Injury

Traumatic injuries to the extra-cranial carotid and vertebral arteries are uncommon occurring in approximately 1% of patients who have sustained blunt trauma [25]. The consequences can be catastrophic as a result of secondary strokes with high morbidity and mortality [26]. Blunt injury to the extracranial internal carotid artery can result in spectrum of injuries including vessel dissection with or without significant luminal narrowing to more serious vessel occlusion. Pseudoaneurysm formation and vessel transection can also occur. Vessel transection requires immediate surgical intervention; it is associated with extremely high mortality [27]. Asymptomatic patients with traumatic carotid dissection are often successfully managed conservatively with antiplatelet therapy and close observation [28]. Indications for endovascular treatment have included failure of medical therapy, impending stroke, and pseudoaneurysm formation for which carotid artery stenting can be performed [29].

Open surgical techniques are considered the gold standard for penetrating internal carotid injury as they have been associated with improved chances of survival and decreased neurological deficits. Whilst stent-grafting has been undertaken in penetrating injuries, relative contraindications include concomitant aerodigestive injury, uncontrolled haemorrhage and infected wounds. Although fewer patients have been treated with endovascular techniques, reported mortality rates between groups treated using endovascular and open surgical techniques are similar [27].

Injury to the external carotid artery can be managed differently as the multiple branches are extremely well collateralized and so, unlike the internal carotid artery, branches can be embolised and sacrificed. Traumatic injuries can manifest as pseudoaneurysms, extravasation, arteriovenous fistulae and vessel occlusion [30]. Embolisation is most often performed with coils, ideally as close to the bleeding point as possible although proximal embolisation of the main external carotid artery can be undertaken. Particulate embolisation should be avoided to decrease the risk of non-target embolisation intracranially via external to internal carotid collaterals. Complications are low; pain can occur up to 2 weeks following embolisation as thrombosis occurs. Partial tongue necrosis has been reported although this was only following bilateral embolisation [31].

Aortic Injury

Traumatic injury to the aorta is often fatal—approximately 20% of road traffic accident deaths in the United Kingdom are due to aortic rupture and up to 90% of patients die at the scene [32].

The mechanism for aortic injury is most often attributed to rapid deceleration. The most common location of aortic injury is at the isthmus where the ligamentum arteriosum inserts and the fixed arch joins the relatively mobile descending thoracic aorta. The differential deceleration at this point between the two regions of the aorta results in significant strain and shearing [33]. Other sites of injury from blunt trauma include the ascending aorta and descending thoracic/abdominal aorta [34].

At a pathological level, injury to the aorta occurs on a spectrum. It varies in severity from small intimal haemorrhages or intimal tears, to tears extending to the media, and complete circumferential aortic laceration involving all layers of the wall, pseudoaneurysm formation and peri-aortic haemorrhage [33, 35].

Historically patients with traumatic aortic injury have been managed with primary surgical repair. However, operative mortality can be up to 30% and the risks of spinal cord injury and paraplegia are also high as the aorta is cross clamped and distal perfusion interrupted [34]. This has called for consideration of delaying surgery with some evidence indicating that this may even be beneficial on mortality, particularly in those who are haemodynamically stable or in those who have profound concomitant injuries that may take precedence [36].

Since the turn of the millennium thoracic endovascular aortic repair (TEVAR) has been a step change in the management of traumatic aortic injuries (Fig. 28.4). Open surgery is a considerable undertaking performed via a thoracotomy, single lung ventilation, aortic cross clamping and replacing the injured aortic segment with a synthetic graft [37]. Endovascular traumatic aortic repair has evolved alongside the stent graft technology developed for aortic aneurysmal disease with the goal of relining and repairing the aorta by a minimally invasive approach. Although no randomised controlled trials have been undertaken comparing open surgical repair to endovascular repair, cohort studies and systematic reviews indicate that endovascular repair is associated with a better survival and few post-operative complications; multinational guidelines now recommend endovascular repair as the first line option [38, 39].

The development of endovascular aortic repair has occurred alongside the increasing availability and rapidity of cross sectional imaging in trauma. Aside from the important role that trauma CT has in diagnosing aortic injury, it is essential for planning an endovascular aortic repair. Meticulous assessment of the vasculature using multiplanar reformatted computed tomography data is of paramount importance in this field. Anatomical suitability is evaluated. The parameters assessed include patency and size of iliac vessels to permit

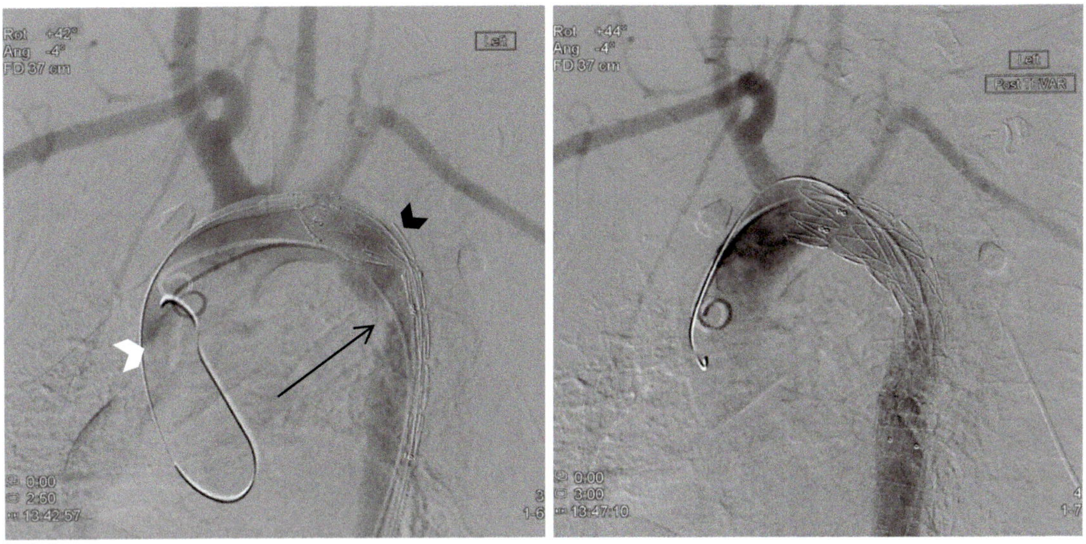

Fig. 28.4 DSA images during (left) and after (right) TEVAR deployment for a traumatic injury. The stent-graft (black arrowhead) is advanced along a support wire (white arrowhead) and deployed. An irregularity in the aortic wall (black arrow) is covered and sealed

insertion of the delivery device, and a satisfactory length of normal aorta to form a seal where the stent-graft opposes the aortic wall at the proximal and distal margin of a defect. The optimum type of device, stent-graft diameter, length and number of pieces will then be selected to best match the patient's anatomy and provide the most durable endovascular repair. Occasionally a combined endovasular and surgical procedure can mitigate difficult anatomy. The most common of these is performed in cases where the left subclavian artery has to be occluded in order to provide a seal zone for the stent-graft; a left carotid to left subclavian bypass may then be required to maintain adequate flow into the distal left subclavian [40].

As with most trauma endovascular procedures TEVAR is usually performed via the common femoral artery (CFA). The procedure can be performed under local anaesthetic although a general anaesthetic may be required if the patient is needing intensive levels of haemodynamic support or is unable to co-operate. Both common femoral arteries are accessed, either through a surgical arteriotomy or percutaneously, with one access site used for device delivery and the other for a catheter to perform angiography. The graft is positioned and deployed under constant fluoroscopy and digital subtraction imaging is used to confirm the final position. Despite TEVAR being a minimally invasive procedure, it is important for the entire trauma team to remember that it is a major undertaking. Complications carrying significant morbidity can occur relating directly to the procedure including cerebrovascular accident, spinal ischaemia, peripheral ischaemia, vessel damage and major bleeding. The patient should therefore be managed in an intensive care environment. The severity of the condition of the patient cohort undergoing stent-grafting is highlighted by an all cause 30 day mortality of 8–9% [41, 42].

Penetrating injury to the aorta is much less commonly encountered, the majority occurring due to stab or gunshot wounds. Whilst endovascular repair of a penetrating injury can be performed (Fig. 28.5) this is much less frequently encountered than in blunt thoracic injury and limited to case reports in the literature [43, 44]. This is in part as most patients will have multiple associated vascular and visceral injuries for which expedient open surgery is usually required [45].

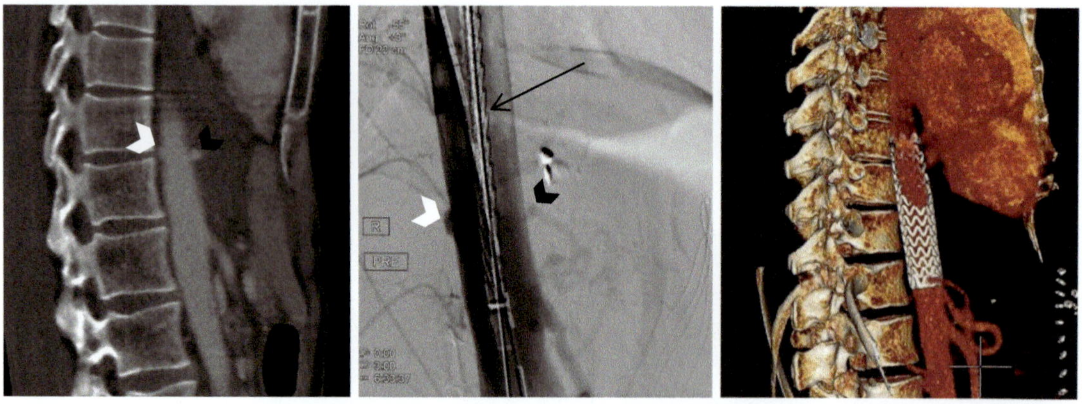

Fig. 28.5 Sagittal CT reconstruction (left) of a patient with an aortic injury as a result of a stabbing. There is aortic wall irregularity posteriorly (white arrowhead) and a small pseudoaneurysm anteriorly (black arrow) with surrounding haematoma. DSA sagittal oblique image (middle) during stent graft (black arrow) positioning similarly demonstrates the injuries. A follow up 3D CT reconstructed image (right) demonstrates the stent graft in situ, sealing the aortic defect

Visceral

Spleen

The spleen is the most commonly injured abdominal organ in blunt abdominal trauma. It is a highly vascular organ that when injured can result in major intra-abdominal haemorrhage. Whilst a person can survive without a spleen, using nomenclature such as a non-vital organ can be misleading as the spleen has an important role in immune function. Surgical splenectomy in the setting of trauma can result in severe post-operative bacterial sepsis and this is now reserved for only the most haemodynamically unstable patients who require an immediate trauma laparotomy [46].

Splenic embolisation is now the preferred splenic preservation management option in trauma and should be considered for any patient with splenic injury who is haemodynamically stable, particularly those with active bleeding detected on CT. In lower grade splenic injuries without evidence of active bleeding on CT (AAST grade I-III) initial conservative and supportive management is reasonable but close observation is required and if there is any deterioration intervention should be considered [47].

Two approaches are generally performed in splenic embolisation. If there is a large laceration or areas of multifocal injury to the spleen, proximal embolisation is performed. The main splenic artery is occluded with coils or a plug just distal to the pancreatica magna artery (Fig. 28.6). This has the effect of decreasing the arterial pressure to the spleen and so inducing haemostasis whilst maintaining perfusion of the spleen via collateral arterial pathways, preventing infarction and preserving immune function [46]. If there is an isolated injury identified, appearing as a focal area of contrast extravasation on digital subtraction angiography, distal embolisation is usually performed. The most distal arterial branch that is bleeding within the spleen is sub-selectively catheterised using a microcatheter and occluded with either a small coil or possibly Gelfoam. Occasionally liquid embolic agents are used for this indication. If a pseudoaneurysm is detected the portion of the artery proximal and distal to the defect must be embolised to prevent backfilling of the pseudoaneurysm [48].

Performing distal embolisation has a higher rate of minor splenic infarcts but lowers the risk of rebleeding compared with proximal embolisation; if there is concern for rebleeding a repeat CT would be an appropriate investigation to help detect any remote sites of injury not apparent on the initial imaging. Major complications which should be considered if the patient deteriorates

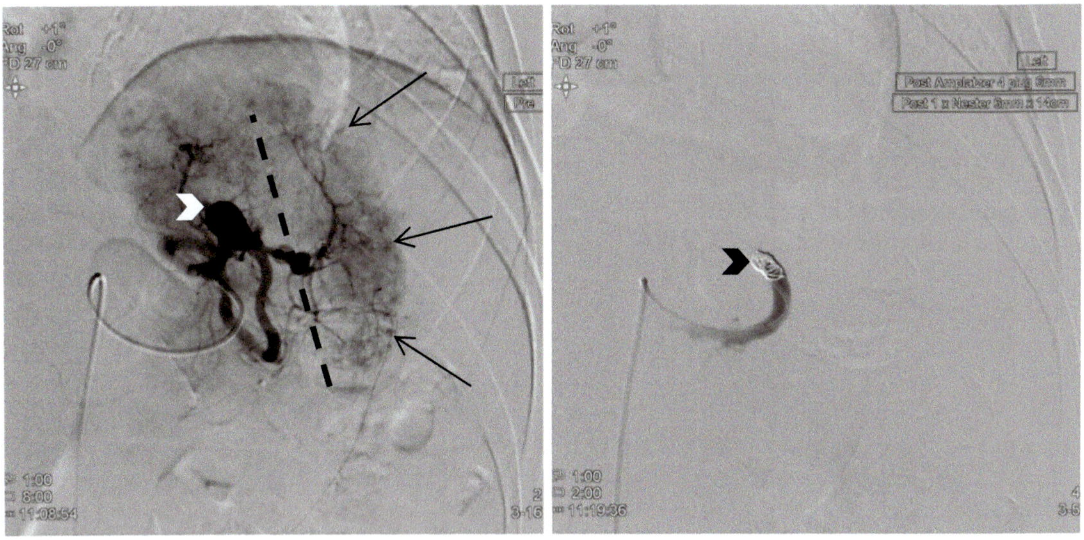

Fig. 28.6 Traumatic splenic injury with a traumatic splenic artery aneurysm (white arrowhead), splenic laceration (dashed line indicating area of non-perfusing splenic parenchyma) and innumerable irregular peripheral hyperdense bleeding foci (black arrows). Coil embolization of the main splenic artery performed with successful occlusion (black arrowhead)

include large volume infarction and infection requiring splenectomy. Such complications are uncommon [49].

Liver

The liver is also frequently injured in both blunt and penetrating abdominal injury. The spectrum of liver trauma is wide and severe injuries causing massive haemorrhage are associated with a high morbidity and mortality. Similar to the practice in splenic trauma, the shift in the last two decades has been towards non-operative management with emergency surgery reserved for haemodynamically unstable patients not responding to emergency fluid resuscitation and those with multiple concomitant injuries [50].

The most common indication for hepatic embolisation is identification of a contrast blush from an arterial source on CT that indicates active bleeding at the time of the scan. As with any imaging finding it is important to take into account the patient's clinical status to avoid interventional procedures which may be unnecessary. Other situations where embolisation is performed include the presence of a pseudoaneurysm and when further haemorrhage control is required following emergency laparotomy [51]. Patients with liver injury on imaging but without a contrast blush/active bleeding and who are haemodynamically stable are now routinely managed conservatively. For those with more severe grade injuries, follow up imaging can be considered to assess for delayed pseudoaneurysm formation or the presence of secondary complications.

The hepatic artery cannot be safely occluded in the same way that proximal splenic artery embolisation is performed as this would result in a very high risk of liver necrosis and fulminant hepatic failure. Although the liver has a dual arterial and portal venous blood supply, arterial embolisation combined with a traumatic insult rendering tissue ischaemic can have a profound effect. Sub-selective catheterisation of the bleeding arterial segmental or segmental branch vessel is therefore necessary using a microcatheter and distal embolisation is performed. Embolic agents commonly used include coils and gelfoam but the use of various other agents has been reported [52].

In addition to hepatic necrosis and liver failure which should be monitored for judiciously other complications that can arise following traumatic liver embolisation include gallbladder ischaemia, abscess formation and bile leak/biloma although in part these could arise as a result of the trauma itself [53].

Renal

Renal injury is present in approximately 1–5% of all trauma. The majority are due to blunt trauma [54]. Lying in the retroperitoneum the kidneys are fixed by the renal pedicle and ureter and so are particularly susceptible to acceleration and deceleration forces that can result in major vascular and parenchyma injury [55]. In addition to renal haemorrhage, damage to the renal collecting system must also be assessed.

One of the main goals of any treatment involving the kidneys is nephron preservation in order to prevent any permanent decline in renal function. The majority of renal injuries are now managed conservatively with evidence indicating that this strategy leads to the best outcomes with low rates of secondary nephrectomy in even the most severe (AAST grade IV and V) injuries. Damage to the main renal artery including arterial thrombosis is also predominantly managed conservatively with intervention usually only performed if there is a single functioning kidney or bilateral injury [56].

The role of embolisation is similar to the other abdominal viscera and is usually the first line management plan in a haemodynamically stable patient with CT findings of active bleeding, pseudoaneurysms or arteriovenous fistulae [57]. With nephron preservation is at the forefront of the radiologist's mind, the smallest possible volume of renal parenchyma is embolised targeting the most distal vessel that is bleeding using a microcatheter. In severe (grade V) injuries the kidney may already be lost due to renal artery avulsion or complete parenchymal shattering in which case the main renal artery or residual stump is embolised rapidly [58]. Attempts at repairing the renal artery and restoring flow are unlikely to be successful as the renal tissue will almost certainly be irretrievably damaged by this point (Fig. 28.7).

Injury to the ureter is rare and seen more frequently in penetrating trauma, particularly gunshot wounds [59]. Ureteric injury may be identified at the time of damage control surgery but is often a delayed diagnosis and should be considered in patients with flank pain, haematuria, urinary obstruction and elevated creatinine.

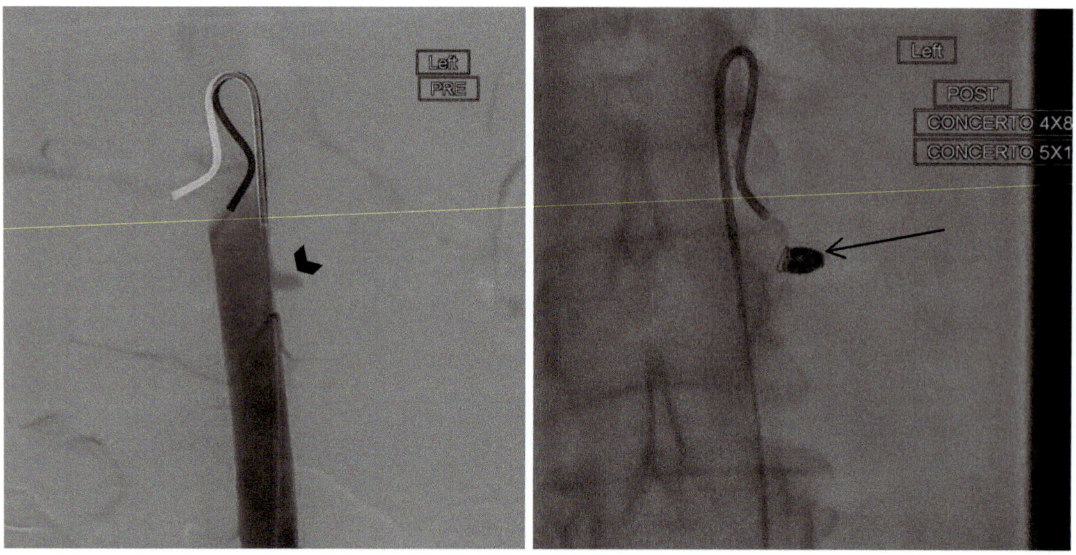

Fig. 28.7 Aortic angiogram demonstrating an avulsed left renal artery with a short residual stump (black arrowhead). This is not actively bleeding at the time of the angiogram but has the potential to spontaneously and catastrophically haemorrhage so was coil embolized (black arrow)

In a minor injury or delayed diagnoses urinary diversion with percutaneous nephrostomy and placement of a ureteric stent may alone be sufficient to allow healing. If identified at the time of damage control laparotomy ureteric repair should be performed [60].

Pelvic

Pelvic fractures occur in 10–20% of high energy blunt traumas. If there is associated bleeding and haemodynamically instability, the mortality rate is high. The retroperitoneal space can hold up to 5 litres of blood and in pelvic ring disruption the ability of this space to tamponade is reduced. Bleeding in pelvic trauma is most often from the presacral venous plexus but there can also be haemorrhage directly from fractured cancellous bone and as a result of iliac arterial injury [61].

If there are clinical features of bleeding but without evidence of arterial bleeding on CT the patient is unlikely to benefit from angiography and embolisation. As it is more likely that the haemorrhage originates from a venous source, surgery including pelvic packing and/or pelvic fixation is more appropriate. If there is CT evidence of arterial pelvic bleeding then embolisation should be considered. Embolisation can be the primary management of both haemodynamically stable and unstable patients with adjunctive stabilising measures including pelvic binder application and/or resuscitative endovascular balloon occlusion of the aorta [62].

Arterial haemorrhage in the pelvis is usually from branches of the internal iliac artery. The CT performed prior to embolisation is used to help navigate quickly to the bleeding vessel during the procedure alongside digital subtraction angiography from the main internal iliac artery and major divisions (Fig. 28.8). If only one distal vessel is demonstrated to be bleeding this can be selectively catheterised and embolised usually with coils. Often in pelvic trauma multiple peripheral branches are injured. In this scenario a more proximal non-selective embolisation can be performed with a temporary agent such as Gelfoam [63]. Internal iliac arterial branches are extensively collateralised and end organ ischaemia and necrotic damage is much less likely to occur compared with solid abdominal viscera.

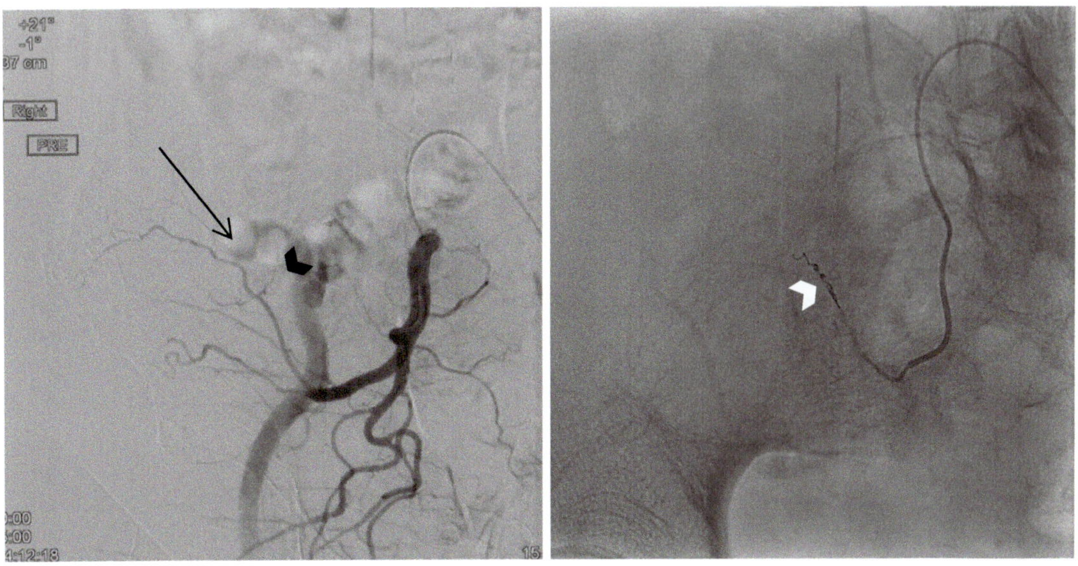

Fig. 28.8 Internal iliac angiogram with active contrast extravasation/haemorrhage (black arrow) from a posterior division branch of the internal iliac artery (black arrowhead). This was selectively cannulated and embolized with a coil (white arrowhead)

Aftercare

Following an endovascular procedure for trauma the ongoing patient care will be largely dependent on the presence of other significant injuries such as intracranial haemorrhage or major musculoskeletal injury. In the first 24–48 h following the procedure the patient should continue to have regular monitoring of their haemodynamic status as any deterioration could indicate re-bleeding. If this is suspected clinically a repeat CT is usually performed with non-contrast, arterial and delayed phases to assess for any active bleeding on imaging and highlight any other potential causes of patient deterioration. Complications relating to embolisation will be largely dependent on the territory embolised but end organ ischaemia and infection/abscess formation should always be considered in a patient with pain and/or fever [64]. Post-embolisation syndrome is a constellation of non-specific signs and symptoms including low grade fever, malaise, non-specific pain and nausea as a result of the body's physiological response to embolisation and tissue ischaemia. This is usually seen following tumour embolisation procedures but has been reported in trauma intervention [65].

The access site in the groin should be monitored following the procedure to assess for the presence of a pseudoaneurysm or persistent bleeding from the arteriotomy. If identified, pseudoaneurysms can be managed conservatively with manual compression or by percutaneous thrombin injection under ultrasound guidance. Surgical repair is rarely required. Follow up imaging is not routinely mandated if the patient is stable except in patients who have undergone aortic stent-grafting who are generally followed up yearly with cross sectional imaging depending on local protocols.

Key Points

- Endovascular techniques can be used as the primary therapy for haemostasis or following damage control trauma surgery when there is ongoing haemorrhage
- Subsequently the target vessel (usually identified on computed tomography in advance) is accessed using a combination of angiographic catheters and wires with a variety of properties based on their intrinsic design [6]
- One of the priorities of any interventional radiologist performing embolisation procedures is to reduce blood flow in or occlude only the intended target vessel and minimise embolisation of healthy tissue (commonly known as non-target embolisation).
- The principle of aortic balloon occlusion is similar to that of cross clamping—blood flow distal to the inflated balloon is halted or significantly reduced preventing further hemorrhage whilst proximally, coronary and carotid flow improve with a raised mean arterial pressure [23]
- Since the turn of the millennium thoracic endovascular aortic repair (TEVAR) has been a step change in the management of traumatic aortic injuries.
- Splenic embolisation is now the preferred splenic preservation management option in trauma and should be considered for any patient with splenic injury who is haemodynamically stable, particularly those with active bleeding detected on CT
- If there is CT evidence of arterial pelvic bleeding then embolisation should be considered.
- Post-embolisation syndrome is a constellation of non-specific signs and symptoms including low grade fever, malaise, non-specific pain and nausea as a result of the body's physiological response to embolisation and tissue ischaemia.

Conclusion

Interventional radiology provides minimally invasive treatments for haemorrhage in haemodynamically stable and unstable patients. Embolisation and stent-graft insertion can be utilised to avoid open surgery. Moreover, the techniques can also be used in cases where open surgery has failed. Effective integration of interventional radiology with the trauma team requires regular multidisciplinary interaction through morbidity & mortality meetings, guideline development and training exercises.

Questions

1. Which of the following equipment is NOT routinely used in the endovascular management of trauma:
   (a) Coils
   (b) Liquid embolics
   (c) Stent-grafts
   (d) Re-entry devices
2. Access for REBOA is normally via the:
   (a) Common Femoral Artery
   (b) Brachial Artery
   (c) Radial Artery
   (d) Common Femoral Vein
3. The commonest site of blunt traumatic aortic injury is:
   (a) Aortic root
   (b) Aortic Isthmus
   (c) At the level of the diaphragm
   (d) Above the aortic bifurcation at the level of T4
4. Proximal arterial embolization is most often utilised in the management of traumatic injuries in which organ.
   (a) Liver
   (b) Spleen
   (c) Pancreas
   (d) Kidney
5. Which of the following is NOT associated with post embolisation syndrome:
   (a) Malaise
   (b) Low grade fever
   (c) Non-specific pain
   (d) Reduced consciousness

Answers

1. d
2. a
3. b
4. b
5. d

References

1. Rösch J, Dotter CT, Brown MJ. Selective arterial embolization. Radiology. 1972 Feb 1;102(2):303–6.
2. Wallis A, Kelly MD, Jones L. Angiography and embolisation for solid abdominal organ injury in adults - a current perspective. World J Emerg Surg. 2010 June 28;5(1):18.
3. Matsumoto J, Lohman BD, Morimoto K, Ichinose Y, Hattori T, Taira Y. Damage control interventional radiology (DCIR) in prompt and rapid endovascular strategies in trauma occasions (PRESTO): a new paradigm. Diagn Interv Imaging. 2015 Aug;96(7–8):687–91.
4. Singh A, Kumar A, Kumar P, Kumar S, Gamanagatti S. "Beyond saving lives": current perspectives of interventional radiology in trauma. World J Radiol. 2017 Apr 28;9(4):155–77.
5. Adnan SM, Romagnoli AN, Madurska MJ, Dubose JJ, Scalea TM, Morrison JJ. Safety and efficacy of radial access in trauma in 65 trauma endovascular cases. J Vasc Surg [Internet]. 2019 Oct 11 [cited 2020 Feb 29];0(0). Available from: https://www.jvascsurg.org/article/S0741-5214(19)32168-8/abstract
6. Northcutt BG, Shah AA, Sheu YR, Carmi L. Wires, catheters, and more: a primer for residents and fellows entering interventional radiology: resident and fellow education feature. Radiographics. 2015 Sep 1;35(5):1621–2.
7. Medsinge A, Zajko A, Orons P, Amesur N, Santos E. A case-based approach to common embolization agents used in vascular interventional radiology. Am J Roentgenol. 2014 Sep 23;203(4):699–708.
8. Vaidya S, Tozer K, Chen J. An overview of embolic agents. Semin Intervent Radiol. 2008 Sep;25(03):204–15.
9. Wang W, Li H, Tam MD, Zhou D, Wang DX, Spain J. The Amplatzer vascular plug: a review of the device and its clinical applications. Cardiovasc Intervent Radiol. 2012 Aug;35(4):725–40.
10. Lopera J. Embolization in trauma: principles and techniques. Semin Intervent Radiol. 2010 Mar;27(01):014–28.
11. Guimaraes M, Wooster M. Onyx (ethylene-vinyl alcohol copolymer) in peripheral applications. Semin Intervent Radiol. 2011 Sep;28(03):350–6.
12. Bauer JR, Ray CE. Transcatheter arterial embolization in the trauma patient: a review. Semin Intervent Radiol. 2004 Mar;21(1):11–22.
13. Pfizer. Gelfoam Product Information [Internet]. Pfizer.com. 2020 [cited 2020 Feb 29]. Available from: https://www.pfizer.com/sites/default/files/products/uspi_gelfoam_plus.pdf
14. Jenkins HP. Present status of gelatin sponge for the control of hemorrhage: with experimental data on its use for wounds of the great vessels and the heart. JAMA. 1946 Nov 16;132(11):614.
15. Barth KH, Strandberg JD, White RI. Long term follow-up of transcatheter embolization with autologous clot, oxycel and gelfoam in domestic swine. Invest Radiol. 1977 May;12(3):273–80.
16. Abada HT, Golzarian J. Gelatine sponge particles: handling characteristics for endovascular use. Tech Vasc Interv Radiol. 2007 Dec;10(4):257–60.
17. Veith FJ, Marin ML, Cynamon J, Schonholz C, Parodi J. 1992: Parodi, Montefiore, and the first abdominal

aortic aneurysm stent graft in the United States. Ann Vasc Surg. 2005 Sep 1;19(5):749–51.
18. Volodos NL, Shekhanin VE, Karpovich IP, Troian VI, Gurev IA. A self-fixing synthetic blood vessel endoprosthesis. Vestn Khir Im I I Grek. 1986 Nov;137(11):123–5.
19. Noori VJ, Eldrup-Jørgensen J. A systematic review of vascular closure devices for femoral artery puncture sites. J Vasc Surg. 2018 Sep;68(3):887–99.
20. Robertson L, Andras A, Colgan F, Jackson R. Vascular closure devices for femoral arterial puncture site haemostasis. Cochrane Vascular Group, editor. Cochrane Database of Systematic Reviews [Internet]. 2016 Mar 7 [cited 2020 Feb 29]; Available from https://doi.org/10.1002/14651858.CD009541.pub2
21. Hughes CW. Use of an intra-aortic balloon catheter tamponade for controlling intra-abdominal hemorrhage in man. Surgery. 1954 July 1;36(1):65–8.
22. Villamaria CY, Eliason JL, Napolitano LM, Stansfield RB, Spencer JR, Rasmussen TE. Endovascular skills for trauma and resuscitative surgery (ESTARS) course: curriculum development, content validation, and program assessment. J Trauma Acute Care Surg. 2014 Apr;76(4):929–36.
23. Moore LJ, Brenner M, Kozar RA, Pasley J, Wade CE, Baraniuk MS, et al. Implementation of resuscitative endovascular balloon occlusion of the aorta as an alternative to resuscitative thoracotomy for noncompressible truncal hemorrhage. J Trauma Acute Care Surg. 2015 Oct;79(4):523–32.
24. Osborn LA, Brenner ML, Prater SJ, Moore LJ. Resuscitative endovascular balloon occlusion of the aorta: current evidence. OAEM. 2019 Jan;11:29–38.
25. Tso MK, Lee MM, Ball CG, Morrish WF, Mitha AP, Kirkpatrick AW, et al. Clinical utility of a screening protocol for blunt cerebrovascular injury using computed tomography angiography. J Neurosurg. 2017 Apr 1;126(4):1033–41.
26. George E, Khandelwal A, Potter C, Sodickson A, Mukundan S, Nunez D, et al. Blunt traumatic vascular injuries of the head and neck in the ED. Emerg Radiol. 2019 Feb;26(1):75–85.
27. Lee TS, Ducic Y, Gordin E, Stroman D. Management of carotid artery trauma. Craniomaxillofac Trauma Reconstr. 2014 Sep;7(3):175–89.
28. Rao AS, Makaroun MS, Marone LK, Cho JS, Rhee R, Chaer RA. Long-term outcomes of internal carotid artery dissection. J Vasc Surg. 2011 Aug;54(2):370–5.
29. Xianjun H, Zhiming Z. A systematic review of endovascular management of internal carotid artery dissections. INE. 2012;1(3–4):164–70.
30. Smith TP. Embolization in the external carotid artery. J Vasc Interv Radiol. 2006 Dec 1;17(12):1897–913.
31. Bynoe RP, Kerwin AJ, Parker HH, Nottingham JM, Bell RM, Yost MJ, et al. Maxillofacial injuries and life-threatening hemorrhage: treatment with Transcatheter arterial embolization. J Trauma. 2003 July;55(1):74–9.
32. Richens D. Rupture of the aorta following road traffic accidents in the United Kingdom 1992–1999. The results of the co-operative crash injury study. Eur J Cardiothorac Surg. 2003 Feb;23(2):143–8.
33. Parmley LF, Mattingly TW, Manion WC, Jahnke EJ. Nonpenetrating traumatic injury of the aorta. Circulation. 1958 June;17(6):1086–101.
34. Nzewi O, Slight RD, Zamvar V. Management of blunt thoracic aortic injury. Eur J Vasc Endovasc Surg. 2006 Jan 1;31(1):18–27.
35. Ayella RJ, Hankins JR, Turney SZ, Cowley RA. Ruptured thoracic aorta due to blunt trauma. J Trauma. 1977 Mar;17(3):199–205.
36. Pacini D, Angeli E, Fattori R, Lovato L, Rocchi G, Di Marco L, et al. Traumatic rupture of the thoracic aorta: ten years of delayed management. J Thorac Cardiovasc Surg. 2005 Apr;129(4):880–4.
37. Von Oppell UO, Dunne TT, De Groot MK, Zilla P. Traumatic aortic rupture: twenty-year metaanalysis of mortality and risk of paraplegia. Ann Thorac Surg. 1994 Aug;58(2):585–93.
38. Lee WA, Matsumura JS, Mitchell RS, Farber MA, Greenberg RK, Azizzadeh A, et al. Endovascular repair of traumatic thoracic aortic injury: clinical practice guidelines of the Society for Vascular Surgery. J Vasc Surg. 2011 Jan;53(1):187–92.
39. Fox N, Schwartz D, Salazar JH, Haut ER, Dahm P, Black JH, et al. Evaluation and management of blunt traumatic aortic injury: a practice management guideline from the eastern Association for the Surgery of Trauma. J Trauma Acute Care Surg. 2015 Jan;78(1):136–46.
40. Uchida K, Nishimura T, Yamamoto H, Mizobata Y. Efficacy and safety of TEVAR with debranching technique for blunt traumatic aortic injury in patients with severe multiple trauma. Eur J Trauma Emerg Surg. 2019 Dec 1;45(6):959–64.
41. Khoynezhad A, Azizzadeh A, Donayre CE, Matsumoto A, Velazquez O, White R. Results of a multicenter, prospective trial of thoracic endovascular aortic repair for blunt thoracic aortic injury (RESCUE trial). J Vasc Surg. 2013 Apr;57(4):899–905.e1.
42. Spiliotopoulos K, Kokotsakis J, Argiriou M, Dedeilias P, Farsaris D, Diamantis T, et al. Endovascular repair for blunt thoracic aortic injury: 11-year outcomes and postoperative surveillance experience. J Thorac Cardiovasc Surg. 2014 Dec;148(6):2956–61.
43. Harris DG, Brenner ML, Ho M, Toursavadkohi S, Lilly MP, Crawford RS. Endovascular repair of an asymptomatic aortic pseudoaneurysm after penetrating injury. Ann Vasc Surg. 2014 Nov;28(8):1933.e15–8.
44. Ghazala CG, Green BR, Williams R, Wyatt MG. Endovascular management of a penetrating abdominal aortic injury. Ann Vasc Surg. 2014 Oct;28(7):1790.e9–1790.e11.
45. Lopez-Viego MA, Snyder WH, Valentine RJ, Clagett GP. Penetrating abdominal aortic trauma: a report of 129 cases. J Vasc Surg. 1992 Sep 1;16(3):332–6.

46. Quencer KB, Smith TA. Review of proximal splenic artery embolization in blunt abdominal trauma. CVIR Endovasc. 2019 Mar 18;2(1):11.
47. Coccolini F, Montori G, Catena F, Kluger Y, Biffl W, Moore EE, et al. Splenic trauma: WSES classification and guidelines for adult and pediatric patients. World J Emerg Surg. 2017 Aug 18;12(1):40.
48. Ahuja C, Farsad K, Chadha M. An overview of splenic embolization. Am J Roentgenol. 2015 Oct;205(4):720–5.
49. Schnüriger B, Inaba K, Konstantinidis A, Lustenberger T, Chan LS, Demetriades D. Outcomes of proximal versus distal splenic artery embolization after trauma: a systematic review and meta-analysis: the journal of trauma: injury. Infect Crit Care. 2011 Jan;70(1):252–60.
50. Gaarder C, Gaski IA, Næss PA. Spleen and liver injuries: when to operate? Curr Opin Crit Care. 2017 Dec;23(6):520–6.
51. Gaski IA, Skattum J, Brooks A, Koyama T, Eken T, Naess PA, et al. Decreased mortality, laparotomy, and embolization rates for liver injuries during a 13-year period in a major Scandinavian trauma center. Trauma Surg Acute Care Open. 2018 Nov;3(1):e000205.
52. Virdis F, Reccia I, Di Saverio S, Tugnoli G, Kwan SH, Kumar J, et al. Clinical outcomes of primary arterial embolization in severe hepatic trauma: a systematic review. Diagn Interv Imaging. 2019 Feb;100(2):65–75.
53. Green CS, Bulger EM, Kwan SW. Outcomes and complications of angioembolization for hepatic trauma: a systematic review of the literature. J Trauma Acute Care Surg. 2016 Mar;80(3):529–37.
54. Serafetinides E, Kitrey ND, Djakovic N, Kuehhas FE, Lumen N, Sharma DM, et al. Review of the current Management of upper urinary tract injuries by the EAU trauma guidelines panel. Eur Urol. 2015 May;67(5):930–6.
55. Erlich T, Kitrey ND. Renal trauma: the current best practice. Ther Adv Urol. 2018 Oct;10(10):295–303.
56. Bryk DJ, Zhao LC. Guideline of guidelines: a review of urological trauma guidelines. BJU Int. 2016;117(2):226–34.
57. Professionals S-O. EAU guidelines: urological trauma [Internet]. Uroweb. [cited 2020 Feb 29]. Available from: https://uroweb.org/guideline/urological-trauma/#4
58. Brewer ME, Strnad BT, Daley BJ, Currier RP, Klein FA, Mobley JD, et al. Percutaneous embolization for the management of grade 5 renal trauma in hemodynamically unstable patients: initial experience. J Urol. 2009 Apr;181(4):1737–41.
59. Siram SM, Gerald SZ, Greene WR, Hughes K, Oyetunji TA, Chrouser K, et al. Ureteral trauma: patterns and mechanisms of injury of an uncommon condition. Am J Surg. 2010 Apr 1;199(4):566–70.
60. Morey AF, Brandes S, Dugi DD, Armstrong JH, Breyer BN, Broghammer JA, et al. Urotrauma: AUA guideline. J Urol. 2014 Aug;192(2):327–35.
61. Mauffrey C, Cuellar DO III, Pieracci F, Hak DJ, Hammerberg EM, Stahel PF, et al. Strategies for the management of haemorrhage following pelvic fractures and associated trauma-induced coagulopathy. Bone Joint J. 2014 Sep;96-B(9):1143–54.
62. Vaidya R, Waldron J, Scott A, Nasr K. Angiography and embolization in the management of bleeding pelvic fractures. J Am Acad Orthop Surg. 2018 Feb;26(4):e68–76.
63. Awwad A, Dhillon PS, Ramjas G, Habib SB, Al-Obaydi W. Trans-arterial embolisation (TAE) in haemorrhagic pelvic injury: review of management and mid-term outcome of a major trauma Centre. CVIR Endovasc. 2018 Dec;1(1):32.
64. Dhand S, Gupta R. Hepatic transcatheter arterial chemoembolization complicated by Postembolization syndrome. Semin Intervent Radiol. 2011 June;28(02):207–11.
65. Ben-Ishay O, Gutierrez IM, Pennington EC, Mooney DP. Transarterial embolization in children with blunt splenic injury results in postembolization syndrome: a matched case-control study. J Trauma Acute Care Surg. 2012 Dec;73(6):1558–63.

Part VI

In-Hospital Speciality Care

29 Decision-Making in Damage Control Surgery

Tim J. Stansfield

Abbreviations

ABRA	Abdominal reapproximation anchor system
ACS	Abdominal compartment syndrome
CNS	Central nervous system
CoA	Course of action
CT	Computerised tomography scan
DAI	Diffuse axonal injury
DCL	Damage control laparotomy
DCR	Damage control resuscitation
ED	Emergency Department
eFAST	Extended Focussed Assessment Sonography in Trauma
$ETCO_2$	End tidal CO_2
EVTM	Endovascular resuscitation and trauma management
GI	Gastrointestinal
GMC	General medical council
ICD	Intercostal chest drain
IIA	Internal iliac artery
IR	Interventional radiology
KDP	Key decision point
MAP	Mean arterial pressure
MTC	Major trauma centre
NPWT	Negative pressure wound therapy
OCEBM	Oxford Centre of Evidence Based Medicine
OT	Operating theatre
P	Pulse
SBP	Systolic blood pressure
SNOM	Selective non-operative management
TAC	Temporary abdominal closure
TARN	Trauma audit research network
TCA	Traumatic cardiac arrest
TTL	Trauma team leader

Overview: Damage control laparotomy is a substantial undertaking in critically unwell trauma patients, and the thought processes and planning behind this procedure has not previously been explicitly explained. This chapter looks at the systemic and logistical setup for performing damage control laparotomy, patient selection and the key decision points before and during the surgical procedure with reference to current literature. Human factors and liaison with the anaesthetist in resuscitating the patient is also explained, and how this factors into pre- and intra-operative management. Common pitfalls are explored, and strategies to avoid them are offered.

Introduction

Major Trauma Centres (MTCs) in England, excluding the Royal London Hospital, perform emergency trauma laparotomies on average less

T. J. Stansfield (✉)
The Leeds Vascular Institute, Leeds Teaching Hospitals NHS Trust, Leeds, UK

Royal Army Medical Corps, Leeds, UK
e-mail: tim.stansfield@nhs.net

P. Lax (ed.), *Textbook of Acute Trauma Care*, https://doi.org/10.1007/978-3-030-83628-3_29

than once per week [1]. Therefore it is likely that the average surgeon providing this MTC capability performs fewer than five such laparotomies per year. Damage control laparotomies (DCLs) for trauma are a subset of these emergency trauma laparotomies and therefore even less frequently performed. For such trauma systems, in order to make similar iterative improvements for those patients undergoing DCL in busier centres, it is likely cognitive rehearsal, collective team training and sharing debrief learning points are of significant importance.

DCR with DCL for trauma may be delivered in a variety of hospital facilities. DCL for trauma performed in Trauma Units is an even rarer procedure than in MTCs. Primarily it is employed in patients whose risk of transfer to an MTC is deemed greater than the risk of delivering a rarely practised intervention. The required infrastructure and system capability to optimally perform DCL is shown in Table 29.1.

DCL is often technically straightforward to perform, and complex reconstruction is rarely required. It is also most often performed on patients with high-quality tissues and baseline physiology. These patients are more likely to have enough physiological reserve to survive from the point of injury to the operating theatre; they are in the younger cohort more likely to get injured, and therefore, as a population, have a lower burden of comorbidity. It is the time-critical nature of DCL in the context of coordinated damage control

Table 29.1 Minimum infrastructure and system requirement to optimally perform DCL for trauma. DCL can be delivered less optimally but still effectively without all these components

Kit	• Verified functional electromedical devices. • Drugs and gases to provide optimal anaesthesia, perioperative and postoperative intensive care. • Surgical instruments familiar to surgeon and scrub staff that allow cavity/junctional access and visceral/vascular surgery. • Blood components and ancillary products and kit to allow a rapid massive blood transfusion to be delivered. • Cell salvage for autologous blood transfusion (red cells or whole blood). • Patient warming devices. • Effective topical haemostatic products.
Hospital personnel (individuals can multi-role if they have the competencies)	• ED: resuscitation team including surgical, anaesthetic and ED key decision makers. • OT: resuscitative surgical team and anaesthetic team. • ICU: intensive care team, surgical team. • Other supporting personnel (at all the above tiers): Haematology team, laboratory staff, radiological staff, portering staff.
Infrastructure	• Capability to perform an eFAST scan. • A clean overall environment with a sterile field for DCL. • Ability to warm environment (probably to at least 20 °C), ability to cool environment if >37 °C.
Processes	• Trauma relevant collective and individual training. • Weekly clinical governance meetings to review major trauma cases and look for iterative improvements. • Code red activation system (this is a communication tool and cognitive aid individually generated by MTCs for exsanguinating trauma patients. It triggers (1) priming and assuring of equipment to a ready state (2) ED resus standby of all senior relevant personnel (3) standby of personnel for patient transfer, blood products, theatre and interventional radiology). • Massive transfusion protocol to allow efficient, safe and coordinated communication between the clinical team and blood bank. • Rapid perioperative and intraoperative checklists to account for the difficult human factors.
Additional capability for broader DCR capability (optimally on site rather than transfer to)	• Multi-speciality clinical and allied health personnel, kit and supporting infrastructure available. • Radiology (plain films and CT) and interventional radiology capability.

resuscitation (DCR) that leads to complexity. The decision-making process involves a balance of accepting risk (through incomplete information or incomplete treatment) to prioritise manoeuvres that will, on the balance of probability, have a more beneficial effect on patient physiology and therefore more likely save a life.

Definitions

A **trauma laparotomy** is a laparotomy with a sequence of manoeuvres to gain access, identify and treat non-skeletal abdominal and pelvic injuries. This may be done with definitive or damage control intent.

A **damage control laparotomy** for a trauma patient is a trauma laparotomy where, by necessity to reduce risk to life, mitigation of deranged physiology is prioritised over definitive anatomical reconstruction. Abdominal wall closure is with temporary intent.

The key features that characterise, although are not necessarily unique to, mitigation of deranged physiology include:

- The time-critical nature of interventions and processes.
- The arrest of haemorrhage through physiological methods in addition to surgical control, i.e. haemostatic resuscitation (appropriately balanced blood product infusion, mitigation of significant hypocalcaemia and targeting normothermia).
- Prioritising perfusion to tissues in this order: (1) myocardial, pulmonary and CNS, (2) other vital visceral tissue (chiefly hepatic, renal, pancreas and foregut/small bowel), (3) other visceral tissue (4) limbs and the remainder of the body.
- Reducing the risk of secondary septic and/or an inflammatory hit by ensuring GI content remains intraluminal for its course within the body, and by providing appropriate drainage of biliary, urinary and pancreatic fluids.

A **definitive laparotomy** for a trauma patient is a trauma laparotomy with repair or resection of injured tissues, anatomical reconstruction of tissue where appropriate and closure of the abdominal wall fascia with permanent intent.

Interpretation of Literature Regarding DCL for Trauma

In appraising the methodology and contextualising the results of literature concerning DCL for trauma, there are several areas of heterogeneity between study and control groups in non-randomised trials (for example, "prospective" registry data studies) that may not be explicitly expressed. These will affect the internal and external validity of the study, potentially to such an extent as to make the conclusions invalid:

1. The denominator of major trauma patients is almost always unknown. In other words: there may be a cohort of patients with a similar injury profile that do not survive to hospital due to pre-hospital factors such as longer timelines, stress from external or environmental factors, or level of intervention delivered. Those that do reach hospital may have already "self-selected" for survival through a favourable premorbid physiological reserve or more survivable injury burden.
2. Shortened pre-hospital timelines can significantly affect in-hospital outcome measurements either positively or negatively by:
   (a) allowing a patient to present with an unsurvivable injury and subsequently die regardless of intervention, or
   (b) having a more favourable outcome due to earlier in-hospital intervention from the point of injury.
3. The variability in energy transfer to various body tissues and associated overall body response to this injury is measured by proxy using chiefly descriptors of injury profile, physiological measures and haematological tests. For matching patients between groups, this is reasonable but cannot be precise.
4. There is likely to be significant intra-group differences in the conduct of DCL. Any two patients that may be logged as having received

the same intervention and similar overall injury burden may have remarkably different treatment, biochemical and physiological course profiles. For example, consider the fictitious two patients who have received a DCL for trauma in Table 29.2. Patient 1 had a DCL from the point of entry of the patient into the trauma network. Patient 2, in the same trauma network, had a damage control strategy as a final OT manoeuvre in the face of deteriorating physiology. Both would meet a registry study inclusion criteria of DCL within an hour of ED arrival and could potentially be propensity matched to similar non-DCL patients. Patient 1 is more likely to demonstrate an outcome in favour of performing for DCL than Patient 2, despite conceivably having a more lethal injury. This example of real-world variability in the delivery of DCL for trauma demonstrates how (a) a result may be weakened in studies with a DCL group and (b) how external validity of DCL study results may be compromised.

Selection of Patients for DCL

As a proportion of Major Trauma calls to ED, **DCL is a very infrequent intervention**. In the UK, the need to perform DCL is probably of the order of 1–2% of all TARN (Trauma Audit & Research Network) registered adult abdominal trauma patients [1, 2]. Many blunt abdominal trauma patients can be managed with selective non-operative management. Managing low energy transfer penetrating abdominal trauma (for example, knife injury) non-operatively in selected cases, is successfully done in many centres. Those patients that require a laparotomy for trauma can often have definitive surgery without the morbidity cost of DCL. Their overall physiology is such that they have a low risk from definitive surgery and are more likely to compensate for this failure in the event it were to occur.

Minimal access techniques have well-established roles in trauma management (for example, laparoscopic hemidiaphragm penetrating injury identification). In the UK, the ratio of laparoscopy: laparotomy for initial management

Table 29.2 Example of differences between two patients characterised as undergoing damage control laparotomy for penetrating abdominal trauma with similar ISS

Patient or DCR characteristic	Patient 1	Patient 2
Age/sex	21-year-old male	21-year-old male
Mechanism of injury	Stabbed with a knife to right upper quadrant	Stabbed with a knife to right upper quadrant, chest and thigh
Prehospital	1 unit packed red cells	Right side ICD, pressure dressing leg
Prehospital time	10 min	90 min
Parameters in ED	SBP 90, P110, pH 7.14, eFAST +ve for abdomen	SBP 90, P110, pH 7.29, eFAST +ve for abdomen
Mental model shared by the team	Damage control resuscitation	Need to identify injuries sequentially and plan definitive repair carefully
Decision	OT	CT then OT
Surgical manoeuvres and events in OT	Focused team brief, prep and drape, induction of anaesthesia, haemostatic resuscitation, four-quadrant packing, liver repacked, 5 min pringle, temporary abdominal closure	Full team brief, induction followed by laparotomy and small bowel repair, thigh wound exposed with proximal/ distal arterial control + haemostasis achieved. After 3 h in OT pH noted to be 7.1, patient temperature 35.8, bowel appears underperfused. Temporary abdominal closure performed.
Injury	ISS = 16, large liver laceration of segments II and IV	ISS = 17, laceration right lung, small bowel laceration, mesenteric laceration, laceration branch of profunda artery
Characterised for data and grouping purposes as:	Damage control laparotomy for penetrating abdominal injury	Damage control laparotomy for penetrating abdominal injury

of the injured abdomen is 1:6, with about one in three laparoscopic approaches converting to open [1]. There is wide variation in its use, with some centres liberally siting an infraumbilical port for peritoneal cavity inspection in those abdominal trauma patients deemed stable enough. There are also clear benefits for patient selection for open surgery in non-trauma situations (for example, laparoscopy to assess whether a tumour is resectable). Extrapolating these applications to a general recommendation for use either in selection or management of very sick trauma patients where DCL is being considered is problematic. Crucially, laparoscopic access is not a route to rapid four-quadrant packing. This may lead to additional hypotensive and bleeding time immediately after induction, with additional trauma team cognitive bandwidth required for assessment and decision to convert to full open access. Even with a team that has rehearsed a minimal access approach in such situations, such disadvantages are unlikely to ever justify its use in sick trauma patients.

An attempt to recognise **Futility** should be made to prevent unnecessary intervention. This also meets an ethical duty to avoid unnecessary opportunity costs associated with wastage of blood product stock, trauma team time, OT use and wider hospital and societal resource. Defining a precise physiological inflection point at which patient care becomes futile is currently unachievable, and forming a national consensus is unlikely to be a workable solution [3]. In the context of the patient lacking capacity (which is very probable in a situation where DCL versus futility is being considered) an approach that is consistent with GMC guidance [4] is as follows:

Futility may be recognised at any stage of the patient care pathway and can be identified as a patient so severely injured, with such a physiological or biochemical profile that leads the trauma team, on consensus, to believe beyond reasonable doubt that further intervention will not either

(a) *allow the patient to survive transfer to the next stage of care or*

(b) *sustain a quality of life that the patient would wish for due to an ensuing devastating disability.*

The situational context and resources available, which are comparatively very favourable in a UK MTC, must obviously be considered. The trauma team in the context of a futility decision must include senior decision makers (chiefly consultants) who have sufficient experience in managing the sickest trauma patients; however, all immediate trauma team staff should be given the opportunity to share their view. To mitigate the emotional impact on the trauma team and to ensure a logical, transparent and justifiable decision, a shared structured ethical decision-making tool is useful, especially for more nuanced decisions. The Defence Medical Services have experience of using the four-quadrant approach (4QA) in severely injured trauma patients and have made efforts to iteratively improve its use through qualitative study and training [5]. The 4QA is a framework to aid discussion and does so by asking the team to consider four domains sequentially: (1) medical implications, (2) patient preferences, (3) quality of life, (4) contextual factors. The aim is to achieve as comprehensive a picture as possible in the circumstances to generate a conclusion and appropriate action. Incomplete clinical information (for example, length of time of low or no cardiac output or unavailability of head cross-sectional imaging) should either default to the most favourable scenario from the known information or be described in terms of a range of probability in predicting outcome. Uncertainty of outcome despite clinical information available, for example an inability to determine if a severe blunt head injury is survivable, is grounds for reasonable doubt. The 4QA can be led by the Trauma Team Leader (TTL) within the space of a few minutes to account for the need for expedited decision-making. Practicing such ethical decision-making tools in simulation settings may facilitate their use in live circumstances.

It is probably helpful to focus on three **key decision points** (KDPs) regarding trauma laparotomy and DCL. This enables a definitive point of logical team communication, shared mental modelling, avoids unnecessary bandwidth expenditure and avoids prevarication in a perpetual decision cycle. Ideally, the process of using KDPs in this way should be consistent with the other Major Trauma team responses—a team process that is only used for the sickest patients will be unfamiliar and more likely confusing. The first such KDP (KDP1) is optimally made on completion of the primary survey, approximately 5 to 15+ min from the patients' arrival in ED depending on interventions required. A more prolonged interval can be expected, for example, if (a) massive transfusion correction of hypovolaemic shock following isolated controlled catastrophic limb haemorrhage is required, (b) a traumatic cardiac arrest protocol is initiated. At KDP1, the trauma team must articulate the next step for the patient: investigation with a view to intervention or primary intervention (e.g. straight to theatre for immediate trauma laparotomy). This first timing balances the need for identification and treatment of immediate life-threatening injuries, sufficient verified information and initiation of time-critical surgical haemorrhage control with reperfusion. The second KDP (KDP2), regardless of the pathway, is at the intraoperative hold phase of the trauma laparotomy, irrespective of how brief the hold is. At this point, the trauma team may wish to alter the operative strategy between definitive surgery and DCL or vice versa, depending on the immediate intraoperative findings. The third KDP (KDP3) is before closure of the trauma laparotomy where the surgeon confirms with the trauma team whether to pursue the original intent of either DCL or definitive surgery or whether an altered strategy is justified.

The **decision process** for use at the KDPs, in patients with an abdominal injury (blunt or penetrating) contributing to their injury burden is schematised in Fig. 29.1. The trauma team first considers the data relating to the patient at the point in time of the KDP. These data are from a wide variety of sources, including:

- prehospital, pre-transfer and premorbid information
- Clinical findings (including additional history)
- Interventions and response
- Trends of vital signs ± invasive monitoring
- Blood gas analysis
- Thromboelastometry results

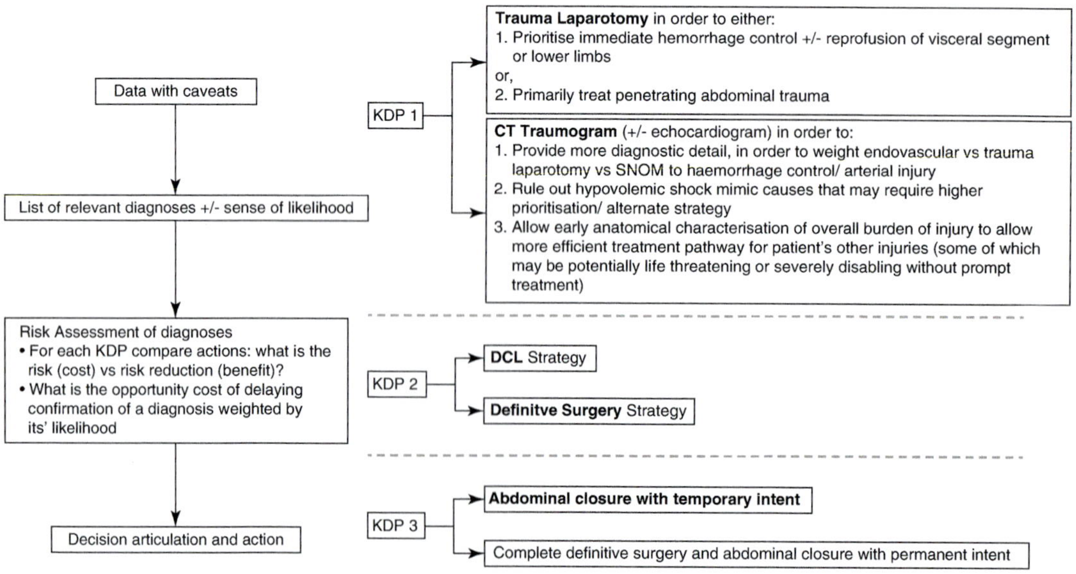

Fig. 29.1 DCL decision making process for a major trauma patient, with specific reference to either blunt or penetrating abdominal trauma at KDP 1 (end of primary survey),2 (intraoperative hold) and 3 (prior to closure)

- Imaging (eFAST, plain film, CT, echocardiography)
- Intraoperative findings.

These individual clinical datum are all caveated; for example (a) pre-hospital information and diagnoses carry uncertainty in accuracy by virtue of the environment [6], and (b) a haemoglobin drop as a marker for significant haemorrhage usually has a much higher specificity than sensitivity [7]. From this data, a written or mental list of relevant differential diagnoses is made. This list should be articulated by the TTL, highlighting the most life-threatening issues, to ensure a shared mental model of the (1) confirmed and unconfirmed injuries and (2) active medical and physiological problems. It may be possible to articulate a sense of likelihood for any one of the unconfirmed diagnoses. At KDP1 the diagnoses are likely to be broad. For example, "life-threatening intra-abdominal bleeding" or "head injury with GCS 3/15 unchanged from paramedic assessment at scene", at KDP3 some are more likely to be detailed "packed 5cm liver laceration at segments 3 and 4 liver with apparent haemostasis".

The next step is to make a risk analysis by comparing the core actions available. As Fig. 29.1 shows, these actions are a binary choice at each KDP. To make this risk analysis:

- Weight the risks of and risk reductions to diagnoses posed by one action compared to the other. Consideration of a risk reduction is probably more understandable than a benefit (although it amounts to the same thing) as it frames the entire process around risk. For example, at KDP2, DCL compared to definitive surgery may be stated to carry the risk of morbidity in (1) potentially unnecessary ICU time, (2) potential bowel discontinuity, (3) complications from laparostomy, (4) thrombosed shunt if thought to be needed) but reduces the risk of (1) sequelae of haemorrhagic shock by minimising the operative time and potential heat loss, (2) failure of tissue reconstruction with associated sequelae, (3) haemorrhage by allowing prolonged packing. The weighting process requires reference to the confirmed and unconfirmed diagnoses. For example, at KDP2, a patient with isolated blunt trauma to the abdomen with massive internal bleeding on laparotomy and a MAP of 60 despite continuing massive transfusion will favour a strategy that reduces the risk of surgery.
- Weight the opportunity cost of one action compared to the other in delaying confirmation of a diagnosis and associated treatment. For example, at KDP2 for definitive surgery compared to DCL, there may be an opportunity cost to delay to head CT that may identify a subdural haematoma requiring surgical decompression. This weighting process involves some sense of the probability of diagnosis. For example, at KDP2 for a patient with a head injury and abdominal trauma the opportunity cost of definitive surgery compared to DCL would be deemed higher for a patient with a pre-anaesthetised GCS of 8 and a unilateral newly dilated pupil to 6 mm compared to a patient with a pre-anaesthetised GCS of 8 and equal 2 mm pupils.

The decision process is then most straightforwardly framed as a question: which action best mitigates the risks presented by the list of diagnoses at an acceptable opportunity cost? This decision process does not imply:

(a) There is a mathematical calculation to make an unassailable correct decision
(b) The team has the luxury of a debated decision covering all the risks, benefits and second-order effects; often pattern recognition and heuristics will be used, especially by experienced teams and clinicians.
(c) A diagnosis must be made with a confidence level of the balance of probabilities (>50%) before intervention or action can occur.
(d) All diagnoses are equally weighted; self-evidently more life-threatening diagnoses carry a higher priority.

The decision process is time-critical, where each minute spent considering a decision or gathering more clinical information to increase diagnostic certainty may represent an additional minute of life-threatening bleeding or tissue hypoperfusion. It is not practical or desirable for the team to discuss in exhaustive detail the risks, risk reduction and opportunity cost of each possible action. Instead, the core options should be articulated and a decision made with a reasonable rationale. It is easy to see the attraction of a simple algorithm for deciding on DCL based on objective, measurable, patient parameters [8–12]. However, use of this more comprehensive risk analysis process at each KDP probably better allows expert clinicians to factor all relevant data, local constraints and patient baseline physiological reserve into the decision-making process. This system, or similar, is the one most clinicians use whether they recognise it as such or not. It is worth noting that a more detailed discussion of risk, risk reduction and the opportunity cost of one action compared to another may be useful in a collective training context or post hoc analysis.

In risk assessing at each KDP, the trauma team will need to consider the local **infrastructure and organisational constraints**. A trauma team in an MTC with an ED resuscitation room equipped with an 80-slice multidetector CT and laparotomy capability will have a different KDP risk analysis compared to a non-UK based, small hospital team with a total of 40 units of blood product, limited ICU holding ability, no higher-level care transfer options, and no access to CT scanning or endovascular options. The former team may justify the risk of delay to laparotomy to acquire a whole-body CT. The latter may justify the risk of definitive surgery as a lesser risk than to managing a temporary abdominal closure with sub-optimal resources. Some trauma systems do not have designated resuscitative or visceral trauma surgeons—to an extent the CT trauma scan is used to determine which speciality or specialities of surgeon to refer to depending on the injury pattern. At a superficial analysis, this system, in contrast to a system with resuscitative surgeons, appears less fluent, less timely and less likely to allow the concentration of surgical trauma experience. This may lead to inconsistencies in the weighting of risk in decision-making, including a definitive vs DCL approach and make rapid adaptability to an intraoperative injury finding more difficult. There is an absence of evidence as to whether outcomes are affected by these different approaches. The real world also often requires clinicians to balance conflicting priorities of treatment and resource use between patients with various clinical need. It is worth noting that this additional dimension of thinking is often forgotten or not recorded for post hoc analysis. A patient requiring lifesaving surgery is of the highest priority; however, without available theatre capacity to surge, immediate DCL is not an option and decision-making will thus be influenced.

Pitfall 1: Trauma Patients with Pathology that Mimics Hypovolaemic Shock

Examples of this phenomenon include cardiac contusion, cardiac valve injury, cardiac tamponade, significant head injury or spinal injury. These injuries may not be immediately apparent to the trauma team and are probably not rare in the most severely injured patients. Ensuring KDP1 is made in a considered manner, with at least some index of suspicion of "shock mimic" pathology, may reduce the risk of a non-therapeutic laparotomy and/ or a higher priority injury treatment being delayed as it remains unidentified until post-op imaging or secondary survey (for example, a decompressive craniotomy or spinal intervention).

Pitfall 2: A "Forced Bailout."

This scenario is where a significant deterioration in patient physiology (e.g. coagulopathy, hypothermia and acidosis) leads to a late intraoperative conversion from a definitive to DCL strategy. This deterioration can manifest to the surgeon by subtle indicators such as bowel or abdominal wall oedema, cold tissues, abdominal wall diffuse bleeding, or to the anaesthetist by the conventional parameters. Such a late change in strategy results in the patient potentially receiving a more significant surgical hit than would otherwise have been necessary if DCL had been chosen from the outset. Such cases should be later discussed in a clinical governance forum. It is important to note that this will be on retrospective analysis; decisions are made on probabilities rather than certainties, and the focus of discussion should be on ensuring KDP2 is made in as considered a manner as possible in the circumstances.

Pitfall 3: Lack of Consideration of Other Surgical Experience

It is probably not a false narrative to state there is a risk of a non-specialist trauma surgeon (experience dependent) tending towards a definitive, non-time-critical approach even if a DCL decision is made. Conversely, a trauma surgeon may not perceive the advantage of specialist help until a late stage, potentially causing a delay in a time-critical environment. Clinicians should aim to become self-aware of any biases in the approach through self-reflection and try to offset such tendencies, without overcorrecting.

Preparation for Trauma Laparotomy

Once a decision to perform a trauma laparotomy (DCL or definitive intent) has been made, regardless of whether this is immediately following primary survey or following CT imaging, the surgeon in collaboration with the trauma team must check several factors. It is therefore sensible to consider these factors before a critical decision point to avoid unnecessary delay. For patients undergoing a trauma laparotomy, treatment is usually time-critical. Consequently, any time expenditure prior to knife-to-skin must be justifiable against the opportunity cost of ongoing bleeding and hypoperfusion. Hirshberg [13] considers the efficiency of a trauma team to be reflected in how the time between arrival on the operating table and skin incision is minimised, calling this time the "black hole". The factors to check are:

1. The ongoing **resuscitative and anaesthetic imperatives** are being addressed and supported. These are addressed elsewhere in this book and other published sources [14]. The trauma anaesthetist and team require space (mentally, physically and temporally) to conduct haemostatic resuscitation and airway management.
2. Whether any more immediate **chest injury management** is required. An untreated pneumothorax with underlying lung injury may tension intraoperatively. The trauma team must decide whether they are willing to tolerate the risk of an intraoperative tension pneumothorax. A small pneumothorax [15] is unlikely to tension even with positive pressure ventilation [16, 17]. If risk toleration is chosen, the team will have to be prepared to recognise that a ventilatory pressure problem or hypotension has a higher than average likelihood of being related to a tension pneumothorax. Treating this during a trauma laparotomy is straightforward. However, such treatment costs team bandwidth and time expenditure; this may

occur at a very inopportune intraoperative moment. A chest injury treated with finger thoracostomies alone may be along a tract of 5 cm or more of soft tissue; effectively making a very high-pressure valve mechanism with a degree of lung collapse. There is level 4 evidence (OCEBM) from the prehospital sphere that these rarely tension with positive pressure ventilation [18, 19]; if in doubt, they can be rapidly re-digitalised. The team must therefore decide whether they will tolerate such an intraoperative risk. Tube thoracostomies have several advantages, including more reliably optimising lung expansion, partially quantifying the volume of thoracic blood loss and identifying an ongoing air leakage. With some chest drainage systems, autologous blood donation by cell salvage may also be an option. However, these must be offset against the time taken to insert and secure the tube, which can be considerable in inexperienced hands. With concurrent thoracic bleeding there may be an indication to perform an open thoracotomy. Without prevarication, the trauma team will need to decide which cavity to access first; the choice should reflect the cavity access that can most rapidly control life-threatening bleeding, given the particular injury profile. Whether or not the choice was "correct", the alternate cavity can be subsequently accessed.

3. **Contingency planning** and **cognitive rehearsal** must include the most likely intraoperative course and findings, but also the worst survivable intraoperative course and findings. The worst survivable injuries at trauma laparotomy will vary depending on the team and resources. These planning considerations should still be made despite the mechanism of injury being incompletely described, not fully witnessed or understood. Such planning will allow the team to concurrently prepare and "stand by" to react to intraoperative difficulties. Examples of the utility of this include:
   (a) A patient who has been stabbed in the RUQ who had a clamshell resuscitative thoracotomy in ED (and no intrathoracic injury seen) before immediate transfer to theatre for a trauma laparotomy is probably going to need management of a liver laceration. The surgeon should cognitively rehearse how this will be managed, so they are prepared to share their mental model with the team at the snap brief (see later).
   (b) For many teams, in patients with an appropriate injury mechanism, a zone 1 retroperitoneal haematoma or freely bleeding retrohepatic caval injury will represent the most difficult to manage and potentially survivable challenges. Any detailed planning for such a scenario is optimally considered in collective training, associated debriefs and other educational or reflective contexts. These could be "actions on" specific intraoperative findings for a department to follow. For the team in action, if a previously discussed core plan is succinctly stated at an opportune moment, they are likely to benefit from reduced stress, preserve bandwidth and have more opportunity for situational awareness.

Pitfall 4: Failure to Consider the Worst-Case Scenario

It is easy to be "dead set" on a diagnosis pre-laparotomy. This may be driven by assuming certainty from imaging. For example, a motorcyclist versus lorry sustaining a blunt head and abdominal injuries has a Bastion protocol trauma CT, initially rapidly reported as diffuse axonal injury (DAI), splenic injury, and right renal lower pole injury with right retroperitoneal haematoma. The patient has a trauma laparotomy and splenectomy. With ongoing massive transfusion and the patient still in shock, the large right zone 2 retroperitoneal haematoma is explored at the level of the right renal hilum with a view to nephrectomy. Perfuse, destabilising, venous bleed-

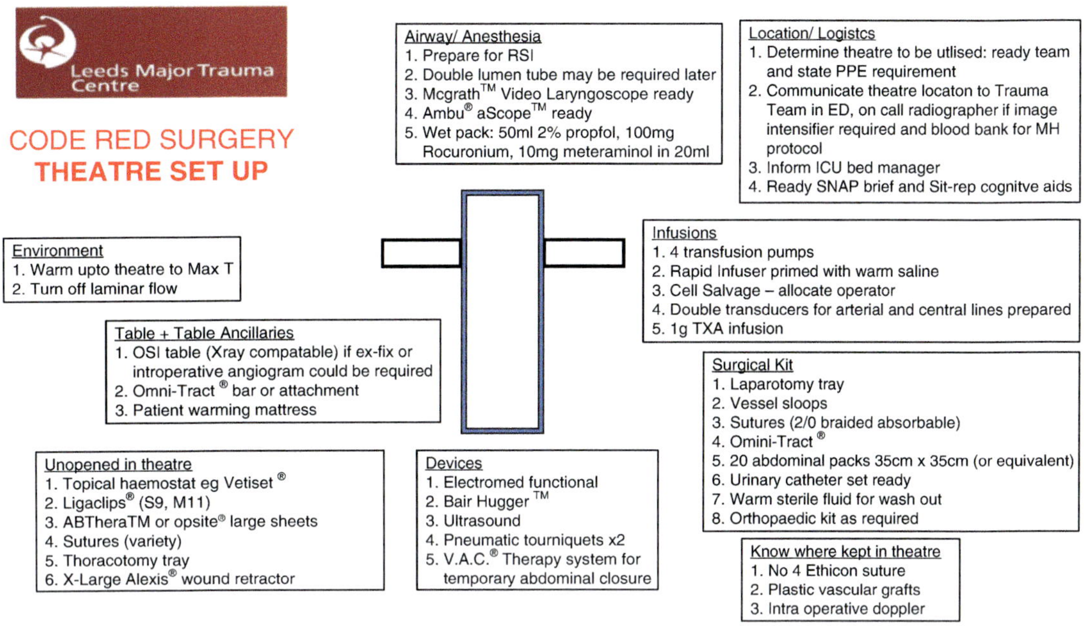

Fig. 29.2 Cognitive aid for theatre preparation in DCL

ing occurs, and the kidney is intact. The team has now to diagnose and react to an infrarenal segment of injured IVC in an unprepared, very time-critical fashion. To avoid such a pitfall, the trauma team should share a mental model that new intraoperative findings should be assessed on their own merits in the context of the patient's physiology.

4. The core plan for **other injury** and **comorbidity management** that has relevance to the operating theatre episode. The details of this planning and whether speciality advice is sought before trauma laparotomy will depend on the infrastructure and systems of the hospital facility. Delay to a trauma laparotomy with the intent to control significant intra-abdominal bleeding cannot be justified to plan for or investigate another injury (non-abdomen, non-chest, airway secure). It may be that the trauma team needs to agree on an adjustment to the plan of manging other injuries with the speciality surgeon, as the patients' overall burden of injury favours tolerating the risk or sequelae of non-treatment. For example, soft tissue wounding may have an initial plan of plastic surgical repair, which is adjusted to wound washout and dressing given a fraught intraoperative course during DCL.
5. Use of **cognitive aids** to prepare for trauma laparotomy. As discussed in human factor considerations below, thought processes and efficiency might be suboptimal in a stressful time-critical environment. The intraoperative trauma team may not be fresh or performing at their best. A cognitive aid used in a challenge-response manner by the theatre team preparing for a trauma laparotomy probably helps to ensure more efficient set up by coordinating concurrent activity amongst members. The details of this will be dependent on the local infrastructure and systems; it may be part of an all-encompassing "code red" SOP. An example of such a theatre preparation cognitive aid that the theatre team can use is given in Fig. 29.2; not dissimilar to cognitive aids [14] used in complex trauma for airway management.

6. Efficient and appropriately safe patient **packaging** and **transfer** from the ED to the operating table. Local infrastructure and systems will determine the nature of the transfer; some hospital facilities have trauma operating rooms within their ED.
    - The process of packaging and transfer to the operating theatre (OT) is probably optimally led by the TTL with appropriate deferral to anaesthetic expertise. Handover of leadership during the transition between ED and OT, especially if immediately after the primary survey, carries the risk of bandwidth overload to the anaesthetic lead. They may potentially end up simultaneously leading the trauma team, coordinating mechanics of transfer, coordinating a massive transfusion and troubleshooting anaesthetic and ventilator problems en-route. The TTL may feel their expertise arbitrarily ends at the exit to the ED, and non-ED team members may feel threatened by a perceived encroachment onto their territory. These expertise and encroachment boundaries are understandable but artificial. The TTL may feel their duty lies with other patients in the hospital or ED requiring their clinical leadership or input. The trauma patient being transferred for DCL could be the sickest survivable patient in the hospital and justify the additional leadership resource.
    - As described above, any intervention or investigation must be justified against the potential cost of ongoing bleeding and hypoperfusion. Improving patient packaging and transfer can probably be gained by
        - a shared mental model where all team members are focused on only essential activity to facilitate the transfer of the patient to theatre for haemorrhage control and reperfusion.
        - effective debriefing of patient cases where all providers being prepared to justify "pre-incision" processes
        - cognitive aids such as checklists
        - collective training
    - Redundancy and ability for staff to multi-role is useful. For example, if Portering staff are not immediately available to transfer a packaged, time-critical patient, trauma team members should be able to take on this role.

Pitfall 5: Task Fixation and Loss of Time Perception

It is possible to enter into a vicious cycle of justifying an extra intervention or investigation by the perceived window of opportunity created by an ongoing procedure. For example, a provider has "one more go" at sheath insertion into a hostile groin for REBOA while the central line is being sutured in. This then has "given time" to set up for a femur plain film radiograph, this then "allows" set up for "one go at a radial arterial line". While none of these steps may seem unreasonable to the individual practitioners, the collective effect may be an additional 30–60 min of bleeding and hypoperfusion before arrival in theatre.

Human Factors in Trauma Laparotomy

Achieving efficient use of human and equipment resources requires a well functioning trauma team and supporting infrastructure. Clinical human factors consider the interface between the healthcare providers and that system they deliver within. These factors can be positively affected "[to enhance] clinical performance through (1) an understanding of the effects of teamwork, tasks, equipment, workspace, culture and organisation on human behaviour and abilities and (2) an application of that knowledge in clinical settings [20]." Trauma laparotomy requires team problem solving and treatment delivery in a time-critical context using multiple system resources. It is therefore a process where the patient outcome is likely to be significantly affected by clinical human factors.

There are several frameworks that assist in a consideration of clinical human factors. All have limitations including overlap in their categorising; however, they offer a systematic approach to system design, implementing and debriefing. The Non-operative-Technical Skills for surgeons (NOTSS) framework [21] is designed for the primary operating surgeon's perspective; it can be adapted for the wider team conducting a trauma laparotomy. NOTSS categorises clinical human factors into situational awareness, decision-making, communication and teamwork, and leadership.

Leeds Major Trauma Centre

CODE RED SURGERY

SNAP BRIEF

Surgeon confirms

- Correct patient
- Clinical and imaging findings
- Surgical intervention so far and plan

Anesthetist states

- Temperature
- Systolic BP
- Blood product given so far
- Clotting (eg TEG)

Team confirms

- Antibiotics given
- TXA given
- Blood available
- Surgical kit ready

EXAMPLE

"This is X, NHS number 12345678, they were a pedestrian hit by a 30mph car 3 hours ago, have a splenic rupture with an open book pelvic fracture. Bilateral tube thoracostomies and a zone 1 RBEOA are in situ. We are going to perform a damage control laparotomy, deflate the balloon and pelvic ex fix."

"Temperature is 35.0, the SBP is 100, blood product given so far is 3 units Oneg and 2 FFP. No clotting results so far."

"We confirm antibiotics and TXA have been/ will be given and 4 group specific red cells are in theatre ready. Is everyone ready?" {allow answer]

"Ok, go." or "ok, wait."

Fig. 29.3 Snap brief prior to commencing a trauma laparotomy for exsanguinating injury

Top Tip: Optimising Bandwidth

In stressful or unfamiliar situations, an individual's bandwidth will narrow. Recall of all necessary perioperative preparation and the required actions may be incomplete. Checklists or aide memoirs (electronic, laminated or paper) by the theatre team preparing theatre before patient arrival, prior to commencement of operating, intraoperatively and before exit from the operating theatre will:

1. save team member bandwidth for more cognitive and decision orientated tasks that do not have such a checklist solution.
2. provide assurance that all salient points have been covered thus probably improving safety.

These checklists should be employed in simulation and scenario-based training, so their existence, location and content are well known to the clinical team.

Situational Awareness

With individual task fixation, tunnel vision from loss of bandwidth, distractions and theatre team members moving in and out of the immediate patient support envelope it is very likely that not all the team in the OT will have a shared understanding of the patient condition and plan. This can be partly mitigated using a briefing tool: the team must choose between a full WHO surgical **safety checklist** or a truncated version, for example, a **snap brief** [22] per Fig. 29.3. The snap brief is designed for patients with a presumed exsanguinating injury. It takes approximately 30–40 s to complete, generates sufficient team understanding, and avoids spending time and bandwidth on extraneous considerations in this select group of Major Trauma patients. The urge for the team (and especially surgeon) to "just to get going" without briefing must be resisted. It is lower risk to let the patient continue with an ongoing life- or limb-threatening insult while baseline information and a plan is shared across the team than to carry the risk in assuming all members of the team have a shared appreciation of the resource available, patient physiology or cavity/ body region priority.

Traumatic Cardiac Arrest Adjustment In the event of traumatic cardiac arrest (TCA) in the OT before the snap brief then the local TCA protocol should be followed, for example, intubation, bilateral finger thoracostomy, ongoing volume filling and confirmation there is a reasonable prospect of non-futility. The team may then decide to proceed to an open thoracotomy to address the management imperatives in non-futile situations of (1) exclusion or release of pericardial tamponade, (2) descending thoracic aorta (DTA) occlusion and (3) haemostatic correction of presumed hypovolaemic shock. If sufficient cardiac output is not restored that will provide reasonable cerebral perfusion, then a shared understanding should be established by the team leader, prior to a futility discussion as described previously. If cardiac output is restored the team should then proceed to a snap brief.

Anticipating Future States The surgeon should share with the scrub team the potential next step (manoeuvre and equipment) to stop the bleeding if the first course of action is unsuccessful. This usually has a calming effect on the surgical team and potentially stops their bandwidth being consumed in sourcing unrequired kit or thinking about their role in manoeuvres that will not be required. If a team member is unfamiliar with trauma laparotomy (and more so DCL), then the surgeon or anaesthetist should briefly explain the process and rationale. This is a procedure that looks vastly different from elective surgery and may be met with trepidation by staff unfamiliar with the idea. By explaining the physiological sequelae and broad plan of the first 48 h post-injury, a shared post-operative mental model will be generated; this may lessen the risk of inconsistencies or missed opportunities in the patient's management.

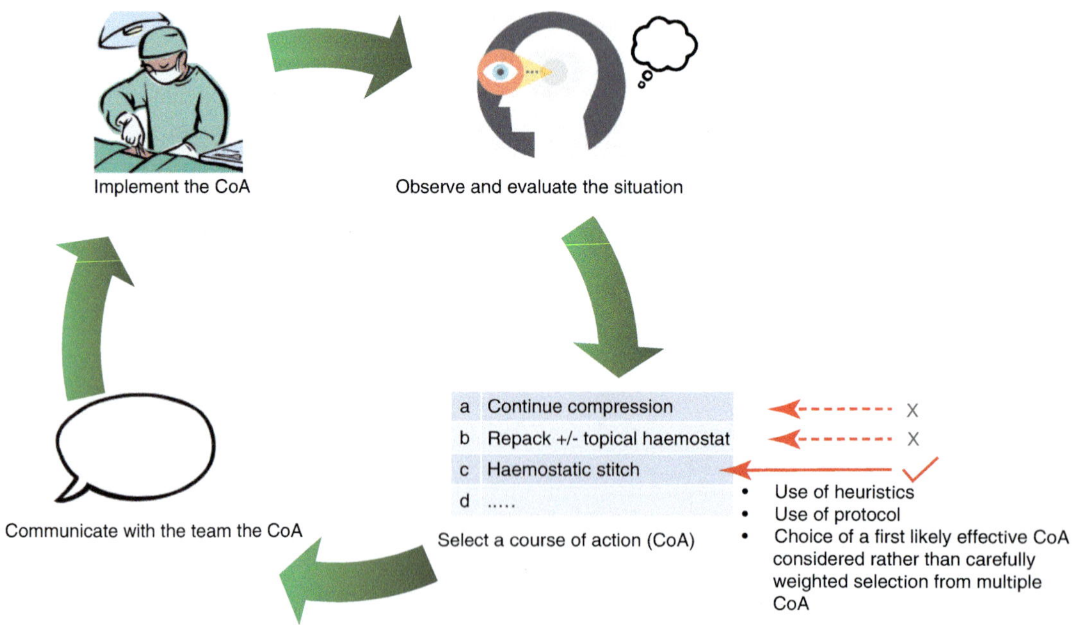

Fig. 29.4 Rapid decision making process in trauma laparotomy

Decision-Making

Intraoperative decision-making by members of the trauma team during a trauma laparotomy can be characterised as either

(a) rapid thinking with a protocol-driven selection of courses of action, or
(b) more nuanced, slow, deliberate thought, weighing up the risk and benefit such as at a KDP.

Team decision-making does require individuals to maintain a sufficient breadth of perspective (mitigating bias in favour of their own niche or role) and attentive listening to understand the imperatives articulated by other members.

Rapid decision-making [23, 24] can be conceptualised as a circular process, as shown in Fig. 29.4. Used efficiently it can iteratively achieve an effective course of action. It carries greater risks of:

- Confirmation bias—this is an unconscious selective processing of information that is then used as confirmation of the held belief
- Incorrect assumptions—that then lead to a sub-optimal decision, regardless of whether the decision process itself was sound.
- Initial selection of a less optimal course of action (CoA)—there has not been sufficient time to fully realise the relative merits of all reasonable courses of action.
- Flailing—this is repeating a surgical manoeuvre or action, expecting a different outcome despite carrying out the same manoeuvre or action without improving the circumstances. It expends time and potentially blood loss without advantage.

The rationale for carrying such risks as these and not opting for slower decision-making is that rapid decision-making probably will arrive, in many circumstances, at a workable solution in a much shorter time. The emphasis on speed in trauma laparotomy is justified by the time-critical need for:

- lifesaving haemorrhage control or resuscitative aortic occlusion
- rapid reperfusion of visceral organs to reduce the risk of multiorgan failure and associated mortality and morbidity
- sequential surgical management of (1) non-abdominal life-threatening injuries such as in the head or chest and (2) limb-threatening injuries.

Some of the rapid decision-making risk can be mitigated, with a low cost to speed, by protocolled information sharing such as the snap brief, and ensuring team members have an opportunity to raise critical concerns openly.

Flailing can be avoided by materially altering the environment in terms of

- better lighting
- better retraction
- better exposure
- improved angle of suture
- optimised technical assistance from an experienced colleague

or by altering the technique, such as

- use of pledgets to reinforce arterial repairs
- repacking in a more compressive alignment for haemorrhage control.

Slow decision-making [23, 24] is a process requiring slower thinking; the provider weighs the risk and benefit of several CoAs logically, before selecting the most favourable course. Using it iteratively is likely to be too inefficient, especially in a time-critical situation. The description of decision-making at KDPs, earlier in this chapter, is an example of slow decision-making in action. Interestingly, it also has a role when rapid thinking and decision-making fails to select a CoA. A brief mental pause followed by a switch to slow decision-making often gives a new perspective and allows weighting of the risk for each CoA logically. Usually, at least one CoA is to call a colleague for assistance in decision-making.

Decision-Making Under Stress Working in time-critical, high stakes, potentially unfamiliar environments where some team members have not worked together previously is stressful. Stress can be significantly exacerbated when something is not going according to plan, mixed with emotions of anger, guilt or embarrassment or there are underlying individual compromising factors involved such as tiredness, hunger, thirst, personal difficulties or personal triggers. It is useful to recognise the symptoms of stress (e.g. impatience, unease, apprehension) which in turn risks illogical thinking and action or freezing (the "fight or flight" response). Protocol familiarisation, personal mental resilience training and collective training offset the difficulty in decision-making under stress. Providing a system where individuals are reasonably well-rested, fed, respected, led and pastorally cared for is likely to reduce stress and promote improved decision-making. If the provider feels at risk of illogical or frozen thought, imagining a "helicopter perspective" of the situation may help. This forces a deliberate switch from fast to the slow decision-making or a reset of their slow decision-making process. Slowing down one's thinking under stress is a sign of mature and highly competent decision-making.

Pitfall 6: Desire Versus Reality
Be careful not to fall into the trap of starting where you would like to be rather than where you are. This may lead to techniques and manoeuvres that are suited for non-time-critical surgery—for example, methodically ensuring haemostasis at the point of laparotomy incision when there is underlying intraperitoneal life-threatening haemorrhage [25].

Communication and Teamwork

Hirshberg's three-tier surgeon support envelope concept [13] for DCL describes a surgeon centric view of staff and equipment supporting the operating effort: within the operative field, otherwise within the theatre and outside the theatre. The anaesthetic lead can also conceptualise a support network in this fashion, the cephalad patient space replacing the operating field. This mental picture helps frame important elements in **coordinating team activities,** especially useful when providers undertake activities requiring task fixation or rapid decision-making. It may be useful to consider several principles to aid efficient coordination and team function:

- All requests for resources have an opportunity cost. For example, an equipment request by the surgeon intraoperatively comes with (1) a cost to time in waiting for the kit to be acquired if non-useful concurrent surgical activity is performed, (2) a cost to human resource in that the specified staff member will be unavailable for other activity and (3) occasionally has a significant distraction effect for the whole team. Be aware that multiple requests for human and equipment resource in time-critical trauma situations will have to be prioritised either by the support envelope or the requester. It is useful to develop the skill of calculating the cost of a resource request to the overall effort against the benefit it may accrue in order to decide whether to proceed. This is not to imply the threshold for an equipment request should be set very high—a marginal gain may make the difference between flailing and not flailing.
- Efficient coordination of team activity can be significantly dependent on team members maintaining situational awareness where possible, and regaining situational awareness after a period of task fixation. This will facilitate the team at all tiers to anticipate the future state and to plan accordingly. For example, the surgeon or support envelope should anticipate the need for surgical equipment to avoid waiting at the point of requirement.
- Each tier and team element will have a potentially useful perspective not seen by other members. No team member must feel hindered in their ability to raise concerns or con-

Leeds Major Trauma Centre

CODE RED SURGERY
SIT REP

At suitable times (approximately every 20 minutes) or 2 units of bloods carry out a situational report (update) between whole team:

T	Time since op started	
S	Systolic BP	
T	Temperature	
A	Acidosis	
C	Coagulopathy	• TEG • Clot formation in operative field
K	Kit/ Blood	• Blood product quantity and type used • Limitations on blood stock

Fig. 29.5 Sit rep, a formalised communication tool for the exchange of information within the operating theatre during trauma laparotomy

tribute to decision-making. Collective training in formal escalatory language to raise concerns, including "STOP" is probably useful to help overcome individual hesitancy induced by a seniority gradient.

- Team coordination is facilitated by a **shared mental model** and an understanding by all team members of the roles and shared responsibilities of others in the team. For example, if the surgeon shares the goal of correction of patient physiology, they are more likely to work in concert with the anaesthetist. This may be to act to temporise haemorrhage or relieve packing pressure on the cava to ensure an adequate end-diastolic volume, rather than insist on prioritising more complex or technical surgical manoeuvres regardless of the resuscitation imperatives.

Situational awareness, decision-making and coordination of team activity all require giving and receiving information in a timely manner amongst team members. This **exchange of information** reduces the risk of counterproductive or irrelevant activity, and is especially important when something is not going to plan. It is generally a constant process during a trauma laparotomy, usually on an informal basis between members within the same tier. A formalised tool is useful to improve exchange of core information amongst all members. An example of a formalised tool is the **sit rep** (situation report) [22], shown in Fig. 29.5. Formal communication avoids the potential pitfall of asking "how is the patient doing?" or "how are you doing?". This seems like an open question that will lead to an open discussion. However, there may be a tendency to understate the patient's condition or, in stressful circumstances, to reply in few words without meaningful detail. The sit rep is designed for use in the operating theatre during a trauma laparotomy at an interval of approximately every 20 min depending on circumstances. A constant stream of dialogue occupies bandwidth, distracts from other activity and is likely to be unnecessary; a balance between doing and communicating is required.

Pitfall 7: Closed-Loop Communication
Avoid always assuming that an explicit request is necessarily followed by an effective action. In relatively low-stress circumstances with an experienced team, where individual capabilities are well known, this is likely to be a safe and efficient assumption. Where experience or capability is unknown, it is likely more efficient to check understanding, ensure or delegate careful explanation of the task and use closed-loop communication—"please let me know when it is done."

Leadership

As discussed in preparation for trauma laparotomy, the resuscitation leadership is probably most effectively continued by the TTL from ED to the operating table and then handed over to the anaesthetist at a suitable pause, usually within 5–10 min of arrival. This arrangement is more pertinent for the more severely injured and is very likely to be more effective if this process is practiced in collective team training. The surgical lead is likely to be entirely task fixated during specific periods of operative activity and temporally lose situational awareness.

The civility saves lives group researches and campaigns on civility in health care [26]. Part of their work includes sharing narrative accounts of the negative impact caused by incivility on patient care; much potentially pertinent to trauma teams. There is level 1b evidence (OCEBM) that incivility in the OT has a significantly negative effect on individual performance [27]. Effective leadership can reduce the risk of incivility in a team by setting an example of courteous and professional behaviour; it is not unusual for the team to copy the leaders' tone and manner. The core tenant to team building, even for new or transient teams is trust [28]. Rudeness or unfairness in approach to a team member can thus have a broader impact than the individual; the team is likely to be more guarded and dysfunctional, and team performance will suffer.

In general terms, a clinical leader should set an example of **high clinical standards** and **support team members** to allow them to give optimal performance. Such support varies depending on the experience and need of the team member. Usually, encouragement and praise are appropriate for performed tasks, and constructive criticism is generally best delivered at post-event debrief in a structured fashion. A friendly demeanour by those in leadership positions is usually the most efficient (but not only) way of mitigating a seniority or perceived power gradient. Such a gradient may avoid uncomfortable challenges from junior members; however, uncomfortable challenges can sometimes be lifesaving. In turn, good followership by team members involves appropriate support to the leader, working towards a common goal and self-control to avoid ego-driven distractions. It is helpful for the surgeon and anaesthetist to maintain an outward calm as this often permeates into the wider team and may help to improve bandwidth and space to think.

Summary

Decision-making during a DCL is characterised by its time-critical nature and based on often incomplete information. It requires a mixed approach of rapid decision-making and slower thought processes weighing the risk and opportunity cost of the available courses of action. The initial phase of DCL generally use the former approach and are more protocol-driven. Decision-making later in the course of DCL, following initial haemorrhage control, generally uses the latter approach.

Questions

1. Damage control laparotomy should only take place after CT scanning so that all diagnostic information is available
   (a) True
   (b) False
2. Once a damage control laparotomy is started, there is no option to convert to a definitive procedure
   (a) True
   (b) False
3. SNAP briefs improve situational awareness for both surgeons and anaersthetic staff
   (a) True
   (b) False
4. Laparoscopic approaches should be considered in haemodynamically unstable patients
   (a) True
   (b) False
5. Pre-theatre rehearsal and the use of cognitive aids can free up bandwidth for intra-operative decision making
   (a) True
   (b) False

Answers

1. b
2. b

3. a
4. b
5. a

References

1. National Trauma Research & Innovation Collaborative. Trauma Emergency Laparotomy Audit 1 Jan 2019 to 30 Jun 2019 (unpublished data) [Internet]. Blizard Institite for Trauma Sciences; [cited 2020 Oct 22]. Available from: https://www.c4ts.qmul.ac.uk/current-natric-studies/trauma-emergency-laparotomy-audit
2. TARN - Home [Internet]. [cited 2020 Oct 22]. Available from: https://www.tarn.ac.uk/
3. Brooks A, Davies B, Richardson D, Connolly J. Emergency surgery in patients in extremis from blunt torso injury: heroic surgery or futile care? Emerg Med J. 2004 July;21(4):483–6.
4. General Medical Council. Treatment and care towards the end of life: good practice in decision making [Internet]. 2010 [cited 2020 Oct 22]. Available from: https://www.gmc-uk.org/ethical-guidance/ethical-guidance-for-doctors/treatment-and-care-towards-the-end-of-life
5. Bernthal EMM, Russell RJ, Draper HJA. A qualitative study of the use of the four quadrant approach to assist ethical decision-making during deployment. BMJ Military Health. 2014 June 1;160(2):196–202.
6. Wilson C, Harley C, Steels S. Systematic review and meta-analysis of pre-hospital diagnostic accuracy studies. Emerg Med J. 2018 Dec;35(12):757–64.
7. Bruns B, Lindsey M, Rowe K, Brown S, Minei JP, Gentilello LM, et al. Hemoglobin drops within minutes of injuries and predicts need for an intervention to stop hemorrhage. J Trauma. 2007 Aug;63(2):312–5.
8. Shapiro MB, Jenkins DH, Schwab CW, Rotondo MF. Damage control: collective review. J Trauma. 2000 Nov;49(5):969–78.
9. Asensio JA, McDuffie L, Petrone P, Roldań G, Forno W, Gambaro E, et al. Reliable variables in the exsanguinated patient which indicate damage control and predict outcome. Am J Surg. 2001 Dec;182(6):743–51.
10. Asensio JA. Has evolution in awareness of guidelines for institution of damage control improved outcome in the management of the posttraumatic open bdomen? Arch Surg. 2004 Feb 1;139(2):209.
11. Mircea B, Florin-Mihail I. Damage control surgery – physiopathological benchmarks - part I. J Med Life. 2008 Apr 15;1(2):96–100.
12. Midwinter MJ. Damage control surgery in the era of damage control resuscitation. J R Army Med Corps. 2009 Dec;155(4):323–6.
13. Hirschberg A. Trauma laparotomy: principles and techniques. In: Moore EE, Feliciano DV, Mattox KL, editors. Trauma. 8th ed. New York: McGraw-Hill Education; 2017.
14. Mercer S, Park C, Tarmey NT. Human factors in complex trauma. Contin Educ Anaesth Crit Care Pain. 2015 Oct 1;15(5):231–6.
15. de Moya MA, Seaver C, Spaniolas K, Inaba K, Nguyen M, Veltman Y, et al. Occult pneumothorax in trauma patients: development of an objective scoring system. J Trauma. 2007 Jul;63(1):13–7.
16. Enderson BL, Abdalla R, Frame SB, Casey MT, Gould H, Maull KI. Tube thoracostomy for occult pneumothorax: a prospective randomized study of its use. J Trauma. 1993 Nov;35(5):726–9.
17. Brasel KJ, Stafford RE, Weigelt JA, Tenquist JE, Borgstrom DC. Treatment of occult pneumothoraces from blunt trauma. J Trauma. 1999 Jun;46(6):987–90.
18. Chesters A, Davies G, Wilson A. Four years of pre-hospital simple thoracostomy performed by a physician-paramedic helicopter emergency medical service team: a description and review of practice. Trauma. 2016 Apr 1;18(2):124–8.
19. Pritchard J, Hogg K. BET 2: pre-hospital finger thoracostomy in patients with chest trauma. Emerg Med J. 2017 Jun;34(6):419.
20. Department of Health. Department of Health Human Factors Referencve Group Inerim Report [Internet]. 2012 Mar [cited 2020 Dec 22] p. 23. Available from: https://www.england.nhs.uk/wp-content/uploads/2013/11/DH-rep.pdf
21. Flin RH, Youngson GG, Yule S. Enhancing surgical performance: a primer in non-technical skills [Internet]. 2016 [cited 2020 Oct 22]. Available from: http://public.ebookcentral.proquest.com/choice/publicfullrecord.aspx?p=4744285
22. Arul GS, Pugh HEJ, Mercer SJ, Midwinter MJ. Optimising communication in the damage control resuscitation—damage control surgery sequence in major trauma management. J R Army Med Corps. 2012 Jun;158(2):82–4.
23. Kahneman D. Thinking, fast and slow. 1st ed. New York: Farrar, Straus and Giroux; 2011. 499 p.
24. Peters S. The chimp paradox: the mind management program to help you achieve success, confidence, and happiness. First Tarcher/Penguin paperback edition. New York: Jeremy P. Tarcher/Penguin; 2013.
25. Hirshberg A, Mattox KL. Top knife: the art & craft of trauma surgery. Shrewsbury, UK: TFM Publishing; 2014.
26. Home | Civility Saves Lives | England [Internet]. civilitysaveslives. [cited 2020 Oct 23]. Available from: https://www.civilitysaveslives.com
27. Katz D, Blasius K, Isaak R, Lipps J, Kushelev M, Goldberg A, et al. Exposure to incivility hinders clinical performance in a simulated operative crisis. BMJ Qual Saf. 2019;28(9):750–7.
28. Lencioni PM. The five dysfunctions of a team: a leadership fable. Boca Raton, FL: Wiley; 2010.

30 Practical Considerations of Damage Control Laparotomy

Tim J. Stansfield

Abbreviations

AAST	The American Association for the Surgery of Trauma
ABRA	Abdominal Reapproximation Anchor System
ACS	Abdominal Compartment Syndrome
CNS	Central Nervous System
CoA	Course of Action
CT	Computerised Tomography Scan
DAI	Diffuse Axonal Injury
DCL	Damage Control Laparotomy
DCR	Damage control resuscitation
ED	Emergency Department
eFAST	Extended Focussed Assessment Sonography in Trauma
$ETCO_2$	End Tidal CO_2
EVTM	Endovascular resuscitation and trauma management
GI	Gastrointestinal
GMC	General Medical Council
ICD	Intercostal Chest Drain
IIA	Internal Iliac Artery
IR	Interventional Radiology
KDP	Key Decision Point
MAP	Mean arterial pressure
MTC	Major Trauma Centre
NPWT	Negative pressure wound therapy
OCEBM	Oxford Centre of Evidence Based Medicine
OT	Operating theatre
P	Pulse
SBP	Systolic Blood Pressure
SNOM	Selective non-operative management
TAC	Temporary Abdominal Closure
TARN	Trauma Audit Research Network
TCA	Traumatic Cardiac Arrest
TTL	Trauma Team Leader

The author composed, revised and approved this manuscript. The work is original. There are no conflicts or relevant disclosures.

T. J. Stansfield (✉)
The Leeds Vascular Institute, Leeds Teaching Hospitals NHS Trust, Leeds, UK

Royal Army Medical Corps, Leeds, UK
e-mail: tim.stansfield@nhs.net

- Universal actions for initiating DCL
- First cavity actions and decisions: initial in-cavity surgical actions dependent on findings
- Targeted cavity actions: identification and control of bleeding sources
- Closure of the abdomen with temporary intent
- Actions on specific injuries: a more detailed consideration of some selected injury profiles

P. Lax (ed.), *Textbook of Acute Trauma Care*, https://doi.org/10.1007/978-3-030-83628-3_30

Introduction

Chapter 29 considered the decision making process surrounding choice of damage control strategies or definitive surgery, and the pre- and intra-operative key decision points. This chapter explores the key manoeuvres of a damage control laparotomy (DCL) and offers exemplars of management strategies for selected specific injuries. It includes some detailed analysis that may be obvious to experienced faculty; such analysis is for those with less practical experience. It aims to provide balanced and nuanced guidance for practitioners involved in the delivery of damage control laparotomy.

DCL is probably best approached as a common stem of initial sequential actions or universal actions. The zero point survey described in Chap. 1 shares similarities to this framework. Attempting to concurrently perform more than one of these actions (given the synchronous cognitive and human resources involved in resuscitation) risks a critical miscommunication or chaotic coordination that impedes the team despite best intentions.

These universal actions, in order, are now discussed.

Universal Actions for Initiating DCL

Optimise Operating Theatre (OT) Setup

This is dependent on the hospital facility and systems; Fig. 29.2 in the previous chapter, offers an example from within a UK Major Trauma Centre. To minimise confusion and priority confliction with patient transfer and ongoing resuscitation, as much OT setup as achievable is completed prior to the patient arrival in the OT. Practiced team coordination usually allows more efficient and concurrent OT setup, patient transfer onto the operating table and patient positioning. If OT setup causes a delay to the patient resuscitation efforts on a regular basis, including commencing trauma laparotomy, then the hospital system and team response should be analysed with a view to reducing such delays. For example, introducing a code red system of notification or other early communication from the receiving trauma team to the OT coordinator no later than the patients arrival in the ED resus bay will allow setup to commence earlier (and continue concurrently to patient ED resuscitation and transfer).

Position Patient

Key Points

The universal initial positioning for DCL is supine and cruciform.

This initial position is a reasonable compromise between surgical and anaesthetic imperatives. Supine positioning is surgically justified for purposes of familiarity of approach, equal four-quadrant access, extensibility into the thorax and vascular access across all torso junctions. Cruciform configuration is where both arms are supported off the main table in a abducted position of approximately 90 degrees. This allows venous access and invasive monitoring usually unconstrained by the surgeons body. If a functional humeral intraosseous access is in situ, and requires preservation, then the ipsilateral upper limb should be internally rotated prior to abduction to reduce the risk of dislodgement.

Modifications

Variations in positioning may benefit access to the surgeon and/ or anaesthetist. Physiological implications and alteration in risk profile, both favourable and unfavourable, should also be considered. Positioning may effect:

- Pulmonary function. For example, an elevated upper body may relatively improve functional residual capacity and lung compliance, and reduce atelectasis risk.
- Cardiovascular function. For example, through venous distribution allowing an auto-

transfusion or risking venous pooling and a reduction in venous return to the right atrium.
- Intracranial pressure. For example, reverse Trendelenburg position may reduce intracranial pressure, whereas Trendelenburg position may increase intracranial pressure.
- Intraocular pressure. For example, significantly increases in the prone position.
- Pressure on soft tissue. For example, risking pressure damage to soft tissues.
- Altering vertebral fracture configuration. For example, risking a de novo or exacerbation of a spinal cord injury.

Specific circumstances may justify subsequent modifications to the initial cruciform supine positioning:

- Some wounding patterns may necessitate peroneal exposure, for example, blast wounds to the pelvis, or pelvic outlet impaling. In this case, the Lloyd Davies position is appropriate, with or without Trendelenburg position.
- Reverse Trendelenburg position (head up) may be appropriate to manage a concurrent head injury. The initial priority is given to the surgeon managing life-threatening haemorrhage. For example, in some circumstances access to a retroperitoneal haematoma (RPH) may be marginally more difficult if the visceral contents are gravitating caudally.
- Arching or "breaking" the operating table at the level of the iliac crests may provide improved access to the central section of the retroperitoneum. This adjustment needs to be balanced against the risk of exacerbating a known or unknown lumbar spine injury.
- Wounds and injuries that the trauma team deem too high a risk to (1) manage conservatively and (2) leave until a later return to theatre, may require, at risk following the imperative DCL manoeuvres, patient repositioning. For example, lateral decubitus positioning for a potentially life threatening oesophageal laceration or for a contaminated wound on the buttock.

Snap Brief

For those patients with potentially exsanguinating haemorrhage, a snap brief is appropriate and an example is outlined in Fig. 30.1. If there is less urgency, then a full WHO surgical safety checklist should be completed. By this stage of the pathway there has very likely been a merger of the resuscitation team with some or all of the OT team. Use of OT scrub caps personalised with the name and role of the individual are likely to be the most efficient and reliable method of sustaining knowledge of who is doing what. Verbal introductions of name and

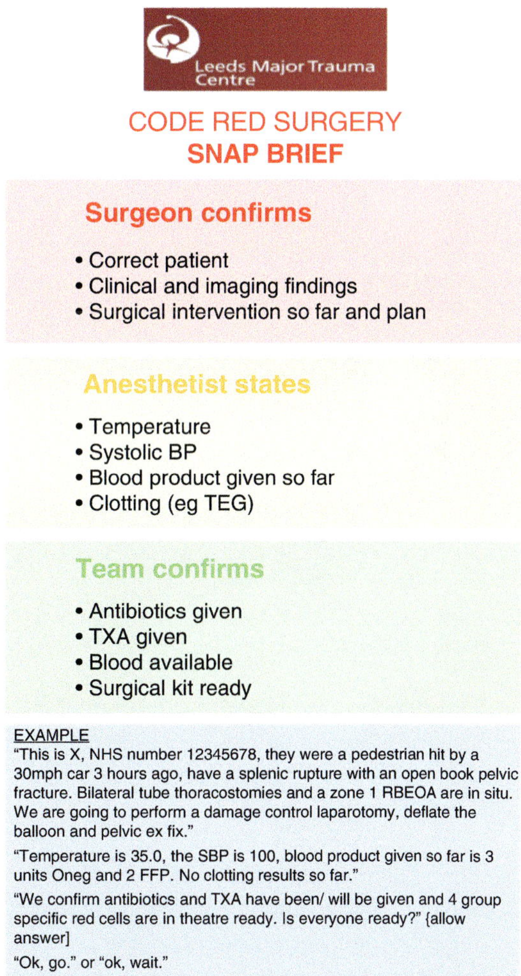

Fig. 30.1 Example of a snap brief for an exsanguinating trauma patient

role are probably much less reliable; for example, 15 people newly forming a team stating who they are is probably unretained and distracting information to most team members.

Key Points

The pre-op brief is the opportunity to ensure the team has sufficient readiness to proceed.

To reduce the risk of miscommunication, the surgeon, anaesthetist and scrub staff lead should individually confirm their readiness to proceed.

Operative Field Preparation

If the surgeon prefers a decision guided by protocol (to conserve their bandwidth for higher priority decisions) then the default surgical field for DCL should be contained within the space from the mid thighs to the chin with the side torso drapes along the posterior axillary lines and drapes covering the arms and shoulders. This allows abdomen, chest access and vascular access across all torso junctions.

Thinking beyond this default approach, increasing the size of the operative field has potential benefits and potential costs:

Potential benefits:

1. Greater access for surgical exposures
2. Risk reduction in needing to redrape (a redrape costs mental bandwidth and may be a threat to the sterile field)

Potential costs:

1. Fewer options for anaesthetic lines (although sheaths and cannula can be covered with a clear sterile dressing and appear in the operative field)
2. Fewer options for anaesthetic team monitoring (including auscultation and palpation)
3. Impaired conservation of core body temperature (the ambient theatre temperature will very rarely be close to body temperature, particularly at global latitudes greater than 45 degrees)
4. Marginally increased delay to knife-to-skin—for example, approximately 2 min for full limb preparation at a time-critical point.

Modifications

Weighting the implications of these effects, it is reasonable to:

- Exclude the chest above the xiphisternum from the operative field if there is a low probability of requiring extra abdominal surgical access. An example of use may be a patient stabbed to the lower abdomen who, through virtue of imaging and physiology, is thought very unlikely to need a resuscitative thoracotomy.
- Exclude the chest (and therefore neck) along a line through the Angle of Louis a patient's handsbreadth below the axillae. This field allows bilateral finger thoracostomy and resuscitative thoracostomy. An example of use may be a exsanguinating multiply injured patient from blunt trauma who may need dual cavity access with no indication for a surgical airway.
- Not include limbs in the initial surgical field, beyond the extant junctional zones of preparation. Rather re-prepare limbs as required post laparotomy.
- Not to include the pelvic binder in the surgical field whether it is in situ for empirical (pelvic fracture not yet excluded) or treatment purposes. Please refer to the text later in this chapter if there is a REBOA in situ.

RSI

If the patient has not already been anaesthetised and intubated, then RSI is the next action. In a patient with suspected life-threatening non-compressible abdominal haemorrhage, the team should share a mental model of anticipated cardiovascular collapse on induction. An appropriate blood product rapid infusion system should be connected and ready to immediately bolus for this eventuality. It is lower risk for a patient to persist with an uncontrolled life threatening haemorrhage than to induce without setting up, priming and attaching such a system. In such a patient and the rare occurrence of blood bank products not being immediately available, it is preferable to use theatre stocks of universal recipient blood product than to wait.

Key Points
The team must have the ability to compensate for a predictable cardiovascular collapse in an unstable patient. Appropriate vascular access, blood product and rapid transfusion capability, all in a ready to use state, is essential.

During RSI the anaesthetic team must not be distracted by extraneous noise or activity. The surgical team can facilitate establishing a secure airway by staying calm, still and quiet. The surgical team should be aware that immediately following RSI the anaesthetic imperatives are still present. In a proportion of patients, their management is more anaesthetically challenging than surgically demanding. The ongoing task of the anaesthetic team is to provide sufficient anaesthesia to ensure the patient is not aware and analgesed, whilst ensuring the same drugs do not worsen cardiovascular collapse. Simultaneously they will be managing a mass transfusion, mitigating the effects of ongoing bleeding, mitigating the effects of surgical therapeutic manoeuvres and consequences of their own anaesthetic interventions. For example, the anaesthetic dosing demands following haemorrhage control and volume filling are likely to increase.

Surgical Access

On confirmation from the anaesthetist ("ok, go") the surgeon makes the laparotomy incision, ("ok, starting").

Key Points
The standard incision for a patient undergoing trauma laparotomy (including DCL) is from the xiphisternum to pubic symphysis.

Compared to other incisions this most appropriately balances the:

- Degree of familiarity to the team
- Degree of visibility of cavity content and retroperitoneal anatomy
- Degree of access for therapeutic manoeuvres
- Time taken for access
- Extent of surgical tissue injury generated
- Integrity of abdominal wall reconstruction
- Surgical wound complication profile
- Post-operative respiratory compromise

For a time-critical, potentially life-threatening injury, the optimal technique [1] for most surgeons is a large scalpel (for example size 22) incision through skin and fat in one bold movement. This is followed by a second single movement incision through the remaining fat onto the fascia. Next, a limited incision of the fascia is made immediately supraumbilically extending down to the preperitoneal tissue. Rapid blunt finger entry through the preperitoneal space into the peritoneum is performed (this is easier when taut from massive haemoperitoneum) or, alternatively, a careful sharp incision is made into the peritoneum. Finally heavy scissor division of the midline fascia and peritoneum is made in a cephalad and caudal fashion. Such entry usually takes about 15 s or less. Use of diathermy to cauterise wound edge bleeding during entry into the abdomen is unlikely to be required in a shocked patient with peripheral vasoconstriction. Such cautery may comfort the surgeon and some of the team due to familiarity; however, it cannot be justified either in terms of overall blood loss, additional time taken or benefit to patient physiology.

Key Points
Division of the falciform ligament is part of the initial access manoeuvre to gain access to the right upper quadrant in order to allow optimal life-saving empirical packing.

The exception to falciform ligament mobilisation is if it is recognised to contain a substantial haematoma tracking to the retrohepatic veins. Such a finding may be containing a potential catastrophic venous bleed. In this case, either:

1. Mobilise only the ligament section where the haematoma will not be released and accept the associated compromise to access and packing, or
2. Pack either side of the falciform haematoma for the anterior liver packing.

If the surgeon feels obliged to enter the falciform haematoma to give sufficient exposure to an active life-threatening liver bleed then they should be prepared to establish total vascular exclusion of the liver following mobilisation. In other words, intentionally converting an unmanageable life threatening circumstance into a marginally more manageable life threatening circumstance.

If a sizeable pelvic haematoma extends from the pelvic retroperitoneum to the anterior preperitoneal fat then, provided access is not critically compromised, avoiding entry into the haematoma during initial incision reduces the risk of releasing the tamponade to freely bleeding pelvic vessels during access and the initial stages of laparotomy.

Surgical Wound Edge Retraction Considerations

The surgical wound edge retraction plan is included in the OT set up action; this may be written into OT set protocol rather than formally discussed by the team. Options generally include a combination of:

- Hand held retraction (e.g. a Morris or Deaver retractor)
- Circumferential wound edge retraction, (e.g. an X-Large or XX-Large Alexis® wound retractor)
- Dual blade self-retaining retractor (e.g. Finochietto or Balfour retractor).
- A multiple bladed retractor on a fixed support to the operating table (e.g. Omni-tract®),

In DCL it is probably most usual to initially use hand retraction due to speed. Siting an Alexis® retractor immediately following the surgical access manoeuvres may justify the 20–30 s of any ongoing blood loss from improved cavity visualisation, particularly in challenging theatre environments. Hand held retraction will need to be used in conjunction with this for optimal visualisation and access to the subdiaphragmatic and pelvic spaces. An in-situ Alexis® retractor has the added utility that it can be rapidly converted to a temporary abdominal closure by unfolding, twisting and clamping the twisted segment. A large Ioban™ dressing can then be placed over the laparostomy for an additional seal to the anterior abdominal wall. The chief utility of the Alexis® retractor used in this fashion is rapid packaging of a patient for onward transfer to a higher level surgical facility. If there is an intent to use hand held retraction followed by an Omni-tract® then an Alexis® retractor is of considerably less use and harder to justify.

Pitfall: Inadequate Exposure

Deciding to make a smaller exploratory incision before committing to a full-length midline incision is a loss of a marginal gain for the surgeon and carries risk. Examples of where such a decision carries more risk than the surgeon may perceive are:

- Trauma laparotomy post-CT, the surgeon should avoid anchoring bias on "known" injury diagnoses prior to laparotomy. A preliminary CT report is precisely that—*preliminary*. A more targeted (smaller) incision to manage renal bleeding may not address concurrent yet unrecognised splenic bleeding.
- Unnecessary haematoma clot disruption may be caused by the surgical team using more force of manipulation or traction to overcome less optimal access.
- Lacerations to the lesser gastric curvature, intraperitoneal lower rectum and ureter may not have associated obvious haematoma or contamination, and a false-negative laparotomy may be declared via a smaller access incision. These untreated injuries will then subsequently evolve, with potential unnecessary morbidity to the patient. Full access and optimal visualisation will reduce such a risk of missed injury.

Hostile Abdomen Considerations

For a trauma laparotomy (including DCL), a hostile abdomen is:

1. Any pre-injury patient condition that materially interferes with access and packing
2. Defined by the surgeon; influenced by their experience and capability.

For example, a patient undergoing trauma laparotomy who has dense intraperitoneal adhesions related to previous multiple laparotomies, chronic enterocutaneous fistulas from inflammatory bowel disease or complex abdominal wall hernias. In the case of profuse adhesions, intraperitoneal bleeding may be more likely to be favourably contained in a compartment segmented by adhesions.

Adhesions and scar tissue along the line of a previous midline laparotomy should be approached via virgin tissue at either end of the scar for safety and rapidity. This requires the previous scar to be less than a full-length incision. If the surgeon suspects a more complex abdominal entry or subsequent fraught dissection through scar tissue then they will need to weigh up the risk for pursuing midline access, packing and surgical management against the risk of alternative strategies:

- Non-midline approach, for example, bilateral subcostal or paramedian
- An extraperitoneal approach to the aortoiliac or cavoiliac segments.
- Endovascular resuscitation and trauma management (EVTM), either in entirety or as a hybrid approach. For example, initial zone 1 partial REBOA or endovascular hepatic branch embolisation.
- Trial of non-operative management allowing a control enterocutaneous fistula to develop; this is not an option where non-compressible haemorrhage control is needed
- Ureteric or biliary covered stent either as temporising control measures or to allow safer intraperitoneal exposure.

Such decisions will be dependent on factors including the nature of the injury burden, the surgeon's experience and the capabilities of the hospital system. For example, in the context of an MTC there are often logistical constraints (particularly out of hours) for EVTM. In such circumstances, in a time-critical situation, it is preferable to move immediately to the operating theatre and create an inadvertent GI, ureteric or solid organ injury than risk patient exsanguination in an isolated location if immediate EVTM intervention is not available.

First Cavity Actions and Decisions

Communicate Assessment of Findings and Begin Decisions

The surgeon must communicate their immediate laparotomy findings with the trauma team leader by using agreed terminology that allows a shared mental model amongst all team members. This rapid assessment may subsequently be shown to have drawn the wrong conclusions. However, it should allow an immediate team reaction in the time-critical circumstance of a large haemoperitoneum and avoid reflex empirical packing if it is not needed. The following is an example of terminology to use with corresponding actions to take:

1. "*big blood in abdomen*": the immediate assessment by the surgeon is that there is a large volume of blood in the peritoneal space. This implies that the view of the contents of the peritoneal cavity is significantly obstructed by blood, whether or not this volume is effected by mixing with GI content ± other fluid. This may be dependent on circumstances, such as the time since the point of injury. There is likely to be ongoing haemorrhage, and potentially the patient will exsanguinate from this. The surgical team is going to proceed to the empirical packing sequence with the aim to temporarily stop or reduce ongoing intra-abdominal bleeding where the source of blood loss is unknown or is potentially coming from more than one quadrant.

2. "*small blood in abdomen*": the immediate assessment by the surgeon is that there is a small volume of blood in the peritoneal space. This implies the view of the contents of the peritoneal cavity is not significantly obstructed by blood and there is unlikely to be significant ongoing haemorrhage. There may be intraperitoneal GI content or other fluid. The surgical team is not going to proceed to empirical packing sequence initially, instead if a source of continuing bleeding is found, it may be temporised through selective packing or application of direct digital pressure.
3. "*no blood in abdomen*": the immediate assessment by the surgeon is that there is no or a trivial amount of blood in the peritoneal space. This implies the injury and physiological hit has not been contributed to by free intraperitoneal haemorrhage. Empirical packing is not initially required but may be used if circumstances change.

Top Tip: Two Pairs of Eyes

When assessing the abdomen, the surgeon and surgical assistant should look and assess together; this is regardless of the surgical experience or seniority gradient. The two-surgeon look is especially pertinent in running the full length of the bowel and in cavity regions prone to missed injury.

Empirical Intraperitoneal Packing Sequence Not Required

In the event of little ("small") or no blood in the abdomen, the surgeon should lead the trauma team in judging whether there is insufficient intraperitoneal blood to explain the patient's physiology that led to the trauma laparotomy decision.

Key Points

The team should briefly pause, in other words conduct an *intraoperative hold*, and agree to deliberately look for and make an alternative working diagnosis.

Alternative Causes of Deranged Physiology

1. Blood loss in a contained haematoma within the retroperitoneum, pelvis or lesser sac. The surgical team should carefully look at these regions to exclude significant findings.
2. Blood loss from an external source. The surgeon and trauma team should reconsider whether external blood loss:
   - during the pre-OT pathway has been adequately replaced
   - is ongoing on the table from a missed penetrating wound (e.g. back or axilla)
   - is occurring from a transfusion which has not reached the intravascular compartment, e.g. line misplacement or disconnection
3. Blood loss into the pleural space. This should be revisited even if clinical findings and chest imaging so far are normal.
4. Hypovolaemic shock mimic from tension pneumothorax. The anaesthetist should rule this out. The surgeon may need to assist the anaesthetist in the assessment of the chest, depending on the draping arrangement. Rapid cardiovascular deterioration and sudden, progressive hypoxia should alert the anaesthetist to this diagnosis. The probability increases if a pneumothorax has previously been identified and there are hard respiratory signs such as surgical emphysema, high airway pressures and differential chest expansion [2, 3].
5. Hypovolaemic shock mimic from sepsis. To make this diagnosis as the chief explanation of the patient's deranged physiology during DCL, requires that:
   - significant haemorrhage is otherwise reasonably excluded
   - the wound carries sufficient overall environmental contamination, or there has been sufficient contamination from a perforated GI viscus
   - there has been a sufficient time interval between the point of wounding and cavity lavage or wound debridement.

For example, a patient undergoing trauma laparotomy in a shocked state 20 h after being stabbed through the abdomen, lacerating the small bowel may have sepsis without significant bleeding.

6. Hypovolaemic shock mimic from cardiac tamponade: The team should revisit whether life-threatening cardiac tamponade has been reasonably excluded with eFAST or other imaging. Note, survivable blunt trauma cardiac tamponade is a rare phenomenon despite isolated case reports [4].
7. Hypovolaemic status exacerbated by significant anaesthetic drug-related vasodilation, for example propofol rather than ketamine use, excess inhalational anaesthetic concentration or anaphylactic reaction.
8. Hypovolaemic shock mimic from blunt cardiac contusion ± cardiac valve rupture. These will be challenging to exclude on the operating table. Usually, the diagnosis is made following an index of suspicion from injury pattern, troponin and ECG with selected patients having an echocardiogram (transthoracic ± transoesophageal).
9. Hypovolaemic shock mimic from a cause that will need cross-sectional imaging to either define or exclude, for example a massive head injury without gross external injury or spinal cord injury above T6.
10. Hypovolaemic shock mimic from a non-trauma related medical cause, for example a myocardial infarction before trauma, an overdose of a hypotension inducing drug before trauma or underlying medical comorbidity.
11. Hypovolaemic shock mimic from hypocalcaemia (either transfusion related [5] or primary medical [6]). High citrate preservative concentrations in FFP and PRBCs will cause a fall in ionised calcium by chelating it in a dose-related fashion. In addition to contributing to coagulopathy (calcium is a clotting cofactor), hypocalcaemia may cause primary hypotension if it has not been replaced as part of the major haemorrhage protocol.

Next Steps

After consideration of blood loss at points 1 and 2, if an alternative working diagnosis has not been reached at this stage, then the trauma team should have a very low threshold for insertion of bilateral tube thoracostomies (if not already done so) to rule out life-threatening bleeding into the pleural space or tension pneumothorax. A significant blood volume may remain undeclared in the pleural space, but ongoing life-threatening haemorrhage will declare itself. If cardiac tamponade with haemodynamic compromise becomes a likely possibility, then a clamshell thoracotomy is usually the optimal access for management. This is particularly true if the tamponade is accompanied by significant pulmonary bleeding. A subxiphoid pericardial window may be a reasonable initial alterative to full thoracotomy if:

- Cardiac tamponade
  - seems an unlikely possibility and,
  - cannot be rapidly ruled out with available imaging and,
- There is no evidence of significant intrapleural blood

Communicate and Decide

The team is now in a position to perform a sit rep [7] per Fig. 30.2 and conduct KDP2; in other words, whether to continue to pursue a DCL strategy or change to a definitive surgery paradigm. Up to this point, DCL and a definitive strategy have shared a common process.

Empirical Intraperitoneal Packing Sequence Required

Hirshberg [1, 8] is unequivocal that en masse small bowel evisceration (to lie on the right abdominal wall) is mandated in trauma laparotomy immediately following access to create a proper working space. The surgeon will probably find this, on balance, helpful. However:

Leeds Major Trauma Centre

CODE RED SURGERY
SIT REP

At suitable times (approximately every 20 minutes) or 2 units of bloods carry out a situational report (update) between whole team:

T	Time since op started	
S	Systolic BP	
T	Temperature	
A	Acidosis	
C	Coagulopathy	• TEG • Clot formation in operative field
K	Kit/ Blood	• Blood product quantity and type used • Limitations on blood stock

Fig. 30.2 Example structure of a sit rep for exchange of pertinent clinical information during a DCL

- such evisceration may result in a marginal loss in ease of packing the liver
- requires repositioning to allow right paracolic gutter packing
- the surgeon should aim to eviscerate within three or four scoops; if a short mesentery or other issue prevents this, then the surgeon must avoid sustained flailing with the small bowel at this time-critical stage.

The surgical team should then scoop free blood or floating clot into a bowl to (sometimes marginally) improve visualisation in order to facilitate more accurate packing. Fixed clot on solid organs or the retroperitoneum should not be deliberately disrupted at this stage, and the team should avoid spending more than about 10–15 s scooping lest they start chasing ongoing bleeding. It is worth noting that packing will often mop up residual blood to allow careful inspection of quadrants at the time of pack removal.

The conditions are now set to begin the process of packing. Packing generally takes about 1 min. Many varieties of sterile textile material could technically be used for packing. The packs referred to in this text are 30 cm × 30 cm or 45 cm × 45 cm laminated gauze pieces with x-ray detectable strips. Packing should start with the quadrant most likely responsible for the chief source of bleeding. This may have been identified by preoperative imaging, by penetrating trauma trajectory, by the mechanism of injury or another form of pattern recognition. Trying to visually identify the bleeding point intraperitoneally diminishes the purpose of empirical packing and is very likely to cost greater blood loss. Therefore, if an agreement has not been made before the skin incision, the surgeons should start packing in the right upper quadrant. A two-surgeon technique is the most effective and efficient. The surgeon on the left retracts the left abdominal wall with a handheld retractor while the surgeon on the right packs the left upper quadrant (spleen/pancreatic tail/splenic flexure/left paracolic gutter) and left lower quadrant (left paracolic gutter/iliac fossa/pelvis). The surgeon on the right retracts the right abdominal wall while the surgeon the left packs the right upper quadrant (liver/gallbladder/right paracolic gutter) and right lower quadrant (right paracolic gutter/iliac fossa/pelvis if not done). The packing surgeon must endeavour to ask for a pack from the scrub staff in a calm and controlled voice. The supracolic spaces are more easily accessible and conceptualised by inferior retraction of the transverse colon with the omentum in the anatomical position. To pack the liver a hand is placed over the dome of the liver, gentle traction is applied obliquely towards the midline and packs are pushed above (anterior superior surface) and below (posterior inferior surface) the liver with the aim of restoring its' "shape". The spleen is packed similarly, with one hand used to gently pull the spleen medially and packs pushed behind (posterior to) and in front of (anterior to) the spleen.

Packing is probably most effective if applied to fully occlude the inflow and outflow of injured vessel segments. It may be at least partially effective if it generates a force greater than the luminal peak pressure of a lacerated vessel segment (provided it is not doing so directly via a porous gauze surface). This concept informs where packing is useful and where it is less useful, and therefore where additional temporising measures may be required.

- Lower pressure vessels with healthy elastic walls are more amenable to occlusion from packing. For example, the portal pressure is usually only 5 mmHg above caval pressure (i.e. the external force required to occlude hepatic vein tributaries usually be between 5 and 25 mmHg), whereas packing is very unlikely to generate enough pressure to control medium to large artery bleeding.
- The force to compress from packing is generated from the exertion of the packs between the peritoneal cavity wall and the tissues underlying the bleeding point. The surgical team should reinforce the compression by pushing the external abdominal wall and packs together manually. Compression of solid organ bleeding is generally best achieved by compression on both sides of the organ where possible; for example, a sandwich packing technique for a liver injury. This is to ensure the tissues underlying the bleeding point do not simply distort in such a way to allow the vessel to remain patent. Retroperitoneal bleeding is probably less amenable to direct packing as the tissues may distort and cannot be "sandwiched".
- If the packing seems in retrospect loose and there is rapid blood strike through add another pack between the peritoneal cavity wall and the bleeding point.

Key Points

After packing, the surgical team should perform an *intraoperative hold*, allowing (1) the anaesthetic team to continue resuscitation and (2) a whole team assessment as to whether a further immediate surgical manoeuvre is required.

Further Surgical Manoeuvres: Caval

If a sudden precipitous loss in end-tidal CO_2 ($ETCO_2$) or blood pressure occurred during packing, then the surgeon should remove packs that may be compressing the cava. Caval compression, including from total vascular exclusion of the liver, should only be performed deliberately if there is no reasonable alternative to assess or repair:

1. a caval injury
2. a caval tributary injury that cannot be otherwise isolated due to its proximity to the cava or due to its inaccessibility.

Further Surgical Manoeuvres: Aortic

An assessment should be made as to whether total or partial supracoeliac or infrarenal aortic occlusion is needed to augment the resuscitative efforts. The technique of aortic occlusion will depend on circumstance. If a REBOA catheter is in situ, then it is probably more favourable to use this rather than to manually compress or expose an aortic segment for clamping. Any temptation to attempt clamping without identification of vessel anatomy, for example blind clamping into a pool of blood, must be resisted at all costs. Extraluminal supracoeliac control for use in DCL is via the lesser omentum, and a clamp should only be applied once the crus has been sufficiently dissected from the aorta. This is usually done bluntly with the thumb and index finger. Most surgeons probably take at least 2–3 min to achieve a suprarenal clamp in such circumstances. In order to make space for this dissection some of the supracolic packing, particularly over the left liver region, may need to be removed, depending on the packing configuration. Manual compression carries less risk of arterial injury than clamping. However, manual aortic compression significantly hampers access to the remainder of the laparotomy and occupies a surgical hand. All aortic occlusion must be clearly communicated with the anaesthetist, including the approximate degree and location of the occlusion. For example "50% supracoealiac aortic occlusion is on, let me know when I can release", or "full infrarenal aortic occlusion is on, I'm planning to move to isolated left common iliac occlusion in 5 min, let's have a sit rep and agreement before I do that."

There are two rationales for aortic occlusion:

1. *As a resuscitative manoeuvre.* If despite empirical packing and ongoing resuscitative efforts there is a persistent low flow cardiac output, then there is a risk of stroke, exacerbation of any concurrent head injury, cardiac arrest or exacerbation of cardiac injury. The aim of aortic occlusion in these circumstances is to increase afterload to improve coronary and carotid perfusion. In essence, the balance of risk between the sequelae of distal hypoperfusion from aortic occlusion versus the risks from a low flow cardiac output should be weighed up. Different patients (and teams) will tolerate different durations of low cardiac output prior to this decision. The patient will have carried a significant burden of injury for some time and will probably be less tolerant of low pressure than in non-traumatic circumstances. As a very rough guide (without an empirical evidence base) if the patients' MAP is <45 for >30 s or <55 for >2 min or <65 for >5 min despite ongoing massive transfusion and ongoing correction of hypocalcaemia (and a mechanical cause such as cardiac tamponade or tension pneumothorax has been excluded), then aorta occlusion at either level is in most circumstances a reasonable step. If the physiological response from an infra-aortic occlusion is inadequate, this can be switched to supracoeliac occlusion.
2. *As haemorrhage control.* Occlusion for haemorrhage control aims to temporise exsanguinating haemorrhage not controlled by empirical packing. The balance of risk between the sequelae of distal hypoperfusion from aortic occlusion versus greater ongoing blood loss should be considered. If there is rapid pack soakage in the pelvis, then a freely bleeding iliac artery transection can be assumed until proven otherwise and infrarenal aortic occlusion performed. It is worth noting that some iliac artery transections rapidly form spontaneous occlusive clot. If there is exsanguinating haemorrhage from a zone 1 RPH despite packing, the surgeons should presume a bleeding aortic injury or bleeding from the root of one or more visceral branches, and proximal control at the supracoeliac aortic segment should be established. Patients with such injuries are unlikely to survive. It should be noted that some experts [8] consider supracoeliac occlusion to be a resuscitative manoeuvre only, whereas they consider the use of infrarenal occlusion to be either as a resuscitative or haemorrhage control manoeuvre. Occluding the aorta distal to a significant bleeding point will probably exacerbate such bleeding from an increased back pressure; this risk should not be tolerated if the level of the bleeding point(s) are unknown. Therefore, given the surgical team may be confronted with blood welling up from an unknown source, supracoeliac aortic occlusion is likely to be the initial default for exsanguinating haemorrhage despite packing.

Further Risk Mitigation in Aortic Clamping

- If there is a known injured segment of the aorta, this may be apparent from aortic wall contusion visable externally, or a CT trauma scan, then direct occlusion of this segment risks:
  (1) perpetuating an intimal dissection causing visceral or limb ischaemia,
  (2) further injuring the aortic wall, which may cause a full laceration or subsequent pseudoaneurysm formation.
- If a zone 1 RPH is extending above the diaphragm, then proximal control will need to be achieved from within the chest cavity. To do otherwise risks an uncontrolled aortic bleed which usually has a fatal outcome.
- When aortic occlusion is performed, the time interval for occlusion should be monitored ("clock on, please"). Every additional minute of total supracoeliac aortic occlusion is likely to increase the risk of mortality and multiorgan failure. The inflection point for survivability will be variable and probably affected by the injury burden and premorbid state of the patient. For general guidance, the team should

share a mental model of no more than 30 min of total supracoeliac aortic occlusion; futility is very likely to have been reached after 45 min. It is unknown to what degree intermittent or partial occlusion of the supracoeliac aorta increases these timelines. Infrarenal aortic occlusion is physiologically far better tolerated. As a general guideline, the team should share a mental model of no more than 90 min of total infrarenal aortic occlusion. Although twice this time will probably be tolerated, a more significant reperfusion hit will be incurred, and lower limb fasciotomies are probably more likely to be needed.

Further Pack Assessment and Action

An assessment should then be made of the packs to identify whether there is a quadrant or specific structure (particularly the liver) that requires repacking or additional packs.

If the liver packs appear sodden, then assess whether additional packs may sufficiently temporise the bleeding, or whether repacking the liver (part or whole) very deliberately would be more effective. For a repack, examine the liver to get a sense of the direction of force required to best restore its shape and therefore provide the best orientation for haemostasis. Look to see if there is a large enough stellate fracture or cavity that may allow packing from within, with a topical haemostatic agent ± small gauze.

The action sequence is:

1. Ready the topical haemostatic agent, a small unfolded gauze and at least 6–7 packs carefully folded in half.
2. Remove the existing packs.
3. Pack from within if there is a large enough cavity.
4. Divide the right or left triangular ligaments only if required to compress a specific injury more effectively. Often, levaing the triangular ligaments intact provides more stability for the liver tissue and packs.
5. Place 2–3 packs below the right lobe including into Rutherford Morrison's pouch.
6. Place 2–3 packs between the liver and the diaphragm over the anterior superior surface.
7. Place one pack around the tail of left lobe.
8. Place further packs as space allows, being aware that unintended caval compression may be counterproductive.

Communicate and Decide

The team is now in a position to perform a sit rep (Fig. 30.2) and conduct KDP2; in other words, whether to continue to pursue a DCL strategy or change to a definitive surgery paradigm. Up to this point, DCL and a definitive strategy have shared a common process. Given empirical packing was chosen, the team should default to DCL unless an agreement and rationale is reached to the contrary. The team should consider whether other injuries have greater imperatives for management. For example, a decompressive craniotomy or whether a chest injury has evolved to take higher priority.

Optimise for DCL

The team can consider and request additional resources not yet acquired:

- Surgical instruments. For example, specific vascular instruments or a vascular tray
- Anaesthetic or surgical assistance can be requested. This deserves emphasis—experienced help can be one of the best ways to optimise challenging circumstances.
- Other kit or additional blood products.

Further DCL action during the intraoperative hold phase requires assessment and the selection of the next priority. This depends on the patient's injury, whether aortic occlusion is in situ, whether the small bowel is accessible/eviscerated, the resource available (for example limitations of blood stock in remote settings) and the patient's current physiological state. A suggested priority order is:

1. *Improve access*. An Omni-tract® retractor or equivalent is probably the most effective way to achieve optimal access via a full-length laparotomy incision.

2. *Accessible mesenteric bleeding*. Definitively control accessible significant small bowel mesenteric bleeding. The temporising manoeuvre is to pinch the arcade between thumb and index finger on either side of the injured vessel. A figure of 8 knot with 4/0 monofilament or 4/0 braided, repeated if required, orientated to be perpendicular to the axis of the artery is generally most effective. Part of the rationale for dealing with this often small bleeding is that it is almost always quick to effectively sort. A rapid intuitive or experienced estimate may be made to further justify such action:

   The rate of ongoing blood loss from all injuries multiplied by the time to definitively stop the mesenteric bleeding plus the sum of subsequent intraoperative blood loss probably equates to less blood loss than that incurred from tackling any other ongoing haemorrhage first.

   Fixing these mesenteric bleeding points may also improve visualisation of other cavity injuries by reducing bleeding that is impracticable to pack. If these rationale are not thought to be extant, then this manoeuvre will hold a lesser priority.
3. *Accessible GI content leakage*. Rapidly temporise ongoing accessible bowel content leakage to improve visualisation of the peritoneal cavity. A constant stream of small bowel content is likely to slow down subsequent manoeuvres. Techniques for this include a wedge or segmental resection of a lacerated small bowel with a linear cutting stapler (e.g. TLC75 Ethicon), using endotracheal tube ties to circumferentially occlude a bowel segment or a suture repair cut to 2 cm when tied to allow subsequent identification.

Agree When to Remove Packs

Key Points

The surgical team must liaise with the anaesthetic team expressing an intent for selective pack removal to improve access and visualisation.

If there is no significant ongoing bleeding, there is no supracoealiac aortic occlusion and ongoing physiological improvement such as rewarming is still required, then it is reasonable to continue to hold. In some cases, this may be for up to 30 min. A patient with a core temperature of 37 °C with adequate functional platelets and a sufficient concentration of red blood cells may spontaneously stop bleeding from multiple sources, rather than unnecessarily chasing every bleeding point with a suture. If a supracoeliac clamp is in situ with no significant ongoing bleeding, then the team will need to weigh the risk of the ongoing distal ischaemic hit and sequelae against the advantages of time spent further resuscitating. It is unlikely that more than a few minutes of hold can be justified in this case. If there is significant ongoing bleeding despite packing and clamping, then further holding to correct physiology is probably a futile act; this a very rare circumstance and the packs should be removed to target the bleed directly. Initiation of pack removal effectively marks the *end of the intraoperative hold phase*.

Targeted Cavity Actions

Pack Removal

Packs should usually be removed, starting with those not thought to be covering bleeding points, then working from the most accessible bleeding regions to the least accessible bleeding areas. This allows more space to deal with the harder to access zones. As active bleeding is encountered it should usually be definitively addressed, repacking is only likely to be successful if done in a more optimal configuration, or if augmented with a topical haemostatic agent (for example, Quikclot, Veriset, Fibular, Floseal, Tachosil). If there is significant ongoing bleeding from a quadrant and adequate access space has already been created, then it is reasonable to deal with this before unpacking more accessible bleeding points that are otherwise temporarily controlled. If a pack is thought to be providing appropriate haemorrhage control, then clearly removal is not mandated, unless the risk from rebleeding prior to second look is thought to outweight the risk of causing further blood loss at this probable physiologically fragile stage. Retained pack(s) are removed at the DCL second look. For example, a liver laceration may be dealt with in this fashion.

If aortic occlusion is in situ, then pack removal is done with an intent to provide proximal control more locally to individual viscera or to move the clamp more distally down the aorto-iliac segments.

Removing Aortic Occlusion

For reasons explained above, this is always a very high priority manoeuvre, especially if supracoeliac occlusion is in situ. There is a danger that, because the proximal arterial pressure and other cardiac output proxy measurements look favourable, the team assumes the situation has become less time-critical. The steps for removal of supracoeliac aortic occlusion are:

1. *Consider pre-emptive left visceral rotation.* If the occlusion is in situ to control haemorrhage from a zone 1 retroperitoneal haematoma, then an aortic injury to the visceral segment should be considered. Of note:
   (a) a haemorrhaging visceral aortic segment is unlikely to be a survivable injury to reach hospital or, indeed, to be survivable at attempted surgical repair.
   (b) Removing supracoeliac occlusion is a time critical manoeuvre.
   (c) Repairing a visceral aortic segment injury requires a left visceral rotation for safe access (rather than an anterior approach or right visceral rotation).

   Therefore, if a visceral aortic injury is definitively known a rapid left visceral rotation augmented with appropriate distal arterial control is justified. If visceral aortic injury is not definitively known then a trial infrarenal aortic occlusion is reasonable in liaison with the anaesthetic team (see below). Supracoeliac control should be rapidly regained if significant ongoing bleeding is the result. Left visceral rotation with an anterior supracoeliac clamp in situ is possible, although self-evidently easier and much likely to inadvertently damage oesophageal, gastric and hepatic tissues if such aortic control is via a zone 1 REBOA. The aorta should be repaired as described further in this chapter.
2. *Localise control as required.* Gain more localised proximal control to any significant aortic branch arterial bleed. Visceral mobilisation, if not already achieved, and/ or arterial exposure will be required to do this. This control may be done in the first instance as an en masse vein and artery bundle. Control of minor vessel injuries at this stage is not required—such bleeding should be tolerated to expedite removal of aortic occlusion. Examples of more proximal control include:
   (a) Pringle manoeuvre for liver haemorrhage despite packing described above,
   (b) Splenic or renal hilar control for ongoing respective solid organ haemorrhage,
   (c) Superior mesenteric artery (SMA) control for a mesenteric root injury or
   (d) Ipsilateral common iliac artery (CIA).
3. *Plan and conduct aortic release.*

Key Points
Aortic release is conducted in continuous communication with the anaesthetist.

The aim is to be sufficiently sequential in patient reperfusion to prevent precipitous cardiovascular collapse. As a very rough guide if supracoeliac aortic occlusion has been less than 10 min and the team have been able to resuscitate the patient to a mean arterial pressure (MAP) > 80 mmHg then a sequential release of occlusion is probably reasonable, targeting full release within the space of 2–3 min. The purpose of this sequential release is to provide some degree of afterload to the heart as the immediate phase of the reperfusion hit occurs, appropriate volume filling and, if appropriate, vasopressors. Re-occlusion of the aorta can be applied if the MAP drops too low, for example <60 mmHg. Reclamping an artery may cause an intimal injury, dissection or worse, and so the surgeon should probably exchange for digital aortic control if more than one reclamping is required. An example of sequential reperfusion is:

- Release the clamp or digital pressure to 50% of the aortic luminal diameter (clearly this is very approximate)
- Re-assess the MAP
- Reapply more or total occlusion as required.

If this strategy does not work, then a more sequential reperfusion should be planned:

- Move the supracoeliac control to an infrarenal position (for example zone 1 to zone 3 REBOA), and reperfuse the visceral segment.
- If any of the visceral segment branches have already been controlled and are ready for reperfusion (in other words, significant bleeding is unlikely to recur), these can be sequentially reperfused as the MAP dictates.
- The common iliac segments can then be sequentially reperfused, one at a time, as the MAP dictates. The additional advantage of sequential leg release is that a confirmatory BP drop and ETCO2 raise reassures that reperfusion is occurring (see below).

Infrarenal aortic occlusion release should be managed following similar principles to supracoeliac aortic occlusion release:

1. *Localise control as required.* This may be done through a right visceral rotation. Further discussion of this follows later in this chapter.
2. *Plan and conduct aortic release.* Infrarenal aortic control generally has much less an effect on the MAP than supracoeliac control and therefore sequential reperfusion is generally achieved more rapidly where required.

Futility

If the patient is unable to tolerate the removal of a complete supracoeliac occlusion after 45 min of constant occlusion time then this is a very clear marker of futility.

Expected Sequelae

If there is no significant $ETCO_2$ or blood pressure change on removing aortic occlusion or selective reperfusion, occlusive luminal arterial thrombus should be excluded. In the first instance, this can be done by checking distal pulses, the intraoperative doppler signal and colour of end organs. In patients with normal doppler signals and leg examination, it may be that the patient has been very well resuscitated. If there is reasonable doubt that an arterial thrombus exists, then the team will need in due course need to decide between

- Revascularisation starting with thrombectomy, or
- In extremis or gross tissue destruction: organ or limb sacrifice.

Supracolic Compartment and Infracolic Compartment Inspection

Following pack removal, the surgeon should aim to perform a full and careful inspection of the abdominal cavity to identify injuries that need action on this index laparotomy.

Reducing Missed Injuries

During inspection, in order to reduce the risk of missed injury:

- Clearly establish the tract or trajectory of the penetrating injury, for example between exit and entry wounds of a gunshot wound; noting that the patient was probably not in the standard anatomical position when wounding occurred.
- For penetrating injuries if an odd number of holes are found in any hollow lumen structure then conduct a second inspection: it is more common to have an even number of holes, and therefore this raises the possibility of a missed injury.
- Visceral rotation may be the safest way to examine a penetrating hole through the retro-

peritoneum. For example, to reduce the risk of missing a ureteric injury.

- Perform rectoscopy for penetrating pelvic injuries or significant pelvic fractures to reduce the risk of missing an extraperitoneal rectal injury. This does not need to be routinely performed if this injury has been excluded by
  - appropriate cross sectional imaging or
  - In penetrating trauma, through clearly identifying that the penetrating tract base lies superficial to the rectum during intraoperative exploration.
- For a penetrating injury or bowel wall haematoma near the origin of the jejunum, mobilise the ligament of Treitz to reduce the risk of missing a proximal jejunal/distal duodenal injury.

In general, the minimum mobilisation should be performed that allows the surgeon to rule out (within a 95% confidence limit, or beyond a reasonable doubt) an underlying injury. Before entering into any retroperitoneal haematoma a surgical plan should be communicated to the team, including how proximal and distal control will be achieved. A full careful sequential inspection of the abdominal cavity may not be possible at the index DCL. This may either be due to preserved packing or more rarely by a judgement on the balance of risk. In other words, if the risk of missed injury is felt to be outweighed by the risk of continuing with a laparotomy when the physiological derangement may be better managed in intensive care. Any region not fully inspected on the index DCL must be documented in the operative note so that a full inspection is made at the DCL second look. Before temporary abdominal closure, adequate drainage must be sited to the peritoneal cavity to account for any risk carried in this regard.

Key Points

A full re-inspection of the intraperitoneal content at the DCL second look is strongly advisable. In the time critical, challenging circumstances of DCL it is possible for the surgical team to miss an injury or defer a possible injury until the second look.

Supracolic Compartment

Principles of examination include:

1. It is mandated to explore the lesser sac. All trauma laparotomies require inspection of the anterior surface of the pancreas and posterior surface of the stomach by entry into the lesser sac via an incision through the gastrocolic ligament. Information may also be gained on the proximal extent of a zone 1 RPH. If the patient has had previous resectional surgery of this region (for example, a Whipple's procedure), then the surgeon should perform enough exposure to rule out significant injury of the reconstructed GI.
2. If there is an anterior stomach wall penetrating injury then a posterior stomach wall full thickness laceration should be presumed until comprehensively ruled out through direct inspection.
3. Careful palpation of the abdominal oesophagus to identify lacerations or other defects is required
4. Careful inspection of the viewable parts of each hemidiaphragm is needed. Those intraperitoneal parts not adequately visualised should be palpated. The surgeon should identify:
   (a) Bulging of a hemidiaphragm into the peritoneal cavity that may be suggestive of air or fluid in the pleural space
   (b) Lacerations of the diaphragm
5. The surgeon should identify zone 1 and zone 2 RPHs. Zone 2 RPHs are likely to be more apparent in the infracolic compartment.

Infracolic Compartment

Principles of examination include:

1. The small bowel should be "run" from the DJ flexure to IC junction with both surgeons looking for injury. Blood or contamination should be progressively wiped from the bowel to allow proper visualisation as the bowel is run. The bowel should be flipped side to side during running so that the entire serosal surface is inspected. The mesentery at the mesen-

teric border interface should be simultaneously examined for lacerations and haematoma. Any haematomas found should be explored to look for underlying bowel injury.
2. The surgeon should identify zone 3 RPHs with inspection and palpation within the true and false pelvis. Zone 1 and 2 RPHs may also be identified from infracolic compartment examination.
3. Recognition of bowel wall colour, warmth and texture. If the whole small bowel is dusky, cool and oedematous, this:
   (a) Is probably indicative of a general perfusion problem. In the absence of another cause, these features may improve with successful ongoing resuscitation.
   (b) May be caused by an injury to the root of the mesentery: double-check this area.
   (c) May, to a degree, be the result of total vascular exclusion of the liver, or portal vein occlusion (including Pringle manoeuvre)

Actions on Identifying Injury

Injuries identified during examination of the supracolic and infracolic compartments will need to be addressed. In the particular context of DCL, some of the actions to be taken for specific injuries are described in the final section of this chapter. Following appropriate management of these injuries the final phase of trauma laparotomy is performed: closing the abdomen with temporary or permanent intent.

Closure of the Abdomen with Temporary Intent

Decision on Closure

KDP 3 for the Major Trauma patient is made immediately before closure of the laparotomy. Regardless of a previous strategy for DCL, a definitive (permanent intent) closure of the abdominal ward should be performed if all the follow criteria are met:

1. No pack is left in-situ
2. There is no definitive luminal, other repair or surgical stoma formation expected to be required within the next 5 days. There maybe an intent to reverse a stoma formation in 3–6 months, however, this is may or may not require a laparotomy incision.
3. There is no plan to re-inspect an injured region or bowel segment thought yet to declare viability; in other words may reasonably thought to require further debridement.
4. Both the risk of and sequelae from an abdominal compartment syndrome (ACS), including the risk of intraabdominal hypertension (IAH) or ACS being suboptimally managed medically and/or surgically, is judged to be lower than the risk of complications from a temporary abdominal closure.

It is not common for such a late stage strategy change in DCL. However, there should be a rationale for temporary abdominal closure rather than using it as a default action.

Method of Temporary Abdominal Closure

Fascial Closure

Partial (superior and inferior portions of a midline laparotomy) or complete fascial closure with temporary intent is reasonable if a second look DCL is planned, and if all the following criteria are met:

1. The patient's respiratory and cardiovascular systems tolerate fascial closure
2. The risk of ACS is tolerable. This is partially dependent on the likelihood of the hospital system recognising and acting on IAH and ACS—initially medically then surgically
3. Rapid transfer to ICU is not imperative; it takes additional time to perform
4. The fascia can be closed without undue tension

Fascial closure will probably lower the risk of fascial retraction and not incur the risk of laparostomy complications. However, if these criteria are not met, then a laparostomy will be needed.

Laparostomy

A laparostomy is best managed with a dressing system that allows:

- A non-adherent material to lie along the length of the paracolic gutters, underneath the abdominal wall superiorly and inferiorly and covers the bowel.
- Drainage via perforations in the non-adherent material into an absorbent system, for example sponge or gauze, that can then be drained into a portable reservoir, with or without a vacuum system.
- An adherent surface dressing to ensure a circumferential seal around the laparostomy.

Such a system will conceivably achieve the goals of visceral protection, removal and quantification of intra-abdominal exudate (including reducing the risk of macerated skin wound edges) and prevention of fascial retraction with a view to facilitating delayed primary closure.

There are many ways to cover and manage a laparostomy wound. For DCL a rapid technique is probably optimal, below are some of the more commonly used methods:

- For rapid transfer purposes, as previously described, an in situ X-Large or XX-Large Alexis® wound retractor can rapidly be converted to a temporary abdominal closure device. The additional advantage of this is that it allows examination of the bowel wall colour through the plastic sheeting.
- An "opsite sandwich" is probably the most commonly used non-proprietary laparostomy dressing option. Use of Opsite™ in this dressing is not mandated. One method of construction is as follows: lay a large 3M™ Ioban™ flat with the sticky side up, place two 30 cm × 30 cm gauze packs (with x-ray detectable strips), overlapping, unfolded and flat on the Ioban™, place a further large Ioban™ sticky side down covering the Ioban/gauze. Next, perforate one side of this construct, cut a hole approximately 5 cm × 10 cm in the opposite side, and lay the perforated side into the laparostomy with the construct edges tucked under the abdominal wall and into the paracolic gutters. Then lay a further one or two 30 cm × 30 cm gauze packs (with x-ray detectable strips) into the abdominal wall wound on top of the construct, ensuring the wound edge is very dry and any body hair is shaved within 5 cm of the wound edge. Finally, stick down a large Ioban™ to the external abdominal wall, covering the gauze in the laparostomy wound. Further strips of Ioban™ may be needed to ensure a seal. A negative pressure wound therapy system can be used to improve the longevity of the vacuum seal, improve the exudate management and reduce the risk of the small bowel prolapsing from underneath the dressing. Similarly, there is more than one way of doing this. An option that is probably more robust than others is as follows: ensure a V.A.C.® pump is charged, switched on and ready to create a vacuum. Make a 3 cm × 3 cm hole in the centre of the Ioban covering the laparostomy wound gauze, attach a V.A.C.® suction port over this hole and confirm the seal by temporarily attaching the wall suction onto the port tube. Finally, exchange the wall suction for the V.A.C.® suction tubing, then connect to the collection canister and pump and switch the V.A.C.® pump on to generate a 100 to 150 mmHg suction pressure.
- An ABThera™ system is a propriety laparostomy dressing that can be rapidly cut to size and probably has a more bespoke positioning in the paracolic gutters than the above options. It is perhaps more effective than the averagely constructed opsite sandwich. It is used in conjunction with a V.A.C.® pump similarly to the opsite sandwich.

Planning a Second Look

In the substantial majority of patients with laparosotomy and/or temporary fascial closure, a second look should be planned for no later than 48 h with an intent to close. This short interval to a comprehensive second look has several technical implications to the index surgery:

- Augmentation of the temporary abdominal closure with a system to mitigate fascial retraction (for example, the abdominal reapproximation anchor system (ABRA) or mesh) is not required
- Prevention of dense adhesions between the viscera and abdominal wall is much less of a relevant consideration at the temporary abdominal closure.
- The risk and consequences of an appropriate negative pressure dressing system used in conjunction with a laparostomy in the presence of stapled or sutured bowel is effectively mitigated. In these circumstances the risk of bowel-laparostomy fistulae caused by a negative pressure system should not prevent use of such a dressing.

Actions on Specific Injuries

The purpose of this final section is to provide an initial framework for core decision-making and the surgical manoeuvres required to enable such decision-making. It is by no means comprehensive for all injuries; this would require a book in itself. Instead, some specific injuries have been selected as exemplars for a "balance of risk" approach to decision-making in DCL. Initial decisions on particular injuries, therefore, often lend themselves more to a "slow" decision-making process described in the human factors section of this chapter.

For more complicated injuries, specialist surgical input will probably be required. However, the resuscitative surgeon and anaesthetist should continue to lead the strategic (rather than technically precise) decision process to ensure it is appropriately weighted. Strategic decisions must account for the patient's injury burden, physiological state and the context of DCL/DCR.

Retroperitoneal Haematoma

Anatomy

The retroperitoneal space is situated posterior to the lining of the peritoneal cavity and envelops visceral and vascular structures including parts of the following systems:

- GI: distal oesophagus, 2nd/3rd/4th part of the duodenum (D2/D3/D4), pancreas, posterior segments of the colon (ascending, descending, flexures) and part of the rectum
- Vascular: chiefly aortocaval and associated branches/tributaries.
- Genitourinary: kidneys, ureters and part of the bladder.
- Musculoskeletal: chiefly—psoas major, quadratus lumborum, iliacus, diaphragm, vertebral bodies and pelvis.
- Endocrine: adrenal glands and pancreas (except the distal tail).
- Nervous.

The tamponade effect (full or partial) created by the retroperitoneum can reduce the risk of exsanguination.

Principles of Management

Retroperitoneal haematomas (RPHs) are neatly traditionally simplified in most general surgical trauma courses, with acknowledgements to Kudsk and Shledon [9], into Zone 1 (midline), Zone 2 (lateral), Zone 3 (pelvis). The standard advice is to explore all RPHs in zone 1 or those caused by penetrating injury and to selectively explore blunt injury aetiology zone 2 or 3 haematomas. This straightforward algorithm is probably sufficient in most circumstances. However, in in selected circumstances there are exceptions. To identify these exceptions, in the particular circumstance of DCL, weight the balance of risk between generating unnecessary severe bleeding in an already sick patient against not missing a critical injury. This also allows the trauma team to account for the particular resource constraints of their system. On this analysis, those RPHs that mandate exploration during DCL are those that:

- may spontaneously lose their tamponade causing either exsanguination or significant morbidity from sequelae of haemorrhage in the context of the overall trauma burden

- may have an underlying occlusive vascular injury that will likely cause a life-threatening burden from tissue infarction or loss of function if not revascularised. An example may be arterial occlusion to a vital organ or lower limb (attempting to sacrifice an entire lower limb carries significant mortality risk, as well as the obvious morbidity implications).
- have a kidney, ureter or bladder (KUB) injury with a balance of risk that favours exploration over the risk of additional haemorrhage and associated physiological hit. This needs to account for the availability and expertise of endovascular intervention either as part of a hybrid or sequential approach.
- have a GI wall injury that includes either a transluminal defect or on the balance of probability will convert to such a defect.

To identify such features includes risk stratification based on available radiological (for example AAST grade), clinical and history findings. Risk of bleeding should be mitigated by appropriate proximal and distal vascular control. Although this appears overly complex, it gives a logical basis for identifying the exceptions to the standard RPH zonal algorithm. Table 30.1 outlines these exceptions, articulates the rationale and comments on the surgical management.

Visceral Rotation for Access

A medial visceral rotation should be the default option for accessing the retroperitoneum in DCL. Right medial visceral rotation (Cattell Braasch) provides rapid access to (in order of exposure) the posterior D2 and head of the pancreas, retropancreatic portal vein, infrahepatic vena cava, the right kidney and hilum, right iliac vessels, (the suprarenal aorta can both be accessed and controlled however this requires more time and dissection), infrarenal aorta, left iliac vessels, D3 and left kidney and hilum. Left medial visceral rotation (Mattox manoeuvre) is unique in providing rapid access to the supracoeliac and visceral aortic segments (the right renal artery origin requires more dissection). It includes access to the infrarenal aorta segment, aortic bifurcation, left iliac artery segments and left kidney and ureter. However, a right medial visceral rotation is more favourable to access these structures.

Pitfall: Left Medial Visceral Rotation Sub Optimal Technique

Left medial visceral rotation should be straightforward, especially if a haematoma has provided some of the dissection. However, there are some points of dissection to be wary of:

- There is often a consistent tributary at the level of the kidney, to the ascending lumbar vein that should be divided in continuity between ties or clips before being avulsed or accidentally divided.
- The final approach to aorta requires division of dense adherent connective tissue; significant delay can be encountered if the surgeon is not familiar with the need to divide this tissue boldy, once the depth of the aortic adventia is identified.
- Leaving the left kidney in situ significantly reduces access to the front of the aorta behind the left renal vein. Mobilisation or division of the left renal vein may be required.
- If the left kidney is included in the rotation, make sure the kidney and hilum are fully mobilised off the posterior abdominal musculature before accessing the aorta; otherwise, the renal hilum is under threat from an iatrogenic injury during division of periaortic tissues.

Kidneys, Ureter, Bladder (KUB)

From the perspective of DCL, the team should select a strategy that balances the risk of additional bleeding, physiological hit and resuscitation imperatives against the following risks:

- Primary risk: to preserve at least some long term renal function to avoid lifelong renal replacement therapy. It may be reasonable to broadly weight this in the same terms as preserving or sacrificing a limb. This accepts that

Table 30.1 RPH management strategy for DCL

Location	Indications to explore RPH (standard zonal algorithm with exceptions)	Rationale of indication	Proximal control and approach	Comments/pitfalls
Midline extending above transverse mesocolon	**All** *Except* • *If contained retrohepatic caval injury likely AND if there is a arterial injury requiring intervention that can reasonably be managed with an endovascular technique. (requires preoperative imaging to determine)* • *Blunt injury AND haematoma extending to the level of or above the lower edge of the diaphragmic crus AND there is reasonable supicion that this represents an aortic injury that may be managed with an endovascular technique.*	• Underlying aortic visceral segment (including lumbar branch) or proximal branch injury likely given location regardless of other findings. • Contained retrohepatic caval injury likely to be transformed from potentially survivable to fatal if opened. • A supra coeliac aorta blunt injury may be manageable with an endovascularly deployed covered stent; this is usually the optimal treatment. • Renal vein avulsion or laceration can be treated from within the RPH during medial visceral rotation, if not identified before exploration. • If pancreatic haematoma this may represent a fractured pancreas and is optimally drained at the index DCL (i.e. regardless of whether there is an underlying vascular injury)	EITHER: • Supracoeliac aorta (± via left crus to target the DTA) via left visceral medial rotation. OR • Zone 1 REBOA AND IF REQUIRED (for vessel laceration or avulsion): • Renal vessel control close to drainage into the aorta or IVC via medial visceral rotation or an anterior approach to the juxtarenal aortic segment. • SMV or SMA control for repair via pancreatic neck division if not otherwise accessible. Aim to transfer to more selective proximal control as soon as possible.	• Some supracolic midline haematomas turn out to be straightforward to manage on exploration (e.g. small branch from proximal SMA) • If the zone 1 RPH coexists with a zone 2 RPH that does not require exploration, then it is reasonable to attempt to do so leaving the zone 2 RPH intact.
Midline not extending above transverse mesocolon	**All** *Except* • *If contained retrohepatic caval injury likely AND if there is a arterial injury requiring intervention it can reasonably be managed with an endovascular technique. (requires imaging to determine)*	• Underlying infrarenal aortic segment injury or lumbar branch avulsion (blunt injury) is likely given location regardless of other findings. • Contained blunt infrarenal caval injury likely to be transformed to significant haemorrhage (total vascular control of this venous segment in trauma is usually not possible due to multiple avulsed lumbar veins).	• Infrarenal aorta and cava via right visceral medial rotation if space above haematoma to clamp. Otherwise supracoeliac aorta via left visceral medial purposes. • Zone 1 REBOA or potentially high zone 3 REBOA may give adequate arterial proximal control: Open approach probably allows a lower level of control for any injury and therefore likely to be a superior option. Will need to be combined with visceral rotation for access purposes.	• Gaining control from within the haematoma is technically possible (e.g. with a Foley catheter) and advocated by some. However, this cannot be recommended as a deliberate manoeuvre. • Note if the surgical team occlude a segment of IVC for control purposes then the reduced venous return may cause a precipitous drop in MAP. This can be mitigated with an infrarenal aortic clamp. • If the zone 1 RPH coexists with a zone 2 RPH that does not require exploration, then it is reasonable to attempt to do so leaving the zone 2 RPH intact.

Location	Indications to explore RPH (standard zonal algorithm with exceptions)	Rationale of indication	Proximal control and approach	Comments/pitfalls
Lateral in the immediate vicinity of the kidney	1. ***All penetrating*** *Except if:* • *No potentially life-threatening vascular (usually arterial) injury on the balance of probabilities i.e do not explore if <u>absence</u> of the following findings:* – *An expansile RPH: a haematoma getting significantly bigger during laparotomy* – *RPH with a thrill or that is pulsatile (false positive sign due to a transmitted pulse very unlikely in this location)* – *RPH freely bleeding into the peritoneal cavity (likely to be the case if DCL for penetrating injury)* – *RPH thought to be significantly contributing to shocked state with imaging demonstrating arterial injury* – *If appropriately phased trauma CT scan available, evidence of vascular injury team consider life threatening if not managed at DCL* • *The risk from haemorrhage sequelae in exploring RPH thought to <u>outweigh</u> the risk and sequelae of long term renal replacement therapy. i.e avoid exploration if <u>absence</u> of the following:* – *Renal artery thrombosis to* (1) *both kidneys (usually only identifiable with appropriate imaging) or* (2) *solitary functioning kidney.* *AND* – *Potential for urine outflow obstruction to* (1) *both kidneys or* (2) *solitary functioning kidney where (assuming there is a possibility of sufficient residual kidney function to justify urinary drainage).* 2. **No blunt** *Except if:* • *<u>Presence</u> of potentially life-threatening vascular (usual arterial) injury on the balance of probabilities as listed above.* • *The risk from haemorrhage sequelae in exploring RPH thought to be <u>less than</u> the risk and sequelae of long term renal replacement therapy.*	• Renal injuries in general heals with reasonably retained renal function. Renal injury that suits reconstruction can often be done so on a delayed basis by a urologist (accepting a higher complication rate). Interventional radiology techniques can provide for nephrostomy, other drainage or angioembolisation. Such non-DCL intervention will mitigates the risk of complication or return to theatre before the second look. • A perirenal injury freely bleeding into the peritoneal cavity, whether mainly venous or arterial, is unlikely to be durably stopped by packing ± topical haemostat • Exploring an isolated renal haematoma is unlikely to generate massive haemorrhage as hilar control can be rapidly achieved. Where the haematoma is more extensive or in conjunction with a zone 1 or 3 RPH, the decision becomes more difficult to balance. However, aiming to preserve at least some renal function is clearly an important consideration, possibly broadly comparable to preserving an upper limb.	Proximal renal pedicle via medical visceral rotation. OR an initial infracolic midline approach for control of the renal pedicle, followed by medial visceral rotation.	Some advocate an anterior approach to the right perirenal aortic and caval segment. Certain injuries make this a potentially unsatisfactory approach. For example, a blunt infrarenal IVC injury can push laterally and manifest as a right perirenal haematoma. On controlling the renal pedicle and opening up the haematoma, the surgeon is confronted with a welling up of a pool blood and a fraught attempt at caval control through distorted anatomy. However, available imaging may sufficiently mitigate this risk to justify the anterior approach.

(continued)

Table 30.1 (continued)

Location	Indications to explore RPH (standard zonal algorithm with exceptions)	Rationale of indication	Proximal control and approach	Comments/pitfalls
Lateral in the immediate vicinity of the duodenum	**1. All penetrating wounds in this location** 2. *Blunt injuries if any index of suspicion of transmural duodenal injury:* • *Bile stained RPH* • *Bile leak from RPH* • *Crepitus overlying RPH*	Requires drainage and repair to prevent a biliary peritonitis or substantial septic hit prior to a second look.	Right renal artery (and exposure for caval control if required) approach via right medial visceral rotation. Right colon will need to be mobilised off the duodenum to expose the anterior deodenal surface.	
Lateral in the immediate vicinity of the colon	1. **All penetrating** 2. *Blunt injuries the haematoma is not clearly tracking up from a gross pelvic haematoma that would otherwise not be explored.*	• Colonic injury requires repair or temporary exclusion to prevent faecal peritonitis or substantial septic hit prior to a second look. • Balance of risk favours not exploring if tracking up from pelvic haematoma that would otherwise not be explored. I.e., in this case, the risk of a simultaneous colonic injury is outweighed by the risk of massive additional blood loss.	Right: Approach via right medial visceral rotation Left: Left paracolic mobilisation of colon and mesentery	

Location	Indications to explore RPH (standard zonal algorithm with exceptions)	Rationale of indication	Proximal control and approach	Comments/pitfalls
Pelvic	**1.** ***All penetrating*** *Except if:* • *No problematic vascular injury identified on imaging if available AND on the balance of probabilities no life threatening vascular injury. i.e <u>absence</u> of the following findings:* *– An expansile RPH: a haematoma getting significantly bigger during laparotomy* *– RPH with a thrill or that is pulsatile (false positive sign due to a transmitted pulse very unlikely in this location)* *– RPH freely bleeding into the peritoneal cavity (likely to be the case if DCL for penetrating injury)* *– RPH thought to be significantly contributing to shocked state with imaging demonstrating arterial injury* *– If appropriately phased trauma CT scan available, evidence of vascular injury team consider life threatening if not managed at DCL* *– Presence of aortic pulse but absent EIA pulse at pelvic brim or equivalent intraoperative Doppler finding.* • *The risk from haemorrhage sequelae in exploring RPH thought to <u>outweigh</u> the risk and sequelae of long term renal replacement therapy, i.e avoid exploration if <u>absence</u> of potential for urine outflow obstruction to* (1) *both kidneys or* (2) *solitary functioning kidney (assuming there is a possibility of sufficient residual kidney function to justify consideration of urinary drainage).* 2. **No blunt** *Except if:* • *Problematic vascular injury identified (e.g. transected CIA) on imaging OR <u>presence</u> of potentially life-threatening vascular (usual arterial) injury on the balance of probabilities as listed above.* *The risk from haemorrhage sequelae in exploring RPH thought to be <u>less than</u> the risk and sequelae of long term renal replacement therapy.*	• A pelvic RPH injury bleeding, whether mainly venous or arterial, into the peritoneal cavity is unlikely to be durably stopped by packing ± topical haemostat. • IIA branch bleeding is usually most expediently and optimally managed endovascularly. Treatment in a hybrid theatre where transfer is not required would make this even more favourable. • In a hybrid setting, it may be possible to site a covered stent to a CIA and EIA injury, the durability of such stents versus an interposition graft or iliofemoral jump graft (± temporised with a shunt) is probably less favourable. Transferring a patient with an occluded iliac artery for revascularisation is probably conferring a much more substantial ischaemic hit to the limb. • A contained pelvic haematoma (i.e. most likely non-penetrating) without evidence of an arterial injury is likely to self tamponade. In contrast, exploration is likely to trigger difficult to control venous bleeding with no higher chance of maintaining venous patency. • Aiming to preserve at least some renal function is clearly an important consideration, possibly broadly comparable to preserving a limb.	Lower infra renal aortic segment from anterior approach	Lack of haematuria does not exclude a renal or ureteric injury. A transected ureter may not generate haematuria into the distal segment.

Notes: (1) This follows the standard zonal algorithm **(in bold)** with exceptions identified (*in italics*); (2) Exceptions listed are not necessarily valid for a definitive surgical strategy.

such an analogy is always going to be problematic and dependent not least on patient characteristics, which limb, limb length and so on. Long term renal replacement therapy carries risks of reduced life expectancy and morbidity. The anatomical injury required to confer this risk is to either a solitary kidney/drainage system or bilateral kidneys/drainage systems.
- Secondary risks: to carry an appropriate level of risk for (1) complications such as extravasation, urinoma, abscess (it should be noted that concurrent GI or pancreatic injuries are likely to carry a higher risk of sepsis from an undebrided injured perinephric region), post-traumatic hypertension from renal artery injury, delayed haemorrhage and (2) problems with delayed reconstruction that immediate reconstruction may not carry.

Such a balance would result in a nephrectomy for a significantly bleeding renal injury where topical haemostat, wrapping/packing the kidney, and selective angioembolisation was deemed to confer too high a risk. Those patients that have had an adequate contrast scan with a sufficiently delayed phase (5–10 min post contrast injection) to visualise the ureters will have had sufficient imaging to reasonably determine how to balance this risk appropriately. Those without such imaging will carry an index of suspicion of KUB injury (ranging from evident, to possible but unlikely) with any of the following features:

- Isolated gross haematuria
- Microscopic haematuria (this may be unknown) with a systolic episode <90 mmHg (probable circumstance for DCL)
- An injury in immediate proximity to the course of the KUB structures, for example, a penetrating injury overlying the kidney or ureter, or a pelvic fracture involving the posterior elements, or a Zone 2 or 3 RPH
- Suboptimal imaging that has provided an index of suspicion of KUB injury

The surgeon should decide whether any existing RPH meets their criteria for exploration. Exploring such RPH may provide definitive identification of an underlying KUB injury. If this is the case, the team (led by the surgeon) should decide whether the primary and secondary risks described above are best:

1. to be tolerated due to extremis and imperatives for resuscitative efforts that can only be delivered in an intensive care setting.
2. to be mitigated by postoperative CT imaging and appropriate endourological or interventional radiological management (such as cystoscopy and double J stent or nephrostomy)
3. to be mitigated by intraoperative investigation such as a one-shot IV pyelogram with the intent for:
   (a) injury management including on table endourological ureteric stenting or open ureteric stenting ± with externalisation ± immediate debridement and delayed reconstruction, or
   (b) injury management including immediate exploration, debridement and reconstruction

Selection of the appropriate course of action will depend on the patient and the hospital system and resources. Note that these strategies should be accompanied by a mitigation strategy for ongoing bleeding that has not sufficiently declared by the criteria for RPH exploration. This can either be in the form of an on-table angiogram or post-operative CT; with the intent for selective angioembolisation.

Posterior Abdominal Wall Musculature

The balance of risk decision for posterior abdominal wall musculature wounds is between the risk conferred by devitalised tissue and/or a contaminated wound and the risk of ongoing bleeding, and the risk of generating haemorrhage from wound exploration including an associated RPH.

- Devitalised tissue and wound contamination: High energy transfer wounds (for example from a high velocity round from a long barrel weapon) or deep wound contaminated with foreign material (particularly dirt or faeces) are likely to carry a risk of fatal sepsis, gas gangrene or tetanus too high to tolerate, regardless of mitigation with antibiotic or immunoglobulin. In low energy transfer wounds, on the balance of probabilities, without an obvious source of contamination, the risk is likely to be low and tolerable. Patient factors, including immunosuppression, and the resource of the hospital system will contribute to this risk assessment. In debridement, there will be a degree of residual devitalised tissue and contamination that will be of tolerable risk to leave, mitigated by the DCL second look in due course. Metal fragmentation (not including radioactive material that is beyond the scope of this chapter) imbedded in the soft tissue, not viewable from within the wound, carries a very low risk. This should be left in situ unless a specific high risk is known; for example, in a war zone, the bomb builder's tactic of defecating on an improvised explosive device after it is laid, thus faecally contaminating the blast fragments.
- For bleeding generated from the primary wound (or post debridement) that appears venous, the surgeon should try to gain haemostasis with a topical haemostat and direct pressure or packing. At the same time, the anaesthetist should ensure that coagulation physiology is being optimally managed. If this is not successful, then small Langenbeck retractors should be used to retract the laceration edges, with suction, to allow visualisation for application of ligaclips. With psoas injuries, dissection and debridement does carry the risk of triggering significant bleeding from an ascending lumbar vein or tributary; hence the aphorism "don't poke a skunk"—particularly for wounds with low risk of contamination and devitalised tissue where such bleeding can be stopped by non-surgical means. The decision making process for bleeding thought to be arterial is by a balance of risk assessment between:
  1. An open surgical approach similar to the venous bleeding management described above, and
  2. Endovascular embolisation.
- The open surgical approach is immediate. However, if the blood loss until effective endovascular embolisation can be achieved is deemed tolerable (which is more likely to be minimal in a hybrid operating suite) then this is probably the most favourable course of action and may confer less blood loss. A methodology that is usually not effective is to gain comprehensive haemostasis only to trigger significant bleeding again through further debridement. Ongoing bleeding should usually be controlled to the extent that allows the surgeon to see what they are debriding before gaining more comprehensive haemostasis.

The surgical team should be cognisant, for patients with penetrating trauma, that there may be hidden ongoing blood loss from an entry/exit wound on the patient's posterior with the tract connected to the posterior abdominal wall laceration.

Summary

The intra-operative management of polytrauma patients can be complex and naunced; in DCL the complexities rarely lie with the technical surgical aspects. Surgical management may impact and be impacted by the patient's physiology and treatment by the anaesthetist, so clear communication is essential in order to optimise patient outcomes.

Questions

1. Which of the following patient circumstances is most likely to require an alternative access approach than a midline abdominal incision for DCL?
   (a) An injury pattern that requires thoracotomy and laparotomy

(b) Multiple previous laparotomies for enterocutaneous fistula
(c) Zone 1 REBOA in situ
(d) Young and Burgess Grade 3 APC pelvic fracture
(e) Hypovolaemic trauma shock

2. The SNAP brief:
   (a) Is a confirmatory brief performed after the WHO surgical safety checklist
   (b) Always replaces the WHO surgical safety checklist in the context of DCL
   (c) Is a truncated version of the WHO surgical safety checklist for time critical situations
   (d) Mandates each team member introduces themselves by name and role
   (e) Is best performed immediately prior to skin incision
3. In DCL where there is little or no intraperitoneal blood on initial findings, a subxiphoid pericardial window may be indicated to:
   (a) Rule out cardiac tamponade
   (b) Control left ventricular bleeding
   (c) Control intrapleural bleeding
   (d) Facilitate total hepatic vascular exclusion
   (e) Improve supracoeliac aortic control
4. In DCL releasing total supracoeliac aortic occlusion:
   (a) Is likely to cause the ETCO2 value to fall
   (b) Requires complete sub diaphragmatic haemorrhage control prior to release
   (c) Should be performed without anaesthetic team awareness
   (d) May require sequential reperfusion
   (e) Between 45 and 60 minutes is likely to be survivable
5. In DCL use of a laparostomy:
   (a) Has significant risk of enterocuntaeous fistulae regardless of whether closed with 48 hrs
   (b) Must never be used in conjunction with a negative pressure dressing
   (c) May not be tolerated due to increased intra-abdominal hypertension
   (d) May not be used in conjunction with liver packing
   (e) May mitigate the risk of abdominal compartment syndrome

Answers

1. b
2. c
3. a
4. d
5. e

References

1. Hirshberg A, Mattox KL. Top knife: the art & craft of trauma surgery. Shrewsbury, UK: TFM Publishing; 2014.
2. Leigh-Smith S, Harris T. Tension pneumothorax—time for a re-think? Emerg Med J. 2005 Jan 1;22(1):8–16.
3. Roberts DJ, Leigh-Smith S, Faris PD, Blackmore C, Ball CG, Robertson HL, et al. Clinical presentation of patients with tension pneumothorax: a systematic review. Ann Surg. 2015 Jun;261(6):1068–78.
4. Rogerson T, Efstratiades T, Von Oppell U, Davies G, Curtin R. Survival after pre-hospital emergency clamshell thoracotomy for blunt cardiac rupture. Injury. 2020 Jan 1;51(1):122–3.
5. Webster S, Todd S, Redhead J, Wright C. Ionised calcium levels in major trauma patients who received blood in the emergency department. Emerg Med J. 2016 Aug;33(8):569–72.
6. Yadav A, Aggarwal R, Kundu R, Soni KD. Unusual cause of hypotension in a polytrauma victim: a case of Fahr's Syndrome. Indian J Crit Care Med. 2018 Aug;22(8):621–3.
7. Arul GS, Pugh HEJ, Mercer SJ, Midwinter MJ. Human factors in decision making in major trauma in Camp Bastion, Afghanistan. Ann R Coll Surg Engl. 2015 May;97(4):262–8.
8. Moore EE, Feliciano DV, Mattox KL, editors. Trauma. 8th ed. New York: McGraw-Hill Education; 2017.
9. Kudsk KA, Sheldon GF. Retroperitoneal hematoma. In: Blaisdell FW, Trunkey DD, editors. Abdominal trauma: with additional revised chapters from Urogenital trauma, volume II. 2nd ed. New York: Thieme Medical Publishers; 1993.

31 Trauma in the Intensive Care Unit (ICU)

James Sira and Peter Lax

- Definition and purpose of the Intensive Care Unit, with examples of care levels
- When and why trauma patients may be cared for in the ICU
- Introduction to the concepts of damage-controlled resuscitation and surgery
- How to approach the resuscitation of a trauma patient, including the importance of correcting the 'lethal triad' of hypothermia, acidosis and coagulopathy
- The importance of attention to adequate nutrition and avoidance of complications such as venous thromboembolism.
- Considerations when coordinating the care of patients with multiple injuries, including those in whom the decision has been made to transition to end of life care.

What Is the ICU?

The Intensive Care Unit (ICU) is a separate and self-contained area of a hospital, by definition dedicated to the monitoring and managing patients with the most serious pathologies. These patient cohorts consist of planned 'elective' cases (such as after major surgery) and emergency 'acute' admissions. The latter are cases such as serious road traffic accidents when the required management exceeds the ability of a standard ward. Increased medical and nursing staff ratios (often one nurse for two patients, or 1:1), greater availability of specialised allied health professionals including physiotherapists and dieticians and advanced monitoring and therapeutic options all contribute to the provision of this care. In the United Kingdom, the majority of Intensive Care doctors (Intensivists) will have a background in Anaesthesia; however, the workforce is evolving to include more doctors with a background in medical specialities such as Respiratory or Renal medicine, and most recently, those who are solely dedicated to intensive care medicine.

Who Is Admitted to the ICU?

Intensive care encompasses all areas that provide Level 2 (high dependency) and/or Level 3 (intensive care) care as defined by the Intensive Care Society document Levels of Critical Care for Adult Patients (2009). While there is some guidance on what constitutes various levels of care, the potential for deterioration, age, comorbidities and frailty, staffing levels and skill mix, and medical support must be factored into patient placement decisions. Therefore ultimately, it is clinical

J. Sira (✉)
Department of Anaesthesia and Critical Care Medicine, Leeds General Infirmary, Leeds, UK
e-mail: jamessira@nhs.net

P. Lax
Tactical Medical Wing, Royal Air Force, Brize Norton, Oxfordshire, UK

P. Lax (ed.), *Textbook of Acute Trauma Care*, https://doi.org/10.1007/978-3-030-83628-3_31

judgement that determines the most appropriate location for ongoing care. Some examples of Levels of Care concerning trauma patients are provided below:

Level 0 Patients

- Require hospitalisation, can be cared for in a regular ward. Observations required less frequently than four hourly, e.g. isolated limb fracture.

Level 1 Patients

- Patients in need of additional monitoring that can be provided on some regular wards or in a High Observations Bed (HOBs) environment. Observations required at least four hourly, e.g. continuous oxygen therapy, chest drain in situ, epidural analgesia or patient-controlled analgesia in use, or those patients with limited physiological reserve or advanced age.

Level 2 Patients

- Patients receiving or likely to require single organ support, which may include non-invasive ventilation or >50% oxygen via face mask.
- Close observation because of the potential for acute deterioration to the point of needing advanced respiratory support, e.g. pulmonary contusions and other chest injuries
- Use of an arterial line for monitoring and/or sampling of arterial blood, e.g. conservatively managed solid organ injuries with a risk of haemorrhage.
- Single intravenous vasoactive drugs to support blood pressure, cardiac output or organ perfusion
- Central nervous system depression, e.g. conservatively managed head injuries.
- Multiple large and complex dressings—limb and head, vacuum dressings

Level 3 Patients

- Advanced respiratory support or multiple organ support
- Invasive mechanical ventilator support alone
- Two or more organ support, e.g. advanced cardiovascular and neurological support.

Trauma Patients in the ICU

Those trauma patients with the most severe injuries are admitted to the ICU following multidisciplinary discussions between Trauma teams (Surgeons, Nurses) and Intensive care teams. There is clearly a subjective element to some of these decisions; however, the increasing experience of high volume trauma centres does improve the assessment and prediction of complications that are unique to this acute cohort, and as a corollary, appropriate placement.

The severity of traumatic injuries can also be assessed using the Injury Severity Score (ISS) [1]. This scoring system has been found to correlate with mortality, morbidity and hospitalisation time after trauma. Advancements in treatments and care, coupled with the limitation of applying a population score to individual patients remain, and its primary utility may be in benchmarking, data collection and research. It is worth noting that a major trauma (or polytrauma) is defined as an ISS of greater than 15. A variety of other trauma scoring systems based on anatomical injuries and/or physiological parameters exist [2, 3], which, when combined with an assessment of the patient's reserve, can provide a starting point for the assessment of outcome.

Trauma patients may present to ICU anywhere along the continuum of their admission (including before, after or between multiple operations), and the approach to trauma patients in ICU must reflect this. The damage control approach to both resuscitation and surgery may result in patients admitted to the ICU. They are deliberately 'incompletely' resuscitated or have not had a definitive surgery to address their injuries. One definition of damage control surgery (DCS) is the "planned temporary sacrifice of normal anatomy to preserve vital physiology" [4]. This is based on the idea that severely injured patients will be unable to tolerate more extensive definitive procedures, and therefore the minimum necessary for stabilisation and haemorrhage control is performed. An example of this is a patient with penetrating abdominal trauma that has had packing of their liver and resection of their small bowel with the ends stapled off and left in discontinuity, the purpose primarily to stop further bleeding or contamination. This patient may have been brought to ICU for further stabilisation before definitive surgery to re-join the bowel and repair any other injuries that are not immediately life-threatening (e.g. closed fractures). With this in mind, the approach to resuscitation and management of the trauma ICU is primarily concerned with the restoration of physiological normality as best as possible to prepare patients for further surgery and/or recovery. In the acute period, this most pertinently consists of correction of hypothermia, acidosis and coagulopathy, often called the lethal triad because of the impact on non-surgical haemostasis and organ dysfunction [5].

Key Points

1. The ICU manages patients with the most severe pathologies
2. The 'Level of Care' relates to how much support they require and helps with staffing, logistics and data collection
3. Trauma scores such as the ISS can help delineate severely ill patients but are more useful for audit and research than to an individual
4. The damage control approach aims to restore homeostasis so that definitive surgery and recovery are likely to be more successful

Initial Assessment & Management

The initial assessment of the trauma patient must always consider two related but independent facets; the physical and physiological consequences of the trauma and the potential of a medical precipitant of or related to the trauma. Some examples include patients who have suffered myocardial infarctions or arrhythmias resulting in road traffic accidents, or patients who have attempted trauma-related deliberate self-harm but have also taken a prescription drug overdose. Each of these may require specific treatments independent of the consequences of the trauma. In addition to an appropriate history, examination and investigations, maintaining a high level of suspicion is essential to ensure treatable pathologies are not missed. A thorough assessment will also allow a more complete picture of comorbidities and physiological reserve.

The initial admission period is also the time to consider a thorough review of all aspects of care that the patient has received. This includes a review of the initial CT reports and any possible addendums, documentation of all injuries including those found when a complete secondary survey is performed, a review of blood tests including viscoelastic measures of coagulation (TEG, ROTEM) and, of course, administration of fluids, drugs and blood products. Discussions with surgeons and reviewing surgical operation notes to see what has been done in theatre, the current state of the patient's anatomy, and plans for further care (including restorative operative management) are also essential.

Resuscitation

Patients may arrive in the ICU from either the emergency department or theatre cold, acidotic, coagulopathic (the so-called lethal triad) and incompletely resuscitated, sometimes in a deliberate attempt to avoid disruption of newly formed clots. This can be an inevitable consequence of large volumes of blood product transfusions, prolonged body cavity surgery, ongoing or new blood loss or organ dysfunction. Despite or because of this, it can be argued that there are few better places for sick patients to be managed than the ICU.

The initial assessment should consider overall stability and the extent of any unresolved or worsening shock. It is helpful to consider shock as a cumulative phenomenon in which the depth and duration determine the total "dose" in an integrative phenomenon [6]. It is, therefore, imperative that it is treated rapidly and appropriately to avoid irreversible organ dysfunction. Resuscitation requires the arrest of bleeding and restoration of haemodynamic stability by adequately replacing the circulating volume and re-establishing macro- and micro-circulatory flow to restore end-organ homeostasis, repaying any "oxygen debt".

Physical haemostasis should be achieved before admission to ICU either through intraoperative surgical control of bleeding such as by vessel ligation and cautery, or via interventional radiological means as is seen with some pelvic injuries. The focus may then begin on achieving physiological haemostasis by aggressively treating the lethal triad mentioned above and subsequent resuscitation.

In simplistic terms, macrocirculation refers to the vessels that transport blood to and from the organs; in contrast, microcirculation refers to terminal arterioles, metarterioles, capillaries and venules. Supranormal and goal-directed therapies presume that attaining macro-circulatory targets such as cardiac output and oxygen delivery will directly lead to perfusion at the level of the microcirculation. However, beyond a minimal level of cardiac output and arterial pressure, there may be considerable disassociation between the micro and macrocirculation which may be worsened by shock. Therefore, normal or low-normal rather than supranormal resuscitative targets may be a more appropriate paradigm to adopt. It is worth mentioning that in some cases, such as those who have sustained traumatic brain injury (TBI), the maintenance of an appropriate cerebral perfusion pressure remains a priority in preventing secondary injuries. The institution of aggressive blood pressure management may be necessary.

In the early phase of traumatic shock, volume loading remains the mainstay of circulatory support. In this context, it must be recognised that while vasopressors may improve macrovascular parameters (particularly arterial blood pressure), they may conversely worsen microvascular perfusion and mask volume depletion. This was demonstrated in a 2008 paper demonstrating that inappropriate vasopressor use in trauma almost doubled mortality in the first 24 h following injury who were inadequately resuscitated [7]. This paper is notable for the aggressive crystalloid resuscitation in both groups (over 16 L in 24 h) in preference to early blood transfusion. Still, it shows a mortality benefit, even with this approach.

A more appropriate tactic may be to consider fluid administration (primarily blood and blood products) to restore circulating blood volume, in combination with analgesia and sedation to dilate constricted blood vessels and improve microvascular perfusion.

Resuscitation targets should be individualised as much as possible depending on age, comorbidities (such as cardiac disease and hypertension) and competing physiological interests (for example co-existing CNS injuries). We must not be overly reliant on arterial blood pressure as a surrogate of blood flow (cardiac output) and organ perfusion. Non-invasive measures of cardiac output based on pulse contour analysis and thoracic bioimpedance have been used to guide fluid, vasopressor and less frequently inotropic therapy in the shocked patient, but concerns about their accuracy remain. The proliferation of critical care echocardiography provides a more modern, non-invasive solution to assess cardiac output and parameters such as stroke volume that may be used to guide resuscitation, calculated using techniques such as velocity-time integrals (VTIs) [8].

Surrogates of end-organ perfusion that may be helpful include changes in conscious levels, respiratory rate, heart rate, mean arterial blood pressure and urine output. Each parameter has limitations and cannot be interpreted in isolation, but trend values are likely to be useful. In the absence of specific goals, a starting point of a mean arterial pressure of 65–70 mmHg in a previously normotensive patient is reasonable, and a target heart rate value under 100 bpm. There may be an argument for targeting a higher MAP in those with known hypertension who demonstrate signs or symptoms consistent with organ hypoperfusion. Although performed in the septic rather than traumatic patient cohort, the SEPSISPAM trial suggested that a MAP of 80–85 mmHg in patients with chronic arterial hypertension may confer some renoprotective effects compared with a lower MAP target. However, this was not associated with a mortality benefit [9].

The normalisation of pH, lactate and base deficit are all suggestive of restored micro-circulatory perfusion. Until definitive haemostasis has been achieved, blood and blood products should provide most if not all of the volume for correction of fluid deficit. Should subsequent fluid management be required, consideration should be given to selecting balanced crystalloids such as Hartmann's solution over 0.9% Saline in the vast majority of situations, with TBIs the obvious exception. This is because there is increasing evidence that balanced crystalloids may be less harmful, particularly with respect to renal dysfunction and or failure [10]. There is absolutely no role for the gelatin or starch-based colloids in modern practice; they confer no advantages and are almost certainly harmful in some capacity [11]. Haemoglobin, electrolytes, static and dynamic clotting profiles may also be targeted for correction in the resuscitation phase. However, as with arterial blood pressure targets, the aim is not to restore complete normality. Transfusion targets should aim for a haemoglobin concentration between 80 and 100 g/L in those patients at risk of bleeding to provide a haematological buffer and to support haemostasis.

Over-aggressive fluid administration can result in hypothermia, clot disruption and haemorrhage exacerbation in the initial period. It is also associated with the development of subsequent organ dysfunction and oedema, contributing to renal failure, cardiac failure and Acute Respiratory Distress Syndrome (ARDS). By giving excess fluids in the first throes of resuscitation, the patient is put at risk of developing potentially life-threatening complications that may have been avoided by more judicious management. Overly aggressive fluid administration also has adverse immunomodulatory effects and adversely affects capillary permeability. This in itself leads to an increased capillary leak (in part via breakdown of the endothelial glycocalyx) and consequently can perpetuate hypotension. This hypotension can be mistakenly treated with further fluids which exacerbate the problem, and the patient may enter into a downward spiral.

Hypotension on ICU

In the hypotensive trauma patient, haemorrhage must always be excluded as the primary cause, especially in the initial management period. Investigation of occult or missed injuries that may now be the source of bleeding will necessitate further imaging in most instances unless there is strong evidence of the source or the patient is physiologically unstable. In this case, immediate resuscitation and operative management may be the more appropriate courses of action. It can be challenging to differentiate between surgical/anatomical/mechanical haemorrhage and bleeding associated with a physiological coagulopathy, especially in the context of conservatively managed injuries. Early involvement of the trauma team may help with future decisions for developing complications and care.

Once haemorrhage and under resuscitation have been excluded as causes for hypotension, the next most likely explanation is the manifestation of the inflammatory response to trauma. A great deal has been written regarding the SIRS (Systemic Inflammatory Response Syndrome) in the context of sepsis. The body's immune system releases multiple cytokines and chemokines in order to combat infection, but occasionally the response can be maladaptive and cause further tissue damage if it is exaggerated. An analogy might be a guard dog—very effective at scaring off intruders, but it may harm its owner if it becomes too aggressive. The SIRS response is caused by Pathogen Associated Molecular Proteins (PAMPs), causing expression of various pro-inflammatory molecules such as interleukins 1, 6, 8 and 12, as well as Tumour Necrosis Factor Alpha (TNFα). Trauma can induce expression of the same factors by releasing Damage Associated Molecular Proteins [12] (DAMPS) into the circulation, such as free haeme molecules and fragments of hyaluronic acid [13]. The same clinical manifestations occur, namely hypotension, fever and organ dysfunction. Both conditions' management strategy is the same—source control of infection or ongoing tissue damage, provision of adequate oxygen delivery to tissues, and cardiovascular support to allow healing to occur. It must be remembered that the SIRS response is a bimodal phenomenon; the initial hyperinflammatory immunologic milieu is later replaced by a relative phase of immunosuppression and risk of secondary infection. In Trunkey's traditional trimodal distribution of traumatic deaths, the late deaths from trauma are usually secondary to infection or multi-organ failure [14]. At a cellular level, the maintenance of the endothelial glycocalyx [15] is key to ensuring that end-organ damage is minimised due to the inflammatory response. Several acute strategies can be employed in the initial mass transfusion and resuscitation phase, such as using blood and FFP in a 1:1 ratio as a resuscitation fluid [16] and use of high dose opiates such as fentanyl [17] to minimise endogenous vasoconstriction. These methods have been associated with good outcomes in severely injured patients. A recently published randomised clinical trial has challenged this paradigm. Infusions of low dose arginine vasopressin during resuscitation of haemorrhagic shock in trauma patients was found to reduce the need for blood transfusions by 1.4 L in the first 48 h. While it is currently a single paper that goes against the extant evidence base, if this study stands up to further scrutiny and the effects confirmed in larger-scale trials, our approach to the bleeding trauma patient may need to change [18].

Blood Products in ICU

Resuscitation with blood products is the expected standard for trauma patients who have bled. However, blood products present additional inherent problems such as Transfusion Associated Circulatory Overload [19] (TACO) and Transfusion Related Acute Lung Injury (TRALI). If the patient is over transfused, TACO can occur and lead to pulmonary oedema via excess left ventricular preload. This is separate from the immunological effects of transfusion of blood products leading to an acute lung injury. It must be noted that although circulatory overload can (and occasionally does) occur with crystalloids, TRALI is a phenomenon specific to blood product transfusion. Certain FFP donor characteristics are associated with a higher rate of TRALI (e.g. female donors with a history of pregnancy), and some studies have looked at only using FFP from lower risk sources [20]. A more pragmatic strategy would be to have a specific endpoint in mind for transfusion (e.g. a normal thromboelastogram such as a TEG or ROTEM) once surgical haemostasis has been achieved. A recent Cochrane review [21] looked at this approach. While a direct mortality reduction was not seen, there was a reduction in the amount of both FFP and platelets given in the groups where therapy was guided by thromboelastography. However, these patients were primarily elective cardiac and liver surgery patients, so the results may not be applicable to the trauma population.

Looking at other evidence, one study [22] suggested that decreasing the mass transfusion ratio away from 1:1 FFP: PRBC to somewhere around 0.3:1 would ensure adequate coagulation while decreasing the risk of respiratory complications. This is an area for much more research, and there are clearly several confounding factors; however, one excellent review [6] highlighted that the Intensivist should aim for adequate rather than normal function. The pursuit of normal values may lead to iatrogenic injury and complications and provide no benefit in the long term. In the context of correcting traumatic coagulopathy, an INR of 1.5 may not be entirely normal, but in the absence of ongoing bleeding it is adequate.

Renal Injury

One recent review [23] has estimated acute renal injury to occur in between 20% and 50% of all intensive care admissions. Trauma patients unwell enough to require critical care have multiple risk factor for the development of renal failure, including direct physical renal or renal tract trauma, rhabdomyolysis from muscle injury, persistent hypotension, poor fluid management including fluid overload, and as a result of medications administered during the critical care admission.

Renal failure may also be precipitated by abdominal compartment syndrome [24]. In this condition, excessive pressure within the abdominal cavity can cause compression of both the kidneys themselves as well as a restriction of their afferent and efferent blood supply, causing them to fail. This pressure can also affect the blood supply to other organs such as the gut and the liver. Abdominal compartment syndrome can also cause difficulty in ventilation due to upward pressure on the diaphragm, and a rise in intracranial pressure due to compression of the vena cava leading to impaired cerebral venous drainage. Abdominal compartment syndrome is common after blunt trauma to the abdomen due to haemorrhage, or secondary to oedema of the abdominal organs or the abdominal wall itself. Intra-abdominal organ and abdominal wall oedema can also result from excessive fluid (particularly crystalloid) administration. Treatment consists of monitoring (usually via an adapted urinary catheter) and, in some extreme cases, a laparostomy to open the abdominal cavity for days or weeks and leave space for the viscera to expand without suffering the effects of pressure. When a damage control laparotomy has been performed, it is not uncommon to leave the abdominal cavity open with a membrane over the wound for at least 48 h to reduce the risk of abdominal compartment syndrome developing.

There will be instances where the cause of any renal injury will be unclear. In addition to standard review and investigations such as a renal tract ultrasound, review of medication charts to exclude nephrotoxic medications and exclusion of infections, it is recommended to monitor serum creatine kinase (CK) levels. If CK levels are raised, this should prompt a search for an occult muscular compartment syndrome, for example, in the gluteal or other less visible regions. The treatment in these instances will be urgent surgical fasciotomy of the affected areas.

Key Points

1. Consideration must always be given to a precipitating medical pathology in any traumatically injured patient.
2. Resuscitation should largely consider replacement of circulating volume with blood products before medications such as vasopressors as started.
3. Competing pathologies such as haemorrhage and head injury require individualised targets for blood pressure management.
4. Acute kidney injury is multifactorial in trauma patients but is common and should be considered in all admissions.

Secondary & Tertiary Survey

It is prudent to complete a secondary and tertiary survey that in the most seriously unwell patients. This may understandably be delayed while life-threatening injuries are managed. Often this will be devolved to the ICU team and may need to be completed within the constraints of a patient's level of consciousness. The tertiary survey is that process by which all injuries are identified and catalogued [25]. Only when this process is complete can a comprehensive treatment plan be formulated. Secondary and tertiary surveys involve a top-to-toe examination to reassess known injuries, confirm suspected injuries, and identify occult injuries by serial re-examination and further diagnostic study. Of particular relevance are injuries that may have long term implications if not dealt with acutely, though they may not be life-threatening.

Consider the example of a fractured wrist in an intubated patient. This injury may lead to a long-term restriction in function or chronic pain if it is not managed correctly, though it will not kill the patient. The initial trauma CT (if performed) is an excellent place to start; by the time a secondary or tertiary survey is performed, it will likely have been peer-reviewed and a formal "cold" report issued. Any region of the body suspected of being injured should be appropriately imaged if it has not already, and in some instances, re-imaged.

Continued Care

Nutrition

Patients who undergo severe trauma can quickly end up in a profoundly catabolic state with profound negative consequences for healing and recovery. Calorific need can be challenging to assess and meet and require expert guidance from critical care dieticians. The optimum way to feed a patient is by the early institution of enteral nutrition [26], in other words, using the patient's own digestive tract. If a patient is unable to maintain oral intake, for example, because of reduced consciousness, then a nasogastric (NG) tube can be passed and the patient can be fed via a pump until they wake up and are safe to swallow. The NG tube can be kept in situ as long as needed. The position should be checked by aspiration and pH assessment to avoid complications, the most significant of which is when feed is inadvertently infused into the lungs.

Both the nutritional state of the patient [27] at the time of their injury and the amount of supplementation [28] have been shown to impact morbidity and mortality in ICU, highlighting the importance of adequate nutritional support. This is especially true if the gastrointestinal (GI) tract has been injured and normal feeding cannot occur, or there is a prolonged ileus. The use of early total parenteral nutrition (TPN—infusing nutrients directly into a large central vein and bypassing the gut altogether) has been the subject of much investigation. Although the idea of supporting nutrition this way seems attractive, in practice the evidence is highly contradictory. In some studies, early initiation of TPN has been shown to prolong ICU stay [29], have no effect in decreasing time on ICU [30] and be prohibitively costly [31] to recommend as a standard therapy.

In contrast, other studies have shown a reduction in ventilator days [30], decreased infection rates and fewer days on antibiotics [32]. What has been agreed in the recent literature is that TPN is safe. Advances in the formulation of TPN have somewhat allayed historical concerns about sepsis and high rates of liver dysfunction. What is not clear is the optimal timing of the introduction of TPN, particularly in the context of major trauma. If the GI tract will not be usable for a prolonged period, there is little to be gained from delaying the establishment of sufficient nutrition; an energy deficit of 1200 k/cal/day has been identified as an independent risk factor for dearth on ICU [33]. If standard enteral feeding is potentially viable, then a period of attempting to establish feeding via this route is appropriate. If it becomes evident after 72 h that enteral feeding is not meeting the patient's calorie requirements, then giving TPN in addition to whatever is being absorbed to 'top-up' the patient's calorie intake is a sound practice. Continuing with small amounts of NG feed is vital in maintaining gut integrity and decreasing the risk of refeeding syndrome [34], which can be a disastrous complication of intensive care admission. Specific guidelines exist [35] to identify patients at risk of refeeding syndrome and its management.

From a practical perspective, maintaining continuous feeding in patients planned for multiple surgeries can be challenging because of the inherent dogma that all patients for theatre require at least 6 h of fasting. Suppose a patient is already intubated (and therefore has a secure airway), and the procedure does not involve the GI tract or manipulation of the airway. In that case, there is no reason to adhere to traditional perioperative fasting practices. The key to preventing this lies in both education of medical and nursing staff, effective scheduling and coordination between specialities timing of operations to ensure multiple procedures are performed at one sitting where possible (see below).

Venous Thromboembolism (VTE) Prophylaxis

Multiple studies have identified the severely injured trauma patient as being at high risk for VTE [36]. Specific factors that increase the risk of VTE in trauma patients include spinal cord injury, head trauma, lower extremity fractures, pelvic fractures and high injury severity scores. Multiple blood transfusions and a delay in pharmacological VTE prophylaxis (especially beyond

72 h) have also been demonstrated to be significant risk factors [37].

The strategies for preventing VTE reduce but do not eliminate the risk entirely. Pharmacological prophylaxis consists of low molecular weight heparin (LMWH) as the first choice agent assuming renal function is adequate. Non-pharmacologic methods consist principally of intermittent compression devices (often in conjunction with compression stockings) and should be instituted in the absence of contraindications (e.g., external fixation, lower extremity fractures, peripheral vascular disease). A Cochrane review found that combined (mechanical and pharmacological) prophylaxis reduced DVT risk relative to pharmacologic prophylaxis alone [38]. Therefore, this should be advocated as the standard of care in all ICU patients.

Early institution of pharmacological prophylaxis is desirable for avoiding the complications of VTE (DVTs & PEs). However, this must be balanced against the risk of bleeding, which will be more pertinent in trauma patients with suspected ongoing bleeding or severe coagulopathy. Data to precisely estimate the risk of bleeding in trauma patients are limited. However, particular mention should be made of patients with traumatic injuries involving the brain (TBI) or spine (TSCI), bleeding from solid organ injuries being managed conservatively, liver injuries that have been packed, and pelvic fractures. In patients with TBI or TSCI, consensus opinion recommends the initiation of LMWH within 72 h of injury if CT imaging and clinical assessments suggest stable pathology. Observational studies have also suggested that LMWH may not increase the rate of bleeding or failure of non-operative management in patients with solid organ injury. Therefore, initiation within 48 h may be appropriate.

The risk of VTE rises sharply if treatment is delayed beyond 72–96 h [39]. If pharmacologic prophylaxis is contraindicated for a period beyond this time frame, placement of a prophylactic inferior vena cava (IVC) filter may be appropriate [40]. The filter serves as a mechanical obstruction to thrombus travelling toward the pulmonary vasculature and may decrease the incidence of pulmonary emboli. However, IVC filters are ineffective at blocking thrombus originating from the upper extremities, chest or neck. Additionally, several complications have been described, including thrombus accumulation potentially leading to IVC thrombosis, filter migration and vena cava perforation. A clear consensus governing the use of prophylactic filters in trauma patients has yet to be reached. It must be stressed that there is a lack of data to support a mortality benefit for prophylactic IVC filter placement, and the American College of Chest Physicians (ACCP) guidelines [41] do not advocate using prophylactic IVC filters in trauma patients routinely. For the time being, prophylactic IVC filter placement should only be considered for the very-high-risk trauma patient with ongoing contraindications to anticoagulation.

Coordinating Further Care

In conjunction with the relevant specialists, the Intensivist must decide on an agenda for further surgeries and treatments to coordinate the best possible care for the patient. In a method analogous to the damage control approach, the intervals between surgeries should allow recovery of physiological normality as much as can be expected to reduce the risk of potential complications and improve healing. However, the schedule should also minimise the interval between surgeries if the injuries to be treated may inhibit recovery or rehabilitation progression. Essential questions to ask are as follows:

- What is the importance of surgical management to waking, weaning, rehabilitation or nursing care? e.g. spinal column fixation and limitations on patient positioning in ICU.
- Which injuries are most important?
- Does the surgery need to be performed in the acute phase of illness? E.g. maxillofacial fractures that do not influence airway management.
- Does the patient have the physiological reserve to tolerate the procedure? Will a delay improve this? E.g. correction of clotting

abnormalities, the institution of RRT, optimising nutrition.

- Can more than one operation be performed at one theatre trip? e.g. fixation of a femoral fracture and surgical tracheostomy.
- What is the expected operative course of an injury? E.g. return for skin grafting or wound closure.
- Does the patient need to remain sedated and intubated before the surgery is complete? E.g. management of agitation and/or extreme pain.
- Can the patient be woken up after the surgery?

Further care of the trauma patient also includes acknowledging the psychological impact critical illness has on patients. Studies suggest that up to 50% of patients or more experience symptoms consistent with post-traumatic stress disorder (PTSD), anxiety or depression following critical care, and expert intervention should be considered [42]. The UK National Institute for Health and Care Excellence guideline on rehabilitation from critical illness recommends early identification and support as part of a recovery plan. Most interventions to reduce psychological morbidity have been implemented in the months following discharge from critical care and hospital. They include follow-up clinics, rehabilitation services, patient diaries and nurse-led psychological recovery sessions [43].

End of Life Care

Trauma patients may be admitted to the ICU even when the multidisciplinary team's consensus is that the injuries are likely to be unsurvivable. This group includes younger patients with TBI or patients with extensive injuries in the context of life-limiting comorbidities. The purpose of these complex decisions can be considered to have two related but distinct reasons. The first is an acknowledgement that early prognostication based on, in many cases, a combination of clinical assessment of injury patterns, clinical experience and imaging reports of brain CTs is very difficult. Therefore, a further assessment period (which may not include aggressive treatments) allows greater prognostic accuracy, which, given the gravity of the decisions to be made, seems eminently sensible. The eventual outcome for such patients is often death or survival with a severe disability. However, there is a greater appreciation that some of our traditional decisions became "self-fulfilling prophecies". This ethos forms the basis for the consensus statement from the FICM & ICS regarding devastating brain injury (DBI) [44], which is unfortunately applicable to many trauma patients. The second reason may be to allow withdrawal of life-sustaining treatments when the family are in attendance, or if the clinician judges the ICU environment to be a more suitable location to provide end-of-life care.

Once the decision has been made that continuation of further life-sustaining therapies is not in the patient's best interests, if appropriate, communication with the Specialist Nurses in Organ Donation (SNODs) can begin. In the UK, SNODs can check the organ donation register to see if the patient has registered to be an organ donor. They can also discuss with the patient's relatives to decide if organ donation would be consistent with the patient's wishes if they were not on the register. Unfortunately, death following trauma (particularly TBI) remains a significant source of organs for donation, primarily because trauma currently disproportionately affects young and otherwise fit people.

Key Points

1. Nutritional support is a fundamental component of recovery from severe trauma injuries, and the involvement of a dietician should begin as soon as possible.
2. VTE is a common complication in traumatically injured patients, and adequate mechanical and chemical thromboprophylaxis must be started when safe. Consideration of an IVC filter should occur if there are contraindications to chemical thromboprophylaxis.
3. Coordinating care is essential to the patient's recovery and rehabilitation, and procedures or operations should be staged and planned as a priority.

4. End of life care is a keystone component of intensive care, and this includes the consideration of organ donation in those patients and families who have consented to this.

Conclusion

The complexity of modern trauma care is mirrored in the requirement for more specialised intensive care. High volume centres with increased experience contribute to better patient outcomes. However, there are still improvements to be made, including advancing treatments, support therapies, and understanding of the trauma patient's pathophysiology. The Intensivist needs to combine attention to detail with particular reference to resuscitative endpoints, fluid and blood administration, occult pathologies with an overarching view of the entire patient journey and coordinate multidisciplinary specialities, including the transition to rehabilitation.

Questions

1. Damage control surgery (DCS) can be described as the following:
   (a) The planned temporary sacrifice of normal anatomy to preserve vital physiology
   (b) Comprehensive surgery to correct all injuries
   (c) Should only occur if admitted overnight
   (d) A surgical technique exclusively for thoracic injuries
2. A Devastating Brain injury describes:
   (a) A patient admitted only for organ donation
   (b) A patient who only has intracranial pathology
   (c) A patient who is dead as assessed using neurological criteria (Brain Stem Tests)
   (d) A brain injury that is likely to be fatal but requires more time for prognostication to occur more accurately
3. Venous thromboembolism prophylaxis:
   (a) Low molecular weight heparin (LMWH) should be started immediately on arrival in ICU.
   (b) Must balance the risks of bleeding versus the risks of thrombosis in each individual case
   (c) Should routinely include IVC filters
   (d) Can always wait over 96 hours before being started
4. In the hypotensive trauma patient:
   (a) Acute haemorrhage should always be considered
   (b) Large volumes of crystalloid fluids should be administered
   (c) Those with a traumatic brain injury can be managed at lower blood pressures
   (d) There is no need for further imaging if performed recently
5. The Intensive Care Unit
   (a) Has a higher ratio of nursing staff to patients
   (b) Aims to provide therapies whilst patients remain on their usual ward
   (c) Cannot provide therapies beyond more accurate monitoring
   (d) Is not for patients over the age of 80 years old

Answers

1. a
2. d
3. b
4. a
5. a

References

1. Linn S. The injury severity score—importance and uses. Ann Epidemiol. 1995 Nov;5(6):440–6.
2. Chawda MN, Hildebrand F, Pape HC, Giannoudis PV. Predicting outcome after multiple trauma: which scoring system? Injury. 2004 Apr;35(4):347–58.
3. Yates DW. ABC of major trauma. Scoring systems for trauma. BMJ. 1990 Nov 10;301(6760):1090–4.
4. Hess J. Blood and coagulation support in trauma care. Hematology. 2007 Feb 1;1:187–91.
5. Roberts DJ, Ball CG, Feliciano DV, Moore EE, Ivatury RR, Lucas CE, et al. History of the innovation of damage control for management of trauma patients: 1902–2016. Ann Surg. 2017 May;265(5):1034–44.
6. Shere-Wolfe RF, Galvagno SM, Grissom TE. Critical care considerations in the management of the trauma

patient following initial resuscitation. Scand J Trauma Resusc Emerg Med. 2012 Sep 18;20:68.
7. Sperry JL, Minei JP, Frankel HL, West MA, Harbrecht BG, Moore EE, et al. Early use of vasopressors after injury: caution before constriction: the journal of trauma: injury. Infect Crit Care. 2008 Jan;64(1):9–14.
8. Orde S, Slama M, Hilton A, Yastrebov K, McLean A. Pearls and pitfalls in comprehensive critical care echocardiography. Crit Care. 2017 Nov 17;21(1):279.
9. Asfar P, Meziani F, Hamel J-F, Grelon F, Megarbane B, Anguel N, et al. High versus low blood-pressure target in patients with septic shock. N Engl J Med. 2014 Apr 24;370(17):1583–93.
10. Semler MW, Self WH, Wanderer JP, Ehrenfeld JM, Wang L, Byrne DW, et al. Balanced crystalloids versus saline in critically ill adults. N Engl J Med. 2018 Mar;378(9):829–39.
11. Perner A, Haase N, Guttormsen AB, Tenhunen J, Klemenzson G, Åneman A, et al. Hydroxyethyl starch 130/0.42 versus Ringer's acetate in severe Sepsis. N Engl J Med. 2012 July 12;367(2):124–34.
12. Marik PE, Flemmer M. The immune response to surgery and trauma: implications for treatment. J Trauma Acute Care Surg. 2012 Oct;73(4):801–8.
13. Volpin G, Cohen M, Assaf M, Meir T, Katz R, Pollack S. Cytokine levels (IL-4, IL-6, IL-8 and TGFβ) as potential biomarkers of systemic inflammatory response in trauma patients. Int Orthop. 2014 Jun;38(6):1303–9.
14. Hadfield RJ, Parr MJ, Manara AR. Late deaths in multiple trauma patients receiving intensive care. Resuscitation. 2001 June;49(3):279–81.
15. Haywood-Watson RJ, Holcomb JB, Gonzalez EA, Peng Z, Pati S, Park PW, et al. Modulation of syndecan-1 shedding after hemorrhagic shock and resuscitation. PLoS One. 2011;6(8):e23530.
16. Dutton RP. Resuscitative strategies to maintain homeostasis during damage control surgery. Br J Surg. 2012 Jan;99(Suppl 1):21–8.
17. Sikorski RA, Koerner AK, Fouche-Weber LY, Galvagno SM. Choice of general anesthetics for trauma patients. Curr Anesthesiol Rep. 2014 Sep;4(3):225–32.
18. Sims CA, Holena D, Kim P, Pascual J, Smith B, Martin N, et al. Effect of low-dose supplementation of arginine vasopressin on need for blood product transfusions in patients with trauma and hemorrhagic shock: a randomised clinical trial. JAMA Surg [Internet]. 2019 Aug 28 [cited 2019 Aug 31]. Available from: https://jamanetwork.com/journals/jamasurgery/fullarticle/2749069
19. Goldman M, Webert KE, Arnold DM, Freedman J, Hannon J, Blajchman MA, et al. Proceedings of a consensus conference: towards an understanding of TRALI. Transfus Med Rev. 2005 Jan;19(1):2–31.
20. Funk MB, Guenay S, Lohmann A, Henseler O, Heiden M, Hanschmann KMO, et al. Benefit of transfusion-related acute lung injury risk-minimisation measures—German haemovigilance data (2006-2010). Vox Sang. 2012 May;102(4):317–23.
21. Wikkelsø A, Wetterslev J, Møller AM, Afshari A. Thromboelastography (TEG) or thromboelastometry (ROTEM) to monitor haemostatic treatment versus usual care in adults or children with bleeding. Cochrane Database of Systematic Reviews [Internet]. 2016 [cited 2019 Aug 3];(8). Available from: https://www.cochranelibrary.com/cdsr/doi/10.1002/14651858.CD007871.pub3/full
22. Lucas CE, Ledgerwood AM. Fresh frozen plasma/red blood cell resuscitation regimen that restores procoagulants without causing adult respiratory distress syndrome. J Trauma Acute Care Surg. 2012 Apr;72(4):821–7.
23. Case J, Khan S, Khalid R, Khan A. Epidemiology of acute kidney injury in the intensive care unit. Crit Care Res Pract [Internet]. 2013 [cited 2019 Aug 3];2013. Available from: https://www.ncbi.nlm.nih.gov/pmc/articles/PMC3618922/
24. Kirkpatrick AW, Roberts DJ, De Waele J, Jaeschke R, Malbrain MLNG, De Keulenaer B, et al. Intra-abdominal hypertension and the abdominal compartment syndrome: updated consensus definitions and clinical practice guidelines from the World Society of the Abdominal Compartment Syndrome. Intensive Care Med. 2013 Jul;39(7):1190–206.
25. Grossman MD, Born C. Tertiary survey of the trauma patient in the intensive care unit. Surg Clin N Am. 2000 Jun;80(3):805–24.
26. Miller KR, Smith JW, Harbrecht BG, Benns MV. Early enteral nutrition in trauma: is there still any doubt? Curr Trauma Rep. 2016 Jun;2(2):73–8.
27. Alberda C, Gramlich L, Jones N, Jeejeebhoy K, Day AG, Dhaliwal R, et al. The relationship between nutritional intake and clinical outcomes in critically ill patients: results of an international multicenter observational study. Intensive Care Med. 2009 Oct;35(10):1728–37.
28. Robinson MK, Mogensen KM, Casey JD, McKane CK, Moromizato T, Rawn JD, et al. The relationship among obesity, nutritional status, and mortality in the critically ill. Crit Care Med. 2015 Jan;43(1):87–100.
29. Casaer MP, Mesotten D, Hermans G, Wouters PJ, Schetz M, Meyfroidt G, et al. Early versus late parenteral nutrition in critically ill adults. N Engl J Med. 2011 Aug 11;365(6):506–17.
30. Doig GS, Simpson F, Sweetman EA, Finfer SR, Cooper DJ, Heighes PT, et al. Early parenteral nutrition in critically ill patients with short-term relative contraindications to early enteral nutrition: a randomised controlled trial. JAMA. 2013 May 22;309(20):2130–8.
31. Vanderheyden S, Casaer MP, Kesteloot K, Simoens S, De Rijdt T, Peers G, et al. Early versus late parenteral nutrition in ICU patients: cost analysis of the EPaNIC trial. Crit Care. 2012 May 25;16(3):R96.
32. Heidegger CP, Berger MM, Graf S, Zingg W, Darmon P, Costanza MC, et al. Optimisation of energy provision with supplemental parenteral nutrition in critically ill patients: a randomised controlled clinical trial. Lancet. 2013 Feb 2;381(9864):385–93.

33. Faisy C, Lerolle N, Dachraoui F, Savard J-F, Abboud I, Tadie J-M, et al. Impact of energy deficit calculated by a predictive method on outcome in medical patients requiring prolonged acute mechanical ventilation. Br J Nutr. 2009 Apr;101(7):1079–87.
34. Mehanna HM, Moledina J, Travis J. Refeeding syndrome: what it is, and how to prevent and treat it. BMJ. 2008 June 28;336(7659):1495–8.
35. NICE. Overview | Nutrition support for adults: oral nutrition support, enteral tube feeding and parenteral nutrition | Guidance | NICE [Internet]. [cited 2019 June 20]. Available from: https://www.nice.org.uk/Guidance/CG32
36. Azarbal A, Rowell S, Lewis J, Urankar R, Moseley S, Landry G, et al. Duplex ultrasound screening detects high rates of deep vein thromboses in critically ill trauma patients. J Vasc Surg. 2011 Sep;54(3):743–8.
37. Meizoso JP, Karcutskie CA, Ray JJ, Ruiz X, Ginzburg E, Namias N, et al. A simplified stratification system for venous thromboembolism risk in severely injured trauma patients. J Surg Res. 2017 Jan;207:138–44.
38. Barrera LM, Perel P, Ker K, Cirocchi R, Farinella E, Morales Uribe CH. Thromboprophylaxis for trauma patients. Cochrane Injuries Group, editor. Cochrane Database of Systematic Reviews [Internet]. 2013 Mar 28 [cited 2019 Aug 3]. Available from: https://doi.org/10.1002/14651858.CD008303.pub2
39. Nathens AB, McMurray MK, Cuschieri J, Durr EA, Moore EE, Bankey PE, et al. The practice of venous thromboembolism prophylaxis in the major trauma patient. J Trauma. 2007 Mar;62(3):557–62.
40. Decousus H, Leizorovicz A, Parent F, Page Y, Tardy B, Girard P, et al. A clinical trial of vena caval filters in the prevention of pulmonary embolism in patients with proximal deep-vein thrombosis. Prévention du Risque d'Embolie Pulmonaire par Interruption Cave Study Group. N Engl J Med. 1998 Feb 12;338(7):409–15.
41. Gould MK, Garcia DA, Wren SM, Karanicolas PJ, Arcelus JI, Heit JA, et al. Prevention of VTE in nonorthopedic surgical patients: antithrombotic therapy and prevention of thrombosis, 9th ed: American College of Chest Physicians Evidence-Based Clinical Practice Guidelines. Chest. 2012 Feb;141(2 Suppl):e227S–77S.
42. Wade D, Als N, Bell V, Brewin C, D'Antoni D, Harrison DA, et al. Providing psychological support to people in intensive care: development and feasibility study of a nurse-led intervention to prevent acute stress and long-term morbidity. BMJ Open. 2018 Jul 1;8(7):e021083.
43. NICE. Overview | Rehabilitation after critical illness in adults | Quality standards | NICE [Internet]. [cited 2019 Aug 3]. Available from: https://www.nice.org.uk/guidance/qs158
44. Harvey D, Butler J, Groves J, Manara A, Menon D, Thomas E, et al. Management of perceived devastating brain injury after hospital admission: a consensus statement from stakeholder professional organisations. Br J Anaesth. 2018 Jan;120(1):138–45.

Spinal and Neurological Trauma

32

Priyank Sinha and Timothy Knight

1. Understand the epidemiology of spinal cord injury and patient presentation.
2. Understand the difference between neurogenic shock and spinal shock
3. Understand why different cord injury patterns manifest with different clinical signs based on the topography of the spinal cord
4. Understand what constitutes a stable vs unstable spinal injury
5. Understand the evidence around indications and proposed benefits of cervical spine immobilisation, and the evidence of harm/complications arising from their use
6. Understand the indications for imaging in cervical spine injury, and common decision making tools that are implemented.
7. Understand specific cervical spine injuries and their operative management.

Introduction

Traumatic spinal cord injury (SCI) is associated with significant mortality and morbidity, it also has a profound effect on the quality of life, mental health, and socio-economic circumstances. Furthermore, it has a major impact on patient's families too.

In recent decades, significant progress has been made in the management of spinal injuries. Improved legislation, public education, infrastructure, and better vehicle designs have reduced the incidence of SCI. There is now a better understanding of the nuances and significance in anatomy, pathophysiology, and biomechanics of the spine and their implications in the management of intrinsic cord injury. Similarly, tremendous progress has been made in prehospital care, transport, management in the Emergency Department (ED), and Intensive Care Unit (ICU) along with improvement in definitive medical and surgical care. There is, however, much that remains elusive and the focus of research. Research is hindered by the implicit challenge of tissue sampling of cerebrospinal fluid for biochemical factors and signalling markers. Litigation from ensuing disability, with both civil causes and iatrogenic, and an adversarial process for financial support in victims make enrolment in clinical trials difficult.

Prehospital spinal immobilisation has (rightly or wrongly) become a universal standard of care for suspected structural spinal injury. Patients are

P. Sinha (✉)
Department of Neurosurgery, Leeds General Infirmary, Leeds, UK

T. Knight
Royal Orthopaedic Hospital, Birmingham, UK

Birmingham Children's Hospital, Birmingham, UK

P. Lax (ed.), *Textbook of Acute Trauma Care*, https://doi.org/10.1007/978-3-030-83628-3_32

supported with a rigid cervical collar with blocks and straps on a backboard or scoop; practice advocated by the Advanced Trauma Life Support (ATLS) guidelines. This is based on the aspiration that spinal immobilisation minimises further spinal movement, thus mitigating secondary spinal cord injury. This is done despite the low incidence of spinal fracture or cord injury, and without level 1 evidence to support such a practice; it may principally be driven by fear of missing a potentially devastating injury and the litigation associated with it. Little consideration is routinely given to the potential harms of cervical collars when applied in this setting. The practice follows on the general principles learnt and influential to trauma management from the Second World War and development of splints such as the Thomas femoral splint that demonstrated tremendous benefit of immobilisation and stabilisation of injuries.

This chapter evaluates the epidemiology of spinal injuries along with classification, assessment, and management of spinal trauma.

Epidemiology

The global incidence of traumatic spinal injury is around 10.5 per 100,000, with traumatic SCI reported from 0.8–24.6 cases per 100,000 [1]. By way of example, 1.7 in Brazil, 19.5 in Ireland, 5.3 in Canada, 3–4 in the United States, and 1.3 in the UK (per 100,000) [2, 3]. The wide variation in the incidence of SCI may be related to several factors such as traffic regulations, socio-economic conditions, geographical distribution, and level of education besides the robustness of data being captured [4]. Perversely, the incidence of traumatic SCI is gradually decreasing in developed countries, which may be related to legislation, improved vehicle design, prevention programmes, improved road safety, and education. However, the overall worldwide incidence of SCI is gradually increasing, with the injury burden primarily carried by low and middle-income countries, factors related to industrialisation and increasing population.

There are approximately 1200 new cases of SCI each year in the UK, and it is estimated that 40,000 people in the UK live with SCI [2, 5]. In the United States, 12,000 cases of SCI occur annually, and it is estimated that 1.3 million people in the US are affected by paralysis secondary to SCI [6, 7]. In the UK, half of SCI is attributable to road traffic accidents, the remainder mainly from falls and less than a tenth occurring in sports [8]. In children, the most common causes are either sports injury or water-related recreational activities. SCI is present in one in twenty severe traumatic brain injuries. (TBI), whereas up to a quarter of the patients with spinal injury will have at least mild TBI [9]. Traumatic SCI is four times more common in males, and the mean age at injury is 33 years [2]. This carries a tremendous economic burden and incapacitates the affected population group who often have yet to amount savings and are thrown into vulnerability.

The incidence of any form of cervical spine injury in blunt trauma is around one in thirty (2–4%) but rises tenfold (34.4%) in obtunded polytrauma patients [10]. Half (56%) of patients with a cervical cord injury have an associated fracture; this is in comparison to all (100%) patients with thoracic cord injury and 85% of patients with injury to the neural tissues in the lumbar spine [2]. In penetrating trauma, the incidence of cervical fracture and SCI is even lower; 1.43% and 0.38% respectively.

Of the fractures causing SCI, half (50%) are located in the cervical spine, a third (37%) in the thoracic spine, and a tenth (11%) in the lumbar spine. In the cervical spine, most commonly the C6/7 (50%) level is affected, and a third (33%) involve C2 [8].

One in ten patients have multi-level spinal involvement; assessment and imaging of the whole spine is of critical importance if a fracture is found. Prospectively collected data from Trauma Audit and Research Network (TARN) from 1988 to 2009 looking at the data from 250,584 patients showed that patients with a GCS of 8 or less, with a fall greater than 2 m, a sports injury or RTA were most at risk of spinal fracture or dislocation. Further to this, predictors of spinal cord injury were patients with their GCS in any way affected (<15), with a fall greater than 2 m, a sports injury, associated chest injury, and gunshot wounds, with both fractures and cord injuries more common in males under 45 years of age [11].

Life expectancy after SCI depends on many factors such as age, co-morbidities, severity, availability of healthcare resources, and is reported from 1.5 years to 52.6 years [2]. The variation from country to country in the incidence of traumatic SCI is telling and underpins the wide, country-specific variation in mortality rate from SCI.

The lifetime cost of care of a patient with SCI is reported to be between £1.2 and 3.6 million (1.6–4.8 million USD), although this figure rises annually. The United States spends around $9.7 billion annually on the treatment of SCI [7, 12]. Cost estimates increase with younger age at the time of injury, and with ever advancing treatment and prosthetic options which are opening doors to the rehabilitation and independence available.

Classification

A number of classification systems have been proposed to explain the type and completeness of injury, spinal stability, and various fracture patterns in the spine to ease communication between treating clinicians, standardise treatment as well as providing consistency for research. An ideal classification system should be easily reproducible and have low inter- and intra-observer variability to be widely accepted [13].

Spinal cord injury can be defined as either primary or secondary. Primary SCI occurs at the time of actual event and may be due to compression, traction, shearing, or haemorrhage. During primary injury, there may be damage to small intramedullary vessels, which can affect blood flow to the grey as well as the white matter. Within minutes of primary injury, secondary injury starts. Several factors have been implicated in secondary traumatic SCI; it may be due to continued compression (mechanical or oedematous), hypoxia, or hypotension secondary to neurogenic or hypovolaemic shock. On a cellular level, free radical-mediated lipid peroxidation and membrane damage, intracellular accumulation of calcium, and disruption of cellular metabolism have been implicated. On a molecular level, reactive oxygen species, activated complement cascade, cytokines, nitric oxide, glutamate, and cytochrome-c have been implicated.

A neurological deficit may occur early (within hours), or late (days or weeks), post primary injury. A primary spinal cord injury cannot be reversed but is preventable [7]. Legislation, public education and improved vehicle designs have been cited as methods for decreasing the incidence of primary SCI. Minimising or preventing secondary SCI is an area of active research, and several strategies have been tried. These include induction of relative hypothermia, CSF drainage, drugs such as methylprednisolone, naloxone, barbiturates, free radical scavengers, and calcium channel blockers. However, these have all met with limited (if any) success that has meant there are no universal recommendations in their use [14].

Another way to classify SCI is complete versus incomplete injuries. In complete spinal injury, there is no motor or sensory function present below the level of the injury, including and notably of the sacral roots. This is due to the structural layout of the spinal cord, with sacral fibres typically in the most vascularised territories lying peripherally, and rostral tracts lying centrally at higher levels (Figs. 32.1 and 32.2). Incomplete injury manifests clinically as sacral sparing, whereby some sacral fibres receive limited blood flow. Complete loss of sacral reflexes, notably the bulbocavernosus, is a poor prognosticator and significant clinical finding. Loss of the sacral roots depicts a cord with the most profound vascular insult.

Level of injury is generally accepted as the most caudal level with motor function on the Medical Research Council (MRC) scale at least grade 3, with intact pain and temperature sensation. An incomplete spinal injury is defined as an injury where there is partial preservation of neurological function more than one level below the level of SCI. There are several recognised patterns of incomplete SCI (Fig. 32.3).

Central Cord Syndrome

- Most common incomplete SCI syndrome
- Usually seen in elderly patients who sustain a hyperextension injury to the cervical spine. The cord is injured between the buckled ligamentum flavum posteriorly and osteophytes anteriorly
- The central area of the cord has a tenuous blood supply, and the upper limb fibres are located more centrally than lower limb fibres

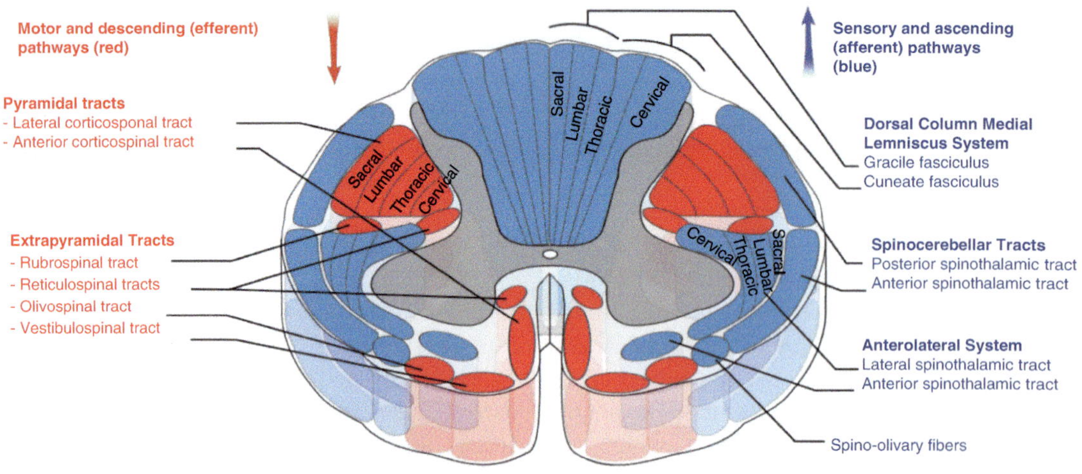

Fig. 32.1 Layout of the motor and sensory tracts in the spinal cord (Courtesy of Mikael Häggström via Wikimedia)

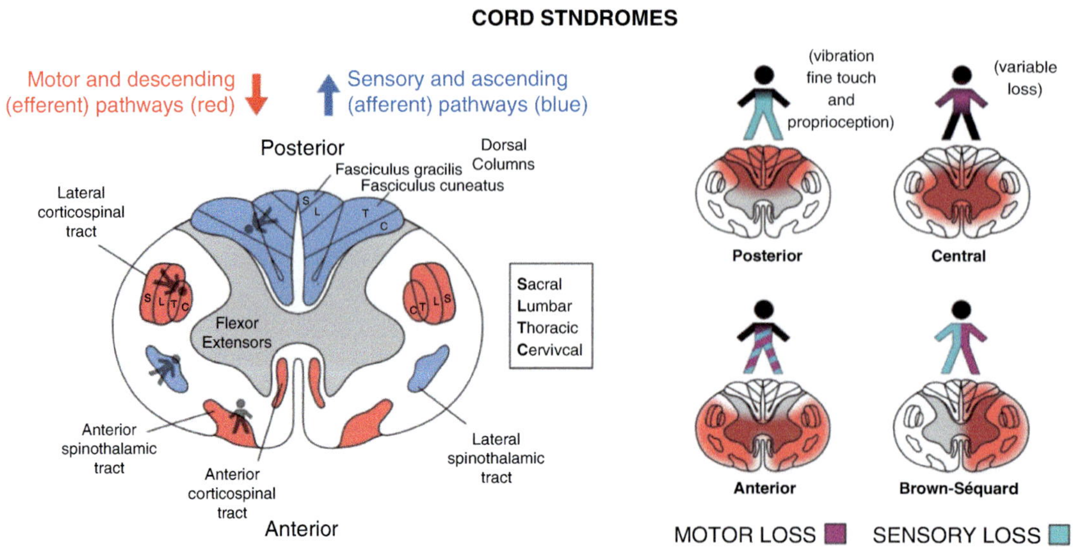

Fig. 32.2 Territorial injuries of the spinal cord. The orientation of the figures on the left explain why sacral sparing occurs in incomplete injury, as sacral tracts are the most lateral. The loss of perineal/peri-anal sensation and the bulbocavernosus reflex indicates that there is damage extending to the periphery of the cord

Syndrome	Mechanism	Clinical	Prognosis
Posterior cord	Hyperflexion or posterior spinal artery infarction	Loss of proprioception and fine touch Preserved motor function and pain sensation.	Variable
Central cord	Hyperextension (forced)	Sensory and motor deficit Upper > Lower extremities	Average
Anterior cord	Vascular insult (anterior spinal artery) Flexion	Complete loss of motor, pain and temperature below the injury. Retained proprioception and vibration sensation	Poor
Brown-Sequard	Penetrating trauma	Ipsilateral loss of motor, vibration and proprioception Contralateral loss of pain and temperature sensation	Good functional prognosis

Fig. 32.3 Clinical manifestations of varying cord syndromes

- The patient presents with weakness which is more pronounced in upper limbs with varying degree of sensory disturbance
- There is usually improvement seen in the initial phase which is followed by plateauing of symptoms followed by a decline
- Indications for surgery include cord compression, neurological deterioration, or persistent motor deficit. The timing of decompressive surgery is controversial and without consensus, as theoretically surgery may worsen the vascular insult and exacerbate the insult it endeavours to improve. Depending on the nature of the compression and curvature of the cervical spine, it can be approached through either anterior, posterior, or a combination of the approaches. Imaging often demonstrates the co-existence of predisposing cervical canal stenosis.

Brown Sequard Syndrome
- Usually as a result of penetrating trauma causing lateral hemisection of the spinal cord
- Patient presents with ipsilateral weakness and loss of posterior column functions along with loss of pain and temperature on the contralateral side

Posterior Cord Syndrome
- Rare syndrome which can be caused by trauma, external compression, demyelination of the spinal cord or posterior spinal artery occlusion/damage. Usually presents with pain and paraesthesia in upper limbs and trunk, with dorsal column signs such as sensory ataxia (decreased coordination, commonly causing poor balance and falls) and decreased sensation of vibration and fine touch

Anterior Cord Syndrome
- May occur as a result of trauma or vascular event
- Presents with weakness and associated sensory loss below the level of the lesion with loss of pain and temperature sensation, but posterior column functions of vibration and proprioception are intact

Classification and Principles of Stability
Historically, Holdsworth in 1963 proposed a two-column theory for spinal stability. In this model, the anterior column is formed by the anterior longitudinal ligament, vertebral body, posterior longitudinal ligament, disc, and annulus. The posterior column is formed by the facet joints, lamina, spinous processes, ligamentum flavum, interspinous, and supraspinous ligaments [15].

A lasting definition of stability was coined in a sentinel paper by White and Punjabi in 1975. They defined instability as "the loss of the ability of the spine, under physiologic loads, to maintain relationships between vertebrae in such a way that there is neither initial damage nor subsequent irritation to the spinal cord or nerve roots and, in addition, there is no development of incapacitating deformity or pain due to the structural changes". This definition remains the mainstay of non-operative management of spinal injuries and underpins the importance of weight bearing imaging and significance of progressive development of neurology [16].

Controversy existed regarding the two-column theory due to its inability to adequately categorise injury stability. This paved the way for Denis in 1983 to propose a three-column theory for spinal stability (Fig. 32.4). This model differs in that the anterior column is now formed by the anterior longitudinal ligament, anterior half of the vertebral body, disc, and annulus. The middle column is formed by the posterior half of the vertebral body, disc, annulus, and posterior longitudinal ligament, and the posterior column is formed by the facets, lamina, spinous process, ligamentum flavum interspinous and supraspinous ligaments. Denis defined unstable fractures as those in which two or more spinal columns were disrupted in an attempt to explain the inherent stability seen in body fractures that could be demonstrated to be stable and managed non-operatively [17].

Neither the two- nor three-column classifications are sufficiently useful to describe injury or guide treatment, and these have become mostly historical.

In 1994 Magerl et al. devised the AO classification for thoracolumbar fractures, dividing them

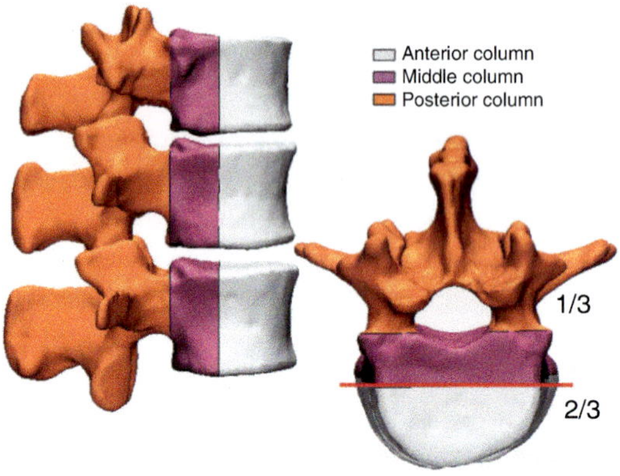

Fig. 32.4 Traditional model of the three-column model of injury (From Su et al.)

into three categories based on mechanism of injury—compression, distraction and rotation [18]. Subsequently, the Thoracolumbar Injury Classification and Severity (TLICS) was proposed in 2005 [19], and the Subaxial Cervical spine Injury Classification System (SLICS) was proposed in 2007 [20]. These scores provide a numerical figure to guide prediction of stability of an injury and guide management.

In 2013, the AO Spine Knowledge Forum on Spinal Cord Injury and Trauma proposed the AO Spine Thoracolumbar Spine Injury Classification System, which combined Magerl's classification with the TLICS system. This looked at not only the mechanism of injury but also the neurological status of the patient along with patient-specific modifiers [21].

The classification splits injuries into type A 'compression', type B 'distraction', and type C 'translational'. Type A includes spinous process and wedge compression fractures which are often stable. A fracture cleft connecting the superior to inferior endplates of two main fragments is highlighted as significant and has a higher risk of collapse than a fragmented burst body fracture. Type B injuries include disruption of the posterior tension band formed by the posterior ligamentous complex (supraspinous ligament, interspinous ligament, facet capsules, ligamentum flavum). Included in this group are Chance fractures, which in distinction to flexion-compression (type-A) fractures are flexion-distraction. Classically they are formed by the fulcrum moment lying anterior to the vertebral body (classically caused by bending the torso around a seatbelt), and the fracture fails through tension alone without collapse or compression of the vertebral body. The significance of this injury is the predictability of uncurtailed progression of kyphotic deformity that is not evident with a burst fracture. The pattern of collapse of the vertebral body is the heralding feature of a less significant injury. Type C injuries are complex, almost always unstable and often associated with substantial neurology.

In 2016, the AO Spine Subaxial Cervical Spine Injury Classification scheme was published [22]. Similarly, type A 'compression', type B 'tension band injuries', and type C 'translational' often have a similar pattern of stability and management to lumbar injures. Two further groups, specific to cervical stability are added, type BL 'bilateral' and type F 'facet injuries' which are by virtue of the mechanical principles of tensegrity likely to lead to neurology through instability and progression of the deformity (available from https://aospine.aofoundation.org/clinical-library-and-tools/ao-spine-classification-systems).

Several SCI assessment scales have also been proposed. The most commonly used scale is the ASIA SCI Scale (Fig. 32.5), which is based on the Frankel Scale. Similarly, muscle strength is assessed by the previously mentioned MRC scale.

Management of Spinal Trauma

The aim of management of patients with SCI in the acute phase is to prevent secondary injury to the spinal cord by avoiding hypoxia, hypotension, hyperthermia, and hyper- and hypoglycemia. In many ways [23], the treatment goals are the same as managing patients with traumatic brain injuries.

Management of the patient with spinal injuries can be divided into three phases—prehospital care and transport, assessment in the Emergency Department, and definitive care. The implications of the MABCD approach described earlier in this book have on spinal cord injury are briefly described below.

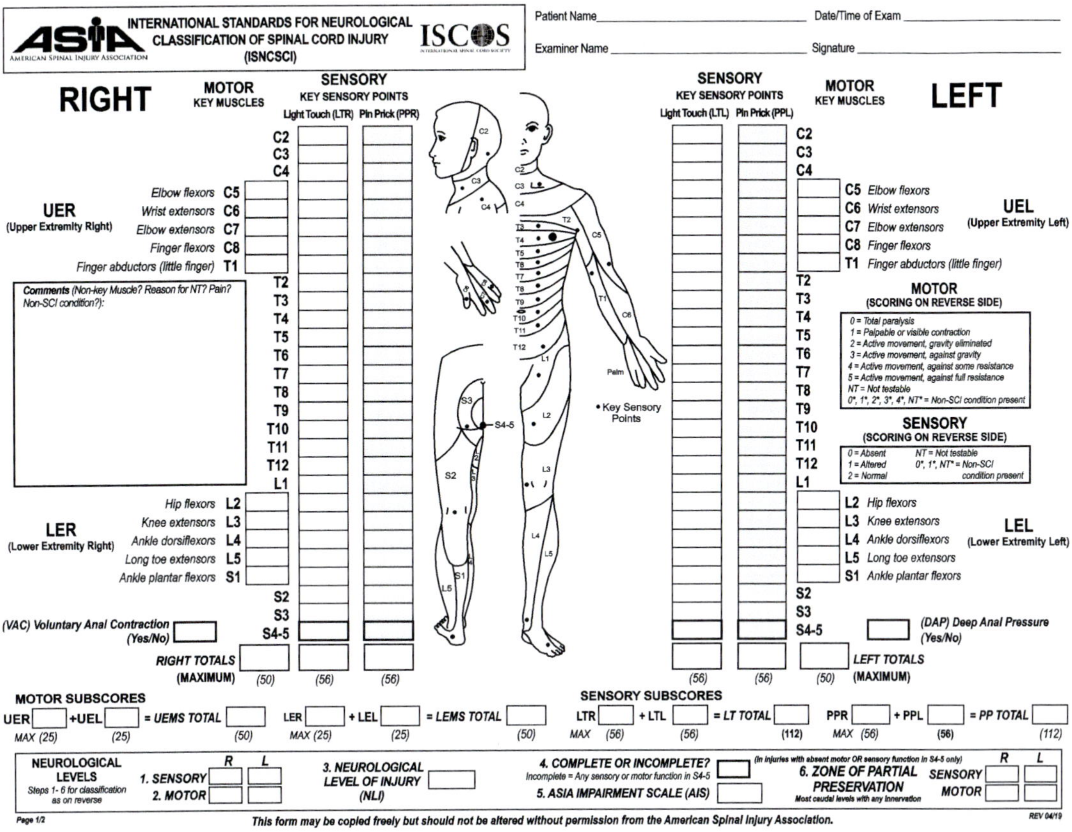

Fig. 32.5 The ASIA SCI scale used to document level of spinal cord injury on initial assessment (© 2021 American Spinal Injury Association. Reprinted with permission)

Massive Haemorrhage

In patients with a spinal cord injury, hypotension may worsen a secondary injury. If this is due to a massive haemorrhage, this must be addressed as the priority. Similarly, in patients with ongoing bleeding who require surgery, the optimum target blood pressure for cord perfusion may be higher than that desired to minimise further bleeding and avoid cyclic hyper-resuscitation. In these patients, haemostasis should be rapidly obtained as the priority, and cord perfusion pressure increased as soon as this has been achieved.

Airway

When managing patients with a spinal cord injury, the clinician should aim to avoid hypoxia and hypercarbia to minimise secondary injury. Patients who have a spinal cord injury may need intubating as a result of this pathology (e.g. high cord lesion with respiratory insufficiency), or due to co-existing injuries. Patients with cervical cord injuries should be monitored carefully in the first few days of their clinical course, as respiration may deteriorate due to ascending cord oedema. Specific issues around cervical spine injuries and airway management are further explored in Chap. 7, Fundamentals of Airway Management, but there is a brief overview below [2].

In cadaveric models with C5/6 ligamentous injury, chin lift and jaw thrust has been shown to increase the disc height by more than 5 mm [24]. Similarly, cricoid pressure to facilitate intubation has been shown to cause a posterior subluxation of more than 5 mm. Manual in-line stabilisation rather than the application of a rigid collar is recommended for airway intervention in patients with a suspected cervical spine injury, as it provides better visualisation of the larynx. In other studies, manual in-line stabilisation with cricoid pressure has not been shown to cause significant spinal movement during intubation [25, 26].

If the patient requires anterior cervical spine surgery, then a reinforced endotracheal tube should be used to prevent kinking of the tube during anterior cervical surgery. Unlike standard ET tubes, reinforced tubes cannot be cut to remove dead space or aid nursing care on ICU due to the reinforcing wire. Therefore, patients may have their ET tube changed after their operation before going to ICU if they are to remain intubated post-operatively. Some reinforced tubes may not have a Murphy's eye and could potentially cause issues with ventilation. This may be especially problematic if the patient has a reinforced ET tube in and is in the prone position for posterior spine surgery.

One in five patients with cervical cord injury may require a tracheostomy due to prolonged mechanical ventilation, poor respiratory drive, and chest infection, as tracheostomy has been shown to reduce dead space ventilation, lower the rate of pneumonia, and aid mechanical weaning. The timing of tracheostomy also depends on other injuries, level of cervical cord injury, and whether or not there has been a trial of weaning from the ventilator that has failed. Due to the loss of baroreflexes, these patients are also at increased risk of hypotension during positive pressure ventilation.

Breathing

The effect of spinal cord injury on breathing depends upon the level of the injury. Cord lesions above C3 lead to apnoeic respiratory arrest. Injuries to C3-5 will lead to paralysis of the diaphragm. In lesions between C5–C8, there is complete intercostal nerve paralysis, leading to paradoxical respiration. In lesions between T1-7, there is impaired chest wall movement and a poor cough. SCI has been shown to reduce forced vital capacity, increase airway secretions, and lead to atelectasis. Hence, such patients need humidified oxygen, frequent change of position, and aggressive chest physiotherapy. Ventilation and perfusion should be assessed by pulse oximetry, arterial blood gas, and end-tidal capnography where required [27]. The effect of hypercapnia on SCI is not well studied, and at present normocapnia or mild hypocapnia is recommended.

Circulation

Neurogenic shock is the cardiovascular manifestation of spinal shock. It is common in cord injury of T5 and above, as cardiac sympathetic fibres emerge from the cord at this level (T1–T5). There is a decrease in systemic vascular resistance and pooling of blood in the periphery, effectively increasing the arterial capacitance and decreasing arterial pressure. This pressure drop also leads to a reduced venous return to the heart, relative hypovolemia, and resultant hypotension. Patients with hypotension secondary to neurogenic shock may need vasopressors as opposed to volume replacement. However, inappropriate use of vasopressors in hypovolaemic shock has been shown to increase mortality, so the correct treatment for the presenting pathology is essential Due to unopposed parasympathetic activity, there is also profound bradycardia which decreases cardiac output and systemic blood pressure further. A fuller explanation of neurogenic shock is found in the Circulation Chap. 10.

Hypotension seen in a trauma patient with SCI may be due to hypovolemia, neurogenic shock or both, and it is essential to differentiate the two pathophysiologies. Patients should be catheterised to monitor intake and output and guide fluid management. Patients with SCI are also prone to postural hypotension due to pooling of blood, reduced blood volume, and altered baroreceptor reflexes. Arterial and central lines should be in place to guide fluid and vasopressor management acutely.

There is level III evidence to show that MAP of 85–90 for the first 7 days is associated with improved neurological outcome. However, this should be balanced with risks related to prolonged vasopressor treatment, and evidence that inappropriate vasopressor administration to under-resuscitated or hypovolaemic patients may increase mortality as previously mentioned.

In the prehospital phase, glucose-containing fluids should be avoided as glucose is rapidly metabolised and produces free water which can worsen oedema. In addition, hyperglycemia can promote anaerobic glycolysis leading to increased lactate formation and acidosis [25].

Disability

Spinal shock is defined as a temporary interruption in the physiological functioning of the cord caudal to the level of an injury. It is thought to be due to loss of excitatory inputs from the higher centres leading to flaccid paralysis. Due to the loss of inhibitory signals from the higher centres this can progress to spasticity, and patients with higher lesions may progress to develop autonomic dysreflexia. Absence of bulbo-cavernous reflex indicates the presence of spinal shock or a complete cord injury rather than an incomplete cord injury. The significance of early assessment and documentation of this reflex is vital for this reason, as it is often subsequently lost, it can become pivotal in the later surgical decision making and prognostication. The reflex is present if there is a contraction of the anal sphincter in response to catheter tug or squeezing of the glans penis. The level of injury cannot be clinically ascertained once spinal shock is established, underpinning the importance of early sacral assessment for completeness of cord injury and neurological function at the time of injury.

The assessment of disability includes recording Glasgow Coma Score, motor and sensory examination, saddle sensation, reflexes, and anal tone. Note should be made of the presence or absence of priapism and a diaphragmatic ("see-saw") breathing pattern. An obtunded or uncooperative patient should be presumed to have a spinal injury until one has been excluded.

Transport

Backboards should only be used for extrication due to concerns over pressure injuries, and a scoop stretcher or a vacuum mattress should be used for transport. Patients with neurological symptoms or signs suggestive of traumatic spinal cord injury should be handled gently, aiming to maintain neutral spinal alignment, and transported to the nearest Major Trauma Centre (MTC). This is irrespective of transfer time unless the patient needs immediate lifesaving intervention, in which case the ambulance should be diverted to the nearest Trauma Unit. A patient with a suspected spinal column injury without suspected spinal cord injury should be taken to the nearest TU if there are no other injuries that require treatment at an MTC.

Role of Collars in Spinal Cord Trauma

From the mid-1960s, cervical spine immobilisation- using a rigid cervical collar and hard backboard was advocated to prevent secondary spinal cord injury during transportation and early management in ED. Since that time, multiple makes and variations in style of cervical collars have entered the market (Fig. 32.6). Geisler et al. in 1966 stated that failure to recognise and protect an unstable cervical spine could lead to catastrophic injury [28]. NICE guidelines (specifically NG41, published February 2016) recommend full spinal immobilisation in any patient with suspected spinal injury. In the prehospital setting, the American Association of Neurological Surgeons/Congress of Neurological Surgeons (AANS/CNS) recommends spinal immobilisation in all trauma patients with suspected cervical spine or spinal cord injury. The committee on Trauma of the American College of Surgeons also recommends that the cervical spine should be immobilised in all trauma patients with multiple blunt injuries. In a telephone survey of 25 general ICUs dealing with Major Trauma in the UK, six units stated that they routinely wait for the patient to regain consciousness before removing cervical collars [29].

From the 1970s to 1980s, there was a significant decline in the number of patients presenting with complete spinal cord injury, and it was during this time that there was an increased empha-

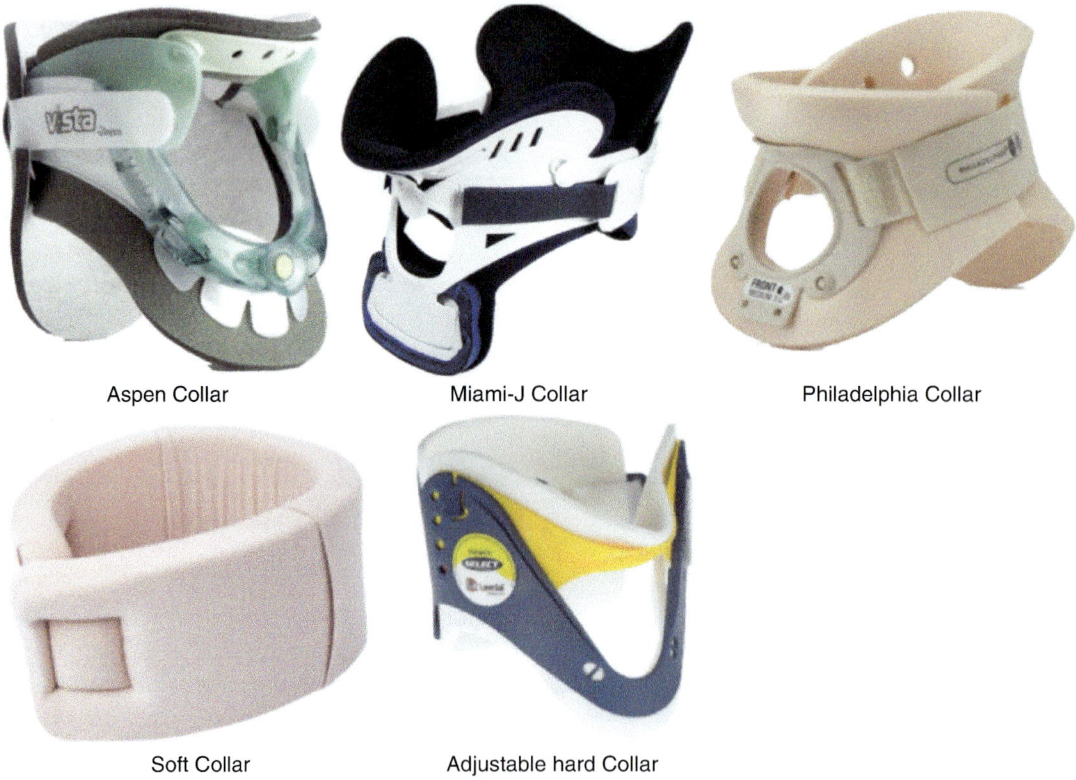

Fig. 32.6 Various types of cervical collars

sis on spinal immobilisation. As a result, several authors have attributed this reduction in patients with complete paralysis to spinal immobilisation. However, correlation is not the same as causation, and there is a lack of high-quality studies that have shown clear benefit of cervical spine immobilisation on neurological outcome or mortality. Changes in vehicle design or other safety features could equally be the cause of this decrease in case incidence. Conversely, there are a number of studies which have shown that rigid cervical collar may be associated with harm. However, because of fear of missing a potentially life-changing injury as well as fear of litigation, more than 5 million people are immobilised each year in the United States. Compensation for missed cervical spine injury can be as high as $3 million. Some authors, on the other hand, feel that prehospital cervical immobilisation may be an overprotective and defensive medical practice, and may even lead to delay in definitive treatment. Sundstrom et al. described spinal immobilisation as a device which creates uncertainty among clinicians and freezes them, thereby limiting adequate clinical examination and leading to overdependence on radiological assessment [9].

Multiple studies have shown that cervical collars may interfere with the assessment and definitive management of life-threatening injuries such as airway compromise. Collars may also be associated with a delay in transfer for definitive treatment, pain and discomfort, increase in ICP, respiratory complications including increased risk of aspiration, pressure ulcers, increased risk of thrombosis, difficulty in performing mouth care and physiotherapy, and gaining central venous access. Cervical collars can also lead to additional radiological assessments in Emergency Departments, increased sedation requirements in ICU, increased time on a ventilator, increased length of ICU stay, and an overall increase in healthcare costs. It is thought that manual in-line stabilisation or traction may be equivalent to collar immobilisation, or even better in certain circumstances such as raised ICP or a compromised airway.

In a systematic review and meta-analysis of prospective studies, cervical collar application was associated with a mean ICP increase of 4.4 mmHg as a result of a decrease in venous return from the brain [30]. The 'closed box' analogy of intracranial pressure (ICP), the Monroe-Kellie doctrine, stating that a change in blood, brain, or CSF volume results in reciprocal changes in one or both of the other two, should be borne in mind. There should also be consideration of the slow production of CSF (0.35 ml/min) which is dwarfed by the dynamic blood delivery and outflow (700 ml/min). Failure of venous efferent flow to precisely match arterial afferent flow will yield immediate and dramatic changes in intracranial blood volume and pressure more than CSF volume manipulation. Interpreting ICP in isolation without interrogating its core drivers may be misleading. Multiple clinical conditions and the cerebral effects of altitude may also relate to imbalances in this dynamic, rather than ICP per se.

The incidence of cervical collar-related pressure ulcers can range from 6.8% to 38% [31]. Pressure ulcers are not only a significant cause of morbidity and mortality; they have also been shown to increase healthcare costs. Studies have shown that the approximate cost of treatment of stage 1 and stage 4 pressure ulcers is £1064 and £24,214 respectively. Schuurman et al. showed that pressure ulcer related healthcare costs constituted 1.21–1.41% of the total health care cost in the Netherlands [32]. Risk factors for the development of cervical collar related pressure ulcers include the length of time spent by the patient in a collar, duration of prehospital transport, decreased level of consciousness, agitation, duration of hospital stay, ICU admission, ICP monitoring, mechanical ventilation, immobility, the requirement for MRI, shock, higher injury severity score, co-morbidities, and poor nutritional status. Cervical collars cause constant pressure on the skin, leading to decreased tissue perfusion, ischemia, necrosis, and cell death. Lien et al. reported that injury to the tissue begins as early as 30 min after the application of a cervical collar [33]. Patients who stay in rigid extrication collars until they reach ICU have a 23.9% incidence of collar-related pressure ulceration [34], and the risk of pressure ulcers increases by 66% for each day patient remains in a cervical collar [35]. To prevent ulceration, strategies include early cervical spine clearance, early replacement of rigid extrication collars with long term cervical collars, regular skin inspection, and meticulous skincare, training of nursing staff for regular skin assessment and care, and frequent change of collar pads [36].

In 1998, Hauswald et al. conducted a 5-year retrospective chart review at two university hospitals (334 patients in New Mexico and 120 patients in Malaysia), comparable in terms of training of clinicians and resources. To account for bias in treatment processes and injury patterns, analysis was limited to patients with cervical injuries. Their conclusion is out-of-hospital immobilisation has little or no effect on neurologic outcome in patients with blunt spinal injuries [23]. A Cochrane review in 2001 of 4453 potentially relevant articles found no definite evidence that spinal immobilisation in patients with a spinal injury is associated with significant improvement in neurological outcome or mortality. The authors concluded that harm from the use of a cervical spine collar is possible [37].

Oto et al. conducted a literature review and identified 41 cases of early neurological deterioration post blunt spinal injury. The authors noted that a precipitating event was only present in only 12 of the cases, of which seven were thought to be iatrogenic such as collar removal and placement of a halo. Of the 41 patients who had deterioration, five had full spinal immobilisation whereas 17 had no or incomplete immobilisation in place when decline occurred. The authors could not find a single instance of sudden, provoked catastrophic neurological deterioration, and hence concluded that early neurological deterioration post spinal injury is a gradual process over minutes to hours rather than an instantaneous catastrophic event. However, the lack of reports of sudden neurological deterioration because of lack of immobilisation or poor handling could be due to the fear of litigation [38]. Lin et al. conducted a retrospective review of 5139 patients with traumatic injury to the cervical spine. The authors showed that there was no significant difference in outcome with or without immobilisation, and concluded that cervical spine immobilisation is an overprotective practice [39].

In 2010, Haut et al. conducted a retrospective review of patients with penetrating trauma registered at US American National Trauma Data bank and found that the mortality rate among the immobilised patients was higher, 14.7% as compared to 7.2% in non-immobilised group. Concerning penetrating trauma, the authors conclude that prehospital spine immobilisation is associated with higher mortality and should not be routinely used in every patient. Spinal immobilisation in patients with penetrating injury is associated with increased time spent at the scene with potential delay in definitive treatment, interference with airway management, masking of important signs and symptoms, and increased mortality rates without any substantial benefit [40]. Vanderlan et al. reviewed 199 patients with penetrating trauma and showed cervical spine immobilisation was associated with an increased risk of death (odds ratio 2.77) [41]. There is level III evidence to show that spinal immobilisation in patients with penetrating trauma is associated with increased mortality. This experience is echoed in military data, which shows that penetrating ballistic trauma to the neck is unlikely to result in an unstable cervical spine in survivors; unstable injuries from penetrating mechanisms are catastrophic and rapidly fatal. In a hazardous environment (e.g. shooting incidents or terrorist bombings), the risk/benefit ratio of mandatory spinal immobilisation is unfavourable and may place medical teams at prolonged risk. In addition, cervical collars may hide potential life-threatening conditions.

At the time of injury, delays due to diagnostic dilemmas identifying patients who would benefit from spinal immobilisation is a risk. In some studies, there is low diagnostic accuracy among medics (31% in one series by Flabouris) in identifying patients with a spinal injury who need spinal immobilisation [42]. Additionally, there is, despite adequate training, evidence of unsatisfactory placement of a collar correctly on mannequins by emergency service personnel; only 11% of collars were placed correctly in one study of trained staff by Kreinest et al. [43]. Tello et al. showed in their retrospective review that nearly half of the patients (101/219) who were not immobilised by pre-hospital clinicians went on to be immobilised in the ED. Subsequently, none of these immobilised were found to have a spinal injury, but incurred delay, increased cost, and excess radiation exposure [44].

To avoid delay in treatment for potentially life-threatening conditions, some authors recommend time-critical patients are transported using the lateral trauma position (LTP) or HAINES manoeuvre (High-Arm-IN-Endangered—Spine—Fig. 32.7) [46]. These have the benefit of providing a degree of spinal support and positional drainage of the airway whilst avoiding the time and morbidity associated with collar application.

It is difficult to predict with certainty the number of spinal cord injuries which have been prevented by spinal immobilisation. This is because of the lack of randomised studies looking at the efficacy of spinal immobilisation in preventing spinal movement in trauma patients. This is understandable, given the ethical and legal issues surrounding such a study design where an accepted standard of practice would not be used. Studies looking at the effects of collars in healthy volunteers have shown contradictory results. These include findings that collars do not effectively reduce movements in unstable spines, rigid collars can *increase* movement in the upper cervical region, and soft collars are as effective as hard collars in restricting cervical spine movements [9].

Similarly, the effect of spinal immobilisation in reducing spinal movement is also not without controversy. Hood et al. in a review identified ten studies which showed that spinal immobilisation

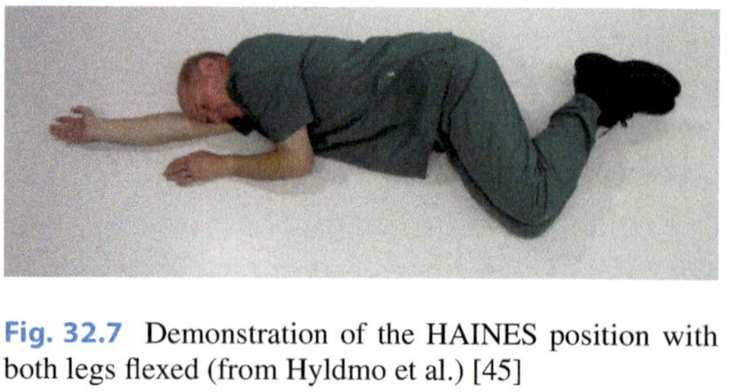

Fig. 32.7 Demonstration of the HAINES position with both legs flexed (from Hyldmo et al.) [45]

was effective in decreasing movement, whereas four studies showed that spinal immobilisation had no effect in reducing spinal movement as compared to no immobilisation [47]. Holla et al. showed that rigid collars did not lead to decreased spinal movement in healthy volunteers who were already strapped to a rigid stretcher with head blocks [48].

Cervical immobilisation remains a controversial area; some authors opine that spinal cord injuries occur during prehospital or early hospital care and may be due to lack of spinal immobilisation or poor handling. However, contrary studies have cast doubts on this suggestion; even with spinal immobilisation neurological deterioration can occur in up to 5% of patients with spinal injury [9]. The force required to fracture the spine is in excess of and dwarfs the subsequent forces generated during movement in prehospital or early hospital care.

Gradually, there is a move towards selective immobilisation of trauma patients, especially those awake and orientated. Blackham et al. in a review concluded that spinal immobilisation is not needed in an alert, conscious patient even if the clinical decision rule is positive unless there is a deterioration in the conscious level. The authors concluded that an awake patient will assume a position of comfort and muscle spasm may be more effective than a collar to maintain stable spinal position [49]. In a study done in Alabama by Gonzalez et al., the authors showed that with judicious use of selective immobilisation, 34% of the cervical spines were cleared at the scene with no missed injuries. It is thought that selective immobilisation can lead to improved outcome, reduced radiation exposure, and reduce healthcare costs [50].

Similarly, several studies have shown that self-extrication with or without a collar results in significantly less cervical spine movement than any other method. NICE guidelines suggest asking alert, orientated patients to self-extricate from motor vehicle collisions if there is no significant distracting injury, abnormal neurology, spinal pain, or high-risk factor (such as age >65 years or a dangerous mechanism), and lay supine once they have self-extricated. In the UK, previous recommendations for immobilising patients included the "standing takedown" method. Using this method, patients who reported neck pain and had self-extricated from cars were strapped on a spinal board as they stood, and then pre-hospital staff would lay them flat. Following consensus guidelines published by the Royal College of Surgeons of Edinburgh Faculty of Prehospital Care, this practice has thankfully been abandoned in UK practice. The risks of mishandling patients and causing further injuries, or causing back or other injuries to ambulance service staff are not acceptable, especially when there is no evidence of patient benefit.

Predominant UK hospital intensive care practice has adopted a pragmatic approach. After a high-quality CT of the cervical spine has demonstrated no apparent unstable injury, in most units the collar is taken off while the patient is sedated. It is then replaced when sedation is weaned to wake the patient up, and the patient is assessed clinically when awake.

Advocates in favour of immobilisation with cervical collars make reasoned arguments. Reid et al. in 1987 showed that the rate of neurological deficit in patients with missed spinal injury was 10.5%, whereas the rate of secondary neurological injury was only 1.4%. The majority of late identified neurological deficit is from missed injuries, but the smaller cohort of secondary deterioration is potentially preventable which raises the question, but leaves unanswered, the role and impact of immobilisation [51]. Tuscano et al. studied 123 patients with significant blunt trauma to the spine. They noted that 32 patients had significant neurological deterioration between the time of injury and time of admission to the trauma unit. The authors concluded that significant neurological deterioration in spinal trauma patients could, idealistically and theoretically, be prevented [52]. Davis et al. looked at 32,117 trauma patients, of which 740 had a cervical injury. Thirty-four injuries were missed, of which ten patients developed permanent neurological deficit [53]. **There is no level I or II evidence to recommend blanket cervical immobilisation after trauma**. Many clinicians have become ensconced with the reassurance that cervical collar use is an effective, time-tested practice, supported by years of cumulative trauma experience with sound anatomical and biomechanical considerations, despite the lack of evidence to this effect.

Imaging

The incidence of cervical spine injury in blunt trauma is approximately 2–4%. Despite this, radiographic evaluation of the cervical spine is very frequently carried out in ED because of apprehension over missed injuries, potential deleterious consequences, or fear of litigation. This leads to increased radiation exposure and excess healthcare cost and can potentially delay definitive treatment of other urgent conditions.

The National Emergency X-Radiography Utilisation Study (NEXUS) advocated that in a trauma patient who is alert and stable, with a normal level of consciousness, no distracting injuries, no midline posterior cervical tenderness, and no focal neurology, imaging of the cervical spine is not indicated. The NEXUS protocol was found to have a sensitivity of 99.6%, a specificity of 12.9%, and a negative predictive value of 99.7% and has been shown to reduce the imaging rate by 30.9%.

The Canadian C-Spine Rule (CCSR) is an alternative to the NEXUS criteria and shown below in Fig. 32.8.

The sensitivity of the CCSR approaches 100%, with a specificity of 42.5% and negative predictive value of 99.98–100%. CCSR has been

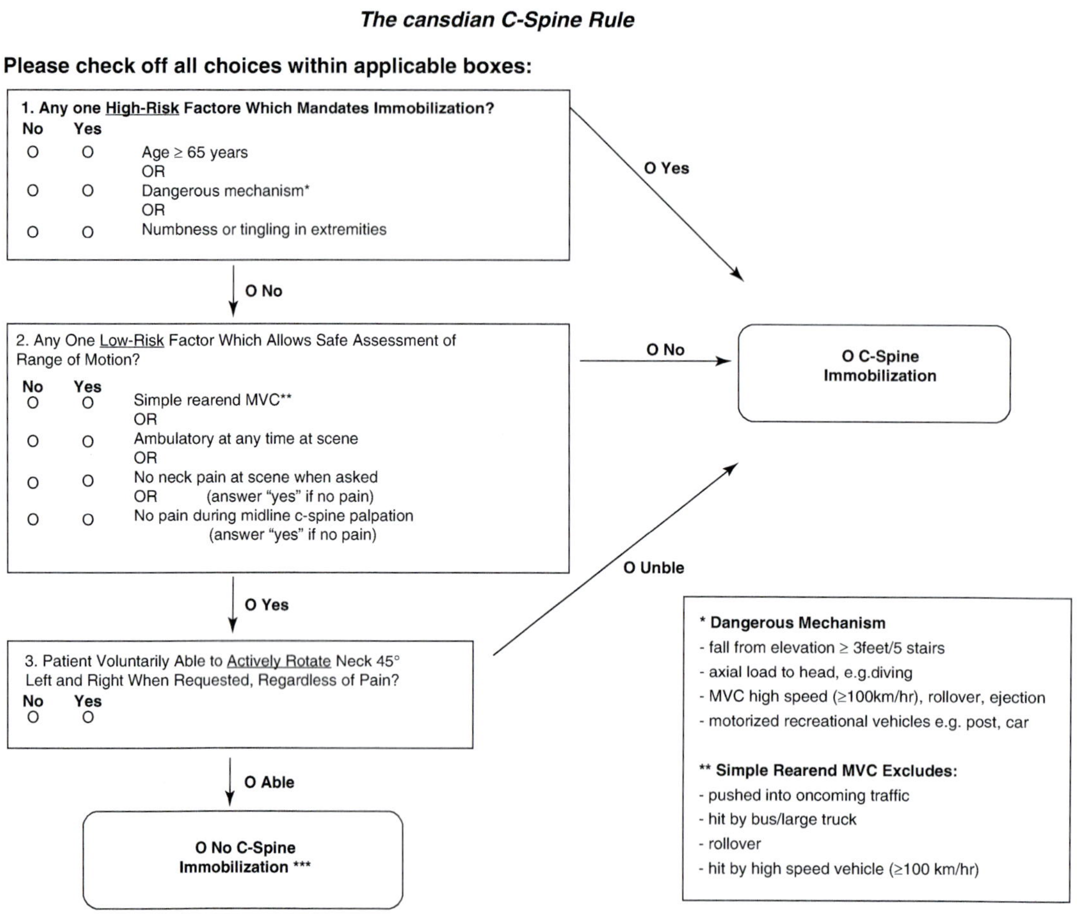

Fig. 32.8 Decision-making tree of the Canadian C-Spine Rule (from Vaillancourt et al. [54])

shown to reduce imaging rates by an average of 44% (compared to 36% for NEXUS) without missing a clinically significant cervical spine injury.

CCSR looks at the mechanism of injury and assesses the range of movement, whereas NEXUS does not. On the other hand, the NEXUS study incorporates distracting injuries which CCSR does not. Stiell et al. [55] compared NEXUS and CCSR studies and showed that 16 cervical spine injuries were missed using the NEXUS protocol, whereas only one was missed using CCSR. NICE guidelines have combined both CCSR and NEXUS and added posterior midline spinal tenderness to CCSR. Thus, in an awake, orientated patient who is not under the influence of alcohol or drugs with no distracting injury, midline posterior cervical tenderness, or focal neurological deficit and who has a full range of movement of the cervical spine, the cervical spine can be cleared clinically. However, some authors feel that even in the presence of alcohol or drugs or distracting injury, the sensitivity of the cervical spine examination is not diminished, and as such these patients should be treated as other patients.

Clearing the cervical spine in obtunded patients remains challenging as these patients cannot be clinically assessed. Cervical spine injury is also more common in obtunded patients as compared to those who are alert and orientated.

Historically, flexion-extension x-rays were used to assess instability in some patients. However, studies have shown that 30–95% of flexion-extension radiographs may be inadequate because of a reduced range of movement as a result of pain or muscle spasm, or because of suboptimal imaging technique. One way to counteract this is to keep the patient immobilised in collar and repeat the imaging in 1–2 weeks. Reitman et al. [56] showed that in up to 16% of normal healthy individuals, spondylolisthesis could be >3.5 mm, which is the cut off for instability. Similarly, cadaveric studies have shown that even after extensive ligamentous damage, flexion-extension radiographs may not show significant instability. Goodnight et al. [57] looked at 379 patients with normal CTs, of which eight patients had abnormal flexion-extension x-rays. In these eight patients, a ligamentous injury was ruled out by normal MRI. Similarly, Mccracken et al. [58] reviewed 1000 patients with normal CT, of which 25 had abnormal flexion-extension radiographs—no patients required any additional intervention. Studies have shown that even passive flexion-extension views are often inadequate. Padayachee et al. [59] looked at the data from 276 patients with normal CTs of the cervical spine, of which 6 had abnormal passive flexion-extension radiographs. In all six patients, a ligamentous injury was ruled out by MRI.

CT cervical spine is now considered imaging of choice in any patient in whom the cervical spine cannot be cleared clinically. This is because up to 25% of plain radiographs of the cervical spine are inadequate. Even when adequate, CT may detect additional injures in 8–14% of these patients. CT is excellent for looking at bony structures but not as good for soft tissues. However, in a meta-analysis by Raza et al. looking at cervical spine clearance in obtunded patients with blunt trauma, based on a normal multi-detector CT scan the sensitivity, positive predictive value and negative predictive value were 93.7%, 93.7%, and 99.7% respectively. As a result, some authors feel that high-quality multi-detector CT is sensitive enough to detect surrogate markers of ligamentous injury such as pre-vertebral swelling, splaying of spinous processes, and distracted facet joints, **with the caveat that the scan must be interpreted by an experienced musculoskeletal or neuroradiologist**. The authors also argue that in adult patients with trauma, unstable ligamentous injury without fracture is extremely rare. Hogan et al. stated that negative predictive value of CT for ligamentous injury is 98.9%, and negative predictive value for unstable injury is 100%.

A normal CT cervical spine with persistent neck pain can be a clinical challenge as immobilisation with a collar is not a benign treatment without consequence. A pragmatic strategy is immobilisation with subsequent re-examination at 1–2 weeks, and if necessary, MRI with a fluid sensitive sequence. This can be helpful in decision making and identification of a discoligamentous injury that can herald instability. A problem with MRI is the high sensitivity with a high false-positive rate of high signal reporting and findings that may be subclinical or not of significance in clinical practice.

MRI can detect haematoma, oedema, cord compression, and provide important prognostic information. However, routine use of MRI in spinal trauma patients is controversial as it can be highly sensitive for ligamentous injury and overestimate instability by 25–40%, according to a study by Taghva et al. [7]. Performing MRI in a trauma patient also has resource, cost, and logistical implications. Como et al. looked at 115 patients with normal CT, and in 6 patients MRI revealed a ligamentous injury but did not lead to a change of management in any of the patients [60]. Similarly, Hogan et al. looked at 366 patients with normal CT, and in four patients MRI showed clinically insignificant ligamentous injury which again did not lead to management change [61]. However, Stassen et al. recommended that MRI should be performed if a patient remains obtunded at day three of admission, as MRI could be positive for ligamentous injury in patients with normal CT cervical spine [62]. Similarly, James et al. reviewed 11 studies and showed that in 4.8% of patients, CT failed to pick up an acute ligamentous injury and 0.7% of the patients with negative CT underwent surgical intervention based on MR findings. From an ICU perspective, a negative MRI in a patient who cannot be woken up is reassuring and allows removal of a cervical collar and mitigation of some of the consequences of their application.

Systemic Complications of Spinal Cord Injury

Autonomic Dysreflexia

Autonomic dysreflexia is usually seen in patients with spinal injury above T6 and occurs as a result of acute sympathetic activity in response to stimulus below the level of the injury. 75–85% of patients with spinal injury level above T6 will demonstrate some form of autonomic dysreflexia. Blocked urinary catheters, constipation, per rectal examination, or even hot or cold stimuli can precipitate autonomic dysreflexia. It is characterised by severe headache, flushing, sweating, blurred vision, hypertension, bradycardia, arrhythmia, and can even lead to seizure and stroke. The afferent impulses from the bladder, bowel, or other stimuli are transmitted via hypogastric, pudendal, and pelvic nerves to the spinal cord, which is free from the influence of higher inhibitory controls leading to acute sympathetic surge [27]. Management of autonomic dysreflexia involves the removal of the precipitating stimulus. Clonidine or beta-blockers (either alone or in combination with calcium channel blockers) have been used to terminate such episodes.

Thromboembolism

Fatal PE can occur in 3% of patients with SCI, whereas the rate of DVT and non-fatal PE are 90% and 10% respectively in patients with SCI as described in a paper by Bonner et al. [2]. After the first three months, the risk of thromboembolism decreases and thromboprophylaxis is usually not needed. In our practice, all patients with spinal trauma are given mechanical thromboprophylaxis initially. Once a decision has been made that surgery is not indicated, prophylactic low molecular weight heparin (LMWH) is started as well, usually after 24–48 h of the initial injury. In patients who have undergone spinal surgery, LMWH is held for 24–48 h as there is a balance of risk between developing spinal canal haematoma and the protective benefit of countering DVT development.

Genitourinary System

Injury to the cord, conus or cauda equina may lead to bladder/bowel incontinence. Patients with SCI may have a neurogenic bladder resulting in reduced bladder capacity, incomplete emptying, and urinary retention leading to recurrent urinary tract infections. There may also be detrusor sphincter dyssynergia leading to vesicoureteric reflux, renal impairment, and stones.

Others

Patients with SCI may initially need a nasogastric tube for paralytic ileus or use of an abdominal binder. Similarly, bowel care or a longer-term bowel program may be required for constipation. Temperature regulation may also be impaired in patients with SCI due to lack of inputs from higher centres and reduced sweating.

Longer-term complications in patients with SCI include chronic pain, spasticity, osteoporosis, pressure ulcer, renal stones, urosepsis, and impaired immune function. Mental health issues are also important to consider in patients with SCI.

Role of Surgery in Patients with SCI

The main indications to operate on spinal trauma are to prevent, reduce, or improve neurological deficit, restore spinal alignment, and to stabilise an unstable spine. Surgery is also indicated in penetrating injury to the spine to explore injuries where there is a deficit. However, the exact timing of surgery in patients with spinal trauma is somewhat controversial. Several factors such as age, co-morbidities, associated injuries, availability of an appropriately trained and senior surgeon/anaesthetist/theatre, and other resources have to be taken into consideration.

Several studies have shown that early surgery may be associated with improved neurological outcome, decreased length of stay in ICU and hospital, fewer days on a ventilator, lower complication rates and lower healthcare costs. Early surgery facilitates early mobilisation and inherently reduces the complications associated with prolonged bed rest such as pressure ulcers, pulmonary complications, and thrombosis. Early surgery also allows early transfer to a rehabilitation unit. Some authors also feel that the severity of initial spinal injury may also play a significant role in determining the timing of surgery; patients with incomplete injury tend to be operated on more urgently than those with complete injury.

Kerwin et al. analysed data of 1.3 million cases from the National Trauma Data Bank and found that 497 patients had surgery within 72 h, whereas 374 patients had surgery after 72 h. The authors showed that early surgery was associated with reduced length in the ICU and lower complication rates and healthcare costs [63]. Papadopoulos et al. prospectively looked at 66 patients who arrived within 9 h of SCI and compared it to 25 control patients outside of the study, demonstrating that 50% of the patients who had early surgery had improvement in neurology as compared to 24% of the control patients [64]. La Rosa et al. studied 1687 patients and showed that patients with complete as well as incomplete spinal injury who had surgery within 24 h had a better neurological recovery [65]. In a systematic review, Dimar et al. showed that early surgery was associated with shorter ICU and hospital stay, fewer days on a ventilator, fewer pulmonary complications, and lower health care costs. The authors also concluded that there is some evidence that early surgery is not associated with increased complication rate [66]. Furlan et al. in a systematic review showed that early surgery is associated with improved patient outcomes, reduced length of stay, lower complications rate, and healthcare cost. The authors recommended surgery within 8–24 h [67]. Verlaan et al. reviewed 132 studies comprising of 5748 patients and concluded that early surgery has acceptable risks and is associated with better functional outcome [68].

Surgical Timing in Acute Spinal Cord Injury Study (STASCIS) was a multicentre, international prospective cohort study of 313 patients which showed a beneficial effect on neurological outcome at six months in patients who underwent surgery within 24 h [69]. Cengiz et al. in their quasi-randomised study of 12 patients who had surgery within 8 h and 15 patients who had surgery after 3 days showed that early surgery was associated with shorter ICU and hospital stay, lower complication rate, and improved neurological recovery [70]. However, both these studies excluded polytrauma patients and had small patient numbers to formalise guidelines.

The timing of surgery in central cord syndrome also remains controversial. In a literature review, Lenehan et al. showed that early surgery in patients with central cord syndrome is associated with improved motor recovery. The authors suggested that it is reasonable and safe to consider early surgical decompression in patients with a profound neurologic deficit (ASIA grade C) and persistent spinal cord compression. The authors also suggested that in patients with a less severe deficit (ASIA grade D), it may be reasonable to wait and watch with a plan for surgery at a later date depending on the neurological recovery of the patient [71].

For incomplete traumatic spinal cord injury with continued compression, surgery should be undertaken once haemodynamic stability is achieved irrespective of the time of the day or night. Werndle et al. in a UK survey conducted in 2012 showed that 30–61% of the surgeons would prefer to perform surgery within 12 h of the injury [72].

However, early surgery may lead to further neurological deterioration as the cord is already inflamed and oedematous. This is very difficult to study due to variance of injury patterns, depth, and no adequate predictive models with which to compare. There is also the consideration of a "second hit" on a medically compromised patient [7, 63]. Mckinley et al. analysed data from 779 patients based on those who were managed conservatively, those who had surgery within 3 days, and those who had delayed surgery. The authors showed that patients who were managed conservatively were more likely to show improvement in motor score, though these patients were more likely to present with an incomplete injury. However, his study also showed that early surgery is associated with shorter ICU and hospital stay. Similarly, he also showed that patients who had late surgery had higher medical complication rates [73].

Fehling et al. in a systematic review showed that in patients with cervical SCI, early surgery was associated with improved neurological recovery, whereas in other SCI evidence supporting early surgery was inconsistent. In a clinical practice guideline Fehling et al. recommended that early surgery should be considered in patients with traumatic SCI irrespective of the initial neurological status.

Blood loss during spinal surgery in a trauma patient can be challenging because of already compromised cord perfusion and physiological alterations. Many studies have looked at ways to minimise blood loss during surgery for SCI. Wong et al. in a randomised study looking at tranexamic acid vs placebo in patients undergoing posterior thoracic or lumbar fusion, showed that the patients who received tranexamic acid had significantly less blood loss compared to those who received placebo. However, there was no significant difference in the amount of blood products transfused between the two groups [74].

Conducting a well-designed randomised control trial to look at the optimum time within which surgery should be performed is extremely difficult because of legal and ethical concerns. Randomisation, consent and resources to operate within a fixed time frame would also be hindrances to conducting such a study [7].

Role of Steroids in SCI

Methylprednisolone (MPS) has been shown to act by stabilising cell membranes by inhibiting lipid peroxidation and neurofilament breakdown, thus protecting the blood: spinal cord barrier. Theoretically, because of its anti-inflammatory properties, MPS reduces the amount of vasoactive products being generated from arachidonic acid metabolism, thereby decreasing cord oedema and improving cord perfusion and impulse generation [6, 7, 14].

The first National Acute Spinal Cord Injury Study (NASCIS I) was a multicentre, double-blinded randomised control study involving 330 patients. Patients were randomised to receive MPS 100 mg IV bolus/day followed by 25 mg every 6 h for 10 days or MPS 1000 mg IV bolus/day followed by 250 mg every 6 h for 10 days. The study lacked a placebo group because of the prevailing belief at the time was that MPS treatment is likely to be beneficial for patients with SCI, and it would be unethical to withhold such a treatment. The study showed no significant difference in neurological outcome at six weeks, six months, and twelve months between the two groups. In contrast, there was a statistically significant increase in the incidence of wound infection in the patient group who received high doses of MPS. There was also a trend towards increased sepsis, pulmonary embolism, and death with 14 days in the high dose MPS group, though it was not statistically significant. A principle and weakness of the study design is the principle that not giving MPS was, at the time, considered to be unethical, and two arms of differing dosages were developed [75].

The second National Acute Spinal Cord Injury Study (NASCIS II) sought to correct the limitations of NASCIS I. A multicentre, double-blinded placebo-controlled randomised study involving 487 patients looking at the safety and efficacy of MPS and naloxone in SCI as compared to placebo. MPS dose used was 30 mg/kg IV bolus followed by 5.4 mg/kg/h IV bolus for the next 23 h. The dose of naloxone used was 5.4 mg/kg IV bolus, followed by 4 mg/kg/h for the next 23 h. No difference in motor or sensory function was noted when the three arms were compared. However, an arbitrary 8-h window from injury to the administration of the drug was chosen for post-hoc analysis. This subgroup of only twelve patients showed that patients who received MPS within 8 h of injury showed an improvement in their motor and sensory functions compared to the placebo group. However, the improvements in this composite outcome did not translate to any functional improvements and the use of steroids has been associated with increased complications per the NASCIS I trial. Naloxone given within 8 h had no significant effect on motor function. After this trial and amidst some criticism, MPS within 8 h became a standard of care in some centres. Criticisms of the study were with methodology including statistical method and outcome measures used, lack of demographic data, lack of widespread reproducibility of the data and post-hoc analysis. Similarly, the study by Berhnard et al. was criticised for the use of raw motor score rather than functional outcome measure. Notably, the rate of complications rose as the dose of MPS escalated to show a threefold rise in pulmonary embolus, two-fold rise in wound infections; and a fivefold increase in gastrointestinal haemorrhage [76, 77].

The third National Acute Spinal Cord Injury Study (NASCIS III) sought to evaluate the effect of a 24- versus 48-h MPS administration protocol with a comparison to another antioxidant, tirilazad. A multicentre, double-blinded randomised control study, NASCIS III involved 499 patients, comparing safety and efficacy of MPS (5.4 mg/kg/h IV bolus for next 24 h) vs MPS (5.4 mg/kg/h IV bolus for 48 h) vs tirilazad (2.5 mg/kg IV bolus followed by 2.5 mg/kg bolus every 6 h for next 48 h). All patients in this study received 30 mg/kg IV bolus of MPS. There was no difference in primary endpoints in the three study arms. However, a post-hoc analysis showed that patients who received MPS within 3–8 h of SCI for 48-h duration had a small but statistically significant improvement in motor function, but not in clinical function, as compared to other arms. However, patients who received 48 h of MPS had more severe sepsis and pneumonia [78, 79].

In a consensus conference of AANS/CNS, it was stated that treatment with MPS for either 24 or 48 h in the treatment of patients with acute spinal cord injury should be undertaken with the knowledge that evidence suggesting harmful side effects is more consistent than any actual clinic benefit [80]. Contentiously, follow-on international studies have not been able to reproduce the NASCIS conclusions. This may be due to flawed statistical analysis in NASCIS-II and NASCIS-III. Multiple t-tests were used with analysis of variance and covariance, which predicates an assumption that the data set follows a Gaussian distribution. There were 66 subgroup comparisons in NASCIS-II and more than 100 in NASCIS-III introducing a high likelihood of type I error, where non-parametric tests could have yielded cleaner results to interpret.

This contention explains the continued uptake of the contentious practice in the United States but is not indicative of best practice recommendations or guidelines in the UK. At the time of writing, there are no UK centres that routinely administer MPS for spinal cord injuries. It is however kept as an adjunct to surgical management in highly select cases where cord oedema may be mitigated by MPS administration.

Specific Spinal Injuries

Atlanto Occipital Dislocation

- Rare and usually fatal injury. Cause of death is usually apnoeic respiratory arrest. The majority who survive have a severe neurological deficit
- Commoner in children due to laxity of ligaments, a larger size of the head compared to the body and smaller/flatter condyles
- Powers ratio is >1 (ratio of the basion (the median (midline) point of the anterior margin of the foramen magnum) to the arch of atlas distance, and opisthion to anterior arch of atlas distance)
- Treated with occipito-cervical fusion

Occipital Condyle Fracture

- The patient usually presents with pain, though occasionally lower cranial nerve deficit may be present.
- May be associated with fracture involving other cervical vertebrae
- Usually stable and treated in a collar. Halo immobilisation or occipito-cervical fusion may be needed in selected cases of instability or atlanto-occipital ligamentous injury

Atlantoaxial Subluxation

- Commonly seen in rheumatoid arthritis, trauma, or with ENT infection (Grisel syndrome).
- Neurological deficit is rare
- Head in "Cock robin" position
- ENT associated subluxation is usually treated with antibiotics, traction followed by Halo
- Subluxations which cannot be reduced or which reoccur following halo immobilisation require C1-2 fusion

Atlas Fracture

- Jefferson fracture involving the arch of C1 fracture is usually due to axial loading
- Patients are usually neurologically intact
- May be associated with a C2 fracture
- Treatment depends upon the integrity of the transverse ligament. If the ligament is intact, then it can be treated in a collar or a halo. Patients with disruption of transverse ligament require C1–C2 fusion
- Rule of Spence—when the sum of the overhang of C1 lateral mass is >7 mm then transverse ligament should be assumed to be disrupted

Axis Fracture

- Peg fracture is usually due to flexion injury and is of 3 types as per Aderson and D'Alonzo classification. They are rarely associated with neurological deficit. In type 1, the fracture line goes through the tip of the peg, in type 2 the fracture line goes through the base of the peg whereas in type 3 the fracture involves the body of the C2. Type 1 and 3 peg fractures can be treated in a collar or a halo. Patient with type two peg fracture may need anterior or posterior fusion surgery.
- Hangman's fracture—It is described as traumatic spondylolisthesis of C2 and is usually due to hyperextension and axial loading. Most patients are neurologically intact. Classified into three types as per Effendi classification. Usually treated with halo immobilisation though surgery may be needed if there is more than 5 mm of subluxation or more than 10 degrees of angulation

Subaxial Cervical Spine Fracture

- Unilateral or bilateral facet dislocations are treated with traction, followed by anterior ± posterior surgery.
- Management is as per SLICS system. Conservative treatment is recommended if score is ≤3 whereas operative treatment is recommended when score is ≥5. Patient with SLICS score of 4 can be managed either operatively or non-operatively (Figs. 32.9 and 32.10)

Morphology	Score
No abnormality	0
Compression	1
Burst	2
Distraction	3
Rotation/Translation	4
Discoligamentous complex	
Intact	0
Indeterminate	1
Disrupted	2
Neurological status	
Intact	0
Root injury	1
Complete cord injury	2
Incomplete cord injury	3
Continuous cord compression with neurological deficit	+1

Fig. 32.9 Cervical SLICS scoring system

Morphology	Score
No abnormality	0
Compression	1
Burst	2
Rotation/Translation	3
Distraction	4
Discoligamentous complex	
Intact	0
Indeterminate	2
Disrupted	3
Neurological status	
Intact	0
Root injury	2
Complete cord injury	2
Incomplete cord injury	3
Cauda equina compression	3

Fig. 32.10 Thoracolumbar TLICS scoring system

Thoracolumbar Fracture

– Management is as per TLICS system. Conservative treatment is recommended if score is ≤3 whereas operative treatment is recommended when score is ≥5. Patient with SLICS score of 4 can be managed either operatively or non-operatively (Fig. 32.10)

Conclusion

In the last few decades, significant advancement has been made in the management of spinal trauma patients with a better understanding of pathophysiology and spinal biomechanics along with improvement in prehospital care, management in ED, and ICU care. There has also been an improvement in the designs of implants used in surgery. However, further research is needed to minimise or prevent secondary injury to the spinal cord. Similarly, further research is required in order to clarify the use of collars in patients with spinal trauma. More studies are also needed to investigate the role and timing of surgery in spinal trauma patients.

A challenge of modern healthcare is to balance the focused and dedicated expertise of individual clinicians with the overall wellbeing and best practice in managing trauma. Selective use of immobilisation collars in the prehospital management trauma may lead to case examples of injury that is attributed to their failure to be immobilised. However, this must be borne with the arguments of this chapter considering the morbidity of immobilisation, the challenge it poses to early responders, and the extent to which the instability is adequately addressed by the application of blocks and tape or a rigid collar. Rather than using rigid cervical collars, identification of patients at risk of cord injury or instability could be by virtue of a marker, visual indicator or application of a soft collar.

Questions

1. Neurogenic shock is the cardiovascular manifestation of spinal cord injury
   (a) True
   (b) False
2. The Canadian C-spine rule for immobilisation can only be used in adult patients under the age of 65
   (a) True
   (b) False

3. Patients who present with central cord syndrome will have a motor loss below the level of the lesion?
   (a) True
   (b) False
4. Loss of the bulbocavernosus reflex early in spinal cord injury is suggestive of severe cord injury
   (a) True
   (b) False
5. Cervical spinal collars are a low risk, benign intervention that should be liberally applied to all trauma patients
   (a) True
   (b) False

Answers

1. a
2. a
3. b
4. a
5. b

References

1. Kumar R, Lim J, Mekary RA, et al. Traumatic spinal injury: global epidemiology and worldwide volume. World Neurosurg. 2018;113:e345–63.
2. Bonner S, Smith C. Initial management of acute spinal cord injury. Continuing education in anaesthesia. Crit Care Pain. 2013;13(6):224–31.
3. Jazayeri SB, Beygi S, Shokraneh F, et al. Incidence of traumatic spinal cord injury worldwide: a systematic review. Eur Spine J. 2015;24:905–18.
4. Oteir A, Smith KL, Stoelwinder JU, et al. Should suspected cervical spinal cord injury be immobilised? A systematic review. Injury. 2015;46(4):528–35.
5. Petsas A, Drake J. Perioperative management for patients with a chronic spinal cord injury. BJA Educ. 2015;15(3):123–30.
6. Dooney N, Dagal A. Anesthetic considerations in acute spinal cord trauma. Int J Crit Illn Inj Sci. 2011;1(1):36–43.
7. Taghva A, Hoh DJ, Lauryssen CL. Advances in the management of spinal cord and spinal column injuries. Handb Clin Neurol. 2012;109:105–30.
8. Connor D, Greaves I, Porter K, et al. Prehospital spinal immobilisation: an initial consensus statement. Emerg Med J. 2013;30:1067–9.
9. Sundstrøm T, Asbjørnsen H, Habiba S, et al. Prehospital use of cervical collars in trauma patients: a critical review. J Neurotrauma. 2014;31(6):531–40.
10. Raza M, Elkhodair S, Zaheer A, et al. Safe cervical spine clearance in adult obtunded blunt trauma patients on the basis of a normal multi-detector CT scan: a meta-analysis and cohort study. Injury. 2013;44(11):1589–95.
11. Hasler RM, Exadaktylos AK, Bouamra O, et al. Epidemiology and predictors of spinal injury in adult major trauma patients: European cohort study. Eur Spine J. 2011;20:2174–80.
12. Bellon K, Kolakowsky-Hayner S, Chen D, et al. Evidence-based practice in primary prevention of spinal cord injury. Top Spinal Cord Injury Rehab.. 2013;19(1):25–30. https://doi.org/10.1310/sci1901-25. *Primary prevention efforts can offer significant cost benefits, and efforts to change behavior and improve safety can and should be emphasised. Primary prevention can be applied to various etiologies of injury, including motor vehicle crashes, sports injuries, and firearm misuse, with a clear goal of eliminating unnecessary injury and its life-changing impact.*
13. Harrop JS, Rymarczuk GN, Vaccaro AR, et al. Controversies in spinal trauma and evolution of care. Neurosurgery. 2017;80(3):S23–32.
14. Grover VK, Tewari MK, Gupta SK, et al. Anaesthetic and intensive care aspects of spinal injury. Neurol India. 2001;49(1):11–8.
15. Holdsworth F. Fractures, dislocations, and fracture-dislocations of the spine. J Bone Joint Surg Am. 1970;52(8):1534–51.
16. White AA 3rd, Panjabi MM. The basic kinematics of the human spine. A review of past and current knowledge. Spine. 1978;3(1):12–20.
17. Denis F. The three column spine and its significance in the classification of acute thoracolumbar spinal injuries. Spine. 1983;8(8):817–31.
18. Magerl F, Aebi M, Gertzbein SD, et al. A comprehensive classification of thoracic and lumbar injuries. Eur Spine J. 1994;3(4):184–201.
19. Vaccaro AR, Lehman RA Jr, Hurlbert RJ, et al. A new classification of thoracolumbar injuries: the importance of injury morphology, the integrity of the posterior ligamentous complex, and neurologic status. Spine. 2005;30(20):2325–33.
20. Vaccaro AR, Hulbert RJ, Patel AA, et al. The subaxial cervical spine injury classification system: a novel approach to recognise the importance of morphology, neurology, and integrity of the disco-ligamentous complex. Spine. 2007;32(21):2365–74.
21. Vaccaro AR, Oner C, Kepler CK, et al. AOSpine thoracolumbar spine injury classification system: fracture description, neurological status, and key modifiers. Spine. 2013;38(23):2028–37.
22. Vaccaro AR, Koerner JD, Radcliff KE, et al. AOSpine subaxial cervical spine injury classification system. Eur Spine J. 2016;25:2173–84.
23. Hauswald M, Ong G, Tandberg D, et al. Out-of-hospital spinal immobilisation: its effect on neurologic injury. Acad Emerg Med. 1998;5(3):214–9.

24. Aprahamian C, Thompson BM, Finger WA, et al. Experimental cervical spine injury model: evaluation of airway management and splinting techniques. Ann Emerg Med. 13(8):584–587. https://doi.org/10.1016/s0196-0644(84)80278-4. *Evaluation of airway manoeuvres with respect to cervical splinting on a cadaver model with unstable C5/6 injury under x-ray. Chin lift, jaw thrust, oesophageal obturator airway (EOA®), and endotracheal intubation can cause extension, widening and anterior subluxation A two-piece, semi-rigid soft cervical collar may minimise flexion but not extension. Take home message: Standard nonsurgical airway management techniques can exacerbate pre-existing injuries. Soft and semi-rigid collars do little to prevent movement, however they remind patients and carers of the injury.*
25. Bernhard M, Gries A, Kremer P, et al. Spinal cord injury (SCI)—prehospital management. Resuscitation. 2005;66(2):127–139. https://doi.org/10.1016/j.resuscitation.2005.03.005. *20% of spinal cord injuries (SCI) die at time of injury. Of the remainder that survive but later deteriorate, 25% occur prehospital. Studies have not demonstrated convincingly that methylprednisolone (MPS) or other pharmacological agents really have clinically significant and important benefits for patients suffering from SCI.*
26. Helliwell, V; Gabbott, DA. The effect of single-handed cricoid pressure on cervical spine movement after applying manual in-line stabilisation: a cadaver study. Resuscitation. 2001;49(1):53–57. https://doi.org/10.1016/s0300-9572(00)00307-5. *Cricoid pressure applied using a cricoid 'yoke' whilst maintaining manual in-line stabilisation of the cervical spine with no other spinal support. Lateral radiographs before and after demonstrated no disruption to the lines formed by the anterior or posterior borders of the cervical bodies. Take home message: Single-handed cricoid pressure does not cause clinically significant displacement of the cervical spine in a cadaver model. This conflicts with previous studies.*
27. Rao GU. Anaesthetic and intensive care management of traumatic cervical spine injury. Indian J Anaesth. 2008;52(1):13.
28. Geisler WO, Wynne-Jones M, Jousse AT. Early management of the patient with trauma to the spinal cord. Med Serv J Can. 1966;22(7):512–23.
29. Gupta KJ, Clancy M. Discontinuation of cervical spine immobilisation in unconscious patients with trauma in intensive care units—telephone survey of practice in south and west region. BMJ. 1997;314(7095):1652–5.
30. Núñez-Patiño RA, Rubiano AM, Godoy DA. Impact of cervical collars on intracranial pressure values in traumatic brain injury: a systematic review and meta-analysis of prospective studies. Neurocrit Care. 2020;32(2):469–77.
31. Ham W, Schoonhoven L, Schuurmans M, et al. Pressure ulcers from spinal immobilisation in trauma patients: a systematic review. J Trauma Acute Care Surg. 2014;76(4):1131–41.
32. Schuurman JP, Schoonhoven L, Defloor T, et al. Economic evaluation of pressure ulcer care.a cost minimisation analysis of preventive strategies. Nurs Econ. 2009;27:390–400.
33. Lien D, Jacques T, Powell K. Cervical spine clearance in Australian intensive care units. Crit Care Resusc. 2003;5(2):91–6.
34. Molano Alvarez E, Pérez M, Mdel A, Salobral Villegas MT, et al. Pressure sores secondary to immobilization with cervical collar: a complication of acute cervical injury. Enferm Intensiva. 2004;15(3):112–22.
35. Ackland HM, Cooper JD, Malham GM, et al. Factors predicting cervical collar-related decubitus ulceration in major trauma patients. Spine. 2007;32(4): 423–8. https://doi.org/10.1097/01.brs.0000255096.52871.4e. *Trauma registry database review of incidence and predictors of cervical collar-related decubitus ulceration. 299 Major Trauma patients admitted over 6-months. Four predictive factors identified: ICU admission, mechanical ventilation, the necessity for cervical MRI, time to cervical spine clearance. Take home message: Time to cervical spine clearance was the major indicator, such that the risk of ulceration increased by 66% for every 1 day increase in cervical collar time.*
36. Lacey L, Palokas M, Walker J. Preventative interventions, protocols or guidelines for trauma patients at risk of cervical collar-related pressure ulcers: a scoping review. JBI Database Syst Rev Implement Rep. 2019;17(12):2452–75.
37. Kwan I, Bunn F, Roberts IG. Spinal immobilisation for trauma patients. Cochrane Database Syst Rev. 2001;2:CD002803.
38. Oto B, Corey JD 2nd, Oswald J, et al. Early secondary neurologic deterioration after blunt spinal trauma: a review of the literature. Acad Emerg Med. 2015;22(10):1200–12.
39. Lin HL, Lee WC, Chen CW, et al. Neck collar used in treatment of victims of urban motorcycle accidents: over- or underprotection? Am J Emerg Med. 2011;29(9):1028–33.
40. Haut ER; Kalish BT, Efron DT, et al. Spine immobilisation in penetrating trauma: more harm than good? J Trauma. 2010;68(1):115–120. https://doi.org/10.1097/TA.0b013e3181c9ee58 *"Prehospital spine immobilisation is associated with higher mortality in penetrating trauma and should not be routinely used in every patient"*.
41. Vanderlan W, Tew B, McSwain N. Increased risk of death with cervical spine immobilisation in penetrating cervical trauma. Injury. 2009;40:880–3.
42. Flabouris A. Clinical features, patterns of referral and out of hospital transport events for patients with suspected isolated spinal injury. Injury. 2001;32(7):569–75.
43. Kreinest M, Goller S, Rauch G, et al. Application of cervical collars: an analysis of practical skills of professional emergency medical care providers. PLoS One. 2015;10(11):e0143409.

44. Tello RR, Braude D, Fullerton L, et al. Outcome of trauma patients immobilised by emergency department staff, but not by emergency medical services providers: a quality assurance initiative. Prehosp Emerg Care. 2014;18(4):544–9.
45. Hyldmo PK, Horodyski MB, Conrad BP, Dubose DN, Røislien J, Prasarn M, et al. Safety of the lateral trauma position in cervical spine injuries: a cadaver model study. Acta Anaesthesiol Scand. 2016 Aug;60(7):1003–11.
46. Maschmann C, Jeppesen E, Rubin MA, et al. New clinical guidelines on the spinal stabilisation of adult trauma patients – consensus and evidence based. Scand J Trauma Resusc Emerg Med. 2019;27:77.
47. Hood N, Considine N. Spinal immobilisaton in prehospital and emergency care: a systematic review of the literature. Australas Emerg Nurs J. 2015;18(3):118–37.
48. Holla M. Value of a rigid collar in addition to head blocks: a proof of principle study. Emerg Med J. 2012;29(2):104–7.
49. Blackham J, Benger J. 'Clearing' the cervical spine in the unconscious trauma patient. Trauma. 2011;13(1):65–79. https://doi.org/10.1177/1460408610385978.
50. Gonzalez RP, Cummings GR, Baker JA, et al. Prehospital clinical clearance of the cervical spine: a prospective study. Am Surg. 2013;79(11):1213–7.
51. Reid DC, Henderson R, Saboe L, et al. Etiology and clinical course of missed spine fractures. J Trauma. 1987;27(9):980–6.
52. Toscano J. Prevention of neurological deterioration before admission to a spinal cord injury unit. Paraplegia. 1988;26(3):143–50.
53. Davis JW, Phreaner DL, Hoyt DB, et al. The etiology of missed cervical spine injuries. J Trauma. 1993;34(3):342–6.
54. Vaillancourt C, Charette M, Kasaboski A, Maloney J, Wells GA, Stiell IG. Evaluation of the safety of C-spine clearance by paramedics: design and methodology. BMC Emerg Med. 2011 Dec;11(1):1.
55. Stiell IG, Wells GA, Vandemheen KL, et al. The Canadian C-spine rule for radiography in alert and stable trauma patients. JAMA. 2001;286(15):1841–8.
56. Reitman CA, Mauro KM, Nguyen L, et al. Intervertebral motion between flexion and extension in asymptomatic individuals. Spine. 2004;29(24):2832–43.
57. Goodnight TJ, Helmer SD, Dort JM, et al. A comparison of flexion and extension radiographs with computed tomography of the cervical spine in blunt trauma. Am Surg. 2008;74(9):855–7.
58. McCracken B, Klineberg E, Pickard B, et al. Flexion and extension radiographic evaluation for the clearance of potential cervical spine injures in trauma patients. Eur Spine J. 2013;22(7):1467–73.
59. Padayachee L, Cooper DJ, Irons S, et al. Cervical spine clearance in unconscious traumatic brain injury patients: dynamic flexion-extension fluoroscopy versus computed tomography with three-dimensional reconstruction. J Trauma. 2006;60(2):341–5.
60. Como JJ, Thompson MA, Anderson JS, et al. Is magnetic resonance imaging essential in clearing the cervical spine in obtunded patients with blunt trauma? J Trauma. 2007;63(3):544–9.
61. Hogan GJ, Mirvis SE, Kathirkamanathan S, et al. Exclusion of unstable cervical spine injury in obtunded patients with blunt trauma: is MR imaging needed when multi-detector row CT findings are normal? Radiology. 2005;237(1):106–13.
62. Stassen NA, Williams VA, Gestring ML, et al. Magnetic resonance imaging in combination with helical computed tomography provides a safe and efficient method of cervical spine clearance in the obtunded trauma patient. J Trauma. 2006;60(1):171–7.
63. Kerwin AJ, Frykberg ER, Schinco MA, et al. The effect of early spine fixation on non-neurologic outcome. J Trauma. 2005;58(1):15–21.
64. Papadopoulos SM, Selden R, Quint DJ, et al. Immediate spinal cord decompression for cervical spinal cord injury: feasibility and outcome. J Trauma. 2002;52(2):323–32.
65. La Rosa G, Conti A, Cardali S, et al. Does early decompression improve neurological outcome of spinal cord injured patients? Appraisal of the literature using a meta-analytical approach. Spinal Cord. 2004;42(9):503–12.
66. Carreon L, Dimar J. Early versus late stabilization of spine injuries: a systematic review. Spine. 2011;36(11):E727–33.
67. Furlan JC, Noonan V, Cadotte DW, et al. Timing of decompressive surgery of spinal cord after traumatic spinal cord injury: an evidence-based examination of pre-clinical and clinical studies. J Neurotrauma. 2011;28(8):1371–99.
68. Verlaan JJ, Diekerhof CH, Buskens E, et al. Surgical treatment of traumatic fractures of the thoracic and lumbar spine: a systematic review of the literature on techniques, complications, and outcome. Spine. 2004;29(7):803–14.
69. Fehlings MG, Vaccaro A, Wilson JR, et al. Early versus delayed decompression for traumatic cervical spinal cord injury: results of the Surgical Timing in Acute Spinal Cord Injury Study (STASCIS). PLoS One. 2012;7(2):e32037.
70. Cengiz SL, Kalkan E, Bayir A, et al. Timing of thoracolomber spine stabilisation in trauma patients; impact on neurological outcome and clinical course. A real prospective (rct) randomised controlled study. Arch Orthop Trauma Surg. 2008;128(9):959–66.
71. Lenehan B, Fisher CG, Vaccaro A, et al. The urgency of surgical decompression in acute central cord injuries with spondylosis and without instability. Spine. 2010;35(21 Suppl):S180–6.
72. Werndle MC, Zoumprouli A, Sedgwick P, et al. Variability in the treatment of acute spinal cord injury in the United Kingdom: results of a national survey. J Neurotrauma. 2012;29(5):880–8.

73. McKinley W, Meade MA, Kirshblum, Set al. Outcomes of early surgical management versus late or no surgical intervention after acute spinal cord injury. Arch Phys Med Rehabil. 2004;85(11):1818–25.
74. Wong J, El Beheiry H, Rampersaud YR, et al. Tranexamic acid reduces perioperative blood loss in adult patients having spinal fusion surgery. Anesth Analg. 2008;107(5):1479–86.
75. Bracken MB, Collins WF, Freeman DF, et al. Efficacy of methylprednisolone in acute spinal cord injury. JAMA. 1984;251(1):45–52.
76. Bracken MB, Shepard MJ, Collins WF, et al. A randomised, controlled trial of methylprednisolone or naloxone in the treatment of acute spinal-cord injury. Results of the Second National Acute Spinal Cord Injury Study. N Engl J Med. 1990;322(20):1405–11.
77. Bracken MB, Shepard MJ, Collins WF, et al. Methylprednisolone or naloxone treatment after acute spinal cord injury: 1-year follow-up data. Results of the second National Acute Spinal Cord Injury Study. J Neurosurg. 1992;76(1):23–31.
78. Bracken MB, Shepard MJ, Holford TR, et al. Administration of methylprednisolone for 24 or 48 hours or tirilazad mesylate for 48 hours in the treatment of acute spinal cord injury. Results of the Third National Acute Spinal Cord Injury Randomized Controlled Trial. National Acute Spinal Cord Injury Study. JAMA. 1997;277(20):1597–604.
79. Bracken MB, Shepard MJ, Holford TR, et al. Methylprednisolone or tirilazad mesylate administration after acute spinal cord injury: 1-year follow up. Results of the third National Acute Spinal Cord Injury randomised controlled trial. J Neurosurg. 1998;89(5):699–706.
80. Hadley MN, Walters BC, Grabb PA, et al. Pharmacological therapy after acute cervical spinal cord injury. Neurosurgery. 2002;50(3 Suppl):S63–72.

Further Reading

Anderson P, Muchow R, Munoz A, et al. Clearance of the asymptomatic cervical spine: a meta-analysis. J Orthop Trauma. 2010;24(2):100–106. https://doi.org/10.1097/BOT.0b013e3181b16494. *A comprehensive review of the literature and subsequent meta-analysis of data regarding appropriate clearance of the asymptomatic cervical spine in blunt trauma patients. Take home message: An* alert, asymptomatic *patient* without a distracting injury *or* neurologic deficit *who is able to complete a functional range-of-motion examination* may safely be cleared from cervical spine *immobilisation* without radiographic evaluation *(sensitivity = 98.1%, negative predictive value = 99.8%).*

Bennett G, Dealey C, Posnett J. The cost of pressure ulcers in the UK. Age Ageing. 2004;33(3):230–235. https://doi.org/10.1093/ageing/afh086 *UK based study: estimated annual cost of treating pressure ulcers. £1,064 (Grade 1) to £10,551 (Grade 4). Costs increase with ulcer grade because the time to heal is longer and because the incidence of complications is higher in more severe cases. The total cost in the UK is £1.4–£2.1 billion annually (4% of total NHS expenditure). Most of this cost is nurse time.*

Branco BC, Plurad D, Green DJ, et al. Incidence and clinical predictors for tracheostomy after cervical spinal cord injury: a National Trauma Databank review. J Trauma. 2011;70(1):111–5.

Dahlquist RT, Fischer PE, Desai H, et al. Femur fractures should not be considered distracting injuries for cervical spine assessment. Am J Emerg Med. 2015;33(12):1750–4.

Dididze M, Green BA, Dietrich WD, et al. Systemic hypothermia in acute cervical spinal cord injury: a case-controlled study. Spinal Cord. 2013;51(5):395–400.

Garfin S, Shackford S, Marshall L, et al. Care of the multiply injured patient with cervical spine injury. Clin Orthop Relat Res. 1989;239:19–29.

Hauswald M. A re-conceptualisation of acute spinal care. Emerg Med J. 2013;30(9):720–3.

Hoffman JR, Mower WR, Wolfson AB, et al. Validity of a set of clinical criteria to rule out injury to the cervical spine in patients with blunt trauma. National Emergency X-Radiography Utilization Study Group. N Engl J Med. 2000;343(2):94–9.

Jaeseong Oh J, Asha SE. Utility of flexion-extension radiography for the detection of ligamentous cervical spine injury and its current role in the clearance of the cervical spine. Emerg Med Australas. 2016;28(2):216–23.

James IA, Moukalled A, Yu E, et al. A systematic review of the need for MRI for the clearance of cervical spine injury in obtunded blunt trauma patients after normal cervical spine CT. J Emerg Trauma Shock. 2014;7(4):251–5.

Ramasamy A, Midwinter M, Mahoney P, Clasper J. Learning the lessons from conflict: pre-hospital cervical spine stabilisation following ballistic neck trauma. Injury. 2009 Dec;40(12):1342–5. *UK Iraq and Afghanistan experience. Penetrating ballistic trauma to the neck is associated with a high mortality rate, penetrating ballistic trauma to the neck will unlikely result in an unstable cervical spine in survivors. In a hazardous environment (e.g. shooting incidents or terrorist bombings), the risk/benefit ratio of mandatory spinal immobilisation is unfavourable and may place medical teams at prolonged risk. In addition cervical collars may hide potential life-threatening conditions.*

Rose MK, Rosal LM, Gonzalez RP, et al. Clinical clearance of the cervical spine in patients with distracting injuries: it is time to dispel the myth. J Trauma Acute Care Surg. 2012;73(2):498–502.

Su Q, Li C, Li Y, Zhou Z, Zhang S, Guo S, et al. Analysis and improvement of the three-column spinal theory. BMC Musculoskeletal Disorders. 2020 Aug 12;21(1):537.

Theodore N, Aarabi B, Dhall S, et al. Transportation of patients with acute traumatic cervical spine injuries. Neurosurgery. 2013a;72(3):35–9.

Theodore N, Hadley MN, Aarabi B, et al. Prehospital cervical spinal immobilization after trauma. Neurosurgery. 2013b;72(3):22–34.

Uchida K, Nishimura T, Hagawa N, Kaga S, Noda T, Shinyama N, et al. The impact of early administration of vasopressor agents for the resuscitation of severe hemorrhagic shock following blunt trauma. BMC Emerg Med. 2020 Dec;20(1):26.

Wilson, M. Monro-Kellie 2.0: The dynamic vascular and venous pathophysiological components of intracranial pressure. J Cereb Blood Flow Metab. 2016. https://doi.org/10.1177/0271678X16648711. *The 'closed box' analogy of intracranial pressure (ICP) doctrine stating that a change in blood, brain or CSF volume resulted in reciprocal changes in one or both of the other two. HOWEVER, The slow production of CSF (0.35 ml/min) is dwarfed by the dynamic blood in and outflow (700 ml/min). Failure of venous efferent flow to precisely match arterial afferent flow will yield immediate and dramatic changes in intracranial blood volume and pressure. Interpreting ICP without interrogating its core drivers may be misleading. Multiple clinical conditions and the cerebral effects of altitude and microgravity relate to imbalances in this dynamic rather than ICP per se.*

33 Limb Trauma

Alexander M. Wood

1. Understanding the management priorities in high energy fractures.
2. Understanding issues caused by mechanism of injury
3. Understanding the anatomy and assessment of a patient with a limb fracture
4. Understanding the importance of Compartment Syndrome
5. Understanding the management of upper limb fractures
6. Understanding the management of lower limb fractures
7. Understanding the management of Open Fractures
8. Understanding the assessment of a Mangled limb and considerations on salvage versus amputation.

Introduction

The involvement of limb injuries in Major Trauma patients varies depending upon the region and injury mechanisms. In the United Kingdom outside of London, the majority of patients classified as having sustained Major Trauma have significant limb injuries. Therefore the understanding of these injuries is critical for anyone involved in trauma. The management of simple fractures is well described, and in minor injury patients it is possible to focus solely on a single fracture. However, in Major Trauma patients there are other considerations which will alter the required approach for the management of these injuries.

In Major Trauma patients, the resuscitation of the whole patient needs to be considered rather than just the limb involved, and this is covered in depth in other chapters. A stepwise approach prioritising the early management of the patient's injuries is also required, and again these considerations are covered in other chapters.

When assessing a high-energy limb injury, it is essential to realise that in these patients the injury is a soft tissue injury with an associated fracture and to tailor the approach in this regard. Therefore, per the BOA/BAPRAS guidelines, it is essential to have a multidisciplinary approach to the management of these injuries. This includes joint surgical planning from the start, including how these injuries will be managed definitively further down the treatment algorithm. This will prevent the figurative "burning of bridges" for the reconstruction of the injuries once the patient has recovered from the initial trauma insult.

High-energy limb injuries involve the whole anatomy of the limb, and key areas of anatomy to aid the decision processes are highlighted in this chapter. Any Major Trauma surgeon needs to know their anatomy in detail as they will be required to approach injuries through different

A. M. Wood (✉)
Orthopaedic Department, John Radcliffe Hospital, Oxford, UK
e-mail: sandy.wood@ouh.nhs.uk

P. Lax (ed.), *Textbook of Acute Trauma Care*, https://doi.org/10.1007/978-3-030-83628-3_33

surgical planes dependent upon the injury they are presented with. They also need to have an in-depth knowledge of the Neurological anatomy so that they can identify if neurological structures have been damaged. Whilst a full anatomical text is out with the purpose of this book, key anatomical knowledge is highlighted within this chapter.

In high energy trauma, all the anatomical structures in a limb may be disrupted from superficial to deep. This includes the skin, facial and adipose tissue, overlying muscular structures and the nervous and vascular structures within the zone of injury. These need to be assessed promptly and accurately, to ensure the rapid appropriate treatment and limb salvage.

Ascertaining if a fracture is open and if there is any vascular compromise to the patient is essential. Limb hypoperfusion limbs and resultant ischaemia can have many causes; locally from damage to the structures around the injury, proximal to the injury, or a systemic cause due to the overwhelming hypotension and condition of the patient. Systemic causes can compromise the overall outcome of the patient and limb, therefore these injuries need a rapid assessment. This is most frequently noted in compartment syndrome or knee dislocations, where it is well documented that delays to intervention and restoration of perfusion in these injuries can have catastrophic effects. These areas are covered within this chapter.

When assessing limbs in Major Trauma, it is also necessary to understand where the energy has passed through the limb and the amount of energy that has dissipated within the tissues. Whilst a fracture may look similar in different energy transfers, the soft tissue injury and periosteal stripping around an injury will be significantly greater in high energy trauma, and the management of these injuries will consequently change. Suppose a limb is axially loaded in a trauma situation and there is a midshaft femoral fracture. In that case, clinicians need to consider where the trauma has come from and assess the structures above and below the injury detected. In axial loading, there is a high proportion of calcaneal and tibial plateau fractures below a femoral fracture, with intracapsular neck of femur fractures, acetabular fractures and spinal fractures above the injury. This demonstrates the path that the energy has taken as it dissipates around the body. The common associated injuries are discussed within this chapter and the considerations required for surgical management.

In high-energy trauma, there is sometimes the requirement to assess a limb regarding the potential for limb salvage or the necessity to perform an amputation. In the UK, this decision should be conducted as a joint approach between Orthopaedics and Plastic surgery as a minimum, with Vascular surgeons and the anaesthetic team. There is conflicting data about which limbs are salvageable, and whilst these tools are discussed, the pre-morbid condition of the patient frequently dictates the management of the limb and its ability to be salvaged. This includes not only their past medical injury, but also their current clinical condition regarding the associated polytrauma injuries, and the surgical resources available for the patient. What is appropriate in a Major Trauma Centre within the UK, will not be applicable in other centres who do not have all the reconstructive solutions available. Likewise, a patient who has been non-ambulatory pre-injury may not have the same reconstructive requirements as a high functioning individual. These considerations are discussed in detail later. There are also cultural reasons that patients may wish to retain their limb, so it is important to understand these considerations within individual areas of practice. In some cultures, patients may prefer to retain a painful, deformed limb rather than have the stigma of a well-functioning amputation. Therefore, in patients who are not able to make a decision at the time of initial injury, it is often beneficial for the patient to defer the decision to amputate until a later surgical episode if clinically safe.

Understanding the Mechanism of Injury

Most major limb injuries in the UK come from fall from heights, motor traffic accidents and industrial accidents, yet these descriptors alone do not help with the understanding of the mechanism of the injury. There is a significant difference to the energy transfer of a person in a modern vehicle who has deflecting collision, to a patient who comes off a motorbike at speed and then has his leg crushed under a passing bus. Whilst the associated bony injury may look the same on radiographs, the soft tissue injuries and energy transfers are significantly different between the two injuries.

Therefore, when understanding the mechanism of injury it is crucial to ascertain what has happened. In patients who have sustained a direct blow to a limb, the energy transfer is likely to be more concentrated; therefore the damage to the soft tissues and bony injury is likely to be a smaller area. However, the degree of periosteal, muscle and skin stripping may be higher due to the energy transfer that has been concentrated in a relatively small area. In contrast, a patient who has sustained a twisting injury may have relatively low focal soft tissue injury as the energy has spread over a significant area, but the energy transfer may affect more than one site as it spirals up a limb. For example, in a Maisonneuve fracture there is an external rotation force through the ankle with transmission of the energy through the interosseous membrane, resulting in a proximal fibular fracture. In these cases the stability of the fracture needs to be assessed, as whilst the osseous component and the soft tissue over the fracture may look insignificant, there may be instability due to disruption up the leg along the interosseous membrane. Bone is very poor at resisting rotational injuries, so twisting injuries may look severe in terms of the length of bone that is disrupted, but the associated soft tissue injury may be relatively small.

In contrast, if a limb is crushed, there may be a relatively small area where the bone is fractured. Still, due to ischaemia and energy from the crushing injury, there can be significant areas of soft tissue damage which will require debridement and assessment for compartment syndrome which is covered later.

Following on from the Afghanistan conflict, there are multiple papers and books which look at the damage that is caused to limbs from blast injuries. Bone is relatively resistant to blast injuries, so initial radiographs may not portray the extent of the injury. Understanding that it is a blast injury and that the fragmentation and energy from the injury have propagated through the muscles, skin, and fascial planes will aid in understanding the required surgical approach. In these injuries, the most significant factor is contamination and necrotic tissue which is often far more dispersed than the osseous injury. Therefore, a staged surgical approach to debride the injured and necrotic soft tissue is required. Even with a thorough debridement, it is necessary to perform a further, staged debridement procedure before progressing to definitive fixation in these patients. Microscopic damage to the tissues is not fully apparent to the naked eye on the initial debridement. As such, a limb which initially looks salvageable due to a relatively simple osseous injury and minimal gross contamination may declare itself unsalvageable at a second surgical visit 72 h later once the full disruption and energy transfer to the limb becomes apparent.

While in the UK the incidence of gunshot wounds is fortunately very low, and most surgeons out-with a few major cities are unlikely to be exposed to many gunshot wounds during their surgical career, this is not the case in other countries. Therefore, an understanding of how gunshot injuries can differ is necessary. When the gunshot goes through the skin and muscle there is little tissue damage out with the track of the bullet. Whilst some studies show cavitation effects, these tissues tolerate this well as they are able to stretch. However, neurological structures do not have the same ability to stretch and recover, in part because they are tethered. While these structures may look normal on inspection, they can be damaged at the axonal level, which highlights the requirement for an accurate pre-operative assessment. Osseous structures are very strong, and so when a bullet hits them there is a significant energy transfer. This will be dependent upon the size and speed of the shell; therefore, higher velocity rounds will cause increased fragmentation and periosteal stripping.

When managing gunshot wounds in the limbs, the priorities are control of haemorrhage, followed by addressing the potential for infection and ultimately, reconstruction of the limb.

At the first surgical sitting vascular injuries need to be addressed. Depending on the location of the injury, this may be by tying off and ligating vessels if required, or placing additional shunts or vascular repairs. This is followed by debriding the wounds, excision of any necrotic tissue and copious irrigation of the wound, and finally stabilising any fracture patterns. Where their fracture is deemed to be a relatively simple injury in a systemically well patient, it may be appropriate to internally fix the fracture definitively. However, a significant number of these fractures will require external fixation initially, followed by a subsequent debridement and definitive fixation and reconstruction either internally or externally at a later date. Patients who have significant bone loss will require further interventions, and this is discussed later.

Assessing a Patient with a Limb Fracture

The mainstay of assessing a patient with a limb fracture is clinical assessment. For example, direct blows to the leg from motor vehicles are associated with other axial injuries. Therefore, when assessing a patient with a limb injury it is vital to assess the other areas of potential damage. These include head injury, chest or abdominal trauma, and any other significant musculoskeletal traumas. It is important to perform a detailed examination as soon as possible to exclude other potential associated injuries.

This assessment can occasionally be performed at the same time as other members of the trauma team are resuscitating the patient. Within the UK, it is practice for Major Trauma patients to be assessed with a CT performed within 30 min of arrival in the emergency department. These CTs are performed from head to mid-femur in most centres due to the inability of the CT to easily scan the whole patient in one go. Therefore, an early assessment of the limbs must be performed to facilitate the acquisition of targeted 3D imaging at the same time as a trauma CT scan is performed to aid surgical planning. In certain circumstances, CT of an area is not possible, and therefore in these cases plain radiographs should be obtained—if possible before going to theatre.

Limb fractures are painful, and where there is a minimal risk of compartment syndrome, then the assessing practitioner should consider regional blocks as soon as possible. For neck of femur patients and proximal femoral patients, the administration of a fascia iliaca block should be considered (Fig. 33.1). In high energy trauma patients with forearm or tibial fractures, in particular, there has been historical concern that regional blocks may mask the early signs of compartment syndrome. This has not been proven, and there is also data that nerve blocks may facilitate earlier detection of compartment syndrome by alerting the surgical teams to new, breakthrough pain which acted as a prompt to investigate further. A though discussion of regional anaesthesia should form part of the team brief and a strategy agreed with surgical and anaesthetic teams before starting the case. A reasonable approach for treating pain in patients who are at risk of compartment syndrome would be to minimise the volume and concentration of local anaesthetics used (0.1–0.25% bupivacaine, levobupivocaine or ropivocaine) as lower concentrations are less likely to mask ischaemic pain. Patients should be followed up by both orthopaedic and pain team staff to look for early signs and symptoms of compartment syndrome, and if suspected, compartment pressures should be measured urgently.

At initial assessment, splints and dressings should be applied after photos have been taken of any wounds that may need surgical management. Traction splintage should also be considered for pain relief and initial treatment of the fracture. Dislocated joints should be reduced (as well as significantly displaced fractures) to prevent neurovascular injury and pressure damage to soft tissue areas. Prior to reduction and immediately post-reduction a neurological assessment should be performed.

In the assessment of neurovascular injuries, it is vital to understand the neurovascular supply of

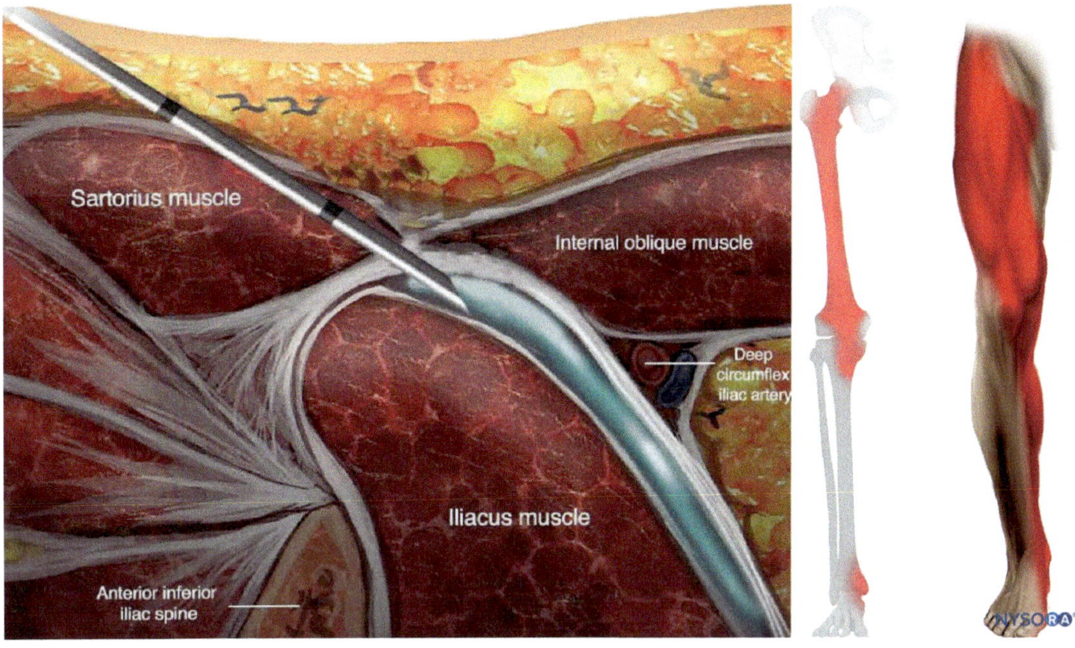

Fig. 33.1 Fascia Iliaca block and anaesthesia distribution (Courtesy of NYSORA.com)

an area and document it. Whilst there is a significant degree of overlap in the assessment of nerve injuries, Table 33.1 gives a suggested algorithm for the evaluation of neurological injuries.

Assessment of Vascular Injuries

To assess vascular injuries in the limb it is important to palpate for the pulses throughout the limb. Where there is an obvious vascular injury, the first priority should be to stem the bleeding. This can be done with either manual compression, either at the site of, or proximal to the injury, or by the use of compressive dressings. Where it is not possible to control the bleeding with manual pressure, then tourniquet use should be considered to allow resuscitation of the patient until an urgent repair can be performed. When there is an obvious vascular injury, urgent surgical intervention is required. The presence of bilateral pulses which are the same is reassuring, however further investigations are still required where there is a suspicion of any vascular injury.

Where there is a requirement to identify the precise level of the vascular disruption, then an arteriogram or duplex ultrasound can provide additional information. In emergency patients, vascular investigations should not delay exploration of the limb as it is necessary to restore perfusion within 6 h of the time of injury.

In patients who have a suspicion of vascular injury but still have normal pulses, further investigation is required. Pulses can be normal in up to 15% of patients with a vascular injury, and vascular damage can be present in up to 25% of patients whom there is a suspicion of injury without obvious vascular signs. The best investigation when there is time is CT arteriography as this has a high level of sensitivity and specificity in the examination of arterial injuries in limb trauma patients.

Assessment of Compartment Syndrome

Compartment syndrome has several different pathophysiological explanations. However, what is not in dispute is that it is relatively common in all tibial fractures and incidence increases with the energy level of the fracture. Compartment

Table 33.1 Neurological assessment of the upper and lower limb

Nerve	Sensory function	Motor function
Suprascapular	N/A	Action: External rotation of shoulder with the elbow at 90 degrees flexion Muscle belly palpated on examination: infraspinatus
Axillary	'Regimental badge' area	Action: Abduction of the arm in 15–90 degree range Muscle belly palpated on examination: deltoid
Musculocutaneous	Lateral aspect of the forearm	Action: elbow flexion in supine arm Muscle belly palpated on examination: bicep
Median	Tip of the index finger	Action: Thumb abduction (thumb to point vertically over base) Muscle belly palpated on examination: Abductor pollicis brevis
AIN	n/a	Action: OK sign Tendon palpated on examination: FPL (palmar aspect of proximal phalanx)
Ulnar	Area tested: tip of the little finger	Action: Abduction of the little finger Muscle belly palpated on examination: Abductor digiti minimi
Radial	Area tested: anatomical snuffbox	Action: thumb up (thumb extension) Tendon visible and palpable on examination: Extensor pollicis longus
Femoral	Area tested: anteromedial thigh	Action: Extension of flexed knee Muscle belly palpated on examination: quadriceps femoris
Obturator	Area tested: middle of the medial surface of the thigh	Action: Adduction of the leg at hip joint Muscle belly palpated on examination: adductor compartment
Tibial	Area tested: sole of the foot	Action: Ankle plantarflexion Muscle belly palpated on examination: gastrocnemius
Deep Peroneal	Area tested: dorsal aspect of first webspace	Action: ankle dorsiflexion Muscle belly palpated on examination: tibialis anterior
Superficial peroneal	Area tested: dorsum of the foot except for first webspace	Action: foot eversion Tendons seen and felt on examination: peroneus longus and brevis

syndrome is not as common in other fractures, but in high energy trauma it can affect any osseofacial compartment. Therefore, a high index of suspicion must be maintained in the assessment of all Major Trauma limb injuries. Major Trauma patients may also develop abdominal compartment syndrome, and this is discussed in the Damage Control Surgery and Trauma ICU chapters.

Regardless of the explanation for the cause of the compartment syndrome, the principle pathophysiology is cellular anoxia due to local ischemia. This ultimately causes cell death and a positive feedback cycle, causing continuous exacerbation of compartment syndrome until the pressure is released. Compartment pressures that are within 30 mm Hg of the diastolic blood pressure cause this ischaemia via capillary and venous congestion and impairment of oxygen delivery despite normal pulses. Consequently, in trauma patients who may have a variation in their diastolic pressure, it is important to continually reassess for the presence of compartment syndrome. There must also be an awareness that in patients with multiple injuries and hypotension there is a higher risk of developing compartment syndrome.

As noted above the most common injury for compartment syndrome is in the lower leg. This has four compartments (Fig. 33.2) which consist

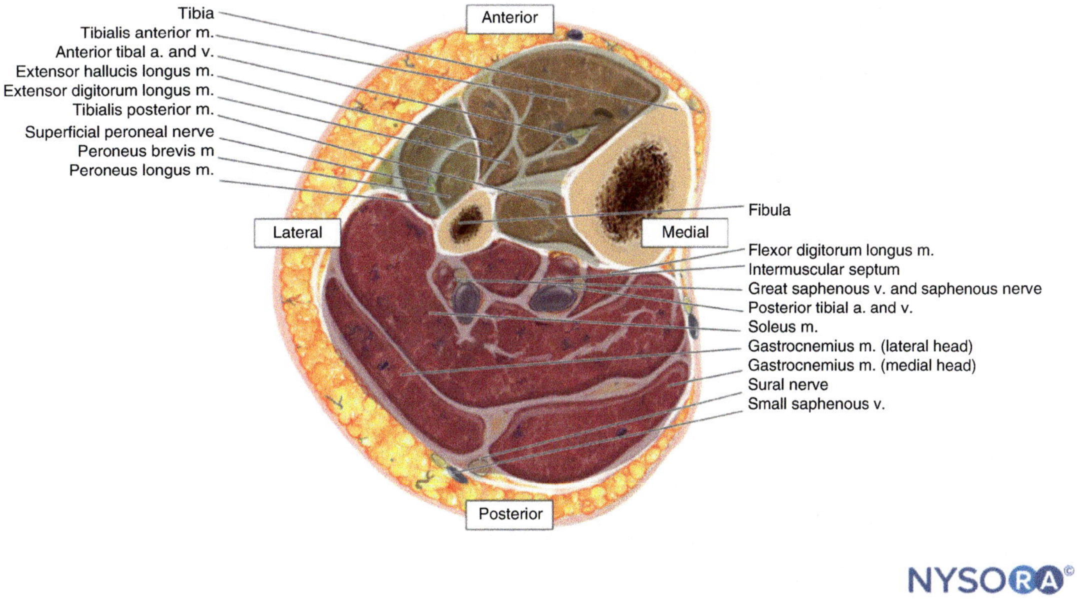

Fig. 33.2 Compartments of the lower leg (Courtesy of NYSORA.com)

of the anterior, lateral, deep posterior, and superficial posterior.

The deep compartment is the most common site for compartment syndrome in the leg. However, due to the accessibility of the anterior compartment, monitors are typically placed here for pressure monitoring. The structures within the four compartments of the leg are listed here:

Compartment	Muscles	Neuro-vascular structures
Anterior compartment	Tibialis anterior Extensor Hallucis longus Extensor Digitorum longus Peroneus Tertius	Deep peroneal nerve Anterior Tibial vessels
Lateral compartment	Peroneus longus Peroneus brevis	Superficial peroneal nerve
Superficial posterior compartment	Gastrocnemius Soleus Plantaris	Sural nerve
Deep posterior compartment	Tibialis posterior Flexor Hallucis longus Flexor Digitorum longus Popliteus	Tibial nerve Posterior Tibial vessels

Late sequelae of compartment syndrome include foot drop, claw foot, and deep peroneal nerve dysfunction.

Another area that is relatively common for compartment syndrome in Major Trauma patients is the forearm. This again has four compartments plus the carpal tunnel (Fig. 33.3). The most common caused for forearm compartment syndrome is paediatric supracondylar fractures and high energy distal radial fractures.

Whilst in general it is rare for acute compartment syndrome to develop in the thigh, it is more common in Major Trauma. The thigh has three large compartments—the anterior, posterior, and medial (Fig. 33.4) with the anterior compartment containing the knee extensors, the posterior compartment the flexors and the medial compartment containing the hip adductors.

Key Learning Point

The main signs and symptoms for compartment syndrome are:

1. Pain that is out of proportion to the injury and pain that is increasing.
2. A burning neurological pain.

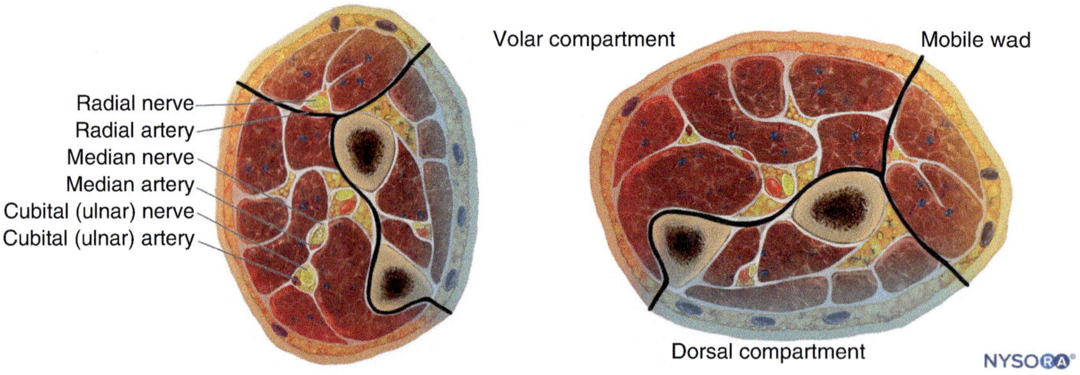

Fig. 33.3 Compartments of the forearm (Courtesy of NYSORA.com)

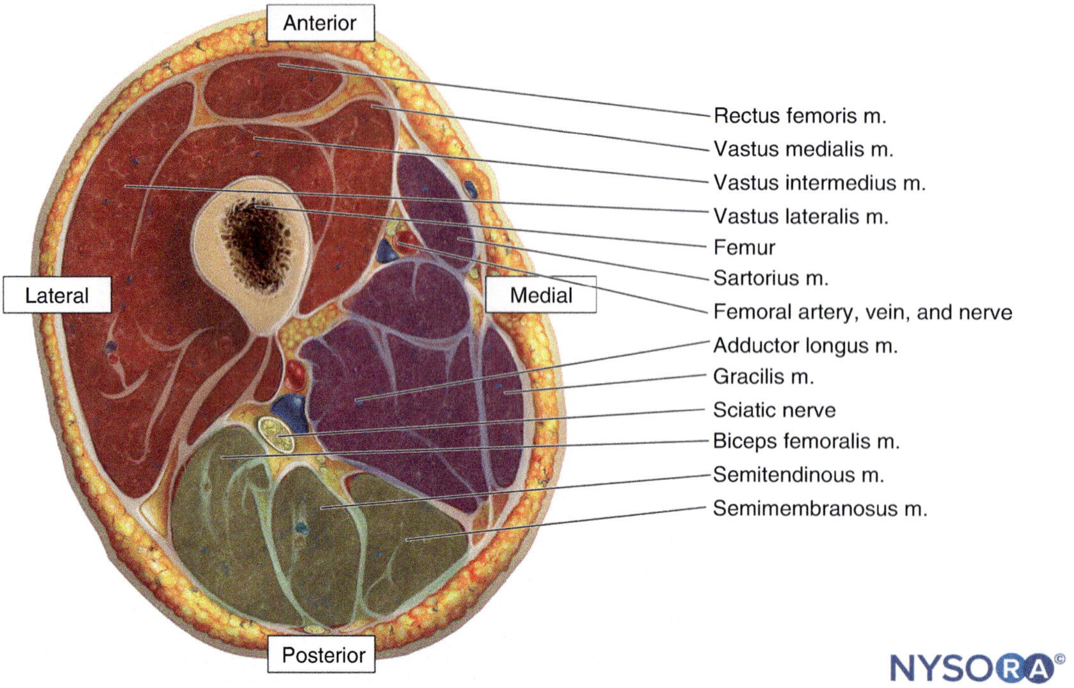

Fig. 33.4 Compartments of the thigh (Courtesy of NYSORA.com)

3. In patients who have presented late, there may also be paresthesia. This is a late sign and suggests that irreversible damage has already been caused.
4. Increased pain when the muscles within a compartment are passively stretched.
5. A firm tense compartment (Not particularly specific or sensitive)

The best of these clinical signs of compartment syndrome is pain out of proportion to injury and analgesia received. This can rapidly increase, and therefore multiple ongoing evaluations are required to ensure that compartment syndrome is picked up early. However, these clinical signs and symptoms have a positive predictive value of between 11% and 19%. The specificity and negative predictive value in lower leg injuries are approximately 98%. This means that "classical" symptoms are more likely to be present in patients without compartment syndrome than those with it. Patients with injuries serious enough to put them at risk of compartment syndrome are highly unlikely to be pain free, so even a 98% negative predictive value is of little use. Compartment pressure measurement is the only objective and accurate test to diagnose and monitor compartment syndrome, and any severe pain should prompt the measurement of pressures unless it is a patently obvious clinical diagnosis that requires urgent treatment. Whilst not a sensitive test, or specific, the presence of a tense compartment should also prompt investigation. In patients that are unable to communicate or have neurological injuries, continual compartment monitoring should be considered in the acute phase of injury and post-surgery. This includes patients who are sedated and ventilated in ICU.

If compartment syndrome is missed, late signs include decreased sensation, muscle weakness, paralysis, diminished pulses and clawing of the digits distally with contractures around joints.

To measure compartment syndrome, either a bespoke compartment pressure monitor like the Stryker compartment monitor can be used (Fig. 33.5), or the introduction of a catheter with multiple slits can be performed. By introducing the catheter into the compartment and then attaching it to a monitor via a pressure transducer in a similar way to measuring the arterial pressure with an arterial line, compartment pressure can be transduced. This method is also useful in moribund patients who cannot complain of pain.

It is essential to maintain a high index of suspicion and continue to reassess for compartment syndrome. If compartment syndrome is suspected, then anything which is increasing the external pressure on a compartment should be removed. This includes reducing a dressing, splint or cast down to the skin for the full length of the limb. The limb should not be elevated or lowered, but should instead be kept level with the heart, which aids arterial blood flow and venous return. It is important to treat the pain; however, care should be employed as to not mask the pain completely which may lead to false reassurance that the compartment syndrome has spontaneously settled. To reduce the hypoxia in the compartment, as a temporary measure the patient should be put on high flow oxygen, and hypotension should be addressed with blood products if appropriate to increase the diastolic pressure and improve the oxygen-carrying capacity of the blood.

The definitive treatment of compartment syndrome is Fasciotomy to decompress all the involved compartments fully. This should be treated as a surgical emergency, as delays in performing fasciotomy increase morbidity, including the need for amputation. In patients who have had a delayed presentation to hospital and the muscle within the compartment is believed to be dead, Fasciotomy should be avoided as it can increase the risk of infection and mortality. In these patients, debridement of the dead tissue should be planned as an elective procedure, particularly if there are systemic metabolic issues due to the dead muscles such as rhabdomyolysis and renal failure. In some cases, amputation may be the only option.

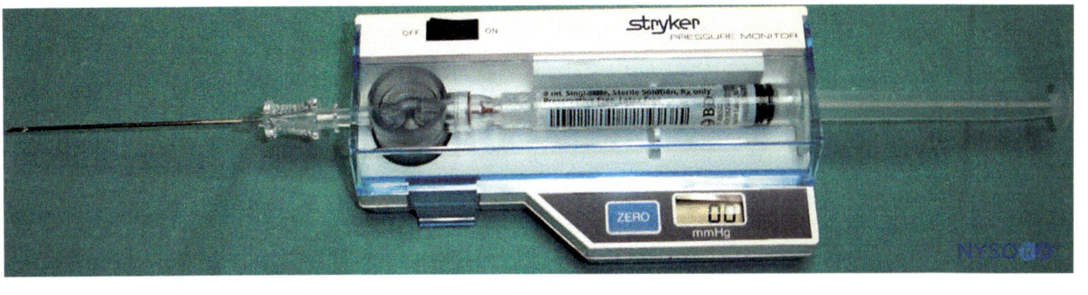

Fig. 33.5 Stryker compartment pressure monitor (Courtesy of NYSORA.com)

All the compartments in the upper or lower part of the limb must be decompressed along the full length. For tibial compartment syndrome, this requires a dual incisional approach. One incision is performed halfway between the fibula and the crest of the tibia for the whole length of the lower leg with the anterior and lateral compartments released through this incision. A second incision is then made 2 cm medial to the posterior border of the tibia along the length of the lower leg to allow the release of the deep and superficial posterior compartments (Fig. 33.6).

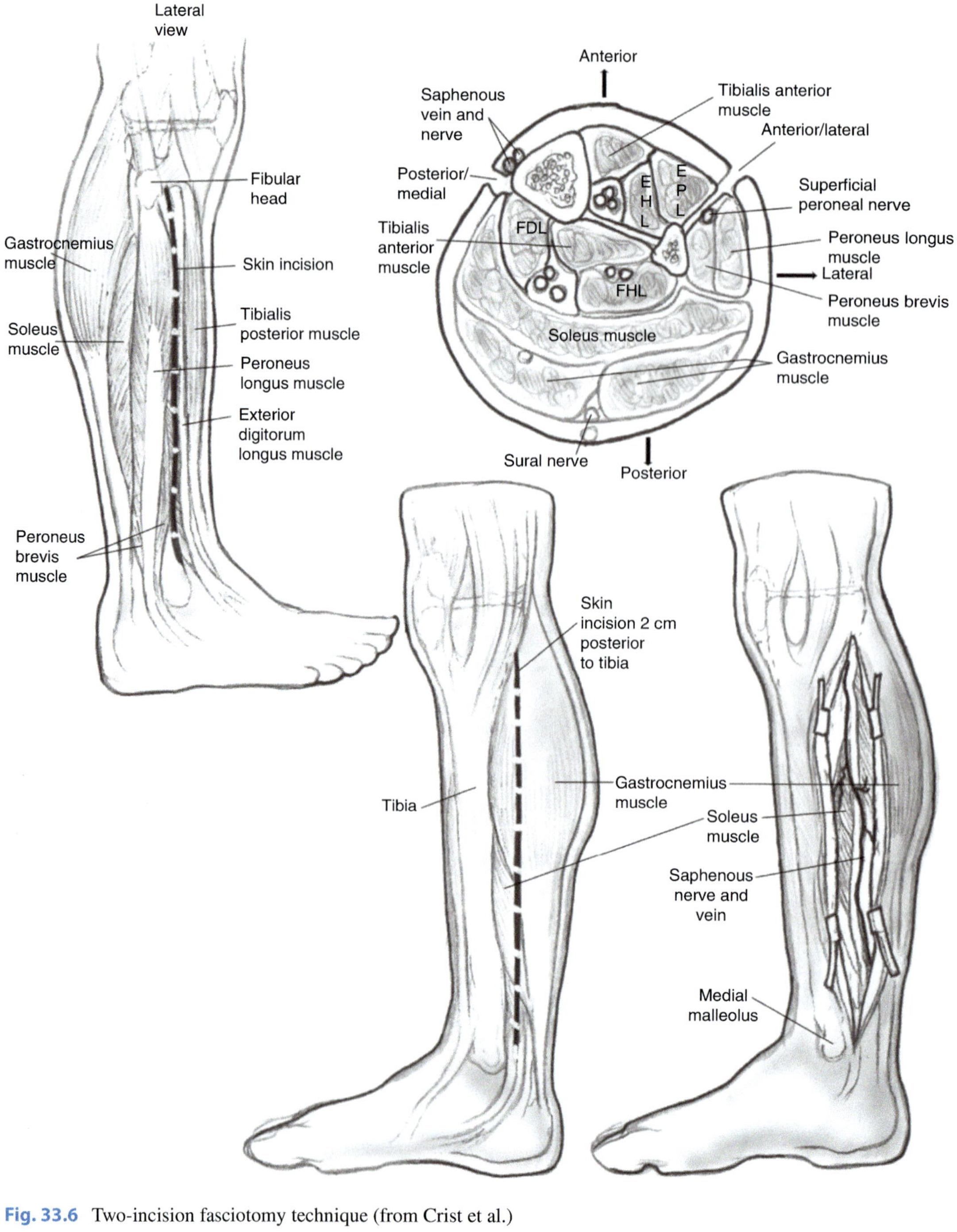

Fig. 33.6 Two-incision fasciotomy technique (from Crist et al.)

Management of Upper Limb Injuries

Upper Limb-Limb Salvage

Limb salvage in the upper limb is attempted in most patients, even when the limb is regarded as mangled. The exception to this rule is in patients who need to have the limb amputated to preserve their life. This is as a result of various studies which have demonstrated that patients who have limb salvage have a higher satisfaction rate than those who have a primary amputation, despite significant improvements in upper limb prosthetics. Even in limbs that only have a few degrees of function and no active movement of digits, patients still report a degree of satisfaction. However, not all limbs are salvageable, and in patients where this is not possible, consideration must be made to keep the length of the residual limb as long as possible following amputation.

In patients who have a severely mangled limb, it is important to perform damage control surgery. This will include the external fixation of the fractures to allow temporary shunting of vascular structures. Where possible, nerves should be identified and flagged for later reconstruction. Initial debridement should include the removal of contaminants and devitalised tissue and decompression of the compartments, including the carpal tunnel. Subsequent surgical episodes should allow internal fixation of fractures and reconstruction of the vascular structures, repair and decompression of the peripheral nerves plus soft tissue coverage.

In upper limb patients, reimplantation of the hand and digits can be performed between 6 and 12 h for warm ischaemia and 12–25 h for cold ischaemia. This is due to the reduced amount of muscle in the hand and fingers which means that they do not suffer the same amount of damage by delayed revascularisation as forearm injuries.

In the upper limb, definitive fixation is generally done with internal fixation, however in cases of significant bone loss and other high energy fractures, Ilizarov fixation can be performed. However, the humerus can be shortened by up to 4 cm without a significant loss of function.

Finger Fractures

Distal phalanx fractures are often associated with a nail bed injury or open fracture. Most of these can be managed by repair of the nail bed and splinting alone, however fractures that are slightly more proximal are rotationally unstable and should be fixed with two or more Kirchner wires to prevent non-union. There is increasing use of screws to fix these fractures, although the outcomes are similar to fixation with Kirchner wires.

In the middle and proximal phalanx, there is an increased complication rate due to the presence of tendons over these bones which can cause adhesions. Where possible these fractures should be managed with K-wires and early mobilization, however in fractures that are more unstable plate and screw fixation may be preferable to allow early mobilisation.

The most common place for metacarpal fractures is at the neck with the fifth metacarpal being the most commonly injured. Most of these fractures can be managed non-operatively with a splint. Where reduction is required these can often be done closed, however where the fracture is unstable, the use of K-wire fixation is advised.

The more proximal the fracture in a metacarpal, the more force is placed over the dorsal aspect of the metacarpal. This can lead to the displacement of fractures along the metacarpal shaft. In these patients, it is often appropriate to place a mini-fragment plate to counteract these forces. A fracture near to the carpal-metacarpal joint is often associated with a dislocation. These dislocations are unstable and cannot typically be managed by splinting alone, so K-wire fixation should be considered to maintain the fracture dislocation in a reduced position.

Carpal Fractures

There are complex forces that transmit through the carpal bones and practitioners managing fractures in this area should also take into account the complex ligamentous structures that give stability in this area.

The most commonly injured carpal bone is the scaphoid, and this has unique challenges in its management due in part to its vascular supply. A branch of the radial artery inserts in the distal portion of the scaphoid, potentially causing avascular necrosis of the proximal fragment and delayed healing if disrupted. This injury pattern is in part due to the complex forces that are transmitted over the scaphoid bone. As a result, many surgeons will internally fix these fractures, although they can also be managed conservatively in a cast for a prolonged period. In higher energy injuries, fractures of the scaphoid can be associated with carpal ligament injuries, including perilunate dislocations. In these fractures, it is vital to repair the ligaments as well as fixing the scaphoid fracture.

Whilst other carpal bones can be injured, due to the complexities in their management, early referral to specialist hand surgeons should be considered.

Radius and Ulnar Fractures

Radius and Ulnar shaft fractures need to be anatomically reduced because they are intimately linked by the interosseous membrane and a combination of ligaments If not reduced correctly, this means that any deformity will severely restrict forearm rotation.

Distal radial fractures have a bimodal distribution, with high energy fractures being recognised as a cause of distal radial fractures in young patients. Most high energy distal radial fractures can be managed with internal fixation, however where there is minimal bone stock available, a combination of bridging external fixation and K-wires can be considered. In lower functioning individuals, bridging the wrist with a metaphyseal plate until union of the fragments may be considered, as well as primary fusion in fractures that are deemed un-reconstructable.

Distal Humeral Fractures

High energy distal humeral fractures in adults can lead to non-union due to the forces that are transmitted across the elbow. These are generally managed with dual plate fixation to afford rotational stability. In lower-functioning adults, it may be preferable to manage the fracture with arthroplasty rather than attempting to hold osteoporotic fragments with plates and screws.

Humeral Shaft Fractures

Most humeral shaft fractures can be managed conservatively, however in the multiply injured patient fixation may be considered to help with rehabilitation. Internal fixation of humeral shaft fractures should also be considered in transverse fractures due to the prolonged healing time. These fractures can be fixed using plates or Intramedullary nails. However, the intramedullary nail disrupts the rotator cuff, and this should be considered before using this as the preferred option.

Management of Lower Limb Fractures

It is essential that good reduction and fixation is achieved in lower limb fractures, as inadequate reduction or fixation may delay rehabilitation and increase morbidity. The principle of treatment should be a stable construct that allows early mobilization and weight-bearing where possible, with minimal surgical insult. The treatment aims should be to restore alignment, length, rotation and function. Whilst this is not exhaustive of all the fractures that can be sustained in the lower limb, the major fracture patterns seen in Major Trauma are discussed. Open fractures are considered later on in the chapter. All lower limb fractures have a high risk of thromboembolism, so chemical or mechanical thromboprophylaxis should be instigated following local guidelines.

Neck of Femur Fractures

To understand the management of neck of femur fractures it is essential to understand the blood

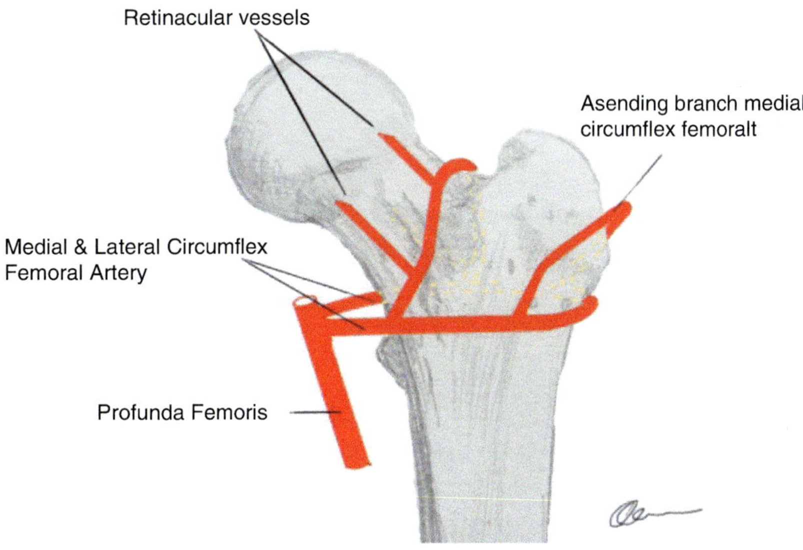

Fig. 33.7 Vascular supply to the femoral head, courtesy of Andre Keenan

supply to the femoral head (Fig. 33.7). In the elderly, there is high mortality in Neck of Femur fractures, and there are comprehensive guidelines on their management which is beyond the scope of this chapter. Initial treatment in the emergency department should contain analgesia and ideally a fascia iliaca block or equivalent.

In inter-capsular fractures, the blood supply is disrupted if the fracture is displaced. Therefore, in the elderly patient, replacement of the femoral head with a cemented prosthesis is the standard treatment protocol. If the patient is higher functioning and would be a candidate for a total hip replacement, then this should be considered as a treatment option in these patients. In frailer patients, a cemented hemiarthroplasty should be the primary treatment option as it is a faster procedure with a lower risk of dislocation. If the fracture is completely undisplaced, internal fixation using cannulated screws into the head is a viable option for the patient and should be considered. In some patients, arthroplasty will remain the preferred treatment option due to the ability to mobilise earlier.

In younger patients who sustain an inter-capsular neck of femur fracture, a CT scan is indicated to assess the degree of displacement and posterior comminution of the neck of the femur. If the fracture is undisplaced, then it should be held reduced using either a combination of cannulated screws or a sliding hip screw and cannulated screw. If there is any displacement to the neck of femur, this should be reduced using the anterior approach to the hip to minimize the risk to the vascular supply to the head, and an open reduction should be performed before the head is stabilized using internal fixation.

For intertrochanteric fractures, the preferred option is to perform a sliding hip screw. This will allow the fracture to compress and has excellent results. In a younger patient, the compression may not be seen as an attractive option and therefore fixing the fracture with an intramedullary nail may be the preferred option. In patients where the fracture is a reverse oblique fracture, meaning that there is no lateral wall for a sliding hip screw to compress the fracture against, the preferred treatment option is an intramedullary nail. Likewise in subtrochanteric fractures, an intramedullary nail is the preferred treatment option (Fig. 33.8).

Femoral Shaft Fractures

In the adult population, femoral shaft fractures are typically managed with intramedullary fixation due to the high rate of success in fracture union using this method. In paediatric populations, there are various considerations which are

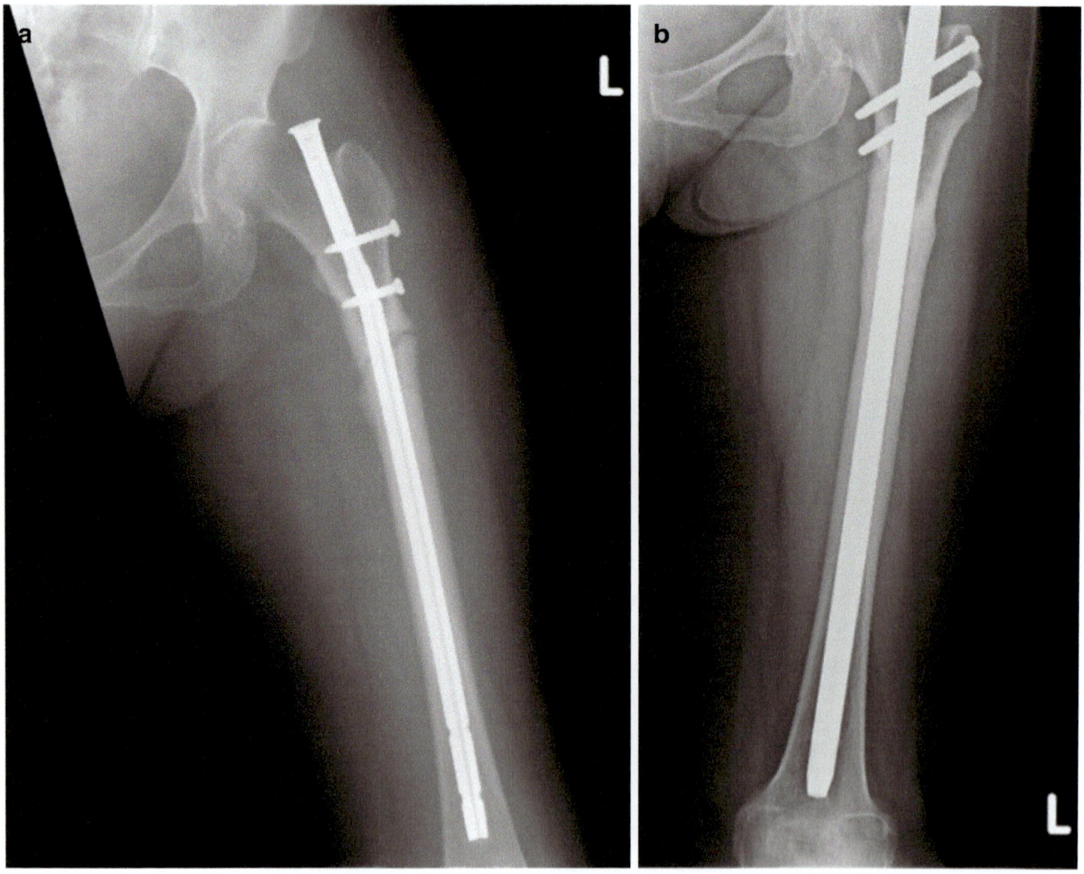

Fig. 33.8 (**a**) Subtrochanteric fracture of the left femur with intramedullary nail fixation, showing poor healing with a broken nail. (**b**) Good union was shown 3 months after the second operation (From Kao et al)

beyond the scope of this chapter. In a closed femoral fracture, the patient should be placed in traction whilst waiting for surgery as this will give them improved comfort, decrease the effective space for blood loss and reduce the risk of fat-embolism. Consideration should be made for utilising a regional block for comfort in these patients, although this should be weighed against the risk of compartment syndrome.

Femoral shaft fractures have a high mortality even in the young patient, and these should be prioritised for fixation within 24 h of arriving in the emergency department. There can be significant blood loss from a femoral fracture; therefore, even in a young adult it is essential to ensure that these patients have been adequately resuscitated. Certain patients will develop fat emboli syndrome which can be fatal, so it is crucial both pre and post-operatively to have regular observations performed on these patients to detect any deterioration.

Where the fracture is open, internal fixation may be considered at the time of debridement as the bone ends are being delivered through a surgical wound. However, most surgeons will then keep the patient partially weight-bearing for a period using this approach. In contrast, in patients managed with intramedullary nailing, there is a tendency to allow full weight-bearing much earlier.

Inter-Articular Distal Femoral Fracture

These patients should be assessed for neurovascular injuries due to the proximity of the neurovascular bundle posteriorly. Along with femoral shaft fractures, these are significant injuries. Therefore they should be fixed as soon as possible (within 24 h) once the patient has been resuscitated. Initial treatment should include the consideration of a nerve block and skin or skeletal traction. This is for pain relief as well as reducing the potential space for blood loss. 3D imaging should be obtained to understand the inter-articular component of the fracture and to establish if there is an associated Hoffa fracture (intra-articular supracondylar distal femoral fracture, characterised by a fracture in the coronal plane).

The surgical management of these fractures is the reduction of the joint surface with absolute stability. This may be achieved by the percutaneous placements of screws across the joint line or may require plating to achieve the fixation of the joint surface. Once this has been achieved, the reduction of the joint surface block onto the shaft of the femur must be established. This can be done either by a combination of plates or by an inter-medullary nail. The nail can be placed either antegrade from the proximal end of the femur, or retrograde from the distal end of the femur through the knee joint.

Knee Joint Dislocations

Knee dislocations refer to disruption of the ligamentous structures around the knee, as opposed to patellar dislocations. Knee dislocations can occur with or without associated fractures. These are catastrophic injuries which have a high level of neurovascular injuries. The dislocation should be reduced as soon as possible to relieve pressure on the neurovascular structures, and placed into a splint. As soon as this has been done a reassessment should be made. Where there is an obvious disruption to the vasculature, the patient should be taken to theatre with a combination of vascular, plastic and orthopaedic surgeons, ideally within 30 min.

If there are equivocal signs of vascular disruption, then a CT angiogram or standard angiogram should be performed if this can be achieved quickly. This should not delay surgery if required, as disruption beyond 6 h has a high incidence of amputation.

Where there is vascular injury, a shunt should be placed immediately with an external fixator applied to reduce the knee, with fasciotomies performed as described previously. Once this has been established, a formal vascular repair should be performed at this operation if the patient is not having a damage control procedure. Pre-operative planning is required to ensure that the fasciotomy wounds and external fixator do not compromise the ability of the vascular surgeons to perform an arterial repair. If there are any neurological symptoms pre-operatively, then the nerves should be inspected in the zone of injury and the common peroneal nerve should be explored to where it crosses the fibular distally. Definitive stabilization of the knee and closure of the fasciotomies should be planned for a subsequent date around 72 h.

Tibial Plateau Fractures

Tibial plateau fractures should be placed in an above-knee cast in the emergency room for comfort. Surgeons are often very concerned around the use of regional blocks in these patients due to the high incidence of compartment syndrome. Some tibial plateau fractures are similar in injury mechanism to knee dislocations; therefore, a high suspicion of neurovascular injury must be maintained. In patients where this is detected, they should be treated with the same urgency as knee dislocations.

Where the patient is too unwell, or the soft tissue injury is extensive, a bridging external fixator across the knee should be placed as a temporary measure using the principles discussed under the external fixator heading.

Definitive fixation of tibial plateau fractures depends upon the severity of the fracture. In fractures which involve both condyles, circular fixation should be considered. This method has a lower infection rate than dual plating, which has a deep infection rate of up to 20%. Where only one condyle is involved, then most fractures will be treated with internal fixation, or in some instances a combination of screws and a nail. As with distal femoral fractures, the principle is to get absolute stability of the joint surface and then connect the joint to the shaft of the tibia, using either a frame, plate or nail.

Tibial Shaft Fractures

These fractures should be stabilised in the emergency department using a splint. Again, there is concern regarding the high incidence of compartment syndrome. The gold standard for mid-shaft tibial fractures in the UK is to manage these injuries with an inter-medullary nail. In proximal third and distal third fractures, it is recognised that it is harder to control these fractures with a nail. Therefore, some centres will manage these with plates, or use pollar screws to control the nail in the proximal or distal fragments. It is the author's preference to use circular frames in proximal third fractures and distal third fractures and in multi-fragmented tibial shaft fractures. This is due to the decrease in the incidence of anterior knee pain, decreased compartment syndrome and the ability to accurately reduce these proximal and distal fragments without the need for soft tissue stripping. Other benefits include improved infection rates compared to those seen with plates or the combination of plates and nails, and the ability to weight bear on a circular frame immediately.

Regardless of how the tibial fractures are reduced, it is essential that the alignment and rotation are corrected and that early mobilisation is achieved.

Distal Tibial Fractures and Pilon Fractures

These fractures have a high incidence of soft tissue complications, and it is essential to document the neurovascular status and have a high suspicion for compartment syndrome as these are high energy injuries with axial loading. Along with tibial plateau fractures, these are associated with other injuries including calcaneal fractures, femoral shaft fractures, occult femoral neck fractures and pelvic and spinal injuries, so a thorough assessment of the patient must be performed.

Pilon fractures are distal tibial fractures that involve the ankle joint and are named after the French word for pestle. The name is a description of the high energy axial compression force of the tibia as it acts as a pestle, driving vertically into the talus in these fractures. The initial management is splintage in the emergency department to allow swelling to occur and for comfort. Again, there is concern in these fractures regarding the high incidence of compartment syndrome.

Pilon fractures will swell quickly, so if definitive fixation cannot be achieved expeditiously, reduction with a temporary external fixator should be performed. This allows the soft tissue to settle, with definitive fixation subsequently performed around 10 days post-injury depending on the resolution of swelling. 3D images should be obtained in the external fixator to aid definitive fixation. As with other interarticular fractures, the main principle of management is to reduce the fracture surface with absolute stability and then reattach the joint surface to the shaft of the tibia.

Definitive fixation depends on the fracture pattern, and there is a significant rate of deep infection with internal fixation where there is a full articular fracture. Therefore, the author manages these predominantly with a circular ring fixator to mitigate this issue and avoid internal metalwork becoming infected. In partial articular fractures, the best management is with internal fixation. In certain patients with significant soft tissue injury and who are low functioning, ankle fusion may be an option. This can be achieved using an intramedullary nail placed into the talus antegrade, or a retrograde nail from the calcaneus through the talus and into the tibia.

Foot and Ankle Fractures

These are frequently missed in Major Trauma, as they are often associated with other more significant injuries, and trauma CT scans may not be distal enough to pick them up incidentally in intubated patients. However, a detailed second and tertiary referral must be made on the foot and ankle, and in moribund patients, any delayed swelling in this area must prompt imaging. In particular, the patient should be investigated for calcaneal or talar fractures and Lisfranc injuries. The management of ankle fractures generally follows the standard principles of ankle fractures, and foot fractures often require fixation to be delayed 7–10 days until swelling has returned to normal. There is an increasing trend to manage calcaneal fractures non-operatively due to the soft tissue complications, and further discussion on these complex fractures is beyond the scope of this book.

Management of Open Fractures

In the UK the method of management of open fractures is currently described in guidelines from the British Orthopaedic Association (BOA) and British Association of Plastic, Reconstructive and Aesthetic Surgeons (BAPRAS) in the British Orthopaedic Association Standards for Trauma (BOAST) Open Fracture Guideline, and national guidelines from the National Institute for Health and Clinical Excellence (NICE). This highlights that the treatment of open fractures requires early antibiotic prophylaxis, tetanus toxoid administration, consultant-led orthoplastic input and early debridement with soft tissue coverage and bone stabilisation within 72 h.

Open fractures are classified using the Gustilo Classification, which classifies and quantifies the degree of soft tissue injury and to guide treatment.

- Type 1 fractures have a wound ≤1 cm, with minimal contamination or muscle damage.
- Type II have a wound 1–10 cm and moderate soft tissue injury.
- Type IIIA have a wound usually >10 cm, high energy, with extensive soft-tissue damage.
- Type IIIB have extensive periosteal stripping, a wound requiring soft tissue coverage (rotational or free flap).
- Type IIIC having a vascular injury requiring vascular repair, regardless of the degree of soft tissue injury.

When an open fracture attends the emergency department, the patient must be assessed in its entirety and managed per standard resuscitative protocols. The limb must be evaluated for neurovascular compromise, and any acute haemorrhage should be controlled with direct pressure plus a tourniquet if required. The wound should be photographed and gross contamination removed, then dressed and protected with a temporary splint. Antibiotics and tetanus prophylaxis must be initiated early, and antibiotics should be continued until definitive wound closure is achieved. As a minimum, x-rays taken at 90 degrees to each other should be obtained and include the joint above and below the fracture. As noted elsewhere, 3D imaging should also be obtained where available to aid surgical planning.

The timing of surgical intervention should be within 24 h by a consultant in orthopaedics and a consultant in plastics who have experience in managing open fractures. The only deviation from this should be if there is significant contamination, impending compartment syndrome, vascular compromise, or in a multi-injured patient the requirement to proceed to surgery earlier for other conditions.

The surgical management of open fractures requires pre-operative planning and should be performed by a combined orthoplastic team. These injuries require a systematic approach to the wound, with debridement performed on necrotic and contaminated tissue from superficial to deep and protection of neurovascular structures. The bone ends should be delivered through the wound and debrided. Once debridement is complete, the wound should be irrigated with a minimum of 9 litres of Normal Saline to ensure that any contamination is flushed out of the wound. Pulse lavage and other pressured delivery systems should be avoided to prevent contaminants from being pushed into clean tissue. Dead bone should be removed (except for metaphyseal fragments which incorporate the inter-articular surfaces), as overall the risk of retention may be outweighed by the benefit. Where soft tissue coverage can be achieved, it is reasonable to internally fix the patient either with screws and plates or inter-medullary nailing. Where is it is not possible to get soft tissue cover at the index operation, the patient should be stabilised using an external fixator and the wound dressed with either a negative pressure dressing or similar. There should be a planned second look and definitive closure within 72 h. When definitive closure has been achieved, internal fixation may be performed. In some cases, a definitive external fixation device like an Ilizarov frame may be applied at this sitting or later on (Fig. 33.9).

The Management of Bone Loss

There are several options available for the management of bone loss following open fractures and debridement. This is particularly relevant in Tibial fractures where there is a high level of infection and non-union following open tibial fractures.

Options available are to acutely shorten the bone and perform a corticotomy proximally, using circular frames or other monolateral external fixators. This can then be used to lengthen the bone through the corticotomy, using osteogenesis to fill in the gap over a period of weeks to months. Alternatively, it is possible to leave a gap and perform a corticotomy proximally and move a fragment of bone down to dock into the distal fragment. Again, this can be done using circular frames, balanced wire transport or monolateral fixators. This should only be done by surgeons specialising in this area. Similar principles can now be employed with telescoping intramedullary nails.

For centres that do not have the ability to perform bone transport, then it is possible to bone graft defects. Due to the high incidence of infec-

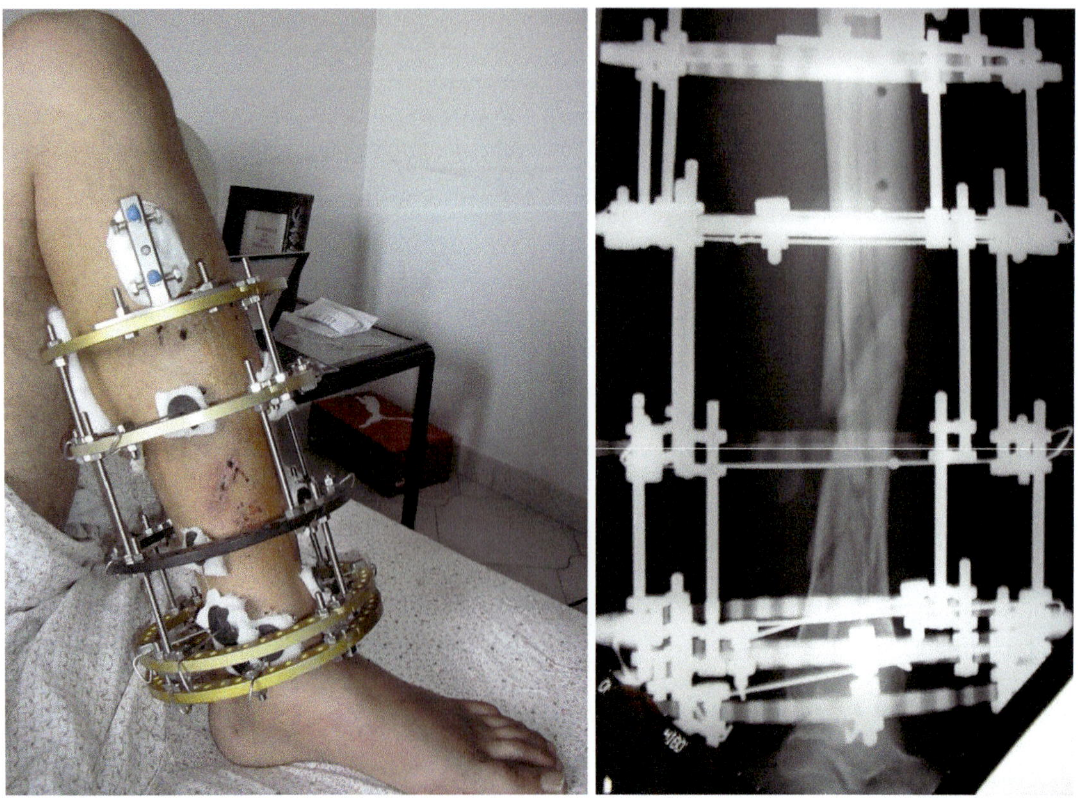

Fig. 33.9 X-ray and photograph of Ilizarov frame in use for a distal tibial fracture (Courtesy of Viapastrengo under Creative Commons Attribution-Share Alike 3.0 license)

tion in open fractures, one of the methods that has the best results is the Masquelet technique. In this technique, the bone defect is filled with cement around the intramedullary nail or plate that is fixing the fracture in position. After around 6 weeks the cement is removed, leaving a membrane that was around the bone cement. This membrane is then packed with bone graft with the intention that this will then remodel and fill the gap.

In certain patients, it is not practical to use bone lengthening and it is reasonable to manage the injury by reducing the length of the limb and getting bone apposition. The limb length discrepancy can then be managed using heel raises.

Decisions on Amputation or Limb Salvage

Whilst it is possible to salvage or reimplant most limbs to one degree or another, it is not always in the patient's best interest to salvage something that does not function or is painful. Likewise, there are general rules for what can be reimplanted. In general, thumbs and multiple digit amputations should be considered for reimplantation. Similarly, injuries to the forearm and more distally should be considered for reimplantation. For injuries proximal to the elbow, results are generally poor unless a very sharp implement has caused an amputation with minimal to no crushing of the tissues. Children do better with reimplantation, and the earlier a limb can be reimplanted, the higher the chance of success. If a limb has been warm and amputated for over 12 h, or if there is significant crushing to the limb or multiple areas of partial amputation then it is not suitable for reimplantation. The pre-morbid and current health of the patient should also be considered.

If it is not possible to salvage or reimplant a limb, then amputation should be performed as early as possible as this decreases the mortality, reduces pain and disability and decreases the length of stay in hospital. It is also important to note that around a quarter of patients who have limb salvage where amputation was being considered undergo amputation within 2 years of initial surgery, even when the initial limb salvage was deemed to be a success. This is due to a variety of factors. Also, patients who have limb salvage will spend longer in hospital than patients who have amputations, require more operative procedures and have more disability than those who undergo amputation. However, over the long term, limb salvage and reconstruction is still seen as beneficial in young patients.

The maxim of "life before limb" is important, and there are some patients who are severely injured where early amputation is essential to save their life due to the metabolic effects of a severely mangled limb. In these patients, even though the limb is technically salvageable, there may be a decision driven by their status at the time which means that there is no choice but to amputate.

Other factors to consider are the level of the injury, the amount of soft tissue injury and contamination and the resultant likelihood of infection and function of a salvaged limb. If the damage is so significant that any salvage option is likely to have a painful, non-functioning or insensate limb, then a well-fitting modern prosthetic on a good amputation may represent a better functional outcome for the patient.

In assessing the viability of a limb, an accurate assessment of the pulses, tissue perfusion, and sensation is essential. The patient should then go to theatre with a minimum of a consultant orthopaedic surgeon and plastic surgeon present. In many cases, a vascular surgeon will also be required to help with the decision making process.

When assessing the limb for salvage, many different scores can be used. The most common trauma score for mangled limbs is the mangled extremity severity score (MESS). In this score, primary amputation is recommended if the cumulative score is over seven.

Skeletal/soft-tissue injury	Points
Low energy (stab; simple fracture; pistol gunshot wound)	1
Medium energy (open or multiple fractures, dislocation)	2
High energy (high-speed vehicular accident or rifle gunshot wound)	3

Very high energy (high-speed trauma + gross contamination)	4
Limb ischemia	
Pulse reduced or absent but perfusion normal	1[a]
Pulseless; paresthesias, diminished capillary refill	2
Cool, paralyzed, insensate, numb	3[a]
Shock	
Systolic BP always >90 mm Hg	0
Hypotensive transiently	1
Persistent hypotension	2
Age (years)	
<30	0
30–50	1
>50	2

[a]Score doubled for ischemia > 6 h

However, all of the systems around do not take into account all the patient variables, and therefore the decision for amputation versus limb salvage should be taken by at least two senior clinicians considering all the potential factors.

Performing a Below Knee Amputation

Whilst there are several different types of amputation available to a trauma surgeon. The most common amputation performed is a below-knee amputation. It is critical to know the anatomy at the level of the desired amputation to understand how to perform a below-knee amputation.

The first stage is to pre-operatively plan where the amputation is going to be performed and if there is enough soft tissue to cover the amputation at the end of the procedure. This needs to be done where possible if time allows with the engagement of the local prosthetic service and a plastic surgeon.

A standard below-knee knee amputation is performed with 10 cm of tibia below the tibial tubercle of the knee. To perform a below-knee amputation, it is necessary to mark out the anterior and posterior flaps, with the posterior flap being 1.5 times longer than the anterior flap. Once the skin flaps are defined, the anterior fascia is divided and the superior and deep peroneal nerves are identified. To decrease problems with the nerve, these are then divided with a new scalpel under gentle traction. The muscle of the anterior compartment is then divided.

The periosteum over the tibia is then elevated into a small flap. Once completed, identify the fibula and cut it a couple of centimetres proximal to the planned tibial cut. Once done, cut the tibia with a saw and saline wash to avoid heat necrosis.

Next, dissect through the posterior structures dividing the muscle and identify the tibial nerve. This should be injected with local anaesthetic, and a nerve catheter may be placed under direct vision to help with immediate post-operative pain. The nerve is divided with a new scalpel under gentle traction then the posterior tibial artery and veins are ligated and divided.

Once this is completed, the tibia is bevelled and drill holes are placed to allow a myodesis of the gastrocnemius. The final step is to close the skin with a drain in situ, and then lots of soft gauze is placed around the residual stump with either wool and crepe or a backslab placed to protect the stump.

Osseous Integration

Whilst prosthetic limbs have improved over the last two decades, trauma patients do not always have a residual limb which is well suited to the traditional method of attaching the limb with a custom-designed socket. This can lead to irritation of the residual stump and periods when the patient is unable to use a prosthesis.

To combat this, new techniques have been developed which enable the prosthesis to be directly attached to the skeleton. This technique is called osseointegration, which is where there is a direct connection between the residual skeleton and the metal implant.

This technique is currently limited to a few centres within the UK with very tight control over which patients fit the criteria for these interventions. It is likely that as the techniques improve and outcomes continue to improve that osseointegration will become more frequently used for patients sustaining amputation as a result of trauma.

Summary

Limb injuries in Major Trauma are best thought of as a soft tissue injury with an associated fracture. The management of fractures can be temporary if required or definitive dependent upon the condition of the patient. It is crucial to have a multidisciplinary approach and peri-operative plan in the management of fractures in a Major Trauma patient. A high suspicion of other injuries is required, and knowledge of the neurovascular anatomy is essential to improve patient outcomes.

Questions and Answers

Question 1. When assessing the sensory function of the lower limb. Which of the following nerves supplies the dorsal aspect of the 1st webspace:

A. A Deep Peroneal
B. Superficial Peroneal
C. Tibial Nerve
D. Femoral Nerve
E. Obturator Nerve

Answer: A. The deep peroneal supplies the dorsal aspect of the 1st Webspace. The superficial peroneal supplies the dorsum of the foot apart from the 1st webspace. The Tibial nerve supplies the sole of the foot, with the obturator nerve supplying the middle of the medial surface of the thigh and the femoral nerve supplying the anteromedial thigh.

Question 2. The Anterior Compartment of the Leg contains the following structure:

A. Deep Peroneal Nerve
B. Superficial Peroneal Nerve
C. Peroneus Longus
D. Tibial Nerve
E. Flexor hallucis Longus

Answer: A. The Deep Peroneal Nerve. The Superficial Peroneal nerve is in the lateral compartment along with peroneus longus. The tibial nerve and flexor hallucis longus is in the posterior compartment.

Question 3. When using the Gustilo Classification, a wound that is 5 cm long sustained after a fracture with moderate soft tissue injury is graded as:

A. Type 1
B. Type 2
C. Type 3A
D. Type 3B
E. Type 3 C

Answer: B Type 2.

Question 4

- Type 1 fractures have a wound ≤1 cm, with minimal contamination or muscle damage.
- Type II have a wound 1–10 cm and moderate soft tissue injury.
- Type IIIA have a wound usually >10 cm, high energy, with extensive soft-tissue damage.
- Type IIIB have extensive periosteal stripping, a wound requiring soft tissue coverage (rotational or free flap).
- Type IIIC having a vascular injury requiring vascular repair, regardless of the degree of soft tissue injury.

When Inserting Local into a fascio-iliaca block. The local anaesthetic should be placed superficial to:

A. Internal Oblique Muscle
B. Rectus Abdominis
C. Iliacus Muscle
D. Sartorius Muscle
E. Quadriceps Femoris Muscle

Answer C. The local is placed anterior to Iliacus Muscle and deep to internal oblique and sartorius muscle.

Question 5. When using a MESS score, a high energy gunshot wound with a cool paralysed insensate numb foot, and in a 60 year old patient with a persistent hypotension for 8 hours scores the following:

A. 9
B. 10

C. 11
D. 12
E. 13

Answer: E

A gunshot wound scores 3, a cool paralysed foot that is insensate and numb for greater than 6 hours scores 6 and persistent hypotension 2 and age over 50 scores 2. Total 13.

Bibliography

1. Alarhayem AQ, Cohn SM, Cantu-Nunez O, et al. Impact of time to repair on outcomes in patients with lower extremity arterial injuries. J Vasc Surg. 2019;69:1519.
2. Allsopp BJ, Hunter-Smith DJ, Rozen WM. Vascularized versus nonvascularized bone grafts: what is the evidence? Clin Orthop Relat Res. 2016;474:1319.
3. Amputations. In: Emergency war surgery: 3rd United States Revision, Chapter 25, Washington, DC: Department of the Army, Office of the Surgeon General, Borden Institute, 2004.
4. Anderson JT, Gustilo RB. Immediate internal fixation in open fractures. Orthop Clin North Am. 1980;11:569.
5. Applebaum R, Yellin AE, Weaver FA, et al. Role of routine arteriography in blunt lower extremity trauma. Am J Surg. 1990;160:221.
6. Arrillaga A, Bynoe R, Frykbert E, et al: Practice management guidelines for penetrating trauma to the lower extremity. EAST practice management work group. Eastern Association for the Surgery of Trauma; 2000.
7. Attebery LR, Dennis JW, Russo-Alesi F, et al. Changing patterns of arterial injuries associated with fractures and dislocations. J Am Coll Surg. 1996;183:377.
8. Baumbach SF, Schmidt R, Varga P, et al. Where is the distal fracture line location of dorsally displaced distal radius fractures? J Orthop Res. 2011;29:489.
9. Bhandari M, Zlowodzki M, Tornetta P 3rd, et al. Intramedullary nailing following external fixation in femoral and tibial shaft fractures. J Orthop Trauma. 2005;19:140.
10. Bishara RA, Pasch AR, Lim LT, et al. Improved results in the treatment of civilian vascular injuries associated with fractures and dislocations. J Vasc Surg. 1986;3:707.
11. Borut LT, Acosta CJ, Tadlock LC, et al. The use of temporary vascular shunts in military extremity wounds: a preliminary outcome analysis with 2-year follow-up. J Trauma. 2010;69:174.
12. Bosse MJ, MacKenzie EJ, Kellam JF, et al. An analysis of outcomes of reconstruction or amputation of leg- threatening injuries. N Engl J Med. 2002;347:1924.
13. Boykin RE, Baskies MA, Harrod CC, Jupiter JB. Intraoperative distraction in the upper extremity. Tech Hand Up Extrem Surg. 2009;13:75.
14. Brown KV, Murray CK, Clasper JC. Infectious complications of combat-related mangled extremity injuries in the British military. J Trauma. 2010;69(Suppl 1):S109.
15. Brumback RJ, Ellison PS Jr, Poka A, et al. Intramedullary nailing of open fractures of the femoral shaft. J Bone Joint Surg Am. 1989;71:1324.
16. Burkhardt GE, Cox M, Clouse WD, et al. Outcomes of selective tibial artery repair following combat-related extremity injury. J Vasc Surg. 2010;52:91.
17. Chung KC, Saddawi-Konefka D, Haase SC, Kaul G. A cost-utility analysis of amputation versus salvage for Gustilo type IIIB and IIIC open tibial fractures. Plast Reconstr Surg. 2009;124:1965.
18. Chung KC, Shauver MJ, Yin H, et al. Variations in the use of internal fixation for distal radial fracture in the United States medicare population. J Bone Joint Surg Am. 2011;93:2154.
19. Crist B, Della Rocca G, Stannard J. Compartment syndrome surgical management techniques associated with Tibial plateau fractures. J Knee Surg. 2010 Aug;23(01):003–7.
20. DaCruz DJ, Slade RJ, Malone W. Fractures of the distal phalanges. J Hand Surg Br. 1988;13:350.
21. Dennis JW, Jagger C, Butcher JL, et al. Reassessing the role of arteriograms in the management of posterior knee dislocations. J Trauma. 1993;35:692.
22. Duncan R, Geissler W, Freeland AE, Savoie FH. Immediate internal fixation of open fractures of the diaphysis of the forearm. J Orthop Trauma. 1992;6:25.
23. Durham RM, Mistry BM, Mazuski JE, et al. Outcome and utility of scoring systems in the management of the mangled extremity. Am J Surg. 1996;172:569.
24. Feliciano DV, Accola KD, Burch JM, et al. Extraanatomic bypass for peripheral arterial injuries. Am J Surg. 1989;158:506.
25. Feliciano DV, Cruse PA, Spjut-Patrinely V, et al. Fasciotomy after trauma to the extremities. Am J Surg. 1988;156:533.
26. Feliciano DV, Mattox KL, Graham JM, et al. Five-year experience with PTFE grafts in vascular wounds. J Trauma. 1985;25(1):71–82.
27. Galano GJ, Ahmad CS, Levine WN. Current treatment strategies for bicolumnar distal humerus fractures. J Am Acad Orthop Surg. 2010;18:20.
28. Gifford SM, Aidinian G, Clouse WD, et al. Effect of temporary shunting on extremity vascular injury: an outcome analysis from the global war on terror vascular injury initiative. J Vasc Surg. 2009;50:549.
29. Glueck DA, Charoglu CP, Lawton JN. Factors associated with infection following open distal radius fractures. Hand (N Y). 2009;4:330.
30. Gopal S, Majumder S, Batchelor AG, et al. Fix and flap: the radical orthopaedic and plastic treatment of

severe open fractures of the tibia. J Bone Joint Surg Br. 2000;82:959.
31. Gordon WT, O'Brien FP, Strauss JE, et al. Outcomes associated with the internal fixation of long-bone fractures proximal to traumatic amputations. J Bone Joint Surg Am. 2010;92:2312.
32. Gustilo RB, Gruninger RP, Davis T. Classification of type III (severe) open fractures relative to treatment and results. Orthopedics. 1987;10:1781.
33. Gustilo RB, Mendoza RM, Williams DN. Problems in the management of type III (severe) open fractures: a new classification of type III open fractures. J Trauma. 1984;24:742.
34. Hancock H, Rasmussen TE, Walker AJ, Rich NM. History of temporary intravascular shunts in the management of vascular injury. J Vasc Surg. 2010;52:1405.
35. Hay RA, Tay SC. A comparison of K-wire versus screw fixation on the outcomes of distal phalanx fractures. J Hand Surg Am. 2015;40:2160.
36. Howe HR, Poole GV, Hansen KJ, et al. Salvage of lower extremities following combined orthopedic and vascular trauma: a predictive salvage index. Am Surg. 1987;53:205.
37. Huh J, Stinner DJ, Burns TC, et al. Infectious complications and soft tissue injury contribute to late amputation after severe lower extremity trauma. J Trauma. 2011;71:S47.
38. Johansen K, Daines M, Howey T, et al. Objective criteria accurately predict amputation following lower extremity trauma. J Trauma. 1990;30:568.
39. Kao C-M, Huang P-J, Chen C-H, Chen S-J, Cheng Y-M. Atypical femoral fracture after long-term alendronate treatment: report of a case evidenced with magnetic resonance imaging. Kaohsiung J Med Sci. 2012 Oct;28(10):555–8.
40. Kaufman SL, Martin LG. Arterial injuries associated with complete dislocation of the knee. Radiology. 1992;184:153.
41. Kendall RW, Taylor DC, Salvian AJ, et al. The role of arteriography in assessing vascular injuries associated with dislocations of the knee. J Trauma. 1993;35:875.
42. Khalil IM, Livingston DH. Intravascular shunts in complex lower limb trauma. J Vasc Surg. 1986;4:582.
43. Khan F, Amatya B, Hoffman K. Systematic review of multidisciplinary rehabilitation in patients with multiple trauma. Br J Surg. 2012;99(Suppl 1):88.
44. Lee FY, Schoeb JS, Yu J, et al. Operative lengthening of the humerus: indications, benefits, and complications. J Pediatr Orthop. 2005;25:613.
45. Lin CH, Aydyn N, Lin YT, et al. Hand and finger replantation after protracted ischemia (more than 24 hours). Ann Plast Surg. 2010;64:286.
46. MacKay BJ, Montero N, Paksima N, Egol KA. Outcomes following operative treatment of open fractures of the distal radius: a case control study. Iowa Orthop J. 2013;33:12.
47. MacKenzie EJ, Bosse MJ, Kellam JF, et al. Factors influencing the decision to amputate or reconstruct after high-energy lower extremity trauma. J Trauma. 2002;52:641.
48. MacKenzie EJ, Bosse MJ, Pollak AN, et al. Long-term persistence of disability following severe lower-limb trauma. Results of a seven-year follow-up. J Bone Joint Surg Am. 2005;87:1801.
49. Marks MW, Friedman RJ, Thornton JW, Argenta LC. The temporal island scalp flap for management of facial burn scars. Plast Reconstr Surg. 1988;82:257.
50. Martinez D, Sweatman K, Thompson EC. Popliteal artery injury associated with knee dislocations. Am Surg. 2001 Feb;67(2):165–7.
51. Mathieu L, Bertani A, Gaillard C, et al. Surgical management of combat-related upper extremity injuries. Chir Main. 2014;33:174.
52. McGuinness B, Ali KP, Phillips S, Stacey M. A scoping review on the use of antibiotic-impregnated beads and applications to vascular surgery. Vasc Endovasc Surg. 2020;54:147.
53. McHenry TP, Holcomb JB, Aoki N, Lindsey RW. Fractures with major vascular injuries from gunshot wounds: implications of surgical sequence. J Trauma. 2002;53:717.
54. McKee MD, Veillette CJ, Hall JA, et al. A multicenter, prospective, randomized, controlled trial of open reduction—internal fixation versus total elbow arthroplasty for displaced intra-articular distal humeral fractures in elderly patients. J Shoulder Elb Surg. 2009;18:3.
55. McNamara JJ, Brief DK, Stremple JF, et al. Management of fractures with associated arterial injury in combat casualties. J Trauma. 1973;13:17.
56. Melvin JS, Dombroski DG, Torbert JT, et al. Open tibial shaft fractures: I. Evaluation and initial wound management. J Am Acad Orthop Surg. 2010;18:10.
57. Melvin JS, Dombroski DG, Torbert JT, et al. Open tibial shaft fractures: II. Definitive management and limb salvage. J Am Acad Orthop Surg. 2010;18:108.
58. Miranda FE, Dennis JW, Veldenz HC, et al. Confirmation of the safety and accuracy of physical examination in the evaluation of knee dislocation for popliteal artery injury: a prospective study. J Trauma. 2000;49:375.
59. Moed BR, Kellam JF, Foster RJ, et al. Immediate internal fixation of open fractures of the diaphysis of the forearm. J Bone Joint Surg Am. 1986;68:1008.
60. Moehring HD, Gravel C, Chapman MW, Olson SA. Comparison of antibiotic beads and intravenous antibiotics in open fractures. Clin Orthop Relat Res. 2000;372:254–61.
61. Mubarak SJ, Hargens AR. Acute compartment syndromes. Surg Clin North Am. 1983;63:539.
62. Nellans KW, Kowalski E, Chung KC. The epidemiology of distal radius fractures. Hand Clin. 2012;28:113.
63. Norman J, Gahtan V, Franz M, et al. Occult vascular injuries following gunshot wounds resulting in long bone fractures of the extremities. Am Surg. 1995;61(2):146–50.
64. Orbay J. Volar plate fixation of distal radius fractures. Hand Clin. 2005;21:347.

65. Palazzo JC, Ristow AB, Cury JM, et al. Traumatic vascular lesions associated with fractures and dislocations. J Cardiovasc Surg. 1986;27:688.
66. Pavey GJ, Formby PM, Hoyt BW, et al. Intrawound antibiotic powder decreases frequency of deep infection and severity of heterotopic ossification in combat lower extremity amputations. Clin Orthop Relat Res. 2019;477:802.
67. Penn-Barwell JG. Outcomes in lower limb amputation following trauma: a systematic review and meta-analysis. Injury. 2011;42:1474.
68. Perkins ZB, De'Ath HD, Sharp G, Tai NR. Factors affecting outcome after traumatic limb amputation. Br J Surg. 2012;99(Suppl 1):75.
69. Possley DR, Burns TC, Stinner DJ, et al. Temporary external fixation is safe in a combat environment. J Trauma. 2010;69(Suppl 1):S135.
70. Rasmussen TE, Clouse WD, Jenkins DH, et al. The use of temporary vascular shunts as a damage control adjunct in the management of wartime vascular injury. J Trauma. 2006;61:8.
71. Romanoff H, Goldberger S. Combined severe vascular and skeletal trauma: management and results. J Cardiovasc Surg (Torino). 1979;20(5):493–8.
72. Rozbruch SR, Pugsley JS, Fragomen AT, Ilizarov S. Repair of tibial nonunions and bone defects with the Taylor spatial frame. J Orthop Trauma. 2008;22:88.
73. Scalea TM, DuBose J, Moore EE, et al. Western trauma association critical decisions in trauma: management of the mangled extremity. J Trauma Acute Care Surg. 2012;72:86.
74. Stannard JP, Sheils TM, Lopez-Ben RR, et al. Vascular injuries in knee dislocations: the role of physical examination in determining the need for arteriography. J Bone Joint Surg. 2004;86A:910.
75. Bhandari M, Guyatt G, Study to Prospectively Evaluate Reamed Intramedullary Nails in Patients with Tibial Fractures Investigators, et al. Randomized trial of reamed and unreamed intramedullary nailing of tibial shaft fractures. J Bone Joint Surg Am. 2008;90:2567.
76. Subramanian A, Vercruysse G, Dente C, et al. A decade's experience with temporary intravascular shunts at a civilian level I trauma center. J Trauma. 2008;65:316.
77. Swithick DN, Benjamin JB, Ruth JT. Timing of vascular and orthopedic repair in mangled extremities: does it really matter? J Trauma. 2003;54:211.
78. Treiman GS, Yellin AE, Weaver FA, et al. Examination of the patient with a knee dislocation: the case for selective arteriography. Arch Surg. 1992;127:1056.
79. Volk I, Gal J, Peleg E, et al. Three-dimensional comparison of alternative screw positions versus actual fixation of scaphoid fractures. Injury. 2017;48:1183.
80. Williams MM, Askins V, Hinkes EW, Zych GA. Primary reamed intramedullary nailing of open femoral shaft fractures. Clin Orthop Relat Res. 1995;318:182–90.
81. Wlodarczyk JR, Thomas AS, Schroll R, et al. To shunt or not to shunt in combined orthopedic and vascular extremity trauma. J Trauma Acute Care Surg. 2018;85:1038.
82. Yamamoto M, Murakami Y, Iwatsuki K, et al. Feasibility of four-dimensional preoperative simulation for elbow debridement arthroplasty. BMC Musculoskelet Disord. 2016;17:144.
83. Yoneda H, Iwatsuki K, Hara T, et al. Interindividual anatomical variations affect the plate-to-bone fit during osteosynthesis of distal radius fractures. J Orthop Res. 2016;34:953.

34 Pelvic Trauma

Kathryn Lowery and Nikolaos K. Kanakaris

- Anatomy of the pelvic girdle—bony, ligamentous and vascular
- Pelvic fracture classification
- Initial resuscitation of the patient with a suspected pelvic fracture
- Resuscitation and Management of haemorrhage control in pelvic fractures
- Emergency skeletal stabilisation in pelvic fractures

Introduction

Pelvic fractures are reported to occur rarely; approximately in 3–8% of all trauma patients [1–4], accounting for just 1–3% of all skeletal injuries [3, 5, 6].

Pelvic trauma is usually the result of high energy blunt forces following motor vehicle accidents, crush injuries, or falls from height. However, the most rapidly growing subgroup of pelvic fracture patients over the last decade is the elderly population, presenting with pelvic fractures following low energy trauma and simple falls [7, 8].

Pelvic fractures are often associated with haemodynamic instability, which can be life-threatening in 1–4% of all pelvic fractures, including the low energy ones [9, 10]. High energy pelvic fractures are generally associated with severe injuries to other body regions and organ systems. The presence of a pelvic fracture should be used as an indicator of severe polytrauma until proven otherwise following appropriate diagnostic investigations [11, 12].

In patients who present with a pelvic fracture and haemodynamic instability, registry studies from multiple countries report mortality rates from 8% to 32% [13, 14]. In these cases, the sources of bleeding are most commonly multiple, and less than 10% have been attributed solely to the pelvic girdle [11, 15].

Furthermore, a fractured pelvis may also result in high morbidity and significant lifelong disability. This can either be associated with complications of fracture healing (malunions/nonunions of the bony pelvis), coexisting urogenital trauma, or chronic pain due to injuries to the lumbosacral plexus and major nerves [14, 16, 17].

An essential prerequisite to the effective management of pelvic fractures is the understanding of the anatomy and mechanical features of the pelvic ring.

K. Lowery (✉) · N. K. Kanakaris
Department of Orthopaedic Surgery, Leeds General Infirmary, Leeds, UK
e-mail: Kathryn.lowery1@nhs.net; n.kanakaris@nhs.net

P. Lax (ed.), *Textbook of Acute Trauma Care*, https://doi.org/10.1007/978-3-030-83628-3_34

Anatomy

Skeletal Components

The pelvic girdle essentially connects the axial skeleton to the lower limbs. The functions of the pelvis are to transmit the forces from the axial skeleton to the lower limbs, protect the pelvic viscera and the large neurovascular bundles of the lower extremities, while it is also a major red marrow reservoir and produces the majority of the 2 million red blood cells per second that the body's bone marrow creates.

The bony pelvis has no inherent stability and is formed by the junction of the two innominate bones (right and left) and the sacrum. These form a bony ring which is joined anteriorly at the symphysis pubis, and posteriorly at the two sacroiliac joints. The innominate bones are composed of three parts: the ilium, the ischium and the pubis, which are interconnected via a Y area of hyaline cartilage at the level of the acetabulum. After the end of puberty, they become fused [9] (Fig. 34.1).

Approximately 60–70% of the stresses during standing/sitting/walking are transferred via the posterior pelvic ring to the sacroiliac joints, then towards the pelvic brim via the thick sciatic buttresses, and finally to the hips at each side (Fig. 34.2). The iliac crests and the pubic rami receive fewer stresses and are mostly relevant to the attachment of the large muscle groups of the torso/abdomen and the lower extremities. These muscle groups also contribute to the stability of the pelvic ring. Furthermore, the rami connected at the symphysis pubis act like struts and resist internal rotation-compression forces during single-leg stance and walking.

The bony pelvis is divided into the false or greater pelvis, and the true or lesser pelvis. The false pelvis is a superior and broader compartment, found between the two iliac blades. This part provides support to the abdominal viscera of the ileum and sigmoid colon. The true pelvis is

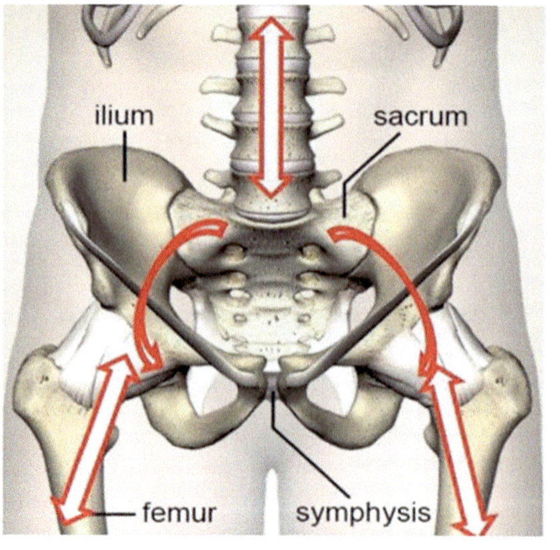

Fig. 34.2 Forces transmitted from axial skeleton to the lower limbs

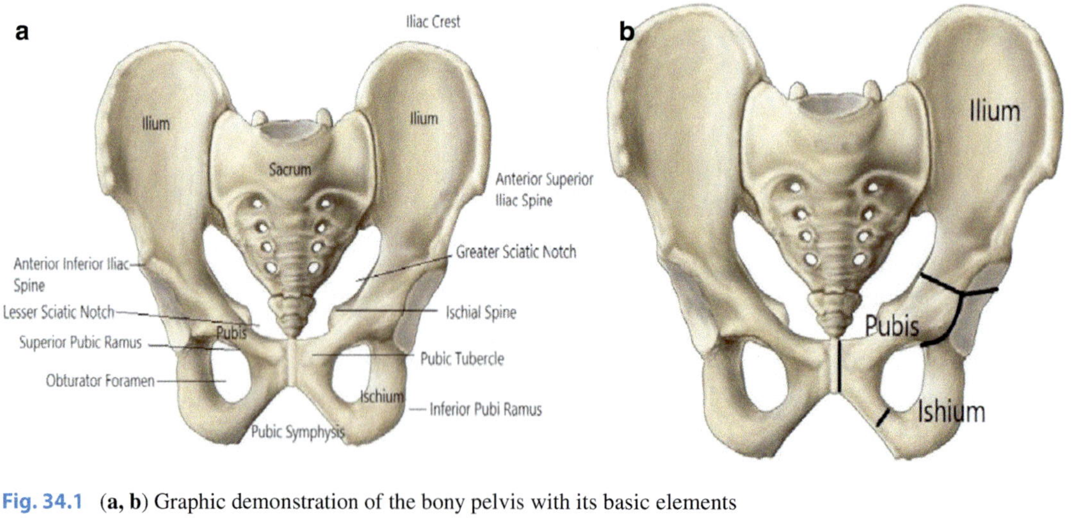

Fig. 34.1 (a, b) Graphic demonstration of the bony pelvis with its basic elements

located more inferiorly and provides support to the pelvic viscera. The border between the two compartments is called linea terminalis or the pelvic brim. This is defined posteriorly from the sacral promontory, anteriorly from the pubic symphysis and laterally from the arcuate line on the inner surface of the two iliums and the pectineal lines of the superior rami.

The exit or outlet of the true pelvis is covered by the pelvic floor muscles (anal sphincter complex and the levator ani muscles), supporting the abdominal and pelvic organs. Between the two genders, there are different anatomical characteristics with the female pelvis being wider and broader, with a shallower true pelvis and less prominent ischial spines than the male pelvis, which has a longer sacrum, deeper true pelvis and a narrow sub-pubic arch.

Ligaments and Joints

The ligaments around the pelvis support and stabilise the bony pelvis and its joints. These are broadly divided into four groups (Fig. 34.3).

The symphysis pubis is a secondary cartilaginous joint. The surfaces are covered by hyaline cartilage and separated by a cartilaginous disc. The ligaments surrounding this joint consist of the anterior pubic ligament, the posterior pubic ligament, the superior pubic ligament, the arcuate pubic ligament, and the interpubic fibrocartilaginous lamina [18]. The "normal" joint space of the symphysis pubis is between 5 and 10 mm.

The sacrococcygeal joint is also a secondary cartilaginous joint, with both an anterior and a posterior ligament. The anterior sacrococcygeal ligament is an extension of the anterior longitudinal ligament. The posterior sacrococcygeal ligament is an extension of the posterior longitudinal ligament [19].

The iliolumbar ligaments represent an additional strong stabilizing component of the spinopelvic elements. They extend bilaterally from the side of the transverse process of the L5 vertebra to the inner lip of the posterior upper iliac crest. These ligaments are responsible for the pathognomonic finding of a mechanically vertically unstable pelvic fracture (i.e. avulsion of the L5 transverse process).

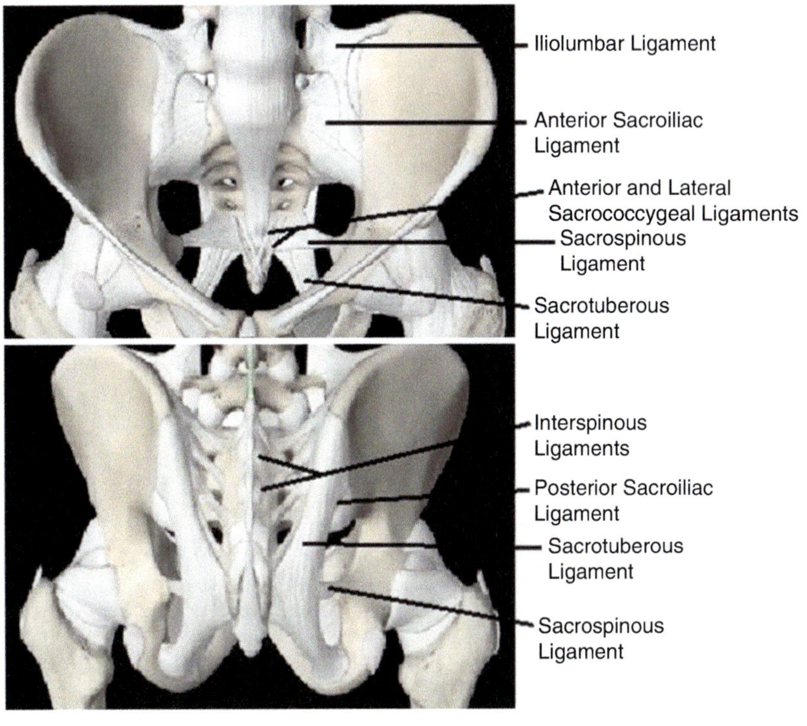

Fig. 34.3 Ligaments of the pelvis, anterior and posterior views

The sacroiliac joints are composed of two parts, the ligamentous part and the articular part. The ligamentous part is located posteriorly, and the articular portion is anterior. The articular part is not truly a synovial joint with the articular cartilage located on the sacral side while the iliac side has fibrous cartilage [20]. The "normal" joint space of the sacroiliac joints is around 2–4 mm.

The main ligaments in this region which are of primary importance to the stability of the pelvic ring consist of:

(a) Anterior sacroiliac ligaments—Not well defined, representing more of a thickening of the anterior capsule of the sacroiliac joints.
(b) Posterior sacroiliac ligaments—These are divided into short and long components. The short posterior sacroiliac ligaments attach from the first and second transverse tubercles on the posterior ridge of the sacrum to the tuberosity of the ilium. The long posterior sacroiliac ligaments attach from the third transverse tubercle on the posterior lateral portion of the sacrum to the superior posterior spine of the ilium.
(c) Sacrospinous ligaments—These attach from the lateral portion of the sacrum to the ischial spines. These ligaments divide the greater and lesser sciatic foramina [20].
(d) Sacrotuberous ligaments—These attach from the posterolateral sacrum and the posterior iliac spines to the ischial tuberosities [20].

Vascular Anatomy

The pelvis is a highly vascular body region which correlates to the high rates of bleeding observed following a pelvic ring injury. The sources of bleeding could be large displaced areas of cancellous bone (mainly the iliac bones or the sacrum), the rich presacral venous plexus or large vessels and their branches.

More specifically, the main arterial tree at the level of the pelvis bilaterally includes the common iliac artery, which is divided into the external and internal iliac arteries at the level of the L4 vertebra. The external iliac artery passes anteriorly along the pelvic brim on the medial side of the psoas muscle and emerges as the common femoral artery distal to the inguinal ligament [21]. The internal iliac artery is divided into an anterior and posterior division at the upper border of the greater sciatic notch [21]. The anterior division gives rise to the inferior gluteal artery, the internal pudendal artery, the obturator artery, the inferior vesical artery and the middle rectal artery [20]. The posterior division gives rise to the superior gluteal artery, the iliolumbar artery and the lateral sacral artery [20].

The common femoral vein (at each side) drains into the external iliac vein at the level of the inguinal ligament, and together with the internal iliac vein form the common iliac vein which eventually drains into the inferior vena cava at the level of the L5 vertebra.

Between them, an extensive plexus of vessels and anastomoses are formed, which are the primary source of haemorrhage in pelvic fractures either due to their proximity to sharp fracture fragments or due to stretching/avulsion at the time of the accident [20]. As previously reported in arteriography clinical studies, the most commonly injured vessels are the branches of the internal iliac arteries, the pudendal and obturator arteries anteriorly and the superior gluteal artery and lateral sacral artery posteriorly [22].

The Corona Mortis (or "Crown of Death") is one of these anastomotic vessels, most commonly between the obturator and the external iliac arterial and/or venous systems. This passes near the superior pubic rami and can easily be injured at the time of the accident or during common surgical procedures such as inguinal hernia repair or the reconstruction of the pelvis and the acetabulum [20, 23, 24] (Fig. 34.4).

Classification of Pelvic Fractures

The Tile classification and the Young and Burgess Classification are both commonly used to classify Pelvic Ring Injuries. The Tile classification

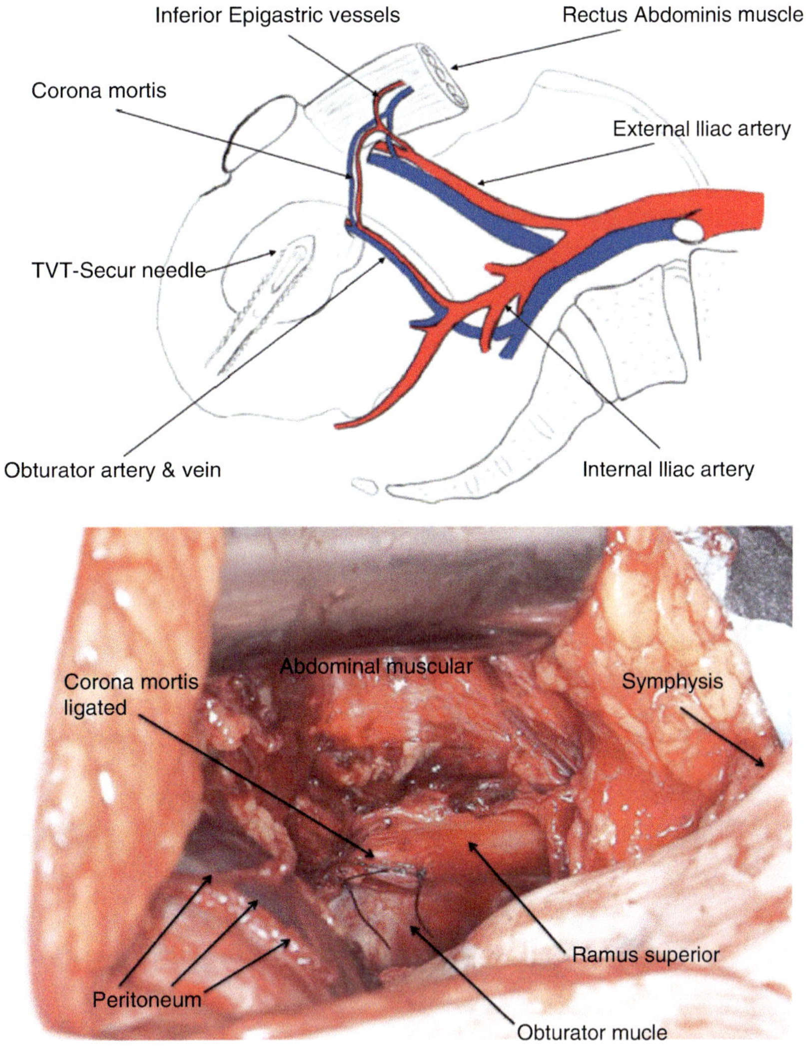

Fig. 34.4 Vascular anatomy in the pelvis with the corona mortis highlighted schematically and in vitro

was first described in 1980 by Tile and Pennal [25]; this classification was based on the force vector involved in the injury. Tile further modified this classification based on the stability of the pelvic ring [26] describing three main types: Type A (stable), Type B (rotationally unstable, vertically stable) and Type C (vertically and rotationally unstable). This classification represents the basis of the widely accepted system of the OTA/AO group [27].

The Young and Burgess classification was introduced in 1986 [28] and is based on the vector of forces/mechanism of injury. It is the most commonly used system by clinicians [28, 29]. In the Young and Burgess classification there are four groups: Lateral Compression (LC), Antero-Posterior Compression (APC), Vertical Shear (VS), and Composite Mechanism of Injury (CMI). These are shown in Table 34.1 and Fig. 34.5.

Management of Pelvic Injuries

As pelvic fractures can be associated with haemorrhage, urogenital trauma and severe injuries in other body regions, they should be treated in hospitals with 24/7 availability of specialists. The ability to provide prompt resuscitation, advanced diagnostic protocols and multidisciplinary expert

Table 34.1 Young and Burgess classification system of pelvic fractures

Types	Subtypes	Anterior pelvic ring lesion	Posterior pelvic ring lesion	Mechanical stability of the pelvic ring
Lateral compression (LC)—"Closed book" Internal rotation vector	LC1	Oblique/buckled rami fracture/s	Compressed sacral wing fracture	Rotationally sometimes unstable Vertically stable
	LC2	Oblique/buckled rami fracture/s	Iliac wing fracture (with disruption of the sacroiliac joint—crescent fracture, or without sacroiliac joint involvement)	Rotationally unstable Vertically unstable
	LC3	Oblique/buckled rami fracture/s	Compressed sacral wing fracture at one side and sacroiliac joint fracture/dislocation at the other side	Rotationally unstable Vertically unstable
Antero-posterior compression (APC)—"Open book" External rotation vector	APC1	Symphysis pubis disruption—widening <2.5 cm	Minimally stressed anterior sacroiliac ligaments but mostly intact sacroiliac joints	Rotationally partially unstable Vertically stable
	APC2	Symphysis pubis disruption—widening >2.5 cm	Disruption of anterior sacroiliac ligaments, partial involvement of sacrotuberous/sacrospinous ligaments and intact posterior sacroiliac ligaments	Rotationally partially unstable vertically stable
	APC3	Symphysis pubis disruption—widening >2.5 cm	Complete disruption of sacroiliac joint/s with rupture of all ligaments	Rotationally unstable Vertically unstable
Vertical shear (VS) Vertical vector	VS	Vertically oriented pubic rami fractures	Sacral wing fractures with or without sacroiliac joint disruptions	Rotationally unstable Vertically unstable
Composite mechanism of injury (CMI)	CMI	Combination of features of fractures/dislocations of the anterior and posterior pelvic ring implying a combination different vectors of forces	Rotationally unstable Vertically unstable	

care for these patients is essential to minimise their morbidity and resulting disability [30].

More specifically for pelvic fractures, the answer to two basic questions dictates the management strategy: Is the patient stable OR unstable haemodynamically? Is the pelvic fracture stable OR unstable mechanically?

Initial Interventions

For patients who are haemodynamically unstable at presentation and have pelvic fractures, death within the first 24 h is commonly due to blood loss [22]. Principles of care in these patients should focus on damage control resuscitation, fracture stabilisation and prevention of secondary complications.

A patient that has a suspected pelvic injury (especially in the presence of hemodynamic instability) should receive a non-invasive circumferential stabilisation of the pelvic ring (pelvic binder) as early as possible, ideally in the prehospital environment [31, 32]. Furthermore, the lower extremities should be bound together unless associated injuries to the lower extremities or deformities of the legs do not allow this (example would be a hip dislocation not allowing mobilisation of the affected limb towards the midline) [33]. Pelvic binders

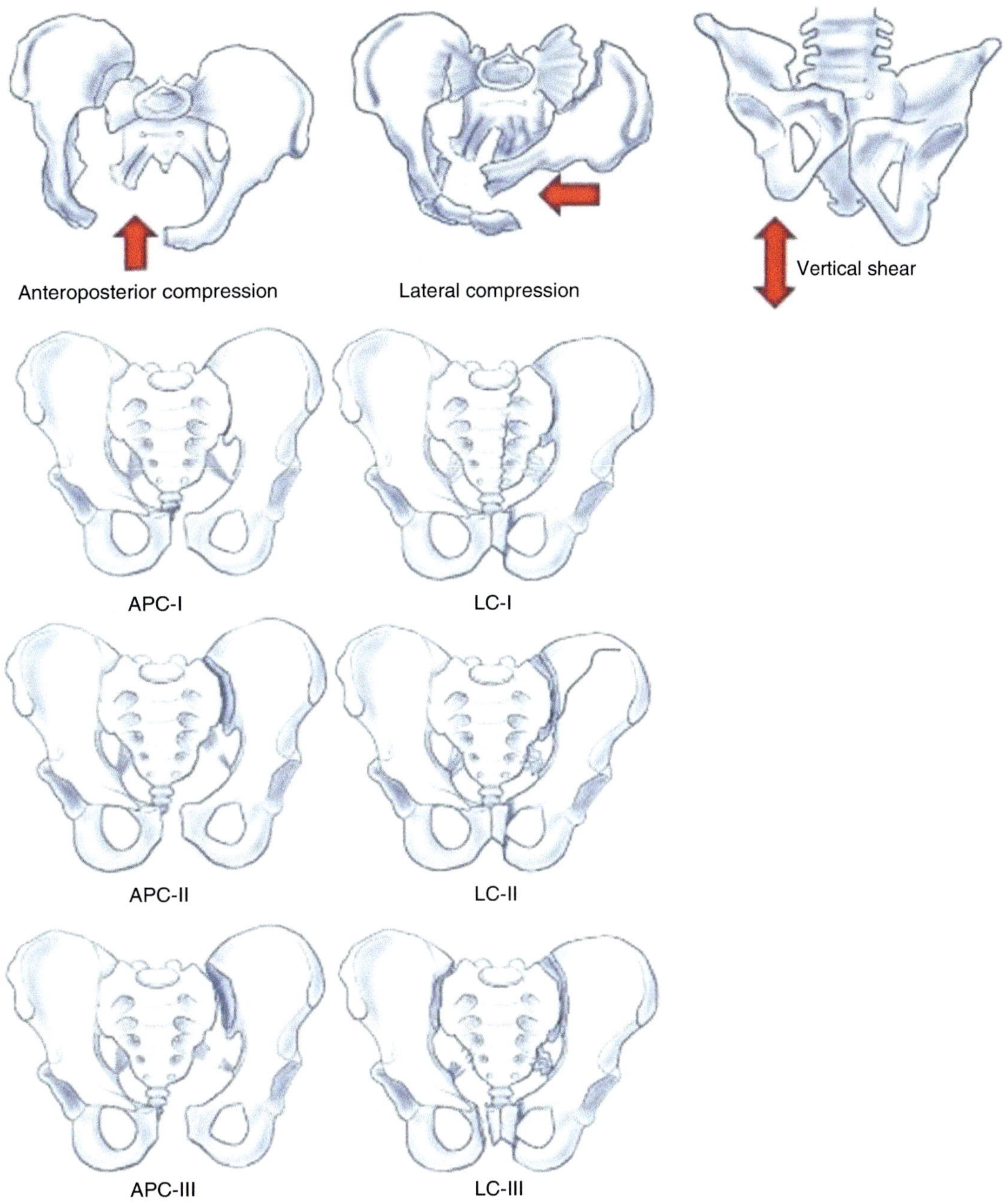

Fig. 34.5 Young and Burgess Classification

are easy to apply. They should be centred at the level of the greater trochanters to apply their effect across the whole pelvic ring symmetrically. A common error in applying pelvic binders is that they are placed too high, typically over the level of the iliac crests. In this position the binder is useless. When correctly positioned, the pelvic binder should cover the genitals as they cross the greater trochanters (Fig. 34.6). One way of recalling this is that correct positioning should look like the patient is wearing a miniskirt as opposed to a belt!

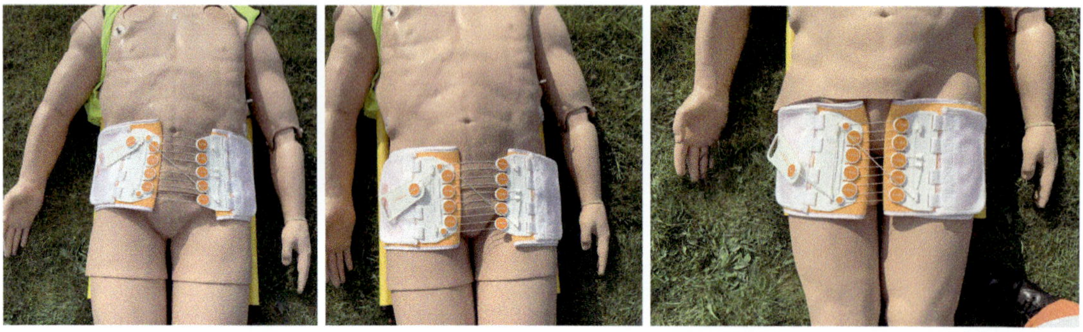

Fig. 34.6 (L-R): Pelvic binder positioned very high, slightly high and in the correct position

Pelvic binders act first by restricting the intrapelvic volume, but most importantly by providing adequate stability to the fractured pelvis allowing the formation of the initial clot of the bleeding bony surfaces, venous plexus and arterial lesions. The pelvic binder should not be removed, unless the patient is both haemodynamically stable, and following imaging, a pelvic fracture is either not identified or is defined as mechanically stable. Contemporary resuscitative strategies of blunt trauma should be applied in all cases of haemodynamically unstable pelvic fractures.

In all patients, an examination of the pelvis should be part of a comprehensive secondary survey of the musculoskeletal examination. This includes attention to the position of the lower extremities, the presence of external rotation or shortening of the injured side. In all pelvic fractures, a thorough examination of the perineum should occur after the restoration of haemodynamic stability and the removal of the binder. Stress examination ("springing") of the pelvis is NOT recommended as this may dislodge any clot that has been formed and cause further catastrophic bleeding. Furthermore, the sensitivity of "springing" in detecting unstable pelvic injuries is only 59%—marginally better than flipping a coin [34–38]. Published guidelines on the Management of Patients with Pelvic fractures and The Management of patients with Urological Trauma associated with pelvic fractures by the British Orthopaedic Association can help to guide management in these patients [30].

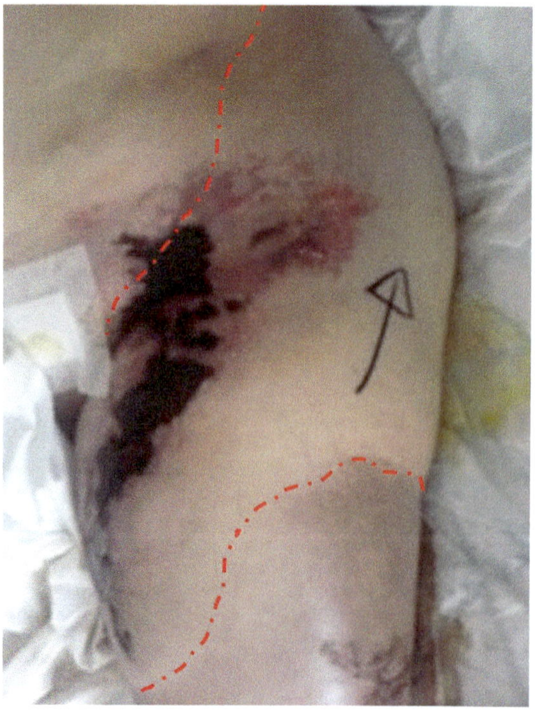

Fig. 34.7 Heavy soft tissue contusion and closed degloving injury to the left (Morell Lavallee—area marked with dotted red line) with underlying lateral compression type 2 pelvic fracture

Attention should be given to the skin condition around the thighs, the sacrum and the perineum to assess for any sign of an open injury, closed degloving trauma suggestive of a Morel-Lavallee lesion or bruising (Fig. 34.7). Examination of the rectum, prostate, scrotum, labia and vagina should also be performed to exclude the presence of an open pelvic fracture with associated perineal/urogenital trauma. Any blood at the urethral meatus should be noted, and an index of suspicion for urethral or bladder injuries should be maintained [20, 21].

A gentle attempt to pass a transurethral Foley catheter should take place during the secondary survey (unless the patient is in extremis and taken to emergency theatres). If following the insertion of the Foley catheter, bloodstained urine is noted, then a transcatheter cystogram should follow, as well as urgent referral to a urologist. If the attempt to pass the catheter fails or clear blood is drained via the catheter, then an urgent retrograde urethrogram should follow and potentially a suprapubic catheter will be required, again with a urological referral. Digital rectal examination (DRE) was traditionally advocated at the early stages of assessment in trauma, as well as a bimanual vaginal examination to assess for disruption of the gastrointestinal or urogenital systems respectively. A "high-riding" or non-palpable prostate in men this was classically taught as being a contraindication to catheterisation, however this is not based on any published data and there is a high rate of false-positive examinations on healthy individuals (up to 25%) especially in the obese [39]. Furthermore, DRE has a poor sensitivity and specificity when compared to other clinical signs for suspicion of index injuries [40] and a high false negative rate in patients who have GI, spinal or urethral injury confirmed either radiologically or at the time of operation [41]. There is no indication for the routine use of DRE in the management of trauma patients at the emergency room as it adds little (if anything) to their management, is time consuming and an unpleasant procedure which can be safely avoided.

It should be performed in selected cases (together with a bimanual vaginal examination (PV)) to assess the presence of blood during the examination which may indicate rectal or vaginal wall trauma which imply an open pelvic fracture (represents a clinical scenario with increased risk for septic complications). The DRE/PV are usually done in theatres prior to the definitive fixation of a confirmed pelvic fracture. In the presence of vaginal bleeding, a speculum assisted gynaecological examination should be employed, whilst in the suspicion of a rectal injury an proctosigmoeidoscopy [30].

If a vaginal, urethral or bowel injury has been identified either on imaging or on DRE/PV examination, then internal fixation usually is avoided at the anterior pelvic ring to minimise the risk of surgical site infections. Other means of fixation can be employed including the infix or the use of external fixation for the definitive management of a pelvic fracture.

Radiological evaluation in a trauma setting involves the use of a CT scan with intravenous contrast to establish potential sources of bleeding for the vast majority of trauma patients. The use of a plain AP pelvic x-ray (together with an AP chest), is useful in the extreme scenario of haemodynamically unstable/in extremis patients, as these patients may get transferred immediately to the operation theatres bypassing the CT scanner.

In the clinical scenario of a patient with no apparent pelvic fracture on the trauma CT scan, a plain AP pelvic radiograph should be taken once the binder has been removed, especially in the unconscious patient scenario, as occasionally an open book (APC) pelvic injury can be fully reduced and masked by a correctly applied binder [42].

Resuscitation

The haemodynamically unstable patient should be managed following the modern principles of damage control resuscitation, which aims to the reverse of the triad of death (hypothermia, coagulopathy, acidosis).

This approach includes:

(a) an initial permissive hypotension phase for the first hour post injury. This refers to restricted volume infusion aiming for blood pressure lower than usual (systolic blood pressure target of 80–90 mmHg—excepting patients with severe brain injury or the elderly) [43];
(b) the early use of tranexamic acid [44] and blood products (haemostatic resuscitation) [45], rather than crystalloid fluids or colloids. The currently recommended ratio of blood products in the exsanguinating patient

scenario is 1:1:1 of RBCs/FFP/PLT within the first 6 h if ongoing haemorrhage;

(c) a damage control surgery strategy aiming to control sources of bleeding, decompress cavities, decontaminate open injuries and restore physiology, rather than achieve anatomical integrity at the initial stage;

(d) attention to hypothermia with rewarming techniques [46, 47].

Most UK Level 1 trauma centres have a Code Red Trauma Call protocol in place. These are triggered by a senior member of staff, as soon as a patient with severe traumatic haemorrhage is identified (even before the arrival to the hospital as part of a pre-alert of a relevant clinical scenario). They refer to additional to the standard trauma call measures, which include the immediate administration of tranexamic acid (1 g bolus and 1 g infusion over the next 8 h) [44], the activation of a massive transfusion protocol (1:1:1 ratio of group O blood products ± cryoprecipitate) [45], mobilisation of the on-call senior members of the interventional radiology, vascular surgery and orthopaedic trauma, as well as of the operating theatres to prepare for potential emergency Code Red surgery (Fig. 34.8).

Haemorrhage Control

Pelvic haemorrhage is attributed to three principle sources (venous, bony, arterial) following a pelvic fracture [11, 34, 48, 49]. Further sources of bleeding should also be considered including bleeding from the pelvic viscera. The finding of haematuria is considered as an indication of associated trauma of the bladder/urethra or less commonly of the kidneys. Advanced radiologic imaging and clinical examination at the early stages of patient management assists their diagnosis and control.

- Venous: the low-pressure pelvic venous plexus (presacral, paravesical, larger pelvic veins, venous iliac branches) is the most common source of bleeding. The venous plexus is reported to account for 80% of blood loss in the presence of unstable pelvic fractures. Cadaveric studies suggest that the posterior vessels around the sacrum and the sacroiliac joints are predominantly responsible.
- Bony: displaced fractures of the pelvic ring expose broad areas of cancellous bone that also can lead to low pressure but significant blood loss.
- Arterial: haemodynamic instability from arterial injuries can be due to vessel dissection or disruption, or secondarily due to pseudoaneurysms or arteriovenous fistula formation. Arterial bleeding occurs in between 10% and 15% of unstable pelvic fractures and the most commonly injured vessels are branches of the internal iliac arteries. Other vessels which are less commonly injured are the external iliacs or the aorta and their anastomotic branches [50]. These injuries are considered as high-pressure haemorrhage and thus the most difficult to control [3, 51].

When considering strategies for managing pelvic haemorrhage, much depends on the effectiveness of the coagulation system of the patient [46]. Extreme instability of the pelvic ring, continuous excessive bleeding, specific comorbidities or use of anticoagulant medication and contribute to the development of acute traumatic coagulopathy and the "triad of death". Early administration of tranexamic acid, haemostatic hypotensive resuscitation, prompt application of circumferential pelvic compression via a binder and gentle patient handling may minimise or mitigate some of the effects of the coagulopathy [3, 52].

Trauma patients are initially evaluated by contrast medium-enhanced multi-detector computed tomography (MDCT), which allows the early detection of injuries across multiple body regions and can identify any active haemorrhage. This enables prompt decision making, therapeutic interventions and ultimately, control of the source of ongoing haemorrhage [3, 46, 52].

Leeds Major Trauma Centre

CODE RED SURGERY

DAMAGE CONTROL SURGERY

Actions to take when a POLYTRAUMA patient is determined to be transferred urgently to theatre-Checklist

P	PREPARTION/ PAUSES	• Inform theatre team (Surgeons, Anaesthetist, Serub team, ODP, Radiographer) • Inform relevant staff of potential injuries and procedures that may occur. • SURGICAL PAUSES led by anaeshetic team every 30min
O	OSI TABLE	• Transfer OSI table to theatre.
L	LOCATION	• Determine theatre capacity. • Notify theatre to be utilised. • Communicate destination theatre to A&E and MTSN case manger.
Y "I"	INFUSION	• 4 transfusion pumps • Rapid infused primed with warm saline. • Cell Salvage-allocate operator. • Double transducers for arterial and central lines prepared. • T&4 infusion.
T	TEMPERATURE	• Warm up Theatre (max^{-T}). • Forced Air warming or Bair Hugger. • Waming mattress. • Warmed fluid ready.
R	RADIOGRAPHY	• Verify if image intensifier is required. • If so contact radiographers (bleep xxx). • Log on at PACS monitor and upload relevant imaging.
A	AIRWAY	• Prepare for RSI. • DLT (double lumen tube). • McGrath, Ambuscope ready.
U	UNIT	• Inform ICU bed manager for postop care. • Urinary catheter set ready. • Ultrasound for central lines.
M	MAJOR HAEMMORHAGE PROTOCOL	• Ensure Blood Bank is aware of MH. • Ensure MH packs are ordered. • 1:1:1 transfusion. • Check Cogulation-TEG. • Tourniquets x2
A	ANAESTHESIA	• Anaesthetist to lead "SURGICAL PAUSES" every 30min. • Ketamine / Opiod / Rocuronium. • TXA infusion. • 50ml 2% Propofol. • 100mg Rocuronium. • 10mg Metaramind in 20ml. • Tourniquets x2. • TXA infusion.
S	SURGICAL EQUIPMENT	• Team Brief – Team Debrief at the end • Communicate with relevant surgical specialities Instrument requirements. • Set up trolleys so kit is readlly accessible if required. • Ligaclips and Hemostatic agents readily available. • Abdominal packs and warmed up Lt of N/S (x12 plus)

Fig. 34.8 Example of the Code Red algorithm for the trauma theatres at the Leeds Teaching Hospital Trust

Pelvic Packing

Pelvic pre-peritoneal packing is typically performed in damage control surgery for a patient who has haemodynamic instability from an unstable pelvic fracture that is not responsive to resuscitative measures and in extremis. Contemporary pelvic packing refers to the insertion of large abdominal gauzes into the pre-peritoneal space of the true pelvis [53].

Pre-peritoneal packing is an emergency procedure. It should be performed after the pelvic ring has been somehow stabilised in order to allow containment of the packs and facilitate the tamponade effect. A pelvic binder or circumferential pelvic sheet can achieve this, or else a quick application of an anterior external fixator/C-Clamp should be performed before damage control laparotomy and packing (Fig. 34.9).

Getting access to the retropubic space of Retzius via a Pfannestiel or vertical midline incision (with limited sub-umbilical extension of the standard midline laparotomy) is the first step (Fig. 34.9). The insertion of lap sponges starts after the quick evacuation of the large clots that are encountered following the entry to the space of Retzius. Usually, the most injured side is packed first with at least three large abdominal gauzes, which are inserted one by one in a meandering fashion as posteriorly as possible. They need to be inserted to the true or lesser pelvis and be advanced as posteriorly possible around the pelvic rim. After one side is fully packed, the procedure is repeated for the contralateral side (in total usually six lap sponges are enough). This technique places the sponges toward the posterior venous plexus and the internal iliac vessels. The tamponade effect simultaneously and non-selectively addresses all sources of bleeding and is a pure damage control procedure, i.e. fast, indicated for unstable patients and requires a secondary procedure in 24–48 h to remove the sponges.

The sponges should be counted at insertion and retrieved carefully at 24–48 h to minimise infection risk. Blood is a perfect culture medium, so once bleeding has been controlled and physiology normalised as far as possible, the risk:benefit ratio moves away from keeping sponges and packs in to minimise bleeding towards favouring their removal to prevent abdomino-pelvic infection. At the time of retrieval, the surgeon should be cautious as developed clots may become dislodged and then repacking with new, clean packs or direct control of the bleeding vessels may become necessary.

Historically, a higher incidence of deep infection (35%) was considered as a problem following pelvic packing. This secondary complication may hinder or alter the subsequent definitive fixation strategy, although recent reports challenge this [14, 54]. When applied for the correct indications, i.e. in the clinical scenario of an exsanguinating patient from pelvic bleeding, these secondary implications are consciously de-prioritised in the initial stages with the intent of saving the patient's life during the initial resuscitation.

Angiography and Embolisation

For the vast majority of trauma patients with a pelvic fracture, a contrast medium enhanced MDCT is performed within the first 30 min of the arrival of the patient [30]. This scan allows the trauma team to identify and diagnose the sources of bleeding rapidly.

When ongoing arterial haemorrhage is present and evident in the trauma scan (arterial blush or contrast extravasation at the arterial phase of the MDCT), angioembolisation is employed to allow direct control of the bleeding vessel [22, 51]. Additional indications for this type of procedure in the presence of a pelvic fracture are all pseudoaneurysms that declare themselves, though this is usually at a later stage. This classically presents as an unexplained slow drop of patients haemoglobin and derangement of haemodynamic parameters. Contraindications to targeted embolisation in the initial phase are the presence of gross haemodynamic instability prior to scan with potential multiple bleeding sites, evidence of massive intraperitoneal bleeding, allergy to iodinated contrast media, or previously altered/unfavourable vascular anatomy (aorto-femoral bypass, stenosis, occlusion, aneurysm repair) [22].

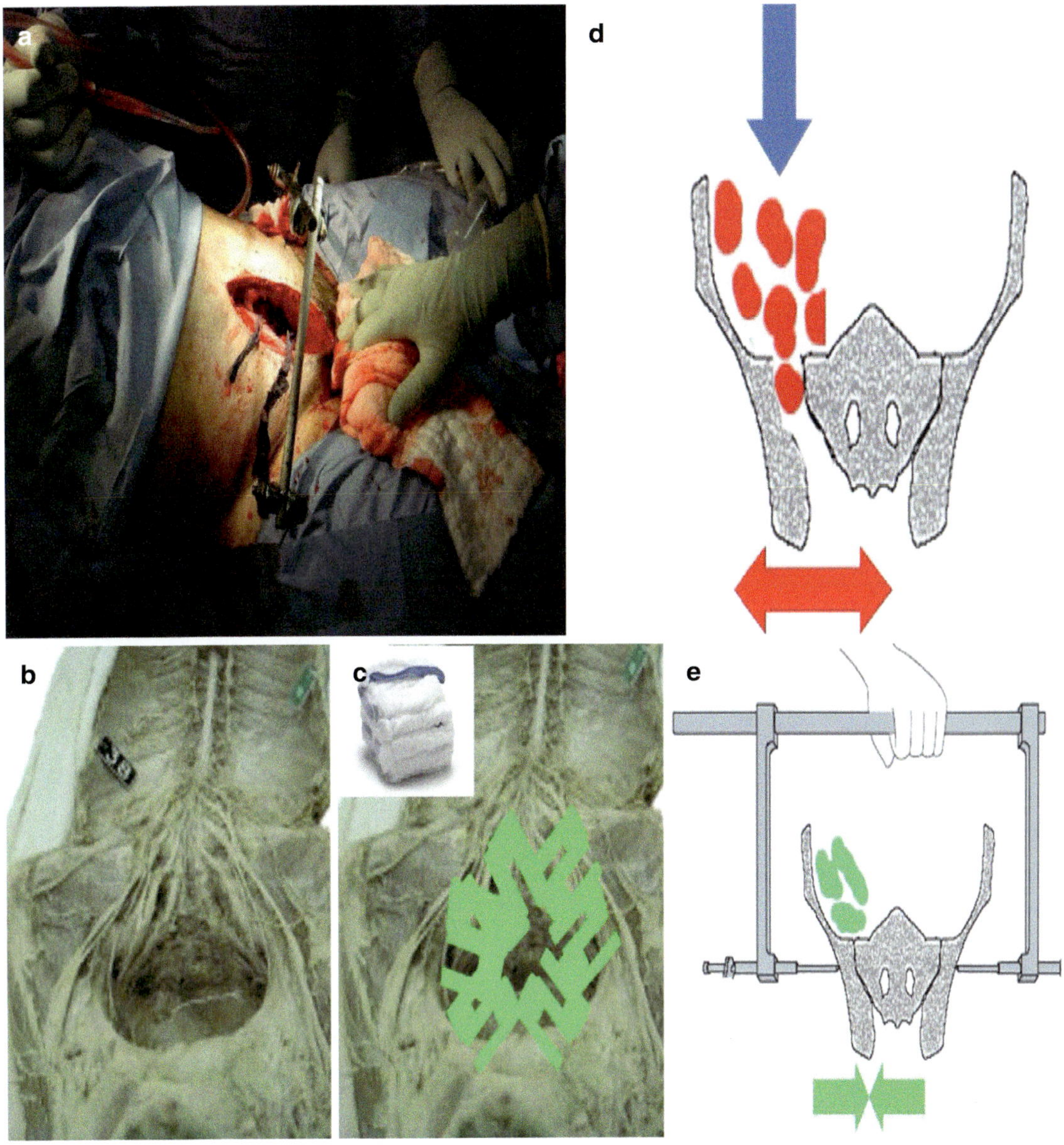

Fig. 34.9 (**a**) Clinical case of packing with anterior pelvic external fixator midline sub-umbilical incision. (**b**) Cadaveric specimen with exposure of the true and false pelvis and the presacral vasculature. (**c**) Same specimen with graphic representation of the position of lap sponges, covering the presacral area and the area below pelvic rim of the true pelvis. (**d**) Graphic demonstration of the effect of packing of a non-stabilised injured pelvic ring. Failure of containment of the lap sponges. (**e**) Graphic demonstration of the effect of packing of a stabilised injured pelvic ring with a C-Clamp. Packing is contained

After the MDCT and the establishment of an access route (usually transfemoral), a diagnostic angiography follows. When a bleeding artery is identified, a selective (4-6F), or super-selective (2.3–2.9 °F) microcatheter is inserted Fig. 34.10. The first-line option in the clinical setting of the bleeding pelvis is that of selective embolisation; targeting the specific bleeding vessel is associated with fewer complications. Non-selective embolisation is preserved as a salvage procedure in patients who are unresponsive to previous measures and “in extremis”, or when the patient

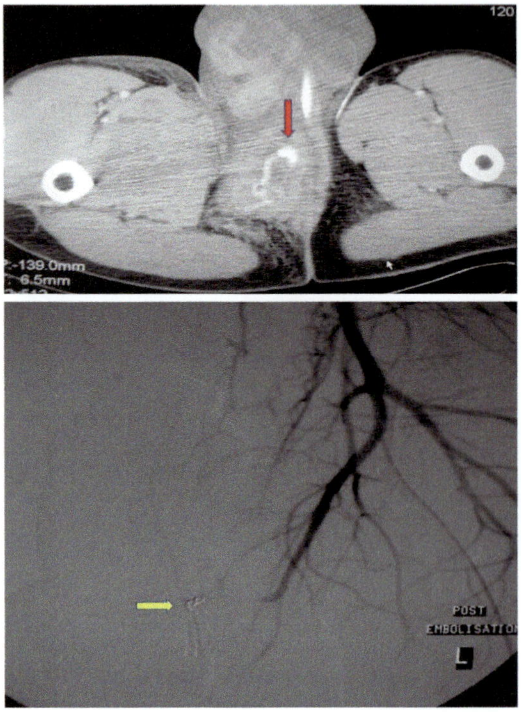

Fig. 34.10 Clinical example of contrast extravasation of the right internal pudendal artery (red arrow) at the arterial phase of the MDCT, and subsequent angiography and super selective embolisation with coils (yellow arrow)

remains unstable without evidence of contrast extravasation or vessel injury. Historically, non-selective embolisations were used more and were strongly associated with severe complications (peripheral ischemic episodes, foot, leg, gluteal, bladder, avascular femoral head necrosis and impotence to name a few) [51]. The embolisation is achieved with the injection of materials (coils, amplatzer, PVA particles, glue, onyx, gelfoam, thrombin) that can produce a permanent (for selective embolisation or pseudoaneurysms) or temporary effect with endogenous vessel recanalization occurring in 4–8 weeks.

The procedure can be repeated if needed, and it is relatively safe. Selective embolisation may also follow an initial pelvic packing procedure in a patient that remains unstable post damage control surgery and has a positive scan for arterial extravasation on repeated contrast CT. The main disadvantage of angioembolisation is that it addresses the arterial sources of bleeding selectively (as opposed to including venous and bony bleeding sites) and is relatively time-consuming. The average procedure times are over 90 min, even in centres that have rapid access to interventional radiologists, staff and equipment so is not appropriate for patients requiring a damage control procedure immediately [51, 55]. All Major Trauma centres should have 24/7 available resources, trained personnel and access to this type of interventions either to an embolisation suite or more recently to hybrid theatres.

It is essential to appreciate that all methods of haemorrhage control can be used in conjunction; they are different and not competitive but rather complementary to each other. Major trauma centres and units should have institutional protocols in place (Fig. 34.11) for the management of these severely injured and compromised patients. Their application should be tailored to the specifics of each clinical scenario and may vary between different hospitals depending on logistics, available resources and local expertise.

Fracture Stabilisation

Non-Invasive Stabilisation (Pelvic Binders and Sheet Wrapping)

Circumferential compression of the pelvic ring has been introduced to all contemporary management protocols over the last 10 years. Either in the form of commercially available binders (e.g. Pelvic Binders such as the SAM pelvic sling or T-POD device), or by wrapping a sheet around the pelvis. These devices should be used as a part of the primary survey as early as possible. In the UK the application of a pelvic binder is usually performed in the prehospital setting following high energy trauma, or with patients who have a mechanism of injury leading to a suspicion of pelvic fracture.

The pelvic binder is applied to reduce the pelvic volume, but most importantly, to provide mechanical stability to the pelvis and encourage tamponade and formation of the primary clot [22, 29]. Of note, the pelvic ring is not a closed compartment. After the first litre of haemorrhage,

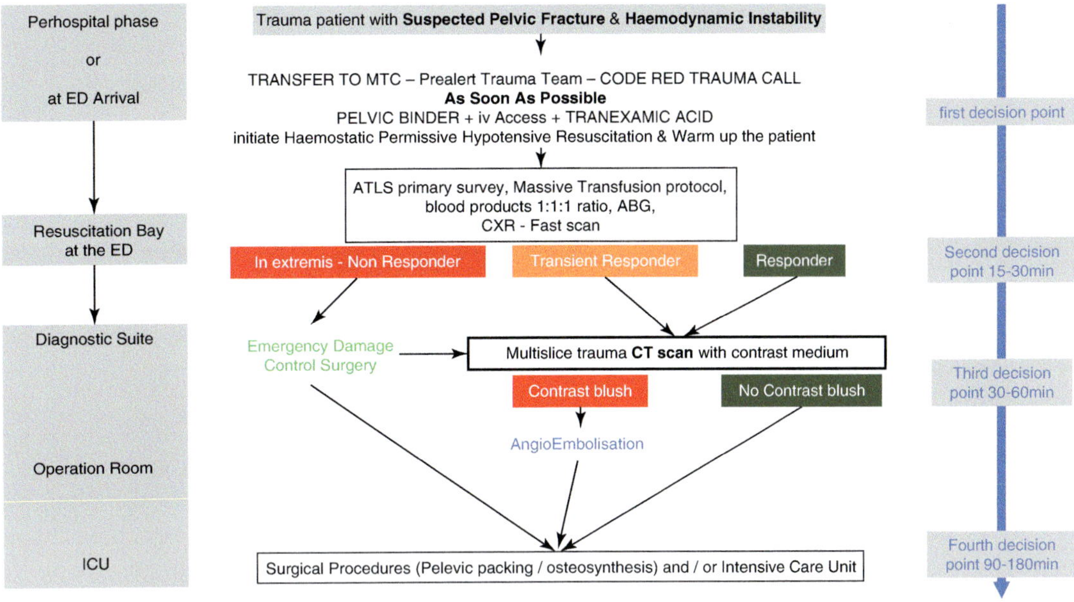

Fig. 34.11 Current algorithm of management of a hemodynamically unstable trauma patient with a suspected pelvic fracture of the Leeds MTC

blood subsequently drains upward to the retroperitoneal space. In the event of rupture of the pelvic floor or the perineum (not unusual in high energy open book or vertical shear fractures), blood can drain externally (Fig. 34.12). The volume of blood that can be contained in the pelvic ring is given by the formula $4/3\pi r^3$. Unless bleeding stops by the formation of blood clots, pelvic fractures can lead to the loss of large volumes of blood in excess of the circulating blood volume of the patient [56, 57].

The binder should be placed at the level of the greater trochanters (Fig. 34.13). At that level, the pressure is applied circumferentially across all the true pelvis and the pelvic girdle; this refers to a virtual ring containing the hip joints, the symphysis pubis, the sciatic buttress and the upper sacrum.

Modern binders allow access to the abdomen and are more lightweight. Their presence allows full access to the pelvis and the abdomen for damage control surgery procedures such as laparotomy, extraperitoneal packing, external pelvic fixation, c-clamp and placement of iliosacral screws without removal of the binder (Fig. 34.13). However, binders still restrict access for examination of the perineum, access for vascular procedures such as the insertion of the REBOA catheter and a complete secondary survey [21, 29].

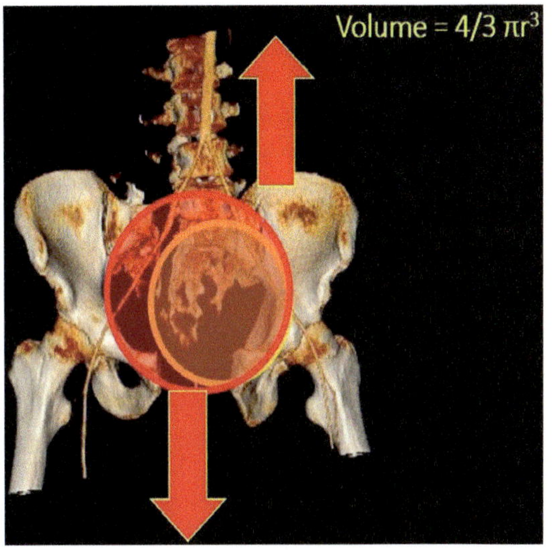

Fig. 34.12 Graphic demonstration of the non-containment of the pelvic volume and the overflow upwards to the retroperitoneal space and downwards after rupture of the pelvic floor

The duration of use of a binder in the presence of a pelvic fracture is relevant to

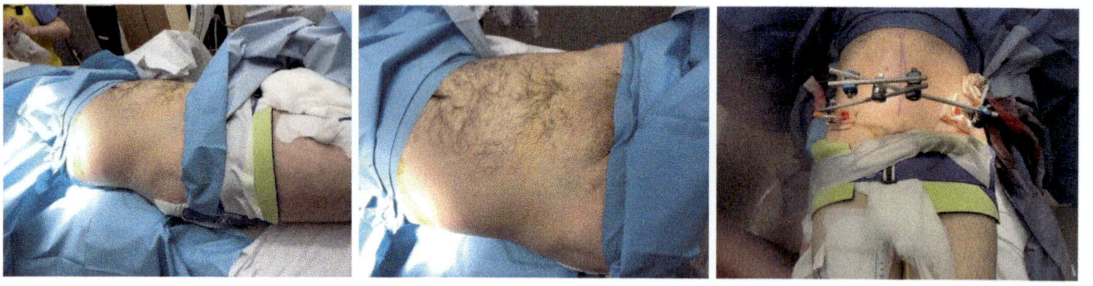

Fig. 34.13 Demonstrates use of binder at the level of the greater trochanters, allowing access to iliac crests for external fixation, the symphysis pubis for packing, the external iliac fossa for the application of c-clamp/iliosacral screws and also clear access to the abdomen for further damage control procedures

1. The hemodynamic stability of the patient and their response to resuscitation
2. The mechanical stability of any identified pelvic fracture, its type and degree of displacement
3. The available resources, skillset and expertise of managing unstable pelvic fractures.

In the vast majority of cases post the initial diagnostics and resuscitation, the binders are removed within the first 24 h. If prolonged use is required, then it is recommended that they are loosened up from time to time to prevent complications in the form of pressure sores and skin necrosis. Any patients who have pelvic injuries outside of a Major Trauma Centre who continue to require the application of a pelvic binder after the primary survey should be urgently discussed with a specialist pelvic surgeon, ideally in the regional Major Trauma Centre. While competing management priorities may mean that immediate pelvic fixation or stabilisation is not possible (or indeed necessary), these patients can have significant morbidity and mortality from delayed surgery and missed or mismanaged injuries [58–61].

Emergency Skeletal Stabilisation

Anterior Emergency Fixation

External fixation devices are minimally invasive systems that are usually applied under fluoroscopic guidance, allow indirect reduction and adequate stability of rotationally unstable pelvic fracture types and can be applied rapidly. These are mostly utilised as standalone, temporary means of stabilisation at the initial damage control procedure, and occasionally as definitive management tools, mostly in association with additional fixation of the posterior pelvic ring.

They consist of a system of interlinked half pins, clamps and rods. Their anchorage and stability is related to the size and number of half pins inserted, the size and configuration of the frame of rods constructed, patient bone quality and the distance of the frame from the area of instability [62]. External fixators restore a degree of stability to the anterior pelvic ring but are inadequate when the posterior ring is completely disrupted (Tile C types of pelvic fractures). Some anterior external fixator systems may provide a degree of stability to the posterior pelvis [63]; however, these have not been widely adopted, mostly due to the availability of more reliable methods of definitive pelvic fixation.

There are two principal types of pelvic anterior external fixators—the iliac crest fixator and the supra-acetabular fixator.

The iliac crest external fixators are the most commonly applied in the trauma setting for damage control resuscitation. They use the iliac crests for insertion of two half pins in each crest which are usually 5 mm diameter and can be placed with or without fluoroscopy (Fig. 34.14). The supra-acetabular external fixator requires fluoroscopy for identification of supra-acetabular bony corridors via the anterior inferior iliac spines (Fig. 34.15). This type of anterior pelvic fixation does offer biomechanical advantages and is considered more stable [64].

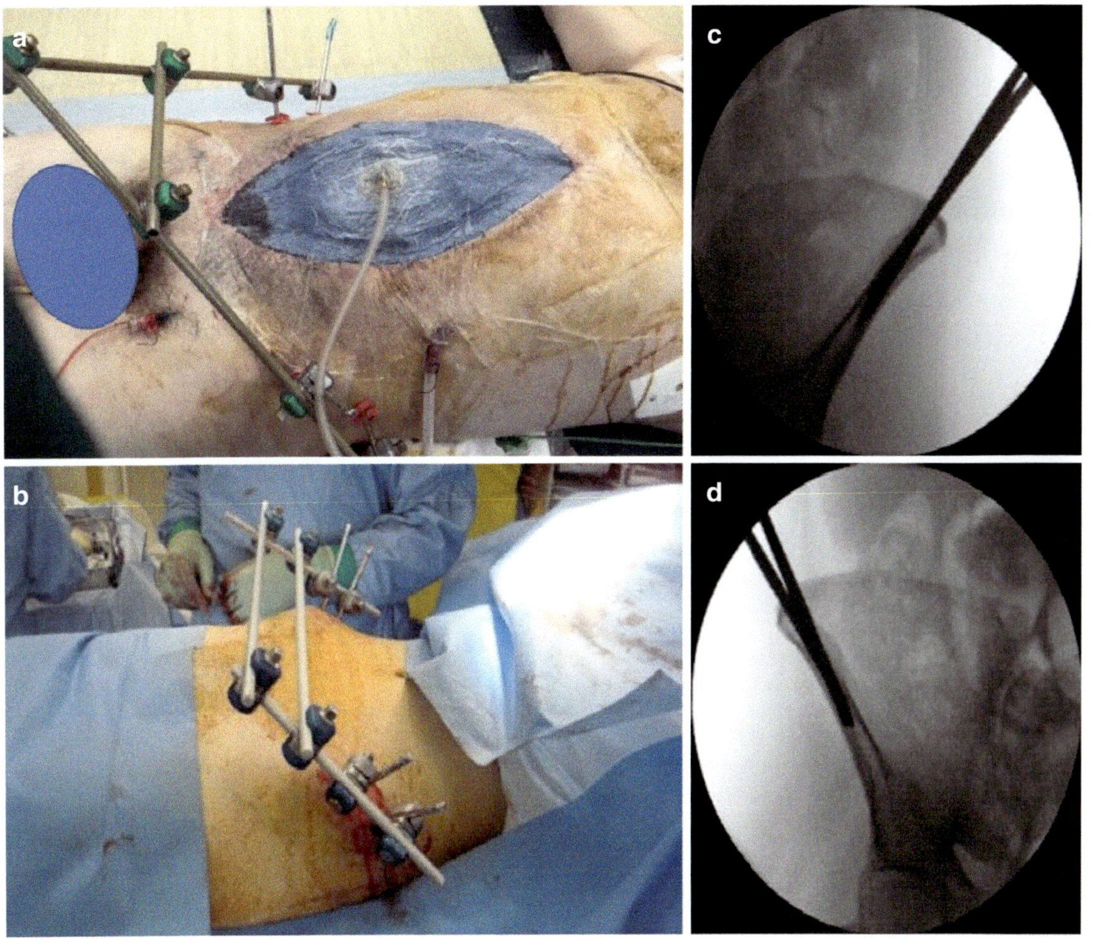

Fig. 34.14 Clinical examples with application of anterior external fixators at the iliac crests. (**a**) Alpha/triangular type of anterior external fixator of the iliac crest. (**b**) Rectangular type of anterior external fixator of the iliac crest. (**c**) Fluoroscopy control of the position of the half pins to the left iliac crest (outlet view). (**d**) Fluoroscopy control of the position of the half pins to the left iliac crest (outlet view)

The two types of rod constructs that are principally employed are either an alpha triangular frame or a rectangular type (Fig. 34.14). Anterior external fixators do stabilise the anterior pelvis but do not control or reduce sufficiently the posterior elements [62, 64].

Posterior Emergency Fixation

The pelvic C Clamp represents the primary invasive method of emergency reduction and temporary stabilisation of the posterior pelvic ring. It is relatively fast to apply and can be used with or without fluoroscopic guidance. This device can compress the pelvic ring posteriorly and maintain reduction until definitive fixation is feasible (Fig. 34.16).

Emergency posterior fixation is predominantly indicated in fractures with rotational and vertical instability (type C per Tile, or else VS or APC-3 and some LC3 injuries per Young & Burgess) [62]. It is contraindicated in the presence of iliac wing fractures (crescent fractures) or comminuted fractures of either innominate bones [65].

The entry points of a C Clamp are very close to those of the "gold standard" method of fixation of the posterior pelvic ring (i.e. percutaneously inserted iliosacral cannulated screws). Therefore,

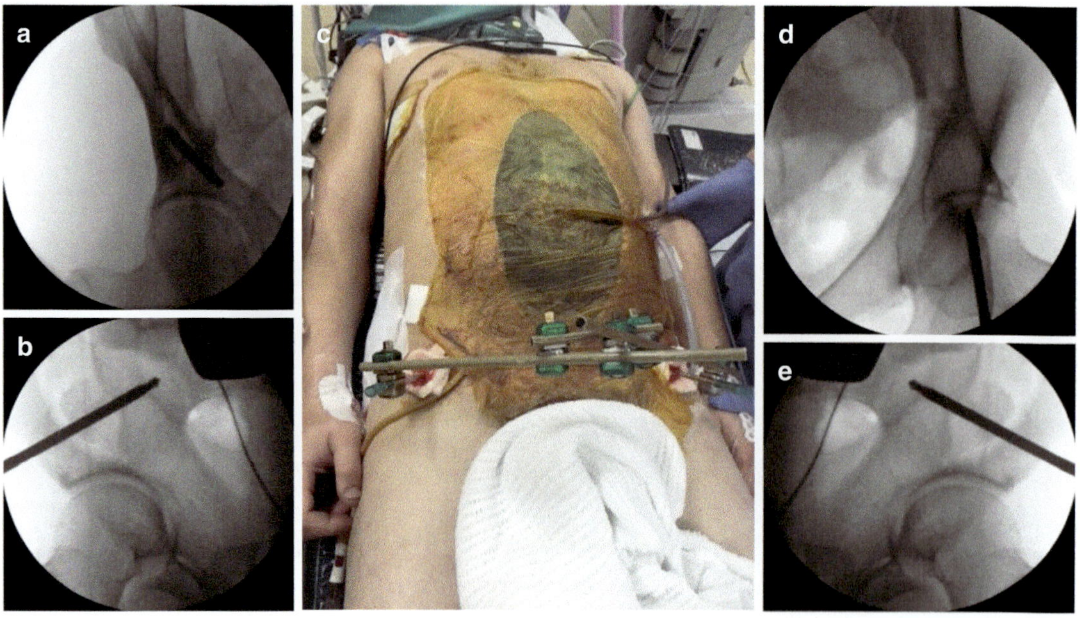

Fig. 34.15 Clinical example with application of anterior external fixator of the supraacetabular type. (**a**) Outlet obturator oblique fluoroscopy view of the left sciatic pilar corridor—teardrop for the half pin of the supra-acetabular external fixator. (**b**) Iliac oblique fluoroscopy view of the left side verifying the entry point at the level of the anterior inferior iliac spine and the trajectory of the half pin above the greater sciatic notch. (**c**) Photo of a patient post anterior pelvis supra-acetabular external fixation (alpha frame), damage control laparotomy, pelvic packing and iliosacral screw fixation. (**d**) Inlet obturator oblique fluoroscopy view of the right side—verification of the starting point at the level of the anterior inferior iliac spine. (**e**) Iliac oblique fluoroscopy view of the right side verifying the entry point at the level of the anterior inferior iliac spine and the trajectory of the half pin above the greater sciatic notch

prolonged use of this device may delay definitive management or increase the risk of surgical site infections. For this reason, C-Clamps are rarely used nowadays, as binders and traction have replaced their role as the principal temporary stabilisation method until definitive fixation can happen. There are also other complications associated with its use which have influenced the move towards increased pelvic splint use (overcompression of the posterior elements, sacral root secondary injuries and injuries of the superior gluteal artery during application).

Another invasive method for temporary fixation of the posterior ring is the so-called "antishock iliosacral screw" [66]. This method aims for a partial reduction and temporary stabilisation of the posterior pelvis and requires fluoroscopic guidance, but is limited by the availability of trained pelvic surgeons and the presence or not of comminution of the innominate bones.

Definitive Skeletal Stabilisation

A comprehensive description of the methods of definitive skeletal stabilisation of the pelvic ring, their indications and contraindications are beyond the scope of this chapter. These methods are principally internal fixation strategies with plates and screws, which can be applied via a variety of minimally invasive techniques or open surgical approaches (Fig. 34.17).

The main contemporary principles of the definitive surgical treatment of fractures of the pelvic ring include:

1. prompt transfer to medical facility with available surgical expertise
2. thorough assessment and management of associated soft tissue and visceral injuries
3. adequate reduction of the pelvic ring

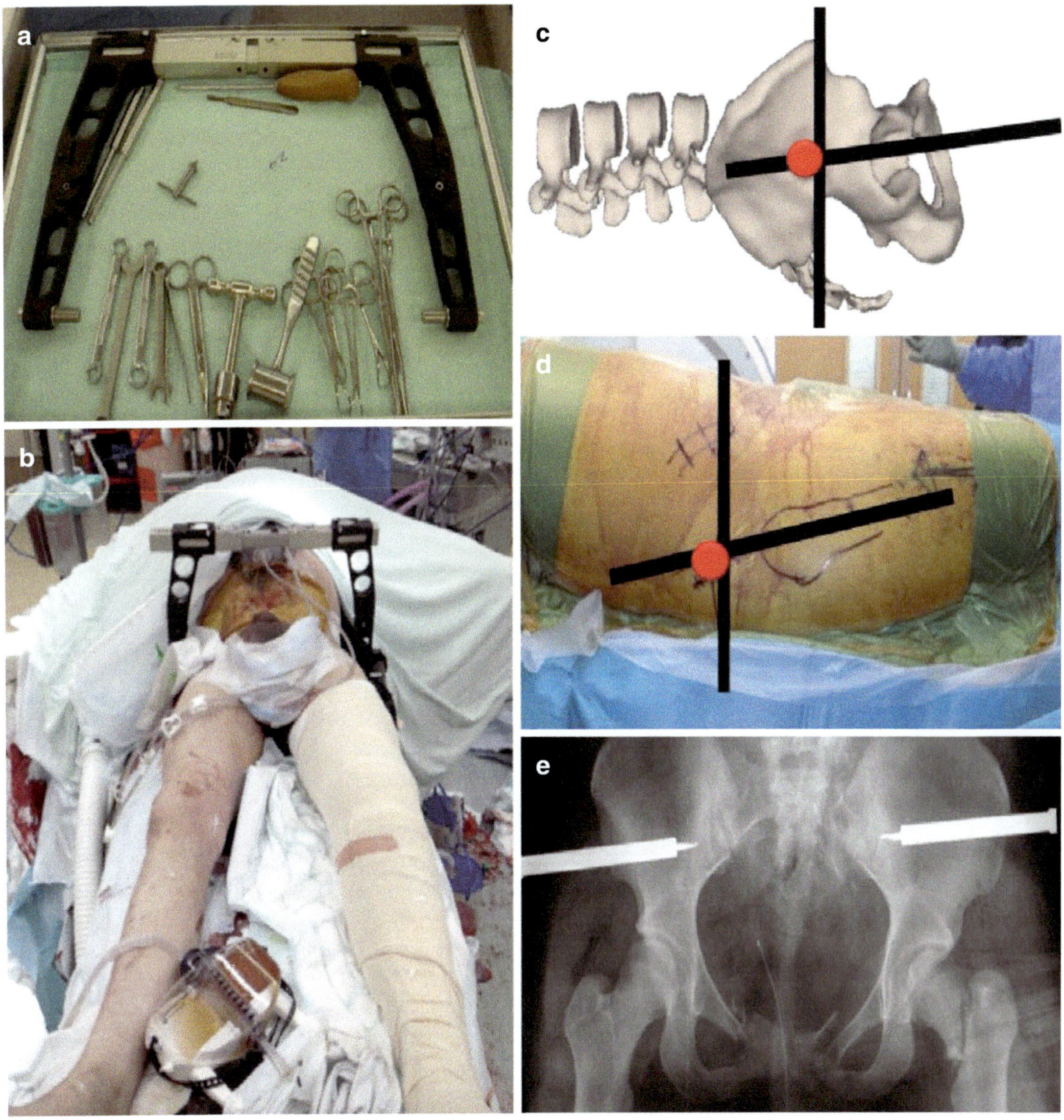

Fig. 34.16 Example of application of the C-Clamp to control an unstable pelvic fracture. (**a**) The C-Clamp kit. (**b**) Clinical photograph of a patient following the application of a C-Clamp. (**c**) Graphic representation of the landmarks for insertion of the compression bolts of the C-Clamp. (**d**) Clinical photograph with demonstration of the entry point for the insertion of the compression bolt of the C-Clamp to the right ilium. It refers to the junction between a vertical line from the anterior superior iliac spine and another line in axis to the femoral shaft. (**e**) Anteroposterior x-ray of the pelvis following the application of a C-Clamp

4. mechanical stabilisation primarily of the posterior and secondarily of the anterior pelvis adequate to allow early mobilization of the patient
5. prevention of secondary complications (i.e. venous thromboembolism, pressure sores, surgical site infections) [14, 16, 67].

Key Points

- The ligaments around the pelvis support and stabilise the bony pelvis and its joints. These are broadly divided into four groups
- The sources of bleeding could be large displaced areas of cancellous bone (mainly the iliac bones or the sacrum), the rich presacral

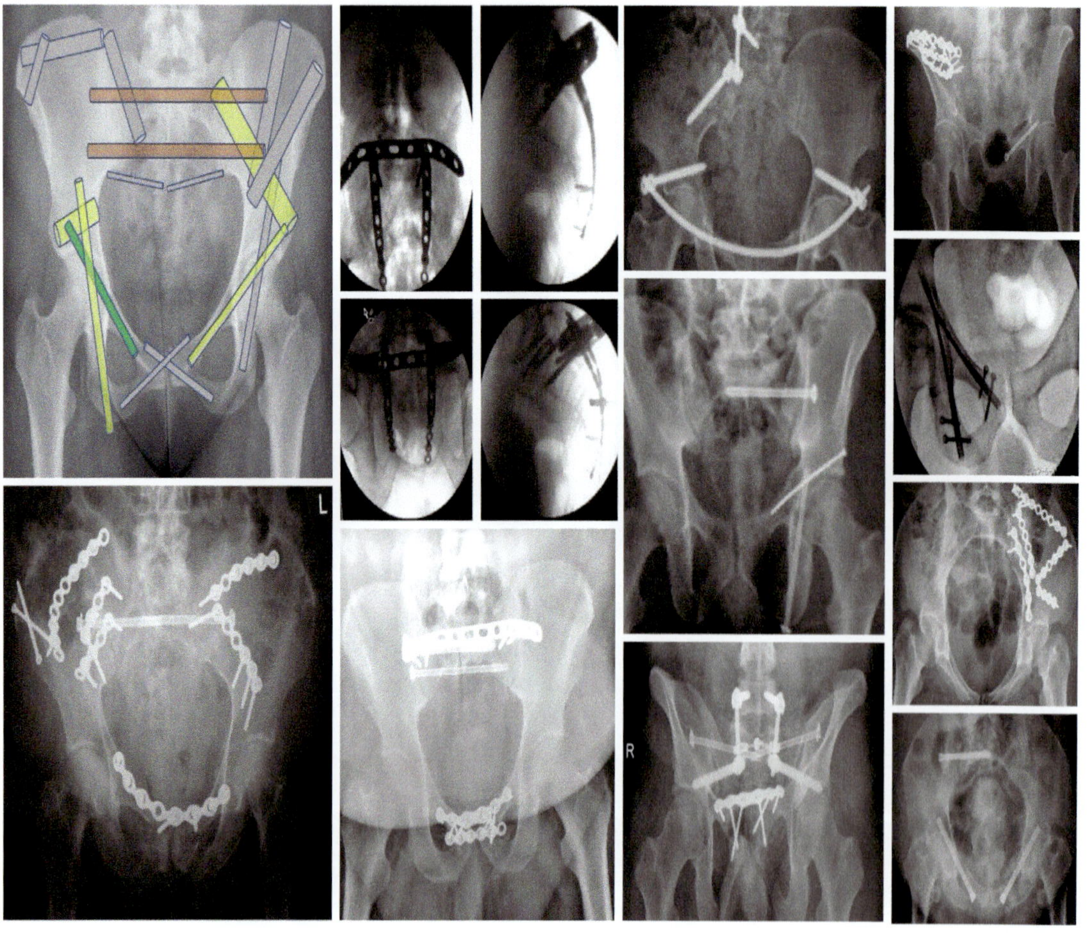

Fig. 34.17 A number of examples with different methods of definitive fixation of the pelvic ring

venous plexus or large vessels and their branches.

- More specifically for pelvic fractures, the answer to two basic questions dictates the management strategy: is the patient stable OR unstable haemodynamically? Is the pelvic fracture stable OR unstable mechanically?
- A patient that has a suspected pelvic injury (especially in the presence of hemodynamic instability) should receive a non-invasive circumferential stabilisation of the pelvic ring (pelvic binder) as early as possible, ideally in the prehospital environment.
- The haemodynamically unstable patient should be managed following the modern principles of damage control resuscitation, which aims to the reverse of the triad of death (hypothermia, coagulopathy, acidosis).
- Pelvic haemorrhage is attributed to three principle sources (venous, bony, arterial) following a pelvic fracture.
- It is essential to appreciate that all methods of haemorrhage control can be used in conjunction; they are different and not competitive but rather complementary to each other.

Summary

Pelvic fractures are a significant injury both in terms of immediate mortality and later stage morbidity. They intrinsically can be responsible for many deaths from exsanguination due to the previously described vascular network, but the presence of pelvic fractures is a marker of a high-energy mechanism of injury in the young or a degree of frailty in the elderly which should encourage a thorough investigation for other potentially occult injuries. While multiple methods of temporary and definitive fixation exist, the underlying principle of them all is to control bleeding and achieve a degree of stability in the acute phase. Pelvic surgeons are not present in every hospital, but regional trauma networks should have referral mechanisms in place in order to deal with complex pelvic injuries, or injuries which require surgical fixation. The acute management of pelvic fractures in non-specialist hospitals can be achieved with pelvic binders, and early discussion with an appropriately qualified trauma team and pelvic surgeon.

Questions

1. At which level should a pelvic binder be applied?
   (a) Umbilicus
   (b) Centred in the Greater trochanters
   (c) Centred on the ASIS
   (d) Below the Greater Trochanter
2. The lethal triad consists of;
   (a) Acidosis, hypothermia and coagulopathy
   (b) Acisosis, hyperthermia and coagulopathy
   (c) Hypothermia, hypotension and acidosis
   (d) Coagulopathy, hypotension and hypothermia
3. Following a failed attempt to pass a urethral catheter in a patient with pelvic fractures, the next step is?
   (a) Repeat attempt with the same catheter
   (b) Urgent retrograde urethrogram with urology input
   (c) Repeat attempt with a larger diameter catheter
   (d) Insertion of a suprapubic catheter
4. A Morel-Lavallee lesion is described as:
   (a) A perineal haematoma
   (b) Avulsion of ASIS
   (c) Avulsion of AIIS
   (d) A Closed degloving soft tissue injury
5. An elderly patient who fell down a flight of stairs underwent a trauma CT scan demonstrating a Lateral Compression Type 2 pelvic injury with an arterial blush demonstrate(d) Following the return to the Emergency department the patient became hypotensive, tachycardic and drowsy. What is the next step:
   (a) Contact the operating theatre for skeletal stabilisation and pelvic packing
   (b) Contact the Interventional radiologist for embolization
   (c) Resuscitation with blood products, Tranexamic acid and ensure pelvic binder is correctly positioned
   (d) Resuscitation with crystalloid and contact vascular surgery

Answers

1. b
2. a
3. b
4. d
5. c

References

1. Brenneman FD, Katyal D, Boulanger BR, Tile M, Redelmeier DA. Long-term outcomes in open pelvic fractures. J Trauma. 1997 May;42(5):773–7.
2. Gänsslen A, Pohlemann T, Paul C, Lobenhoffer P, Tscherne H. Epidemiology of pelvic ring injuries. Injury. 1996;27(Suppl 1):S-A13–20.
3. Mauffrey C, Cuellar DO, Pieracci F, Hak DJ, Hammerberg EM, Stahel PF, et al. Strategies for the management of haemorrhage following pelvic fractures and associated trauma-induced coagulopathy. Bone Joint J. 2014 Sep;96-B(9):1143–54.
4. Pohlemann T, Gänsslen A, Schellwald O, Culemann U, Tscherne H. Outcome after pelvic ring injuries. Injury. 1996;27(Suppl 2):B31–8.
5. Grotz MRW, Allami MK, Harwood P, Pape HC, Krettek C, Giannoudis PV. Open pelvic fractures: epidemiology, current concepts of management and outcome. Injury. 2005 Jan;36(1):1–13.
6. Mardanpour K, Rahbar M. The outcome of surgically treated traumatic unstable pelvic fractures by open reduction and internal fixation. J Inj Violence Res. 2013 July;5(2):77–83.
7. Kanakaris NK, Greven T, West RM, Van Vugt AB, Giannoudis PV. Implementation of a standardized protocol to manage elderly patients with low energy pelvic fractures: can service improvement be expected? Int Orthop. 2017;41(9):1813–24.
8. Prieto-Alhambra D, Avilés FF, Judge A, Van Staa T, Nogués X, Arden NK, et al. Burden of pelvis fracture: a population-based study of incidence, hospitalisation and mortality. Osteoporos Int. 2012 Dec;23(12):2797–803.

9. Rommens PM, Ossendorf C, Pairon P, Dietz S-O, Wagner D, Hofmann A. Clinical pathways for fragility fractures of the pelvic ring: personal experience and review of the literature. J Orthop Sci. 2015;20:1–11.
10. Bramos A, Velmahos GC, Butt UM, Fikry K, Smith RM, Chang Y. Predictors of bleeding from stable pelvic fractures. Arch Surg. 2011 Apr;146(4):407–11.
11. Papadopoulos IN, Kanakaris N, Bonovas S, Triantafillidis A, Garnavos C, Voros D, et al. Auditing 655 fatalities with pelvic fractures by autopsy as a basis to evaluate trauma care. J Am Coll Surg. 2006 July;203(1):30–43.
12. Holtenius J, Bakhshayesh P, Enocson A. The pelvic fracture - indicator of injury severity or lethal fracture? Injury. 2018 Aug;49(8):1568–71.
13. Skitch S, Engels PT. Acute management of the traumatically injured pelvis. Emerg Med Clin North Am. 2018 Feb;36(1):161–79.
14. Papakostidis C, Kanakaris NK, Kontakis G, Giannoudis PV. Pelvic ring disruptions: treatment modalities and analysis of outcomes. Int Orthop. 2009 Apr;33(2):329–38.
15. Poole GV, Ward EF. Causes of mortality in patients with pelvic fractures. Orthopedics. 1994 Aug;17(8):691–6.
16. Kanakaris NK, Angoules AG, Nikolaou VS, Kontakis G, Giannoudis PV. Treatment and outcomes of pelvic malunions and nonunions: a systematic review. Clin Orthop Relat Res. 2009 Aug;467(8):2112–24.
17. Harvey-Kelly KF, Kanakaris NK, Obakponovwe O, West RM, Giannoudis PV. Quality of life and sexual function after traumatic pelvic fracture. J Orthop Trauma. 2014 Jan;28(1):28–35.
18. WiseGEEK. What Are the Pelvic Ligaments? (with pictures) [Internet]. wiseGEEK. [cited 2020 Mar 6]. Available from: http://www.wisegeek.com/what-are-the-pelvic-ligaments.htm
19. Standring S, Ananad N, Gray H, editors. Gray's anatomy 41st Edition: the anatomical basis of clinical practice [Internet]. 41. ed. Philadelphia, PA: Elsevier; 2016. 1562 p. Available from: https://www.bartleby.com/107/57.html
20. Brinker MR. Review of orthopaedic trauma. 2nd ed. Philadelphia, PA: Lippincott Williams & Wilkins; 2013.
21. Ellis H, Mahadevan V. Clinical anatomy: applied anatomy for students and junior doctors. 13th ed. Wiley-Blackwell: West Sussex; 2013.
22. Vaidya R, Waldron J, Scott A, Nasr K. Angiography and embolization in the management of bleeding pelvic fractures. J Am Acad Orthop Surg. 2018 Feb 15;26(4):e68–76.
23. Bataduwaarachchi VR, Thillainathan S. Bilateral indirect inguinal hernia with bilateral corona mortis: A case study from a laparoscopic perspective. International Journal of Anatomical Variations [Internet]. 2011 Sep 9 [cited 2020 May 4];4(1). Available from: https://www.pulsus.com/abstract/bilateral-indirect-inguinal-hernia-with-bilateral-corona-mortis-a-case-study-from-a-laparoscopic-perspective-1648.html
24. Darmanis S, Lewis A, Mansoor A, Bircher M. Corona mortis: an anatomical study with clinical implications in approaches to the pelvis and acetabulum. Clin Anat. 2007 May;20(4):433–9.
25. Pennal GF, Tile M, Waddell JP, Garside H. Pelvic disruption: assessment and classification. Clin Orthop Relat Res. 1980 Sep;151:12–21.
26. Alton TB, Gee AO. Classifications in brief: Young and Burgess classification of pelvic ring injuries. Clin Orthop Relat Res. 2014 Aug;472(8):2338–42.
27. Meinberg E, Agel J, Roberts C, Karam M, Kellam J. Fracture and dislocation classification compendium. J Orthop Trauma. 2018;32:S1–S10.
28. Young JW, Burgess AR, Brumback RJ, Poka A. Pelvic fractures: value of plain radiography in early assessment and management. Radiology. 1986 Aug;160(2):445–51.
29. Lasanianos NG, Kanakaris NK, Giannoudis PV, editors. Trauma and Orthopaedic Classifications [Internet]. London: Springer London; 2015 [cited 2020 Mar 6]. Available from: https://doi.org/10.1007/978-1-4471-6572-9
30. BOA. BOAST - The Management of Patients with Pelvic Fractures [Internet]. 2018 [cited 2020 Mar 6]. Available from: https://www.boa.ac.uk/resources/boast-3-pdf.html
31. Routt MLC, Falicov A, Woodhouse E, Schildhauer TA. Circumferential pelvic antishock sheeting: a temporary resuscitation aid. J Orthop Trauma. 2002 Jan;16(1):45–8.
32. Chesser TJS, Cross AM, Ward AJ. The use of pelvic binders in the emergent management of potential pelvic trauma. Injury. 2012 Jun;43(6):667–9.
33. Gardner MJ, Parada S, Chip Routt ML. Internal rotation and taping of the lower extremities for closed pelvic reduction. J Orthop Trauma. 2009 May;23(5):361–4.
34. Heetveld MJ, Harris I, Schlaphoff G, Balogh Z, D'Amours SK, Sugrue M. Hemodynamically unstable pelvic fractures: recent care and new guidelines. World J Surg. 2004 Sep;28(9):904–9.
35. Scalea TM, editor. The Shock Trauma Manual of Operative Techniques [Internet]. New York, NY: Springer New York; 2015 [cited 2020 Mar 6]. Available from: https://doi.org/10.1007/978-1-4939-2371-7
36. Grant PT. The diagnosis of pelvic fractures by 'springing'. Arch Emerg Med. 1990 Sep;7(3):178–82.
37. White CE, Hsu JR, Holcomb JB. Haemodynamically unstable pelvic fractures. Injury. 2009 Oct;40(10):1023–30.
38. Lee C, Porter K. The prehospital management of pelvic fractures. Emerg Med J. 2007 Feb 1;24(2):130–3.
39. Johnson MH, Chang A, Brandes SB. The value of digital rectal examination in assessing for pelvic fracture–associated urethral injury: what defines a high-riding or nonpalpable prostate? J Trauma Acute Care Surg. 2013 Nov;75(5):913–5.
40. Esposito TJ, Ingraham A, Luchette FA, Sears BW, Santaniello JM, Davis KA, et al. Reasons to omit digital rectal exam in trauma patients: no fingers, no

rectum, no useful additional information. J Trauma. 2005 Dec;59(6):1314–9.
41. Docimo S, Diggs L, Crankshaw L, Lee Y, Vinces F. No evidence supporting the routine use of digital rectal examinations in trauma patients. Indian J Surg. 2015 Aug;77(4):265–9.
42. Fagg JAC, Acharya MR, Chesser TJS, Ward AJ. The value of 'binder-off' imaging to identify occult and unexpected pelvic ring injuries. Injury. 2018 Feb;49(2):284–9.
43. Spahn DR, Bouillon B, Cerny V, Duranteau J, Filipescu D, Hunt BJ, et al. The European guideline on management of major bleeding and coagulopathy following trauma: fifth edition. Crit Care. 2019 Mar 27;23(1):98.
44. Roberts I, Shakur H, Coats T, Hunt B, Balogun E, Barnetson L, et al. The CRASH-2 trial: a randomised controlled trial and economic evaluation of the effects of tranexamic acid on death, vascular occlusive events and transfusion requirement in bleeding trauma patients. Health Technol Assess [Internet]. 2013 Mar [cited 2019 May 7];17(10). Available from: https://www.journalslibrary.nihr.ac.uk/hta/hta17100/
45. Holcomb JB, Tilley BC, Baraniuk S, Fox EE, Wade CE, Podbielski JM, et al. Transfusion of plasma, platelets, and red blood cells in a 1:1:1 vs a 1:1:2 ratio and mortality in patients with severe trauma: the PROPPR randomized clinical trial. JAMA. 2015 Feb 3;313(5):471.
46. Giannoudi M, Harwood P. Damage control resuscitation: lessons learned. Eur J Trauma Emerg Surg. 2016 June;42(3):273–82.
47. Pape H-C, Halvachizadeh S, Leenen L, Velmahos GD, Buckley R, Giannoudis PV. Timing of major fracture care in polytrauma patients – an update on principles, parameters and strategies for 2020. Injury. 2019 Oct;50(10):1656–70.
48. Baqué P, Trojani C, Delotte J, Séjor E, Senni-Buratti M, de Baqué F, et al. Anatomical consequences of "open-book" pelvic ring disruption. A cadaver experimental study. Surg Radiol Anat. 2005 Dec;27(6):487–90.
49. Huittinen VM, Slätis P. Postmortem angiography and dissection of the hypogastric artery in pelvic fractures. Surgery. 1973 Mar;73(3):454–62.
50. Scemama U, Dabadie A, Varoquaux A, Soussan J, Gaudon C, Louis G, et al. Pelvic trauma and vascular emergencies. Diagn Interv Imaging. 2015 Aug;96(7–8):717–29.
51. Papakostidis C, Kanakaris N, Dimitriou R, Giannoudis PV. The role of arterial embolization in controlling pelvic fracture haemorrhage: a systematic review of the literature. Eur J Radiol. 2012 May;81(5):897–904.
52. Langford JR, Burgess AR, Liporace FA, Haidukewych GJ. Pelvic fractures: part 1. Evaluation, classification, and resuscitation. J Am Acad Orthop Surg. 2013 Aug;21(8):448–57.
53. Filiberto DM, Fox AD. Preperitoneal pelvic packing: technique and outcomes. Int J Surg. 2016 Sep;33:222–4.
54. Stahel PF, Moore EE, Burlew CC, Henderson C, Peña AJ, Harry D, et al. Preperitoneal pelvic packing is not associated with an increased risk of surgical site infections after internal anterior pelvic ring fixation. J Orthop Trauma. 2019 Dec;33(12):601–7.
55. Jarvis S, Orlando A, Blondeau B, Banton K, Reynolds C, Berg GM, et al. Variability in the timeliness of interventional radiology availability for angioembolization of hemodynamically unstable pelvic fractures: a prospective survey among U.S. level I trauma centers. Patient Saf Surg. 2019 June 20;13(1):23.
56. Grimm MR, Vrahas MS, Thomas KA. Pressure-volume characteristics of the intact and disrupted pelvic retroperitoneum. J Trauma. 1998 Mar;44(3):454–9.
57. Köhler D, Sellei RM, Sop A, Tarkin IS, Pfeifer R, Garrison RL, et al. Effects of pelvic volume changes on retroperitoneal and intra-abdominal pressure in the injured pelvic ring: a cadaveric model. J Trauma. 2011 Sep;71(3):585–90.
58. Li P, Zhou D, Fu B, Song W, Dong J. Management and outcome of pelvic fracture associated with vaginal injuries: a retrospective study of 25 cases. BMC Musculoskelet Disord. 2019 Oct 22;20(1):466.
59. Zong Z-W, Bao Q-W, Liu H-Y, Shen Y, Zhao Y-F, Hua X, et al. Diagnosis and treatment of rare complications of pelvic fractures. Chin J Traumatol. 2016 Aug;19(4):199–205.
60. Cano-Luís P, Giráldez-Sánchez MÁ, Andrés-Cano P. Pelvic post-traumatic asymmetry. EFORT Open Rev. 2018 May 1;3(5):335–46.
61. Sen RK, Goyal T, Tripathy SK. Neglected pelvic fractures: an overview of literature. J Orthop Traumatol Rehab. 2014 Jan 1;7(1):43.
62. Stahel PF, Mauffrey C, Smith WR, McKean J, Hao J, Burlew CC, et al. External fixation for acute pelvic ring injuries: decision making and technical options. J Trauma Acute Care Surg. 2013 Nov;75(5):882–7.
63. Sellei RM, Schandelmaier P, Kobbe P, Knobe M, Pape H-C. Can a modified anterior external fixator provide posterior compression of AP compression type III pelvic injuries? Clin Orthop Relat Res. 2013 Sep;471(9):2862–8.
64. Kim WY, Hearn TC, Seleem O, Mahalingam E, Stephen D, Tile M. Effect of pin location on stability of pelvic external fixation. Clin Orthop Relat Res. 1999 Apr;361:237–44.
65. Gänsslen A, Krettek C, Pohlemann T. Emergency stabilization of pelvic instabilities with the pelvic C-clamp. Eur J Trauma. 2004 Dec 1;30(6):412–9.
66. Gardner MJ, Chip Routt ML. The antishock iliosacral screw. J Orthop Trauma. 2010 Oct;24(10):e86–9.
67. Tosounidis TH, Sheikh HQ, Kanakaris NK, Giannoudis PV. The use of external fixators in the definitive stabilisation of the pelvis in polytrauma patients: safety, efficacy and clinical outcomes. Injury. 2017 June;48(6):1139–46.

Part VII

Special Populations

35 Trauma in Pregnancy

Rashmi Menon and Thomas Irving

- Epidemiology and mechanisms of trauma in pregnancy
- Anatomical and physiological changes of pregnancy and its implications in trauma
- Approach to a pregnant trauma patient
- Primary survey and its modifications in pregnancy
- Imaging in the pregnant trauma patient
- Specific obstetric complications in trauma
- Management after trauma
- Special considerations

Introduction

Trauma in pregnancy is a leading non-obstetric cause of maternal mortality. The mechanism of trauma is most commonly blunt and caused by motor vehicle accidents (MVA), assaults (often intimate partner violence) and falls [1]. Even relatively minor maternal trauma can result in significant fetal injury. Trauma in the pregnant woman presents unique challenges and requires early involvement of the multidisciplinary team to achieve the best possible outcomes for the mother and the fetus.

R. Menon (✉)
Department of Anaesthesia and Critical Care Medicine, Leeds General Infirmary, Leeds, UK
e-mail: Rashmi.Menon@nhs.net

T. Irving
Liverpool University Hospitals NHS Foundation Trust, Liverpool, UK
e-mail: Tom.Irving@liverpoolft.nhs.uk

Epidemiology

Trauma is a leading cause of mortality in the younger population accounting for approximately 10% of all deaths annually [2]. In the United States, 6–8% of pregnancies are complicated by some degree of trauma [3]. In the United Kingdom, estimates suggest that 1 in 100 women of childbearing age having major trauma will be pregnant [4]. Trauma is reported as the single most common cause of maternal death with 20% of maternal deaths directly related to injury [5]. No single other diagnosis (e.g. Pulmonary Embolus, Sepsis, Haemorrhage) accounted for as many deaths, with a maternal mortality rate due to trauma in some series in the range of 1.5/100000 live births [6]. Accidental injury occurs in line with the baseline population, however there a disproportionate incidence (8%–17%) of domestic violence in the pregnant population and a 7% increased risk of suicide [3].

The United Kingdom has seen a progressive decline in mortality and morbidity from trauma since the establishment of the regional trauma networks in 2012 (2010 in London). Trauma patients who reached hospital alive in 2017 had

P. Lax (ed.), *Textbook of Acute Trauma Care*, https://doi.org/10.1007/978-3-030-83628-3_35

a 19% increase in odds of survival compared with patients in 2008 [7]. This improvement is believed to be due to coordinated care by experienced personnel in major trauma centres and clinical advances such as the routine use of tranexamic acid (TXA) and the concept of damage control resuscitation (DCR). It is not known at present if the increased survival odds apply to pregnant trauma patients. The rate of fetal loss in trauma is variously described as between 3.4% and 56% with the majority of fatalities being secondary to placental abruption. An Injury Severity Score of more than 9 and a fetus of less than 24 weeks gestation are shown to be independent risk factors for fetal loss [8].

Injury in Pregnancy

Trauma in pregnancy may be blunt or penetrating. The majority of all traumatic injury is blunt. In pregnant women, there is a higher incidence of penetrating trauma as compared to non-pregnant women (5–10% vs 2%) [3, 4]. Penetrating trauma is associated with higher fetal and maternal mortality rates as compared to blunt trauma [9].

Motor Vehicle Accidents (MVA)

MVAs remain the most frequent cause of trauma in pregnancy, accounting for about half of all maternal trauma [4]. Incorrect placement of or failure to wear seat belts in the later stages of pregnancy can lead to significant injury following even minor accidents.

Falls

Falls are common in the late second and third trimester of pregnancy. The combination of an altered centre of gravity due to an enlarging uterus, increased joint laxity due to raised progesterone levels and altered proprioception predispose pregnant women to falls [3]. The majority do not cause significant injury.

Assaults

According to the Office for National Statistics, 8% of women experience domestic violence at some point in their lives [10]. Domestic violence may first present in pregnancy or if pre-existent, may escalate during pregnancy [3]. Violence is usually perpetrated by the partner or a family member. The body areas most commonly targeted in pregnant women are the abdomen, breasts and genitalia [11]. Trauma may be blunt or penetrating. Repeated attendances and inconsistent history of the mechanism of injury should raise suspicion of domestic abuse and trigger local safeguarding protocols.

Burns

Burn injury is fortunately rare in pregnancy. All pregnant burn patients must be treated in a tertiary burns centre with adequate access to obstetric services. The pregnant abdomen represents an increased proportion of total body surface area, and this should be taken into account while calculating the percentage of burns. Airway burns will compound the difficulty associated with the obstetric airway, and a relatively lower threshold for early intubation of the patient by rapid sequence induction (RSI) before further deterioration occurs is recommended. The major fluid shifts occurring with extensive burns will negatively affect uteroplacental perfusion if the patient is not adequately resuscitated. Burns affecting over 40% body surface area in pregnancy are associated with a poor maternal and fetal prognosis [3].

Anatomical and Physiological Changes of Pregnancy

During pregnancy, there are hormonal influences on the mother's body to create an ideal environment for fetal growth and to prepare for childbirth. These changes become more noticeable as pregnancy advances and abate a few weeks after delivery of the fetus. The anatomical and physiological changes in pregnancy are well described. They may have a significant impact on the presentation of trauma in pregnant patients (Table 35.1) and necessitate specific modifications of the initial management of the pregnant trauma patient [12].

Approach to a Pregnant Trauma Patient

Legal Position of the Fetus

Under current UK law, the fetus has no intrinsic rights until it is born. Recent high profile cases have highlighted this [13], so it must be reinforced that all clinical decisions are made with the needs of the mother in mind rather than the needs of the fetus.

Recognising Pregnancy

The possibility of pregnancy must be considered in all women of childbearing age presenting with trauma. In most cases, the patient will be able to communicate, and the possibility of pregnancy can be discussed directly with the patient. Examination during the primary survey may also reveal pregnancy if the uterus has reached the intra-abdominal level. Neither history nor examination can safely exclude pregnancy, and urinary pregnancy testing or an ultrasound examination of the abdomen must be performed if doubt exists. In time-critical major trauma, pregnancy may first be identified on a trauma CT.

The anatomical and physiological changes that are associated with pregnancy must be taken into account when managing the pregnant trauma patient [12]. Knowing the gestational age of the fetus is essential as it will affect subsequent management of the patient as well as the fetus.

Initial management must focus on maternal resuscitation and stabilisation. As in any trauma patient, a MABCDE (Major haemorrhage, Airway, Breathing, Circulation, Disability and Exposure) approach should be followed. Fetal assessment should only be performed once life-threatening maternal injuries have been addressed [14]. Prompt and effective maternal resuscitation will aid in ensuring favourable fetal outcomes.

Massive Haemorrhage

Maternal blood volume is increased at term by up to 50%, there is a physiological dilutional anaemia of pregnancy and cardiac output is increased by 28 weeks to 40% greater than pre-pregnancy levels. This hypervolaemic, haemodiluted state is intended to protect the mother during haemorrhage associated with childbirth. As a consequence, up to 40% of maternal circulating volume may be lost before the clinical signs of shock become manifest.

By term the uterus and placenta receive 800 ml/min of blood (a significant portion of the cardiac output). Placental abruption or direct utero-placental injuries can result in catastrophic haemorrhage either externally (per vaginum) or concealed within the abdomen. Early involvement of an obstetrician is therefore recommended.

Airway and Cervical Spine

Assess and ensure a patent maternal airway while maintaining immobilisation of the cervical spine. It is well known that obstetric airway management is challenging due to increased upper airway oedema and vascularity, increased adiposity, patients being positioned with a lateral tilt and a higher risk of gastric aspiration [12]. In the obstetric trauma patient, this difficulty may be increased further by cervical spine immobilisation, the urgent nature of the intervention and the presence of airway trauma or burns [15].

If airway problems are anticipated, early intubation is recommended for airway protection and to assure good maternal oxygen delivery. An RSI by an experienced operator, following the obstetric airway management guidelines of the Difficult Airway Society (DAS) is recommended (Fig. 35.1) [16].

The patient should be positioned 30° head up to improve the functional residual capacity (FRC), reduce the risk of aspiration of gastric contents and cause downward movement of the breasts, making laryngoscope insertion easier. The cervical collar should be removed, and man-

Table 35.1 Anatomical and physiological changes in pregnancy and its implications in trauma

System	Changes in pregnancy	Implications in trauma
Airway	• Increased airway mucosal vascularity and oedema • Weight gain	• Increased incidence of difficult intubation; early RSI by an experienced operator recommended in case of airway compromise • Avoid nasal interventions • Use of videolaryngoscopes and bougies as first line
Respiratory system	• FRC decreased by 30% due to cephalad displacement of the diaphragm • $PaCO_2$ decreased • Oxygen consumption increased by 60% • Minute ventilation increased by 50% [tidal volume 45% and respiratory rate 5%] due to respiratory stimulant effects of progesterone • Diaphragm raised 4 cm due to gravid uterus	• Increased oxygen requirements and decreased stores can rapidly cause hypoxemia during apnoea (such as with RSI) or airway obstruction. Hence, oxygen supplementation is essential. • 30° head-up tilt will increase FRC and oxygen stores. • The raised diaphragm pushes abdominal organs upwards and can cause abnormal injury patterns. • Thoracostomy tubes, if indicated, should be placed 1–2 spaces higher than normal
Circulatory system	• Decreased systemic vascular resistance • Decreased preload • Increased heart rate • Increased stroke volume • Increased cardiac output • Increased circulating blood volume • Aortocaval compression by the gravid uterus becomes significant after 20 weeks gestation • Uterine autoregulation is lost, so uterine perfusion depends on maternal blood pressure	• Due to increased blood volumes, signs of hypovolaemia appear late, and a high index of suspicion must be maintained at all times • Uterine displacement (manual displacement of uterus preferred over left lateral tilt as it better maintains spinal alignment) in all patients over 20 weeks gestation • Dilated uterine and pelvic vasculature can cause catastrophic bleeding in pelvic fractures. • Maternal hypotension (such as with permissive hypotension) can affect uteroplacental perfusion
Haematological system	• Increased clotting factors • Increased fibrinogen levels • Decreased haemoglobin (physiological anaemia of pregnancy) • Decreased anticoagulant factors • Decreased fibrinolytic activity • Decreased platelet count	• Be aware of altered normal values in pregnancy • Hypercoagulable state; VTE prophylaxis to be considered for all pregnant trauma patients
Gastrointestinal system	• Reduced gastric emptying and 'full-stomach' state • Reduced motility throughout the GI tract due to the effects of progesterone • Anatomical displacement of pylorus by the gravid uterus • Decreased LOS tone • Increased intraabdominal pressure	• Increased risk of aspiration of gastric contents with loss of airway reflexes; early RSI if airway reflexes are compromised
Musculoskeletal system	• Increased joint laxity towards term • Altered centre of gravity with enlarging uterus, causing exaggerated lumbar lordosis	• High incidence of falls towards the latter stages of pregnancy
Renal system	• Increased renal blood flow • Increased GFR • Increased urinary protein excretion • Increased hydronephrosis and hydroureter • Reduced creatinine values	• Altered 'normal' values

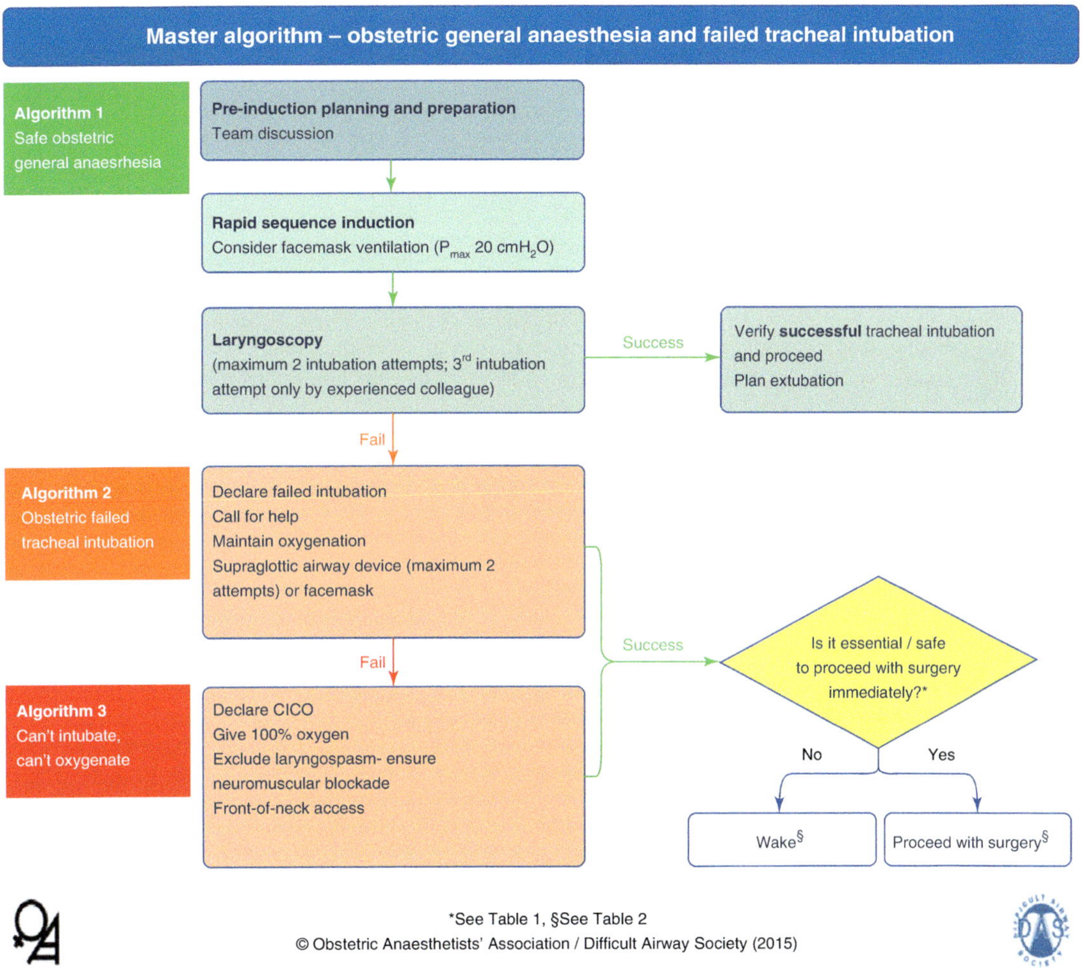

Fig. 35.1 Reproduced from Mushambi et al. [16] with permission from Obstetric Anaesthetists' Association/Difficult Airway Society

ual in-line stabilisation (MILS) used instead to immobilise the cervical spine, in order to facilitate laryngoscopy. Apnoeic oxygenation techniques such as nasal high-flow may be used to maximise oxygen stores and delay desaturation during RSI. Use of video laryngoscopes as the first line, with a bougie and a smaller diameter endotracheal tube may increase first-pass intubation success rates. In cases of difficult intubation, the DAS guidelines should be followed, namely releasing cricoid pressure, gentle bag and mask ventilation, and prioritisation of oxygenation [15]. A second-generation supraglottic airway device (SAD) may be used for rescue, and front of neck access (FONA) will be required in a 'Can't Intubate, Can't Oxygenate' (CICO) scenario. Neck adiposity may make FONA challenging; an open approach with longitudinal neck incision and finger dissection down to the trachea is recommended [15].

Breathing

High maternal oxygen requirements, coupled with low oxygen stores, cause rapid desaturation with respiratory compromise. High flow supplemental oxygen should be administered as for any trauma patient in the first instance. Once stable, the oxygen should be titrated down to achieve maternal saturations of over 94% as this will ensure the maintenance of the uteroplacental oxygen gradient and adequate fetal oxygen delivery [17, 18]. If mechanically ventilated a target $PaCO_2$ of 4–4.5 kpa should be aimed for, as is normal in pregnancy. Further falls in $PaCO_2$ will shift the oxygen dissociation curve to the left and reduce fetal oxygen delivery. The gravid uterus causes upward displacement of the diaphragm. Intercostal drain (ICD) insertion should thus be performed two spaces above the usual fifth intercostal space within the safe triangle, to avoid damage to abdominal viscera [3, 14]. If the mother is stable, imaging is recommended prior to ICD insertions to determine definite clinical need as well as to confirm the suitability of the insertion site. CT scans have more sensitivity than ultrasound in the diagnosis of haemopneumothorax if there is doubt surrounding the diagnosis [18].

Circulation

As discussed above, the increased blood volume of pregnancy results in a significant degree of compensation in trauma, with hypovolaemia presenting late and catastrophically [12]. A high index of suspicion for hypovolemia must be maintained in the injured pregnant patient. Uterine causes (such as rupture or placental abruption) must be actively considered as sources of bleeding, and in these cases serious pathology can often be concealed.

After 20 weeks' gestation, aortocaval compression is significant, and uterine displacement must be maintained; either manually or by a lateral tilt of the trauma board. Large-bore intravenous (IV) access must be obtained as for any trauma patient, and ideally, the access should be above the diaphragm so that drugs and fluids reach the central circulation without being impeded by compression of abdominal vessels due to the gravid uterus (Fig. 35.2).

Pelvic fractures are of concern as the pelvic vasculature is maximally dilated in late pregnancy and can cause catastrophic bleeding [12].

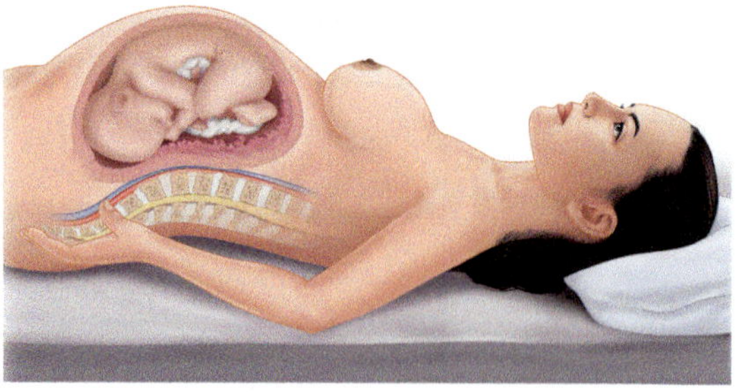

Fig. 35.2 Supine Hypotensive Synddrome by Bonnie Gruenburg via Wikimedia Commons under Creative Commons attribution share-alike4.0 license

Pelvic binders must be used if the mechanism of injury is significant [14].

A full set of trauma blood tests should be performed, being mindful of altered values in pregnancy. A Kleihauer-Betke blood test (KBT) should also be sent in all pregnant trauma patients. This test measures the amount of fetal haemoglobin in the maternal circulation and is a marker of the degree of fetomaternal haemorrhage and uteroplacental injury. In women who have a Rhesus negative blood group but are carrying a Rhesus positive baby, the KBT result also allows calculation of the correct dosing of anti-D immunoglobulin. Fetomaternal haemorrhage has been used as a surrogate marker of the severity of trauma and a KBT assists in fetal prognostication, independent of the Rhesus status [3, 18, 19].

Damage Control Resuscitation is an integral part of contemporary trauma care and advocates a restrictive fluid replacement strategy with permissive hypotension and controlled resuscitation to a palpable central pulse until definitive control of bleeding is achieved [14]. This approach raises concerns in pregnant patients as maternal hypotension may cause decreased uteroplacental perfusion and compromise the fetus. However, the primary consideration is maternal stability, and fetal prognosis will depend on several other factors such as fetal gestation and uterine injury. These decisions should thus be made with multidisciplinary team input and be well documented.

The use of vasopressors to maintain blood pressure is not ideal in trauma or obstetrics patients as they may increase the risk of clot dislodgement and cause further bleeding. Most commonly used vasopressors intrinsically reduce uteroplacental perfusion in healthy individuals, so the problem will be compounded in trauma patients. Hence, they must only be used if aggressive volume resuscitation fails and for the shortest time possible.

If the patient does not respond to volume resuscitation, plans must be made to transfer to theatre. Damage control surgery may be needed, potentially including delivery of the fetus if there is obstetric bleeding. Limited imaging such as plain X-rays or ultrasound can be performed in the trauma bay without delaying transfer to theatre and may provide vital information to guide surgery. If stability is achieved with volume resuscitation, then a trauma CT is recommended [14].

Tranexamic acid (1 gram IV) is considered safe in pregnancy and must be administered within the first 3 h to confer survival benefit [20].

Disability

Assessment and management of disability is the same as in the non-pregnant patient.

Cervical collars may not fit properly due to increased neck adiposity. In such cases, manual in-line stabilisation should be used. The spine board or scoop stretcher (if used) can be tilted 30° to the left using a wedge beneath to reduce aortocaval compression.

In the case of traumatic head injury, control of ICP may require maternal hyperventilation. Maternal alkalosis can shift the oxygen dissociation curve to the left and reduce fetal oxygen delivery [12]. Blood sugars must be measured, and care is taken to prevent hypoglycaemia as it can impair glucose transport to the fetus.

Exposure

During exposure and examination of the patient, particular attention should be paid to excluding vaginal blood loss [3, 18] and maintain normothermia.

Specific Obstetric Complications

Preterm Labour

The most common obstetric complication of trauma is the onset of contractions. This results from several mechanisms: Placental abruption, prostaglandin release from damaged myometrial cells and premature rupture of membranes. Contractions may be accompanied by cervical dilatation and/or rupture of membranes. Contractions often stop spontaneously but may require treatment with tocolytics. Advice from obstetric team is crucial and patients with a viable fetus should ideally be cared for in a centre with a neonatal unit. Depending on fetal gestation, the patient may need steroids (for fetal lung maturity) and magnesium sulphate (fetal neuroprotection) for optimal fetal outcomes [18].

Placental Abruption

Some degree of placental abruption occurs in up to 50% of cases of major trauma and may occur with little or no signs of external injury. Fetal mortality is high at 20–35%. The placenta is devoid of elastic tissue while the myometrium is very elastic predisposing to shearing. Blunt trauma will deform the elastic and flexible myometrium which is sheared from the relatively inflexible placenta. It usually presents between 2 and 6 h after trauma, with clinical signs of abdominal pain, contractions, vaginal bleeding, uterine tenderness or a uterus larger than would be expected for gestational dates, features of maternal hypovolaemia and fetal distress. Abruption (occult or concealed—see Fig. 35.3) may lead to major maternal bleeding and consumption coagulopathy. Diagnosis is mainly by history and clinical examination. Diagnosis may be confirmed on ultrasound scan (USS) however management of suspected abruption should not be delayed for USS as it is not a sensitive tool for diagnosis [18]. It is particularly vital to monitor fetal status as this will guide obstetric led management.

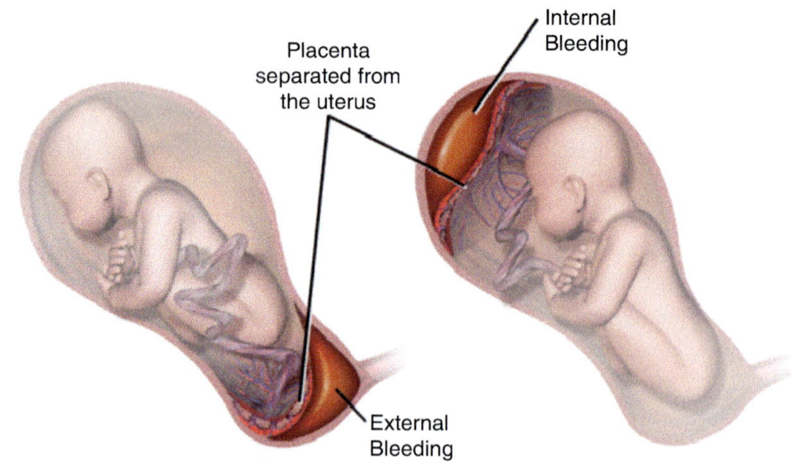

Fig. 35.3 Blausen.com staff (2014). "Medical gallery of Blausen Medical 2014". WikiJournal of Medicine 1 (2). DOI:https://doi.org/10.15347/wjm/2014.010. ISSN 2002-4436. - Own work under Creative Commons BY 3.0 license

Uterine Rupture

Rupture of the uterus is a rare complication of direct abdominal trauma in late pregnancy, occurring in 1.6% of patients. Severity ranges from serosal haemorrhage to a complete avulsion of the uterus. 75% of cases involve the fundus. Presentation is with severe abdominal pain and tenderness, features of shock, palpable fetal parts and maternal collapse. There is almost universal fetal mortality and maternal mortality approaches 10%. Urgent maternal resuscitation and surgical intervention is required (often hysterectomy in the traumatic setting) to control haemorrhage [21].

Fetal-Maternal Haemorrhage

Transfer of fetal blood to the mother is common in trauma and is a predictor for the severity of trauma. A Kleihauer test (Acid elution test) estimates the amount of fetal haemoglobin transferred to the mother. In high risk patients (Rhesus negative mother, Abdominal or Major Trauma and Kleihauer positive) Anti-D immunoglobulin should be administered. Dosing recommendations vary from unit to unit. Treatment with Anti-D is aimed at preventing Haemolytic Disease of the Newborn in future pregnancies. Whilst Anti-D Administration is important, it is not an immediate priority in acute resuscitation. As long as it is administered within 72 h of the sensitising event then it will be effective.

Amniotic Fluid Embolism

Amniotic Fluid Embolism (AFE) is a rare event precipitated by entry of amniotic fluid into the maternal circulation. The pathophysiology remains unclear, however AFE is characterised by a sudden onset of dyspnea, cyanosis, cardiovascular collapse with subsequent organ dysfunction, coagulopathy and potentially death. Although classically described in labour and delivery, trauma may expose the maternal circulation to amniotic fluid and thus the risk of AFE [22]. Treatment remains supportive, often requiring multiple organ support in an intensive care setting.

Maternal Cardiac Arrest

Cardiac arrest in the pregnant patient is managed in a similar way to the non-pregnant patient, with a few modifications. Manual uterine displacement is recommended to avoid aortocaval compression; this is preferred over a left lateral tilt which causes chest compressions to be less effective. Resuscitative hysterotomy is a significant addition to advanced life support algorithms for pregnant patients and is time-critical and logistically challenging.

Resuscitative Hysterotomy

Resuscitative hysterotomy is performed in the event of maternal cardiac arrest, ideally within 4 min of confirmed arrest, with the baby delivered within 5 min of arrest to achieve the best outcomes [3, 18], though survival has been reported with arrest times up to 15 min [23]. The primary aim is to aid maternal resuscitation; emptying the uterus removes aortocaval compression, provides placental autotransfusion and improves respiratory dynamics. The procedure is straightforward and can be done with minimal equipment. Most emergency departments store a basic caesarean tray, but the procedure can be performed with a basic surgical tray containing a knife, retractors and clamps. The obstetrician, who should be asked to attend the trauma call immediately once pregnancy is suspected, is the best person to perform this procedure. If the fetus is of sufficient gestation, a hysterotomy offers it the best chance of survival, but this is a secondary objective. If there is return of spontaneous circulation (ROSC), the patient must then be taken to theatre to control bleeding and close the abdominal wound. If an obstetrician is not available, Emergency Department physicians and Pre-Hospital physicians are increasingly being taught to perform the procedure via a vertical laparotomy incision, rather than the traditional Pfannenstiel incision.

A retrospective review of 94 cases of resuscitative hysterotomy has shown a maternal survival rate of 54%, with 80% of these having good neurological outcome for the mother. It is shown that time to delivery following arrest is key to outcome and should be performed as soon as possible. Fetal survival was reported at around the 60% level; the earlier the fetus is delivered following arrest, again the better the outcomes [23].

Technique for Perimortem Section

Decision to Operate

Often the most difficult step—With an obviously pregnant patient with an easily palpable uterus, a hysterotomy within 15 min of the arrest can still result in over 50% favourable fetal outcomes [23] and beyond that time, even though fetal survival decreases, it is still indicated as an intervention that may aid maternal resuscitation.

Adult cardiac arrest management must be continued during the procedure and a separate team must be tasked to resuscitate the baby once delivered. In the event of pre-hospital hysterotomy, additional crews should be requested as soon as the procedure is being considered in order to provide additional resources for neonatal resuscitation.

Preparation

This is a resuscitative intervention and therefore there is no role in delaying to perform skin preparation or application of surgical drapes. Urethral catheterisation will introduce delay and should not be performed, care should be taken therefore to avoid surgical injury to the bladder.

Surgical Technique

1. **Laparotomy**—A midline incision from xiphisternum to pubic symphysis. Rapid but careful dissection through all layers of the abdominal wall and peritoneum
2. **Hysterotomy**—Expose the uterus, a careful scalpel incision is made then extended in the midline using scissors to avoid injury to the baby.
3. **Delivery of Baby**—Rupture the amnion (if intact). Deliver baby, clamping the umbilical cord in two places and dividing. Pass the baby out to the allocated team for resuscitation.
4. **Delivery of Placenta**—Gentle traction of the cord and scoop the placenta out. Consider administration of Syntocinon (Oxytocin) if maternal circulation restored.
5. **Haemostasis**—Will depend on prognosis of patient. Abdominal packing will allow for ongoing resuscitation with temporary haemostasis. Following ROSC meticulous haemostasis is required to prevent subsequent haemorrhage when cardiac output improves.

6. **Closure**—Following ROSC the patient should be transferred to an Operating Theatre for formal closure of the uterus and laparotomy.

Imaging in the Pregnant Patient

X-Rays

Radiological investigations, if indicated, should be undertaken promptly. The gold standard in trauma imaging is computerised tomography (CT), which should be performed straight after the primary survey in stable patients and aids in timely diagnosis and directed management of injuries [14]. Delayed imaging due to concerns relating to fetal radiation and IV contrast exposure may result in a delay in treatment and cause harm to both mother and fetus (Fig. 35.4).

According to the guidelines of the Royal College of Radiologists [24], the dose of radiation associated with standard diagnostic trauma imaging is not believed to increase the risk of miscarriage, teratogenesis, growth retardation or neurological abnormalities in the fetus. A trauma CT uses a radiation dose between 10 and 50 mGy, which may result in a slight increase in the incidence of childhood cancers, but in absolute terms the risk remains low. Radiation effects are cumulative and repeated scans should be avoided. A consultant radiologist's opinion should be sought early to aid in planning the scans and radiation dosages. Intravenous iodine or gadolinium-based contrast agents are considered safe in pregnancy.

Ultrasound

Extended Focused Assessment of Trauma (eFAST) and plain radiographs may be used in unstable patients for rapid identification of intraabdominal or intrathoracic injuries that are amenable to immediate intervention. These investigations are, however, inferior to a CT scan in diagnosis. Diagnostic peritoneal lavage has now been replaced by CT and eFAST due to risks of visceral injury and leading to unnecessary surgery [3, 14].

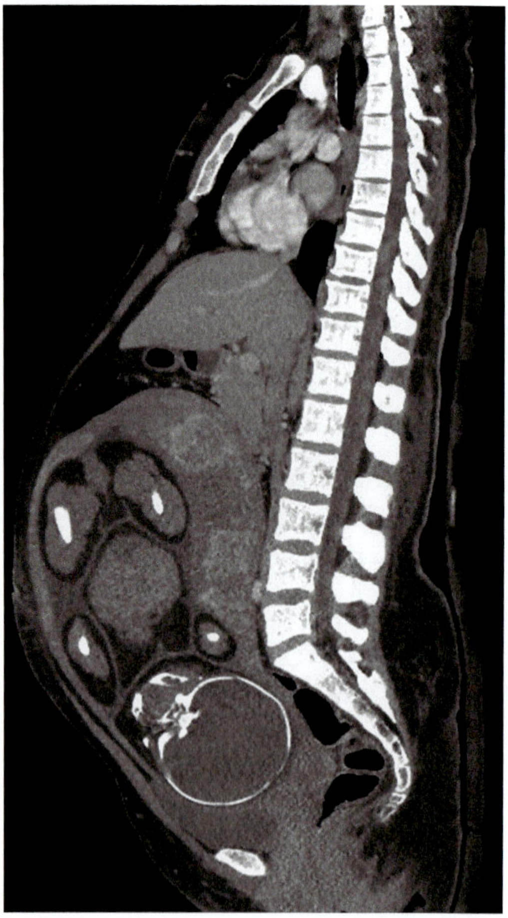

Fig. 35.4 By Mikael Häggström via wikimedia, used with permission (see https://commons.wikimedia.org/wiki/User:Mikael_H%C3%A4ggstr%C3%B6m#Attribution)

Obstetric Assessment

After initial assessment and stabilisation of the mother, a full obstetric assessment must be performed to assess the fetus and to identify any maternal obstetric complications that were not obvious during the primary survey [3, 18]. Fetal survival can be determined rapidly by auscultating the fetal heart rate (FHR, normally between 110 and 160 bpm), and further information on fetal well-being and uterine activity can be obtained by continuous cardiotocographic (CTG) monitoring (Fig. 35.5). Non-reassuring fetal heart rate patterns on CTG may be the first indicator of uterine pathologies such as placental abruption or uterine rupture. The ideal period of

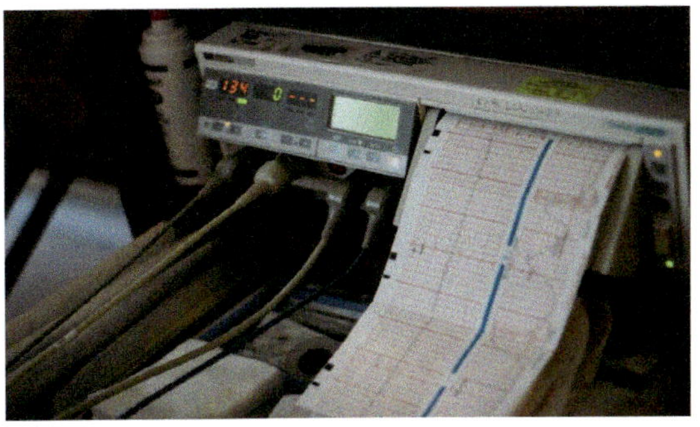

Fig. 35.5 Via pexels.com under Creative Commons 0 license (https://www.pexels.com/photo/business-commerce-computer-delivery-263194/)

CTG monitoring is unclear. A practical approach suggested by the American College of Obstetrics and Gynecology (ACOG) [3] is to monitor CTG for 4 h initially, and if there are any non-reassuring signs present in this time, to continue monitoring for a further 24 h. The non-reassuring signs are uterine contractions more than one every 10 min, significant abdominal pains, uterine tenderness, rupture of membranes, vaginal bleeding or an abnormal antenatal FHR pattern.

An ultrasound scan of the abdomen will provide more accurate information on fetal wellbeing and help in the estimation of gestational age, which has an important bearing on management. It may also help in the diagnosis of uteroplacental pathology and localisation of the placenta.

Patient Management After Trauma

The decision to continue a pregnancy or deliver urgently after trauma depends on multiple factors. The degree of fetal maturity, presence of uterine injury, the nature of the maternal traumatic injury and the effect of continuing pregnancy on the mother's prognosis should all be taken into account while making this decision.

Maternal traumatic injuries should be managed as for the non-pregnant patient. If the continuation of pregnancy prevents optimal treatment of the mother, then difficult decisions such as termination of pregnancy may have to be discussed. These decisions should be made on a case by case basis and after MDT discussion. If continuation of pregnancy does not interfere with maternal treatment, then the pregnancy should be continued for as long as possible to give the fetus the best possible outcome.

Obstetric complications, if present, should be treated appropriately (see section on "specific obstetric complications"). The patient may need joint obstetric and trauma surgery. If there are no obstetric complications, the patient may be discharged after 24 h with advice to return for urgent assessment if worrying signs or symptoms develop [3]. Obstetric follow up should be as for any other patient. The eventual mode of delivery will depend on patient choice, obstetric considerations and the residual effect of any trauma, such as a pelvic fracture. If the patient has a significant period of decreased mobility due to the trauma, such as a plaster cast on a broken ankle, VTE prophylaxis must be considered as pregnancy and trauma are both pro-thrombotic states [14].

Those who suffer pregnancy loss or pre-term delivery as a result of trauma or to facilitate maternal treatment should be offered psychological support and counselling.

Special Considerations

Pelvic Fractures

Pelvic fractures may have an increased incidence in the pregnanct population due to hormonal and biomechanical changes (Fig. 35.6). Pelvic fractures in pregnancy are associated with high maternal and fetal mortality [25, 26]. There is limited guidance on the management of these conditions. If the mechanism of trauma is suggestive of pelvic injury, pelvic binders can be life-saving and must be applied as soon as possible [14]. The pelvic binder, when correctly applied, sits over the greater trochanters and can be applied effectively even in term pregnancy.

In stable pelvic fractures, a conservative approach may be followed. If pelvic fractures cause pelvic arterial bleeding, the treatment is by embolization of the pelvic vessels in the interventional radiology suite. High radiation doses are needed for this procedure which may have detri-

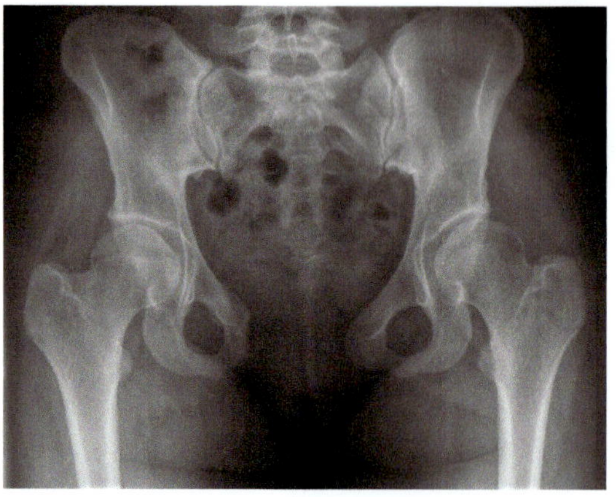

Fig. 35.6 © Nevit Dilmen via wikimedia under Creative Commons Attribution-Share Alike 3.0 Unported license

mental effects on the fetus. There is also a risk that pelvic vessel embolization may reduce utero-placental blood flow and cause fetal distress.

In the case of complex, unstable pelvic fractures, an open reduction and internal fixation of the pelvis will be indicated. This surgery is usually performed via a lower abdominal approach and may be challenging to perform in the heavily pregnant patient. Prone positioning may be required for posterior pelvic fractures. Intraoperative imaging is essential, and radiation exposure can be significant. Modifications to the surgical technique and radiation doses may be needed if fetal preservation is planned [26].

In rare cases, if the fetal head is engaged in the pelvis, a pelvic fracture can also cause a fetal skull fracture.

The above scenarios cause difficult treatment dilemmas. The care of each patient should thus be individualised and the multidisciplinary team involved in decision making. In significant pelvic injury, the fetus may already be compromised and hence may need to be delivered simultaneously with pelvic surgery. If the continuation of the pregnancy is not conducive to maternal treatment, pregnancy may have to be terminated prematurely in maternal best interest.

If pregnancy is continued to term after a pelvic fracture, the eventual mode of delivery will depend on the type of fracture and its treatment, patient choice and obstetric considerations. Pelvic fractures do not automatically mandate a caesarean delivery.

Penetrating Injury

Penetrating trauma is rare in pregnancy but has a high morbidity for the mother and a higher mortality rate for the fetus as compared to blunt trauma [3, 18, 19]. Trauma may be in the form of knife or gunshot injuries. Injury patterns will vary depending upon the period of gestation. In late pregnancy, the gravid uterus and the fetus take the brunt of any anterior abdominal injury, protecting the maternal viscera. Approximately 60–70% of penetrating injuries affect the uterus and fetus, while only 20% affect maternal viscera [18]. Abnormal injury patterns may also be seen as the abdominal viscera are pushed upwards and backwards. In the case of gunshot injuries, there is transmission of kinetic energy to the viscera, causing a higher amount of damage. Fetal mortality in gunshot injuries of the abdomen can be as high as 75%.

The management of penetrating trauma to the abdomen is similar to the non-pregnant patient. Pregnancy should not deter exploratory laparotomy if needed. The pregnancy may be preserved if there is no damage to the uterus and the fetus is not distressed. If the fetus has reached an appropriate gestational age, then delivery may be considered at the time of laparotomy. A dead or injured fetus does not necessarily need caesarean section as vaginal delivery may be more appropriate.

Obstetric vs Traumatic Blood Loss

It is crucial to distinguish obstetric haemorrhage (placental abruption, uterine atony) from traumatic haemorrhage. In traumatic haemorrhage, a 1:1:1 transfusion strategy is recommended [14], while in obstetric haemorrhage, the management should be based on the aetiology of haemorrhage. In uterine atony, coagulation may stay normal despite large volume blood losses due to the hypercoagulable state of pregnancy. In the case of placental abruption, consumption of clotting factors can occur even with minimal bleeding. Fibrinogen concentrations are most important in pregnancy as they fall early, and low normal values may indicate the onset of coagulopathy.

Recent review articles and guidelines [27, 28] suggest treating obstetric bleeding different from trauma. Early use of point of care coagulation tests and involvement of haematologists will aid appropriate management. Use of coagulation factors is recommended after four units of red blood cell transfusion, and after that in a 1:1 ratio of red cells and fresh frozen plasma. Early fibrinogen replacement, when values fall below 3 g/L is vital, and this is achieved by using fibrinogen concentrate or cryoprecipitate.

Summary

Trauma in the pregnant individual presents unique challenges requiring modifications in standard trauma management principles and early multidisciplinary input for best possible maternal and fetal outcomes.

Questions

1. Which of the following is the commonest cause of trauma during pregnancy?
   (a) Domestic violence
   (b) Falls
   (c) Burns
   (d) Motor vehicle accidents
   (e) Self-harm attempts
2. Which of the following are not true regarding the airway management of a pregnant trauma patient?
   (a) There is increased vascularity and mucosal oedema making airway management challenging
   (b) Supraglottic airway devices should be used as first-line as endotracheal intubation can be difficult
   (c) Adequate pre-oxygenation is essential to prevent desaturation during rapid sequence intubation (RSI)
   (d) The cervical collar should be removed and manual inline stabilisation applied during an RSI
   (e) The patient should be positioned flat on the table
3. Which of these is not an obstetric complication of traumatic injury?
   (a) Amniotic fluid embolism
   (b) Preterm labour
   (c) Fetal macrosomia
   (d) Feto-maternal haemorrhage
   (e) Placental abruption
4. Which of the following are not steps in resuscitative hysterotomy?
   (a) Catheterisation to empty the bladder to prevent bladder injury
   (b) Lower abdominal transverse incision
   (c) Hysterotomy
   (d) Delivery of baby
   (e) Delivery of placenta
5. Management of the pregnant patient after major traumatic injury involves all the below except
   (a) Immediate management of the traumatic injury
   (b) Trauma CT to determine nature of injuries
   (c) Delivery of the baby to facilitate maternal care
   (d) Thromboprophylaxis as trauma and pregnancy are both prothrombotic conditions
   (e) Continued obstetric follow-up until delivery

Answers

1. d
2. b, e
3. c
4. a, b
5. c

References

1. Cantwell R, Clutton-Brock T, Cooper G, Dawson A, Drife J, Garrod D, et al. Saving mothers' lives: reviewing maternal deaths to make motherhood safer: 2006-2008. The Eighth Report of the Confidential Enquiries into Maternal Deaths in the United Kingdom. BJOG. 2011 Mar;118(Suppl 1):1–203.
2. Saving lives, improving mothers' care - surveillance of maternal deaths in the UK 2011-13 and lessons learned to inform maternity care from the UK and Ireland Confidential Enquiries into Maternal Deaths and Morbidity 2009-13 [Internet]. Oxford: National Perinatal Epidemiology Unit, University of Oxford; 2015 [cited 2019 Sep 18] p. 94. Available from: https://www.npeu.ox.ac.uk/downloads/files/mbrrace-uk/reports/MBRRACE-UK%20Maternal%20Report%202015.pdf
3. Mendez-Figueroa H, Dahlke JD, Vrees RA, Rouse DJ. Trauma in pregnancy: an updated systematic review. Am J Obstet Gynecol. 2013 Jul;209(1):1–10.

4. Battaloglu E, McDonnell D, Chu J, Lecky F, Porter SK. Epidemiology and outcomes of pregnancy and obstetric complications in trauma in the United Kingdom. Injury. 2016 Jan;47(1):184–7.
5. Hill CC, Pickinpaugh J. Trauma and surgical emergencies in the obstetric patient. Surg Clin N Am. 2008 Apr;88(2):421–40.
6. Rusen ID, Liston R. Special report on maternal mortality and severe morbidity in Canada: enhanced surveillance: the path to prevention. Ottawa: Health Canada, Public Health Agency, Maternal and Infant Health Section; 2004.
7. Moran CG, Lecky F, Bouamra O, Lawrence T, Edwards A, Woodford M, et al. Changing the system - major trauma patients and their outcomes in the NHS (England) 2008–17. EClinicalMedicine. 2018 Aug;2–3:13–21.
8. Theodorou DA, Velmahos GC, Souter I, Chan LS, Vassiliu P, Tatevossian R, et al. Fetal death after trauma in pregnancy. Am Surg. 2000 Sep;66(9):809–12.
9. Deshpande NA, Kucirka LM, Smith RN, Oxford CM. Pregnant trauma victims experience nearly 2-fold higher mortality compared to their nonpregnant counterparts. Am J Obstet Gynecol. 2017 Nov;217(5):590.e1–9.
10. Office for National Statistics. Domestic abuse in England and Wales year ending March 2018 [Internet]. 2018 Nov [cited 2019 Sep 18] p. 69. Available from: https://www.ons.gov.uk/peoplepopulationandcommunity/crimeandjustice/bulletins/domesticabuseinenglandandwales/yearendingmarch2018
11. World Health Organisation. Intimate partner violence during pregnancy [Internet]. World Health Organisation; 2011 [cited 2019 Sep 18] p. 4. Available from: https://www.who.int/reproductivehealth/publications/violence/rhr_11_35/en/
12. Bedson R, Riccoboni A. Physiology of pregnancy: clinical anaesthetic implications. Contin Educ Anaesth Crit Care Pain. 2014 Apr;14(2):69–72.
13. Collins K. 'Too hard to convict people of harming unborn babies' [Internet]. BBC Newsbeat. 2015 [cited 2019 Sep 20]. Available from: http://www.bbc.co.uk/newsbeat/article/32332040/too-hard-to-convict-people-of-harming-unborn-babies
14. NICE. Major trauma: assessment and initial management [Internet]. 2016 [cited 2019 Sep 18]. Available from: https://www.nice.org.uk/guidance/ng39/evidence/full-guideline-2308122833
15. Kinsella SM, Winton AL, Mushambi MC, Ramaswamy K, Swales H, Quinn AC, et al. Failed tracheal intubation during obstetric general anaesthesia: a literature review. Int J Obstet Anesth. 2015 Nov;24(4):356–74.
16. Mushambi MC, Kinsella SM, Popat M, Swales H, Ramaswamy KK, Winton AL, et al. Obstetric anaesthetists' association and difficult airway society guidelines for the management of difficult and failed tracheal intubation in obstetrics. Anaesthesia. 2015 Nov;70(11):1286–306.
17. O'Driscoll BR, Howard LS, Earis J, Mak V. British Thoracic Society guideline for oxygen use in adults in healthcare and emergency settings. BMJ Open Respir Res. 2017 May 1;4(1):e000170.
18. Jain V, Chari R, Maslovitz S, Farine D, Bujold E, Gagnon R, et al. Guidelines for the management of a pregnant trauma patient. J Obstet Gynaecol Can. 2015 June;37(6):553–71.
19. Brown S, Mozurkewich E. Trauma during pregnancy. Obstet Gynecol Clin N Am. 2013 Mar;40(1):47–57.
20. Roberts I, Shakur H, Afolabi A, The CRASH-2 Collaborators. The importance of early treatment with tranexamic acid in bleeding trauma patients: an exploratory analysis of the CRASH-2 randomised controlled trial. Lancet. 2011 Mar;377(9771):1096–1101.e2.
21. Sisay Woldeyes W, Amenu D, Segni H. Uterine rupture in pregnancy following fall from a motorcycle: a horrid accident in pregnancy—a case report and review of the literature. Case Rep Obstet Gynecol. 2015;2015:1–3.
22. Rudra A, Chatterjee S, Sengupta S, Nandi B, Mitra J. Amniotic fluid embolism. Indian J Crit Care Med. 2009 Sep;13(3):129–35.
23. Einav S, Kaufman N, Sela HY. Maternal cardiac arrest and perimortem caesarean delivery: evidence or expert-based? Resuscitation. 2012 Oct;83(10):1191–200.
24. Wall BF, Health Protection Agency (Great Britain), Royal College of Radiologists (Great Britain), College of Radiographers (Great Britain), Health Protection Agency (Great Britain), Centre for Radiation C and EH. Protection of pregnant patients during diagnostic medical exposures to ionising radiation: advice from the Health Protection Agency, the Royal College of Radiologists and the College of Radiographers, 2009.
25. Leggon RE, Wood GC, Indeck MC. Pelvic fractures in pregnancy: factors influencing maternal and fetal outcomes: the journal of trauma: injury. Infect Crit Care. 2002 Oct;53(4):796–804.
26. Almog G, Liebergall M, Tsafrir A, Barzilay Y, Mosheiff R. Management of pelvic fractures during pregnancy. Am J Orthop. 2007 Nov;36(11):E153–9.
27. Collis RE, Collins PW. Haemostatic management of obstetric haemorrhage. Anaesthesia. 2015 Jan;70:78–e28.
28. Klein AA, Arnold P, Bingham RM, Brohi K, Clark R, Collis R, et al. AAGBI guidelines: the use of blood components and their alternatives 2016. Anaesthesia. 2016 Jul;71(7):829–42.

36 Paediatric Trauma

Edward Rothera, Clare Thompson, and Rebecca Powell

Overview and Epidemiology

Paediatric trauma can be an emotive and challenging aspect of major injury management even for the experienced clinician. The potential of parental presence during the resuscitation and the prospect of less familiar anatomy and physiological parameters can compound an already stressful situation. This being said, a well-trained and practised trauma care provider can safely and proficiently manage these scenarios by applying the same principles that they would use in an adult. The underlying approach remains the same—**<M>**assive haemorrhage control, **A**irway (with cervical spine protection), **B**reathing, **C**irculation, **D**isability and **E**xposure. Where differences exist in the paediatric population physiologically, anatomically, and due to the mechanism of injury, the intricacies of management are appropriately modified while maintaining the structured approach.

E. Rothera (✉)
Department of Anaesthesia and Critical Care Medicine, Leeds General Infirmary, Leeds, UK

Leeds Children's Hospital, Leeds, UK
e-mail: erothera@nhs.net

C. Thompson
West Yorkshire Deanery, Yorkshire, UK

Leeds Children's Hospital, Leeds, UK
e-mail: clare.thompson32@nhs.net

R. Powell
Leeds Children's Hospital, Leeds, UK
e-mail: rebecca.powell7@nhs.net

In the UK, traumatic injury is second only to childhood neoplasms as the leading cause of death amongst children aged 1 to 15 [1]. Half of all emergency department paediatric attendances are injury-related and place a significant burden on the health system. Major trauma in childhood is most common in infancy (age under 1 year) with a preponderance within the first 3 months of life, resulting from non-accidental injury (Fig. 36.1). Pedestrian road traffic collisions remain the most significant cause of trauma in children over one; 39% of all injuries are pedestrians, rising to 47% of all trauma cases in the UK when pedestrians, cyclists and motor vehicle passengers are considered together. Asphyxiation and drowning, while not common, carry the highest fatality rate [2]. Knowledge of the mechanisms of trauma and associated patterns of injury in childhood are pertinent to direct not only a team's initial management of the injuries, but also the subsequent examinations, investigations and family discussions.

The epidemiology of presentation and mode of arrival of paediatric major trauma patients can be considered in three distinct groups; 60% are brought in by ambulance, 15% by air ambulance and 25% by parents or other means without any pre-hospital care. Despite the establishment of paediatric Major Trauma Centres (MTC), only 37% of paediatric major trauma patients present to a paediatric MTC initially, with the majority (63%) presenting at non-specialist trauma units or adult MTCs [2]. The majority of paediatric major trauma patients (73%) present with iso-

P. Lax (ed.), *Textbook of Acute Trauma Care*, https://doi.org/10.1007/978-3-030-83628-3_36

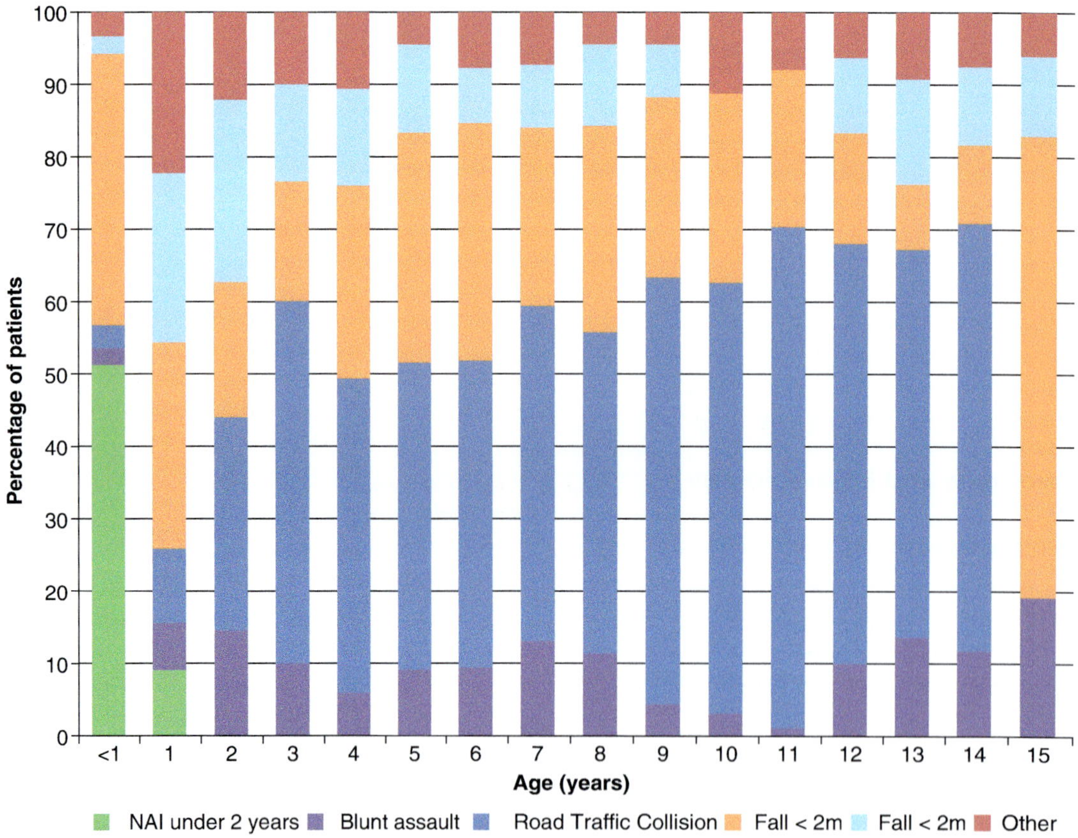

Fig. 36.1 From The Trauma Audit & Research Network (TARN) [2]

lated head injuries, 21% with isolated thoracic injuries, 14% with isolated intra-abdominal injuries and only 9% of paediatric trauma patients have polytrauma. Consequently, the commonest presentation of a paediatric major trauma patient would be an isolated head injury which attends a non-specialist hospital (though 50% of paediatric major trauma cases are subsequently transferred to a paediatric MTC). Despite this, in the UK paediatric trauma patients have lower risks of death than their adult counterparts (5 times lower when considering pedestrian vs car, 1.5 times lower in bicycle vs car and 4.5 times lower when occupants of a car involved in a collision) [2].

Much of the anxiety regarding managing children's trauma can be related to uncertainty surrounding appropriate drug dosing and equipment size. While in adults, drug dosing remains reasonably constant and equipment is based mostly on gender and size, in children there is a broad spectrum based on age and (estimated) weight. Although in experienced hands this information may be commonplace, for the majority, the use of charts and apps to guide one's practice is a much safer approach. The advanced life support group (ALSG) teaches a weight formula based on three distinct age groups (Table 36.1).

Table 36.1 Weight estimation formulae in different age groups [3]

Works best for	Formulae
0–12 months	Weight (in kg) = (0.5 × age in months) + 4
1–5 years	Weight (in kg) = (2 × age in years) + 8
6–12 years	Weight (in kg) = (3 × age in years) + 7

While this can provide an accurate weight estimation, particularly when there is preparation time before a patient's arrival, it is more complicated than the formulae still employed by the resuscitation Council of the UK (RCUK). The RCUK formula provides a safe and quick weight estimation for children over 1 year in an emergency (Table 36.2).

Table 36.2 Alternative weight estimation formulae

Works for	Formulae
1 year +	Weight (in kg) = (age (in years) + 4) × 2

Weight-based calculations clearly apply to fluid and blood product resuscitation as well. As with many of the paediatric algorithms, due to a paucity of data, they are downward extrapolations from adult algorithms where there is a far greater body of evidence and research.

In a bleeding patient, aggressive crystalloid administration can exacerbate coagulopathy [4] and so in children, sensible aliquots of 10 ml/kg followed by constant reassessment is key. It is worth noting that, in trauma patients, it is common practice to resuscitate with blood products in the first instance and the use of crystalloid is reserved for situations where blood products are not immediately available. Once major haemorrhage has been recognised, or circulatory shock has not been controlled with 20 ml/kg of crystalloid, a major transfusion protocol (MTP) should be initiated. This constitutes blood products administered initially in a 1:1:1 ratio of packed red blood cells (PRBC), pathogen inactivated fresh frozen plasma (FFP)and platelets. Patients born after 1996, which will now include all paediatric cases, should be treated with plasma products sourced from variant Creutzfeldt–Jakob disease (vCJD) free countries. These products have been exposed to both prion and viral pathogen reduction steps. In the UK, the available products are Methylene Blue photosensitised FFP (Theraplex®) and solvent-detergent FFP (Octaplas® LG) [5]. These products should be considered equivalent to standard FFP dosing. It should be noted that the ratio of 1:1:1 is of dose and not product bags (PRBC 10 ml/kg, FFP 10 ml/kg, Platelets 10–15 ml/kg) [6] Further treatment should be guided by point of care coagulation studies (such as ROTEM ™ or TEG™) or formal lab-based coagulation assays.

Product replacement should be closely followed by the administration of antifibrinolytics. The CRASH-2 study [7] has mandated the use of tranexamic acid (TXA) in the adult bleeding trauma patient, and that has been assimilated into paediatric practice as a weight-based dose of 15 mg/kg (up to 1 g) as a bolus followed by an infusion of 2 mg/kg/h (up to 125 mg/h) [8, 9]. A useful aide memoire for the bolus dose of TXA in children is that it is the same as the intravenous paracetamol/acetaminophen dose once over 1 month of age. The use of cryoprecipitate, calcium, potassium control and temperature management should not be overlooked. The above should coincide with the involvement of surgical and interventional radiological advice on the control of haemorrhage. As adult practice moves more towards using blood and blood products, paediatric trauma may follow, notwithstanding the previous observation that the commonest paediatric major trauma presentation is an isolated head injury which may not require blood transfusion.

The remainder of this chapter is dedicated to looking more closely at some of the unique challenges posed by the paediatric trauma patient.

Physiological and Anatomical Considerations

Airway

The priority in managing a trauma patient (once catastrophic haemorrhage has been addressed) is assessing, supporting and securing the airway—this is as true in children as adults. There exist, however, subtle physiological and anatomical differences that mandate a slightly different approach to airway management in children. From the neonatal period through infancy into childhood, the shape and structure of the airway develops, slowly approaching its adult form towards the beginning of adolescence. A relatively larger occiput and cranial vault with a smaller midface and jaw in infancy create a natural flexion of the neck when laid supine on a flat surface. This, combined with a large tongue, can quickly lead to obstruction in the incapacitated child. Support placed behind the shoulders while maintaining cervical-spine alignment allows the face to be maintained parallel to the surface the child lies on and make airway manoeuvres far more effective. As age and size increase the position for optimum airway management becomes similar to that of an adult, although in all cases the sequence of airway manoeuvres remain constant; jaw thrust, removal of debris under direct vision, airway adjuncts, tracheal intubation, and finally the "can't intubate can't oxygenate" (CICO) scenario. Traditionally the paediatric larynx has been considered conical compared to its adult cylindrical counterpart. *In vivo* CT and MRI studies in recent years have dispelled some of these myths [10, 11]. The narrowest portion in the majority of paediatric patients is the level of the glottis or subglottis and not the cricoid cartilage. The airway has also been shown to be elliptical rather than circular [12]. With this new information combined with the development of paediatric specific cuffed endotracheal tubes, there is now a suitable and sensible option to place cuffed endotracheal tubes in children down to 3 kg (where experience allows) providing superior airway protection and ventilation profiles. This is in contrast to previous practice which suggested that non-cuffed tubes should be used to prevent long term tracheal sequalae in children. The high-volume/low-pressure microthin polyurethane cuff allows placement in the subglottis while reducing the risk of endobronchial intubation in the shorter paediatric trachea. Cuff pressure monitoring using a maximum pressure of 20 cmH_2O should be employed.

Evidence suggests that non-syndromic, anatomically normal children do not have difficult airways. Difficult paediatric airways are reasonably predictable with midface and mandibular hypoplasia syndromes creating the mainstay of anticipated difficult airways [13]. Oral, maxillofacial and neck trauma can, however, make a previously normal airway into a more complex one. Supraglottic airways are an effective tool for clinicians less confident in tracheal intubation or as airway rescue in difficult airway management. Sizes are available to suit the vast majority of patients, with the smallest laryngeal mask airway (size 1) appropriate for children up to 5 kg and the iGel™ (size 1) suitable for children over 2 kg.

Although not providing a traditional 'secured airway' they can offer an effective means of ventilating and oxygenating a difficult airway, especially in the presence of intubating inexperience. Failing to maintain oxygenation with these options and in the face of CICO scenario, the final common pathway is front of neck access. Airway anatomy, internal and external, is also a factor in the choice of approach in this situation. A short neck and indistinguishable surface anatomy make any technique fraught with difficulty. Experience within paediatrics is limited, and where adult guidelines have moved away from needle cricothyroidotomy it remains a primary option in children under eight [14]. 18-gauge cannula in infants to 14-gauge in larger children are used. The neck is extended, using a shoulder roll where appropriate and the larynx stabilised with the non-dominant hand. Access the cricothyroid membrane with the cannula aimed slightly caudad. Confirmation of entering the trachea is through aspiration of air in to an attached saline primed syringe. Traditional ventilation techniques are unsuitable and cautious pressure limited jet ventilation [15] or a 4 Bar O_2 source with a flowmeter must be employed. Although this will allow oxygenation, ventilation is significantly impacted by the narrow diameter of the cannula and a long expiratory phase must be used, especially in the face of complete upper airway obstruction. This is a short term solution and must be converted to a definitive airway as soon as possible. In the older child where anatomy is clearer, a scalpel-bougie-endotracheal tube technique should be used in the first instance. Where a difficult airway is encountered or indeed predicted, an experienced (ideally paediatric) anaesthetist should be sought, and the presence of ENT surgical expertise is desirable. There remains, however, no clear consensus on which technique results in the highest chance of success. What is clear, however, is that given the inability to oxygenate by any other means, failure to commit to a 'surgical' airway will result in death.

Breathing

The infant chest has several anatomical and physiological differences from its adult counterpart. Soft, cartilaginous, horizontal ribs combined with poorly developed intercostal muscles and a flattened diaphragm create a respiratory system that is rate-dependent rather than tidal volume dependent. Not only is the system prone to rapid exhaustion (the diaphragm in childhood lacks fatigue-resistant type 1 oxidative fibres), but the protective aspect of a fully formed and ossified rib cage is lost. This results in a more significant transfer of energy to the lung parenchyma and mediastinal contents with trauma to the thorax, which may not be highlighted due to a lack of rib fractures. The presence of rib fractures signifies a substantial impact has been received. An analogy may be to dropping an orange (a child's thorax) or an egg (an adult's thorax). The egg shell may crack, protect the internal contents and show externally visible signs of damage. The orange skin, however, will remain intact but energy would be transmitted to the inside of the fruit with few (if any) external signs of damage. This compliant chest wall, combined with a functional residual capacity (FRC) that is reduced in both actual and relative size, creates a small respiratory reserve. This is compounded by the fact that the closing capacity (CC) (the volume of the lungs during expiration when the small airways begin to close) of a child's lung up to 6 years old is greater than the FRC. The impact of a CC encroaching or exceeding the FRC (effectively the reserve tank of the lungs) means that areas distal to closure and within the FRC will have a worsening ventilation/perfusion relationship which when exacerbated by decreased consciousness, apnoea and anaesthesia will all result in rapid desaturation. Where major thoracic trauma is present and intervention required, the anatomical landmarks for needle decompression (second intercostal space, midclavicular line) and thoracostomy or intercostal drain placement (fifth intercostal space, mid axillary line) remain the same as in adults. Care must be taken in the choice of both size and depth of insertion of the cannula and drain to prevent further parenchymal injury.

Circulation

At birth, the heart is composed of immature myocytes with an underdeveloped sarcoplasmic reticulum that has a high proportion of fibrous compared to contractile tissue. Although this re-orientates over time, it leaves the infantile cardiac output (CO) more reliant upon heart rate than stroke volume. Although actual CO may be low in a child, when adjusted for weight, it is at its highest at birth (300 ml/kg/min) reducing to adult levels (100 ml/kg/min) by the age of 16. This leads to an oxygen consumption of 6 ml/kg/min in infancy compared to 3 ml/kg/min in adulthood, and explains why children tolerate hypoxia less than adults.

Children have a good physiological cardiac reserve and can maintain systolic arterial pressures even in the face of 25–40% blood volume loss [16]. This complicates matters as children will compensate for significant blood loss for a large period and then rapidly and catastrophically decompensate. Fluid resuscitation should begin with cautious aliquots of 10 ml/kg warmed isotonic crystalloid, swiftly moving to the administration of blood products as discussed in the introduction. There is a move towards permissive hypotensive resuscitation in adult trauma practice, and it has been suggested for paediatric trauma resuscitation too, though the evidence for this is limited [16]. Given the difficulty in assessing hypovolemic shock in children compared with adults, where systolic hypotension and tachycardia are often late signs and an indication of imminent cardiovascular collapse, extreme vigilance must be applied to the practice of permissive hypotensive resuscitation in children and if used, a lower threshold for fluid administration adopted in comparison to adults [17, 18]. Rather, a patient-specific end-organ perfusion directed practice should be employed utilising indicators such as lactic acidosis and urine output (Table 36.3).

Disability

Children are particularly vulnerable to traumatic brain injury (TBI) as a result of their size, mechanism of injury and composition of the cranial vault. Road traffic pedestrian collisions remain a leading cause of major trauma in children, and

Table 36.3 Normal physiological parameters in childhood

Age (years)	Respiratory rate (breaths min^{-1})	Pulse (beats min^{-1})	Systolic BP (mmHg)	Urine output (ml h^{-1})
<1	30–60	110–160	65–90	2
1–2	25–40	110–150	70–95	1.5
3–5	25–35	95–140	70–100	1
6–12	20–25	80–120	80–110	1
>12	15–20	60–100	90–120	0.5

75% of all major trauma admissions will have some form of TBI [19]. TBI is still the leading cause of death associated with trauma [2]. A fragile neck, larger head- to-torso ratio and a more compliant skull mean the consequences of acceleration-deceleration injuries and transfer of force to the brain parenchyma are more significant. There is also limited brain atrophy and a smaller subarachnoid space in children. Subsequently, they are less able to compensate for a rise in intracranial pressure (ICP) [20].

Following trauma, there is a trimodal pattern of death. Half of all deaths occur within minutes and are often due to the primary brain injury (PBI) received. The second group comprises 20% of the deaths and occurs within hours as a result of circulatory and respiratory collapse or secondary brain injury (SBI). The final peak is in the days and weeks after injury as a result of TBI, infection and multi-organ failure [19]. It is in the second group and the prevention of SBI where the difference can be made. The mainstay of managing SBI is the prevention of hypotension and hypoxia [21] and providing time-critical neurosurgical intervention where indicated. '*Guidelines for the Acute Medical Management of Severe Traumatic Brain Injury in Infants, Children, and Adolescents*' [22] first published in 2003 and updated in 2012 and 2019 provides a systematic review of best practice for managing TBI in children. The recent updates include advice on a minimum cerebral perfusion pressure of 40 mmHg in children aged 1–5 years and 50 mmHg aged 6 years and over with a systolic blood pressure equal to or greater than the 75th centile for that age group. Hyperosmolar therapy using hypertonic 3% saline in boluses over 5 to 10 minutes (2–5 ml/kg) and subsequent infusion (0.1–1.0 ml/kg/hr) should be used for raised ICP. Hyperventilation should be used for refractory raised ICP only in the presence of advanced cerebral ischemia monitoring and failure of other therapies, as over vasoconstriction can decrease cerebral oxygen delivery. Moderate hypothermia, if employed for ICP control, should be continued for >24 h and <48 h, and corticosteroids no longer have a role in the management of TBI or raised ICP [23, 24]. The best induction agent and neuromuscular blocking agent (NMBA) for the initial management of TBI where intubation and ventilation are required remains a source of debate. The previously held beliefs that ketamine is inappropriate due to its deleterious effect on ICP have been questioned [25] and its use is now becoming commonplace. Short-acting potent opioids such as alfentanil or fentanyl offer a useful adjunct in obtunding the physiological response to laryngoscopy and preventing ICP surges in the cardiovascularly stable patient. Thiopentone and midazolam remain viable alternatives given the necessary conditions are met (i.e. no significant blood loss or cardiovascular instability). Regarding NMBA's, suxamethonium still has a role due to its rapid onset, quality of intubating conditions and potentially short half-life, despite its adverse effects of muscle fasciculations on ICP. With the widespread availability of sugammadex, rocuronium now seems to be the NMBA of choice. In any case, one must consider carefully the haemodynamic stability of the patient as well as the teams' experience and expertise in the use of the selected drug combinations before a decision is made.

Exposure

The changing size of children as they grow has a significant impact on their thermoregulation as well as the estimation of burn extent. In infancy, children have a much greater surface area (SA) to mass ratio with a reduction in subcutaneous tissue placing them at much higher risk of heat loss through conduction, convection, evaporation and radiation. For this reason, they must be cared for in a warmed environment with the addition of warmed fluids, forced air warmers and overhead heaters where appropriate. Exposure should be kept to a minimum, allowing only for assessment and interventions. Failure to do so will adversely affect the efficacy of resuscitative treatment, promote coagulopathy and increase the risk of morbidity and mortality. Bearing these changes in body dimensions in mind, assessment of the paediatric burn patient cannot follow the same rules as in an adult. The 'rule of 9s' is unsuitable for children less than 14. The safest method is to use a Lund-Browder chart (Fig. 36.2) for reference which considers variation in SA of the head and limbs with age or app-based calculators such as the Mersey Burns app [26].

If no charts or apps are available, the palm of the child's hand, including their fingers may be used as an estimation for 1% total body SA. Fluid resuscitation should follow the Parkland formula with isotonic crystalloid, but with close attention to urine output which should be kept at ≥2 ml/kg/h. Maintenance and replacement fluids should be in addition to this. Although appropriately managing and resuscitating burns is essential, the impact of smoke inhalation cannot be overlooked. Most fire-related deaths are attributable to smoke and its related toxins. Carbon monoxide (CO) and to a lesser, but not insignificant extent, cyanide contribute to significant morbidity and mortality from enclosed space fires involving the combustion of many common fabrics and plastics.

Estimating percent Total Body Surface Area in Children Affected by Burns

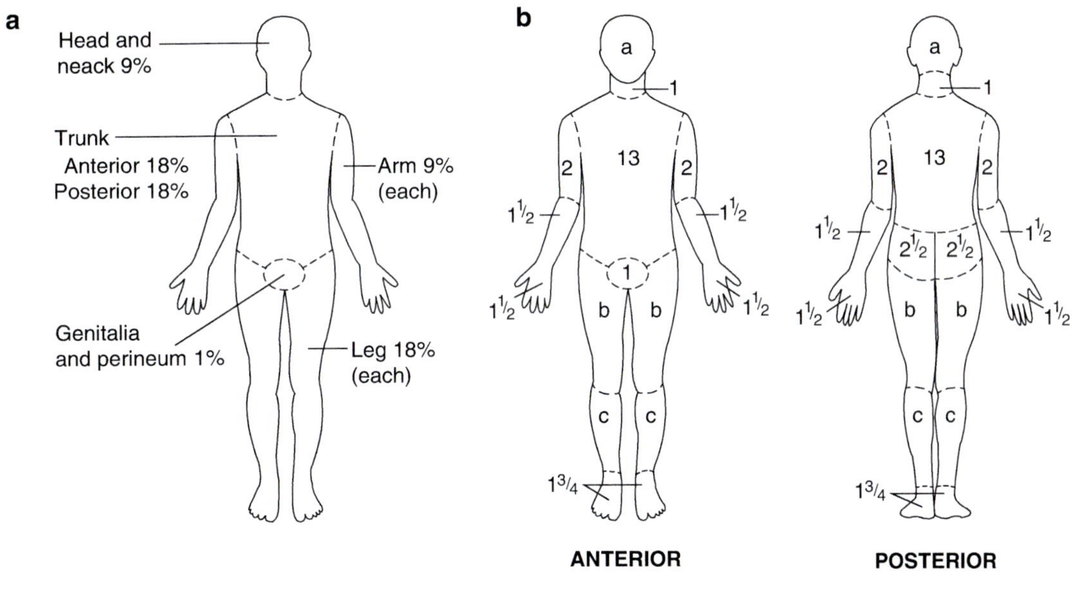

Relative percentage of body surface areas (% BSA) affected by growth

	0 yt	*1 yt*	*5 yt*	*10yt*	*15yt*
a— *½ of head*	9½	8½	6½	5½	4½
b— *½ of 1 thigh*	2¾	3¼	4	4¼	4½
c— *½ of 1 lower leg*	2½	2½	2¾	3	3¼

Fig. 36.2 Burns calculations charts in children (**a**) Rule of 'nines' (**b**) Lund-Browder chart

Children are particularly vulnerable due to their high respiratory rate, reduced mass and juvenile metabolism. Treatment strategies follow the established structure MABCD, with a high fraction of inspired oxygen the key treatment for CO poisoning, while antidotes, such as hydroxocobalamin, are the therapy of choice for cyanide toxicity [27].

Assessing the Traumatised Child

As with all emergencies, communication and preparation are fundamental to success. Assembly of a team with the most experienced available staff and task allocation before patient arrival should be the goal, although circumstances may dictate that this is not always possible. This allows for the preparation of key equipment, estimation of weight and calculation of subsequent drug doses based on the established Advanced Life Support Group (ALSG) formulas outlined above [3].

Assessing the Child in Trauma

Hospital attendance for any child is a daunting experience—even more so when they are in pain and have been through a traumatic injury. One should be mindful of this in their approach and try to minimise the team to only essential staff with support (at a distance) if needed from others. The presence of their caregiver can be the key to keeping both the child and caregiver calm during what is a stressful time. Peri-traumatic stress is a risk factor for the development of post-traumatic stress disorder (PTSD) and parental separation, even in the time following a traumatic event, is a powerful determinant of post-traumatic phenomena [28].

Distraction techniques may be helpful to allow access for measurement of physiological parameters and facilitate a more detailed examination of less severe injuries, and Play Specialists are being utilised to assist with this in some major trauma centres.

Analgesia

The management of pain after paediatric trauma is treated well in high acuity patients, but in those with less visible or detrimental injuries, there is often a substantial delay in administration or inadequate analgesia given. It is difficult to identify specific barriers to this and likely multifactorial [29].

Pain scoring in children is very subjective, especially when anxiety and fear are confounding factors affecting the ability to perform the child's self-assessment of pain. An observational scoring system is recommended—one example is The Alder Hey Triage Pain Scoring chart [3] (Table 36.4). In the conscious child, in practice, visual analogue scales or facial representation scales are more useful (Fig. 36.3).

Once the child's pain has been assessed, it is essential to address pain management. This begins with basic interventions and strategies such as splinting, realignment of normal anatomy and dressings. Anxiety can often contribute to perceptions of pain, and it is vital to have a caregiver present for reassurance and to offer explanations when able.

Using the WHO analgesic ladder [30] treatment can be directed according to the level of pain experienced, beginning with simple analge-

Table 36.4 The Alder Hey Triage Pain Scoring Chart

	Response	Score 0	Score 1	Score 2
1	Cry or voice	No complaint/cry Normal conversation	Consolable Not talking, negative	Inconsolable Complaining of pain
2	Facial expression	Normal	Short grimace <50% of the time	Long grimace >50% of the time
3	Posture	Normal	Touching/rubbing/sparing	Defensive/tense
4	Movement	Normal	Reduced or restless	Immobile or thrashing
5	Colour	Normal	Pale	Very pale/ "green"

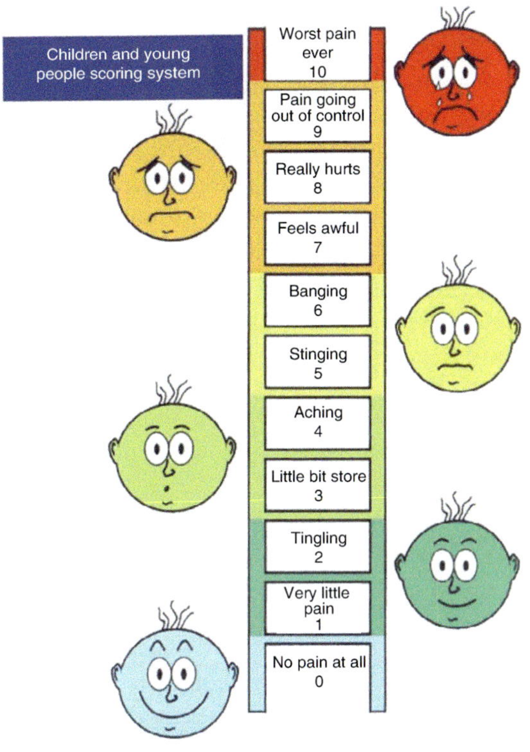

Fig. 36.3 Faces scale and pain ladder (from Gandhi M, Thomson C, Lord D, Enoch S. Management of Pain in Children with Burns. Ratnapalan S, editor. Int J Pediatr. 2010 Sep 16;2010:825657)

sia and escalating as necessary. In the critically injured but haemodynamically stable patient, intranasal diamorphine (or Entonox in the compliant older child) may allow time to get intravenous access for other agents or complete a painful procedure [31].

Another option that may be considered is intramuscular S-Ketamine in the young child. S-Ketamine has a concentration of 25 mg/ml allowing smaller volumes to be used for those less than 18 kg. This may be utilised to allow joint manipulation, simple suturing or a more definite vascular access.

Intranasal diamorphine has a well established role in the management of moderate to severe pain in trauma. The main benefit is the rapid route of administration and onset of action. The College of Emergency Medicine and Advanced Paediatric Life Support Guidelines recommend the use of intranasal diamorphine in the acute management of pain at 0.1 mg/kg in children [32]. Where diamorphine is unavailable, intranasal fentanyl at a dose of 1.5 mcg/kg is a suitable alternative.

In specific cases, such as femoral fractures requiring splinting, consideration should be given to a regional technique such as a femoral nerve block administered by an experienced practitioner.

Scoring Systems

Scoring systems that help guide management decisions and predict mortality and morbidity play an essential role in the assessment and treatment of major trauma. A scoring system specifically used in major paediatric trauma, the Paediatric trauma score [33], is modified to adjust for body weight and airway diameter and combines subjective and objective data to aid quantifying trauma severity.

Pulses and Blood Pressure

Depending on the age and body habitus of the child, appropriate sites for palpation of pulses can vary considerably. Most babies will have little to no neck with chubby arms and legs. The best place to palpate a pulse peripherally is the brachial artery in the antecubital fossa. To reflect a central pulse, the femoral artery in the groin is the best choice in a child.

Resting pulse rates in children are higher and normal physiological parameters show significant variation with age. It is often difficult to recall exact values, especially when under stress and so the use of standardised paediatric advanced warning scores (PAWS) charts offers a visual safe and reliable repository of this information.

Blood pressure is an important marker but not the first indicator of deterioration in a child, as their cardiovascular reserve is often good. Respiratory reserve is poor, and so respiratory rate is a much more sensitive gauge of impending collapse. In a patient that has been intubated and ventilated, the onus is shifted towards cardiovascular parameters for monitoring.

Blood Pressure is best monitored on a PAWS chart or guided using standardised Royal College of Paediatric and Child Health (RCPCH) blood pressure reference charts based on centile growth. Consider carefully signs of shock, such as end-organ perfusion, combined with clinical assessment rather than hypotension alone [34]. Due to variance in height and weight affecting blood pressure, a standardised formula to estimate blood pressure is no longer endorsed and should not be applied in the critically ill child. There are various apps (discussed later in this chapter) which can be used for estimation of height and weight based on age, drug dosing and recall of centile-adjusted vital signs. These can be incredibly useful in resuscitation and onward care, but all values should be agreed on by the team rather than using the outputs from multiple apps on one patient!

Blood Products

Fluids in children should be used judiciously as per all trauma and given in 10 ml/kg/min aliquots. The blood product administration of 1:1:1 ratio of packed red blood cells (PRBC), Fresh Frozen Plasma (FFP) and platelets is still applicable and utilised within all departments. Isotonic crystalloids help with volume expansion but have no oxygen-carrying capacity.

Massive Transfusion can be initiated in the presence of major trauma and haemodynamic instability in keeping with hypovolaemia. Blood volume decreases with increasing age. At birth it may be as high as 90 ml/kg/min, reducing to 80 ml/kg/min in infancy, 75 ml/kg/min in childhood and reaching adult levels of 65–70 ml/kg/min in the early teens. Remember, when haemorrhage is evident, what appears to be a small volume visually may be comparatively significant to the child.

While transfusion is continuing, every effort should be made to identify and control ongoing bleeding. This may involve surgical control in theatre or interventional radiology, however a definitive plan to do so must imminently be put in place. Efforts to prevent hypothermia should be implemented, using warmed fluids, preventing unnecessary exposure and forced-air warming devices such as a Bair hugger™.

Activating or continuing a massive transfusion should not be based on blood results alone but ongoing assessment and need for blood product resuscitation. A definition or specific numerical trigger is difficult to identify in the acute situation. However, the British Committee for Standards in Haematology (BCSH) 2015 and NICE advise the following [5]:

- Massive blood loss may be defined as either 80 ml/kg/min in 24 h, 40 ml/kg/min in 3 h or 2–3 ml/kg/min
- In clinical practice, the usual triggers are haemodynamic changes compatible with hypovolaemia accompanying evidence or suspicion of serious haemorrhage
- A senior doctor (middle grade or above) authorises blood component use to ensure that scarce resources are used appropriately.

Communication Is Critical with Transfusion

As with much of medicine and especially in the trauma situation, although chaotic, clear communication and labelling of samples is paramount. Where possible, pre-alert the Transfusion lab, provide available patient details and request a Major Haemorrhage Pack. Content will vary slightly between hospitals in numbers of each blood product provided, but are largely similar and contain documentation as well as guidance for administration. As soon as possible, a correctly labelled transfusion sample should be urgently transported to the lab (identify a member of staff to do this).

Red Blood Cells

Time permitting; the gold standard is to administer fully cross-matched blood. Failing this, type-specific blood is the next choice. If the clinical situation demands the immediate administration of blood and any delay with cross-matching would be detrimental to the patient, then readily available O negative blood must be considered.

Group O Rhesus negative red blood cells can be used, but the decision must be made by the most senior doctor present and only if a delay of up to 10 min would be a danger to life. Type-specific blood can be available relatively quickly by most blood banks with an aim of 10–15 min to supply if needed (Table 36.5). Type Specific blood is ABO and rhesus compatible; however, other autoantibody incompatibilities may exist.

Fresh Frozen Plasma (FFP)

FFP must be thawed and takes time to defrost (approximately 40 min), similar to the emergency crossmatch timeframe. Ongoing coagulation tests (ideally near-patient tests such as TEG™ or ROTEM™ due to their quick availability and accurate reflection of clot formation) usually guide further administration. If fibrinogen levels remain critically low (<1.5 g/l), cryoprecipitate therapy should be considered.

Platelets

Communicate early with the blood transfusion laboratory to highlight the requirement for platelets. Be aware of stock levels within the hospital. In some areas, platelet stock is held regionally and will need to be transported. Request 20 ml/kg/min platelets after approximately 50% blood volume has been transfused (40 ml/kg/min if there is on-going blood loss). Platelets are also given in 10 ml/kg aliquots.

Table 36.5 A comparison of blood products and their estimated time of availability

Blood product	Urgency	Availability
Group O Rh negative blood	Immediate	Immediate
Grouped but not crossmatched	Very Urgent	5–10 minutes
Type-specific blood-ABO and Rh compatible (not crossmatched)	Urgent	15 minutes from sample and prewarned
Emergency crossmatch	Expedited	Minimum 40 minutes

Cryoprecipitate

Again, communication and early decision making are paramount. Cryoprecipitate takes approximately 40 min to thaw and should be administered aiming to maintain fibrinogen level > 1.5 g/l in aliquots of 10 ml/kg.

Be wary of waiting for blood results before initiating further treatment. In the face of an ongoing need for blood component resuscitation, be guided by the clinical assessment.

Temperature Control

Temperature control in the child is primarily affected by body surface area (BSA). Body surface area decreases with age and weight. It is vital to keep the child warm and covered. In a small baby they have a comparatively large head, around 20% of their BSA, so consider using a hat, often stored in the resuscitaire.

Head Injuries

As mentioned in the introduction, head injury is a major presenting complaint in the paediatric trauma population. Time-critical head injuries should be scanned within 30 min of presentation and discussed with the local neurosurgical centre as soon as possible.

The definition of severe traumatic brain injury (TBI) is a post-resuscitation Glasgow Coma Score (GCS) of 8 or less. All children with a GCS of less than 8 should be deemed to have a potentially unprotected airway, and this is an indication for intubation and ventilation. Nasal intubation and the use of nasal adjuncts such as nasopharyngeal airways and nasogastric tubes are strictly contraindicated in the presence of head injury due to the associated risk of a base of skull fracture.

Glasgow Coma Scale (GCS)

GCS is frequently misquoted in children due to their verbal communication being variable with age [35], and should only be used only for those over 2 years of age. There is a modified paediatric GCS [36] for those less than 2 years, however the AVPU score (graded on their best response to stimuli—alert, to voice, to pain, unresponsive) is an easy, repeatable and useful assessment in these children.

Head injury management is categorised into two stages. The primary head injury, which is the initial insult to brain tissue caused at the moment of impact. This may comprise of subarachnoid, subdural or extradural bleeding, intracranial or intraventricular haemorrhage, acute obstructive hydrocephalus, vascular injury or diffuse axonal injury and shearing. Secondary brain injury is further neurological injury caused by failure to maintain normal blood or oxygen delivery to at-risk brain tissue following injury, or metabolic disturbances such as hypoglycaemia.

Many public health strategies have been initiated to decrease primary brain injury—bicycle helmets, seatbelts, airbags and road safety initiatives—but the aim in hospital is to prevent secondary brain injury. This is achieved by preventing hypoxia, hypotension, hypoglycaemia and precluding a rise in intracranial pressure as detailed in the head injury chapter.

Injuries, Interventions and Imaging

Immobilisation and C-Spine Control

In the prehospital setting, if the paediatric trauma patient is a passenger in a motor vehicle collision and in a correctly fitted car seat with tight straps, if the child is pink and breathing well, they can be immobilised in the car seat [37].

C-spine immobilisation in children is difficult and can cause much distress. Small babies have limited head control and very short necks so c-spine collars may cause an abnormal head position, overextending the neck and obstructing the airway. If a c-spine collar has been fitted but is causing the child a significant degree of distress and agitation, wriggling and crying of discomfort may be more detrimental than beneficial and the collar should be removed.

Significant paediatric neck injuries are thankfully rare, though can be devestating if not picked up early. Whilst the routine use of cervical collars is being increasingly questioned given a substantial complication rate and no trial evidence to support their use [38], cervical spinal injuries should be aggressively excluded and a low threshold for CT or MRI imaging maintained in at-risk patients.

In most circumstances, allowing the child to be immobilised using only blocks will suffice with verbal reminders to remain still. In most cases, if the child does have severe neck pain, they will lie surprisingly still to compensate. The spine should always be kept in alignment during transfers, rolls and airway manoeuvres. Aim for a neutral position and look for evidence of airway obstruction. Using jaw thrust rather than a head tilt/chin lift in a compromised cervical spine is mandatory. Use all the equipment available to help manage a compromised airway including airway adjuncts (avoiding a nasopharyngeal airway in suspected head injury) and a second person if required.

The Royal College of Emergency Medicine (RCEM) has issued a position statement referencing both Advanced Paediatric Life Support (APLS) and the National Institute for health and Care Excellence (NICE) guidance:

- In conscious children, use manual in-line stabilisation (MILS) whenever possible
- In unconscious children, or when MILS cannot be maintained, immobilisation should be with a properly fitting collar, blocks and tape
- If no properly fitting collar is available, then blocks or rolled blankets should be used to provide an immobilisation device [39].

The vast majority of traumas presenting to the emergency department will be on trauma scoops which can be opened at both ends and divided, reducing movement required in the unstable patient, to transfer to the trauma board. Ongoing moving and handling of the actual or suspected Spinal Cord Injury (SCI) should be kept to a minimum, but when needed, log rolling continues to be the method of choice [40].

Spinal Injuries

It is important to be alert to spinal cord injury in children as they are less able to articulate symptoms and pain. Clinical suspicion and observation are key tools in eliciting back pain in a child. Although the cervical spine is covered in the MABCD approach, it is crucial to be mindful of the spine as a whole entity. Consider spinal cord injury if the child complains of back or neck pain, is guarding those areas or if they complain of any sensation changes remembering they may describe these in a myriad of ways. Difficulty micturating or motor weakness should also be sought out in the clinical examination. An elevated level of suspicion should remain in significantly high-risk mechanism of injuries. These include road traffic accidents, fall from a height, multi-trauma accidents or loss of consciousness.

It is essential to carefully and systematically document a neurological examination in all trauma patients. This can be difficult to perform in young children, especially with distracting injuries and the heightened emotional state of the child. The neurological examination should be performed by an experienced team member, including perianal sensation; however, deep anal tone is not always possible or reliable in a child. When not performed, the reasoning should be documented. Sacral involvement can be challenging to ascertain immediately but does aid in prognostic factors, such as long-term bowel and bladder dysfunction.

Although imaging is important, it is not always conclusive and pathology can be diagnosed in children based on clinical examination when CT scans initially are reported as normal (spinal cord injury without radiological abnormality—SCIWORA). A lower threshold for MRI in children compared to adults should be maintained. Spinal cord injury, depending on the spinal level, can be complex involving multidisciplinary teams, including intensive care, respiratory, orthopaedics, urology and neurosurgery acutely with prolonged rehabilitation needs.

Truncal Injuries

Traditional teaching for major trauma focuses on six life-threatening injuries; airway obstruction or disruption, tension pneumothorax, open pneumothorax, massive haemothorax, flail chest and cardiac tamponade. The same principles apply in children, and immediate treatment is similar.

Due to chest physiology and rib compliance to pressure as covered in paediatric chest physiology section, there is a higher incidence of pulmonary contusion in children. Flail segments are rare due to rib elasticity, but if present suggests high force injury and are tolerated poorly by the child. Pulmonary contusions may be evident on the initial chest x-ray seen as non-segmental opacification but are not always apparent. As oedema and haemorrhage take time to develop the clinical picture may well deteriorate as the pathology evolves.

Infants rely heavily on diaphragmatic breathing which will be problematic in patients with high cervical cord injuries affecting the phrenic nerve. Vigilance, early intubation and ventilation may well be required to prevent secondary injury. If diaphragmatic rupture has occurred through blunt injury, or more commonly through penetrating trauma, this also can have a deleterious effect on breathing and likewise must be mitigated early by intubation and ventilation.

Blunt abdominal trauma is common in children and can carry high morbidity—the anatomy of the ribs and flattened diaphragm means the rib cage offers less protection to the abdominal viscera. The abdominal organs lie lower and more anteriorly and are thus exposed to greater insult. The urinary bladder is intra-abdominal rather than pelvic, meaning it too is at higher risk from damage having lost its bony shield. Compounding this is the comparative lack of muscle and subcutaneous tissue in a child's abdominal wall, allowing significant transmission of blunt force.

Pelvic fracture is rare, again as the result of more cartilaginous bone allowing for greater flex in a crush injury. If a fracture is present, it too indicates a high force injury has occurred. Due to the pelvic rim being narrow, pelvic organs are offered less protection and are more susceptible to injury. Immediate treatment involves splinting the pelvis, minimal handling and instigating major haemorrhage protocols until definitive management is prepared.

Access Options

Intravenous (IV) cannulation in the paediatric population is always challenging, but in a scared, peripherally shocked child this can be especially difficult. Fortunately, there are other viable alternatives.

Firstly, "the best person should attempt the task the first time" is a core principle that must be remembered in paediatric trauma. Vein viewers and other options are available to the stable patient, but the critically unwell child needing blood, fluids or analgesia may require intraosseous (IO) access. The American College of Surgeons Committee on Trauma recommends IO access should be attempted after two failed IV attempts [41].

Intraosseous access is best obtained using a drill, EZ-IO® branded sizing is below [42] (Fig. 36.4) and should be used based on the appropriate age and weight. Insertion points can vary depending on the injury site—for example, there is no value in inserting IO access in the tibia if the patient has an ipsilateral femoral fracture.

When choosing an insertion site for intraosseous access, the most common option is the proximal tibia. Aim for the flat anteromedial bony surface approximately 2 cm below the tibial tuberosity. This location is favoured to avoid the tibial growth plate. In very small children less than 2 years old there is an underdeveloped tibial tuberosity, so aiming approximately 3 cm below and 1 cm medial to the lower margin of the patella is recommended. The distal femur may also be chosen with landmarks being the anterolateral surface of the femur approximately 2–3 cm above the lateral condyle.

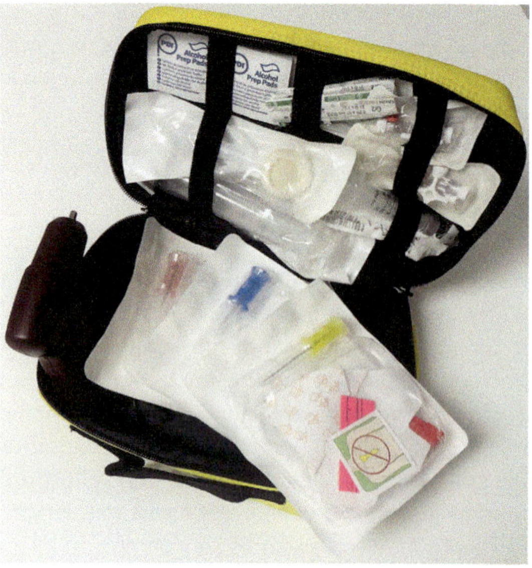

Fig. 36.4 EZ-IO needles of varying sizes. Pink is 15 mm long and for tibial insertion in children 3–39 kg, blue is 25 mm long and for tibial insertion in all patients over 39 kg, and yellow is 45 mm long and for patients over 40 kg with excessive tissue, or for humeral insertion

Due to concern of pelvic fractures or femoral fractures, prehospital trauma teams often use the humeral head as an alternative site. For this, place the patient's hand on their stomach, if able, allowing for internal rotation and adduction of the shoulder joint, exposing the most prominent aspect of the greater tubercle. In children less than 40 kg this will be difficult to palpate due to underdevelopment of the greater tubercle and is not a suitable option.

There is often a reticence from clinicians to resort to intraosseous access in children believing it is a painful and distressing procedure. Aside from the fact that it is frequently a lifesaving intervention, it is usually well-tolerated. This is particularly true in a shocked patient, and little more uncomfortable than multiple attempts at peripheral IV cannulation. Subcutaneous lidocaine infiltration or intranasal diamorphine, fentanyl or ketamine can be used before insertion but is usually unnecessary. In a conscious patient, it is often the infusion of fluids or drugs that is painful, and this may be mitigated by injection of 0.5 mg/kg lidocaine IO, slowly, beforehand.

The Use of Imaging in Paediatric Trauma

One key difference in paediatric trauma is the use of imaging. Whole-body computed tomography (CT) is readily used in trauma centres for adults however in children a more injury specific approach is used [43]. The aim is to reduce ionising radiation exposure and lifelong sequelae due to extended life expectancy and the higher radiation sensitivity of organs. Although weight-based paediatric protocols are used for scanning, radiosensitive areas such as thyroid and breast tissue should be avoided or appropriate shields employed. The ALARA principle has been introduced to safeguard exposure to ionising radiation. ALARA stands for "As Low as Reasonably Achievable". The aim is to minimise radiation exposure while maintaining safe assessment and detection of injury [44].

It is important in children to utilise the full range of imaging modalities available to answer the clinical question. Ultrasound is useful for interventional procedures such as central venous access peripheral cannulation and regional anaesthetic techniques in the hands of a skilled operator. However, FAST (Focused assessment with sonography for trauma) has no place in the paediatric emergency department [45]. Current guidelines from the Royal College of Radiologist's (RCR) do not advocate the use of ultrasound in the paediatric trauma setting to aid diagnostics- "in the acute trauma setting there is currently no role for ultrasound outside of assisting in interventional procedures". The primary reason for this current view is that attempted FAST scanning may delay transfer to CT without additional clinically useful information. This is justified by the RCR by citing FAST's low Negative Predictive Value and poor sensitivity in paediatric trauma. However, in the adolescent may still hold some value [46]. Plain Radiographs are utilised readily in the paediatric patient, and in blunt trauma to the chest should be part of the primary survey.

NICE Guidelines recommend performing magnetic resonance imaging (MRI) for children under 16 years of age if there is a strong clinical suspicion of cervical cord or spinal column injury indicated by assessment or abnormal neurological signs [37]. However, access to MRI, timing, haemodynamic stability, requirement for general anaesthesia and multi-trauma patients requiring CT for other injuries means MRI is not always the pragmatic choice.

CT can be used in a targeted modality to aid clinical decision making. As previously mentioned, the chest radiograph is the primary investigation for blunt chest trauma and is part of the primary survey in children of major trauma. However, if the mechanism of injury, clinical condition or finding on plain radiograph requires further evaluation, an isolated chest CT can be performed. Penetrating trauma such as stabbing, ballistic or impaling incidents are an indication for a contrast-enhanced CT due to risk of vascular injury.

Head injury, both isolated and as part of a multi-trauma is a common presentation to the Emergency Department. NICE has a defined guideline for imaging in these circumstances. The Royal College of Radiologists has specific guidance which states "CT is the primary investigation for cranial imaging in the child who has suffered head trauma. It displays high sensitivity and specificity for identification of traumatic brain injury and is readily available in most centres. However, the dose of ionising radiation required for cranial CT has been demonstrated to be associated with an increased incidence of cancer and it should not be used for all children with a head injury." [47].

Abdominal CT is indicated in trauma but must be a senior decision based on clinical findings. Some clinical features may be compelling factors in the choice to perform an abdominal CT, which should be elicited on the primary survey (e.g. abdominal wall bruising or tenderness, handlebar injuries/lap belt injuries, abdominal distension and rectal or nasogastric blood).

Mobile Apps

There now exists an extensive collection of medical-based apps available to the clinician, online and to download, to assist in the management of paediatric trauma and resuscitation. There are both free to use and purchasable content, although many of the good ones are free, such as:

The British National Formulary (BNF) which also includes the BNFc for all medication types and doses.
Toxbase—for Information and management of toxins following ingestions, contaminations and inhalations.
Paediatric Companion Online—Access for Paediatricians for references to child protection manual and links.
Mersey Burn App—Useful information and calculations for burns patients.
PediREF App—References for normal physiological parameters, weight-based drug doses and other useful information.

Other apps have limited free access and then a one-off fee for full access:

Neonatology—Calculation of tubes and drugs based on gestation and weight.
Paediatric Emergency—This links to all the resus council guidelines and allows input of an age with a subsequent estimation of weight and calculation of drug doses needed for different situations.

Psychological and Safeguarding Considerations

Parental Involvement

The attitude towards parental presence during resuscitation attempts has evolved over time [48] and historically, parents were kept at distance. However, research and feedback, particularly following unsuccessful resuscitations, have suggested that psychologically it may be beneficial for the parents to watch resuscitative attempts [48, 49], with a dedicated member of the team to support them and explain the steps the clinical team are taking. This allows the parents/carers a greater understanding of the processes involved and also permits the real-time exchange of information with the opportunity to prepare them if the situation is looking grave.

Where the trauma is unlikely to be life-threatening, and the child is conscious and distressed, having the caregiver (where able) next to the head or holding the child can significantly reduce the child's anxiety. Trying to minimise the number of people in the room to only essential personnel also reduces fear. It is good practice to step down the trauma team as soon as the team leader can do so, allowing streamlining of staff and freeing up of the team for other clinical responsibilities.

If a procedure is required that may be painful or distressing, having a parent or carer present to comfort and reassure the child can be a useful adjunct to analgesia, as well as providing a valuable distraction from other activities occurring around them.

Parents and carers should be allowed near to or to hold their child, even in the case of suspected non-accidental injury. This ought to be the default, unless directed otherwise by police or if their presence is making attempts at resuscitation problematic. Clinicians are not there to attribute blame; their responsibility is to treat the patient. The medical team provide facts to police and social care; providing detailed documentation of the examination and injury pattern. The further actions and ultimate decision making surrounding a non-accidental injury case involves a multidisciplinary (medical/social care/police) approach with careful consideration of the evidence ensuring the safety and best interests of the child are maintained at all times.

The impact of psychological trauma on parents and carers can vary significantly depending on their resilience and previous exposure to traumas. For this reason, all families must have access to bespoke psychological support [50]. A significant proportion of the post-traumatic stress is thought to be associated with guilt following the event, whether the caregiver is directly responsible or not.

Psychological Input and the Mental Wellbeing of the Team

Paediatric trauma can have an amplified psychological and emotional impact on the team compared to adult trauma. There is increasing evidence that teams involved in traumatic events and resuscitations benefit from a "hot" debrief (within the shift) to discuss how everyone is feeling following the case and acknowledge thoughts and responses to the incident. This can then be followed, if necessary, a few weeks later by a "cold" debrief where ongoing concerns can be raised, lessons learnt and emotional support sought [51].

The natural reactions to being involved in traumatic events are important to recognise as they enable an understanding that grief, stress and anxiety can be within the normal spectrum of responses. Rather than dwelling and ruminating in solitude over decisions made, talking them through and developing mechanisms and strategies to try and move forward is the healthier approach.

The evidence suggests that first responders and the subsequent teams involved in paediatric traumatic events are particularly vulnerable to post-traumatic stress disorder (PTSD) [52]. Recognition and proactive management of this is essential for preserving long term psychological health and reduction in burnout [51, 53].

Safeguarding

With every case of paediatric trauma, safeguarding must be considered. Extensive studies have shown that wearing a helmet reduces the risk of intracranial injury, morbidity and mortality in accidents involving cyclists [54], but not every parent/carer enforces this. Although there are recommendations, there is currently no law in the UK which mandates the provision of protective headgear in children. Conversely, where UK law exists surrounding the use of seatbelts and car seats, a child correctly restrained in an appropriate seat is far less likely to have less significant injuries than an unrestrained child. As a result of the compulsory introduction of restraints in the 1970s and their subsequent use mandated by law in 1989, there has been a 50% reduction in the number of paediatric passenger fatalities of road traffic collisions [55].

Failure to enforce the use of protective equipment in a child cycling, in isolation, would not prompt a social services referral. Instead, a collection of signs of neglect or several small incidents (such as inappropriate clothing, a child who is not mature enough to be out alone or inadequate supervision etc.) suggest that a referral or, at the very least, discussion of the case with the local safeguarding team may be necessary. Referral and raising of safeguarding concerns can vary from area to area but if the child is in hospital then referrals normally include involvement of the consultant general Paediatrician on call, the Duty and Advice team or Emergency Duty Team from social care and in some cases the police. Not all referrals involve immediate involvement of the police but severe cases do. There are initial decisions made about whether action needs to be taken immediately to safeguard other children in the household. All decisions are made in collaboration with the different agencies so not one takes the whole burden of the decisions.

The role of the medical team is to present the facts of the case (injury documentation) backed up with statistics of injury patterns and to write a report stating so. There are normally strategy meetings following the initial assessment where the child's GP and school nurse/health visitor are also invited along with the medical team, social care and police (if involved) to discuss the case and make plans for the future.

Highlighting the possibility of non-accidental injury or raising safeguarding concerns should be something that every member of the multidisciplinary team should feel able to do. By empowering every team member, safeguarding is always considered, and ultimately children's safety and interests are at the forefront of care. There have been previously high profile cases such as Baby P and Victoria Climbie, which showed failings from services and led to changes. The Victoria Climbie case lead to the formation of the Every Child Matters initiative and then the Children's Act 2004 which stated that every child should be entitled to "stay safe, be healthy, enjoy and achieve, make a positive contribution, achieve economic well-being" [56]. This states that all agencies should work together for the benefits of the child.

Although one should continually remain vigilant, there are specific injury mechanisms where safeguarding concerns should be triggered [57].

- A fall from a first-floor window or above.
- A road traffic incident where the child was not appropriately restrained.
- An injury without a credible history or where the history is changing or inconsistent with the injuries.
- Any injury/bruise in an immobile child or injuries inconsistent with the child's age or development.

Sudden Unexpected Death in Childhood

Sudden unexpected death in childhood (SUDIC)—every child who dies unexpectedly (under the age of 18 years), which includes traumatic deaths, mandates a referral to the coroner and the local SUDIC team. Examinations and investigations are carried out to identify the cause of death and the situation surrounding it. There is often a multidisciplinary team meeting, including community members such as health visitors and school nurses to review the case.

Conclusions

Paediatrics is a challenging aspect of trauma management. Unfamiliarity with anatomy and physiology can cause apprehension for the clinicians involved, although following the recognised structured approach can provide confidence in dealing with these scenarios. Making use of reference sources, paediatric specific charts and utilising local expertise will ensure the safest care is delivered. While many of the practical interventions remain the same as in adults, it is worthwhile familiarising one's self with the nuances posed by this population. Parental presence is both beneficial and encouraged during resuscitation and subsequent management, although consideration to safeguarding of a child's health under your care is crucial and must not be overlooked.

Questions

1. The most common mechanism of trauma in an infant (less than 1 year old) is:
   (a) Fall from a height < 2 m
   (b) Thermal injury
   (c) Road traffic collision
   (d) Non-accidental injury
2. The most accurate formulae to estimate a 7 year old child's weight in kilograms is:
   (a) (0.5 × age in months) + 4
   (b) (2 × age in years) + 8
   (c) (3 × age in years) + 7
   (d) (Age in years + 4) × 2
3. The narrowest portion of a child's airway is:
   (a) The supraglottis
   (b) The glottis/subglottis
   (c) The cricoid cartilage
   (d) The carina
4. The best position to palpate a central pulse in an infant (less than 1 year old) is:
   (a) Carotid Artery
   (b) Femoral Artery
   (c) Brachial Artery
   (d) Radial Artery
5. The estimated circulating blood volume of a 5 year old child is:
   (a) 90 ml/kg
   (b) 80 ml/kg
   (c) 75 ml/kg
   (d) 65 ml/kg

Answers

1. d
2. c
3. b
4. b
5. c

References

1. Patel V. Child and infant mortality in England and Wales [Internet]. Office for National Statistics; 2019 June [cited 2019 Dec 9] p. 19. Available from: https://www.ons.gov.uk/peoplepopulationandcommunity/birthsdeathsandmarriages/deaths/bulletins/childhoodinfantandperinatalmortalityinenglandandwales/2017
2. TARN. Severe Injury in Children January 2015–December 2016 [Internet]. The Trauma Audit and Research Network; 2016 [cited 2019 Dec 9] p. 11. Available from: https://www.tarn.ac.uk/content/downloads/3572/SevereInjuryinChildren15-16.pdf
3. Samuels M, Wieteska S, editors. Advanced Paediatric Life Support: The Practical Approach [Internet]. The Atrium, Southern Gate, Chichester, West Sussex, PO19 8SQ, UK: John Wiley & Sons, Ltd; 2011 [cited 2019 Dec 9]. Available from: https://doi.org/10.1002/9781118369784
4. Spinella PC, Holcomb JB. Resuscitation and transfusion principles for traumatic hemorrhagic shock. Blood Rev. 2009 Nov;23(6):231–40.
5. Hunt BJ, Allard S, Keeling D, Norfolk D, Stanworth SJ, Pendry K, et al. A practical guideline for the haematological management of major haemorrhage. Br J Haematol. 2015 Sep;170(6):788–803.
6. Cooper S, editor. Yorkshire and Humber Paediatric Major Trauma Dec 2018 [Internet]. The West Yorkshire Major Trauma Network; 2018 [cited 2019 Dec 9]. Available from: https://www.networks.nhs.uk/nhs-networks/yorkshire-humber-paediatric-critical-care-odn/guidelines/draft-y-h-paediatric-major-trauma-guidelines
7. Roberts I, Shakur H, Afolabi A, The CRASH-2 Collaborators. The importance of early treatment with tranexamic acid in bleeding trauma patients: an exploratory analysis of the CRASH-2 randomised controlled trial. Lancet. 2011 Mar;377(9771):1096–1101.e2.
8. Royal College of Paediatrics and Child Health. Evidence Statement: Major trauma and the use of tranexamic acid in children. November 2012 [Internet]. 2012 [cited 2019 Dec 9]. Available from: https://www.tarn.ac.uk/content/downloads/3100/121112_TXA%20evidence%20statement_final%20v2.pdf
9. Norfolk D. United Kingdom blood services. Handbook of transfusion medicine. London: H.M.S.O; 2013.
10. Litman RS, Weissend EE, Shibata D, Westesson P-L. Developmental changes of laryngeal dimensions in unparalyzed, sedated children. Anesthesiology. 2003 Jan;98(1):41–5.
11. Wani TM, Bissonnette B, Rafiq Malik M, Hayes D, Ramesh AS, Al Sohaibani M, et al. Age-based analysis of pediatric upper airway dimensions using computed tomography imaging: upper airway dimensions in children. Pediatr Pulmonol. 2016 Mar;51(3):267–71.
12. Tobias JD. Pediatric airway anatomy may not be what we thought: implications for clinical practice and the use of cuffed endotracheal tubes. Paediatr Anaesth. 2015 Jan;25(1):9–19.
13. Cook TM, Woodall N, Frerk C. Major complications of airway management in the UK: results of the Fourth National Audit Project of the Royal College of Anaesthetists and the Difficult Airway Society. Part 1: anaesthesia. Br J Anaesth. 2011 May;106(5):617–31.
14. Black AE, Flynn PER, Smith HL, Thomas ML, Wilkinson KA. Development of a guideline for the management of the unanticipated difficult airway in pediatric practice. Paediatr Anaesth. 2015 Apr;25(4):346–62.
15. Bolton P. Emergency jet ventilation in children. Pediatr Anesth. 2009 May;19(5):425–7.
16. Blain S, Paterson N. Paediatric massive transfusion. BJA Educ. 2016 Aug;16(8):269–75.
17. Jones N, Ee M, Fenton E. Permissive hypotension in paediatric trauma: letters to the editor. ANZ J Surg. 2012 July;82(7–8):567–8.
18. Tosounidis TH, Giannoudis PV. Paediatric trauma resuscitation: an update. Eur J Trauma Emerg Surg. 2016 Jun;42(3):297–301.
19. Hiu Lam W, Mackersie A. Paediatric head injury: incidence, aetiology and management. Pediatr Anesth. 1999 Sep;9(5):377–85.
20. Bhalla T, Dewhirst E, Sawardekar A, Dairo O, Tobias JD. Perioperative management of the pediatric patient with traumatic brain injury: perioperative management of the pediatric patient with neurotrauma. Pediatr Anesth. 2012 Jul;22(7):627–40.
21. Pigula FA, Wald SL, Shackford SR, Vane DW. The effect of hypotension and hypoxia on children with severe head injuries. J Pediatr Surg. 1993 Mar;28(3):310–6.
22. Kochanek P. Guidelines for the acute medical management of severe traumatic brain injury in infants, children, and adolescents-second edition. Pract Guidelines. 2012;13:S1–2.
23. Hardcastle N, Benzon HA, Vavilala MS. Update on the 2012 guidelines for the management of pediatric traumatic brain injury - information for the anesthesiologist. Paediatr Anaesth. 2014 July;24(7):703–10.
24. Kochanek PM, Tasker RC, Carney N, Totten AM, Adelson PD, Selden NR, et al. Guidelines for the management of pediatric severe traumatic brain injury, third edition: update of the brain trauma foundation guidelines, executive summary. Neurosurgery. 2019 June 1;84(6):1169–78.
25. Bar-Joseph G, Guilburd Y, Tamir A, Guilburd JN. Effectiveness of ketamine in decreasing intracranial pressure in children with intracranial hypertension. PED. 2009 July;4(1):40–6.
26. Barnes J, Duffy A, Hamnett N, McPhail J, Seaton C, Shokrollahi K, et al. The Mersey Burns App: evolving a model of validation. Emerg Med J. 2015 Aug;32(8):637–41.
27. Mintegi S, Clerigue N, Tipo V, Ponticiello E, Lonati D, Burillo-Putze G, et al. Pediatric cyanide poisoning by fire smoke inhalation: a European expert consensus. Pediatr Emerg Care. 2013 Nov;29(11):1234–40.

28. Kolaitis G. Symptoms of posttraumatic stress, depression and anxiety among youths exposed to a massive fire disaster in Greece. BJMMR. 2011 Jan 10;1(4):320–32.
29. Day LM, Huang R, Okada PJ. Management of pain after pediatric trauma. Pediatr Emerg Care. 2019 Jan;36(2):e33–7.
30. Ventafridda V, Saita L, Ripamonti C, De Conno F. WHO guidelines for the use of analgesics in cancer pain. Int J Tissue React. 1985;7(1):93–6.
31. Cuomo A, Bimonte S, Forte CA, Botti G, Cascella M. Multimodal approaches and tailored therapies for pain management: the trolley analgesic model. JPR. 2019 Feb;12:711–4.
32. The College of Emergency Medicine Clinical Effectiveness Committee, London. The College of Emergency Medicine [Internet]. The College of Emergency Medicine; 2010 [cited 2020 Jan 8]. Available from: https://www.surreyandsussex.nhs.uk/wp-content/uploads/2013/04/2-College-of-Emergency-Medicine.pdf
33. Tepas JJ, Mollitt DL, Talbert JL, Bryant M. The pediatric trauma score as a predictor of injury severity in the injured child. J Pediatr Surg. 1987 Jan;22(1):14–8.
34. Haque IU, Zaritsky AL. Analysis of the evidence for the lower limit of systolic and mean arterial pressure in children. Pediatr Crit Care Med. 2007 Mar;8(2):138–44.
35. Ciurea AV, Sandu AM, Popescu M, Iencean SM, Davidescu B. Neurotrauma pediatric scales. J Med Life. 2008 Dec;1(4):403–14.
36. Tatman A, Warren A, Williams A, Powell JE, Whitehouse W. Development of a modified paediatric coma scale in intensive care clinical practice. Arch Dis Child. 1997 Dec 1;77(6):519–21.
37. National Institute for Health and Care Excellence. Spinal injury: assessment and initial management [Internet]. NICE; 2016 [cited 2019 Dec 10]. Available from: https://www.nice.org.uk/guidance/ng41/resources/spinal-injury-assessment-and-initial-management-pdf-1837447790533
38. Sundstrøm T, Asbjørnsen H, Habiba S, Sunde GA, Wester K. Prehospital use of cervical collars in trauma patients: a critical review. J Neurotrauma. 2014 Mar 15;31(6):531–40.
39. The Royal College of Emergency Medicine. Paediatric Trauma - Stabilisation of the Cervical Spine (Aug 2017).pdf [Internet]. RCEM; 2017 [cited 2019 Dec 10]. Available from: https://www.rcem.ac.uk/docs/RCEM%20Guidance/Paediatric%20Trauma%20-%20Stabilisation%20of%20the%20Cervical%20Spine%20(Aug%202017).pdf
40. The Spinal Cord Injury Centres of the United Kingdom and Ireland. Moving and Handling Patients with Actual or Suspected Spinal cord Injuries [Internet]. 2015 [cited 2019 Dec 10]. Available from: https://www.mascip.co.uk/wp-content/uploads/2015/02/MASCIP-SIA-Guidelines-for-MH-Trainers.pdf
41. American College of Surgeons, Committee on Trauma. Advanced trauma life support: student course manual - 10th Edition. Chicago, IL: American College of Surgeons; 2018.
42. Teleflex. Arrow-EZ-IO-Intraosseous-Vascular--Access-Needles.pdf [Internet]. Teleflex; 2015 [cited 2019 Dec 10]. Available from: https://www.teleflex.com/en/usa/ezioeducation/documents/Arrow-EZ-IO-Intraosseous-Vascular-Access-Needles.pdf
43. Abe T, Aoki M, Deshpande G, Sugiyama T, Iwagami M, Uchida M, et al. Is whole-body CT associated with reduced in-hospital mortality in children with trauma? A nationwide study. Pediatr Crit Care Med. 2019 June;20(6):e245–50.
44. Uffmann M, Schaefer-Prokop C. Digital radiography: the balance between image quality and required radiation dose. Eur J Radiol. 2009 Nov;72(2):202–8.
45. Holmes JF, Gladman A, Chang CH. Performance of abdominal ultrasonography in pediatric blunt trauma patients: a meta-analysis. J Pediatr Surg. 2007 Sep;42(9):1588–94.
46. The Royal College of Radiologists. Paediatric trauma protocols [Internet]. 2014 [cited 2020 Jan 8]. Available from: https://www.rcr.ac.uk/system/files/publication/field_publication_files/BFCR%2814%298_paeds_trauma.pdf
47. National Institute for Health and Clinical Excellence. Selection of children for a CT head scan CG176 Head injury: assessment and early management [Internet]. NICE; 2014 [cited 2019 Dec 10]. Available from: https://www.nice.org.uk/guidance/cg176/resources/head-injury-assessment-and-early-management-pdf-35109755595493
48. Brasel KJ, Entwistle JW, Sade RM. Should family presence be allowed during cardiopulmonary resuscitation? Ann Thorac Surg. 2016 Nov;102(5):1438–43.
49. Cowley A, Durge N. The impact of parental accompaniment in paediatric trauma: a helicopter emergency medical service (HEMS) perspective. Scand J Trauma Resusc Emerg Med. 2014 Dec;22(1):32.
50. McGarry S, Girdler S, McDonald A, Valentine J, Wood F, Elliott C. Paediatric medical trauma: the impact on parents of burn survivors. Burns. 2013 Sep;39(6):1114–21.
51. Grundlingh H, Knight L, Naker D, Devries K. Secondary distress in violence researchers: a randomised trial of the effectiveness of group debriefings. BMC Psychiatry. 2017 Dec;17(1):204.
52. Hollingsworth CE, Wesley C, Huckridge J, Finn GM, Griksaitis MJ. Impact of child death on paediatric trainees. Arch Dis Child. 2018 Jan;103(1):14–8.
53. Gunasingam N, Burns K, Edwards J, Dinh M, Walton M. Reducing stress and burnout in junior doctors: the impact of debriefing sessions. Postgrad Med J. 2015 Apr;91(1074):182–7.
54. Dodds N, Johnson R, Walton B, Bouamra O, Yates D, Lecky FE, et al. Evaluating the impact of cycle helmet use on severe traumatic brain injury and death in a national cohort of over 11000 pedal cyclists: a retrospective study from the NHS England Trauma Audit and Research Network dataset. BMJ Open. 2019 Sep;9(9):e027845.

55. Weaver NL, Brixey SN, Williams J, Nansel TR. Promoting correct Car seat use in parents of young children: challenges, recommendations, and implications for health communication. Health Promot Pract. 2013 Mar;14(2):301–7.
56. UK Government. Children Act 2004 [internet]. Statute Law Database; 2004. Available from: http://www.legislation.gov.uk/ukpga/2004/31/contents
57. Brandon M, Brivio S, Glaser D, Lushey C. Missed opportunities: indicators of neglect – what is ignored, why, and what can be done? [Internet]. 2014 Nov [cited 2019 Dec 10] p. 46. Available from: https://assets.publishing.service.gov.uk/government/uploads/system/uploads/attachment_data/file/379747/RR404_-_Indicators_of_neglect_missed_opportunities.pdf

37 Silver Trauma

Peter Lax

Overview: This chapter deals with the effects of trauma in the elderly population with specific mention of the physiology of ageing, modifications to the primary survey, considerations when prescribing drugs and treatment of common complications such as delirium.

Introduction

The elderly population has traditionally been defined as any patient over the age of 65 [1]. This has been further divided into the "young-old" (ages 65–74), the "middle-old" (ages 75–84), and the "old-old" (aged 85 and older) [2, 3]. These definitions are purely age-based and do not consider differences in functional or physiological capacity; some patients in their 50s with chronic disease may have less reserve than a fit and active person in their 70s.

While it is well noted that trauma is a disease that disproportionately affects younger people, it remains the seventh highest cause of death in the USA for people over the age of 65 [4]. The 2017 Major Trauma in Older People report from TARN has shown that the age of the average Major Trauma patient has increased since 2005, primarily driven by an increase in elderly trauma patients out of proportion to changes in the UK population demographics (Fig. 37.1) [5]. While part of this change may be due to increased reporting, it does not explain the whole picture, especially when this report excluded common injuries such as isolated neck of femur fractures and single fractures distal to the elbow or knee. As treatments improve for diseases that may have killed patients earlier in life, patients are now living longer and more actively. These later years bring with them the physiological changes associated with ageing (as discussed below), consequently leading to patients who are still active but generally frailer than their younger counterparts. The most common mechanism of injury in UK elderly Major Trauma patients is a fall from less than two metres; the proportion of patients who present with this mechanism increases almost linearly with age (Fig. 37.2). This is likely reflective of behavioural changes (people become less active as they age) and increased frailty associated with ageing, requiring less physical insult to cause significant injury.

What is also apparent from these data is that the elderly population is underserved by major trauma services. They are less likely to be transported to a Major Trauma Centre, less likely to be seen by senior medical staff and more likely to have a delay to initial treatment or definitive surgery if required. Part of these observations may be due to the change in risk: benefit analysis of

P. Lax (✉)
Tactical Medical Wing, Royal Air Force, Brize Norton, Oxfordshire, UK

The Air Ambulance Service (TAAS), Rugby, Warwickshire, UK
e-mail: p.lax@NHS.net

P. Lax (ed.), *Textbook of Acute Trauma Care*, https://doi.org/10.1007/978-3-030-83628-3_37

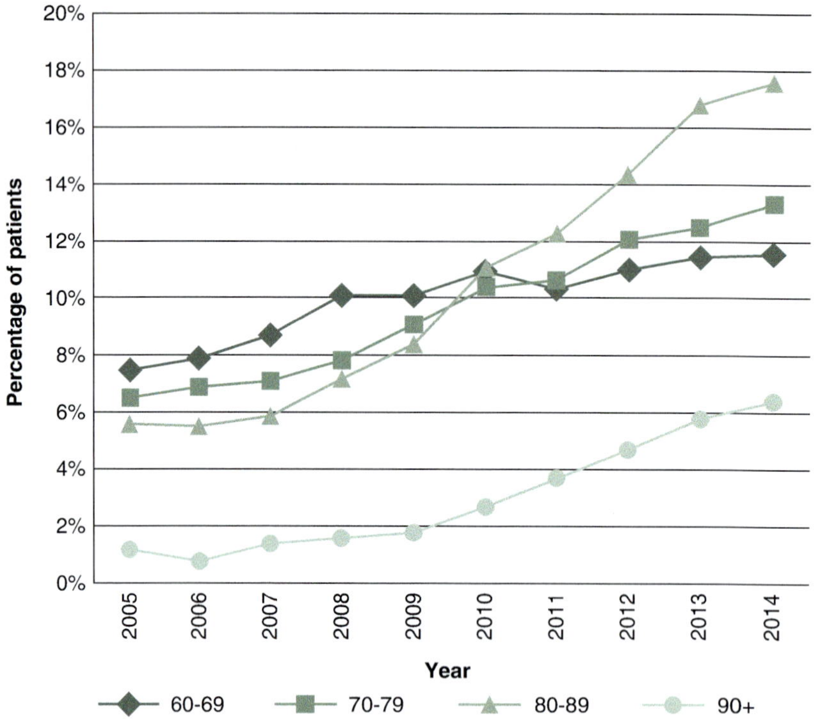

Fig. 37.1 Severely injured patients since 2005 by age (from TARN)

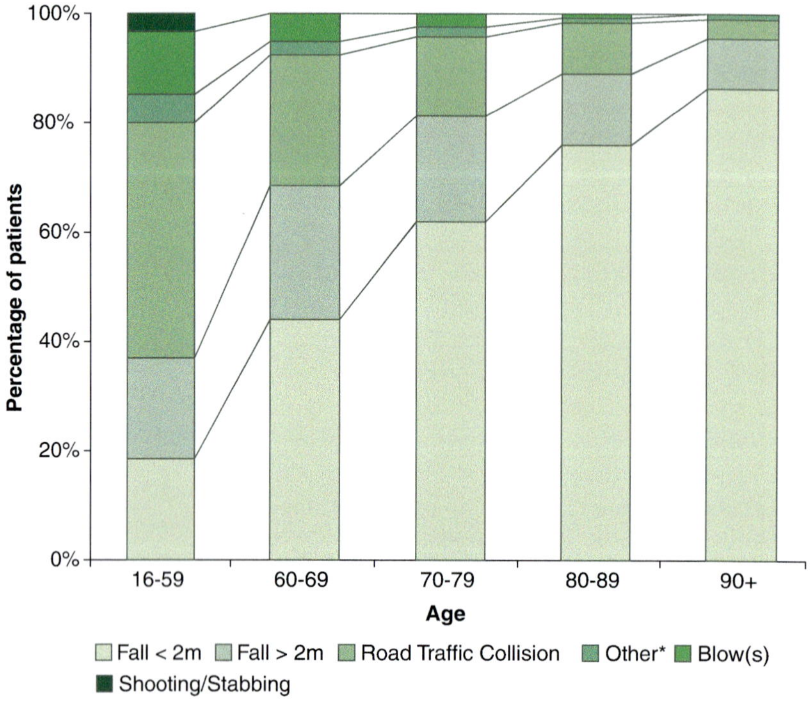

Fig. 37.2 Mechanism of Injury of ISS > 15 patients by age

anaesthesia and surgery as patients age, increased difficulty in assessing patients with multi-system co-morbidities and undertaking stabilisation, or older patients being seen as being a lower priority than younger ones; there are currently insufficient data to say whether these delays are justified. Elderly trauma patients are also a relatively under-investigated group in terms of international research priorities [6, 7].

This leads to a paradox wherein available data shows that the elderly who receive intensive early management of their injuries have better outcomes [8]; however, they are less likely to receive that monitoring than their younger counterparts and may be more complex to diagnose [9]. This age-related selection bias may result in therapeutic nihilism, as potentially salvageable patients are not actively managed, fuelling a perception of futility in this cohort. This self-fulfilling expectation is not challenged as the research in this area is scarce. While some available data show a *relative* increase in mortality in the over 80's, increased costs and length of stay, the *absolute* numbers do not indicate as poor an outcome as many practitioners expect [10, 11].

The Physiology of Ageing

Age-related changes occur in all tissues, with function steadily decreasing throughout adulthood. These changes may be exacerbated or diminished by lifestyle factors such as diet and exercise. However, it is fair to say that most patients over the age of 65 will have less overall physiological reserve than those in their 20s. Some of the principal changes in each system that may be relevant in the context of Major Trauma are outlined in Table 37.1.

As patients age, applying "normal" physiological parameters as a screening test to detect pathology becomes increasingly more problematic. This is for several reasons:

Key Learning Points

- Patients who have a "normal" systolic blood pressure may be relatively hypotensive if they suffer from hypertension
- Patients may be taking medication that masks physiological signs or changes that would otherwise be concerning (e.g. patients taking beta-blockers or some calcium channel block-

Table 37.1 Common physiological changes with ageing

Body system	Physiological changes
Cardiovascular	Decreased cardiac reserve [12], increased atherosclerosis Decreased VO_2Max leading to earlier decompensation Higher incidence of hypertension means "normal" blood pressures may reflect hypoperfusion Decreased maximal physiological response (e.g. decreased maximum heart rate) [13] Coronary atherosclerosis limits blood flow—tachycardia causes unmet myocardial oxygen demand and type 2 MI.
Respiratory	Stiffer ribcage with weaker muscles and impaired parenchymal function [14] Impaired responses to hypercapnoea, hypoxia and exercise Decreased gas transfer and functional residual capacity
Neurological	Visual problems and slower reflexes—more prone to trauma? Higher background incidence of cognitive impairment as age increases—history taking may be difficult Higher rates of postoperative delirium, with increased 30-day mortality
Renal	Decreased GFR Impaired drug excretion/metabolism Drug accumulation More prone to renal dysfunction and complications/electrolyte disturbances
Musculoskeletal	Decreased muscle mass, decreased muscle: fat ratio, altered volume of distribution for drugs Higher incidence of osteoporosis and fragility fractures Fractures as a marker of frailty and underlying reserve
GI	Decreased liver function Decreased metabolic rate and impaired thermogenesis
Immune	Decreased immune response leading to higher rates of infection and impaired wound healing

ers may not be able to mount a tachycardic response)

- The degree of injury to provoke a stress response may be comparatively lower than a younger individual
- Medications for chronic conditions may make a comparatively minor injury into a catastrophic one (e.g. a minor intracranial bleed may become severe if the patient is taking anticoagulants/anti-platelet agents)

Traditional targets used for hypotensive resuscitation in younger patients (80–90 mmHg) may be insufficient in the elderly and need to be revised upwards (e.g. 100–110 mmHg). It is important to note that this is still relative hypotension in this group, as their "normal" blood pressures are likely to be higher than younger patients.

The higher incidence of chronic conditions and use of medications in the elderly also causes further diagnostic problems for practitioners. Consider a patient admitted as the driver following a road traffic collision with a sternal injury and mild confusion/hypotension. If they have signs of ST changes on their ECG with hypotension, this could either be a cause or consequence of the injury; did they have an MI, become unconscious and crash the car, or hit their chest on the steering wheel and develop a myocardial contusion? Is the hypotension due to heart failure following an MI, bleeding, or an exaggerated response to IV opiates given for analgesia before arriving in hospital? Is this an aortic dissection rather than an MI? Is it primary or secondary? The pre-test probability of medical events precipitating trauma in the elderly is much higher, and the degree of compensatory response they can mount is likely to be lower, with poorer tolerance of hypotension and hypoxia.

Medication and Prescribing in the Elderly

It follows from the increased incidence of chronic conditions in the elderly that there will be an increased incidence of patients taking medications before suffering a traumatic injury. Approximately 20% of the UK population are 60 years or older, but they account for 59% of all prescriptions and over 50% of all NHS drug expenditure [15]. In the USA, one study found that 87% of all people over the age of 60 took at least one prescription medication, with 36% of people taking at least five classes of medication [16]. This may be further compounded on discharge from hospital; another study found that elderly patients discharged to nursing homes following hospitalisation were prescribed an average of 14 medications, with one-third of these prescriptions for drugs with side effects that could exacerbate underlying geriatric symptoms [17].

Analgesia is more fully discussed in the relevant chapter, but specifically regarding the elderly, many of the analgesic drugs commonly prescribed in trauma may cause additional problems. Control of pain is an end in itself and may be necessary for physiological optimisation, such as allowing effective breathing in chest trauma. It is also important to note that inadequate analgesia will also increase the rate of delirium and potentially lead to prescriptions of other drugs to treat this [18, 19]. However, in the elderly, analgesic drugs are a double-edged sword as medications such as opiates may also cause or contribute to delirium or acute confusional states, either as a direct effect or by inducing side effects such as urinary retention or constipation [20, 21]. While other medications such as non-steroidal anti-inflammatories can alleviate pain, they remain at risk of causing other problems with prolonged use (such as acute kidney injury or gastric ulceration). The use of regional anaesthesia, either in "single-shot" nerve blocks at the time of operation or via continuous catheter infusion techniques (e.g. peripheral nerve catheters or epidurals) is an attractive alternative to avoid these drugs. However, using these techniques depends on the availability of an appropriate nursing skill mix to be used safely outside of a HDU/ICU environment.

Prescribing in the elderly can be problematic. Age-related changes affect both pharmacokinetic (effects of the body on the drug) and pharmacodynamic (effects of the drug on the body) parameters [22, 23]. Several criteria can be used to identify potentially inappropriate drugs in the elderly outside of trauma, for example, the Beers criteria [24] and the STOPP/START criteria [25]. Ensuring regular administration of some medications is essential, even when patients are nil-by-mouth (e.g. levodopa and decarboxylase inhibitors in Parkinson disease). Certain medications will be subject to an individual risk: benefit discussion about their continuation or cessation, a typical example being anti-platelet medications in patients with a recent history of coronary angioplasty who are at risk of both in-stent thrombosis and ongoing traumatic/surgical bleeding.

Many trauma services that deal with elderly patients have dedicated orthogeriatric physicians. These doctors can assess and manage some of the complex medical problems that may have been the cause or result of hospital admission and acute medications required for traumatic injuries. They are highly useful regarding medicines management in the perioperative period, as management of longer-term medications (such as antihypertensives) in an acute illness can be challenging. This approach also allows a dedicated care of the elderly physician to optimise medications on discharge and may prevent potentially inappropriate medication use [26, 27]. This shared care model has been implemented in some centres internationally with improvements in both short and longer-term outcomes [28, 29].

Key Learning Point
As a general principle, the minimum number of additional drugs that are necessary should be prescribed for the shortest duration possible.

Changes in Assessment of the Elderly Trauma Patient

The fundamental principles of MABCD outlined throughout this textbook are the same. However, some subtleties need to be borne in mind when treating elderly patients. As mentioned, elderly patients are more likely to take medication that will affect vital signs such as pulse and blood pressure at baseline. The use of clinical and biochemical markers as signs of organ hypoperfusion such as level of consciousness, urine output and serum lactate levels should be considered earlier than perhaps they would be in a younger patient. There is also evidence that cardiac output monitoring in the elderly may help improve outcome, but whether this is a marker of the effect of closer observation improving outcomes rather than an endorsement of specific goal-directed therapy is unclear [30–33].

Mechanisms of Injury

As previously stated, falls from a standing height contribute to a significant burden of major trauma in this age group. Falls account for 60% of injuries and half the traumatic deaths in the over 65 [5, 34], and is likely indicative of the relative frailty of this group of patients. Hence, a high index of suspicion for significant injuries in any elderly trauma patient is appropriate. Motor vehicle collisions account for 20–25% of injuries, with the patient as either driver, passenger or pedestrian, and approximately 1% of injuries resulting from assault or elder abuse.

Key Learning Point
Mechanisms that are particularly concerning in the elderly are falls from height or down stairs, motor vehicle collisions at over 30 mph or where the patient is a pedestrian or ejected vehicle occupant, or any penetrating chest/abdominal injury.

Specific Differences in the Primary Survey

Airway and Cervical Spine

A combination of osteoporosis and frailty means that upper c-spine injuries (especially C1–C2 fractures) are more common, even in the context of a relatively minor mechanism of injury. There should be a low threshold to CT the cervical spine as it has a higher sensitivity and specificity than plain films for detecting cervical spine injuries. This is especially true in the context of patients who may have degenerative changes that make plain film interpretation more complex, making CT the investigation of choice in this population. There is also data that cervical spine injuries are more common in the elderly, with the incidence doubling with each decade over the age of 60, justifying the additional radiation exposure [35, 36]. If the CT shows a fracture, then subsequent MRI imaging is necessary to assess for cord, disc and ligamentous injuries.

Elderly patients are also more likely to wear dentures which may complicate airway management initially. If they are secure and well-fitting, it may be best to leave them in situ until the airway is secure to assist in forming a good seal for ventilation, but have a low threshold for removing them if damaged or loose. Dentures should be kept with the patient so they can eat following trauma; it is surprisingly common how insufficient oral intake after trauma can be caused by misplacing them!

Breathing

An initial saturation target of 94–98% is appropriate unless there is pre-existing evidence of type 2 respiratory failure that may mean a target of 88–92% is better. Thoracic trauma is considered in the dedicated chapter, however it is worth pointing out that elderly patients may start from a more precarious position and have the most to gain from adequate analgesia and early rib fixation. More than two unilateral rib fractures have been shown to increase the risk of respiratory failure, hypoxia and delirium, so consideration should be given to admission to a HDU environment where effective analgesia, close monitoring and chest physiotherapy can be instituted in the first 48–72 hours. Other predictors of complications in this group are the presence of haemothorax or pneumothorax, age >85 years, or underlying pulmonary contusions/pre-existing chest pathology.

Circulation

Where possible, patient and collateral history should be taken, the possibility of a precipitant cardiac event causing trauma should be considered, and all elderly trauma patients should have a screening ECG taken. A systolic blood pressure of less than 110 mmHg increases mortality and should be regarded as significant hypotension, and a heart rate of 90 bpm or higher should be regarded as a significant tachycardia [13]. Elderly patients with a history of cardiovascular disease are also more likely to take medication which may alter their physiological response or increase their bleeding risk. Adequacy of resuscitation may be more guided by improvements in base deficit and lactate rather than restoration of a specific blood pressure [37]. Tranexamic acid should be used for the same indications in younger people following the CRASH-2 and CRASH-3 trials.

Disability and Head Injury

Baseline neurological function and any history of pre-existing delirium or cognitive impairment should be documented, ideally with a scoring system such as the 4AT [38]. If there is an advanced care directive or medical power of attorney then this should also be noted with contact details. If the patient is from a residential care home, then any accompanying carers should have relevant details of the patient's medical history and medications if the patient cannot communicate these themselves. Any glasses or hearing aids should also be kept with the patient to ease communication.

As patients age, they undergo cerebral atrophy and the volume of the brain decreases. This can prove advantageous in some senses, as patients with head injuries may have more capacity in their skull vault to accommodate blood before suffering the effects of raised intracranial pressure. Conversely, this may be a problem as it may lead to undertriage, as patients with significant head injury may have a higher than expected GCS. In the case of subdural haematomas, they may have a delayed presentation with neurological symptoms weeks after their initial trauma. As with other injuries, a higher index of suspicion and low threshold for CT should be encouraged if any concerning features are present in the context of head injury, such as:

- Decreased GCS from baseline or new-onset headache

- Antiplatelet or anticoagulant use
- Significant/concerning mechanism of injury
- Traumatic epistaxis
- Loss of consciousness at any point or amnesia of events

The CRASH score includes age as part of its calculations and may also aid in estimating the trajectory of illness and recovery in head-injured patients [39].

Abdominal/Pelvic Injuries

Surgery in the elderly comes with more risk, so there may be a higher threshold for operative vs conservative management of solid organ injuries, but vascular injures will need definitive management [8]. Interventional radiology is even more attractive an option in the elderly compared to the young trauma population as it avoids much of the morbidity and mortality associated with a major laparotomy. Any elderly patients with significant abdominopelvic injuries should have a whole-body CT to pick up other occult injuries.

Burns and Extremity Trauma

Decreased dermal thickness and a lower collagen/elastin content of the skin as patients age mean that wound healing is delayed. As the incidence of type 2 diabetes and use of medications that may impair the immune response increases (e.g. steroids, DMARDs), the risk of infection also increases. Patients with open fractures or soft tissue injuries such as pre-tibial lacerations may need input from specialist teams such as tissue viability or plastic surgery in addition to orthopaedics to best effect wound closure.

Safeguarding and Elder Abuse

Patients who present with traumatic injuries may do so as a result of elder abuse, or abuse may become apparent during their hospital stay. Elder abuse is likely underreported as those most prone to it may be more deprived, dependent on others for care or have physical or cognitive disabilities [40]. In similar fashion to paediatric non-accidental injuries, the clues may come from an inconsistent history of events, a suggested mechanism of injury that may be physically impossible for the patient, radiographic appearances of multiple injuries occurring at different times, other discrepancies that cannot be adequately explained or signs of neglect [41, 42]. However, there are some dissimilarities with paediatric practice, as both the victim and perpetrator are more willing to disclose abuse when directly asked despite the potential legal consequences [43]. Another difference is that even when elder abuse is identified, most patients are discharged back into the care of their abusers as they have the capacity to make this decision, rather than a "best interests" decision that may be made on behalf of a child [44]. Abuse should be reported to the local safeguarding lead in hours (or the Social Services Emergency Duty Team or Police out of hours) as it is a statutory duty [45].

Blood Management in Elderly Trauma

As highlighted in the circulation chapter, haemoglobin is essential for oxygen transport around the body. There may be pre-existing pathology that causes anaemia in the elderly before any acute blood loss (e.g. anaemia of chronic disease from any cause, dietary iron or folate deficiencies, impaired haemopoietic function), so DO_2 may be reduced at baseline in some patients. The cardiac output is the other important factor in this equation, and due to age-related changes cardiac output and reserve may drop. This could be due to impairment of flow through stiffened and atherosclerotic vessels, decreased myocardial contractility/valvular disease and reduced ejection fraction. Consequently anaemia is not as well tolerated in the elderly as in younger patients.

The classical definition of anaemia by the WHO in 1968 was based on gender and pregnancy status, with different haemoglobin cutoffs from men (130 mg/dl), non-pregnant women (120 mg/dl) and pregnant women (110 mg/dl) [46]. While this does reflect the impact of the physiological changes of pregnancy, this definition of anaemia is outdated and was subsequently revised in 2017. A haemoglobin concentration of <130 mg/dl in either sex is now considered diagnostic of anaemia based on international consensus [47].

Anaemia has a high prevalence in the elderly, and it appears to increase with advancing age [48]. Approximately a third of elective patients for hip or knee replacement were anaemic preoperatively in one systematic review. The proportion of patients for emergency hip and knee surgery that were anaemic was found to be as high as 87%, depending on the definition of anaemia used [49]. Of note, patients presenting for emergency surgery were more likely to be older, more likely to be anaemic and have a lower haemoglobin level than elective patients. While there may have been a degree of blood loss due to trauma, the significant discrepancies between these group suggest that this cannot be the only factor. On average, men have a higher body mass and consequently a larger circulating volume, so a 500 ml blood loss is a higher proportion of total circulatory loss in women compared to men. While there has been a trend towards accepting lower haemoglobin levels in younger patients before transfusion (especially in critical care where a trigger of 70 mg/dl is used [50]), the same transfusion triggers should not be used in the elderly. To compensate for anaemia, cardiac output will need to be increased, and hence myocardial workload increased. If there is coronary arterial disease present, the delivery of blood to the myocardium may be impaired to begin with. The discrepancy between myocardial oxygen supply (due to anaemia and restriction of coronary flow) and increased demand (the physiological drive to increase cardiac output) may cause a type 2 myocardial infarction.

What Is the Optimum Haemoglobin Concentration?

Guidance from the Association of Anaesthetists of Great Britain and Ireland on hip fracture patients supports a more liberal transfusion threshold, aiming to keep a haemoglobin concentration of 90–100 mg/dl [51]. This would seem a sensible compromise in most elderly trauma patients, with the caveat that haemoglobin levels in acute trauma may not necessarily drop quickly and so the degree of blood loss may be underestimated. This has to be offset against the increased risk of transfusion-associated circulatory overload (TACO) in elderly patients who may not tolerate large volume infusions.

A 2016 meta-analysis of elderly orthopaedic patients demonstrated that this higher transfusion target led to a decreased incidence of complications in the first 30 days post-operatively [52]. This target is concordant with other published literature showing the benefit of a more liberal strategy in the elderly [53, 54].

A paper that heavily weighted earlier reviews debating liberal or restrictive strategies was published by Carson et al [55], however, the methodology was flawed. This trial favoured a restrictive approach, but patients were not randomised into their groups until the third postoperative day. Therefore, blood management advice is not directly applicable to a silver trauma patient at hospital presentation, nor any immediate perioperative journey. Furthermore, a liberal strategy (90–100 g/L) is supported by another 2016 systematic review and meta-analysis in patients with pre-existing cardiovascular disease to prevent MI, acute coronary syndrome, and cardiac arrest [56]. Further evidence also suggests that a liberal strategy is helpful in terms of early functional recovery and re-enablement [57]. Therefore, there should be a low threshold for blood transfusion in the initial stages of trauma management and any perioperative care. A baseline transfusion strategy aiming to keep haemoglobin concentration in the range of 90–100 mg/dL should be employed before subsequent patient tailoring by orthogeriatricians.

Anti-Platelet Agents and Their Reversal

Medications such as aspirin, clopidogrel and ticagrelor are commonly used following a variety of stenting procedures and for secondary prevention in peripheral and cerebrovascular disease. In trauma, consideration needs to be given to the risk and benefit of continuing these medications, usually in conjunction with a consultant from the speciality that started them or haematology. There are essentially no blanket rules, but some principles should be borne in mind:

- Anti-platelet agents irreversibly bind to platelets, so the only way to reverse their effect is to transfuse new platelets or wait for the bone marrow to produce more.
- Monotherapy with any agent does not need to be stopped for the sole purpose of spinal anaesthesia [51].
- Dual anti-platelet therapy (DAPT) is not an absolute contraindication to spinal anaesthesia if the patient is in a higher risk group for complications following a general anaesthetic (e.g. active pneumonia or other reason for poor preoperative respiratory function). The increased relative complication rate will need to be discussed with the patient preoperatively, but the absolute incidence of vertebral canal haematoma remains low [58]. However, higher risk patients should be monitored for signs of vertebral canal haematoma in the postoperative period (back pain, numbness, motor weakness, bladder/bowel incontinence) [51].
- Drug-eluting stents (DES) are more at risk for early in-stent thrombosis than bare-metal stents (BMS) if DAPT is stopped, so determining the kind of stent fitted and its insertion date is vitally important [59, 60]. The most significant risk is in the first 30 days, and after 6 months, the risks in both groups appear equivalent.
- DAPT can occasionally be rationalised to a single agent for the perioperative period, though this is more for elective surgery and needs to be done in conjunction with the relevant speciality [61].
- If stopped, DAPT or monotherapy should be restarted as soon as possible after surgery when the bleeding risk is acceptable (this will largely vary on speciality and kind of surgery or injury), and local guidelines should be developed.
- If immediate anti-platelet agent reversal is required, two packs of platelets (8 pooled units) will be sufficient to return to adequate function. However, for patients with intracranial bleeds, there may not be a benefit for platelet transfusion [62], and platelets may increase mortality [63].

The management of patients on anticoagulants is discussed elsewhere in this textbook. However, in the elderly, consideration should be given to the reasons for anticoagulation, the absolute bleeding risk, risks of reversing anticoagulation and the need for some form of bridging therapy to cover the perioperative period.

Delirium

Delirium is defined as an acute disorder of mental functioning over hours or days. This is rarely a linear trajectory as the course of illness can fluctuate over this period, not uncommonly with patients becoming more agitated or confused at night. Delirium can be triggered by either a primary illness or the drugs used to treat it, and can be distressing for patients, carers and staff. In addition to this, delirium has been linked with increases in morbidity, mortality, increased length of stay, increased risk of falls and increased likelihood of discharge to a care home rather than the patient's home. Risk factors for delirium include patients with pre-existing cognitive impairment, severe illness, age over 65, and those presenting with hip fractures or other acute trauma.

The diagnosis of delirium is often subjective in the early stages, with family or carers describing the patient as "not acting like their usual self." Several risk factors have been noted in delirious patients—sleep disturbance or insomnia, reduced mobility and under- or untreated pain. Symptoms may include agitation, withdrawal, lack of cooperation or changes in mood or the presence of audiovisual hallucinations. The presence of reversible organic pathologies such as hypoxia, hypoglycaemia, hypotension or any drug intoxication or withdrawal should be sought in the first instance. If no immediate life-threatening causes are found, a review of systems should be undertaken to look for other treatable causes.

Respiratory

Hypoxia should be treated and saturations of 94–98% targeted in most people. For those with chronic hypoxia, saturations of 88–92% may be more appropriate.

CNS

Patients admitted with traumatic injuries should have been adequately imaged before coming to the ward. Occasionally this is not the case, or injuries may evolve over a longer period. In elderly patients with a history of head trauma, a low threshold for CT examination should be held in the context of new confusion or behavioural changes. Subdural haematomas may present as acute confusion or unusual neurological symptoms and have implications for acute and subacute management, i.e. anticoagulation management and discussion with neurosurgical colleagues regarding conservative management or optimisation for surgery.

Anaesthetics/Analgesia

Non-anaesthetists often blame the effects of anaesthesia for postoperative problems. Some anaesthetic medications are rightly identified as deleriogenic (for example, midazolam, cyclizine, ketamine and atropine). However, awareness of the deleterious effects of these drugs amongst anaesthetists has improved, and their use decreased in the elderly population. A review of the anaesthetic chart to see if these medications have been given may confirm or refute this assumption. In addition, using depth of anaesthesia monitoring or age-adjusted targets when using volatile anaesthesia will further decrease this risk, as will increased use of regional anaesthesia and procedural sedation with an agent such as propofol rather than a formal general anaesthetic [64]. Postoperative analgesia with paracetamol is helpful in treating delirium [65, 66] and is additionally supported by evidence from community settings and cardiac surgery [67]. Pain itself causes delirium, so it must be controlled. Weak opioids are contentious in older people as they can both cause delirium and treat pain contributing to it. Vigilance is vital when starting older people on opioids. However, the risk of pain causing delirium is probably higher. In terms of more potent opioids, oxycodone is preferable to morphine. Compared to morphine, oxycodone is associated with less delirium and does not have active metabolites that accumulate in renal failure. Regional anaesthesia techniques (e.g. single-shot blocks) are excellent adjuncts to analgesia and are opioid-sparing. However, unless fed by a continuous infusion via a catheter, they will only last for approximately 12 hours, so they must not be seen as a panacea but as part of a multi-modal approach to analgesia.

Medication Pre-admission medication, plus medication that is omitted once admitted to hospital, can contribute to delirium. If any of the following have been started (or abruptly ceased), they could be causative [68]:

- Antihistamines (e.g. cyclizine)
- Antimuscarinics (e.g. oxybutynin, atropine, hyoscine) can cause confusion, delirium, urinary retention.
- Benzodiazepines (e.g. midazolam)
- Gabapentin
- H2 receptor antagonists (e.g. ranitidine)
- Opioids (particularly codeine, dihydrocodeine, morphine, tramadol) can cause delirium but do remain a vital class of drug for treating pain.
- Theophylline

Long-standing medications may also contribute to the development of delirium. Attention should be paid to the total anticholinergic burden of all the patient's medication. Withdrawal from non-prescription medications or other substances (i.e. drug/alcohol withdrawal) must be considered and treated.

Sedation If pharmacological restraint is necessary, then it should be used at the lowest possible dose for the shortest time possible. NICE recommends haloperidol in the first instance and lorazepam if there is a contraindication to haloperidol (e.g. Parkinson's disease, cardiovascular disease such as recent MI, arrhythmias, prolonged QTc, second- or third-degree block, hypokalaemia) [69]. Olanzapine might have a role, but expert help should be sought before using this medication. The expected treatment length is 24–48 h and should be reviewed daily.

Infection/Host Defence

Infections (specifically urinary tract infections) are overdiagnosed and overtreated in hospitals [70]. Urinary dipstick testing and cultures are unreliable due to the high rate of asymptomatic bacteriuria. UTI can be a difficult diagnosis to make in elderly patients admitted with trauma, as other systemic markers of infection/inflammation (CRP and white cell count, for example) may be raised due to trauma [71–73]. If there is specific diagnostic information available that is highly suggestive of infection (e.g. visible pneumonia on a chest x-ray with compatible findings on examination or purulent/discharging wounds), then these should be treated. Empirical "trial by antibiotics" is not an appropriate treatment strategy in these patients as it puts them at risk of developing side effects, selective resistance of organisms and other complications from antibiotics that may not be indicated.

Fluid Balance and the Renal System

Patients should have an assessment of their volume status, with a caution that an acute stress response such as trauma will promote retention of water and decreased urine output. Just because a patient has a low urine output does not mean they are underfilled! If patients do not have water within reach (if immobile), they will not be able to drink. Similarly, delirious or over-medicated patients may forget to drink, so dehydration could be either a cause or effect of delirium. Any consequent acute kidney injury may further worsen delirium, so it should be actively treated.

Trauma patients may have been dehydrated before admission if they have been immobile/lying on the floor before being found, or may have been kept nil by mouth for a prolonged period without IV fluids (especially if the operating list order is repeatedly changed or patients are cancelled). Once pre- or post-op blood loss is factored in, there are many reasons that patients can become dehydrated. If patients are to be given IV hydration, a balanced crystalloid such as Hartmann's solution, Ringer's lactate or Plasmalyte should be given as the default, unless specific electrolytes are being actively replaced. Excessive chloride load is dangerous; hyperchloremia is independently associated with an overall twofold increase in morbidity, mortality and hospital stay [74]. Therefore, "normal" saline should be avoided unless treating hyponatraemia.

Urinary retention may also cause delirium and can be caused by pain, constipation or trauma. Urinary catheterisation is useful in trauma patients to help monitor fluid balance accurately. In patients who cannot mobilise to the toilet or use other continence aids, they also provide some dignity. In uncatheterised patients, bladder scans should be used to provide objective data to assess retention. Patients with retention may still pass small volumes of urine but have large post-void residual volumes best treated with catheterisation. Catheters should be used for the shortest period possible, and a plan for their removal thought through before insertion.

Gastrointestinal

Constipation is a common side effect of opiate medication and cause of delirium. Patients who have decreased oral intake of food and water are at risk, and enquiries into bowel habit should be part of the ward round with laxatives given if there has been no bowel movements for 24–48 hours. Delirious patients may also eat less, so high-calorie meals and supplementary build-up drinks should be offered where possible with dietetic input. A nutritional scoring tool such as MUST should be used [75].

Several tools are available to aid in the diagnosis of delirium, with the 4AT [76] probably being one of the best. It performs well for sensitivity and patient completion rate, does not require specific training and can be easily used in the Emergency Department [38, 77]. For these reasons, it is the test advocated by the National Hip Fracture Database in the UK. Once delirium has been diagnosed, the diagnosis should be communicated to the rest of the medical and nursing team in addition to carers and relatives. Familiar faces such as family and friends can help calm patients and may avoid the use of medications that may have side effects. National guidelines exist to help in the management of delirium, with the aims of decreasing the rates of falls, dehydration, pressure sores, malnourishment and isolation [69].

Rehabilitation and Re-Enablement

Elderly patients who suffer a traumatic injury may be at risk of not regaining their previous state of independence. It may be that depending on their injury and any complications that they are not safe to be discharged back to their own home, even with a medical and social care package in place.

Re-enablement refers to the process of patients getting back to their activities of daily living (such as washing and dressing) with the assistance and assessment of specialist rehabilitation clinicians, physiotherapists and occupational therapists. These assessments are usually between 2–5 days following surgery depending on their clinical course. For this reason, attention to detail in minimising some of the avoidable complications described above is paramount in the early postoperative period. The longer patients take to start making progress, the more challenging and less successful it may ultimately be [51].

Rehabilitation refers to the resumption of everyday living as a whole, and returning to their place of residence after discharge from the hospital. There may be some non-clinical organisational factors that delay discharge, but clinical reasons for delay in getting home may include postoperative complications such as undertreated delirium or pneumonia. This focus on restoring function and capability must be central, even from the beginning of the patient's hospital admission. Evidence-based interventions that have been shown to improve re-enablement and rehabilitation include [78]:

- Prompt surgery
- Mobilisation the day of or day after surgery
- Physiotherapy assessment the day after surgery
- Geriatrician review within 72 h of admission
- Nutritional risk assessment
- Falls assessment
- Bone health assessment

Conclusion

Elderly patients may be more complicated to manage than their younger counterparts due to their limited reserve, generally poorer background health and specific challenges posed by physiological changes in ageing and difficulties in diagnosis. They may also have the most to gain from early investigation and intervention, even when the mechanism of injury appears relatively innocuous. Of note, "normal" vital signs may not be normal for these group of patients, so a systolic blood pressure of <110 mmHg or a heart rate of >90 bpm should be concerning. There are specific courses available for those managing elderly trauma patients on a regular basis (such as the HECTOR course [13]). However, the fundamental focus should be on re-enablement from an early stage for all clinicians working with this patient group.

Questions

1. Most elderly trauma patients present following a fall from less than 2 meters.
   (a) True
   (b) False
2. Elderly patients will benefit from a restrictive transfusion strategy and should not be given blood until their haemoglobin level drops to 70 mg/dl.
   (a) True
   (b) False

3. Cyclizine is not recommended as an anti-emetic in the elderly population
   (a) True
   (b) False
4. If an elderly patient or their carer discloses that they are being abused, they cannot be discharged home.
   (a) True
   (b) False
5. Patients taking anti-platelet agents cannot have spinal anaesthesia
   (a) True
   (b) False

Answers
1. a
2. b
3. a
4. b
5. b

References

1. World Health Organisation. Men ageing and health - achieving health across the life span. WHO; 2001.
2. Forman DE, Berman AD, McCabe CH, Baim DS, Wei JY. PTCA in the elderly: the "young-old" versus the "old-old". J Am Geriatr Soc. 1992 Jan;40(1):19–22.
3. Lee SB, Oh JH, Park JH, Choi SP, Wee JH. Differences in youngest-old, middle-old, and oldest-old patients who visit the emergency department. Clin Exp Emerg Med. 2018 Dec 31;5(4):249–55.
4. Centers for Disease Control and Prevention. Leading Causes of Death and Injury [Internet]. CDC Injury Prevention and Control. 2021 [cited 2021 May 11]. Available from: https://www.cdc.gov/injury/wisqars/LeadingCauses.html
5. TARN - Major Trauma in Older People [Internet]. The Trauma Audit and Research Network; 2017 [cited 2019 Dec 30] p. 40. Available from: https://www.tarn.ac.uk/content/downloads/3793/Major%20Trauma%20in%20Older%20People%202017.pdf
6. Newgard CD, Caughey A, McConnell KJ, Lin A, Eckstrom E, Griffiths D, et al. Comparison of injured older adults included in vs excluded from trauma registries with 1-year follow-up. JAMA Surg. 2019 Sep 18;154(9):e192279.
7. Ho VP, Reider L, Haut ER. The true outcomes of geriatric trauma—if we do not count them, we will never know. JAMA Surg. 2019 Sep 18;154(9):e192324.
8. Victorino GP, Chong TJ, Pal JD. Trauma in the elderly patient. Arch Surg. 2003;138:6.
9. Griffiths E, Torrance A, Powell S. Emergency surgery in the elderly: challenges and solutions. Open Access Emerg Med. 2015 Sep;7:55.
10. Oshima K, Murata M, Aoki M, Nakajima J, Sawada Y, Isshiki Y, et al. Efficacy of the treatment of elderly trauma patients requiring intensive care. Emerg Med Int. 2018 Dec 30;2018:1–6.
11. Hashmi A, Ibrahim-Zada I, Rhee P, Aziz H, Fain MJ, Friese RS, et al. Predictors of mortality in geriatric trauma patients: a systematic review and meta-analysis. J Trauma Acute Care Surg. 2014 Mar;76(3):894–901.
12. Frankenfield D, Cooney RN, Smith JS, Rowe WA. Age-related differences in the metabolic response to injury. J Trauma Inj Infect Crit Care. 2000 Jan;48(1):49.
13. Raven D. The Heartlands' elderly Care trauma & ongoing recovery programme (HECTOR) course manual. 1st ed. Birmingham, UK; 2014. 197 p.
14. Schwab CW. Trauma in the geriatric patient. Arch Surg. 1992 June 1;127(6):701.
15. Milton JC, Hill-Smith I, Jackson SHD. Prescribing for older people. BMJ. 2008 Mar 15;336(7644):606–9.
16. Qato DM, Wilder J, Schumm LP, Gillet V, Alexander GC. Changes in prescription and over-the-counter medication and dietary supplement use among older adults in the United States, 2005 vs 2011. JAMA Intern Med. 2016 Apr;176(4):473–82.
17. Saraf AA, Petersen AW, Simmons SF, Schnelle JF, Bell SP, Kripalani S, et al. Medications associated with geriatric syndromes and their prevalence in older hospitalized adults discharged to skilled nursing facilities. J Hosp Med. 2016 Oct;11(10):694–700.
18. Sampson EL, West E, Fischer T. Pain and delirium: mechanisms, assessment, and management. Eur Geriatr Med. 2020 Feb 1;11(1):45–52.
19. Feast AR, White N, Lord K, Kupeli N, Vickerstaff V, Sampson EL. Pain and delirium in people with dementia in the acute general hospital setting. Age Ageing. 2018 Nov;47(6):841–6.
20. Clegg A, Young JB. Which medications to avoid in people at risk of delirium: a systematic review. Age Ageing. 2011 Jan;40(1):23–9.
21. Rosen T, Connors S, Clark S, Halpern A, Stern ME, DeWald J, et al. Assessment and management of delirium in older adults in the emergency department: literature review to inform development of a novel clinical protocol. Adv Emerg Nurs J. 2015;37(3):183–E3.
22. Mangoni AA, Jackson SHD. Age-related changes in pharmacokinetics and pharmacodynamics: basic principles and practical applications: age-related changes in pharmacokinetics and pharmacodynamics. Br J Clin Pharmacol. 2003 Nov 14;57(1):6–14.
23. Mallet L, Spinewine A, Huang A. The challenge of managing drug interactions in elderly people. Lancet Lond Engl. 2007 July 14;370(9582):185–91.
24. 2019 American Geriatrics Society Beers Criteria® Update Expert Panel. American Geriatrics Society 2019 updated AGS Beers criteria® for potentially

inappropriate medication use in older adults. J Am Geriatr Soc. 2019 Apr;67(4):674–94.
25. O'Mahony D, O'Sullivan D, Byrne S, O'Connor MN, Ryan C, Gallagher P. STOPP/START criteria for potentially inappropriate prescribing in older people: version 2. Age Ageing. 2015 Mar 1;44(2):213–8.
26. Hudhra K, García-Caballos M, Casado-Fernandez E, Jucja B, Shabani D, Bueno-Cavanillas A. Polypharmacy and potentially inappropriate prescriptions identified by Beers and STOPP criteria in co-morbid older patients at hospital discharge. J Eval Clin Pract. 2016 Apr;22(2):189–93.
27. Lester E, Dykstra M, Grant C, Fawcett V, Tsang B, Widder S. High-risk medications in older patients with trauma: a cross-sectional study of risk mitigation. Can J Surg. 2019 Apr;62(2):100–4.
28. Schuijt HJ, Kusen J, van Hernen JJ, van der Vet P, Geraghty O, Smeeing DPJ, et al. Orthogeriatric trauma unit improves patient outcomes in geriatric hip fracture patients. Geriatr Orthop Surg Rehabil. 2020 Jan 1;11:2151459320949476.
29. Gosch M, Hoffmann-Weltin Y, Roth T, Blauth M, Nicholas JA, Kammerlander C. Orthogeriatric co-management improves the outcome of long-term care residents with fragility fractures. Arch Orthop Trauma Surg. 2016 Oct;136(10):1403–9.
30. Scalea TM, Simon HM, Duncan AO, Atweh NA, Sclafani SJ, Phillips TF, et al. Geriatric blunt multiple trauma: improved survival with early invasive monitoring. J Trauma. 1990 Feb;30(2):129–34.
31. Trauma Resuscitation of the Elderly Patient [Internet]. Consultant 360. [cited 2021 May 11]. Available from: https://www.consultant360.com/articles/trauma-resuscitation-elderly-patient
32. Kuster M, Exadaktylos A, Schnüriger B. Non-invasive hemodynamic monitoring in trauma patients. World J Emerg Surg WJES [Internet]. 2015 Mar 8 [cited 2021 May 11];10. Available from: https://www.ncbi.nlm.nih.gov/pmc/articles/PMC4359395/
33. Ziegler D, Blackburn K, Eisenstein C, McReynold D, Garcia F, Webber C, et al. Need for cardiac output monitoring in elderly trauma patients determined by base deficit. Crit Care. 2001 Mar 2;5(1):137.
34. Richmond TS, Kauder D, Strumpf N, Meredith T. Characteristics and outcomes of serious traumatic injury in older adults. J Am Geriatr Soc. 2002 Feb;50(2):215–22.
35. Hu R, Mustard CA, Burns C. Epidemiology of incident spinal fracture in a complete population. Spine. 1996 Feb 15;21(4):492–9.
36. Sadro CT, Sandstrom CK, Verma N, Gunn ML. Geriatric trauma: a radiologist's guide to imaging trauma patients aged 65 years and older. Radiographics. 2015 June 12;35(4):1263–85.
37. Callaway DW, Shapiro NI, Donnino MW, Baker C, Rosen CL. Serum lactate and base deficit as predictors of mortality in normotensive elderly blunt trauma patients. J Trauma. 2009 Apr;66(4):1040–4.
38. Shenkin SD, Fox C, Godfrey M, Siddiqi N, Goodacre S, Young J, et al. Delirium detection in older acute medical inpatients: a multicentre prospective comparative diagnostic test accuracy study of the 4AT and the confusion assessment method. BMC Med. 2019 Dec;17(1):138.
39. MRC CRASH Trial Collaborators. Predicting outcome after traumatic brain injury: practical prognostic models based on large cohort of international patients. BMJ. 2008 Feb 23;336(7641):425–9.
40. World Health Organization. Regional Office for Europe. European report on preventing elder maltreatment. World Health Organization, Regional Office for Europe: Copenhagen; 2011.
41. Pereira C, Fertleman M. Elder abuse: a common problem, commonly missed in trauma and orthopaedics. Eur Geriatr Med. 2019 Dec;10(6):839–41.
42. Lachs MS, Pillemer K. Abuse and neglect of elderly persons. N Engl J Med. 1995;332(7):7.
43. Cooper C, Selwood A, Livingston G. The prevalence of elder abuse and neglect: a systematic review. Age Ageing. 2008 Mar 1;37(2):151–60.
44. Rosen T, Bloemen EM, LoFaso VM, Clark S, Flomenbaum NE, Lachs MS. Emergency department presentations for injuries in older adults independently known to be victims of elder abuse. J Emerg Med. 2016 Mar 1;50(3):518–26.
45. NHS England, NHS Improvement. NHS Safeguarding Policy [Internet]. NHS; 2014 [cited 2021 May 11]. Available from: https://www.england.nhs.uk/publication/safeguarding-policy/
46. WHO Scientific Group on Nutritional Anaemias & World Health Organization. Nutritional anaemias: report of a WHO scientific group [meeting held in Geneva from 13 to 17 March 1967] [Internet]. World Health Organization; 1968 [cited 2021 May 12]. Available from: https://apps.who.int/iris/handle/10665/40707
47. Muñoz M, Acheson AG, Auerbach M, Besser M, Habler O, Kehlet H, et al. International consensus statement on the peri-operative management of anaemia and iron deficiency. Anaesthesia. 2017 Feb;72(2):233–47.
48. Randi ML, Bertozzi I, Santarossa C, Cosi E, Lucente F, Bogoni G, et al. Prevalence and Causes of Anemia in Hospitalized Patients: Impact on Diseases Outcome. J Clin Med [Internet]. 2020 Mar 30 [cited 2021 May 12];9(4). Available from: https://www.ncbi.nlm.nih.gov/pmc/articles/PMC7230611/
49. Spahn DR. Anemia and patient blood management in hip and knee surgery: a systematic review of the literature. Anesthesiology. 2010 Aug 1;113(2):482–95.
50. Hébert PC, Wells G, Blajchman MA, Marshall J, Martin C, Pagliarello G, et al. A multicenter, randomized, controlled clinical Trial of transfusion requirements in critical care. N Engl J Med. 1999 Feb 11;340(6):409–17.
51. Griffiths R, Babu S, Dixon P, Freeman N, Hurford D, Kelleher E, et al. Guideline for the management of hip fractures 2020: guideline by the Association of Anaesthetists. Anaesthesia. 2021 Feb;76(2):225–37.
52. Hovaguimian F, Myles PS. Restrictive versus liberal transfusion strategy in the perioperative and acute care settings: a context-specific systematic review and meta-analysis of randomized controlled trials. Anesthesiology. 2016 Jul;125(1):46–61.

53. Simon GI, Craswell A, Thom O, Fung YL. Questioning the benefit of restrictive transfusion practice in older adults. ISBT Sci Ser. 2019 Feb;14(1):58–66.
54. Pelavski AD, de Miguel M, Villarino L, Alcaraz G, Buendía P, Rochera MI, et al. Audit of transfusion among the oldest old: treading the fine line between undertransfusion and optimum trigger. Transfusion (Paris). 2019;59(9):2812–9.
55. Carson JL, Terrin ML, Noveck H, Sanders DW, Chaitman BR, Rhoads GG, et al. Liberal or restrictive transfusion in high-risk patients after hip surgery. N Engl J Med. 2011 Dec 29;365(26):2453–62.
56. Docherty AB, O'Donnell R, Brunskill S, Trivella M, Doree C, Holst LB, et al. Effect of restrictive versus liberal transfusion strategies on outcomes in patients with cardiovascular disease in a non-cardiac surgery setting: systematic review and meta-analysis. BMJ. 2016 Mar;29:i1351.
57. Lawrence VA, Silverstein JH, Cornell JE, Pederson T, Noveck H, Carson JL. Higher Hb level is associated with better early functional recovery after hip fracture repair. Transfusion (Paris). 2003 Dec;43(12):1717–22.
58. Cook TM, Counsell D, Wildsmith JAW. Major complications of central neuraxial block: report on the third National Audit Project of the Royal College of Anaesthetists. Br J Anaesth. 2009 Feb;102(2):179–90.
59. Philippe G, Rutledge DR, Tullio P, Adriano C, Elvin K, Hermiller JB, et al. Stent thrombosis and dual antiplatelet therapy interruption with Everolimus-Eluting stents. Circ Cardiovasc Interv. 2015 May 1;8(5):e001362.
60. Weaver JM. Caution: maintain anti-platelet therapy in patients with coronary artery stents. Anesth Prog. 2007;54(4):161–2.
61. Spahn DR, Howell SJ, Delabays A, Chassot P-G. Coronary stents and perioperative anti-platelet regimen: dilemma of bleeding and stent thrombosis. Br J Anaesth. 2006 Jun;96(6):675–7.
62. Batchelor JS, Grayson A. A meta-analysis to determine the effect on survival of platelet transfusions in patients with either spontaneous or traumatic antiplatelet medication-associated intracranial haemorrhage. BMJ Open. 2012;2(2):e000588.
63. Baharoglu MI, Cordonnier C, Salman RA-S, de Gans K, Koopman MM, Brand A, et al. Platelet transfusion versus standard care after acute stroke due to spontaneous cerebral haemorrhage associated with antiplatelet therapy (PATCH): a randomised, open-label, phase 3 trial. Lancet. 2016 Jun;387(10038):2605–13.
64. Gogarten W, Vandermeulen E, Van Aken H, Kozek S, Llau JV, Samama CM. Regional anaesthesia and antithrombotic agents: recommendations of the European Society of Anaesthesiology. Eur J Anaesthesiol. 2010 Dec;27(12):999–1015.
65. Mian P, Allegaert K, Spriet I, Tibboel D, Petrovic M. Paracetamol in older people: towards evidence-based dosing? Drugs Aging. 2018 Jul;35(7):603–24.
66. Dixon J, Ashton F, Baker P, Charlton K, Bates C, Eardley W. Assessment and early management of pain in hip fractures: the impact of paracetamol. Geriatr Orthop Surg Rehabil. 2018 Jan;9:215145931880644.
67. Subramaniam B, Shankar P, Shaefi S, Mueller A, O'Gara B, Banner-Goodspeed V, et al. Effect of intravenous acetaminophen vs placebo combined with propofol or dexmedetomidine on postoperative delirium among older patients following cardiac surgery: the DEXACET randomized clinical trial. JAMA. 2019 Feb 19;321(7):686.
68. British Geriatrics Society. 14. CGA in Primary Care Settings: Patients presenting with confusion and delirium | British Geriatrics Society [Internet]. British Geriatrics Society; 2019 [cited 2019 Dec 30]. Available from: https://www.bgs.org.uk/resources/14-cga-in-primary-care-settings-patients-presenting-with-confusion-and-delirium
69. Young J, Murthy L, Westby M, Akunne A, O'Mahony R, on behalf of the Guideline Development Group. Diagnosis, prevention, and management of delirium: summary of NICE guidance. BMJ. 2010 July 28;341(2):c3704.
70. Rousham E, Cooper M, Petherick E, Saukko P, Oppenheim B. Overprescribing antibiotics for asymptomatic bacteriuria in older adults: a case series review of admissions in two UK hospitals. Antimicrob Resist Infect Control. 2019 May 2;8(1):71.
71. Ferroni M, Taylor AK. Asymptomatic bacteriuria in noncatheterized adults. Urol Clin North Am. 2015 Nov;42(4):537–45.
72. Woodford HJ, George J. Diagnosis and management of urinary tract infection in hospitalized older people. J Am Geriatr Soc. 2009;57(1):107–14.
73. Quality statement 1: Diagnosing urinary tract infections in adults aged 65 years and over | Urinary tract infections in adults | Quality standards | NICE [Internet]. NICE; [cited 2021 May 12]. Available from: https://www.nice.org.uk/guidance/qs90/chapter/quality-statement-1-Diagnosing-urinary-tract-infections-in-adults-aged-65-years-and-over
74. McCluskey SA, Karkouti K, Wijeysundera D, Minkovich L, Tait G, Beattie WS. Hyperchloremia after noncardiac surgery is independently associated with increased morbidity and mortality: a propensity-matched cohort study. Anesth Analg. 2013 Aug;117(2):412–21.
75. Frank M, Sivagnanaratnam A, Bernstein J. Nutritional assessment in elderly care: a MUST! BMJ Open Qual. 2015 Jan 1;4(1):u204810.w2031.
76. Bellelli G, Morandi A, Davis DHJ, Mazzola P, Turco R, Gentile S, et al. Validation of the 4AT, a new instrument for rapid delirium screening: a study in 234 hospitalised older people. Age Ageing. 2014 July 1;43(4):496–502.
77. Macharouthu A, MacLullich A. SIGN Guideline 157: Risk Reduction and Management of delerium [Internet]. Scottish Intercollegiate Guidelines Network; 2019 [cited 2019 Dec 30]. Available from: https://www.sign.ac.uk/assets/sign157.pdf
78. Royal College of Physicians. National hip fracture database annual report 2018. London: RCP; 2018. p. 32.

38 Ballistics and Blast Injury

Jowan Penn-Barwell

Introduction

The fundamental nature of ballistic and blast injuries is no different from other mechanisms of traumatic injury: the transfer of kinetic energy resulting in tissue damage. However, the *character* of blast and ballistics is often distinct from other traumatic injury mechanisms. Blast injuries are less frequently seen outside of military conflict; the kinetic energies involved (and therefore the potential for tissue damage) is often massive, and the resultant wounds are often heavily contaminated and have the potential to evolve over several days.

This chapter will provide an overview of the pathophysiology of blast and ballistic injury mechanisms, enabling clinicians to assess wounds and anticipate likely complications. While every wound—and every patient—is unique, the general principles and clinical priorities for managing these injuries will be discussed.

Wound Ballistics

The study of ballistic science that examines the interaction between a bullet and tissues is termed *Wound Ballistics*. Reduced to its fundamental form for clinical context, wound ballistics concerns the work done by the transfer of kinetic energy (KE) from the projectile leading to crushing, lacerating, stretching and shearing of body tissues. The KE transferred into tissues is simply the difference between the KE of the projectile as it strikes the body and that which remains should it exit the tissues. If the round does not exit the tissues, all of its KE will be transferred into the body.

The severity of a Gun Shot Wound (GSW) is not just dependent on the total amount of KE that is transferred into the tissues. The *rate* at which

J. Penn-Barwell (✉)
Royal Navy, Portsmouth, UK

Department of Orthopaedic Surgery, John Radcliffe Hospital, Oxford, UK
e-mail: Jowan.penn-barwell@ouh.nhs.uk

P. Lax (ed.), *Textbook of Acute Trauma Care*, https://doi.org/10.1007/978-3-030-83628-3_38

energy is transferred to the tissues also dictates severity: the more quickly a bullet slows, the faster its KE is transferred into the tissues, and the more damage is caused.

There are two principal mechanisms by which bullets injure tissue: the formation of a temporary cavity and the creation of a permanent cavity or tract.

Permanent Cavity

The permanent cavity is a simple concept; as the bullet crushes, cuts and shears the tissue in front of it, it creates a tract that is typically of a similar size to that of the contact area of the projectile. The permanent cavity is usually a continuation of the trajectory of the projectile. However, it must be remembered that this trajectory can be deflected by tissue planes, bone strike or otherwise from the instability of the round itself as it traverses the tissues.

If the bullet fragments, each fragment will create its own permanent cavity before leaving the body or coming to rest. Similarly, if the bullet strikes and fractures bone, these bone fragments can be accelerated through tissue, creating their own permanent cavity.

Temporary Cavity

The temporary cavity is formed by the stretching of tissue radially away from the path of the bullet and occurs in its wake as it passes through tissue [1]. When a projectile strikes tissue it starts to decelerate rapidly. This deceleration involves the rapid transfer of KE from the round into the surrounding tissues, causing those tissues to radially accelerate away from the path of the bullet. As the tissues accelerate away from the passage of the round, a temporary space or cavity at sub-atmospheric pressure is formed, creating a vacuum which potentially draws air and surface contaminants into the cavity via the entrance (or exit) wound. As the tissues are stretched those tissues which stretch beyond their capacity to absorb such deformation will tear or fracture.

Assessing the Severity of Ballistic Wounds

The purpose of wound assessment is to determine:

- ***The functional effect*** of the wound on physiology, i.e. the potential for bleeding, intestinal contamination and organ damage.
- ***The quantity of tissue destruction,*** i.e. the amount of non-viable tissue and contamination with the potential for infection.

An assessment of the amount of energy transferred to a limb by a GSW is essential. High-energy wounds are associated with a greater risk of infection and therefore warrant a more aggressive surgical approach. Conversely, avoiding excessive debridement and 'laying-open' of low-energy wounds avoids unnecessary morbidity. The amount of energy transferred to a limb can be estimated with a combination of clinical assessment and plain x-rays. The factors associated with higher energy transfer are [2]:

- A **large exit wound** implying a large temporary cavity and tissue damage.
- **Bone strike:** this will be associated with sudden slowing of the bullet and large energy transfer, as shown in Fig. 38.1.
- **Bullet fragmentation** indicates a rapid transfer of nearly all the KE of the bullet and the potential for complex wounds, as shown in Fig. 38.2.

An example of an injury associated with high-energy transfer is shown in Figs. 38.1 and 38.2

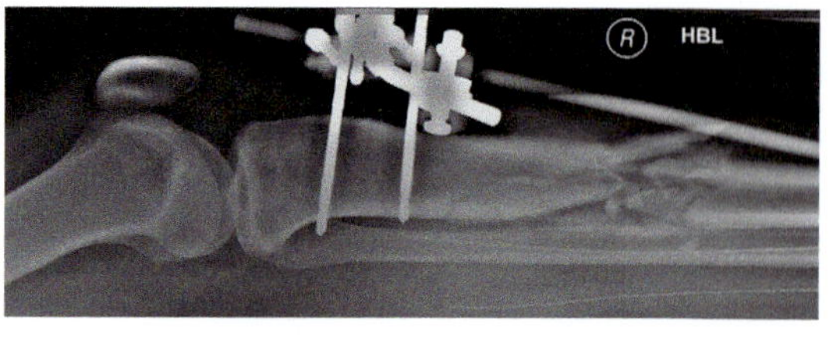

Fig. 38.1 A lateral X-ray of a knee and proximal tibia with external fixator stabilising a multi-fragmentary diaphyseal fracture predictive of a high-energy transfer wound. Crown Copyright 2021

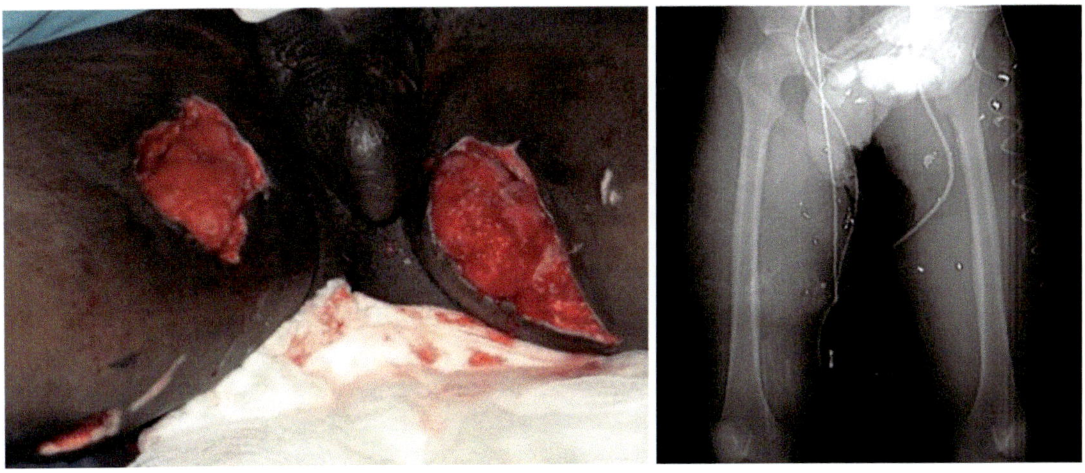

Fig. 38.2 Clinical photograph taken 2-days post-injury and CT scout view showing a GSW to bilateral thighs. The wound was caused by a military 5.56 mm SS109 round which fragmented despite not hitting bone. Fragments passed from the right thigh into the left with high energy transfer and tissue destruction

below. The surgical management of these wounds is discussed in more detail later.

In addition to clinical examination and plain X-ray to assess wound severity, injuries to the head and torso will need CT imaging which can readily identify the likely physiological effect of a GSW.

Blast Pathophysiology

Explosions are complicated processes that occur exceptionally rapidly with the release of energy and the generation of large volumes of gaseous products. Their precise nature depends on the type of explosive. Industrially manufactured military or mining grade explosives will behave differently to 'home-made' munitions, e.g. 'fertiliser bombs', which behave technically more like rapid combustions.

A vast range of different weapons are based on explosives to generate a destructive effect. Industrially manufactured military explosive weapons are typically called munitions and include indirect fire weapons, i.e. mortars and artillery—rockets, mines and grenades. Improvised 'home-made' or 'cottage industry' weapons include improvised explosive devices (IEDs) [3].

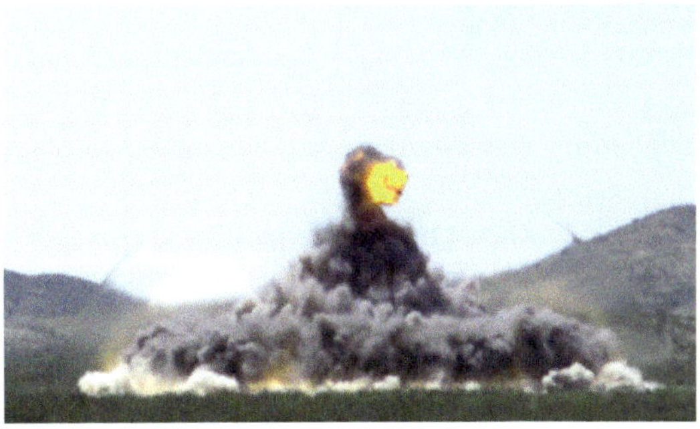

Fig. 38.3 An explosion with the shock wave visible and separating from the rest of the explosion as it travels faster

The process of an explosion can be divided into three main phases, which correspond to the different mechanisms of injuries that they can cause.

The first component is the **shock wave**. This is analogous to a sound wave in that it passes through substances rather than moves them. A shock wave, as shown in Fig. 38.3, is only produced as a result of a true explosion and is typically not a feature of 'home-made' explosives.

The shock wave travels much faster than the speed of sound and produces a virtually instantaneous rise in pressure for milliseconds. The energy of the shockwave rapidly dissipates as it propagates away from the source explosion, proportional to the radius to the power of three (r^{-3}) [4].

As the shock wave moves through the casualty's body, energy is transferred into tissues, particularly at interfaces between gases and tissues. This is analogous to the 'absorption' of sound energy by the foam in ear-defenders. As the sound wave travels through the foam, it encounters multiple air-plastic interfaces of the foam cells, and the energy of the wave is dissipated.

The organs particularly affected unsurprisingly are those with gas-tissue interfaces, i.e. the lungs, ears and bowel. This is known as the **Primary Blast Injury** [5]. The pressure generated by the shockwave typically must be >35 KPa to produce ear injuries and >250 KPa to produce lung or bowel injuries [6].

Primary blast injury to the lung can result in disruption at the alveolar-capillary interface, resulting in lung parenchymal haemorrhage, pneumothorax and alveolar-venous fistulae as shown in Fig. 38.4 [7]. The incidence of blast lung in terrorist bombings varies enormously depending on proximity and enclosure but has been reported as high as 14% of casualties [8, 9]. Enclosed spaces prevent dissipation of the shock wave, which can 'echo' off walls and buildings leading to multiple episodes of energy transfer from a single blast.

Blast intestinal injury is rare in land-based explosions but very common in submerged victims because water is a superior medium for the transmission of the shockwave compared to air [10]. The blast wave causes intermural haemorrhage and even perforation, which may occur several days after injury [11].

Ear injuries typically range from tympanic membrane rupture to ossicle dislocation and can be seen in up to half of blast casualties [8]. It has been noted that the presence of ear injuries varies significantly depending on the position of the head relative to the blast and even though the threshold pressure for ear damage is theoretically an order of magnitude less than that for lung injury, the absence of ear injuries is a poor surrogate for the absence of visceral injury [12].

The gas created by the explosion expands outward at high velocity known as the **blast wind**. It is this blast wind that carries objects, e.g. fragments and shrapnel. The effect of the blast wind has a much greater range than the shock wave.

The majority of injuries are due to secondary blast effects, i.e. the effect of pre-formed projectiles (as shown in Fig. 38.5), fragmentation, debris (as shown in Fig. 38.6) and even tissue from other victims being accelerated by the blast wind into the victim's tissue. These projectiles are accelerated radially away from the blast epicentre and follow an arced trajectory due to the effect of gravity. Injuries caused in this manner are classed as **Secondary Blast Injuries.**

Fragments and debris behave exactly as projectiles discussed earlier, with the caveat that they are often irregularly shaped and are subject to

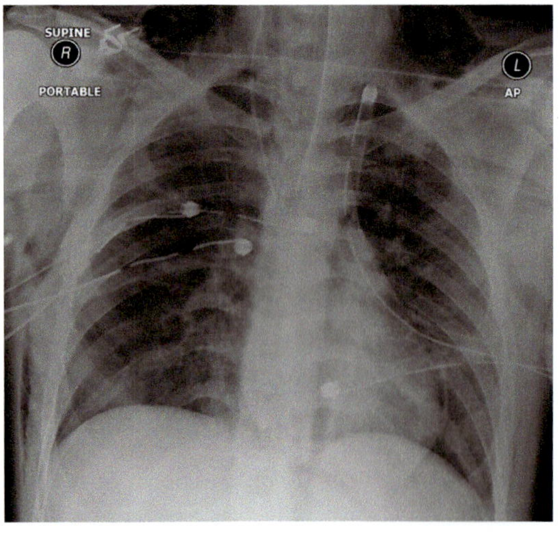

Fig. 38.4 X-ray image of a chest showing parenchymal haemorrhage and pleural drains for treatment of the pneumothorax

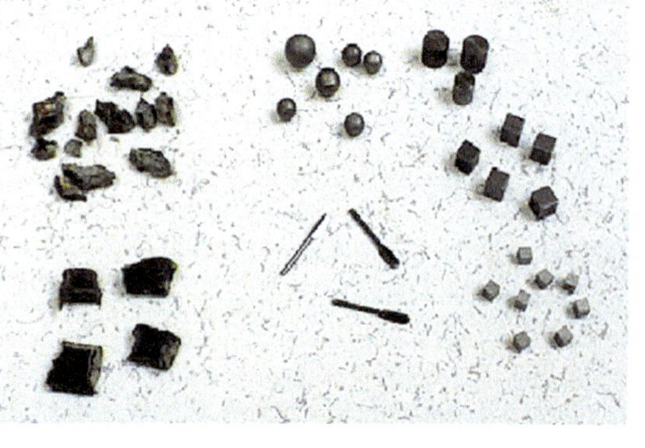

Fig. 38.5 Pre-formed fragmentations from industrially manufactured munitions, typically multiple small similarly-sized projectiles

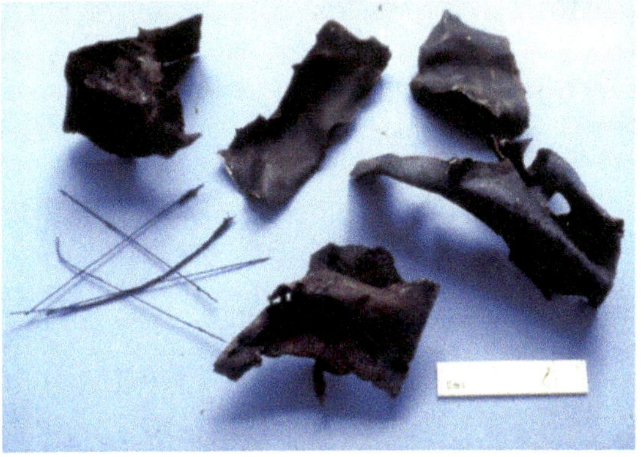

Fig. 38.6 Examples of debris and fragments from IED explosions-typically irregular, larger fragments from casing or object used to disguise the IED

greater drag and therefore do not travel as far. Victims are often struck by multiple projectiles along with the tissue stripping effect of large numbers of small pieces of debris. Each fragment and piece of debris will create its own permanent cavity as it penetrates the victim and travels through them.

Clinical Priorities

The clinical priorities in assessing patients injured through blast and ballistic mechanisms do not differ to those outlined elsewhere in this book. The priorities are:

- **Haemorrhage Control**. This may well require damage control resuscitative surgery.
- **Infection Prevention**. The surgical exploration of wounds with incision and excision of necrotic tissue and contamination.
- **Stabilisation**. The temporary stabilisation of fractures e.g. with plaster casts, traction or external fixation, allows the resuscitation of tissue in the wound and reduces the risk of infection. It also provides pain relief.
- **Fixation**. The definitive fixation of fractures, especially around joints, permits rehabilitation and restoration of function, but can only occur when the wound is healthy and free from contamination.
- **Coverage and Closure**. Definitive fixation can only occur when wounds can be covered or closed. In complex injuries with significant tissue loss, this may require more complex plastic surgical techniques in the form of local or free tissue 'flaps'.

While many injuries will require surgical reconstruction, this can only occur after successful resuscitation, which itself can necessitate resuscitative surgery. Once life-threatening haemorrhage has been arrested, surgical attention can turn to preventing infection and reconstruction following the steps outlined above.

Ballistic and blast injuries are heterogeneous, and few surgeons deal with them frequently. Discussed below are some potential difficulties and mistakes that can occur.

As previously stated, ballistic injuries evolve. A common mistake is for the surgeon to perform primary closure after wound excision. Even if the wound bed looks clean and healthy after initial excision, further tissue necrosis and swelling will occur, with deep infection the likely result. This is a lesson that has been learnt and re-learnt over the course of several generations of military surgeons [13].

Judging how aggressively to excise tissue is challenging, and not all ballistic wounds need surgical treatment. Ballistic injuries that can be managed without surgery are those with only minimal haemorrhage and without features of high-energy transfer. For example, a 'through-and-through wound' with no significant visible soft tissue damage, no bone strike and no round fragmentation suggests minimal energy transfer and therefore little tissue damage [2]. These wounds, more typically seen from handgun injuries, may be managed non-operatively. Typically this would involve non-restrictive, absorbable dressings to permit wound drainage, oral antibiotics for 48 h and consideration to splintage to prevent excessive movement of the injured limb. Wounds should be followed-up closely to watch for the development of infection [14].

Conclusion

Traumatic injuries from ballistic or explosive weapons should be approached using the same fundamental principles and techniques described in this book. However, clinicians should realise that the unique characteristics of these injury mechanisms are the potential for enormous tissue damage and the evolution of wounds. A lack of familiarity with these injuries may result in failure to appreciate their true severity, which may take several days to manifest.

Questions

1. The severity of the gunshot wound most closely relates to:
   (a) The calibre of the firearm
   (b) The speed of the bullet
   (c) The rate of energy transfer into the tissues
   (d) The distance between the firearm and the casualty
   (e) The length of the barrel of the firearm
2. Which of the following is false about blast injuries:
   (a) Wounds can evolve over hours and days
   (b) Intact tympanic membranes precludes a blast lung injury
   (c) Gas containing organs are vulnerable to primary blast injury
   (d) Secondary blast injury usually has a greater range than primary blast injury
   (e) A shock wave travels faster than the speed of sound
3. Which of the following is not predictive of a more severe ballistic wound?
   (a) The casualty being able to identify the weapon
   (b) Bone strike
   (c) Bullet fragmention
   (d) Retention of bullets or fragments
   (e) A large wound cavity
4. Which of the following statements are true?
   (a) Fracture fixation is a priority and must not be delayed if concurrent coverage or closure is not possible at the same surgical episode
   (b) Early primary closure of ballistic wounds to the forearm is a priority
   (c) All ballistic wounds require at least one surgical operation
   (d) Ballistic fractures should never be fixed with plates and screws
   (e) Delayed primary closure of ballistic wounds should occur around 48hrs after initial surgical treatment

Answers

1. c
2. b
3. a
4. e

References

1. Krauss M. Studies in wound ballistics: temporary cavity effects in soft tissues. Mil Med. 1957 Oct 1;121(4):221–31.
2. Penn-Barwell JG, Sargeant ID. Severe lower extremity combat trauma (SeLECT) study group. Gun-shot injuries in UK military casualties - features associated with wound severity. Injury. 2016 May;47(5):1067–71.
3. Ramasamy A, Hill AM, Clasper JC. Improvised explosive devices: pathophysiology, injury profiles and current medical management. J R Army Med Corps. 2009 Dec;155(4):265–72.
4. Taylor G. The formation of a blast wave by a very intense explosion I. Theoretical discussion. Proc R Soc Lond A. 1950 Mar 22;201(1065):159–74.
5. Guy RJ, Kirkman E, Watkins PE, Cooper GJ. Physiologic responses to primary blast: the journal of trauma: injury. Infect Crit Care. 1998 Dec;45(6):983–7.
6. Ritenour AE, Baskin TW. Primary blast injury: update on diagnosis and treatment. Crit Care Med. 2008 Jul;36(7 Suppl):S311–7.
7. Guy RJ, Glover MA, Cripps NP. The pathophysiology of primary blast injury and its implications for treatment. Part I: the thorax. J R Nav Med Serv. 1998;84(2):79–86.
8. Mellor SG, Cooper GJ. Analysis of 828 servicemen killed or injured by explosion in Northern Ireland 1970-84: the hostile action casualty system. Br J Surg. 1989 Oct;76(10):1006–10.
9. Ritenour AE, Blackbourne LH, Kelly JF, McLaughlin DF, Pearse LA, Holcomb JB, et al. Incidence of primary blast injury in US military overseas contingency operations: a retrospective study. Ann Surg. 2010 June;251(6):1140–4.

10. Huller T, Bazini Y. Blast injuries of the chest and abdomen. Arch Surg. 1970 Jan;100(1):24–30.
11. Sg M. The pathogenesis of blast injury and its management. Br J Hosp Med. 1988 June 1;39(6):536–9.
12. Hill JF. Blast injury with particular reference to recent terrorist bombing incidents. Ann R Coll Surg Engl. 1979 Jan;61(1):4–11.
13. Ogilvie WH. Lessons of the war that are already being forgotten. Guys Hosp Gaz. 1956;51(10):401–5.
14. Ordog GJ, Wasserberger J, Balasubramanium S, Shoemaker W. Civilian gunshot wounds—outpatient management. J Trauma. 1994 Jan;36(1):106–11.

Part VIII

Environmental Trauma

Immersion and Submersion

39

Paul Savage OBE

This chapter clarifies the differences between Immersion and Submersion, and reviews the timeline of physiological events that occur when entering cold water; from Cold Shock, through Peripheral Cooling to Hypothermia. It analyses how these are related to the pathology created by cold water immersion and details potential causes and outcomes for the patient.

Introduction

In recent years the International Liaison Committee on Resuscitation (ILCOR) and the World Congress on Drowning have re-defined drowning. Terms such as near drowning, dry drowning, secondary drowning etc. are now obsolete. The agreed definition of drowning is

The process of experiencing respiratory impairment following submersion in liquid.

P. Savage OBE (✉)
Health Sciences Department, Bournemouth University, Bournemouth, UK

UK Search and Rescue Medical Group, London, UK
e-mail: paul@saviourmedical.com

It can be seen from this that the major issue is a respiratory one and thus all treatment should be aimed at the alleviation of hypoxia and its sequelae.

Epidemiology

Key Points
Understand difference between Immersion and Submersion.

Understand the timeline associated with key physiological changes.

Understand the challenges at the point of rescue.

Drowning accounts for >500,000 deaths worldwide annually [1]. Mortality from drowning in Europe shows two peaks:

- Children <5 years old
- Adult males 14–35 years old

Alcohol and drugs clearly play a significant role in incidents involving the latter. Unsupervised access to water is one of the biggest risk factors among children; unfenced swimming pools, ponds, rivers and ditches being the biggest killers worldwide.

There is an unfortunate association with child abuse in drownings amongst the under-fives and

P. Lax (ed.), *Textbook of Acute Trauma Care*, https://doi.org/10.1007/978-3-030-83628-3_39

clinicians in these cases should consider the possibility of intentional drowning or severe neglect. The NICE guidelines state that any child drowning is a safeguarding issue and should be reported.

Pathophysiology

The process of drowning is a less simple one than is imagined. Drowning can be the primary pathology in straightforward submersion, but is often secondary to other physiological processes, and in this chapter we will focus on the additional complications associated with cold water immersion.

A fundamental misunderstanding exists around drowning. It has been established that the whole process usually occurs in seconds to minutes—yet what is puzzling is that 67% of victims were deemed to be good swimmers and 55% of drownings occur within 3 m of safety [2]. To understand these figures, an understanding of the different physiology that is associated with cold water immersion compared to submersion is required.

Immersion vs Submersion

Video—immersion in cold water—sudden death and prolonged survival [https://www.youtube.com/watch?v=bwvFhmr5nis].

Immersion in this context is defined as the body entering cold water but with the airway remaining clear of the water, as would be achieved when wearing a correctly fitted lifejacket. Submersion is defined as the airway being kept under the surface of the water, in which case the inability to breathe is obvious (Fig. 39.1).

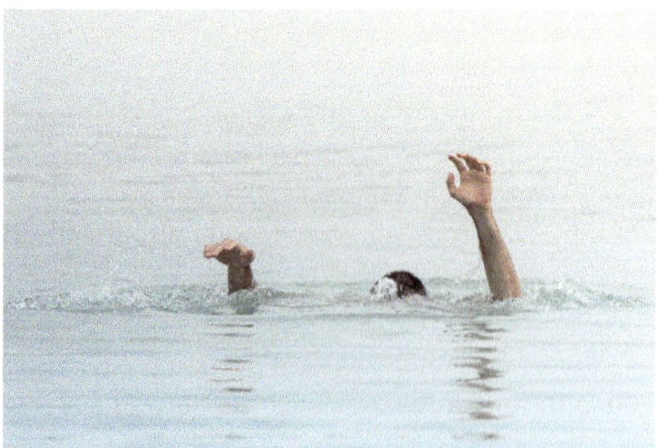

Fig. 39.1 Submersed body—the airway is under the surface of the water

Submersion

If a casualty is not wearing a lifejacket, is a non-swimmer, or is held under the surface for a variety of reasons (for example trapped, full stomach, waterlogged clothes), an initial breath hold will eventually give way to swallowing and coughing. In a 1951 experiment on dogs, Fainer et al. [3] demonstrated that after this point, around 70 seconds of uncontrolled respiration occurred once submerged and led to mass aspiration.

In cases of salt water drowning the alveolar space will fill with water and prevent oxygen transport, whereas in cases of fresh water drowning, there is a tendency to cause oedema of the alveoli wall because the fresh water is hypotonic. This, combined with surfactant washout as fresh water crosses the lung membrane and entering the bloodstream, leads to alveolar collapse. Either route will cause rapid hypoxemia leading to loss of consciousness and apnoea. The casualty proceeds to hypoxic cardiac arrest with rhythm disturbance -usually tachycardia followed by bradycardia then PEA and finally asystole. At this point, classically the casualty will be found floating face down just on or below the surface.

A submersed, drowned casualty should be rapidly removed from the water by any means, assessed and given CPR in line with standard Advanced Life Support (ALS) protocols. In the UK, protocols that have been drawn up in agreement with the Joint Royal Colleges Ambulance Liaison Committee (JRCALC) [4] state that CPR is not started if there is evidence of extreme trauma incompatible with life, decomposition or proven submersion time of more than 60 or 90 min, dependent on water temperature as explained in the following text.

Prolonged Submersion and Survival

New evidence has clarified the reasons behind prolonged submersion survival. Patients drowning in cold water can swallow litres of cold water (the stomach and mediastinum via oesophagus will be in contact with cooling effect). In addition rinsing the oropharynx and external cold water on the neck leads to rapid cooling of the brain. If the brain/body cools prior to cardiac arrest it is "protected" from the cell death cascade to an extent. At lower body temperatures, brain survival can therefore theoretically increase. Once active respiration ceases any further cooling will only occur due to conduction of heat from the warm body to the cold water.

Adults do not conduct heat well into the water due to the average amount of body fat, and therefore it appears never really pass a 20 min survival time that initial cooling during active respiration brings.

However, children and slim adults can continue to cool as they have greater surface area to mass ratios, at a rate of 2.5 °C every 10 min. Therefore they drop their core temperature an additional 5 °C in the first 20 min of brain survival time, resulting in potential core temperatures as low as 25 °C by the end of the first 20 min. This confers another 20 min of brain survival at this point, which allows further cooling of 5 °C. The process continues until about a maximum known survival time of 65 min.

It should be noted that coastal waters of the UK rarely fall below 5 °C, and therefore it is now strongly believed that survival times in excess of 30 min of true submersion and drowning at sea are virtually impossible for a variety of factors [5]. Still lakes and lochs do have the potential to drop below 5 °C, and therefore survival times for children and slim adults may potentially reach as high as 60 min. In an attempt to protect rescuers from risking life to rescue a non-viable patient, a new algorithm was created to assist on scene management decisions (Fig. 39.2). This has formed part of the 2016 UK Resus Guidelines [6].

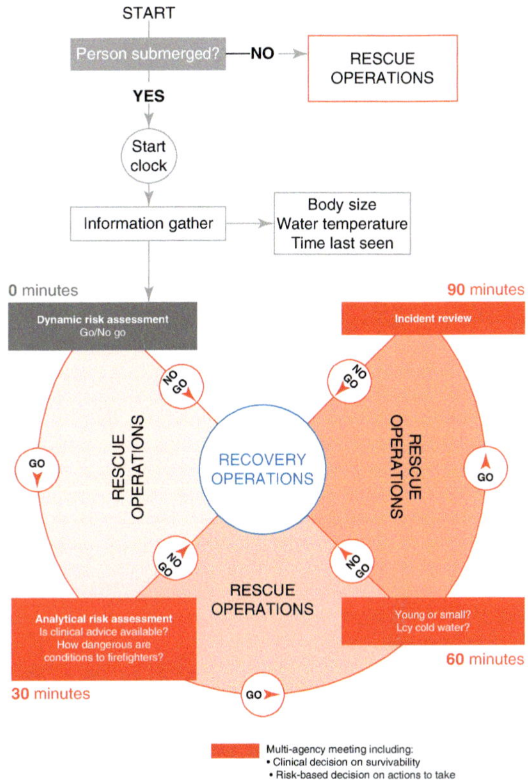

Fig. 39.2 UK risk assessment for submersion

The Conscious Drowned Patient

This describes the casualty that is just on the surface of the water, but may have aspirated wave splash or had a period of brief submersion—the previous nomenclature for this has included "near drowning". The aspiration of salt or fresh water may cause coughing, spluttering with associated wheeze or crackles/crepitations on auscultation with a stethoscope. The patient may complain of chest pain, vomiting and in serious cases have difficulty breathing with rapid shallow respirations and an associated rapid thready pulse. This can then lead to a reduction in conscious levels.

Pre-hospital management will need to focus on oxygenation and care of the unconscious airway. Any patient who has been at risk of aspiration must clinically assessed, as the latent effects of this aspiration can cause serious later complications as described below.

Complications of Drowning

Previous nomenclature for this collection of symptoms has included “secondary drowning” or “late onset near drowning”.

Water (especially salt water) irritates the lung tissue and causes a localised inflammatory response, causing inflammatory damage to lung membrane leading to pulmonary oedema. The victim may initially appear well but may rapidly deteriorate. This usually occurs in the first 12 h, but can take up to 72 h. Clinicians should look out for excessive coughing, chest pain, crackling or wheezy chest sounds. Initial white frothy sputum can start to become blood speckled and then blood stained.

2–4 ml/kg of water in the lungs has the potential to impair gas exchange directly and remove surfactant. Water can block the small airways due to surface tension and cause bronchospasm in others. Pulmonary oedema is common from the irritant and osmotic effects of the water (disrupting the basement membrane) and Adult Respiratory Distress Syndrome (ARDS) can often be precipitated. Casualties who aspirate will develop a large ventilation-perfusion mismatch with as much as 75% of pulmonary blood reported to flow through unventilated lungs (increased right to left shunt). This, coupled with impaired gas exchange in ventilated alveoli from pulmonary oedema and inhaled fluid, will result in a profound hypoxia.

Much has been made of the differences between fresh and seawater in animal models but it seems to have no appreciable effect on outcome in humans [7, 8]. However, there exists a reported excess of disseminated intravascular coagulation (DIC) in cases of freshwater immersion. Contaminated water can cause either microbiological or chemical injury to the lung parenchyma, and serious thought should be given to any specific complications from immersion in these media.

Non invasive ventilation (eg; BiPAP and CPAP) have been used to good effect in awake patients with worsening hypoxia following drowning, and mortality seems to follow that of other forms of non- cardiogenic pulmonary oedema [9, 10]. If evidence of ARDS is established then the usual protocols and lung protective ventilation strategies should be followed.

Immersion

First 0–3 Minutes of Rapid Immersion: Cold Shock

Cold shock results from a sudden cooling of a large area of skin following sudden contact with cold water. It occurs in water below 25 °C, reaching a maximum effect in water at 10 °C or less. It predominantly affects the respiratory and cardiovascular systems via a huge sympathetic nervous system response.

Respiratory system effects are an initial large gasp, which can lead to drowning. This is followed by rapid respiration (up to an eightfold increase in respiratory rate). As it is uncontrolled it can also lead to drowning if there is any subsequent wave splash. There is also an inability to breath-hold voluntarily. If the victim is trapped in rising water, this may render a casualty unable to hold a breath to effect an escape [11]. Cold shock also leads to impaired ability to coordinate breathing with swim stroke, potentially causing even experienced swimmers to drown if not wearing a lifejacket.

The effects on the circulatory system are a generalised peripheral vasoconstriction, weakening skeletal muscle in limbs, an increase in venous return leading to pulmonary artery hypertension and significant increase in heart rate and cerebral hypertension, impairing cerebral function and potentially precipitating CVA in susceptible patients.

These cold shock effects account for 56% of open water deaths in the UK within the first 3 min of immersion. If cold shock leads to cardiac arrest via a stroke or arrhythmia, the casualty may present as drowned and should be treated per the submersed protocol. However these patients usually have dry lungs with minimal aspiration if the route to arrest was arrhythmic. This is because there may have been no opportunity for rapid, uncontrolled respiration whilst submerged if the patient entered cardiac arrest due to cold shock or its sequelae at the point they first hit the water. These patients also tend to present in VF rather than the classic Tachy-Brady-PEA of submersed drowned patients. The Cold Shock response can be reduced and even eradicated by acclimatisation or by warming the skin past 40 °C which is why going from a sauna to an ice-hole is not a fatal event!

Next 3–30 Minutes of Immersion: Extremity Cooling

If a casualty survives the cold shock effects, their extremities (but not their core) cool rapidly. As extremities cool to 25–29 °C, muscle and superficial nerve function deteriorate resulting in ineffective attempts at swimming. If no flotation aids are worn, the casualty will quickly be unable to support themselves in the water, leading to inhalation of water and drowning as previously described [12].

The small muscles of the hands are also affected quickly, so any simple lifesaving tasks are impossible (for example, using lifejacket buckles or firing signalling flares). If extremity cooling leads to drowning and subsequent cardiac arrest, the casualty will present as drowned and should be treated as a submersed casualty. Note, at this stage core temperature is still above 35 °C and the casualty is not yet hypothermic.

30+ Minutes of Immersion: Hypothermia in Water

Hypothermia starts when the bodies' core temperature drops from the norm of 37 °C to below 35 °C. This is very different to limb temperature, which will have cooled much quicker to well below 30 °C by that time through extremity cooling.

In the coldest of coastal UK and Republic of Ireland waters, due to protective body responses, core hypothermia still takes around 30 min to occur. As the core temperature reduces from 35 °C, shivering increases in intensity until the body adopts an almost rigid foetal position. The level of consciousness drops steadily with a fall in temperature, resulting in confusion and an inability speak or give a history due to muscle

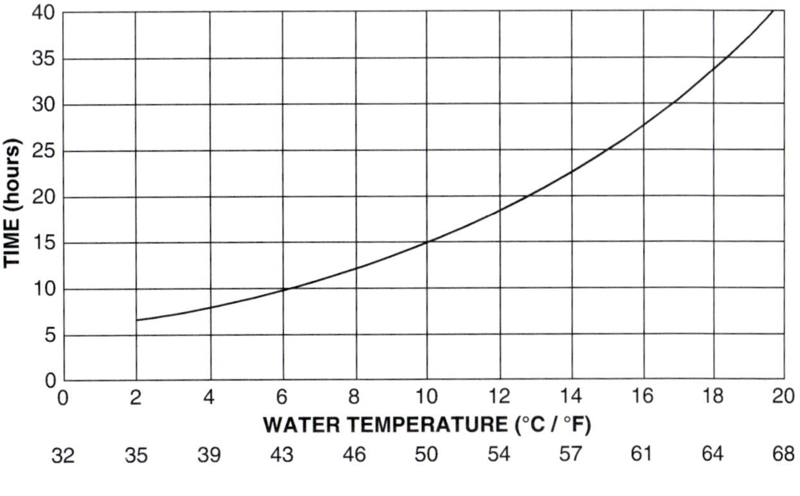

Fig. 39.3 Maximum Survival time of a lightly clad male from entry into water with normal clothing whilst wearing a lifejacket (from IAMSAR Guidelines volume 3, International Maritime organisation)

spasm. As the core temperature reaches 30 °C the casualty will become unconscious.

At this stage if they are not wearing a lifejacket, the patients' face will enter the water and they will drown. If they are in a lifejacket and continue to cool, as core temperature reaches 28 °C the heart enters ventricular fibrillation (VF) and the casualty goes into cardiac arrest.

Figure 39.3 shows the realistic upper limit of survival time for people in the water wearing normal clothing and a lifejacket, from time of entry into the water. Water temperatures around the British Isles typically range from 4 to 19 °C. The graph indicates the maximum survival time of casualties in different water temperatures. This is used by the UK Coastguard as an aid in determining appropriate search durations. Whilst many factors can reduce this maximum survival time, it is worth noting that in optimal survival conditions in water of 2 °C it can take up to 7 hours for a patient's core to drop from 37 °C to 28 °C and VF arrest occur. In summer, in inshore waters off the south coast of the UK with the potential for an average water temperature of 19 °C, it can mean possible maximum survival times of 37 hours before 28 °C is reached and VF arrest occurs. To further complicate matters, there is no reliable pre-hospital temperature measurment as tympanic thermometers do not work in cold wet ears and give readings far lower than the actual core temperature. Conscious, lucid, shivering talking patients with immersion times less than 30 min are not hypothermic but are cold.

Mammalian Dive Reflex

As described above, the cold shock response is driven by a huge sympathetic nervous system response triggered by large areas of bare skin in contact with cold water. There is also another autonomic driven response to cold water immersion driven by the parasympathetic nervous system, called the mammalian dive reflex.

This reflex is evoked by stimulation of the cold receptors of the face in isolation, innervated by Cranial nerves V, VII, X and XII [13], and may happen in people protected by PPE on their body but with an exposed face. This reflex drives a large parasympathetic response causing profound sinus bradycardia driven by excitation of cardiac vagal motor neurones, expiratory apnoea ("breath hold") by reflex inhibition of central respiratory neurones, excitation of sympathetic vasoconstrictors and stimulation of vagal receptors in the pharynx and larynx further enforcing these responses.

Autonomic Conflict

Very rarely would a situation occur where either cold shock, or the mammalian dive reflex happened in pure isolation, and Tipton et al. [14] have studied the effects of both reflexes being simultaneously or sequentially stimulated causing an "autonomic conflict" (Fig. 39.4). What has been elucidated is that when both the parasympathetic and sympathetic nervous systems are triggered together, a significant arrhythmia is caused at the break of breath hold. While this may be not too catastrophic in young fit individuals, if the casualty happened to have any predisposing cardiac pathology, the arrhythmia produced could be fatal.

This evolving concept could explain the high death rates in the first 3 min of immersion, previously thought to be purely accountable to cold water shock. However, as arrhythmias are not detectable at post mortem it is hard to prove, but certainly accounts for a significant number of casualties having dry lungs and no signs of drowning as described previously.

Rescue from Water

Simply being immersed in water for a prolonged length of time will cause cardiovascular instability. External hydrostatic pressure causes redistribution of the circulating volume towards the thorax and then intracellularly, and hormonal responses cause a forced diuresis (up to 2 L in the first 2 h) and subsequently a profound relative hypovolaemia.

Hydrostatic squeeze is the pressure the sea exerts on the casualty when they are vertical in

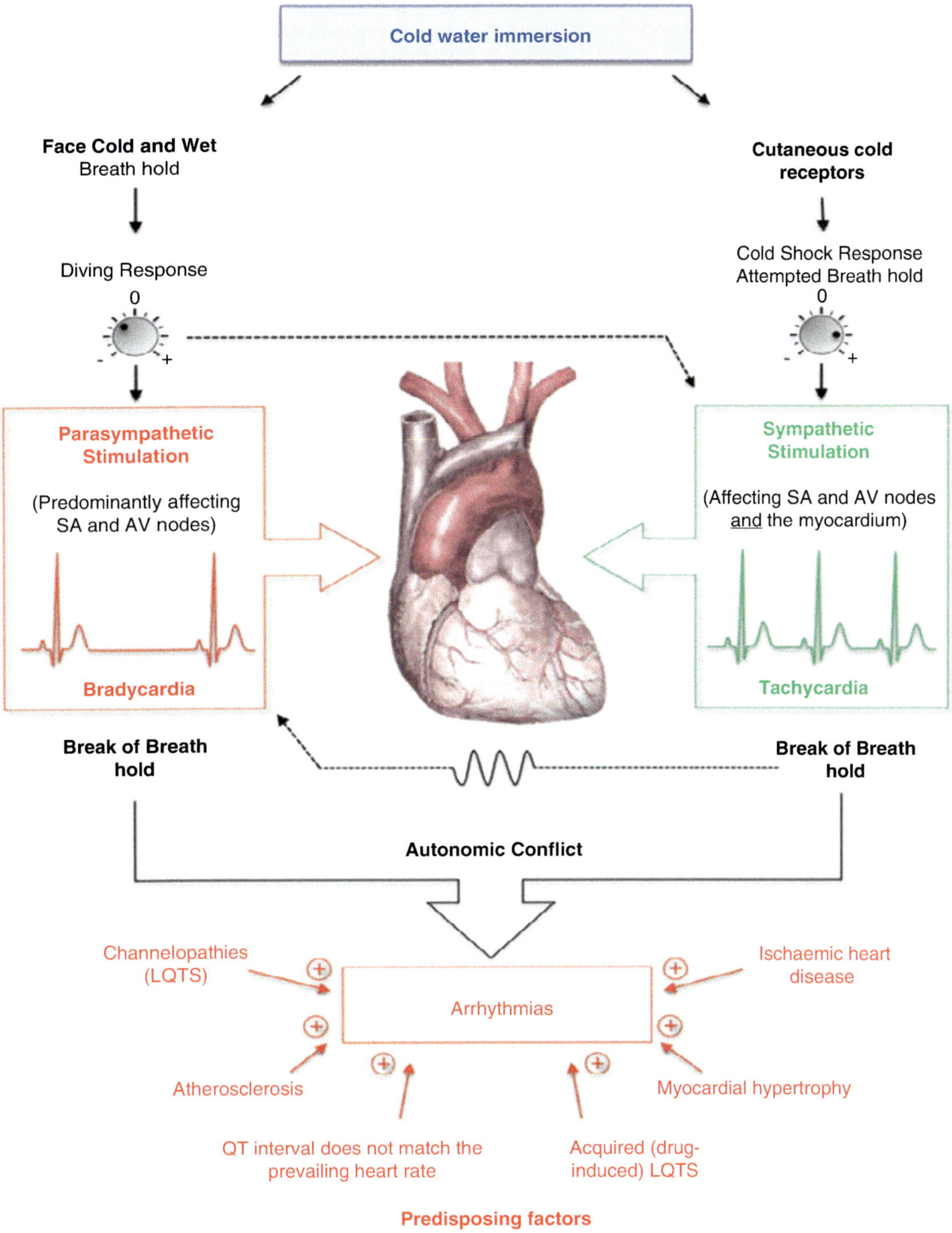

Fig. 39.4 Mechanism of autonomic conflict (from Shattock and Tipton [14])

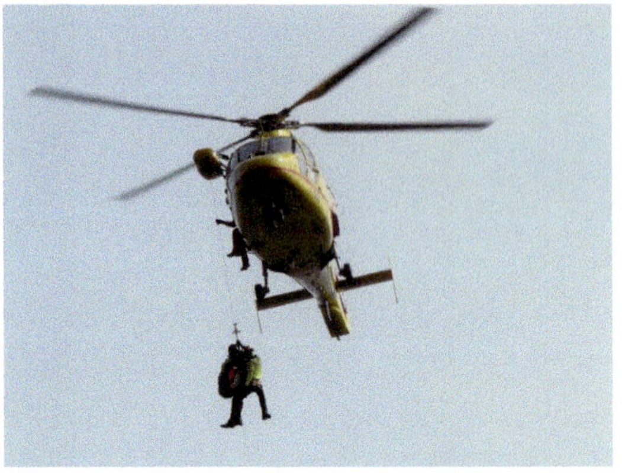

Fig. 39.5 Helicopter winch rescue may cause potential cardiovascular collapse if the patient is not lifted horizontally after a prolonged immersion

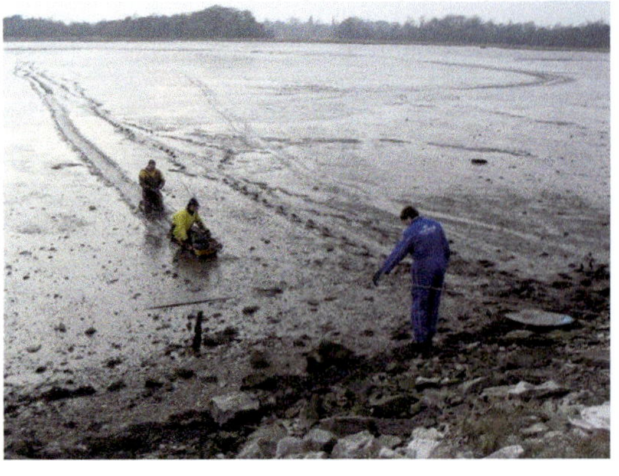

Fig. 39.6 Mud rescue (Stephen Williams/*Coastguard mud rescue exercise in Holes Bay*/CC BY-SA 2.0)

the water. This pressure maintains a blood pressure within the core. If the casualty is removed vertically from the water and suspended for several minutes (e.g. by winching into a helicopter as seen in Fig. 39.5), there is a rapid loss of the supporting hydrostatic pressure and reintroduction of gravity. This creates significant effects in the body and the potential for hypovolaemic cardiac arrest can occur. Therefore, it is important to remove the prolonged immersed casualty (30 min plus) from the water horizontally to minimise the potential for collapse. This controls the removal of hydrostatic squeeze and the re-introduction of gravity. There are a number of ways to achieve this. But remember—this is for immersed casualties. The submersed patient should be extricated rapidly in any fashion so CPR can commence.

Mud Rescue

Casualties trapped in mud are subject to the same physiology as casualties immersed in water for a period of time (Fig. 39.6). Therefore once released from the mud they should, ideally, be transported lying down where practical, especially if trapped to a depth above their knees. Concepts based on either crush injuries or suspension trauma and the use of tourniquets etc. are not relevant to the mud environment.

Concomitant Injury or Medical Conditions

Remember that drowning is usually the result of an underlying event or condition that contributes to unintentional immersion or immersion with incapacitation, such as trauma, intoxication, seizure, hypothermia, dysrhythmia, shallow-water blackout, and for divers, a lost or improper breathing source. It is important to search for and treat any underlying triggering factors or complications.

Infection

Prophylactic antibiotics are not recommended in all cases though in the case of contaminated water inhalation they do seem to be of some use. Clearly the possibility of an unusual organism being involved is high and early involvement of microbiologists would be advisable. Other interventions such as steroids have not been evaluated specifically in drowning, but have roles defined in other related conditions.

In summary it is vital to always have a high sensitivity to risk around water and remember that all submersed casualties need rapid removal, assessment and treatment if appropriate, whilst immersed casualties may benefit from horizontal extrication. All casualties who have aspirated need to be seen in hospital. Rescuers should be aware of the effects of sudden immersion in cold water for themselves or their casualties and make allowances for peripheral cooling and hypothermia. There should always be the consideration of autonomic conflict as a cause of cardiac arrest.

Conclusion

The physiological changes to the human body when placed in cold water are well proven and once understood can be used to map the patient's journey against the time of immersion or submersion, and the expected pathological outcomes that are associated with this.

Questions and Answers

1. Which is the most lethal phase of Immersion
   (a) Hypothermia
   (b) Swim Failure
   (c) Cold Shock
   (d) Circum-Rescue Collapse

   Answer c

2. Mammalian Dive Reflex is a rare occurrence caused by stimulation of:
   (a) Parasympathetic Nervous System
   (b) Sympathetic Nervous System
   (c) Somatic Nervous System
   (d) Cerebellum

   Answer a

3. True or False – Submerged casualties need to be carefully removed from the due to the risks of the reduction in hydrostatic squeeze and the reintroduction of gravity

   Answer False

4. What might be the upper realistic survival time of an adult in light clothing in 6 degree C water
   (a) 2 hours
   (b) 4 hours
   (c) 8 hours
   (d) 10 hours

   Answer d

5. True or False – Rescue Operations become body recoveries in all cases after 60 minutes

   Answer False

Acknowledgement Produced with thanks to Prof. Mike Tipton and Dr. Patrick Morgan.

References

1. Weltgesundheitsorganisation, editor. The injury chartbook: a graphical overview of the global burden of injuries. Geneva; 2002. 75 p.
2. Great Britain, Working Party on Water Safety. Report of the Working Party on Water Safety [Internet]. London: H.M.S.O.; 1977 [cited 2019 Sep 15]. Available from: http://books.google.com/books?id=Z36upFXAaV8C
3. Fainer DC, Martin CG, Ivy AC. Resuscitation of dogs from fresh water drowning. J Appl Physiol. 1951 Jan;3(7):417–26.
4. Brown SN, Kumar D, James C, Mark J, Association of Ambulance Chief Executives (Great Britain), Joint Royal Colleges Ambulance Liaison Committee, et al. JRCALC clinical guidelines 2019 [Internet]. 2019 [cited 2020 May 15]. Available from: https://search.ebscohost.com/login.aspx?direct=true&scope=site&db=nlebk&db=nlabk&AN=2293957
5. Golden F, Tipton M. Essentials of sea survival. Champaign, IL: Human Kinetics; 2002.
6. Nolan J, Resuscitation Council (Great Britain). Advanced life support. London: Resuscitation Council, UK; 2016.

7. Bierens JJLM, Lunetta P, Tipton M, Warner DS. Physiology of drowning: a review. Physiology. 2016 Feb 17;31(2):147–66.
8. Michelet P, Dusart M, Boiron L, Marmin J, Mokni T, Loundou A, et al. Drowning in fresh or salt water: respective influence on respiratory function in a matched cohort study. Eur J Emerg Med. 2019 Oct;26(5):340–4.
9. Michelet P, Bouzana F, Charmensat O, Tiger F, Durand-Gasselin J, Hraiech S, et al. Acute respiratory failure after drowning: a retrospective multicenter survey. Eur J Emerg Med. 2017 Aug;24(4):295–300.
10. Ruggeri P, Calcaterra S, Bottari A, Girbino G, Fodale V. Successful management of acute respiratory failure with noninvasive mechanical ventilation after drowning, in an epileptic-patient. Respir Med Case Rep. 2016 Feb 21;17:90–2.
11. Parkes MJ. Breath-holding and its breakpoint: breath-holding and its breakpoint. Exp Physiol. 2006 Jan;91(1):1–15.
12. Tipton M, Eglin C, Gennser M, Golden F. Immersion deaths and deterioration in swimming performance in cold water. Lancet. 1999 Aug;354(9179):626–9.
13. Guz A, Noble MI, Widdicombe JG, Trenchard D, Mushin WW, Makey AR. The role of vagal and glossopharyngeal afferent nerves in respiratory sensation, control of breathing and arterial pressure regulation in conscious man. Clin Sci. 1966 Feb;30(1):161–70.
14. Shattock MJ, Tipton MJ. 'Autonomic conflict': a different way to die during cold water immersion? Autonomic conflict and cardiac arrhythmias. J Physiol. 2012 Jul;590(14):3219–30.

Further Reading

Giesbrecht GG. Prehospital treatment of hypothermia. Wilderness Environ Med. 2001 Mar;12(1):24–31.

Nasrullah M, Muazzam S. Drowning mortality in the United States, 1999–2006. J Community Health. 2011 Feb;36(1):69–75.

Tipton M, Wooler A. Science of beach lifeguarding, Chapter 6. Boca Raton, FL: CRC Press; 2016.

Tipton M, Eglin C, Gennser M, Golden F. Immersion deaths and deterioration in swimming performance in cold water. Lancet. 1999 Aug;354(9179):626–9.

Burns and Thermal Injuries

40

Brendan D. R. Sloan

Learning Objectives

- Understand and describe the early management of hypothermia and other cold injuries
- Understand and describe initial assessment and management of the burnt patient
- Understand and describe the assessment and initial management of airway and inhalation burns
- Understand and describe the early management of chemical burns and electrocution
- Understand medium to long-term issues in the severely burnt patient

Hypothermia

Hypothermia is defined as a reduction in core temperature below 35 °C (see Table 40.1). It is associated with significant morbidity and mortality, both independently and in conjunction with trauma, where temperatures below 34 °C are associated with coagulopathy and increased bleeding. In health, the body maintains temperature homeostasis between 36.5 °C and 37.5 °C, with a degree of diurnal variation. The thermoneutral zone for resting humans is generally between 21 °C and 30 °C, whereby core temperature is maintained without the need to use energy above normal basal metabolic rate. At any temperature below this, there needs to be some degree of additional thermogenesis or heat preservation to maintain a normal core temperature [1].

Table 40.1 Physiological changes in hypothermia [1]

Core temperature	Physiological changes
35 °C	Shivering begins
33 °C	Progressive confusion
32 °C	Shivering reduces
30 C	Shivering ceases, bradycardia and reduced cardiac output, dysrhythmias (AF, premature atrial and ventricular beats)
28 °C	Unconsciousness, increased risk of VF/asystole, hypoventilation
25 °C	Pulse undetectable, areflexia, fixed pupils
13.7 °C	Lowest recorded core temperature with full neurological recovery

Hypothermia is a common complication of trauma and injury, occurring in up to 37% of patients presenting to trauma centres with critical injuries [2]. There are many predisposing factors relating to the environment, the patient, and the injuries sustained. Heat is lost through four main

B. D. R. Sloan (✉)
Departmentof Anaesthesia and Critical Care Medicine, The Yorkshire Regional Burns Centre, Pinderfields Hospital, Wakefield, UK
e-mail: brendan.sloan1@nhs.net

P. Lax (ed.), *Textbook of Acute Trauma Care*, https://doi.org/10.1007/978-3-030-83628-3_40

routes; conduction, convection, evaporation and radiation. Hypothermia is most likely to develop when there is increased heat loss, a reduced ability to produce new heat, or a combination of both.

Increased Heat Loss

Factors include reduced air temperature, moisture, wind chill, increasing altitude, increased length of exposure, reduced body fat, type of clothing, vasodilatation (e.g. medication, spinal injury), major haemorrhage, use of cold fluids, significant burn injury, and young infants/neonates (high surface area to weight ratio).

Reduced Heat Production

Factors include increasing age, alcohol/drug use, reduced muscle mass, immobility, inadequate nutrition, spinal injury (impaired shivering), and concomitant medical disease.

Physiology of Hypothermia

There are several physiological responses following exposure to cold, regulated by the hypothalamus. Shivering and active movement both involve contraction of skeletal muscle, producing significant amounts of heat as a byproduct. There is also an increase in cardiac output and basal metabolic rate secondary to catecholamine release, while vasoconstriction of the peripheries reduces heat loss. Other adaptive responses include seeking shelter and applying more clothing.

Once core temperature drops below 32 °C, these mechanisms cease to be effective. Shivering stops, along with a reduction in basal metabolic rate. There is progressive myocardial irritability, with bradycardia and a reduction in cardiac output, along with an increased risk of arrhythmias (principally atrial fibrillation). Pathognomonic J waves appear on the ECG. The respiratory rate falls in association with the reduced metabolic activity, and cerebral activity decreases, resulting in confusion and eventual unconsciousness at around 28 °C. Platelet function is impaired, resulting in coagulopathy, and the oxygen-haemoglobin dissociation curve shifts to the left, reducing oxygen release. Central pooling of blood due to vasoconstriction, along with a reduction in antidiuretic hormone secretion result in a diuresis. Ileus and pancreatitis are also common [3].

Staging of Hypothermia

Hypothermia can be staged using several methods, but one of the most commonly used is the Swiss staging system for hypothermia (Table 40.2). Hypothermia is staged from I to IV, depending on core temperature. This requires accurate measurement of core temperature, which can be extremely challenging. There may be significant variation on the measured temperature depending on the site used, environmental conditions, and perfusion. The 'gold standard method' for an intubated patient is an oesophageal temperature probe in the lower third of the oesophagus. Epitympanic temperature measurement is accurate if there is good contact with the tympanic membrane. However, it may be obstructed with snow in the ear canal and is extremely unreliable in the presence of water. Cutaneous and oral thermometers are often inaccurate in hypothermia due to peripheral vasoconstriction. Rectal temperature requires good contact with mucosa but often lags behind core temperature during the rewarming process. If the measurement of core temperature is not feasible, treatment should be based on clinical scoring systems [1].

Table 40.2 Swiss clinical staging system for hypothermia [4]

Swiss hypothermia stage	Core temperature	Clinical symptoms
I	32–35 °C	Conscious, shivering
II	28–32 °C	Reduced conscious level, not shivering
III	24–28 °C	Unconscious, not shivering, vital signs present
IV	<24 °C	No vital signs present

Pre-Hospital Management

Patients with significant hypothermia require extremely careful handling to avoid precipitating life-threatening arrhythmias. They should be positioned horizontally to minimise the effect of hydrostatic pressure. Preventing further heat loss is also essential. Removal of wet clothing and replacement with blankets and a vapour barrier will minimise heat loss via evaporation and convection. Reflective blankets help reduce radiation. Use of heat packs may cause problems, either from burning skin which is intensely vasoconstricted, or by inducing peripheral vasodilatation which can result in the return of more cold blood to the core, and a worsening of core temperature. In practice, rewarming casualties in the prehospital setting is extremely challenging, and the main aim should be a rapid but smooth transfer to hospital while attempting to minimise further heat loss [5].

Investigations

Electrocardiography is useful, and there is a broad range of arrhythmias that may occur. J waves are pathognomonic but of no clinical significance. There is also temperature-dependent prolongation of the PR, QRS and QT intervals. Bradycardia and atrial fibrillation are common in moderate hypothermia, but as core temperature decreases, increasing conduction times can lead to more malignant arrhythmias, particularly VF.

A full series of blood tests is also essential. Electrolyte derangement is common due to both hypothermia and rhabdomyolysis with subsequent renal failure. Pancreatitis is a recognised complication, and amylase/lipase should be measured. Volume depletion due to diuresis may result in increased haematocrit. DIC and thrombocytopenia also commonly occur. Blood gas analysis can be challenging to interpret and should be performed both with and without temperature correction. Normal values for pH and $PaCO_2$ should be targeted on the uncorrected gas, but PaO_2 monitored with temperature correction due to alterations in the oxygen-haemoglobin dissociation curve.

Treatment

The principle treatment of hypothermia is rewarming. Patients with Stage I hypothermia can be managed with warm clothing, nutrition and encouragement of active movement if appropriate. Stage II–IV hypothermia requires active rewarming. Forced-air warming, warmed fluids and other non-invasive techniques can be used, but rewarming rates are variable (0.1–3.4 °C/h). External rewarming has been linked with peripheral vasodilatation and worsening core temperature (referred to as 'afterdrop') due to cold peripheral blood returning centrally. This can result in a drop in core temperature of up to 5–6 °C, and continuous core temperature measurement is recommended during the rewarming process.

Peritoneal lavage, thoracic lavage and haemodialysis have all been used with variable effect. In Stage III or IV hypothermia ECMO has been used, with survival rates of up to 63% without neurological injury [3]. Warming rates of up to 9 °C/hour have been achieved with ECMO. In extremely severe cases, a degree of therapeutic hypothermia (32–34 °C) for neuroprotection may be of value rather than aiming for normothermia, although there is a lack of definitive evidence. The potential use of ECMO depends on availability, and any contraindication to the anticoagulation required. It should be noted that the cases of survival in extreme hypothermia have been in patients involved in cold water submersion or avalanche burial where cooling was rapid and there were no other significant injuries.

Other management is principally supportive. Airway support may be required, and any intubation should be done as gently as possible to avoid precipitating arrhythmias. Fluid resuscitation is often needed due to hypothermia-induced diuresis. Any fluids should be warmed, and solutions containing dextrose will help provide energy for endogenous thermogenesis. If central lines are required, the femoral route is preferable to minimise the risk of myocardial irritation with the guidewire during insertion. Atrial fibrillation usually resolves as core temperature increases, although magnesium may be of use. Bradycardia, ventricular ectopics and other atrial arrhythmias are physiological responses to hypothermia and require no specific treatment.

Management of Cardiac Arrest

Severe hypothermia can lead to ventricular fibrillation or asystole. It may also be extremely difficult to detect vital signs in patients with severe hypothermia (<32 °C) with a potentially perfusing rhythm. In patients with severe hypothermia and no vital signs or a cardiac arrest rhythm, and the absence of an overtly lethal injury (e.g. decapitation), cardiopulmonary resuscitation should be started. This should be continued in conjunction with rewarming. Chest wall and myocardial compliance will be reduced, making chest compressions more difficult. Use of an automated CPR device (such as a Lucas or Autopulse device) should be considered, especially as resuscitation may be prolonged. Defibrillation is often ineffective at core temperature below 30 °C. Current resuscitation guidelines recommend that if there is no response to three initial shocks, further defibrillation should be deferred until the core temperature is above 30 °C. Due to reduced drug metabolism, medications (e.g. adrenaline) are usually only given once the core temperature is over 30 °C. Above 30 °C, drug administration frequency should be halved (e.g. adrenaline every four cycles of CPR) [6].

Potential indications to stop CPR include serum potassium of >12 mmol/L, core temperature < 7 °C, incompressibility of the chest (i.e. the patient is physically frozen), pH <6.5, or persistent asystole with a core temperature > 32 °C. During rewarming, other problems may become evident (e.g. severe coagulopathy with uncontrollable haemorrhage) which may make continued resuscitation efforts futile.

Key Points

Hypothermia is a common and serious complication of trauma, increasing morbidity and mortality.

Core temperature should be measured, but clinical staging is of use where this is not possible.

Rewarming can be extremely challenging, especially in severe hypothermia, and may require specialist centres.

Cold Injury

A reduction in temperature can easily damage tissues. Cold injury can be divided into freezing and non-freezing injuries. The main difference between these is the presence of ice crystals within the tissues in freezing injury, resulting in physical tissue disruption and cell death. Risk factors include environmental conditions, duration of exposure, inadequate clothing, peripheral vascular disease, alcohol and substance use, and neuropathies.

Non-freezing Injury: Trench Foot/Frostnip

Non-freezing cold injury occurs when tissues are exposed to prolonged low temperatures, but without freezing of tissue fluid. Typically, the affected area has been cold and wet for prolonged periods, hence the name trench foot. The principal issue is sensory neuropathy, with severity related to the duration of exposure. After rewarming, the affected areas become extremely painful; much more so than in freezing injuries, and this is commonly the reason for presentation. This pain can last for months, and result in chronic pain syndromes. There is also an increased sensitivity to cold, which may be profound. Treatment includes slow rewarming, analgesia (including neuropathic agents), and careful management of the neuropathic areas to prevent ulceration and further tissue damage. However, there are often long-term sequelae, and prevention is preferable.

Frostnip refers to superficial non-freezing cold injury. It occurs on exposed skin (typically fingers, cheeks, ears and nose) due to extremely low ambient temperature. Ice crystals form on the skin, and there is significant peripheral vasoconstriction resulting in pallor and numbness. However, ice crystals do not form within tissues, and the condition is entirely reversible with shelter and warming. With continued exposure, frostnip will progress to frostbite.

Freezing Injury: Frostbite

Frostbite occurs when temperatures are so low that ice crystals form within body tissues. Injury occurs via several mechanisms. Before ice crystal formation, there is intense vasoconstriction with resultant tissue ischaemia—the 'pre-freeze phase'. Ice crystal formation then causes cell membrane damage resulting in electrolyte and protein shifts, ultimately causing cell death. This is referred to as the 'freeze-thaw phase'. As the tissue thaws, there is a release of inflammatory mediators leading to microcirculatory damage and platelet aggregation—the 'vascular stasis phase'. This can result in further tissue infarction, as well as thrombus formation and release of microemboli—the 'late ischaemic phase'. Refreezing results in worsening of the initial cell damage [7].

Frostbite initially results in oedema and paraesthesia as nerve tissue becomes frozen, preventing neural transmission. As it deepens blisters develop, which may become haemorrhagic if freezing occurs within deeper dermal tissue. Severity of damage is divided into four tiers, from superficial to full-thickness injury, comparable with thermal burns severity grading (Table 40.3).

Management is ideally preventative, as once freezing occurs some degree of tissue injury is almost inevitable. Prevention includes adequate awareness of symptoms, along with appropriate clothing, nutrition and hydration. The cornerstone of treatment is rapid rewarming, which is best achieved via water bath immersion at 37–39 °C. Once thawed, it is essential that the tissue does not refreeze as this can result in a significant extension of the injury. Thawing may result in significant swelling, and fasciotomy may be required. Other therapeutic options include NSAIDS to reduce thromboxane and prostaglandin production, rehydration, tetanus vaccination, and analgesia. If available, there is evidence to suggest thrombolysis using intravascular or intra-arterial tPA may help reduce amputation in patients with deep frostbite [8]. Iloprost has also been shown to reduce amputation rates. Ultimately, surgical debridement or amputation may be required for severe injuries.

Table 40.3 Classification of frostbite [5]

Depth	Classification	Clinical picture
Partial skin	1st degree	Erythema, oedema, hyperaemia, no blisters
Full-thickness skin	2nd degree	Erythema, significant oedema, blisters
Skin, subcutaneous tissue	3rd degree	Blue/grey discolouration, haemorrhagic blisters, necrosis
Skin, subcutaneous tissue, muscle, bone	4th degree	Mottling, cyanosis, progressing to dry mummification

Key Points

Direct cold injury can cause significant tissue damage, and prevention is key.

Non-freezing injury should be rewarmed slowly.

Freezing injury (frostbite) should be rewarmed rapidly, and often requires specialist management.

Hyperthermia

Hyperthermia is defined as a core body temperature above 37.5 °C. It can result from several causes, most commonly related to heatwaves (classical heatstroke), or excessive exercise in high ambient temperatures (exertional heatstroke). A variety of medications can also result in hyperthermia, both prescribed (MAOI, tricyclic antidepressants, SSRIs, sympathomimetics) and illicit (amphetamines, MDMA, LSD, cocaine). Other diagnoses to consider include metabolic syndromes such as thyroid storm, phaeochromocytoma, and serotonin syndrome. Mortality of heatstroke is over 35% if combined with hypotension, and correlates with the duration and magnitude of hyperthermia [9].

Hyperthermia develops when the body's production of heat outweighs the ability to dissipate it. This is a normal response to exertion, and core temperature alone does not imply heat illness. Pathological manifestations include heat cramps, usually associated with dehydration and electrolyte disturbance, and heat syncope, which generally resolves with rest and rehydration. Heat exhaustion is a more serious condition, with weakness, fatigue, thirst and muscle aches. Heatstroke occurs at a core temperature over 40 °C and requires an element of neurological disturbance (e.g. encephalopathy, seizures, or coma).

Significant hyperthermia triggers a profound inflammatory reaction similar to SIRS. This progresses into multiorgan dysfunction, with ARDS, circulatory failure, DIC, rhabdomyolysis, renal and liver dysfunction. Brain activity becomes progressively disturbed, with confusion, seizures and decreased consciousness above 40.5 °C. Excessive heat is also directly cytotoxic.

Rapid and effective cooling is the critical treatment, aiming to reduce core temperature to below 39 °C as quickly as reasonably possible. Effective methods include cold-water immersion, infusion of cold fluids, use of ice packs, and haemofiltration. Management of resultant organ dysfunction is supportive. There are no effective pharmacological agents to accelerate cooling. Both traditional antipyretics (aspirin, paracetamol), and dantrolene (used for anaesthesia-related malignant hyperthermia) act on different pathways to those in heatstroke, and should not be used [10].

Key Points

Hyperthermia can be life-threatening, especially above 40 °C.

Rapid and effective cooling is essential, aiming for a core temperature of <39 °C.

Burn Injury

Epidemiology

Annually, around 11 million people suffer a burn severe enough to require medical attention. Worldwide, burns are the fourth highest cause of death due to injury [11]. The majority of these happen in lower and middle-income countries, often relating to the use of open fires for heating and cooking. High-income countries have seen a reduction in incidence related to public health and prevention strategies, but in the UK there are over 250,000 burn injuries per annum. Of this number, around 25,000 attend hospital, and around 5000 require inpatient management by specialist burn centres.

Within the UK, the majority of burns occur in the home. Common risk factors include extremes of age, alcohol or drug intoxication, smoking, and sensory disability. Over a third of burns in the UK are related to carelessness [12].

Types of Burn

Burn injury and tissue damage can occur as a result of exposure to a variety of noxious substances. These can be divided into several categories, each with their own specific considerations.

Thermal Burns

These occur as a result of exposure to extreme temperature, with the degree of tissue damage directly related to the temperature and duration of exposure. Exposure to cold is discussed above. Exposure to heat is usually divided into dry heat and scald burns. Dry heat includes both flame injury, and contact burns (e.g. radiators). With flame burn, there is a risk of inhalation injury related to smoke and fumes produced during combustion, which may be more severe than the cutaneous burn. Scald injuries occur from exposure to hot liquids. These are commonly associated with either hot drinks or bathing. Scald injuries are particularly common in toddlers and the elderly. Scalds are often less severe due to the lower temperature than flame burns. The

Table 40.4 Time-surface temperature thresholds at which cutaneous burning occurs [13]

Temperature (°C)	Time for cutaneous burning to occur
44	6 h
50	5 min
54	30 s
60	5 s
70	<1 s

temperature and time required to develop a burn is illustrated in Table 40.4 below [13].

Chemical Burns

Chemical burns are injuries to the skin or mucous membranes caused by caustic substances. Typically, strong acids or bases cause protein denaturation and cell death. Acid burns are typically painful, with tissue coagulation. Alkali burns can be more insidious, with tissue liquefaction resulting in deeper tissue damage. The extent of damage is related to the type, amount, and concentration of the agent, as well as the duration of exposure. The burning process will continue until the agent is neutralised, and is generally longer than for thermal injury. Some agents also cause systemic toxicity, including renal failure, electrolyte abnormalities, and methaemoglobinaemia. The majority of injuries result from domestic, laboratory and industrial accidents, as well as deliberate assault. Common causative agents include.

Household

- Alkalis: drain cleaners, cement, paint remover
- Phenols: deodorants, sanitizers, disinfectants
- Sodium hypochlorite: disinfectants, bleach
- Sulphuric acid: toilet cleaner

Industrial

- Acids: sulphuric, hydrochloric, hydrofluoric, tannic, acetic (etching, electronics)
- Alkalis: ammonia, sodium hydroxide, cement, calcium hydroxide (washing powder, drain cleaner, paint remover)

Decontamination is ***essential*** to the management of any chemical burn. Dry chemicals should be brushed off, and contaminated clothing removed. Constant irrigation with water should be started as soon as possible (except for burns from elemental sodium, potassium or lithium which may worsen injury), and continued until the tissue pH reaches 8. Diphoterine is a non-specific buffer that can also be used to neutralise most caustic agents [14]. Healthcare staff should take all possible precautions to avoid becoming contaminated during treatment, and any accidental exposure treated promptly with irrigation.

Electrical Burns

Electrical burns result from heat generation as electrical energy passes through body tissues. The amount of heat generated is dependent on the electrical current, the duration, and the tissue resistance. Skin resistance is relatively high, but varies depending on thickness and moisture, with thin, moist skin the most conductive. High current concentrations at the point of contact result in intense heat and charring of tissues. Once the skin is breached, an increased current can flow, preferentially via nerves, blood vessels and muscles. This can result in deeper tissue damage and swelling, which may be remote from the point of entry. Electrical burns can be grouped according to voltage.

Low Voltage Injury

This is classified as less than 1000 V and includes UK standard domestic (240 V) and industrial (415 V) supplies. These can cause significant local contact injury, but rarely deep tissue damage. However, the path taken by the electrical current can cause significant morbidity. In the UK, household supply is 50 Hz alternating current, which is particularly dangerous to the human body, even at low currents. At 15 milliamperes (mA), muscles spasm and become tetanic, which may prevent release of the source. If the current runs across the chest, it can result in diaphragmatic paralysis and apnoea. A current of 60 mA in an adult or 30 mA in a child can induce ventricular fibrillation. Higher frequency current is safer, with medical diathermy operating at 100,000 Hz.

High Voltage Injury

This includes anything above 1000 V, with high tension power lines operating at 11,000 or 33,000 V, and substations even higher. At these levels, injury can occur via two methods. A high tension discharge or 'flash-over' ignites clothing and can result in deep dermal injury but without the formation of contact sites. High voltage current transmission results in full-thickness contact burns, along with deep tissue damage along the course of transmission. Muscle damage can be extensive and may result in the development of compartment syndrome requiring urgent fasciotomy. The damaged muscle also releases myoglobin, along with haemoglobin from red cell haemolysis. Both precipitate in renal tubules, and acute renal failure is a common complication.

Lightning Strike

This is an extremely high voltage, high amperage direct current of ultra-short duration. A direct strike is usually fatal, but a secondary deflection (e.g. from a tree) can result in injury. The current flows over the surface of the victim, typically resulting in partial-thickness burns, but little deep tissue damage. There may be deep exit burns on the feet. However, respiratory and subsequent asystolic cardiac arrest is common as a result of stunning of the medullary respiratory centres. This is potentially reversible, but resuscitation may be prolonged as paralysis can last up to 30 min [15].

Scene safety is of paramount importance, as high voltage electricity can arc several metres through soil, and several centimetres through air. Practitioners should confirm that the power source is inactive before attending to the casualty. A detailed history of the event and examination for contact points can give useful information as to the likely course of the current, and therefore tissues at risk. ECG changes are common, and patients should have three-lead monitoring for 24 h post-electrocution, as cardiac damage may take time to become evident [16]. Serial troponins can help identify true myocardial damage.

Pathophysiology

Burn injuries can be divided into different zones, reflecting the changes to the tissues involved. The standard description is Jackson's Burn Wound Model, which breaks an injury down into 3 regions (see Fig. 40.1) [17]. The central area is the *zone of coagulative necrosis*. There is immediate coagulation of cellular proteins, resulting in cell death and irreversible tissue damage. Surrounding this is the *zone of stasis*. Microcirculatory blood flow in this region is impaired, with reduced oxygen delivery resulting in tissue which is at risk of ischaemia. Much of the initial resuscitation, including fluid management, is directed at maintaining blood supply to this region and preventing extension of the injury. If inadequately treated, this will become necrotic due to the inflammatory reaction resulting from cellular injury. Beyond this is the *zone of hyperaemia*, with inflammatory mediators resulting in vasodilatation. In small injuries this will be evident as a warm, erythematous area around a burn. However, in burn injuries of >25% TBSA sufficient mediators are released that the zone of hyperaemia covers the rest of the body. Patients become generally vasodilated, which, if uncorrected, can result in significant hypoperfusion and extension of the burn injury.

Burns are classically classified by depth, as this describes the structures damaged by the injury [18]. Superficial partial-thickness injuries involve damage to the epidermis, with homogenous erythema, blistering, and pain. Deep partial-thickness burns have a lighter appearance, blisters, and a lower level of pain due to the destruction of some nerve fibres. These injuries have the potential for spontaneous healing as the dermis is at least partially preserved. Full-thickness burns involve the destruction of epidermis and dermis, including hair follicles, nerve endings and glands. The tissue is often white and leathery in texture. The wound is not painful due to neural destruction. Deep full thickness injuries include injury to deeper structures, including muscle, tendon and bone.

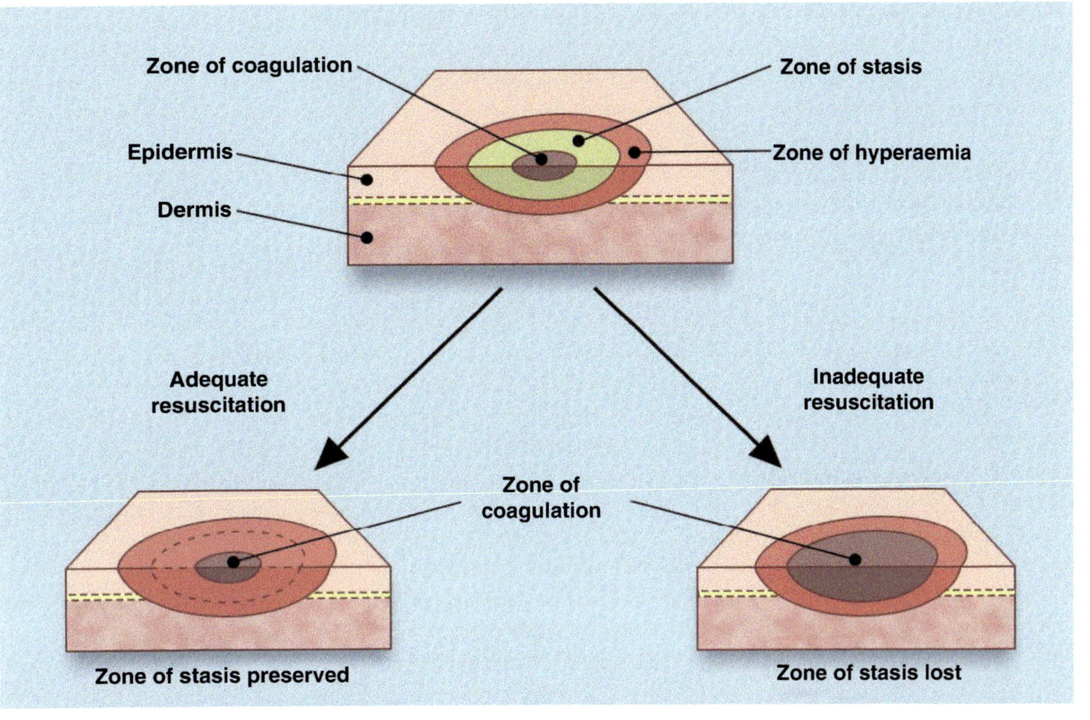

Fig. 40.1 Jackson's burns zones. Resuscitation may diminish the amount of tissue damage by restoring flow to the zone of stasis, but inadequate resuscitation may increase overall tissue damage

Burn Area Assessment

It is important to calculate the total body surface area affected by a burn, as well as estimation as to the amount of partial and full-thickness injury. Erythema is not burn, and should not be included in the calculation. There are several methods used for surface areas calculations.

- Serial halving allows rapid assessment of extensive confluent burns. For example, a 25% TBSA injury involves half of one half of the body.
- The Rule of Nines [19] divides the body into 11 areas of 9%: head, front and back of the chest, front and back of the abdomen, both thighs, both lower legs and both arms. The perineum makes up the remaining 1%. In children, this is modified depending on age. In younger children, the head is proportionally larger while the limbs are proportionally smaller.
- Palmer area can also be used, where the area covered by the patient's palm and closed fingers equates to ~1% of their TBSA. This is useful in more patchy injuries, although it tends to overestimate injury size [20].

Ideally, the extent of injury should be recorded on a dedicated burn assessment chart. The Lund Browder chart (Fig. 40.2) [21] uses a similar technique to the Rule of Nines, but with modifications for different age groups. Increasingly, novel technology is being used, including the Mersey Burns App [22], where the areas affected are coloured onto a template, and a TBSA automatically derived. It is vital to reassess the burn area on arrival at definitive care, as overestimation is common [23].

Referral Criteria for Specialist Review/Care

Within the UK, the British Burn Association has produced a list of burns requiring referral for review or discussion with a specialist burn ser-

Estimating percent Total Body Surface Area in Children Affected by Burns

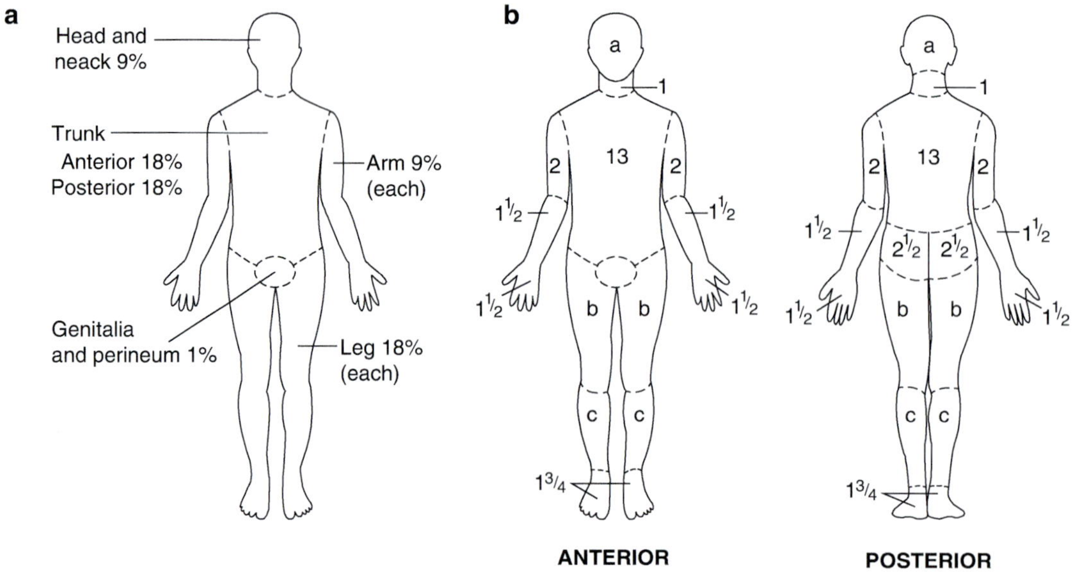

Relative percentage of body surface areas (% BSA) affected by growth

	0 yt	*1 yt*	*5 yt*	*10yt*	*15yt*
a— ½ *of head*	9½	8½	6½	5½	4½
b— ½ *of 1 thigh*	2¾	3¼	4	4¼	4½
c— ½ *of 1 lower leg*	2½	2½	2¾	3	3¼

Fig. 40.2 Lund Browder Chart for burn estimation (U.S. Department of Health and Human Services) (**a**) Wallace Rule of Nines burn estimation for adults (**b**) Lund and Browder chart for use in children

vice [24]. These centres can offer input across the full range of burns multi-disciplinary care, not just surgical services.

- All burns ≥2% TBSA in children or ≥3% TBSA in adults
- All full-thickness burns
- All circumferential burns
- Any burn not healed within 2 weeks
- Any burn with suspicion of non-accidental injury
- All burns to hands, feet, face, perineum or genitalia
- Any chemical, electrical or friction burn
- Any cold injury
- Any unwell/febrile child with a burn
- Any concerns regarding burn injuries and co-morbidities that may affect treatment or healing of the burn

Key Points
Burns are a common cause of injury and death worldwide.

Accurate assessment of the depth and size of injury helps determine treatment.

Patients with large or complex injuries should be referred to specialist burn centres.

Immediate Management

Initial Assessment

Scene safety is of paramount importance in the pre-hospital environment, and instructions from the fire and rescue services should be followed. Structures may be severely weakened by fire or explosion, and appropriate PPE should be worn.

An accurate history of the event is essential to help management. The nature of the burn, as well as the duration, allows estimation of the likely degree of injury. A history of entrapment or unconsciousness may suggest potential inhalation injury. Explosion, or jumping from height to escape can result in multiple other injuries, and these should be actively sought out. Exposure to chemicals may require formal decontamination, as well as enhanced PPE for the managing team, as well as notifying the receiving hospital.

Immediate first aid involves stopping the burning process and cooling with water for injuries up to 10% TBSA. This can effectively reduce the progression of the injury if undertaken within the first 3 h. In injuries over 10% TBSA, irrigation can result in profound hypothermia and is therefore discouraged. Burnt clothing, jewellery and piercings should be removed, and any burn covered in a non-adhesive sterile dressing. Clingfilm is an acceptable option.

Airway and Breathing: Assessment and Management

Inhalation of hot vapours, gases and products of combustion can result in injury to any level of the respiratory tract. It can also result in poisoning due to toxic gases, most notably carbon monoxide and cyanide. Explosions and rapid combustion, for example using petrol on a bonfire, often result in facial burns. A significant number of patients with facial burns also have an inhalation injury, but external blistering and superficial burns to the face do not themselves cause airway obstruction. Smoke inhalation is the most common cause of death within the first hour of a burn injury, and significant inhalation injury doubles burn mortality [25]. Of note, while 70% of inhalation injury patients present with facial burns, 70% of patients with facial burns do not incur significant pulmonary injury [26].

Airway Injuries Above the Larynx

These are generally related to inhalation of steam, or hot gases. Typically these are a result of an injury in an enclosed space, or entrapment. The major complication is related to tissue swelling and oedema, either following direct tissue injury or as a consequence of extensive volume fluid resuscitation for a large TBSA injury. Oedema reaches a peak 12–36 h post-injury. Management is principally supportive, with airway protection the priority.

Endotracheal intubation should be undertaken early, as delay may result in oedema making later attempts impossible. Laryngoscopy can be challenging, and a range of small, uncut tubes should be available. Swelling may cause compression or migration of ET tubes, so consideration should be given using a reinforced, uncut tube early. The laryngeal mucosa can be extremely fragile, so early use of a bougie can reduce the risk of airway obstruction. Suxamethonium is safe to use in the first 24 h post-injury. After this period, extra-junctional acetylcholine receptors develop with the risk of significant hyperkalaemia with subsequent suxamethonium administration. This risk can persist for up to a year following burn injury. Acutely, tissues may remain swollen for several days and head up positioning may be useful to reduce this. The upper airways are very efficient at heat conduction, so direct heat damage to the lower airways is rare.

Features that raise suspicion of an upper airway injury include

- Burns to the mouth, nose and pharynx
- Singed nasal hairs
- Carbonaceous sputum
- Change of voice
- Stridor
- Drooling
- Hoarse, brassy, productive cough
- Hypoxia and respiratory failure
- Extensive neck burns—these may cause external compression

Airway Injuries Below the Larynx

The inhalation of products of combustion produces these injuries. Fires produce multiple chemical compounds, including carbon monoxide and dioxide, ammonia, cyanide, hydrogen chloride, sulphur dioxide and complex organic compounds. Many of these are irritant and toxic and can produce acids or alkalis when they dissolve in lung tissue fluid. This can result in chemical burns to the lung parenchyma. Small soot particles damage airway mucosa, producing inflammatory mediators and reactive oxygen species. This can result in plugging of small airways, with distal collapse, as well as significant ulceration and mucosal sloughing. Lung parenchymal damage can also occur, with loss of surfactant, interstitial oedema, and development of acute respiratory distress syndrome (ARDS). Explosions can also result in pneumothorax and pneumomediastinum, and chest x-ray +/− CT is mandatory [27].

Patients with significant lower airway injuries are likely to require intubation and mechanical ventilation to manage their respiratory failure. Definitive diagnosis is by bronchoscopy, noting the presence of contamination, ulceration or sloughing (Table 40.5). If contamination is seen, the area should be irrigated with saline. This removes potentially irritant and obstructive material, as well as allowing assessment of the underlying mucosa. In severe injuries with extensive contamination, this may need to be repeated several times. Ventilation should follow ARDSnet principles, with tidal volumes of 6 ml/kg ideal body weight, and limited peak pressures. Nebulised heparin is used to prevent cast formation, while nebulised N-acetylcysteine helps mobilise secretions [29, 30]. Salbutamol is also used.

Table 40.5 Grading of inhalation injury by bronchoscopy [28]

Grade of injury	Severity of injury	Bronchoscopic features
Grade 0	No injury	Absence of carbonaceous deposits, erythema, oedema, bronchorrhoea or obstruction
Grade 1	Mild injury	Minor or patchy areas of erythema, carbonaceous deposits in proximal of distal bronchi
Grade 2	Moderate injury	Moderate degree of carbonaceous deposits, erythema, oedema, bronchorrhoea or obstruction
Grade 3	Severe injury	Severe inflammation with friability, copious carbonaceous deposits, bronchorrhoea, bronchial obstruction
Grade 4	Massive injury	Evidence of mucosal sloughing, necrosis, endoluminal obliteration

Carbon Monoxide Poisoning

Carbon monoxide (CO) is a colourless, odourless gas produced as a result of incomplete combustion of organic material. It avidly binds to haemoglobin, with an affinity 240 times that of oxygen. This results in reduced oxygen-carrying capacity and delivery of oxygen to tissues, with subsequent tissue hypoxia. CO also binds to the intracellular cytochrome system, resulting in abnormal cell functioning. Patients with an altered mental state after a burn injury should be assumed to have CO toxicity until proven otherwise (Table 40.6). Normal pulse oximeters cannot distinguish between oxy- and carboxyhaemoglobin and are of little use. Dissolved oxygen is unaffected, and PaO_2 remains normal. Co-oximeters are required for a formal diagnosis.

Carboxyhaemaglobin dissociates slowly, with a half-life of 250 minutes in air, and 40 minutes in 100% oxygen. Treatment is principally supportive, with 100% oxygen until carboxyhaemoglobin levels return to normal. Hyperbaric oxygen can be used but is rarely practical due to the scarcity of centres and the challenge of managing associated injuries. While scientifically attractive from first principles and some positive studies showing improvement of acute neurologi-

Table 40.6 Symptoms associated with varying levels of carboxyhaemaglobin [31]

Carboxyhaemaglobin in blood, %	Symptoms
0–10	None (may be normal for smokers)
20	Headache, shortness of breath on moderate exertion
30	Headache, irritability, fatigue, dizziness, impaired judgement
40–50	Severe headache, confusion, collapse
60–70	Unconsciousness, convulsions, death if exposure continues
>80	Rapidly fatal

cal symptoms [32–34], a 2011 Cochrane review concluded that there is insufficient evidence to support the use of hyperbaric oxygen for treatment of patients with carbon monoxide poisoning [35].

Cyanide Poisoning

Hydrogen cyanide is produced by burning plastics. Cyanide is rapidly absorbed, and binds to the cytochrome system, resulting in anaerobic metabolism. Symptoms of toxicity include loss of consciousness, cardiac instability, and convulsions. Blood cyanide levels are not readily available, so diagnosis is clinical. A persistently raised lactate despite adequate fluid resuscitation, along with a reduced arterial-venous oxygen gradient is suspicious for cyanide toxicity. Several antidote options exist for treatment, using one of three main methods.

Methemoglobin-Forming Agents

Cyanide has a higher affinity for ferric iron (Fe^{3+}) in methaemoglobin than ferrous iron (Fe^{2+}) in haemoglobin. Agents such as amyl nitrite, sodium nitrite and 4-dimethylaminophenol (4-DMAP) induce methaemoglobinaemia, chelating cyanide, and forming cyanomethaemoglobin. This is then excreted by the kidneys. These agents can have significant side effects including hypotension, cardiovascular instability and worsening hypoxia.

Sulphur Donors

The liver enzyme rhodanese converts cyanide into thiocyanate, which is much less toxic and is renally excreted. This reaction is accelerated by administration of sodium thiosulphate, which acts as a substrate. However, thiosulphate does not readily penetrate cells and mitochondria, and so its effectiveness is limited by delayed onset of action and short half-life.

Cobalt Compounds

Cyanide has a high affinity for cobalt, with rapid chelation. Dicobalt edetate is effective but is associated with severe hypertension, arrhythmias and anaphylaxis. It can also cause cobalt toxicity if administered with a false diagnosis of cyanide toxicity. Hydroxycobalamin combines with cyanide to form cyanocobalamin (Vitamin B12), which is renally excreted (Fig. 40.3). This is generally well tolerated, acts rapidly, and is the first choice in many centres, at a dose of 100 mg/kg. It can result in allergic reactions, headache, and skin discolouration.

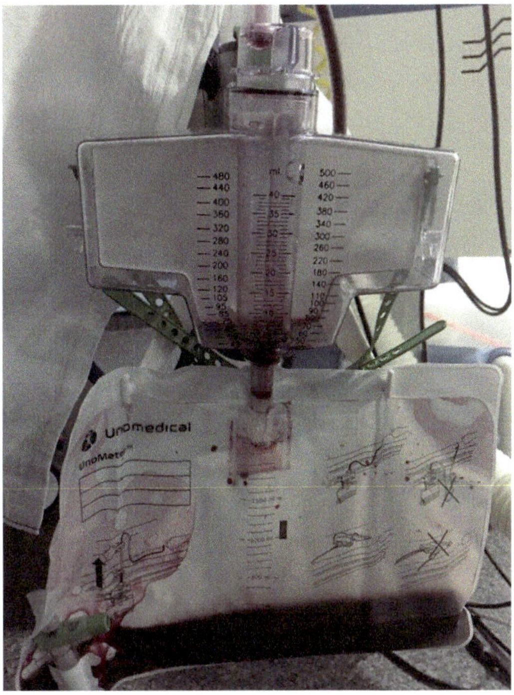

Fig. 40.3 Purple urine discolouration from treatment with hydroxycobalamin

Circulation

Burns do not cause immediate hypotension, so if present, the patient should be assumed to be bleeding until proven otherwise. Hypovolaemia does develop over several hours, partly due to fluid loss through burnt tissue, and partly as a result of inflammatory vasodilatation. Mediators including histamine, prostaglandins and bradykinin cause increased vascular permeability, with subsequent oedema formation. If the intravascular hypovolaemia is uncorrected, it can result in organ failure, particularly acute kidney injury.

Formal fluid resuscitation is required for all burns over 10% TBSA in children and 15% TBSA in adults. The most commonly used formula is the Parkland Formula, which gives a fluid volume for the first 24 h.

- 2–4 ml Hartmann's solution/kg/%TBSA burn
  - The first half is given in the first 8 h FROM THE TIME OF THE BURN
  - The second half is given in the remaining 16 h

In children, this should be in addition to maintenance fluids, which should be 5% glucose in 0.45% saline, with the volume calculated using the 4:2:1 rule.

The volume recommended for resuscitation is a guide. The most reliable measure of adequacy is urine output, which should be 0.5 ml/kg/h in adults, and 1 ml/kg/h in children. Accurate fluid balance is essential, and urinary catheterisation is required in injuries >10% TBSA. Hypotension, acidaemia or oliguria should be treated with fluid boluses. Initially these can be crystalloid, but in the event of refractory hypotension and oliguria, boluses of 20% human albumin may be of use. Vasopressors, typically noradrenaline, can also be used, but there is a suggestion this may lead to deepening of burn wounds, particularly if there is ongoing hypovolaemia. In major burns (>40% TBSA) both albumin and noradrenaline are usually required, but as long as there is an adequate urine output, a mean arterial pressure of 60 mmHg is often satisfactory. After the first 24 h, fluid therapy should be guided by urine output and end-organ perfusion. Excessive fluid administration can result in worsening oedema, ARDS, and intra-abdominal hypertension, which significantly increases mortality. Nasogastric feeding should be instigated early, and administration of extra crystalloid should be kept to a minimum.

Intravenous access and monitoring can be challenging in major injuries. Intraosseous devices are often used in prehospital care, but should be removed as soon as reasonably possible to minimise the risk of osteomyelitis. Intravenous lines should ideally be placed through unburnt skin, but this is not always possible. In large injuries, central venous access is often required. Groin creases are often relatively spared, although anatomy can be challenging. Ultrasound should be used for central access, and can be extremely helpful for peripheral access; however, visualisation through unexcised burn can be very poor. Venous cutdown may be necessary, most commonly using the saphenous veins. Securing lines is also important. Most adhesive dressings do not stick well to burnt skin, and suturing may be required, even for peripheral access. Poor adhesion is also a challenge with ECG monitoring, and skin staples may be required to gain electrical contact. Non-invasive blood pressure monitoring is inaccurate if there is significant oedema, and invasive arterial monitoring is often required. There is little evidence for the use of cardiac output monitoring in the management of major burns [36].

Circumferential Burns

Circumferential burns have the potential to constrict the underlying tissue. This typically occurs 12–48 h after the injury, due to shrinking of the burn eschar combined with generalised tissue oedema. Any circumferential injury must be carefully and regularly inspected for any sign of impaired distal perfusion. Circumferential chest burns can lead to respiratory failure, which may present as increasing ventilator pressures (these patients are highly likely to be intubated). Circumferential abdominal injuries can lead to intraabdominal compartment syndrome, renal and gut failure, and death. If there are signs of compression, then an escharotomy should be performed. This involves incision down onto healthy tissue, releasing the pressure within the tissues. These are emergency procedures and may be required in a non-specialist centre before transfer.

Analgesia

Burns are painful, and adequate analgesia is essential, using a multimodal method. Pain occurs both form the somatic damage, and from the re-innervation of damaged tissues. Paracetamol and NSAIDs are useful as baseline analgesia. Opioid drugs are often the mainstay of treatment, although somatic pain is not always responsive. Gabapentin and pregabalin are extremely useful, both with pain and itch, which is a common complication of burn healing. Dressing changes and physiotherapy often require a degree of procedural sedation or analgesia. Entonox and methoxyflurane (Penthrox) can both be used with good effect, although side effects limit the duration of use [37].

Thermoregulation

Major burn injury results in significant alterations to temperature regulation, compounded by a failure of normal temperature homeostasis. Burnt skin loses its insulating properties, which, when combined with excess fluid loss through the wound, results in rapid heat loss. Hypothermia is a common complication of major injuries, both in the pre-hospital environment and during hospital admission. This should be aggressively treated, as the development of hypothermia is associated with worse outcome. All efforts should be made to insulate patients, particularly during transfer, and active rewarming used if hypothermia does occur. Intravenous fluid should be warmed, particularly the large volumes given during initial resuscitation. It is essential to measure core temperature in patients with major burn injury, with appropriate methods including oesophageal or bladder thermometers. Invasive warming methods are sometimes used, with intravascular and oesophageal devices available.

The impaired ability to preserve heat is compounded by the resetting of the hypothalamic temperature above normal levels. In severe burns, core temperature will reset to 38–38.5 °C and is associated with increased catecholamine and cytokine production. Attempts to lower this temperature will result in excess heat loss and an increased metabolic rate. For this reason, patients should be cared for in thermally controlled environments, with the ambient temperature kept around 28–30 °C.

Nutrition

Major burn injury induces a profound catabolic state, with the body breaking down healthy muscle in an attempt to provide amino acids for healing. If nutritional demands are not met, patients lose lean body mass, their wounds do not heal, and mortality is dramatically increased [38–40]. It is essential to establish enteral feeding early, both to meet the nutritional demands, and to protect the gut mucosa. Curling's ulcers [41] are acute stress ulcers following major burn injury, and, if untreated, carry high mortality from associated haemorrhage. Early enteral feeding, combined with proton pump inhibitors, has massively reduced the incidence.

Patients with severe burns should have a nasogastric tube inserted and feed started as soon as possible. Ileus is common, and prokinetics may be required. Patients should be weighed on admission, and this should be repeated regularly. Patients are often nutritionally depleted before their injury, and supplementation of B-vitamins and trace elements are frequently required. It is essential to calculate the caloric requirements, which are higher than non-burn patients. Several formulae are used, with the Harris-Benedict equation being most commonly used for adults [42]. It is essential to get early dietician involvement, as the consequences of inadequate nutrition can be disastrous.

Infection

Sepsis is the primary cause of death in patients with burns who survive over 48 h [43]. Burn wounds rapidly become colonised with micro-organisms. Common pathogens include *Streptococcus, S. aureus, Pseudomonas, Enterobacter, Enterococcus, Acinetobacter* and *Stenotrophomonas. Streptococcus* is of particular concern as it produces streptokinase, which results in skin graft failure. Swabs should be taken from all wounds on admission and repeated regularly. Diagnosis of infection (as opposed to colonisation) can be extremely challenging, as features such as tachycardia, neutrophilia, pyrexia and raised inflammatory markers all occur as a response to major burn injury. Concerning features include worsening pyrexia or hypothermia, progressive tachycardia or tachypnoea, thrombocytopenia, and hyperglycaemia. Wounds should be regularly examined for overt evidence of infection, with fluid and tissue cultures sent if there is a clinical concern. Antibiotic therapy should be targeted towards positive culture results, as the development of antibiotic resistance is common.

Hypermetabolism

Significant burn injuries induce a profound hypermetabolic state, which can last for months to years. The resting metabolic rate increase by 160–200% and patients become persistently tachycardic, pyrexial, and catabolic. While early excision of burn wounds attenuates this response, it is essential to ensure adequate nutrition [44]. Propranolol is used to reduce resting heart rate, energy expenditure and muscle catabolism [45, 46]. Oxandrolone, an anabolic steroid, is also shown to improve outcomes [47].

Definitive Management

The principle treatment of full-thickness burns is excision and grafting. Partial-thickness injuries may heal spontaneously, but for extensive deep partial-thickness burns surgery is usually required. Modern methods involve early excision, aiming to completely remove the burn eschar within the first 5 days [48]. Removal of the burn reduces the inflammatory load, as well as removing a focus for infection. This has traditionally been done using surgical knife excision, but newer techniques include the use of bromelain-based enzymatic dressings to selectively debride dead tissue [49]. Excision of extensive burns results in significant blood loss and is often complicated by hypothermia. The wounds are generally covered with cadaveric skin, xenograft or skin substitutes, with split skin autografting being used later to provide definitive coverage. In extensive injuries (>70% TBSA) this process can be prolonged over several weeks.

Longterm Sequalae

Burn injury is a significant cause of morbidity, with the risk of permanent disability around ten times the risk of death. Hospital stay following a significant burn is usually around 1 day per %TBSA, although it may be much longer. Recovery from a major burn is often protracted and may require lifelong input from burns services. Scar management can require multiple operations, particularly if sustained in childhood before growth is complete. Burn survivors may require ongoing input from occupational and physiotherapists, as well as psychological support. Prompt and effective management of the acutely burnt patient can help reduce this burden of disease.

Key Points

It is essential to assess for signs of inhalation injury, and, if required, the airway should be secured early.

Carbon monoxide and cyanide poisoning should be considered in patients with significant smoke inhalation.

Appropriate fluid resuscitation (e.g. using Parkland formula) should be started in burns over 10% TBSA in children and 15% TBSA in adults.

Escarotomies may be required for circumferential burns, and are a surgical emergency.

Patients with significant burn injury should be transferred to specialist burn centres once initial stabilization is completed.

Summary

Thermal injuries are an important cause of morbidity and mortality worldwide. When they occur, prompt assessment and treatment are essential to give patients the best chance of a good outcome. A good understanding of the pathophysiology of thermal injury helps guide the management of these complex patients. While many of them may require specialist care, appropriate pre-hospital and primary facility treatment can help reduce long term sequalae.

Questions

1. The following are all features of severe hypothermia except:
   (a) bradycardia
   (b) increased urine output
   (c) atrial fibrillation
   (d) tachypnoea
   (e) coagulopathy
2. Concerning rewarming in hypothermia
   (a) Active warming methods are usually required for Stage 1 hypothermia
   (b) Central rewarming causes afterdrop
   (c) Forced air warming is highly effective
   (d) Fluid resuscitation is rarely required in severe hypothermia
   (e) ECMO can rewarm patients at up to 9°C per hour
3. Concerning frostbite
   (a) affected areas should be slowly rewarmed
   (b) cell damage is caused by ice crystal formation in the tissues
   (c) amputation of affected areas is inevitable
   (d) it is exquisitely painful as it occurs
   (e) affected areas become coagulopathic as they thaw
4. The following burns all require referral to a specialist centre except
   (a) a burn to the perineum
   (b) circumferential burns
   (c) a burn that has not healed within 1 week
   (d) a chemical burn
   (e) an electrical burn
5. Concerning inhalation injuries
   (a) ARDS is a rare complication
   (b) cyanide poisoning is treated with hyperbaric oxygen
   (c) most patients with facial burns have a significant lung injury
   (d) broncheo-alveolar lavage should be avoided
   (e) bronchoscopy provides definitive diagnosis

Answers

1. d
2. e
3. b
4. c
5. e

References

1. Zafren K, Giesbrecht GG, Danzl DF, Brugger H, Sagalyn EB, Walpoth B, et al. Wilderness medical society practice guidelines for the out-of-hospital evaluation and treatment of accidental hypothermia: 2014 update. Wilderness Environ Med. 2014 Dec;25(4):S66–85.
2. Balvers K, Van der Horst M, Graumans M, Boer C, Binnekade J, Goslings JC, et al. Hypothermia as a predictor for mortality in trauma patients at admittance to the intensive care unit. J Emerg Trauma Shock. 2016;9(3):97.
3. Brown DJA, Brugger H, Boyd J, Paal P. Accidental hypothermia. N Engl J Med. 2012 Nov 15;367(20):1930–8.
4. Durrer B, Brugger H, Syme D. The medical on-site treatment of hypothermia: ICAR-MEDCOM recommendation. High Alt Med Biol. 2003 Mar;4(1):99–103.
5. McIntosh SE, Freer L, Grissom CK, Auerbach PS, Rodway GW, Cochran A, et al. Wilderness medical society practice guidelines for the prevention and treatment of frostbite: 2019 update. Wilderness Environ Med. 2019 July;30:S19–32.
6. Nolan J. Resuscitation council (Great Britain). Advanced life support. 2016.
7. Handford C, Buxton P, Russell K, Imray CE, McIntosh SE, Freer L, et al. Frostbite: a practical approach to hospital management. Extrem Physiol Med. 2014;3(1):7.
8. Gonzaga T, Jenabzadeh K, Anderson CP, Mohr WJ, Endorf FW, Ahrenholz DH. Use of intra-arterial thrombolytic therapy for acute treatment of frostbite in 62 patients with review of thrombolytic therapy in frostbite. J Burn Care Res. 2016;37(4):e323–34.
9. Epstein Y, Yanovich R. Heatstroke. N Engl J Med. 2019 June 20;380(25):2449–59.
10. Lipman GS, Gaudio FG, Eifling KP, Ellis MA, Otten EM, Grissom CK. Wilderness medical society practice guidelines for the prevention and treatment of heat illness: 2019 update. Wilderness Environ Med. 2019 June;30(4S):S33–46.
11. Mathers C, Fat DM, Boerma JT, World Health Organization, editors. The global burden of disease: 2004 update. Geneva, Switzerland: World Health Organization; 2008.
12. Stylianou N, Buchan I, Dunn KW. A review of the international burn injury database (iBID) for England

and Wales: descriptive analysis of burn injuries 2003-2011. BMJ Open. 2015 Feb 27;5(2):e006184.
13. Moritz AR, Henriques FC. Studies of thermal injury: II. The relative importance of time and surface temperature in the causation of cutaneous burns. Am J Pathol. 1947 Sep;23(5):695–720.
14. Alexander KS, Wasiak J, Cleland H. Chemical burns: diphoterine untangled. Burns. 2018 Jun;44(4):752–66.
15. Muehlberger T, Vogt PM, Munster AM. The long-term consequences of lightning injuries. Burns. 2001 Dec;27(8):829–33.
16. Pfortmueller CA, Yikun Y, Haberkern M, Wuest E, Zimmermann H, Exadaktylos AK. Injuries, sequelae, and treatment of lightning-induced injuries: 10 years of experience at a Swiss trauma center. Emerg Med Int. 2012;2012:1–6.
17. Hettiaratchy S, Dziewulski P. Pathophysiology and types of burns. BMJ. 2004 June 12;328(7453):1427–9.
18. Jackson DM. The diagnosis of the depth of burning. Br J Surg. 1953 May;40(164):588–96.
19. Knaysi GA, Crikelair GF, Cosman B. The role of nines: its history and accuracy. Plast Reconstr Surg. 1968 Jun;41(6):560–3.
20. Amirsheybani HR, Crecelius GM, Timothy NH, Pfeiffer M, Saggers GC, Manders EK. The natural history of the growth of the hand: I. Hand area as a percentage of body surface area. Plast Reconstr Surg. 2001 Mar;107(3):726–33.
21. Minimas D. A critical evaluation of the Lund and Browder chart. Wounds UK. 2007;3(3):58–68.
22. Barnes J, Duffy A, Hamnett N, McPhail J, Seaton C, Shokrollahi K, et al. The Mersey burns app: evolving a model of validation. Emerg Med J. 2015 Aug;32(8):637–41.
23. Hammond JS, Ward CG. Transfers from emergency room to burn center: errors in burn size estimate. J Trauma. 1987 Oct;27(10):1161–5.
24. National Network for Burn Care (NNBC). National Burn Care Referral Guidance-2012.pdf [Internet]. 2012 [cited 2019 Aug 30]. Available from: https://www.britishburnassociation.org/wp-content/uploads/2018/02/National-Burn-Care-Referral-Guidance-2012.pdf
25. Smith DL, Cairns BA, Ramadan F, Dalston JS, Fakhry SM, Rutledge R, et al. Effect of inhalation injury, burn size, and age on mortality: a study of 1447 consecutive burn patients. J Trauma. 1994 Oct;37(4):655–9.
26. Moylan JA. Inhalation injury—a primary determinant of survival following major bums. J Burn Care Rehab. 1981 Mar;2(2):78–85.
27. Foncerrada G, Culnan DM, Capek KD, González-Trejo S, Cambiaso-Daniel J, Woodson LC, et al. Inhalation injury in the burned patient. Ann Plastic Surg. 2018 Feb;80:S98–S105.
28. Albright JM, Davis CS, Bird MD, Ramirez L, Kim H, Burnham EL, et al. The acute pulmonary inflammatory response to the graded severity of smoke inhalation injury. Crit Care Med. 2012 Apr;40(4):1113–21.
29. Miller AC, Rivero A, Ziad S, Smith DJ, Elamin EM. Influence of nebulized unfractionated heparin and N-acetylcysteine in acute lung injury after smoke inhalation injury. J Burn Care Res. 2009 Mar;30(2):249–56.
30. Endorf FW, Gamelli RL. Inhalation injury, pulmonary perturbations, and fluid resuscitation. J Burn Care Res. 2007 Jan;28(1):80–3.
31. Winter PM. Carbon monoxide poisoning. JAMA. 1976 Sep 27;236(13):1502.
32. Coric V, Oren DA, Wolkenberg FA, Kravitz RE. Carbon monoxide poisoning and treatment with hyperbaric oxygen in the subacute phase. J Neurol Neurosurg Psychiatry. 1998 Aug 1;65(2):245–7.
33. Weaver LK, Hopkins RO, Chan KJ, Churchill S, Elliott CG, Clemmer TP, et al. Hyperbaric oxygen for acute carbon monoxide poisoning. N Engl J Med. 2002 Oct 3;347(14):1057–67.
34. Weaver LK. Hyperbaric oxygen therapy for carbon monoxide poisoning. Undersea Hyperb Med. 2014 Aug;41(4):339–54.
35. Buckley NA, Juurlink DN, Isbister G, Bennett MH, Lavonas EJ. Hyperbaric oxygen for carbon monoxide poisoning. Cochrane Injuries Group, editor. Cochrane Database of Systematic Reviews [Internet]. 2011 Apr 13 [cited 2019 Dec 7]; Available from: http://doi.wiley.com/10.1002/14651858.CD002041.pub3
36. Holm C, Mayr M, Tegeler J, Hörbrand F, Henckel von Donnersmarck G, Mühlbauer W, et al. A clinical randomized study on the effects of invasive monitoring on burn shock resuscitation. Burns. 2004 Dec;30(8):798–807.
37. Griggs C, Goverman J, Bittner EA, Levi B. Sedation and pain management in burn patients. Clin Plast Surg. 2017 July;44(3):535–40.
38. Newsome TW, Mason AD, Pruitt BA. Weight loss following thermal injury. Ann Surg. 1973 Aug;178(2):215–7.
39. Mosier MJ, Pham TN, Klein MB, Gibran NS, Arnoldo BD, Gamelli RL, et al. Early enteral nutrition in burns: compliance with guidelines and associated outcomes in a multicenter study. J Burn Care Res. 2011 Jan;32(1):104–9.
40. Rousseau A-F, Losser M-R, Ichai C, Berger MM. ESPEN endorsed recommendations: nutritional therapy in major burns. Clin Nutr. 2013 Aug;32(4):497–502.
41. Curling TB. On acute ulceration of the duodenum, in cases of burn. Med Chir Trans. 1842 Jan;25(1):260–81.
42. Harris JA, Benedict FG. A biometric study of human basal metabolism. Proc Natl Acad Sci. 1918 Dec 1;4(12):370–3.
43. Greenhalgh DG, Saffle JR, Holmes JH, Gamelli RL, Palmieri TL, Horton JW, et al. American Burn Association consensus conference to define sepsis and infection in burns. J Burn Care Res. 2007 Nov;28(6):776–90.
44. Hart DW, Wolf SE, Chinkes DL, Beauford RB, Mlcak RP, Heggers JP, et al. Effects of early excision and aggressive enteral feeding on hypermetabolism, catabolism, and sepsis after severe burn. J Trauma. 2003 Apr;54(4):755–64.

45. Herndon DN, Hart DW, Wolf SE, Chinkes DL, Wolfe RR. Reversal of catabolism by Beta-blockade after severe burns. N Engl J Med. 2001 Oct 25;345(17):1223–9.
46. Arbabi S, Ahrns KS, Wahl WL, Hemmila MR, Wang SC, Brandt M-M, et al. Beta-blocker use is associated with improved outcomes in adult burn patients. J Trauma. 2004 Feb;56(2):265–71.
47. Wolf SE, Edelman LS, Kemalyan N, Donison L, Cross J, Underwood M, et al. Effects of oxandrolone on outcome measures in the severely burned: a multicenter prospective randomized double-blind trial. J Burn Care Res. 2006 Mar;27(2):131–9.
48. Janzekovic Z. A new concept in the early excision and immediate grafting of burns. J Trauma. 1970 Dec;10(12):1103–8.
49. Cordts T, Horter J, Vogelpohl J, Kremer T, Kneser U, Hernekamp J-F. Enzymatic debridement for the treatment of severely burned upper extremities – early single center experiences. BMC Dermatol. 2016 Dec;16(1):8.

Environmental Trauma: CBRN Incidents

41

Sam Todd, Steven Bland, and Jonathan Ritson

1. To introduce the general principles of CBRN casualty care.
2. Appreciate the 'all hazards' approach to CBRN casualties.
3. Discuss the challenges of providing casualty care in a CBRN environment.
4. Highlight specialist resources available to the general clinician.

Introduction

The threat of chemical, biological, radiological and nuclear (CBRN) agents present challenges to clinical care both in the rare syndromes they cause patients to suffer in isolation or combined with injury, and in the limitations that the use of personal protective equipment (PPE) causes responders. The latter is due to the residual risk from a contaminated or contagious patient.

Historically, the threat from CBRN agents has been mainly within the military context. The release of the nerve agent sarin on the Tokyo underground in 1995 [1], the 2001 Anthrax letters [2] and the use of CBRN substances as a method for assassination [3] mean civil responders should also be aware of these threats and the risk from them. Despite different military and civilian operational environments, the principles of CBRN casualty care are the same. In addition, the same principles and use of PPE can also be applied during non-malicious events such as hazardous material (HAZMAT) incidents including chemical suicide [4], and outbreak response, e.g. Ebola (2014-5) and COVID-19 reflecting the all-hazards approach.

Learning Objective
The objectives of civilian and military CBRN casualty (patient) care can be described as:

1. The management of any casualty, including trauma, in a CBRN environment.
2. The management of a CBRN casualty from the point of exposure through to rehabilitation.

This chapter seeks to describe the general principles that can be applied by any medical response to a CBRN incident, namely:

S. Todd (✉)
Emergency Medicine Department, Addenbrookes Hospital, Cambridge, UK

Tactical Medical Wing, Royal Air Force, Brize Norton, Oxfordshire, UK
e-mail: samuel.todd@nhs.net

S. Bland
Queen Alexandra Hospital, Portsmouth Hospitals NHS Trust, Portsmouth, UK

Royal Navy, Portsmouth, UK

J. Ritson
Addenbrooke's Hospital, Cambridge University Hospitals NHS Foundation Trust, Cambridge, UK

Royal Navy, Portsmouth, UK
e-mail: J.ritson@nhs.net

P. Lax (ed.), *Textbook of Acute Trauma Care*, https://doi.org/10.1007/978-3-030-83628-3_41

1. Recognise a CBRN incident has occurred.
2. Enable responders to protect themselves and others.
3. Provide clinical care effectively.

Types of Hazard

The main groups of hazards that will be discussed in this chapter are:

- Chemical
- Biological, including biological warfare agents, endemic and emerging diseases
- Radiological (i.e. any non-nuclear hazards causing ionising radiation)
- Nuclear
- Explosives and blast (where these overlap with CBRN)

The military all-hazards (CBRNE3T) approach describes CBRN and explosives within the broader context of environmental hazards including extremes of temperature, endemic disease and conventional trauma [5].

General Considerations of CBRN Casualty Care

There are two principle considerations in the management of a casualty within a CBRN environment.

1. The impact this has on what immediate care can be provided safely and effectively, and the subsequent limitations placed on medical responders.
2. The management of casualties who are exhibiting signs and symptoms of CBRN exposure (toxidrome), this includes specific clinical care (including antidotes) and also hazard management to protect staff and other patients in downstream care.

Casualty Management Within a CBRN Environment

Principles of CBRN Casualty care [6]

The central tenets of CBRN casualty care are:

- Recognition of a CBRN casualty or incident
- Personal safety including cordons and personal protective equipment (PPE)
- First aid
- Triage
- Life-saving interventions
- Casualty hazard management including decontamination and isolation
- Advanced medical care
- Rehabilitation

Recognition of CBRN Incidents

This can be challenging in isolation but even more so in the context of the injured patient where physiology is likely to be abnormal, and the exact history of events may not be immediately apparent.

Overt CBRN incidents (e.g. incidents involving vehicles carrying hazardous material) are more likely to be chemical incidents with early symptoms and signs. In contrast, covert incidents are more likely to be radiological (unless detected) and biological with delayed onset features due to a longer latency or incubation period.

Scenario A: Chemical Suicide

You have been called as part of the statutory emergency response to a person unresponsive in a car. When approaching the vehicle, you notice a number of large plastic containers in the front passenger seat, some of which have labels that show UN label 6 'Poison' (below).

Using the all-hazards approach, you reflect that the patient shows signs of *Intoxication* and that the closed atmosphere in the car represents a hazard to you as the rescuer.

You call for assistance from specialist rescuers who are able to use positive-pressure respiratory equipment that protects them from the atmosphere within the car whilst removing the casualty for assessment.

Consider: In your area, who would the specialist rescuers be and how would you get ask them to attend an incident?

On recognition, consider the six C's:

- Confirm (hazard and type of incident)
- Clear (upwind and uphill)
- Cordon (set up hazards zones (see below) and clean/dirty line)
- Control (control of the scene, cordon entry and exit and hazard spread)
- Communicate (tell Command, responders and receiving hospitals)
- Contain (contain the hazard, risk assess for casualty hazard management)

The critical step is to always consider a CBRN incident in the list of differential diagnoses, even if subsequently discarded as more likely causes of illness and injury come to light.

Throughout the patient's clinical course, recognition will rely on the close working between different agencies (law enforcement, healthcare, fire and rescue, military etc.) and various clinical specialities within the hospital and after discharge.

In the initial phases, the term 'STEP 1-2-3 plus' has been coined to provide an *aide-memoire* for the recognition of CBRN events.

1. If one patient incapacitated with no apparent cause, proceed as usual (see below)
2. If two patients incapacitated with no apparent cause, approach with caution
3. If three or more patients incapacitated use caution and adopt the following approach:
   (a) Evacuate people from the scene
   (b) Communicate and advise the patient what is happening
   (c) Disrobe
   (d) Decontaminate

When assessing a patient, the following signs or symptoms should cause clinicians to consider CBRN incidents within the differential diagnosis:

- Airway irritation or cough
- Difficulty in breathing
- Eye pain, altered vision or altered pupil size
- Headaches
- Seizures (especially in multiple patients)
- Non-thermal burns

Later in the clinical pathway, it may be that laboratory investigations highlight pathology or that a pattern of illness or injury is identified that raises concern for a CBRN incident.

Case Study 1: Novichok, Salisbury [7, 8]

In March 2018, two Russian nationals were admitted to hospital in Salisbury UK having been found unconscious in a public area.

The initial presentation was of depressed conscious level and respiratory failure, which failed to respond to treatment for opiate overdose (naloxone).

As the clinical picture evolved, it became clear that poisoning with a novel nerve agent (Novichok, A-234). This was partly due to the clinical toxidrome, supported by laboratory investigations including measuring serum anti-cholinesterase levels.

Learning point: Some toxidromes are difficult to identify without specialist tests, but a generic approach using the CRESS assessment tool allows prompt supportive treatment.

For some incidents, the agent may be obvious due to the route of exposure, rapid onset and obvious toxidrome. Some agents, however, especially if ingested or absorbed through the skin, have a slower onset and the toxidrome may not be initially obvious or may be non-specific (e.g. ricin). In these cases, environmental (scene) detection, identification and monitoring (DIM) or clinical investigations such as laboratory investigations are vital both for clinical management and collecting evidence for the criminal investigation.

Safety Considerations

In general, the multiply injured trauma patient presents a low hazard to treating clinical staff. This is in contrast to the CBRN casualty, who may be either contaminated or contagious and therefore may represent a considerable danger to other patients and staff.

To manage this hazard, as well as the conventional major incident zones (see Mass Casualty Incidents Chapter) used to control the scene, and marshal personnel including media and onlookers, CBRN incidents are typically divided into three hazard zones (see Fig. 41.1):

- *Hot zone*
  There is a direct hazard from the environment.
- *Warm zone*
  There is a residual risk from personnel, equipment and casualties (alive or dead). The warm zone is the area in which decontamination is carried out.
- *Cold zone*
  This is considered 'clean', where decontamination has been carried out and hazard is low. The cold zone is separated from the warm zone by a clean-dirty line (CDL), which requires careful management.

Decontamination of patients will be discussed later in 'Casualty Hazard Management'.

Management of CBRN Casualties

First Aid

This will vary according to the patient's context. In civilian practice it may be limited to providing reassurance or following instructions from an emergency call handler.

Treatment by specialist teams, emergency responders or in military practice may include administering an antidote and other medications intra-muscularly using devices such as autoinjectors (Fig. 41.2). This may be by non-

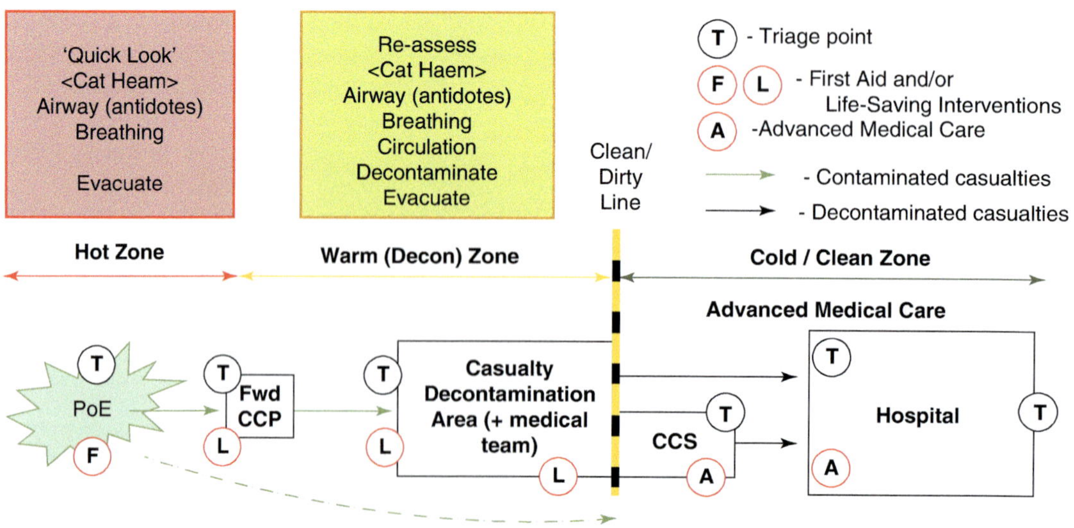

(Fwd) CCP – (Forward) Casualty Collection Point **CCS** – Casualty Clearing Station
Role 2/3 MTF – Medical Treatment Facility (including R2-Afloat, R2-Light Manoeuvre and R2-Enhanced)

Fig. 41.1 Configuration of an incident with hot, warm and cold zones for treatment

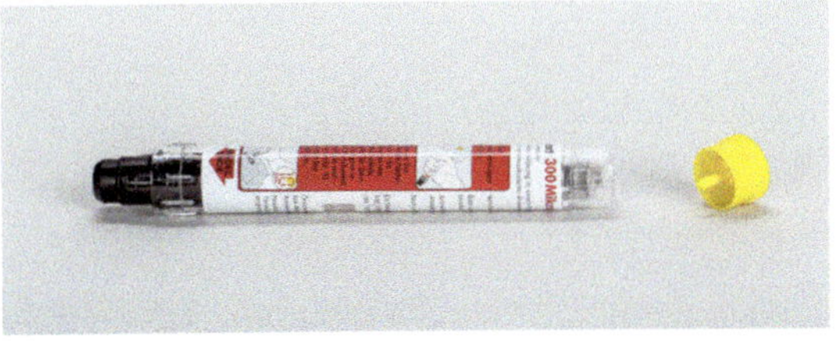

Fig. 41.2 Example of an Autoinjector which may be self-administered or given by rescuers in CBRN incidents (© CEphoto, Uwe Aranas)

medical personnel (e.g. military or law-enforcement personnel) under emergency use medicines regulations or other regulatory frameworks.

Being aware of treatments given prior to medical care is vital to allow individualised care.

Primary Survey (Identification of Life-Threatening Conditions)

Conventional medical education describes a stepwise approach to the injured patient. This can be carried out sequentially (vertical resuscitation) in resource-poor environments or by multiple practitioners simultaneously (horizontal resuscitation) in resource-rich environments, led by a team leader who directs overall clinical care [9].

There is no need to deviate from standard clinical practice for CBRN casualties; however, some additional points arise that are worth considering when using this adapted 'MABCDE' approach, highlighted in bold below.

M—Massive haemorrhage
A—Airway management

- **a—Antidote administration**

B—Breathing
C—Circulation **(including fluids for sepsis management)**
D—Disability, **especially seizures**

- **d—Decontamination**

E—Evacuation to warm or clean zone

In CBRN events, there are several toxidromes and conditions that are of significance due to lethality and/or the fact that they may be treatable. These are:

- Nerve agents (cholinergic syndrome)
- Blistering agents
- Pulmonary agents
- Chemical asphyxiants including cyanide and hydrogen sulphide
- Mental incapacitants such as opioids including high potency narcotics (similarities to nerve agent toxidrome), and some psychotropic agents
- Physical incapacitant including short-acting riot control agents (e.g. CS or pepper spray)
- Iatrogenic (antidote overdose or misuse)
- Heatstroke (especially if wearing PPE)
- Sepsis
- Botulinum (anticholinergic type toxidrome)
- Acute radiation syndrome—prodromal stage

These can all be identified by focusing on five key clinical signs; **CRESS**—Conscious level, Respiratory pattern, Eyes (pupils), Secretions and Skin as well as some other associated features. The relevant findings and associated toxidromes are included in Fig. 41.3, below. Key management points for significant agents are addressed later in the chapter.

Life-Saving Interventions

In CBRN casualties there are four groups of signs and symptoms to be alert to and provide treatment for. These are grouped as the 'four Is':

- **Intoxication** caused by chemical agents or toxins (chemical agents of biological origin)
- **Infection** caused by a live micro-organism
- **Irradiation**
- **Injuries** (as part of the all-hazards approach and combined casualties)

In terms of life-saving intervention, for CBRN casualties this includes antidote administration (discussed later), and supportive medical care. Supportive care includes the same approach that one may take with any medically unwell patient; opening the airway, reversing hypoxia and supporting the circulation.

Extended CRESS	Nerve agent	Vesicants (blistering agents)	Pulmonary agents	Cyanide / Hydrogen sulphide	Met-Hb	Opioids	Atropine	Sepsis	Botulinum toxin	Heat stroke
	THIS LIST IS NOT EXHAUSTIVE AND ALL FEATURES MAY BE PRESENT									
Consciousness	Convulsions	Normal	Normal / Agitated	Unconscious / Convulsions	Agitated	Reduced → Unconscious	Agutated / Confused	Normal, reduced or altered	Normal	Altered
Respiration	Increased or reduced → stopped	Normal / Increased	Increased	Increased or stopped	Normal / Increased	Reduced → stoppped	Increased	Increased	Reduced	Increased
Eyes	Pinpoint pupils*	Normal / Inflamed	Normal / Inflamed	Normal / Diated pupils	Normal	Pinpoint pupils	Dilated pupils / Blurred vision	Normal	Dilated pupils / Blurred vision	Normal / Diated pupils
Secretions	Increased*	Normal / Increased	Increased / Pink tinged sputum	Normal	Normal	Normal	Dey mouth / Thirsty	Normal / Sputum	Dey mouth / Thirsty	Normal
Skin	Sweaty	Red / Blistered	Cyanosed	Pink → cyanosed	Cyanosed	Normal / Cyanosed	Flushed / Dry	Warm → pale Non-blanching rash	Flushed / Dry	Varied
Other features	Altered vision headache Vomiting Incontinence Slow pulse	**Rapid:** Caustic agent, Lewisite **Delayed (6-24h):** Sulphur mustard		Sudden onset Arterialised venous blood Raised lactate	Chocolate coloured blood No improved cyanosis or O_2 saturations with oxygen	Chest wall rigidity / myoclonus associated with fentanyis	Tachycardia	Fast pulse Fever (>38.3°C) Bio-syndrome ♦ Hypotension (>100mmHg) / No radial pulse	Descending paralysis incl. ptosis and dysphagia	High temperature (>38°C)
Initial treatment	Astropine Oxime Benzodiazepine	**Lewisite:** Chelating agents **HF:** Calcium	Supportive	See local guidance	Methylene blue	Naloxone	Supportive (physostigmine)	Sepsis Six	Botulinum antitoxin	Urgrnt cooling Supportive

* Pinpoint pupils (and/or increased secretions) may be delayed if skin absorption or eye protection worn.
♦ 'Bio-syndromes' include: respiratory, cutaneous (skin), lymphadenopathy, haemorrhagic, gastrointestinal, and neurological (central & peripherall).
2016 Criteria for sepsis: 2 of 3 - altered conscious level; respiratory rate ≥ 22; or systolic blood pressure < 100mmhg ± non-blanching rash (additional NATO criterion)
[see AmedP-7.1 Part 4]. Consider SEPTIC SHOCK if blood pressure < 90mmHg or no radial pulse.

Fig. 41.3 Common clinical signs of toxidromes that may be encountered in CBRN

Casualty Hazard Management

A generic approach to staff safety and clinical care will mitigate much of the risk to rescuers and other patients to allow first aid and immediate resuscitation to be carried out.

Standard contact precautions (apron, nitrile gloves, hand hygiene) with additional respiratory eye protection may be required, or alternately, specialised PPE. The removal of the patient's clothing will reduce any potential hazard from the casualty by around 90% [10]. This will permit CBRN emergency medical treatment of patients triaged as severe and requiring life-saving interventions. PPE choice and method of casualty decontamination for HAZMAT incidents may be informed by transportation/carrier information or manifest. It is better to assume the worse and then step down in the level of PPE and decontamination requirements. In vehicles which are carrying hazardous material, a four-digit UN number must be displayed prominently [11]. There are multiple applications and databases that can give specific information on what the chemical is, hazards associated with it and the necessary PPE and decontamination requirements for operating around it.

Beyond this, and after life-saving interventions have been carried out, a risk: benefit analysis should be performed between the benefits of 'full' decontamination versus the delay this may introduce before further medical care. Additional decontamination may be achieved using absorbing material and wet decontamination (rinse) methods. However, the technique used will depend on the agent's characteristics (e.g. chemical, caustic, live biological) and physical properties (e.g. volatility, particulate).

Decontamination can be considered to have three phases in the clinical setting:

Dry decontamination

Use absorbent material, such as paper towels, to carefully dab or brush off liquid or solid contaminant.

Wet decontamination

Use copious amounts of water at 35 °C to shower for up to 90 s. Pay particular attention to wounds to dilute any contamination.

*Surgical debridement*Remove devitalised tissue from wounds to reduce the bacterial load and any residual hazard from CBRN agents.

Advanced Medical Care

Advanced medical care is divided into:

- Supportive (non-specific and symptomatic-related); and
- Definitive (agent-specific and include antidotes, specific antibiotics and anti-toxins).

This will be outlined for some specific threats (chemical vs biological vs radiological and nuclear) in a later part of the chapter.

Rehabilitation

CBRN rehabilitation includes physical, mental and social elements. The physical rehabilitation of patients following CBRN exposure is very individual. It will relate to the type of exposure that they had and consequences of treatment (e.g. prolonged stay on critical care).

As an example, the long-term management of chemical burns and eye lesions after exposure to sulphur mustard will require a multi-disciplinary approach similar to that required for thermal burns.

Any CBRN exposure may also have a significant psychological impact on the patient. There is limited evidence to support any particular strategy, and so conventional care should be offered.

Given the low frequency of CBRN events, patients who have been affected are likely to be the subject of increased media and public attention, and this should be considered when planning care to minimise additional harm to the patient or their family.

Learning Objective
Assessing the Scene and the All-Hazards Approach

Many large international bodies recommend the all-hazards approach as a means to allow a generic response to a wide range of potential threats; the acronym CBRNE3T acts as an aide-memoire and is discussed earlier in the chapter.

It allows responders to rehearse how they may respond to any number of different threats, which is particularly helpful in rare but high consequence events such as a CBRN incident. As a result, the differentiation between HAZMAT and CBRN is less relevant.

The use of the term 'hot zone' is also used in some tactical situations to describe an area where there remains an active hazard whether that is from CBRN, explosives or an armed perpetrator. An 'exclusion zone' is used to describe a hot zone where PPE will not mitigate the hazard present. Therefore, exclusion by distance is recommended (e.g. a cordon due to a bomb or radiation hazard).

A common way that one may group CBRN threats in the all-hazards approach is by the observed effect on the human casualty, that is:

- Lethal
- Damaging
- Incapacitating
- Iatrogenic

The points highlighted earlier about 'Step 123 plus' provide healthcare responders with some clues as to when a CBRN event may have occurred. Other sources of information are likely to come from specialist teams, for example law enforcement or fire and rescue services. Steps should be taken to ensure that each emergency service or military sub-units share information to improve situational awareness. It is likely that CBRN events will only be recognised once many, seemingly disparate, pieces of information are collected together and appreciated as a whole.

Key Management Points

Chemical Incidents

Below is information to supplement Fig. 41.3, particularly the pathophysiology and suggested treatment for each toxidrome. Medical treatment for associated trauma is in addition to this, and occasionally diagnosis of specific toxidromes can be difficult because the physiological response to trauma may mask or mimic other signs and vice versa.

Nerve agents and other organophosphorus compounds (e.g. Sarin, VX, Novichok, pesticides)

Pathophysiology:

Overstimulation of the cholinergic parts of the nervous system due to excess acetylcholine caused by the inhibition of the enzyme acetylcholinesterase [8] (see Fig. 41.4):

- Parasympathetic nervous system (pinpoint pupils, bradycardia, excessive secretions, bronchospasm)
- Neuromuscular junctions (depolarising muscle paralysis)
- Central nervous system (confusion, coma, convulsions).

Key management including antidotes:

Oximes—reactivate the acetylcholinesterase enzyme inhibited by nerve agent binding.

Atropine—reverse excess cholinergic (muscarinic) drive

Benzodiazepines—neuroprotection and anti-convulsant.

Chemical Asphyxiants: Including Hydrogen Cyanide and Hydrogen Sulphide (H_2S)

Pathophysiology:

- Causes paralysis of aerobic respiration within the mitochondria [12].
- Leads to a sudden loss of consciousness, initial respiratory stimulation (due to lactic acidosis) followed by respiratory arrest and cyanosis.

Key management including antidotes:

- Oxygen and respiratory support
- Cyanide antidotes include sodium nitrite/thiosulphate, cobalt-chelation therapy (including hydroxocobalamin).
- H_2S management is sodium nitrite (and oxygen) in isolation.
- Note: Nitrite (methaemoglobin-forming) antidotes should be avoided in cases of trauma and carbon monoxide due to the potential loss of haemoglobin.

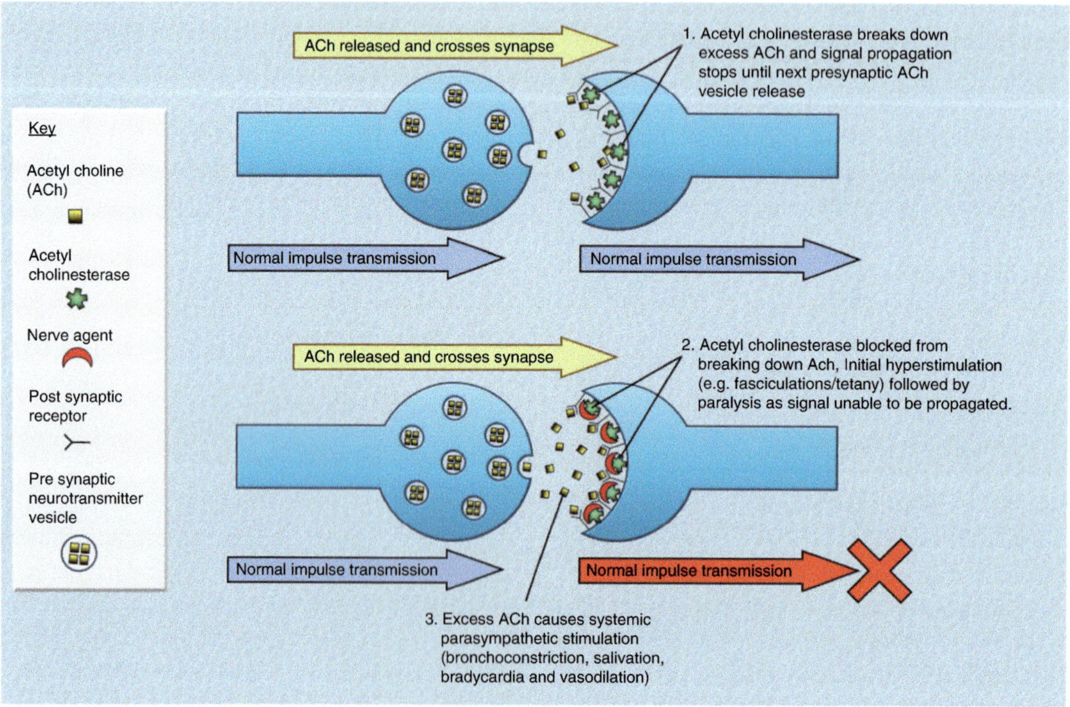

Fig. 41.4 Diagram of normal nerve conduction (top) and effect of nerve agent (bottom)

Mental Incapacitating Agents (Sedating): Opioids

Pathophysiology:

- Stimulate mu-opioid receptors causing euphoria, sedation, coma and respiratory depression as well as pinpoint pupils.
- Some opioids also cause chest wall rigidity and myoclonus, leading to confusion with nerve agent poisoning.

Key management including antidotes:

- Respiratory support is vital in the case of severe opioid toxicity.
- Naloxone is a highly effective antidote, but in the case of some highly potent fentanyl-analogues, may be required in very high doses. Due to its relatively shorter half-life compared to some opioids, naloxone may also need to be given repeatedly, or as an infusion. Naloxone can be given by a variety of routes (intranasally, IV, IM or IO).

Case Study 2: Opiates, Moscow [13]

In October 2002, a theatre with 850 people inside was held hostage in Moscow, Russia by Chechen separatists. Russian security services used aerosolised opiates delivered through the building's ventilation system in order to subdue the hostage takers. Casualty estimates vary, but the Russian federation lists the cause of death as 'terrorism'. During the casualty evacuation phase, several people deteriorated *en route* to hospital, possible due to a lack of basic airway manoeuvres as the toxicant took its effect.

Learning point: Basic life support and clinical care needs to be maintained throughout the patient pathway, from point of exposure to definitive care.

Mental Incapacitating Agents (Psychotropic): Anticholinergics Including BZ (and Atropine Overdose)

Pathophysiology: This group has anticholinergic effects and crosses the blood-brain barrier causing tachycardia, confusion, hallucinations and increasing the risk of heat illness [14]. The anticholinergic effects can be remembered by the *aide-memoire* "Hot as a hare, blind as a bat, dry as a bone, red as a beet, mad as a hatter".

Key management including antidotes: Supportive management, sedation and potentially physostigmine [15].

Blistering Agents: Sulphur Mustard

Pathophysiology:

- Penetrating alkylating agent—causes damage to the skin, eyes, airway and, in severe cases, lungs. It is generally considered to have low lethality (<5%).
- The effects are usually slow with features appearing over hours—eye irritation (3–6 h), erythema (6–12 h), blistering including bullae formation (12–24 h).
- Systemic features may include bone marrow suppression and acute respiratory distress syndrome (ARDS).

Key management: Similar to thermal burns, including the deroofing of the blisters and removal of any necrotic tissue.

Eye management is initially supportive with cycloplegics for pain relief and topical chloramphenicol eye ointment; specialist ophthalmological review is advised.

Scenario B: Sulphur Mustard Shells

On duty in the Emergency Department, a 34-year-old Police officer presents with painful burns and blisters on both forearms.

They work as a Police diver, and earlier in the day had been involved in the retrieval of spent munitions (artillery shells) that had been illegally discarded in a reservoir.

Considering that the blisters appeared around 12 h after exposure to the munitions, you suspect that these may have contained sulphur mustard.

The blisters are deroofed and the skin injury managed in the usual manner with dressings and burns clinic follow-up.

Consider: Where you work, how would you raise your concerns about this patient's exposure to chemical agent, and who would you take clinical advice from?

Blistering Agents: E.g. Lewisite [16]

Mechanism of action:

An arsenic-based blistering agent with initial acid-like effects causing immediate pain and grey coloured chemical burns.

Also systemic arsenic toxicity and death, due to inhibition of glucose metabolism leading to haemolysis, renal failure, distributive hypovolemia and lung damage if inhaled.

Key management including antidotes:

- Supportive care, including correction of any hypovolaemia and antidote treatment based on the chelation of arsenic (e.g. dimercaprol, succimer, unithiol).

Pulmonary Agents: Including Chlorine, Phosgene, Ammonia, Sulphur Dioxide

Mechanism of action:

- Varies between the agents and depends on their water solubility (ammonia > chlorine > phosgene).
- The more water-soluble agents have immediate effects (eye and upper airway irritation) due to their reaction with moisture. In contrast, phosgene has a more insidious onset which may be delayed up to 12–24 h [17]. The lung effects range from non-cardiogenic pulmonary oedema through to ARDS.

Key management:

- Essential supportive therapy is the use of continuous positive airway pressure (CPAP) and potentially invasive ventilatory support with positive end-expiratory pressure (PEEP) and fluid resuscitation.

Biological Incidents

Biological agent can cause issues either due to infection with the live agent (e.g. anthrax, plague-*Yersinia pestis*) whether that is bacteria virus or fungi, or due to toxins (chemical agents of biological origin, e.g. ricin, venom or botulinum toxin).

In the context of any trauma, an open wound is automatically considered biologically contaminated, and empirical antibiotic prophylaxis is given.

Most biological agents are found in the environment and cause disease having breached host defence in one manner or another. Alternatively, some biological agents can be weaponised or have a mass effect if deliberately released.

Case Study 3: Salmonella, Oregon USA [18]

In August 1984, a religious movement led by Bagwan Shree Rajneesh in Oregon, USA, used *Salmonella enterica* in a number of restaurants in order to incapacitate voters and manipulate the results of a local election.

Identifying the causative agent relied on samples from local hospitals, contact tracing from public health officials and finally law enforcement action before being able to identify the deliberate nature of the release.

Learning point: Biological hazards take time to diagnose and recognising deliberate release relies on multiple agencies working and sharing information.

The Syndromic Approach

Patients unwell due to biological agents rarely present to a clinician complaining of a specific agent. Instead, they present with a group of signs and symptoms (bio-syndromes) often preceded by a flu-like prodrome (fever, tiredness, muscle pain).

The type of syndrome often reflects the route of exposure even for the same causative agent (e.g. inhalational, intestinal and cutaneous anthrax).

Below are natural and deliberate release examples for each of the seven syndromes.

Respiratory

Symptoms: dyspnoea, cough, chest pain, sputum and/or haemoptysis.

Natural examples: influenza, coronavirus, streptococcal pneumonia.

Deliberate release examples: inhalational anthrax, pneumonic plague.

Cutaneous

Symptoms either a generalised rash which may be maculopapular, vesicular or petechial/purpuric, or localised lesion(s) including localised infection ± necrosis and abscesses.

Natural examples: maculopapular rash (measles, rubella), vesicular rash (chickenpox), petechial/purpuric rash (meningococcal disease).

Deliberate release examples: tularaemia, smallpox (vesicular/pustular rash), anthrax (cutaneous).

Non-infectious disease or other CBRN causes include caustic and blistering agents (chemical), bites or local radiation injury.

Lymphadenopathy

Symptoms painful swellings, typically in confluences of lymph nodes such as the axillae or groins called buboes.

Natural examples: Rubella (occipital lymphadenopathy), HIV seroconversion illness (generalised lymphadenopathy).

Deliberate release examples: Bubonic plague (although this is more typical of the natural presentation).

Gastrointestinal

Symptoms

- Upper GI (nausea, vomiting, potentially early onset <6 h), e.g. toxins, viruses.
- Lower GI (abdominal pain, diarrhoea, delayed onset >6 h, fever), e.g. bacteria, viruses.

Natural examples: Salmonella, Shigella, norovirus, cholera.

Deliberate release examples: Any deliberate contamination of food or water chain with enteric pathogens.

Food deliberately contaminated with a toxin may cause early vomiting and upper abdominal cramps within hours. In some cases (e.g. campylobacter), the abdominal pain may be severe enough to mimic a surgical emergency.

Haemorrhagic

Symptoms: blood loss, thrombocytopenia, disseminated intravascular coagulopathy (DIC). May also include bruising, petechia/purpura, microscopic and macroscopic bleeding, and hematomas.

Natural examples: Haemorrhagic viral diseases.

Deliberate release examples: Any biological agent causing DIC (e.g. plague).

Non-infectious disease causes include haemopoietic syndrome of snake (viper) envenomation and acute radiation syndrome (ARS-H).

Neurological: Central

Symptoms inflammation of the brain itself (encephalitis), the meninges (meningitis) or from a mass-effect.

Natural examples: Herpes encephalitis, meningococcal meningitis.

Deliberate release examples: Equine encephalitides, anthrax (haemorrhagic 'cardinal cap' meningitis, usually a post-mortem pathognomonic finding).

Neurological: Peripheral

Symptoms A peripheral neurological syndrome characterised by paralysis and autonomic dysfunction.

Natural examples: Wound botulism due to *Clostridium botulinum* anaerobic infection, Guillain-Barre disease.

Deliberate release examples: Botulinum toxin (in the absence of live agent).

Non-infectious disease or other CBRN events include tickborne neurotoxin, elapid envenomation (e.g. cobra, mamba) and pharmaceutical-based agents.

Antimicrobial Chemotherapy

An empirical approach to antimicrobial chemotherapy is to use broad-spectrum agents against a particular syndrome initially, whilst waiting for laboratory investigations to identify narrow-spectrum agents to which the causative agent is sensitive. Some epidemiological data will be required to know what the common causative organisms are and their antimicrobial sensitivity to establish appropriate initial treatment guidelines. An example in the UK is the National Institute for Clinical Excellence (NICE) published guidelines for common infections on their website [19].

Diagnosis as part of source identification and subsequent narrowing of antibiotic selection includes diagnostic imaging, near-patient testing or laboratory facilities. Testing may include:

- Microscopy
- Cultures and sensitivity
- Molecular biology, e.g. polymerase chain reaction (PCR).
- Serology, e.g. antibody testing.

Sepsis and Abnormal Host Response to Infection

Sepsis is defined by consensus, most recently in 2016 [20] where sepsis is considered to be a "life-threatening organ dysfunction caused by a dysregulated host response to infection" and septic shock "a subset of sepsis in which profound circulatory, cellular and metabolic abnormalities are associated with a greater risk of mortality than sepsis alone".

The principles of managing sepsis include the six key interventions:

- Fluids
- Oxygen therapy as required
- Antibiotics
- Source identification
- Biochemical analysis (serum Haemoglobin and lactate in particular)
- Fluid balance measurement

In practice, this moves the clinical definition towards a more severe spectrum of disease than has been considered in previous consensus statements. This highlights the importance of Sequential Organ Failure Assessment (SOFA) and identifying any significant change potentially due to sepsis as time progresses and infection has an opportunity to take hold.

Radiological and Nuclear Incidents

Radiological hazards are those that may present a risk to patients, responders and hospital staff due to ionising radiation, including contamination and irradiation. This may also compromise trauma management due to contamination, concurrent trauma especially following an explosive radiological disposal device ('dirty bomb') and, in rare occasions, high dose radiation exposure and risk of acute radiation syndrome (ARS).

Ionising Radiation

Three types of radiation are described, all caused by unstable nuclei disintegrating. They are:

- *Alpha particles*—two protons and two neutrons (helium nucleus) and carry a double positive charge. They can only travel a few centimetres in air and can be shielded by paper or the dead layer of skin. However, alpha particles are 20 times more damaging compared to beta and gamma radiation and therefore, a significant hazard if injected. Examples of alpha emitters include polonium-210, uranium-238 and americium-241.

- *Beta particles*—these are electrons emitted from the nucleus. They can travel further than alpha particles but are less ionising. Damage may include 'beta burns' to the skin. Examples of beta emitters include hydrogen-3 (tritium), carbon-14 and strontium-90.
- *Gamma (and X) rays*—These types of ionising radiation are a form of high-energy electromagnetic (EM) radiation. They have no mass and behave like other forms of EM radiation including visible light. Gamma rays are generated from the atomic nucleus while x-rays are usually lower energy and generate from the electron shells. Gamma (and X) rays may travel for millions of miles, are more difficult to shield and will penetrate the human body easily.
- *Neutron particles*—neutrons are a form of ionising radiation but are only associated with nuclear fission (splitting of the atom).

The hazard to a patient (and potentially medical staff) from ionising radiation includes:

- Irradiation due to energy transfer to biological tissue from direct exposure to ionising radiation.
- Contamination due to the deposition of radioactive material which will continue to irradiate local tissue. Contamination may be external, internal or in a wound.

Nuclear Incidents

A nuclear incident involves the process of splitting the atom (fission) usually either as a controlled process (power production) or nuclear weapon/detonation on its own or for nuclear weapons is more commonly combined with a nuclear fusion reaction.

The result of a nuclear incident including an explosion is the potential for contamination, blast, thermal and irradiated casualties, and a combination of all of the above. The combined effect of this will result in higher morbidity and mortality than otherwise expected, including psychological casualties.

The presence of radioiodine, a fission product of the nuclear process, carries a specific risk of thyroid cancer due to concentration in the thyroid gland. This can be mitigated by very early administration of stable iodine.

Overview of the Management of Radiological Casualties

The management of radiation casualties includes:

- Primary survey and resuscitation (including some decontamination)
- Damage control surgery
- Full external decontamination including the oral and nasal cavities
- Assessment and management of any internal contamination (decorporation)
- Assessment and management of any significant irradiation and potential radiation illness.
- Restorative surgery, following the return of bone marrow function

Decontamination

The first stage of decontamination is the removal of clothing while preventing internalisation through the mouth and nose.

Further decontamination will depend on the urgency for damage control surgery and the physical properties of the contaminant. At the same time, consideration should be given to the estimation of absorbed dose and the presence of internal contamination. This is summarised in Fig. 41.5 and is based on an adaption of the casualty algorithm from the Radiation Emergency Assistance Centre/Training Site (REACT/TS) [21].

The principles behind radiological decontamination are almost identical to the chemical casualty, except with less urgency. The advantage to the rescuer is that radioactive contamination is readily identified with a handheld detector such as a Geiger-Muller tube. Once further decontamination is appropriate; prioritise wounds, then orifices then intact skin.

Using a baby wipe initially followed by fluid for irrigation will achieve a good effect. Draping around the area and being careful to direct and collect fluid run-off is critical, as this will be contaminated. All fluid, sheets etc. used in decon-

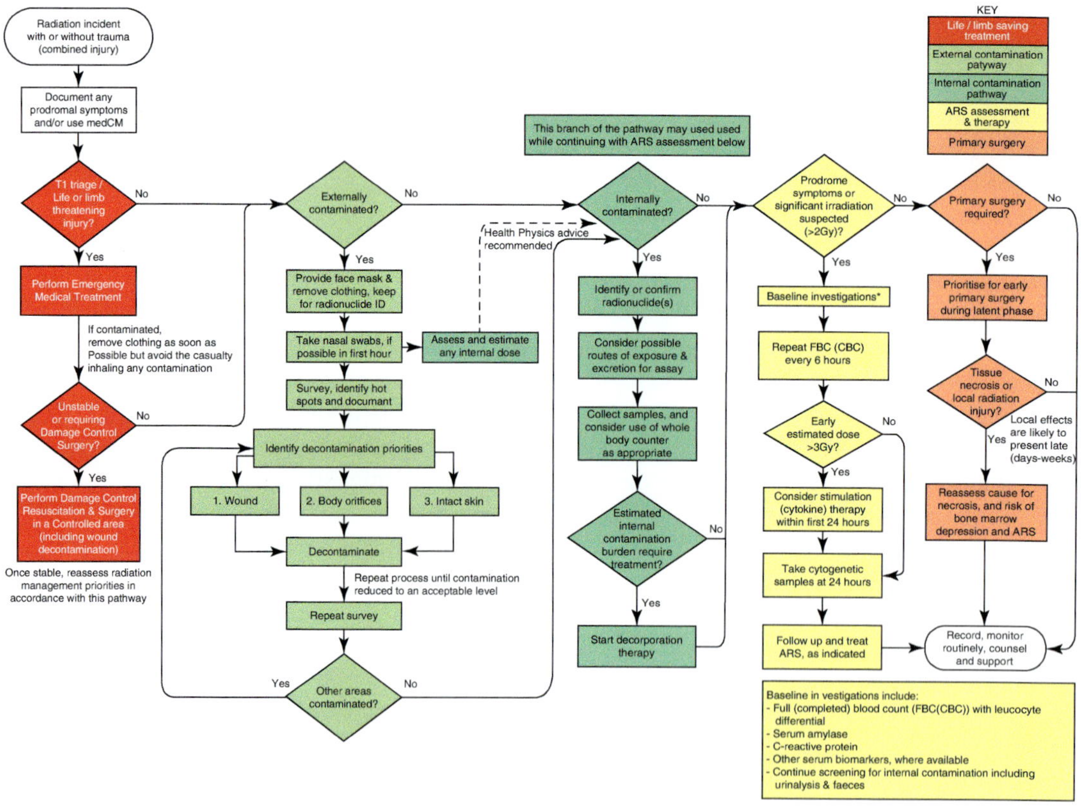

Fig. 41.5 Radiological considerations in mass casualty incidents (Taken from NATO AMedP-7.1 Medical Management of CBRN Casualties (Ref. [6] for this chapter), and adapted from REAC/TS (Ref. [21] from this chapter)

tamination should be saved and sent for analysis as this may help identify unknown agents and estimate dose.

Exposure and Dosimetry

The medical response to a patient who has been irradiated depends very much on the amount of ionising radiation they have been exposed to and whether this exposure is external or internal. In industrial accidents, the patient and their line management will likely have an intimate knowledge of the material involved and be able to assist with dose estimation etc.

In most healthcare settings, health physicists work in radiology or oncology departments. They will be an excellent source of advice when attempting to estimate the dose of radiation experienced by a patient. Also, any country with a civil or military nuclear programme will have access to radiation medicine specialists. The means of accessing this advice will vary between countries, in the UK, for example, this is via the Toxbase™ service (www.toxbase.org).

Information that will assist them in giving appropriate advice:

- **History**—is the source material known? How far away was the patient from the source and for how long were they exposed to it?
- **Examination**—time to vomiting can provide a rough guide to the amount of absorbed dose, or any anti-emetic given. As a rule of thumb—vomiting in <1 hour suggests an absorbed dose of 4–6 Gray (Gy), in <2 h a dose around 3 Gy and between 8 and 10 h an absorbed dose of <1 Gy [21].
- **Investigations**—serial full blood counts and absolute and relative changes/ratios of leukocytes and platelets every 6 h. Further specialist tests are available and advice should be sought.

Acute Radiation Syndrome (ARS)

Acute radiation syndrome describes the illnesses experienced in the first few hours to weeks of exposure to radiation.

It typically follows the pattern of a prodrome, latent period and then manifest illness.

ARS can be sub-divided into:

- *Haematopoietic syndrome (ARS-H)* (>1 Gy) occurs due to bone marrow suppression causing infection, neutropenic sepsis and coagulopathy.
  Clinical signs can be expected over the first few weeks, and the duration of the latent period is shortened by increased initial dose.
- *Gastrointestinal syndrome (ARS-G)* (>6–8 Gy) characterised by gut failure leading to fluid loss, hypovolaemia, malabsorption, translocation of bacteria and GI bleeding. An associated ARS-H compounds these effects and increases the risk of fatal infection and bleeding.
- *Neurovascular syndrome (ARS-N)* (>20 Gy) this has a particularly poor prognosis and is characterised by very early (within minutes) vomiting and nausea followed by a brief period of improvement before deterioration towards coma, hypotension and loss of homeostasis.

Treatment of Acute Radiation Syndrome

- Supportive care, including anti-emetics (ondansetron or granisetron), fluid replacement and continuing hydration until early enteral feeding is started.
- Blood therapy, including platelets early on and later packed red cells.
- Prophylactic antimicrobials including antibiotics, antivirals and antifungals.
- Stimulation therapy using cytokines to stimulate bone marrow recovery.

With effective treatment, the median lethal dose for 50% of an exposed population at 60 days ($LD_{50/60}$) can be increased from 3.5–4 Gy to 5–6 Gy. With intensive care and cytokine therapy, this can be further increased to 6–8 Gy.

In the case of combined trauma, the threshold for cytokine therapy may be lowered. This is different in mass casualty events, which are discussed in the algorithm at reference 21.

Localised Radiation Injury

This is due to local damage, usually with the preservation of some bone marrow even with relatively high doses. With increasing doses, one may see local erythema, hyperpigmentation, dry leading to moist desquamation and ulceration.

The surgical consideration of the potential damage should take into account the absorbed dose, different tissue sensitivities and their distance from the source. E.g. external irradiation to the pelvis may have a significant effect on pelvic organs while the pelvic wall itself may be relatively intact.

Treatment is focussed on ensuring adequate tissue oxygenation, and imaging to assess perfusion may be of assistance in the long-term management of these injuries.

Timing of Surgery

The principles of damage control resuscitation and surgery still apply in general. ARS and the presence of contamination may mean that definitive surgery needs to be considered earlier than in the non-irradiated patient. This window of opportunity for further surgery during the latent phase of illness occurs before immunosuppression and coagulopathy are present. The duration of this window depends on the size of the initial radiation dose.

During the manifest illness stage of ARS, surgery may have to be deferred until recovery, when the chance of healing and recovery is optimal.

Learning Objective

Where to go next

When caring for a patient, clinical advice exists at three levels:

1. Within the hospital
   - Microbiology/Infectious Diseases
   - Intensive Care Medicine

2. Local/Regional
    - Radiation physics
    - Haematology/Oncology
    - Local/Regional Health Protection teams
    - Toxicology
3. National
    - National Poisons Centres or Information Services
    - Centres of Excellence for Radiation Medicine
    - National Public Health/Centres for Communicable Disease Control

Summary

It is unlikely that many clinicians will encounter a CBRN incident; however, the risk exists, and many of the standard treatment options from general clinical practice apply.

In the context of trauma, clinical care priorities follow familiar paradigms—control bleeding and support normal physiology with surgical and intensive care techniques. The additional consideration is that injuries may be compounded by exposure to unfamiliar substances that require unfamiliar treatments, such as antidotes.

Early consideration and therefore, recognition allows patients to receive optimal care immediately in the emergency phase, but also later from a wider multi-disciplinary team in the definitive care and rehabilitation phases.

Questions

1. On recognising a CBRN incident, the '6 Cs' are:
    (a) Confirm, Cordon, Control, Clear, Communicate, Collapse
    (b) Confirm, Clear, Cordon, Control, Communicate, Contain
    (c) Control, Clear, Cordon, Communicate, Clean, Contain

2. The following are all examples of biological syndromes
    (a) Neurological, Respiratory, Cutaneous
    (b) Respiratory, Gastrointestinal, Haemorrhage
    (c) Cutaneous, Radiation, Neurological

3. You see a 40 year-old male who has been involved in an incident at a pharmaceutical production plant.

    His MABCDE assessment demonstrates:

    M: No signs of massive haemorrhage.

    A: He is maintaining his own airway with no increased secretions.

    B: No signs of chest wall injury with a respiratory rate of 34 and oxygen saturations of 88% on 15 L/min high flow oxygen.

    C: His heart rate is 110 with a palpable radial pulse.

    D: He is agitated with normal pupils.

    E: He is cyanosed and has no signs of external injury.

    The most likely cause for his signs and symptoms is:

    (a) A vesicant
    (b) A pulmonary agent
    (c) Methaemoglobinaemia
    (d) Atropine

4. The following are all features of the 'CRESS' assessment
    (a) Consciousness, Radiation signs, Skin
    (b) Respirations, Eyes, Syndromes (biological)
    (c) Consciousness, Skin, Eyes

5. A 23 year-old fire fighter is brought to the Emergency department having responded to a fire at a garage 'lock up', wearing standard fire service breathing apparatus and PPE. She found 2 dead males on scene with no external signs of injury, who themselves were wearing basic PPE. Whilst disrobing she came into contact with a liquid and has become increasingly unwell. Her initial MABCDE assessment shows:

    M: No massive haemorrhage.

    A: Requiring jaw thrust to maintain airway. No added sounds or secretions.

    B: Respiratory rate of 8. Oxygen saturations 92% on 15 L/min high flow oxygen.

    C: Her heart rate is 50. Her blood pressure is 76/ 42.

D: She is unconscious. Her pupils are size 2 and responsive.

E: She is fully exposed and her skin is normal. She is noted to have sporadic jerking of her limbs.

The most likely cause of her signs and symptoms is:

(a) A nerve agent
(b) Smoke inhalation
(c) Cyanide
(d) A synthetic opioid

Answers

1. b
2. a
3. c
4. c
5. d

References

1. Okumura T, Hisaoka T, Yamada A, Naito T, Isonuma H, Okumura S, et al. The Tokyo subway sarin attack—lessons learned. Toxicol Appl Pharmacol. 2005 Sep 1;207(2):471–6.
2. Bush LM, Perez MT. The anthrax attacks 10 years later. Ann Intern Med. 2012 Jan 3;156(1):41–4.
3. McFee RB, Leikin JB. Death by Polonium-210: lessons learned from the murder of former Soviet spy Alexander Litvinenko. Semin Diagn Pathol. 2009 Feb;26(1):61–7.
4. Anderson AR. Characterization of chemical suicides in the United States and its adverse impact on responders and bystanders. West J Emerg Med. 2016 Nov;17(6):680–3.
5. NATO. AJP-4.10, Allied Joint Doctrine for Medical Support, Edition C Version 1 [Internet]. NATO Standardisation Office; 2019 [cited 2020 Sep 10]. Available from: https://assets.publishing.service.gov.uk/government/uploads/system/uploads/attachment_data/file/841686/doctrine_nato_med_spt_ajp_4_10.pdf
6. NATO. Allied Medical Publication (AMedP) 7.1: The Medical Management of CBRN Casualties. Edition A Version 1 [Internet]. NATO Standardisation Office; 2018 [cited 2020 Sep 10]. Available from: https://www.coemed.org/files/stanags/03_AMEDP/AMedP-7.1_EDA_V1_E_2461.pdf
7. Chai PR, Hayes BD, Erickson TB, Boyer EW. Novichok agents: a historical, current, and toxicological perspective. Toxicol Commun. 2018;2(1):45–8.
8. Hulse EJ, Haslam JD, Emmett SR, Woolley T. Organophosphorus nerve agent poisoning: managing the poisoned patient. Br J Anaesth. 2019 Oct 1;123(4):457–63.
9. Rasmussen TE, Tai NRM, Rich NM, editors. Rich's vascular trauma. 3rd ed. Philadelphia, PA: Elsevier; 2016. 350 p.
10. Chilcott RP, Larner J, Matar H. UK's initial operational response and specialist operational response to CBRN and HazMat incidents: a primer on decontamination protocols for healthcare professionals. Emerg Med J. 2018 Dec 1;2018:1–7.
11. Yılmaz Z, Erol S, Aplak HS. Transportation of hazardous materials (hazmat) a literature survey. Pamukkale Univ J Eng Sci. 2016;22(1):39–53.
12. Beasley DMG, Glass WI. Cyanide poisoning: pathophysiology and treatment recommendations. Occup Med. 1998;48(7):427–31.
13. Wax PM, Becker CE, Curry SC. Unexpected "gas" casualties in Moscow: a medical toxicology perspective. Ann Emerg Med. 2003 May;41(5):700–5.
14. Dawson AH, Buckley NA. Pharmacological management of anticholinergic delirium - theory, evidence and practice. Br J Clin Pharmacol. 2016 Mar;81(3):516–24.
15. Beaver KM, Gavin TJ. Treatment of acute anticholinergic poisoning with physostigmine. Am J Emerg Med. 1998 Sep;16(5):505–7.
16. Goldman M, Dacre JC. Lewisite: its chemistry, toxicology, and biological effects. In: Ware GW, editor. Reviews of environmental contamination and toxicology [Internet]. New York, NY: Springer New York; 1989 [cited 2020 Sep 10]. p. 75–115. (Reviews of Environmental Contamination and Toxicology; vol. 110). Available from: https://doi.org/10.1007/978-1-4684-7092-5_2
17. Hardison LS, Wright E, Pizon AF. Phosgene exposure: a case of accidental industrial exposure. J Med Toxicol. 2014 Mar;10(1):51–6.
18. Török TJ, Tauxe RV, Wise RP, Livengood JR, Sokolow R, Mauvais S, et al. A large community outbreak of salmonellosis caused by intentional contamination of restaurant salad bars. JAMA. 1997 Aug 6;278(5):389–95.
19. NICE. Antimicrobial Prescribing Guidelines [Internet]. NICE; 2019 [cited 2020 Sep 10]. Available from: https://www.nice.org.uk/Media/Default/About/what-we-do/NICE-guidance/antimicrobial%20guidance/summary-antimicrobial-prescribing-guidance.pdf
20. Singer M, Deutschman CS, Seymour CW, Shankar-Hari M, Annane D, Bauer M, et al. The third international consensus definitions for sepsis and septic shock (Sepsis-3). JAMA. 2016 Feb 23;315(8):801.
21. Radiation Emergency Assistance Center/Training Site (REAC/TS), US Department of Energy. The Medical Aspects of Radiation Incidents, 3rd Edition [Internet]. QuickSeries Publishing; [cited 2020 Sep 10]. Available from: https://www.semanticscholar.org/paper/The-Medical-Aspects-of-Radiation-Incidents-Site-Ts/fedfc0ea7a87d16e698693ad2981ee610f55f801

42 Decompression Illness and Diving Medicine

Alice Roberts and Chris Press

- Physiological changes during diving
- Gas mixtures and nitrogen absorption
- Bubble formation and decompression illness
- Cerebral arterial gas embolus (CAGE)
- Treatment of decompression illness
- Drowning
- General principles when managing divers

Introduction

The Professional Association of Diving Instructors (PADI) is the world's most popular diving teaching organisation and has provided approximately 27 million people with certificates around the world [1], equating to approximately 500,000 certificates per year [2]. As the popularity and accessibility of recreational scuba diving continues to increase, it is becoming increasingly relevant to understand the fundamentals of dive medicine as the sport is still associated with significant health risks. Unlike previous years where the Divers Alert Network (DAN) has reported a decline in diving fatalities, in 2016, DAN was notified of 169 diving fatalities worldwide. This was 33% higher than the previous year [3]. Furthermore, in 2018, the British Sub Aqua Club documented 215 diving accidents. The most common accident was injury followed by decompression illness (DCI) [4]. This chapter covers the basic principles of diving physiology, the pathophysiology and acute management of life-threatening diving accidents, including decompression illness and drowning. The recommendations for hyperbaric chamber use are discussed in detail in addition to hospital care and rehabilitation. Overall, this chapter aims to provide healthcare workers with the knowledge needed to be confident and useful when faced with a patient who has been involved in a diving accident.

What Are the Different Types of Diving?

There are three main types of diving: "bounce" diving, breath-hold or "free diving" and saturation diving. The various diving methods are designed for different purposes with the majority of recreational and occupational divers engaging in bounce or breath-hold diving. The expense and logistical challenges associated with saturation

A. Roberts
Department of Anaesthesia and Critical Care Medicine, Sheffield Teaching Hospitals, Sheffield, UK
e-mail: aliceroberts1@doctors.net.uk

C. Press (✉)
Department of Anaesthesia and Critical Care Medicine, Sheffield Teaching Hospitals, Sheffield, UK

The Air Ambulance Service (TAAS), Rugby, Warwickshire, UK
e-mail: chris@strategicmedicalservices.co.uk

P. Lax (ed.), *Textbook of Acute Trauma Care*, https://doi.org/10.1007/978-3-030-83628-3_42

diving mean that it is more often reserved for divers working within the oil industry [5].

As it sounds, breath-hold diving involves diving without breathing apparatus and dates back to when Neanderthals would use breath-hold diving to hunt for food. Nowadays, breath-hold diving continues to be used to gather seafood and has also emerged as a competitive sport [6].

"Bounce diving" is when a diver descends and then "bounces" back up to the surface in a single short episode. The invention of the self-contained underwater breathing apparatus (SCUBA) is responsible for the rise in recreational bounce diving popularity. When diving using SCUBA, the diver breathes via a mouthpiece which is attached to a highly-pressurised gas cylinder by a hose [5]. Similar to a tap, a two-stage valve system controls the flow of breathing gases. The valve opens on inspiration, allowing gas to flow to the mouthpiece. Once the negative pressure associated with inspiration ceases at end inspiration, gas flow is terminated [6]. The diver inhales and exhales gases at ambient pressure which vary by only a few centimetres of water. The design varies according to its purpose with occupational divers having more complex apparatus known as surface-supply breathing apparatus (SSBA) which receives gas from the surface [5]. Rebreathers are systems which recirculate exhaled gas via a carbon dioxide absorption system. They are increasing in popularity among recreational divers, and confer several advantages, but they are technically more complicated and increase the risks of carbon dioxide or oxygen toxicity over open circuit SCUBA [7].

Saturation diving is when divers spend a more extended period underwater at great depths, often contained in a pressure chamber found on a diving support vessel (DSV) or an oil platform. Saturation divers often work in the oil or gas industry and as a team descend to great depths via a "diving bell" to work on the infrastructure necessary to maintain underwater oil or gas reserves. The team is gradually brought back to the surface over several days to minimise the risk of decompression illness [6].

How Does a Diver's Physiology Change Whilst Underwater?

Whilst underwater, a diver's physiology adapts to a hyperbaric environment. In particular, respiratory and cardiovascular systems undergo significant changes.

Respiratory Adaptations Whilst Diving

Inspiration is dependent on overcoming two forces; firstly, the elastic forces that prevent the chest from expanding and secondly, the frictional resistance caused by air flowing through the respiratory tract. Whilst underwater, ventilation is more difficult as there is higher resistance to airflow, and the air within the respiratory tract becomes denser with increasing depth. As the respiratory rate rises, a greater amount of work is needed to overcome these forces as the airflow becomes increasingly turbulent and stimulates more friction throughout the lungs [6]. Additionally, at depth the molecules breathed in are denser, which further increases resistance to flow. The density of the air molecules is directly proportional to depth. Increased gas density causes more frictional resistance throughout the airway, for example at 30 m, resistance to airflow is double that at the surface. Hence, it was found that at 30 m, the maximum volume of air inspired and expired in a given period (known as the maximum breathing capacity) is half the volume breathed at the surface [8].

There is a risk of hypercapnia can as the rate of gas exchange is unable to meet the demands caused by the increased work of breathing. This is worsened by restrictive scuba diving equipment that increases the amount of dead space in the lungs, where certain alveoli are perfused but not ventilated, allowing the blood to accumulate carbon dioxide [8].

Cardiovascular Adaptations Whilst Diving

When immersed in water, the higher ambient pressure causes the peripheral circulation to be compressed, causing an increase in central blood volume around the heart, head and neck. The increase in blood volume is detected by baroreceptors located in the aortic arch and carotid sinus. To maintain homeostasis, the pituitary gland inhibits the release of anti-diuretic hormone (ADH) causing an "immersion diuresis". This explains why many divers often experience the urge to urinate whilst underwater. If this response is excessive, divers can become dehydrated. To avoid this issue, some divers deliberately restrict their fluid intake before diving, exacerbating dehydration [7].

Rarely, divers can experience "immersion induced pulmonary oedema". The pathophysiology of this process is not fully understood, but some cases are related to the heart's inability to adapt to the increase in preload caused by immersion and peripheral vasoconstriction in cold water. Additionally, peripheral vasoconstriction increases systemic vascular resistance which makes it harder for the heart to pump blood efficiently. In most healthy divers, these challenges are normally overcome; however, for patients with pre-existing heart disease such as hypertension, coronary artery disease and valvular problems, the heart can become inefficient and pulmonary oedema can occur. This can cause symptoms of hypoxia and characteristically pink frothy sputum, which tend to resolve quickly once the diver is removed from the water and given oxygen [8].

The diving reflex is stimulated when a mammal dives underwater. Specifically, the reflex is triggered when a mammal holds their breath, and the face is immersed in cold water. The trigeminal parasympathetic nerve is activated, which causes bradycardia and peripheral vasoconstriction. This redistributes blood towards the brain and heart and away from organs not essential for immediate survival, such as the skin and kidneys. Although the reflex is more profound in diving mammals such as seals and whales, reflex bradycardia has been demonstrated in breath-hold divers with heart rates been shown to decrease up to 50% upon immersion. The overall effect of the diving reflex is that the myocardial oxygen demand is reduced. This helps to optimise cardiovascular function in diving mammals swimming in hyperbaric conditions. However, research has not yet proven this effect in diving humans. Significantly, the parasympathetic response associated with cold water immersion has triggered several deaths in elderly humans with pre-existing cardiac disease [8].

Gas Mixtures and Diving

Whilst underwater, divers using breathing apparatus can breathe a range of gas mixtures via a system of demand valves and pressure regulators. These gases are contained in highly pressurised cylinders and are delivered at ambient pressure. Alternative gas mixtures include enriched air ("nitrox") which contains nitrogen and a higher oxygen concentration than air. Heliox contains helium and oxygen, and trimix contains oxygen, helium and nitrogen. Diving with pure oxygen is also possible for several hours. Many diving accidents are associated with the absorption or elimination of inhaled inert gases [8].

For example, under hyperbaric conditions, pure oxygen is toxic; hence it is usually delivered in a mixture of gases. Oxygen toxicity is dose-dependent with long term use of pure oxygen whilst diving can cause pulmonary oxygen toxicity. Exposure to an oxygen partial pressure greater than 1.6 atmospheres (equivalent to >70 m of sea water (MSW) breathing air or six MSW breathing 100% oxygen) can cause acute CNS toxicity. The signs and symptoms of this are non-specific and vary according to the region affected; however, loss of consciousness and tonic-clonic seizures are common. The mnemonic VENTIDC (Fig. 42.1) can be useful to remember the clinical features of acute oxygen toxicity. The removal of oxygen will terminate seizures, but drowning is likely to occur in divers who lose consciousness and are not quickly rescued [5].

Nitrogen results in narcosis when breathed in under hyperbaric conditions. This results in feelings of euphoria, intoxication and CNS dysfunction. The onset of nitrogen narcosis is gradual and can cause poor judgment, illogical and overconfident behaviour and impaired risk assessment. The severity of narcosis increases with the partial pressure of nitrogen. For example, exposure to 4 to 6 atmospheres can cause overconfidence and mathematical errors, and exposure to more than 10 atmospheres can result in hallucinations, loss of consciousness and death. It is believed that the risks associated with nitrogen narcosis are underestimated, and an Australian

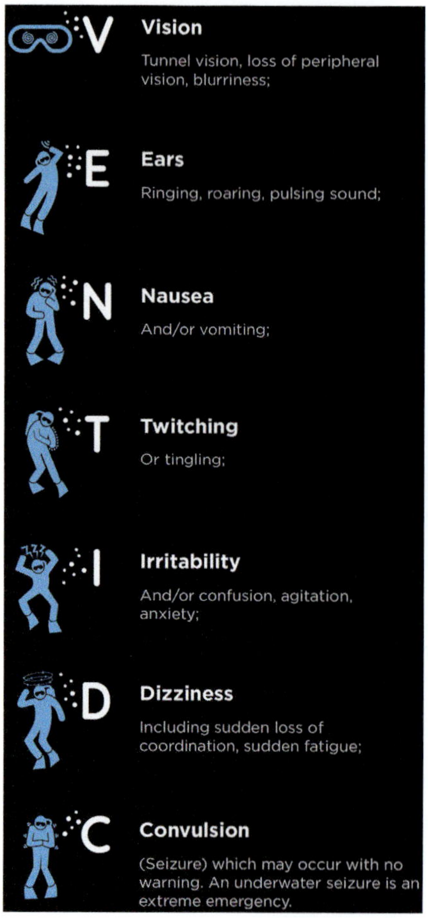

Fig. 42.1 Clinical features of oxygen toxicity (courtesy of Shearwater research/Barbara Shykoff)

database showed that nitrogen narcosis contributed towards 9% of diving-related deaths [5].

Helium is used for deep diving as it does not result in narcosis. However, under 120 m divers are at risk of "high-pressure neurological syndrome" (HPNS) and develop features of neurological hyper-excitability such as tremor, myoclonic jerks and irritable behaviour. It is believed that the effects of high pressure on the neurotransmitters and synapses result in HPNS and that its effects are reversed when the diver reaches normal atmospheric pressure. The use of trimix can help minimise HPNS and maximise divers' ability to explore extreme depths [5].

Additionally, contaminants such as carbon monoxide and low molecular weight volatile hydrocarbon contamination have been suggested as potential causes of underwater "incapacitation and post-dive malaise" [5].

Most importantly, decompression illness is caused primarily by the ineffective elimination of dissolved nitrogen. Therefore, it is essential to understand how nitrogen is absorbed and eliminated to appreciate why things can go wrong [8].

Nitrogen Absorption

Whilst underwater, a diver is exposed to a hyperbaric environment. As the ambient pressure increases with depth, the partial pressure of inhaled gases also increases. This can be conceptualised by imagining each breath containing more gas molecules while occupying the same volume. For example, at 10 m, divers are subjected to 2 atm of pressure compared to 1 atm at sea level. As a result, at 10 m, the partial pressure of nitrogen is 1.6 atm compared to 0.75 atm at sea level. Unlike at sea level, when the body is in a state of equilibrium, at depth, nitrogen diffuses across the alveolar membrane and into the blood from an area of high tension to low tension. According to Henry's Law, "*The amount of gas that will dissolve into a liquid is proportional to the partial pressure of the gas above the liquid*". As the ambient pressure increases, more gas molecules are available to dissolve into a liquid. Therefore, when the ambient pressure doubles at 10 m deep, twice the volume of gas can dissolve into the blood. The deeper the dive, the more nitrogen molecules dissolve into the blood. *black book*

Once absorbed into the bloodstream, nitrogen-rich blood travels around the body and diffuses into unsaturated tissues down the pressure gradient. If a diver remained at a specific depth, this would continue until a state of equilibrium was reached, and all body tissues were equally saturated with nitrogen. At this stage, no further diffusion can occur, and the body is described to be in a state of saturation [8].

Factors Influencing the Absorption of Nitrogen

Various bodily tissues absorb nitrogen (and other inert gases) at different rates. The rate of absorption depends on the tissue's blood supply and the solubility of nitrogen in that particular tissue. This means that different tissues take various amounts of time to reach a stage of saturation, where the maximum amount of nitrogen has been absorbed.

Nitrogen is far more soluble in fat than water; therefore, tissues with high fat content can absorb greater volumes of nitrogen compared to tissues containing minimal fat. Subsequently, tissues such as fat and cartilage will take longer to reach saturation point as they can absorb high quantities of nitrogen.

As previously mentioned, the rate of absorption is also dependent on the tissue's blood supply; hence highly vascular tissues such as the brain, heart and kidneys will receive nitrogen faster than poorly perfused tissues.

Overall, highly vascular tissues with a low fat content saturate quickly and are referred to as "fast tissues". In contrast, "slow tissues" are poorly perfused, contain a high fat content and therefore take a long time to reach saturation. As most recreational dives tend to be characterised by their short "bottom time", divers' slow tissues will never reach saturation [8]. *black book*

In addition to fast and slow tissue types, exercise and temperature also influence the rate of nitrogen absorption. Exercise is a risk factor for decompression illness as it increases cardiac output and the rate of nitrogen diffusion from the blood and into the tissues. This explains why divers are encouraged to minimise effort whilst underwater. Conversely, cold temperatures trigger vasoconstriction, which reduces the rate of diffusion. However, if a diver becomes progressively colder throughout the dive, their vasculature shifts from vasodilation to vasoconstriction. This will limit the amount of nitrogen that can be eliminated during decompression and also increasing the risk of decompression illness [8].

It is important to note that although divers absorb more nitrogen during deep dives, the various tissue saturation times remain constant at different depths. For example, if a tissue becomes saturated after 30 min at 1 atm, it will also saturate after 30 min at 2 atm, despite the volume of inhaled nitrogen doubling [8].

Nitrogen Elimination

As a diver ascends, the process occurs in reverse. When approaching the surface, the ambient pressure declines, causing the partial pressure of nitrogen to decrease. The drop in surrounding pressure encourages nitrogen to diffuse from nitrogen-rich tissues back into the bloodstream. Similarly to absorption, fast tissues eliminate nitrogen quicker than slow tissues. Nitrogen-rich blood in the lung's capillary network diffuses down the pressure gradient and across the alveolar membrane to be exhaled. This process continues to occur whilst ascending until all tissues are devoid of nitrogen. Dive computers can help plan a gradual ascent that allows sufficient time for the majority of absorbed nitrogen to be eliminated in this way. The ascent is deliberately gradual to avoid supersaturation, a high-risk state that can trigger DCI and is described in more detail below.

Bubble Formation

During ascent, harmful bubbles can form as the body attempts to eliminate nitrogen. The formation of bubbles is believed to occur when certain tissues reach a state called "supersaturation". As with nitrogen absorption, different tissues take varying amounts of time to eliminate gas, depending on whether they are a fast or slow tissue. During ascent, the partial pressure of nitrogen decreases as the ambient pressure drops and nitrogen is removed from the blood and tissues. However, the decline in ambient pressure occurs at a faster rate than the rate that certain tissues can eliminate nitrogen. Hence, at certain points during ascent, the partial pressure of the gas in tissues will exceed ambient pressure; this describes a state called "supersaturation" [8].

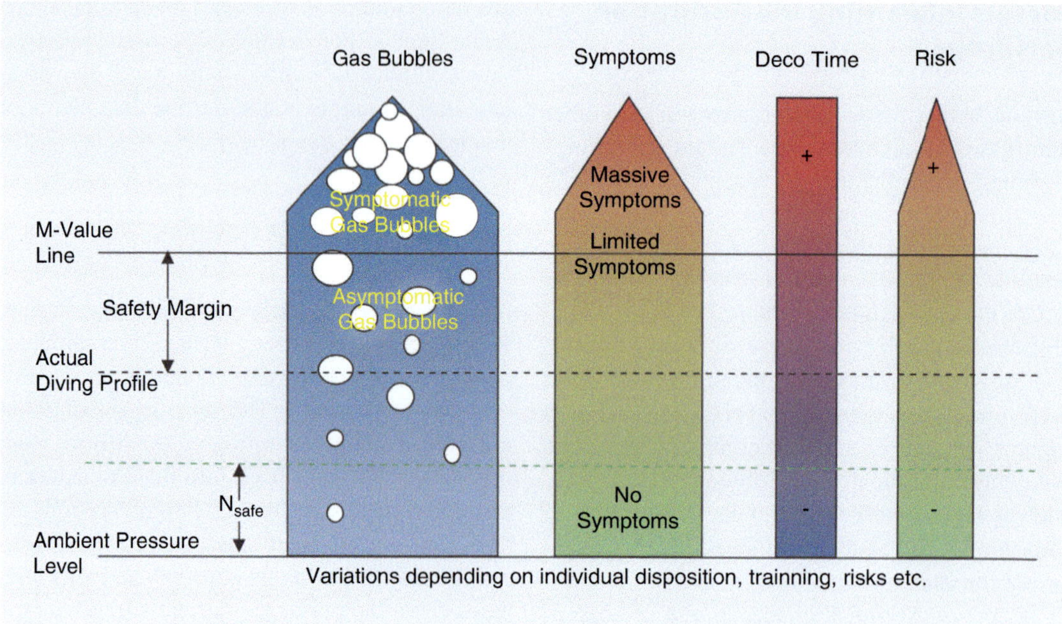

Fig. 42.2 Gas bubble formation and the likelihood of symptoms (from Rusoke-Dierich [7])

Although supersaturation encourages nitrogen elimination by creating a steep diffusion gradient, it promotes the formation of bubbles. After every dive, a certain number of bubbles are inevitable; however, if an excessive quantity are created (for example, during a rapid ascent), decompression illness can occur, which can be life-threatening (Fig. 42.2). To help prevent bubble formation and DCI, dive computers recommend maximum depths, bottom time and ascent rate. Meticulously following the advice from a dive computer will not eliminate the risk of bubble formation, but will help reduce the likelihood of harmful symptoms. If DCI is suspected, it is essential to note that Doppler ultrasound only detects bubbles present in the circulation and not in the tissues. Users must be aware that this tool may underestimate the extent of bubble formation after diving [8].

During recreational diving, certain types of tissue are more likely to form bubbles than others. If ascending at a safe rate, very fast tissues such as the brain and heart are unlikely to be the source of any bubbles. This is because fast tissues rapidly absorb and eliminate nitrogen before bubbles have time to form. Similarly, very slow tissues such as tendons and lipid stores are unlikely to be associated with bubble formation as their poor blood supply limits the amount of nitrogen they can absorb and use to develop bubbles. However, slow tissues become increasingly affected as the length of dive increases and the tissue is given adequate time to become saturated with nitrogen. Above all, bubbles are most likely to form from medium-fast tissues such white matter in the spinal cord. This can occur during short dives, as these tissues absorb nitrogen reasonably quickly. However, the ascent rate may not allow enough time for the gas to diffuse into the blood [8].

Decompression Illness

Definitions

Before launching into the subject, it is essential to define several terms commonly used when describing decompression illness. Firstly decompression illness (DCI) is defined as a disorder caused by bubbles forming in blood or tissues, or being introduced into or in the blood. The umbrella term "decompression illness" is used when the mechanism of bubble formation is unknown or not relevant. If known and relevant, the mechanism of bubble formation can be used to describe the two types of DCI which are discussed separately in this chapter. Firstly, the confusingly similar term "decompression sickness" (DCS) is used when excessive nitrogen in the veins has caused bubble formation. Secondly, cerebral arterial gas embolism (CAGE) occurs in divers who experience pulmonary barotrauma causing arterial bubble formation. Note that DCS and CAGE are used when the specific mechanism of damage is known and relevant to the discussion [8].

Decompression Sickness

DCS or "the bends" occurs when a diver ascends, nitrogen comes out of solution and forms bubbles in the venous system. The presentation, natural history and severity of decompression sickness is highly variable and depends on the location of gas bubble formation.

In the acute situation, bubbles cause direct damage by obstructing venous return, occluding arteries and/or causing endothelial damage. Secondly, in severe cases of DCS, the activation of the inflammatory response can cause delayed damage [7]. This is mediated by the activation of the platelets, complement, leucocytes and the clotting cascade. Those affected typically present with flu-like symptoms, such as fatigue and malaise, up to 72 h after resurfacing.

The spinal cord is vulnerable to the acute and latent effects of DCS. As previously mentioned, the spinal cord's white matter is a medium-fast tissue which is at higher risk of bubble formation during ascent. Additionally, a serious consequence of inflammatory activation is "venous infarction" of the spinal cord when activation of the clotting cascade impairs venous drainage [8].

Usually, the lungs act as an effective filter for venous bubbles; however, if the lung capillary filter becomes overwhelmed, pulmonary DCS or "the chokes" can develop [9]. Pulmonary DCS is characterised by shortness of breath, cough and chest pain shortly after resurfacing from a dive. These symptoms suggest severe DCS and indicate that bubbles are likely to be present elsewhere. It is essential to treat these patients urgently to prevent further damage, for example in the spinal cord [8].

Due to the expansion of gases during ascent (in addition to the dissolved nitrogen in the blood), air-filled cavities of the body—ears and sinuses in particular—must be able to equalise the pressure with the environment and allow air to escape. In conditions such as ear infections or sinusitis, this may not be possible at all or be impeded, causing severe pain. These have been termed "squeezes", and can occur in spaces that are usually air-filled, or have an abnormal collection of gas (e.g. teeth with caries or infection) [10]. Any acute condition which predisposes divers to these effects means that they should not enter the water in the first instance. The expansion of gases also means that Entonox should not be given to anyone who has been diving within the previous 24 h. Nitrous oxide can diffuse into bubbles of nitrogen or air-filled cavities and increase their size. This may cause either vascular compromise, or in the case of a patient with sinus pain following a dive, may paradoxically increase pain by increasing the pressure in the cavity.

Cerebral Arterial Gas Embolism

CAGE is a type of DCI that occurs when nitrogen bubbles enter the arterial system and cause cerebral ischaemia. For completeness, it is important to note that arterial gas emboli can also affect the musculoskeletal system and the skin. If present in the joint capsule, tendons or ligaments, divers can complain of painful "achy joints," typically affecting the shoulders, hips, elbows and knees. Bubbles that form in the skin commonly manifest as an erythematous and itchy rash. Less frequently, the skin can look blue or violet with a mottled appearance, supposedly caused by bubbles in the skin's blood vessels (Fig. 42.3).

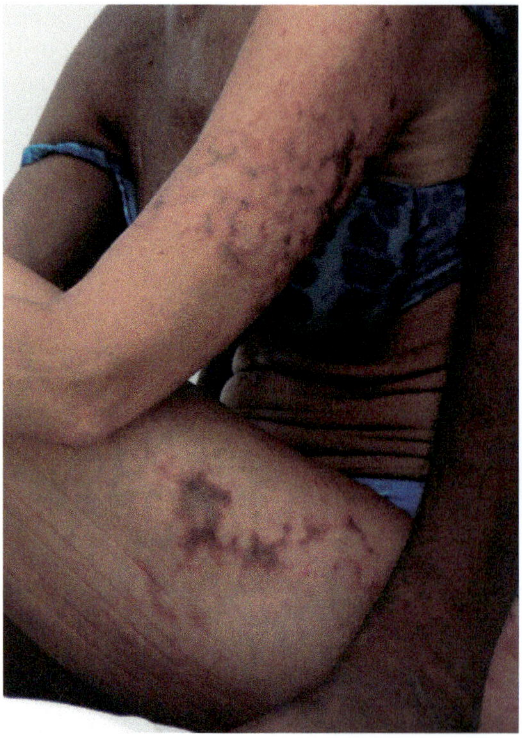

Fig. 42.3 Cutaneous manifestation of DCI (otherwise called livedo reticularis or cutis marmorata). From Vann et al [11]

Although these presentations are important as they indicate the presence of harmful circulating bubbles, their consequences are less severe than neurological DCI.

Presentation of CAGE

In an upright diver, the location of the brain coupled with its rich blood supply makes it particularly vulnerable to the presence of arterial bubbles. Although certain tissues can withstand a limited quantity of bubbles, the capillaries in the brain and spinal cord are not included in this category and bubbles can be life-threatening [6–8].

Divers with CAGE tend to present within minutes after surfacing from with signs and symptoms similar to a stroke. These signs include the immediate loss of consciousness, uncoordinated movements, visual and speech disturbance, cognitive impairment, muscle weakness and sensory changes, which can be ipsilateral or bilateral [8].

A proportion of affected patients may spontaneously recover, as the arterial bubble(s) responsible for causing symptoms pass through the cerebral circulation, and blood flow is restored. However, despite their apparent recovery, these patients remain at high risk for future events as other arterial bubbles are likely to be present. Additionally, the original bubble may have caused significant damage to previously contacted arteries. Therefore, any patient who has a history suggesting neurological DCS should be given 100% oxygen and transferred to a hyperbaric chamber, regardless of their current state. Patients should be placed in a supine position, to minimise the risk of bubbles ascending towards the brain [8].

The spinal cord has a poorer blood supply than the brain, and therefore gas bubbles are less likely to be eliminated via the circulation. Two main theories explain spinal cord damage in DCI—venous infarction following DCS and arterial gas embolism. The "arterial embolism" hypothesis suggests that gas bubbles form in spinal arteries and cause damage by obstructing blood flow and applying direct pressure on surrounding nerves. This hypothesis provides a mechanism for spinal DCI in patients with a patent foramen ovale, approximately 25% of the population [12]. Patients affected with spinal DCI frequently present with a varying degree of sphincter dysfunction, limb weakness and sensory changes, depending on which part of the spine is affected. If the cervical spinal cord is involved, the nerve supply to the diaphragm can be compromised, and this can cause life-threatening breathing problems [8].

Causes of CAGE

CAGE occurs in the setting of pulmonary barotrauma, divers with a patent foramen ovale (PFO) or arteriovenous malformation, and when the lung capillary filter becomes ineffective at removing bubbles [4].

One of the first learning points taught to new divers is to "never hold your breath" whilst diving. Diving used breathing apparatus does not cause drastic changes in lung volume during descent; however, the expansion of compressed gases can trigger problems during ascent. As the diver ascends, time must be given for the expanded gases to escape the pulmonary system to avoid high trans-pulmonary pressures and the rupture of blood vessels and alveoli. Released gas can enter the pleural cavity, mediastinum, pericardium and pulmonary veins which can cause pneumothoraces, subcutaneous and retroperitoneal emphysema, pneumopericardium and arterial gas emboli respectively. This is known as pulmonary barotrauma and can cause air to enter the arterial system via the left side of the heart [5, 11].

However, pulmonary barotrauma is not the only cause of arterial gas emboli. Divers with a PFO provide venous gas bubbles with a direct route into the arterial system. Usually, the lung capillary filter can effectively filter out gas bubbles that can then diffuse into the alveoli to be exhaled (Fig. 42.4). However, a PFO allows bubbles to bypass the lungs and enter the arterial system directly via the right atrium [7].

Research strongly supports PFOs as a leading cause of DCI and in particular, the severe neurological form of DCI. One study found that out of 91 patients evaluated for DCI, 39 were found to have a PFO. Of the 64 patients in this study who had more severe neurological symptoms, 32 of them had a PFO [13]. The prevalence rate of 50% of patients in the severe group is double that of the background population. To help prevent DCI, it has been suggested that divers should be screened for PFOs, given the high population prevalence. A British study found that 24% (15/63) of divers with no history of DCI had a PFO that they were unaware of, but in divers who had neurological symptoms attributed to DCI, the rate of PFO was higher [14]. The counter-argument is that the rate of severe neurological DCI is uncommon and usually caused by large PFOs; therefore, screening may unnecessarily restrict the number of people deemed medically fit to dive. A Swiss study found that in 230 experienced scuba divers, the overall rate of DCI was 5 cases per 10,000 dives. However, while the prevalence of PFO was close to that of the background population (27 vs 25%), the rate of DCI was five times higher in divers with a PFO than those without even when following recommended dive tables [15]. The decision to refer divers for screening for a PFO is best discussed in an article by Sykes and Clark [16], and sumarised in Fig. 42.5, below.

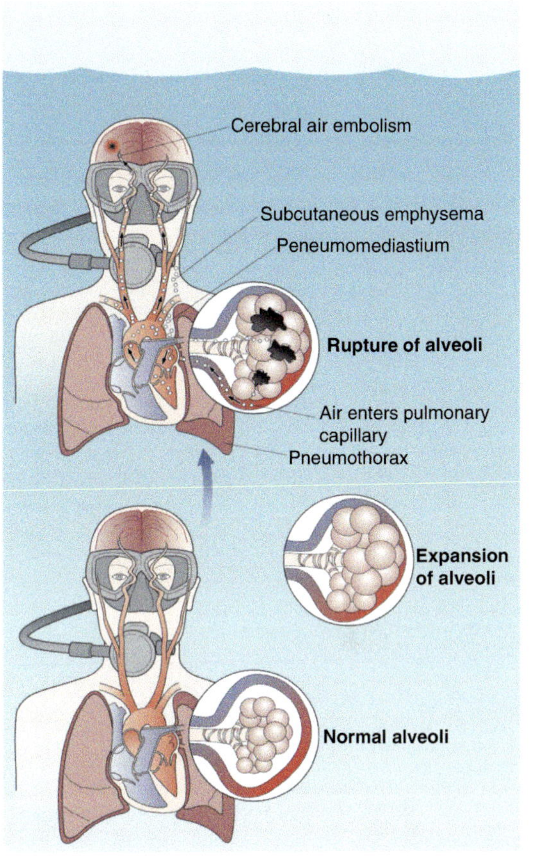

Fig. 42.4 Mechanism of barotrauma on ascent (from Vann et al [11])

PFO's can be closed via a straightforward procedure, or divers may elect to dive using more conservative dive profiles safely, however this latter option may not be possible for commercial divers [17, 18].

Preventing DCI

The use of dive computers, widely accessible dive tables and software have helped prevent decompression sickness for the majority of divers, with only 1:5000 divers experiencing signs and symptoms. However, it is well recognised

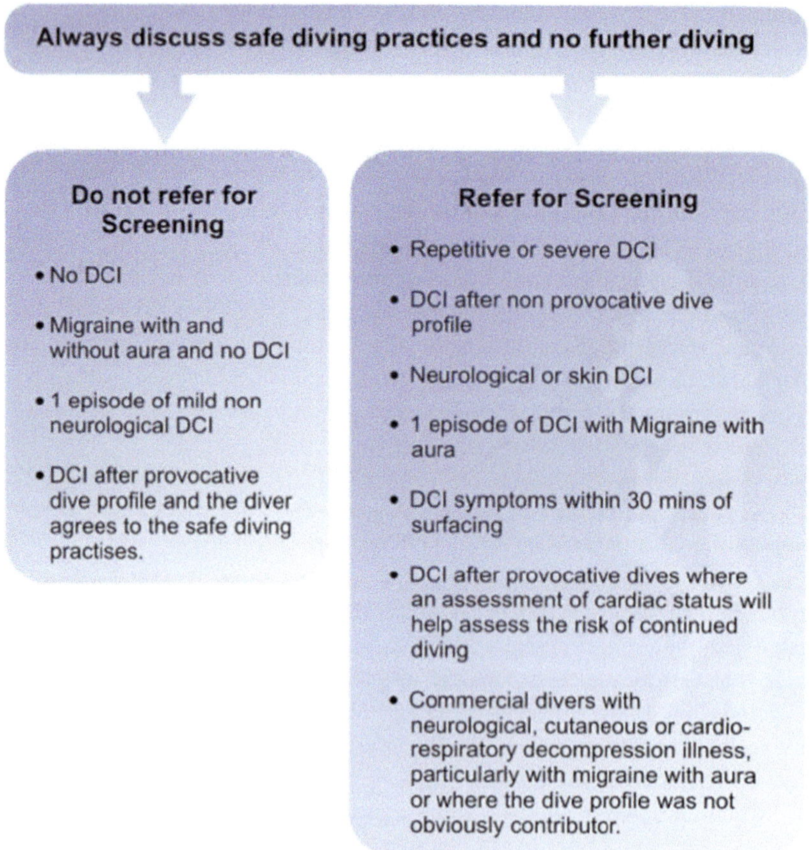

Fig. 42.5 When to refer for PFO investigation (from Sykes and Clark [16])

that certain individuals with specific risk factors will be more susceptible to decompression sickness and may experience illness despite following the correct precautions. Obesity, tiredness, cold temperatures, dehydration and suffering illness at the time of diving are factors that have been shown to increase the risk of decompression sickness. Apart from modifying known risk factors, recent research has explored whether regular divers can develop tolerance and the role of intense exercise pre-dive to "pre-condition" the body [19].

Management of DCI

The definitive treatment for DCI involves recompression in a hyperbaric chamber and inhalation of 100% oxygen. Intravenous fluids may be beneficial, and research has also highlighted the advantages of adjunctive medications. An urgent referral to a hyperbaric unit should be made in any patient who is suspected of having DCI. All units have 24 h contact numbers that can be found on the Divers Alert Network website or by dialling 999 and asking for the coastguard.

Recompression resolves DCI by reducing the size of gas bubbles. This improves symptoms by decreasing the amount of tissue hypoxia caused by bubble obstruction, stops structures being compressed by large bubbles and increases the likelihood of bubbles bursting. Symptoms usually improve quickly when re-pressurised, and this can be termed a "trial of pressure". There are various categories of recompression chambers depending on the facilities that are available in the chamber itself and the immediate vicinity. Category 1 chambers can provide advanced life support whilst re-compressing patients [20].

For this reason, patients with acute DCI who require repressurisation should, where possible, be taken to a Category 1 chamber. However, some areas (e.g. oil rigs) may have temporary level 2 or 3 chambers available for emergency recompression given the transfer distances to Category 1 chambers. Category 4 chambers can only accept patients who are unlikely to require any other medical treatment during repressurisation, and such patients are usually having hyperbaric oxygen therapy for indications unrelated to diving or decompression illness.

Various schedules can be used for recompression [21] with the majority following a similar pattern; rapid recompression at a given pressure followed by a more extended period of milder, graded recompression. During recompression, the diver inhales oxygen but will be given specific "air breaks." For the majority of divers, one to three treatments are required until symptoms resolve [8]. Hyperbaric chambers and recompression will be discussed in more detail later on in this chapter. In-water recompression, the practice of returning a patient underwater instead of transferring them to a hyperbaric chamber, is sometimes discussed as a potential treatment option. This is a dangerous approach with a myriad of risks associated with managing a sick patient underwater. The traditional teaching has always been that it should never be attempted, but in particularly remote settings it may sometimes be the only option open to medical teams, who should plan and prepare for the eventuality to minimise the grave risks involved [22].

Administering 100% oxygen is useful for several reasons; hypoxic tissues receive oxygen, the inflammatory response is attenuated, but most importantly 100% oxygen helps to eliminate circulating nitrogen as it diffuses down the created steep pressure gradient and into the alveoli to be exhaled. An example can help demonstrate how the pressure gradient is formed. At sea level, a diver with DCI will contain bubbles which have the same pressure as the surrounding atmosphere. The partial pressure of nitrogen in the alveoli is lower than ambient pressure as the alveoli contain other gases such as water vapour and carbon dioxide. Therefore, without additional oxygen, nitrogen will slowly diffuse out into the alveoli across a small pressure gradient. By inhaling 100% oxygen partial pressure of nitrogen is further reduced, which increases the rate of nitrogen diffusion from the blood into the alveoli. The hyperbaric conditions of a chamber enhance this effect [6]. Modern emergency and critical care medicine are, appropriately, moving away from high concentration oxygen for all unwell patients. Still, this acceleration of nitrogen "wash-out" means it is crucial that diving casualties continue to be treated with 100% oxygen as a high priority.

Additionally, intravenous fluids are advised, targeting euvolaemia, as patients are usually hypovolaemic as the cold and hyperbaric underwater environment suppresses anti-diuretic hormone (ADH) release and causes a diuresis, while most divers will also be breathing dry gasses compounding fluid loss. Additionally, endothelial injury and increased capillary permeability contribute towards the divers' hypovolaemia [7].

Research focusing on adjunctive treatments for decompression sickness have looked at the administration of non-steroidal anti-inflammatory drugs (NSAIDs) and lignocaine [23]. A double-blind, randomised controlled trial showed that use of NSAIDs reduced the number of recompression appointments, but there was no difference in symptoms [24]. Additionally, after successful animal studies, case reports have documented the beneficial effects of lignocaine, even if it is administrated late or given to patients who haven't responded to initial treatment [25]. Neither of these, however, are yet core tenets of pre-hospital management.

Drowning

Introduction

Drowning is defined as "a process resulting in primary respiratory impairment from submersion/immersion in a liquid medium. Implicit in this definition is that a liquid/air interface is present at the entrance of the victim's airway, preventing the victim from breathing air. The victim may live or die after this process, but whatever the outcome, he or she has been involved in a drowning incident."

Drowning is responsible for 72–84% of all recreational scuba diving fatalities [26]. Despite drowning being the most common cause of death in divers, the topic of drowning is often underplayed when studying dive medicine, especially when compared to other less frequent accidents such as decompression illness.

Out of 100 cases of diving fatalities, 38% did not have any known diving qualifications. In contrast, 81% of divers who survived near-drowning episodes had obtained at least basic dive qualifications. Additionally, more than 50% of the fatalities involved the diver being exposed to an unfamiliar situation. Surprisingly, more than half of drowning incidents occurred in tranquil water. There were marginally more fatalities in divers facing strong currents.

However, it is important to note that drowning is infrequently the primary cause of death in divers. Divers often drown as a result of becoming unconscious after suffering a primary event rather than drowning being the foremost cause. Drowning frequently occurs as a result of an accident occurring in the underwater environment rather than on land, where the diver may have survived.

The Pathophysiology of Drowning

Several animal experiments studying the effects of drowning found that on average, consciousness is lost 3 min after submersion and death occurs after 4–8 min, due to cerebral hypoxia.

This timescale is believed to be similar in humans and causes death by the following mechanism: When a human drowns, there is an initial panic response followed by fighting and instinctive swimming movements. As normal breathing is impossible, there may be voluntary breath-holding. The individual becomes hypoxic, acidotic and hypercapnic. The rise in serum carbon dioxide levels stimulates involuntary inspiration. Automatic laryngospasm can occur as water contacts the epiglottis, preventing the initial aspiration of water. This is eventually overcome as the individual becomes progressively hypoxic, unconscious and aspirates water into their lungs. The fluid-filled alveoli prevent effective gas exchange, and their surfactant is diluted, leading to atelectasis and progressive hypoxaemia. Eventually, cerebral hypoxia triggers bradycardia and death is attributed to asystolic cardiac arrest, shortly followed by hypoxic brain injury.

Unlike other drowning deaths, only one-third of drowning divers exhibited a panic response. This could potentially be explained by the relaxing narcotic effect experienced at depth or due to pre-existing hypoxia caused by aspiration. The fact that 63% of divers showed no unusual behaviour further supports these theories [3]. The pathophysiology and management of drowning in non-diving incidents are further considered in the immersion and submersion chapter.

Management of the Drowning Diver

Immediate Management of a Drowning Diver

Recognition

The first step in drowning management is to quickly recognise that a diver is drowning. Typically a drowning diver will be unconscious, not swimming and unresponsive to hand signals or tactile stimuli.

Immediate Ascent

Once a diver has been recognised to be drowning, it is imperative that they are brought to the surface as soon as possible. If the diver's regulator has remained in his/her mouth, the rescuer should hold it in place but should not place it into the mouth in the more likely event that it has fallen out. The rescuer must judge whether they need to prioritise their own decompression with a safety stop. If this is necessary, they should make the victim buoyant and send them to the surface. Generally, all drowning divers should be brought immediately to the surface with one exception; a seizing diver with their mouthpiece in place. In this situation, hold the mouthpiece in place and wait until the seizure has terminated before bringing the diver to the surface. In this group of patients, the risk of pulmonary barotrauma outweighs the risk of drowning, providing the airway is secure.

In-Water Rescue Breaths

At the surface, ensure the diver has positive buoyancy and is facing upwards. Mouth-to-mouth or mouth-to-nose rescue breaths have been shown to be effective to stimulate spontaneously breathing [27, 28].

Get to a Surface

If a surface, such as a shore, boat or floating platform is immediately available, remove the victim from the water and commence resuscitation. If the rescuer believes it would take less than 5 min of towing to access a suitable surface, they should begin towing the victim towards the surface and provide intermittent rescue breaths during the journey. However, if the rescuer estimates a longer tow, they should continue to give rescue breaths for 1 min and then begin to tow to the nearest surface, either land or a dive boat.

The Practical Approach to the Diving Patient for Emergency Medical Services (EMS)

In the early phases of the assessment and management of victims of diving accidents, it is often unclear what pathologies are afoot. Drowning pathophysiology often coexists with decompression illness, barotrauma and hypothermia. In one series, it was suggested 27% of all recreational diving fatalities were primarily caused by a cardiovascular event occurring underwater. This diagnostic uncertainty and complex physiology make this group of patients distinct from others in the pre-hospital arena.

While following a standard MABCD approach, high priority should be given to delivering the highest possible fraction of inspired oxygen, regardless of oxygen saturation. Where the skills are available, patients in cardiac arrest should be positively pressure ventilated with either a supraglottic airway or, ideally, endotracheal intubation. Those with reduced consciousness or severe hypoxia will benefit from early Rapid Sequence Induction (RSI) to facilitate invasive ventilation, and consideration should be given to activation of an advanced pre-hospital team who can provide this service at the scene.

Pneumothorax should be considered, as a rapid ascent from even a few metres can cause enough proportional change in pulmonary gas volume to cause alveolar rupture. Patients in cardiac arrest should be assumed to have bilateral tension pneumothoraces, and these should be decompressed according to training and local standard operating procedures for traumatic cardiac arrest.

IV access should be obtained and fluid bolus given. The aim should be euvolaemia rather than anything more. A number of these patients will develop pulmonary oedema from a range of causes, and this should be anticipated and treated.

Hypothermia is common in many patients who have been immersed or submersed, and care should be taken to prevent further heat loss during transfer. Active patient warming may be appropriate during prolonged transfers, but caution should be exercised, as vasodilation during rewarming may cause haemodynamic instability.

Exposure and a thorough examination are essential. Rashes may imply decompression sickness, and evidence of myocardial infarction or other medical condition will influence treatment or hospital destination.

As much information as possible should be gathered about the dive. Critical information is dive profile in terms of time and depth, as well as what gas mixes were in use. Thermal protection and the history available from any witnesses is also helpful in narrowing the differential diagnosis. The patient's dive computer (where available) should be taken to the hospital or hyperbaric chamber.

Transfer the Patient to Hospital

Diving incidents often involve prolonged transfer to a suitable medical facility, and this should form a routine part of dive planning. All dive boats should be equipped with oxygen, to be given in all cases. Choosing the appropriate facility can be challenging and needs to take into account how stable the patient is, the proximity of the nearest medical facility vs the nearest hyperbaric facility and the patient's other medical requirements. It will also depend on the skill and capabilities of the transferring medical team and whether the patient is being transported by land, air or water. Specialist advice is available from local expert units, or internationally from the Diver's Alert Network (DAN).

Helicopter or fixed-wing aircraft transfer needs to consider the pressure changes associated with altitude. Although these differences are relatively small compared with those encountered underwater, it can make a difference to the pathophysiology of already compromised patients. Most guidelines suggest maintaining an altitude below 1000 feet (330 m) or using an aircraft with a cabin pressurised to 1 atmosphere. A head down or supine position is often described in an effort to minimise migration of gas bubbles to the head. The author's experience is that taking meticulous care around patient position, or concerns around a few feet of extra altitude, sometimes lead to marked delays in the treatment of serious pathology or can extend the time taken to reach hospital. These factors need to be carefully balanced.

Hospital Management

Management in the Emergency Department

Further hospital management depends on how clinically stable the patient is. The immediate priority is to reverse any respiratory failure. Patients who are asymptomatic with a normal respiratory examination, chest X-ray and oxygen saturations/arterial blood gas are unlikely to deteriorate and can be discharged after a period of observation (6 h would be reasonable). However, if any of these investigations show abnormal findings, the patient should be admitted and any respiratory deficit managed appropriately. Patients who are moderately hypoxic yet alert and breathing can be considered for continuous positive airway pressure ventilation (CPAP) if there is no pneumothorax, but endotracheal intubation may be required. Patients that are critically hypoxic or are in a state of fluctuating consciousness should be transferred to the high dependency or intensive care unit. Consideration should be given to emergency induction, endotracheal intubation and ventilation.

A secondary survey is important to reveal any other injuries endured during the drowning accident, and to establish the primary cause of the incident. Therefore, a 12-lead electrocardiogram is an essential investigation to diagnose myocardial infarction in divers. Additionally, the rapid ascent to the surface may have caused pulmonary barotrauma or the formation of arterial gas emboli that may require specific treatment discussed earlier.

Summary

Diving is a safe sport, however physiological changes can cause severe morbidity and mortality if safety standards are not adhered to or in an emergency. Certain divers may be more prone to developing neurological complications due to undiagnosed cardiac defects such as PFO's, so appropriate investigation and modification of diving profiles may be necessary in some cases. While recompression is the mainstay of treatment for decompression illness, logistically this can be challenging due to the distances between appropriate dive chambers and their ability to care for critical care patients. Treatment with oxygen, and a high index of suspicion for injuries due to barotrauma as well as complications including relative hypovolaemia and hypothermia for any divers who suffer a traumatic injury or medical event while diving are prudent.

Questions

1. Patients suffer decompression illness due to the rapid expansion of nitrous oxide when they surface too quickly.
   (a) True
   (b) False

2. The mnemonic VENTIDC can be used to recall the signs of oxygen toxicity.
   (a) True
   (b) False
3. Oxygen toxicity only occurs at depths approaching 70 metres
   (a) True
   (b) False
4. Patients who have been diving in the last 24 hours should not be given Entonox for analgesia
   (a) True
   (b) False
5. Helicopter transfer of patients suspected of having decompression illness is contraindicated
   (a) True
   (b) False

Answers

1. b
2. a
3. b
4. a
5. b

References

1. About PADI [Internet]. PADI. [cited 2020 Sep 10]. Available from: https://www.padi.com/about-padi
2. Kafil-Hussain N. Scuba diving. BMJ. 2007 Dec 8;335(7631):s209.
3. Buzzacott P, Moore JP, Bennett CM, Caruso JL, Nelson C, Denoble PJ. Diving fatalities [Internet]. DAN Annual Diving Report 2018 Edition: A Report on 2016 Diving Fatalities, Injuries, and Incidents [Internet]. Divers Alert Network; 2018 [cited 2020 Sep 10]. Available from: https://www.ncbi.nlm.nih.gov/books/NBK540496/
4. Clayton S, Walklett C. Decompression Illness [Internet]. RCEMLearning. [cited 2020 Sep 10]. Available from: https://www.rcemlearning.co.uk/reference/decompression-illness/
5. Levett DZH, Millar IL. Bubble trouble: a review of diving physiology and disease. Postgrad Med J. 2008 Nov 1;84(997):571–8.
6. Edmonds C, Bennett M, Lippmann J, Mitchell S. Diving and subaquatic medicine. 5th ed. Boca Raton, FL: CRC Press; 2016.
7. Rusoke-Dierich O. Diving medicine [internet]. Cham: Springer; 2018 [cited 2020 Sep 10]. Available from: https://doi.org/10.1007/978-3-319-73836-9
8. Lippmann J, Mitchell DS. Deeper into diving. Carnegie, VIC: J.L. Publications; 2005.
9. Kondo Y, Shiohira S, Kamizato K, Teruya K, Fuchigami T, Kakinohana M, et al. Vascular hyperpermeability in pulmonary decompression illness: 'The chokes'. Emerg Med Australas. 2012 Aug;24(4):460–2.
10. Battisti AS, Haftel A, Murphy-Lavoie HM. Barotrauma. In: StatPearls [Internet]. Treasure Island (FL): StatPearls Publishing; 2020 [cited 2020 Sep 10]. Available from: http://www.ncbi.nlm.nih.gov/books/NBK482348/
11. Vann RD, Butler FK, Mitchell SJ, Moon RE. Decompression illness. Lancet. 2011 Jan;377(9760):153–64.
12. Atianzar K, Casterella P, Zhang M, Gafoor S. Update on the management of patent foramen ovale in 2017: indication for closure and literature review. Journal - Update on the Management of Patent Foramen Ovale in 2017: Indication for Closure and Literature Review [Internet]. 2017 Aug 22 [cited 2020 Sep 10]. Available from: https://www.uscjournal.com/articles/patent-foramen-ovale-2017
13. Moon RE, Rorem D. Patent Foramen Ovale—DAN | Divers Alert Network—Medical Dive Article [Internet]. 1995 [cited 2020 Sep 30]. Available from: https://www.diversalertnetwork.org/medical/articles/Patent_Foramen_Ovale
14. Wilmshurst PT, Byrne JC, Webb-Peploe MM. Relation between interatrial shunts and decompression sickness in divers. Lancet. 1989 Dec;334(8675):1302–6.
15. Torti SR, Billinger M, Schwerzmann M, Vogel R, Zbinden R, Windecker S, et al. Risk of decompression illness among 230 divers in relation to the presence and size of patent foramen ovale. Eur Heart J. 2004 Jun 1;25(12):1014–20.
16. Sykes O, Clark JE. Patent foramen ovale and scuba diving: a practical guide for physicians on when to refer for screening. Extrem Physiol Med. 2013 Apr 1;2:10.
17. National Institute for Health and Clinical Excellence. Interventional procedure overview of percutaneous closure of patent foramen ovale for the secondary prevention of recurrent paradoxical embolism in divers [Internet]. 2010 [cited 2020 Sep 30]. Available from: https://www.nice.org.uk/guidance/ipg371/documents/percutaneous-closure-of-patent-foramen-ovale-for-the-secondary-prevention-of-recurrent-paradoxical-embolism-in-divers-overview2
18. Dowse MSL, Waterman MK, Penny CE, Smerdon GR. Does self-certification reflect the cardiac health of UK sport divers? Diving Hyperb Med. 2015;45(3):184–9.
19. Gempp E, Blatteau J-E. Preconditioning methods and mechanisms for preventing the risk of decompression sickness in scuba divers: a review. Res Sports Med. 2010 June 30;18(3):205–18.
20. Chamber Categories – British Hyperbaric Association [Internet]. [cited 2020 Sep 10]. Available from: https://www.ukhyperbaric.com/hbot/chamber-categories/

21. Hyperbaric treatment schedules. In: Wikipedia [Internet]. 2020 [cited 2020 Sep 10]. Available from: https://en.wikipedia.org/w/index.php?title=Hyperbaric_treatment_schedules&oldid=951263411
22. Department of Anaesthesiology, University of Auckland, Auckland, New Zealand, Doolette D, Mitchell S, Department of Anaesthesiology, University of Auckland, Auckland, New Zealand. In-water recompression. Diving Hyperb Med. 2018 June 30;48(2):84–95.
23. Bennett MH, Lehm JP, Mitchell SJ, Wasiak J. Recompression and adjunctive therapy for decompression illness: a systematic review of randomized controlled trials. Anesth Analg. 2010 Sep;111(3):757–62.
24. Bennett M, Mitchell S, Dominguez A. Adjunctive treatment of decompression illness with a non-steroidal anti-inflammatory drug (tenoxicam) reduces compression requirement. Undersea Hyperb Med. 2003;30(3):195–205.
25. Mitchell SJ. Lidocaine in the treatment of decompression illness: a review of the literature. Undersea Hyperb Med. 2001;28(3):165–74.
26. Denoble PJ, Caruso JL, de Dear GL, Pieper CF, Vann RD. Common causes of open-circuit recreational diving fatalities. Undersea Hyperb Med. 2008 Dec;35(6):393–406.
27. Leclerc T, Canabal J, Leclerc H. The issue of in-water rescue breathing: a review of the literature. IJARE [Internet]. 2008 Feb [cited 2020 Sep 10];2(1). Available from: http://scholarworks.bgsu.edu/ijare/vol2/iss1/5/
28. Mitchell SJ, Bennett MH, Bird N, Doolette DJ, Hobbs GW, Kay E, et al. Recommendations for rescue of a submerged unresponsive compressed-gas diver. Undersea Hyperb Med. 2012 Dec;39(6):1099–108.

Part IX

Post-Incident Care

43 Rehabilitation After Trauma

Oliver O'Sullivan, Jill Neale, and Alan Mistlin

- How are rehabilitation services designed and how it is best delivered?
- Who makes up the trauma rehabilitation team and what do their job roles entail?
- How is musculoskeletal rehabilitation delivered?
- What factors need to be consider regarding amputation, and how are patients rehabilitated following this
- How do brain injuries impact on patients, and what can be done about them?
- What needs to be done following a spinal cord injury, and what are the specific complications to monitor for?
- What lessons can be learnt from recent conflicts in Iraq and Afghanistan?

Learning Outcomes

- To gain an understanding of the trauma rehabilitation pathway.
- To understand the roles of the rehabilitation multidisciplinary team.
- To get an insight into the key aspects of musculoskeletal, amputation and neurological rehabilitation.

Introduction

The field of rehabilitation aims to improve the function of those with illness, injury or impairment (a structural or functional deviation or loss), often leading to a disability (the result of an impairment on a persons life). Rehabilitation following trauma is critical to restore choice and independence to patients, even if full health is unachievable. This chapter will outline how, and by whom, trauma rehabilitation is delivered, discuss some of the specific areas of rehabilitation that relate to trauma patients, and share some lessons learnt from military related trauma rehabilitation.

How Is Trauma Rehabilitation Delivered?

Rehabilitation should begin as soon as possible, ideally in intensive care—even if the patient is intubated. Understanding the injury mechanism, sever-

O. O'Sullivan · A. Mistlin (✉)
Royal Army Medical Corps, Defence Medical Rehabilitation Centre Stanford Hall, Loughborough, UK
e-mail: oliver.o'sullivan@nhs.net; Alan.mistlin@nhs.net

J. Neale
Regional Rehabilitation Unit, RAF Cranwell, Sleaford, Leicester, UK

University Hospitals of Leicester NHS Trust, Leicester, UK
e-mail: Jill.neale@doctors.org.uk

P. Lax (ed.), *Textbook of Acute Trauma Care*, https://doi.org/10.1007/978-3-030-83628-3_43

ity and types of injures can allow the correct team to be identified. Discussions can be held regarding psychosocial factors, peer support and an understanding of the patients pre-morbid state can be drawn up. This leads to early targets for rehabilitation being identified. Whilst initial management will be under the trauma team, this should be transitioned into rehabilitation pathway with regular communication between the two teams.

In the post-acute phase, patients need to be medically stable to make good progress. This often requires them to be not undergoing frequent medical or surgical procedures, infection free and with good pain relief. The latter is an area requiring particular focus, and often requires a multimodal approach. An early assessment by all members of the multi-disciplinary team (MDT) will identify a problem list, enabling goals to be set and a treatment plan to be devised.

A successful treatment plan involves communication between the patient, family and treatment team, with ideas, concerns and expectations of all parties explored by the MDT. In turn, they can use their expertise to guide the patient through the initial stages, providing some realistic goal setting with timelines to either encourage or rein back under- or over-aiming. Successful goals should be jointly created by patients and clinicians and follow the SMART criteria (Specific, Measurable, Achievable, Realistic, Time-limited). Furthermore, they should be mapped against short, medium and long term—with often the latter feeding into the former.

Short-term goals can often be useful to demonstrate progress and encourage buy-in, and long-term goals give everybody a common target to aim for. Successful rehabilitation is built on active participation by all parties, and achieving regular goals promotes engagement. An idea of what and where the long-term target is likely to be will guide early discharge planning, reintegration into the community and vocational rehabilitation if suitable.

Key Points

- Early assessment and commencement of the rehabilitation pathway is essential
- Communication between acute trauma team, specialist services and the rehabilitation team is vital
- A joint treatment plan, using short, medium and long term goals, is draw up between the rehabilitation team, the patient and their families.

Who Is Involved in the Multi-Disciplinary Team?

The MDT should be led by a consultant in Rehabilitation Medicine, providing over-arching direction and coordinating the team managing a patient with complex, multi-system injury patterns, as well as providing specialist medical knowledge. Other members of the MDT include physiotherapists, exercise therapists, podiatrists, prosthetists/orthotists, occupational therapists, speech and language therapists, psychologists, social workers, mental health workers, dieticians, nurses and administrative support. Clearly, with such a large team, communication is critical, as is regular updates of progress and goals.

Physiotherapists often provide one-to-one support, backed up by exercise therapists, working on the physical goals and helping the patient regain as much physical function as possible. They perform multiple roles including assessment of gait, addressing muscle imbalance, creating specific strength and conditioning programmes, supporting the prosthetists and orthotists in the assessment and fitting of aids, and preventing contractures.

Occupational therapists (OTs) can enable independence in the home environment with targeted plans addressing the activities of daily living (ADLs), the need for adaptions and aids, as well as providing specific input for with specific OT roles in cognitive, vocational and mental health needs.

Speech and Language Therapists aid the dietician in nutrition, and are experts in communication, both verbal and non-verbal, helping to develop alternative strategies, tools and environmental controls to communicate.

Psychology services, alongside the mental health team, plus any pastoral support, can aid in the psychological recovery essential to good long-term outcomes. Depression, anxiety and post-traumatic stress disorder (PTSD) are very common in this patient population, as is the grief reaction of sustaining a life changing injury, and these members of the MDT will support this adjustment. Successful long-term outcomes are strongly correlated to successful adaptation to physical, cognitive and psychological change.

The nursing team have a vital role in supporting the patient through the rehabilitation journey. Good nursing will promote independence in ADLs; prevent complications such as pressure sores, infections (commonly urinary tract and chest) and bowel problems; ensure good nutrition and hydration; prevent deep vein thrombosis; as well as providing input for tissue viability, wound dressing and other specialist areas.

Social workers, alongside the key worker, liaise with and update the family and address patient and family concerns as they appear. They also can assist with discharge planning, community support, benefits application and any legal proceedings.

Regular Treatment Planning Meetings ensure that progress is on track, any outside referrals have been made and goals are being regularly reviewed and updated—a Key Worker can be invaluable to act as a single point of contact between the MDT and family to communicate the outcomes of these meetings.

For those who are able, vocational rehabilitation is very important. Work is central to patient's lives and the lack of it is exceedingly detrimental for mental and physical health. A disability might impact on the ability to work, however, schemes exist to encourage people back to work, supported by legislation. The process of re-integration into work, 'work-hardening', is overseen by a vocational rehabilitation specialist (often an OT), supported by the employer and occupational health, and will continue, often for months, to ensure that it is successful.

Key Points

- The rehabilitation MDT is large with each discipline providing a specialist role. Not all disciplines will be required for every patient, it depends on their rehabilitation needs. Good communication is essential between the MDT, patient and family
- Once the treatment plan has been developed, regular treatment planning meeting are held to update the team and patient on progress and update the plan accordingly
- Vocational rehabilitation is critical to ensure the patient is able to successfully integrate back into the work place

Specific Areas of Rehabilitation Following Trauma

Musculoskeletal Trauma

Patients with significant musculoskeletal trauma should be initially managed in an acute care setting with the involvement of the MDT. The overall rehabilitation plan will be dependent on the primary diagnosis and initial management (i.e. non-surgical versus surgical). Early mobilisation is important in reducing thromboembolic events and deconditioning and the patient should be encouraged to mobilise as able, often partial weight-bearing in the first instance. Short and long-term goals should be defined for each patient and reviewed regularly, with appropriate clinical markers selected to monitor progress. There are three main stages of rehabilitation;

- Early—POLICE (Protection, Optimal Loading, Ice, Compression, Elevation) and normalisation of gait
- Middle—Restoration of full range of movement and muscle length, stretching of all major muscle groups, early proprioceptive and strength and conditioning exercise to improve motor control, strength, power and endurance
- Late—Functional activities, progressing strength and conditioning to include plyometrics and any vocational or sport-specific activities

All the above exercises should be done alongside activities which maintain cardiovascular fitness. Generally, rehabilitation will be led by a physiotherapist, and whilst some sessions are with the physiotherapist or exercise therapist in person, the patient will also be given an independent programme (IP) to complete on their own to promote progression and function. Regular reassessment by the physiotherapist and tailoring of the IP to the patient's needs and improvements will ensure that the patient remains engaged with the process, with the focus on what they can do, not what they can't. The patient should also receive education on pain management and recognise that as the rehabilitation progresses, they may require increases in analgesia (which should then taper and ideally stop as the healing process finishes).

Key Points

- Early mobilisation is important for minimising further complications following trauma (such as VTE and deconditioning)
- Musculoskeletal rehabilitation is typically divided into early, middle and late stage, with different aims, to allow patient progression
- The use of an independent programme allows the patient to make improvements outside of the medical setting

Amputee Rehabilitation

Amputee care is constantly evolving, with improvements in both medical and functional outcomes as a result of advances in surgery, the development of improved prosthetics and increased awareness of the importance of stump care.

Patients who undergo an amputation following trauma are more likely to be younger adults, with increased future functional demands and a longer period of prosthetic usage, meaning it is especially important to limit complications and promote function in this patient group. An MDT approach involving experienced surgical and rehabilitation teams is important to ensure optimal patient care in the acute and later stages, with early involvement of both teams in pre-operative assessment if possible. Important considerations include time to surgery, level of amputation, creation of a good quality stump, pain management, appropriate post-operative mobilisation as well as mental health promotion to reduce potential complications [1]. Early involvement of the prosthetics team can promote acceptance and aid adjustment to the prosthetic, even before the prosthesis has been fitted and improve long-term outcomes.

There is emerging evidence that amputations performed due to trauma can offer improved outcomes compared to limb salvage procedures, with reduced complications and enhanced function, although this area is still debatable. In situations where limb salvage is attempted, it is recommended to counsel the patient on the possibility of amputation should it not be successful. In the acute stages it is advisable to involve the patient in decision making as much as possible and to delay amputation until they are able to make an informed decision about the possible management options available to them, with the least restrictive option selected in the first instance if possible. Prior to surgery, it is imperative that the level of amputation is carefully considered as this influences future prosthetic selection as well as the overall function, energy requirements and cosmetic appearance. The length of the distal residual limb is also significant as it provides sensory feedback, force transmission and is the interface between the remaining limb and the prosthetic. Whilst a longer length can provide more stability, if too long it can make fitting prosthetics difficult. Furthermore, recent research has shown that the higher the level of amputation (above knee vs below knee), and the greater the number of limbs amputated (uni vs bilateral) have a higher metabolic cost of walking and a reduction in ambulatory physical activity [2].

In the post-surgical period, appropriate early mobilisation can help to reduce complications such as contractures and thromboembolic events, and improve strength and wound healing. Patients may find adjusting to the amputation difficult and involvement of the clinical psychologist should be facilitated. Following amputation, there are three recognised pain categories; phantom limb pain, residual limb pain and phantom sensations

[3]. Patients can experience one or several of these pain types and the management can prove complex, requiring a combination of pain education, alongside pharmacotherapy, injectables, alternative therapies and surgery—it is recommended that the pain team are involved throughout all stages of care.

Once the surgical wound has healed, the patient is taught to care for their stump, as any irritation or infection can prevent use of any prosthesis, alongside strengthening, desensitisation programmes and 'doning-doffing' techniques. The socket and limb fitting follows, with multiple stages of adjustment, before patients progress to walking using parallel bars initially, followed by aids. Patients are encouraged to build up the time wearing a prosthetic, before eventually, aiming to walk independently without any aids.

Key Points

- When time allows, amputations should involve an MDT approach with the experienced surgical team and the rehabilitation team (including prosthetics, pain team and mental health support) to ensure the best outcomes
- The level of amputation and length of residual limb impacts on the energy expenditure, prosthetic fitting and cosmetic appearance post amputation
- Progression to independent walking with a prosthesis is rarely straightforward

Neurological Rehabilitation

Traumatic Brain Injury

Neurorehabilitation provides care for patients who have sustained a neurological deficit from a variety of pathologies, from congenital to acquired brain injury. Traumatic brain injury (TBI), classified as mild, moderate or severe, can result from assaults, falls and road traffic accidents, with gun shot wounds being less common but having the highest fatality rates.

Once the brain has been injured, it results in a series of well-recognised events including tissue damage, reduced cerebral blood flow and altered brain metabolism, most of which demonstrate minimal reversibility, and ultimately a secondary injury resulting in cell death and cerebral oedema. The goal in the management of acute TBI is to reduce ischemia and hypoxia in order to minimize the impact of the primary injury, reduce development of secondary injury and improve long-term outcomes [4]. The overall deficits seen in TBI are dependent on which part of the brain has been affected and whether the injury is focal, non-focal, diffuse or multi-focal. In the acute stages it is important for the patient to be managed in a multi-disciplinary unit prior to transfer to a neurorehabilitation setting once medically stable.

Patients with TBI should be assessed regularly by the MDT, especially in the early stages, to identify any deficits; categorised into physical, communication, cognitive and behavioural. Once an assessment has been completed, goals should be agreed, with as much patient involvement as possible, to enhance their ability to perform daily physical, vocational and social activities. The Glasgow Outcome Score is a validated tool which has been widely used to monitor rehabilitation progress.

An individualised rehabilitation programme should be created involving the patient's family and carers to promote optimal recovery. A structured schedule should be initiated with distractions limited, as patients with TBI can struggle if there is a lack of routine. There should also be planned rest periods in the programme to ensure that the patient does not become cognitively overwhelmed. Neurorehabilitation can be a long process, with support often needed for years after the initial injury, therefore a key-worker should be assigned to co-ordinate care and communicate with family members. It is essential to consider the mental capacity of the patient following TBI and depending on the severity, a deputy can be appointed to assist in decision making.

Mild traumatic brain injury (mTBI) has attracted increasing attention over recent years with the initial belief that behavioural changes were limited and transient, with no long-term neuropsychiatric sequalae in the majority of patients. However, with increased understanding, particularly from blast-related mTBI in the military and in sports men and women, the effects of mTBI are now recognised to be potentially more longstanding. The diagnosis and monitoring of mTBI can be challenging, with the Glasgow Coma Scale (GCS) and the Sport Concussion Assessment Tool being used commonly in the UK, although it is now recognized that the GCS has limited discriminative or prognostic value in mTBI [5]. Post-concussion syndrome is divided into four main categories; cognitive, somatic, affective and sleep-arousal complaints and, should these be identified, the patient should be referred to a specialist centre, as although they commonly resolve in the year post-injury, they can be persistent and result in significant functional limitations.

Key Points

- Traumatic brain injuries can complicate any trauma, and should be actively looked for to minimise secondary damage
- Once recognised, specific assessments should be performed to identify deficits and develop structured rehabilitation with periods of cognitive rest
- Mild TBI can lead to persistent symptoms and have a life changing impact,

Spinal Cord Injury

Spinal cord injury (SCI) can result from infections, vascular injury, malignancy and trauma, such as road traffic accidents, falls and sports injuries. The incidence in the United Kingdom is estimated to be 12–16 per million with about 75% of cases secondary to trauma, with most traumatic SCI affecting younger individuals. Although relatively rare, SCI can result in significant long-term neurological compromise.

Following acute trauma, the patient should be assessed in a major trauma centre by the surgical and SCI teams to determine whether a surgical intervention is required. In the early stages, spinal shock is evident before the extent of neurological function becomes apparent and regular American Spinal Injuries Association (ASIA) assessments are recommended. Once medically stable, the patient should be transferred to a spinal cord injury centre for multi-disciplinary management, in order to promote functional outcomes and reduce the chance of potential complications.

The ASIA scoring system is a standardised assessment tool which aids in predicting prognosis by characterising the neurological deficit. Ultimately the level of SCI is the most important influence on outcome, but regular assessment is useful to identify any clinical change or complications early so that they can be managed. Common complications following SCI depend on the level of injury but can include bowel and bladder dysfunction, pressure sores, delayed wound healing, spasticity and life-threating events such as autonomic dysreflexia. The most significant increases in mortality are seen in tetraplegics and those with ASIA grade A-C lesions, with standardised mortality ratios between 5.4 and 9.0 for people under 50, reducing with advancing age [6].

Specific areas of management for this group of patients compared to other trauma related patients include spasticity management and autonomic dysreflexia. Spasticity and the development of muscle contractures can be a significant source of impairment to the patient and can be managed often with simple measures such as regular stretching and attention to posture, however if these are not successful, patients may require pharmacological management with agents such as baclofen, botulinum toxin, or even surgery. In patients with a SCI at or above T6, autonomic dysreflexia is a potential complication which can lead to a life-threatening medical emergency. A stimulus, such as a blocked catheter, causes reflex sympathetic over-activity below level of cord lesion resulting in vasoconstriction and hypertension. This stimulates the carotid and aortic baroreceptors, leading to increased vagal tone and bradycardia. Peripheral vasodilatation, which would normally reduce blood pressure, cannot occur because of the injured cord. Rapid assessment and identification of the underlying cause is vital as well as addressing the hypertension, with sublingual glyceryl trinitrate or nifedipine. Patients and their families are taught how to recognise early symptoms and what immediate action is required.

Key Points

- Patients with a spinal cord injury (SCI) have increased mortality and need to be transferred to specialist centres
- Repeated use of the American Spinal Injuries Association (ASIA) assessment is used as a prognostic indicator to identify any changes.
- Many complications can result from a SCI, some of which are life threatening, requiring vigilance from the MDT, patient and their families

Lessons from Military Rehabilitation

The recent conflicts in Iraq and Afghanistan have driven a lot of change in the field of trauma rehabilitation. Whilst the military model for rehabilitation is specific to the needs of its users, lessons that have been learnt that map across to other victims of trauma. It is true that the psychological component of trauma influences outcomes, so involving professionals, peers and patients further down the rehabilitation pathway can be helpful to mitigate this. Co-existing traumatic brain injury and other injuries need to be screened for and identified as they impact on physical outcomes, especially if missed early in the rehabilitation pathway. Aggressive management of pain, including neuropathic and phantom, using both pharmacological and non-pharmacological techniques, is essential.

Other lessons have been learnt about trauma surgery, and constant feedback from the teams back in the UK treating the repatriated patients during these conflicts led to adaptations and changes in surgical techniques for the deployed surgical teams throughout the conflicts. These recommendations included that limb salvage should be attempted (amputation could always be performed later in the patient pathway), but if required to save life, amputation should be performed with operating team taking heed of the importance of residual stump lengths, locations of amputation (including through-knee) and the formation of stumps with the knowledge of how this would aid prosthetics and orthotics. It is hoped the long term follow up ADVANCE study will provide evidence on outcomes of these decisions made during the Iraq and Afghanistan conflicts.

Key Points

- Recent conflicts, and the polytrauma resulting from it, have meant changes in the field of military rehabilitation, many of which have been adopted in civilian practice.
- In particular, screening for brain injuries, aggressive use of multi-modal pain relief and trauma surgical techniques have been key lessons adopted
- The 20 year longitudinal study ADVANCE study will report on the long term outcomes of trauma victims from these conflicts.

Conclusion

A trauma patient often has multiple injuries requiring an individualized, complex trauma pathway and a large MDT to deliver this. This journey begins at the point of initial resuscitation—those involved in the patient's early care can shape the later stages, such as the type of prosthetic following amputation or the psychologically challenging commencement of identity change management. Different patients with the same injuries can have markedly different outcomes based on many factors, including the residual limb and stump formation as well as the emotional response to the event. Further injuries, both physical and mental, may become more apparent as rehabilitation commences.

For some trauma patients, an ideal outcome following successful rehabilitation is living independently in the community and back in the workplace. This is not possible for everyone, so the art of rehabilitation is identifying what is possible, what is desired, and creating a treatment plan to get there. This can take different forms depending on the number, severity and type of injury, but in every case, and for everyone involved, it requires patience, perseverance and communication.

Questions

1. Rehabilitation following a traumatic injury is critical for regaining independence, improving function and returning to as full as life as possible. When should the rehabilitation pathway begin with the initial rehabilitation assessment and early management?
   (a) When the patient is discharged from hospital
   (b) Once the patient is discharged from the intensive care unit
   (c) As soon as practically possible, including whilst on the intensive care unit

2. In conjunction with the patient and the rehabilitation team, regular goals should be set for the short, medium and long term. These enable an objective way to measure progress and promote investment in the rehabilitation journey. By what criteria should these goals be set?
   (a) SMART – Simple, Motivating, Agreed, Relevant, Timely
   (b) SMART – Specific, Measurable, Achievable, Realistic, Time-limited
   (c) SMART – Sensible, Meaningful, Attainable, Resourced, Time-bound

3. Musculoskeletal injury is a very common confounder factor in all types of trauma and can impact on the delivery of rehabilitation and subsequent recovery. In order to mitigate the impact of injury, early intervention is critical, and can easily be remembered by which acronym?
   (a) POLICE – Protect, Optimal Loading, Ice, Compression, Elevation
   (b) PRICE – Protect, Rest, Ice, Compression, Elevation
   (c) PRINCE – Protect, Rest, Ice, Non-weight bearing, Compression, Elevation

4. In the case of a non-life saving amputation following a traumatic injury, the site and level will impact on the future functional ability, cosmetic appearance and energy expenditure for the individual patient. With this in mind, how should amputations be performed?
   (a) After discussion with the surgical team, it soon as possible to allow the patient to get used to it
   (b) The surgical, rehabilitation, prosthetic, and psychological teams should decide when between them to avoid distressing the patient.
   (c) The least restrictive option should be taken initially with the patient involved in the decision and subsequent reviews

5. Traumatic brain injuries can be caused by a multitude of events and lead to significant impairments, with initial management is aimed at minimising primary injury, preventing any secondary injury and improving outcomes. By which international criteria are are Traumatic Brain Injuries classified?
   (a) Mild, Moderate, Severe
   (b) Physical, Communication, Cognitive, Behavioural
   (c) Cognitive, Affective, Somatic, Sleep-arousal

Answers

1. c
2. b
3. a
4. c
5. a

References

1. Noblet T, Lineham B, Wiper J, Harwood P. Amputation in trauma—how to achieve a good result from lower extremity amputation irrespective of the level. Curr Trauma Rep. 2019;5(1):69–78.

2. Ladlow P, Nightingale TE, McGuigan MP, Bennett AN, Phillip RD, Bilzon JLJ. Predicting ambulatory energy expenditure in lower limb amputees using multi-sensor methods. PLoS One. 2019;14(1):1–18.
3. Hsu E, Cohen SP. Postamputation pain: epidemiology, mechanisms, and treatment. J Pain Res. 2013;6:121.
4. Vella MA, Crandall ML, Patel MB. Acute management of traumatic brain injury. Surg Clin. 2017;97(5):1015–30.
5. Mayer AR, Quinn DK, Master CL. The spectrum of mild traumatic brain injury: a review. Neurology. 2017;89(6):623–32.
6. Middleton JW, Dayton A, Walsh J, Rutkowski SB, Leong G, Duong S. Life expectancy after spinal cord injury: a 50-year study. Spinal Cord. 2012;50(11):803.

44 Preventing and Treating Trauma-Related Mental Health Problems

Samantha K. Brooks and Neil Greenberg

- Many people will experience a potentially traumatic event (PTE) in their lifetime.
- Everyone reacts differently to potentially traumatic events and some may experience no distress at all while others experience a range of emotional, cognitive, behavioural, sleep-related or physical symptoms.
- While these symptoms improve on their own for the majority of people, a minority may require professional help.
- Professionals recommend that trauma-exposed individuals do 'active monitoring' of their symptoms for the first 4 weeks after the event, during which time they should engage in self-care and reach out to those close to them for support.
- Factors predicting whether someone might develop mental health problems after a PTE include lack of social support and poor coping strategies.
- Those still struggling to cope 4 weeks after the PTE may benefit from professional help such as cognitive behavioural therapy.

Introduction

Potentially traumatic events, which are experiences that put an individual (or someone close to them) at risk of serious injury, death or sexual violence [1], are unpredictable by nature. Throughout their lives, many people experience such incidents such as road accidents, natural disasters, war or terrorist attacks and interpersonal violence such as sexual assault and prolonged abuse. Indeed in the UK, around one in three people report having been exposed to traumatic events [2]. However, specific occupational populations such as military personnel [3] and emergency services workers [4] are more likely to be exposed and thus are at particular risk of trauma-related mental health disorders. Rates of post-traumatic stress disorder (PTSD) within the English population are around 4.5% [2] although rates of PTSD amongst trauma-exposed populations are higher. For instance, approximately 7.5% of UK military veterans report symptoms consistent with PTSD and studies of ambulance workers suggest that over 20% may experience PTSD [5].

Experiencing a potentially traumatic event can be extremely distressing in the short-term and can lead to a range of longer-term health consequences, both physical and psychological. In fact, it has been suggested that after experiencing a major traumatic event such as a disaster, the psychological injuries actually outnumber the physical injuries [6]. It is important to note that

S. K. Brooks · N. Greenberg (✉)
Health Protection Research Unit,
King's College London, London, UK
e-mail: samantha.k.brooks@kcl.ac.uk; neil.greenberg@kcl.ac.uk

P. Lax (ed.), *Textbook of Acute Trauma Care*, https://doi.org/10.1007/978-3-030-83628-3_44

not everyone will react in the same way—while many people will be distressed, some will be unaffected, and only a minority will go on to develop mental health problems [7]. For those who do suffer long-term psychological effects, the impact can be wide-reaching, affecting their relationships with others, physical health, personal and professional lives and the lives of people close to them. It is therefore imperative to establish best practice for the prevention, early detection and treatment of trauma-related mental health disorders.

This chapter aims to provide information about the potential psychological impact of a traumatic incident and the prevention and treatment of trauma-related mental health disorders.

Immediate and Short-Term Responses to Potentially Traumatic Events

No two potentially traumatic incidents are exactly the same, and no two people will react to a trauma in exactly the same way, either. There is not one specific reaction to a traumatic incident which could be considered 'the norm'—rather, a wide range of different responses are all considered normal. It is also normal for people to show a variety of different reactions at different times; there is no usual flow, or pattern, to symptoms. This is why such events are referred to as *potentially* traumatic—because not everyone will be traumatised by their experience. What one person thinks is traumatic may not be to someone else and vice versa. Indeed, some people become more resilient after exposure to a traumatic event; this has been termed post-traumatic growth [8].

It is natural to feel fear during a traumatic event itself. When faced with a potentially traumatic event, we are evolutionally programmed to either fight or to run away; Cannon [9] coined the phrase 'fight or flight' to describe this response. When experiencing such an incident, the body creates the 'fight or flight' response which includes the secretion of many substances, including adrenaline, which prepare the body for an emergency—either to defend it against danger or to run away from it. This response includes physical symptoms such as muscle tension, sweating and increased heart rate. More recent research has considered an additional 'freeze' response, where the body 'freezes up' and is unable to either fight or run away [10].

Over the days and weeks following the event, people may experience other physical responses such as changes in appetite, fatigue, aches and pains, being easily startled, and difficulties sleeping or sleeping too much. In addition to these physical symptoms, it is common for people to experience immediate psychological reactions. While some people may experience no symptoms whatsoever after experiencing a potentially traumatic event, many will experience some level of distress symptoms in the short term. There are a wide range of potential psychological responses; these include shock, numbness, confusion, disorientation, feelings of helplessness, anger, guilt, shame, fear, anxiety, sadness and grief, intrusive thoughts, inability to concentrate, irritability and difficulty making decisions. People who have existing mental health problems may also find their usual symptoms exacerbated by the event. Experiencing any, all, or none of these symptoms in the immediate aftermath is normal in the short term. They are simply the mind's way of trying to process, make sense of and come to terms with such an extreme, unfamiliar and often unexpected event.

Key Points
Common stress reactions include *emotional; cognitive*; *behavioural*; *sleep-related*; and *physical.* These reactions can be further categorised into intrusive reactions, avoidant reactions, and physical arousal reactions.

It is entirely normal to experience such symptoms of distress after a traumatic incident. More often than not, these do not lead to serious long-term psychological consequences and improve on their own over the days and weeks following the incident.

Common stress reactions include *emotional* (such as fear, worrying, feeling depressed, feeling helpless, denial, hopelessness, anxiety, and guilt); *cognitive* (such as confusion, poor attention, flashbacks, preoccupation with the event, intrusive thoughts, feeling on-edge, being vigilant, and memory problems); *behavioural* (such as anger, emotional outbursts, irritability, withdrawal, isolation, and antisocial acts); *sleep-related* (such as insomnia, nightmares, waking frequently during the night, and poor quality sleep); and *physical* (such as fatigue, nausea, dizziness, indigestion, chest tightness, dry mouth, chills, sweating, trembling, difficulty breathing, and racing heart).

These reactions can be further categorised into intrusive reactions, avoidant reactions, and physical arousal reactions. *Intrusive reactions*—that is, continuing unwelcome and unavoidable thoughts of the event—include disturbing or upsetting thoughts, images or dreams of the traumatic incident; continuing to experience physical or emotional reactions to reminders of the event; and flashbacks or feelings of re-experiencing the event all over again. *Avoidant reactions* include wanting to avoid all reminders of the incident (such as talking or thinking about the event, specific people or places, and media coverage); feelings of numbness; feelings of detachment from other people. *Physical arousal reactions* may also occur, including feeling jumpy or 'on edge'; being easily startled (for example by loud noises), feeling irritable or angry, difficulties sleeping and difficulties concentrating. More recent classifications of trauma symptoms have also described *negative alterations in cognition and mood* which include feelings of guilt or shame, persistent and distorted perceptions of themselves, others or the world and becoming socially withdrawn; and loss of interest in usual activities.

It is entirely normal to experience such symptoms of distress after a traumatic incident. More often than not, these do not lead to serious long-term psychological consequences and improve on their own over the days and weeks following the incident without any need for professional help [11]. It is important to differentiate between *distress,* a 'normal' and common response to an abnormal situation, or a *disorder*—a clinically significant behavioural or psychological syndrome which occurs less commonly. There are fundamental differences between the two and merely suffering feelings of sadness or worry as a natural response to a stressful situation is not a mental disorder [12]. In the following section, the best ways to support people experiencing distress after a potentially traumatic event are outlined to prevent (as much as is possible) that distress becoming a disorder.

Post-Incident Care: What Should Be Done in the Immediate Aftermath of a Potentially Traumatic Event to Prevent Mental Health Disorders Developing?

There is, unfortunately, some controversy concerning the best ways to support those exposed to potentially traumatic events, particularly in the days and weeks immediately following the incident.

As far back as World War I, the term debriefing was used to refer to a meeting of military personnel and their commanders after potentially traumatic incidents (such as major battles) when they would talk through the episode. In the late twentieth century, psychological debriefing, sometimes referred to as critical incident stress debriefing, was suggested as a useful way to alleviate acute stress responses and reduce the risk of delayed stress reactions [13]. This type of debriefing generally involves a trained counsellor, or another mental health professional, speaking to those affected, either individually or as a group, to discuss their feelings towards what they have just experienced. This was with the aim of allowing them to process the event and reflect on its impact and provide psychoeducation about traumatic stress responses.

Key Points

It was also believed that a one-off session with a counsellor/mental health professional—discussing the experience, personal reactions and emotions, symptoms experienced since the event, and seeking reassurance about symptoms and education about what might be expected—would be helpful in processing the event. The idea behind this was to promote emotional processing of the event and the venting of emotions, intending to reduce distress and prevent long-term mental health problems (like post-traumatic stress disorder) from setting in. However, despite the laudable aims of preventing the development of post-traumatic stress and similar disorders, there is little evidence to suggest this approach is effective. In fact, the majority of high-quality research in this area indicates that debriefing is ineffective at best and harmful at worst [14–16].

A systematic review of early interventions for post-traumatic stress disorder [17] found that not only did debriefing not prevent the disorder, but it actually increased the likelihood of such symptoms as a result of interfering with the natural recovery process. One particular study demonstrating the potentially detrimental effects of debriefing [18] involved randomly assigning burn victims to either a debriefing session or a no-treatment, assessment-only condition. At initial assessment, there were no significant differences between the two groups in terms of depression, anxiety or post-traumatic stress. After 3 months, the debriefed group had non-significantly higher levels of post-traumatic stress disorder than the assessment-only group, and after 13 months, the debriefed group had *significantly* higher levels of post-traumatic stress disorder. Similar findings were found in a study of road traffic accident victims [19], with debriefed participants reporting significantly more symptoms of post-traumatic stress disorder in the long term.

As a result of the lack of evidence for debriefing being helpful, and the increasing amount of evidence suggesting it is ineffective and can even be harmful, the publication of National Institute for Health and Care Excellence (NICE) guidelines in 2018 [20] emphasised that this kind of psychological debriefing, or immediate trauma counselling where initial symptoms are not severe, is unhelpful and not recommended. It is worthwhile noting that where evidence in support of a particular intervention is lacking, NICE ordinarily do not provide any recommendation on the intervention at all. As such, NICE's recommendation that psychological debriefing should not be used is a testament to NICE's view that it has the potential to cause harm. Explicitly, the guidelines state: "**Do not offer psychologically-focused debriefing for the prevention or treatment of PTSD…** Evidence on psychologically-focused debriefing, either individually or in groups, showed no benefit for children or adults, and some suggestion of worse outcomes than having no treatment."

So, if psychologically-focused debriefing cannot be provided, what *can* be done in the immediate aftermath of a potentially traumatic event? A variety of other psychosocial interventions have been explored, with limited evidence [17]. For example, memory-structuring interventions which help people who have experienced trauma to organise their memories of the traumatic event have yielded inconsistent results in terms of preventing post-traumatic stress disorder [21]. Self-help psychoeducation—that is, providing people who have experienced potentially traumatic events with self-help booklets describing likely responses and suggesting coping strategies—also have not been found to be particularly helpful [22]. Rather than any type of immediate mental health-focused intervention, the evidence suggests that offers of practical support, a temporary reduction in exposure to stress and remaining vigilant for how someone is coping appears to be the best approach unless initial symptoms are very severe and impairing.

Key Points

The National Institute for Health and Care Excellence 2018 guidelines for the management of post-traumatic stress disorder recommend a period of 'active monitoring' for the first 4 weeks after the trauma if symptoms are mild [23]. To put it simply, this means that trauma-exposed people (and/or those close to them) just need to monitor their symptoms.

The majority of people will recover on their own within this period, without requiring any formal intervention. This active monitoring period was previously referred to as 'watchful waiting' in earlier versions of the guidelines but is changed to active monitoring in the 2018 guidelines. This change is in order to be more explicit that individuals should not be passive about their symptoms, but should actively keep an eye on them. Healthcare professionals, in some cases, can perform active monitoring. However, more realistically family, friends, colleagues and line managers are often better placed to actively monitor as well as ensuring that appropriate support is offered. Some routinely trauma-exposed organisations, such as the media or emergency services, have implemented trauma risk management (TRiM) as a method of actively monitoring trauma-exposed staff members. TRiM is a peer support system which was developed in the UK military and has been widely researched since [24]. While TRiM is certainly not a panacea for trauma, there is good evidence that it is well accepted and improves social support and help-seeking [25] as well as being associated with a decrease in trauma-related sickness absence [26].

Consequently, if no professional treatment or intervention is recommended during the immediate aftermath of a potentially traumatic event, it falls to the individual and those close to them to manage their wellbeing while they come to terms with their experience. It can be challenging to cope with the experience of a traumatic event and adapt to life afterwards. Still, there are many simple things that trauma-affected people and their loved ones can do [27].

Recommendations for Self-Care

- It is recommended that people exposed to traumatic incidents stick to their regular, pre-incident routines as much as possible (where appropriate); stability is important, and people should get 'back to normal' as soon as they can.
- People should make particularly sure that they engage in activities which have previously made them feel good and which distract them from overthinking about the event. These activities will naturally differ from person to person but may include playing sports, reading, writing, doing arts and crafts, doing puzzles or participating in social activities with friends or family.
- Relaxation techniques may help calm the mind and lessen feelings of distress or anxiety—for example, yoga, meditation, deep breathing exercises, massage or calming self-talk. Relaxation techniques have been cited as being helpful by people involved in providing disaster mental health services [28].
- It is vital that people pay attention to their physical needs—they should ensure they get adequate rest (even if they may be struggling to sleep), sufficient healthy food (even though their appetite may be diminished) and fluid.
- Since feelings of helplessness are common in the aftermath of a potentially traumatic event, it helps if people focus on practical things they can do that may give them a sense of purpose or accomplishment.
- Exercise can be extremely beneficial; there is a wealth of literature on the benefits of physical activity for our mental health and general wellbeing [29], and a growing body of research on the positive effects of exercise for symptoms of distress after a trauma [30].
- Expressing feelings is often important. While some people may not feel ready or able to talk to other people, expressing emotions does not need to involve another person. It can be helpful just to write things down on paper whenever they feel the need to, keep a journal, or express themselves in other ways such as through art [31].
- Spending time with people they trust and seeking social support are particularly important and will be discussed more detail in the next section.
- It must also be noted that while participating in hobbies and interests, exercising, and taking part in activities which distract them are useful ways of taking one's mind off the potentially traumatic event and helping people to cope, individuals should not rely on distracting themselves to the point of altogether avoiding thinking or talking about the traumatic event they have experienced. Extreme avoidance can be just as harmful as focusing too much on the event—a balance is needed.

Social Support

Key Points

A good level of social support is one of the key factors increasing the chances of a positive outcome after a potentially traumatic event; that is, social support promotes resilience and positive adaptation despite adversity [32]. Social support can come from many different sources—it may be from friends, partners, family members, colleagues, or other people who experienced the same incident and may be dealing with similar feelings.

Reaching out to whoever people feel comfortable talking to can help individuals to gain clarity about the situation, and indeed merely sharing can lessen the psychological 'load'; the old adage of *a problem shared is a problem halved* holds true. However, some people may prefer to talk to someone they are less close to in order to have a more neutral space for talking—a colleague, religious leader, teacher, manager, or support group. Talking to other people who experienced the same event can be extremely helpful in terms of reflecting on the experience, gaining clarity and coming to terms with it. Indeed, evidence from military studies shows that military personnel favour speaking with colleagues who have had similar experiences and doing so is associated with better mental health [33]. It is important to note that people sharing their feelings with others who experienced the same incident should not compare their emotions, reactions or coping methods—because, as discussed, everyone reacts in different ways. Neither party should leave that interaction feeling that their response is 'abnormal' or that they are not coping as well as the other person.

People should make sure that the person they talk to is supportive, non-judgmental, and understanding. It is normal to feel anxious about talking to someone about feelings, so choosing a person they feel comfortable and calm with is essential. Before reaching out to someone—whoever that someone may be—it may be helpful for people to plan ahead of time what areas and aspects they want to discuss. This may even involve making some notes before any conversation begins. This can reduce feelings of anxiety about saying the wrong thing or not knowing what to say.

Recommendations for Trauma-Exposed People: Reaching Out

- The individual should not be afraid to tell others what kind of support they think they need, or how they think the other person can help. It may be that they want empathy, input, suggestions of how to cope, someone to simply listen while they talk about their experience or even just company in a comfortable environment. Also having typical, everyday conversations—not related to the event—with someone can be helpful.
- People must not feel pressured to talk about painful memories or feelings before they feel ready, or even to talk about details of the event itself if they do not feel comfortable to at first. Some people may be prepared to talk about it straight away, while others may feel unable to for some time. Again, everybody reacts to potentially traumatic events in different ways, and so naturally, their needs in the immediate aftermath are different.
- If someone *does* want to express their thoughts or feelings, they should do so; bottling them up is not helpful.
- If someone does not want to (or feel able to) discuss the event with their friends or family, they may find it useful to join a support group. Local community groups on social media and noticeboards in the local area are excellent ways of finding out about such groups; also, GPs can recommend any local groups that may be appropriate. 'Informal support groups' can also be created by those who experienced the same potentially traumatic event together, arranging to spend time with each other. However, it is not clear if these are always helpful. NICE recommends that such groups are facilitated or supervised to help ensure that they are of benefit to attendees' mental health.

Recommendations for Those Close to Trauma-Exposed People: How to Communicate

Key Points

The people who trauma-exposed individuals turn to are most often not trained mental health professionals. However, in most cases they do not need to be: anyone can help simply by listening, understanding and supporting. There are several things they can do, such as acknowledging the experience that the other person has been through; asking how they are and how they have been doing since the incident, maintaining an air of calm interest and engagement. It may seem like common sense, but simply showing interest in the person and their wellbeing can help, as it lets the trauma-exposed person see that they are valued.

The person they turn to should be careful to focus on the trauma survivor's own interpretation of their experience and should communicate calmly and efficiently, using neutral language to avoid creating extra anxiety or fear. They should engage in *active listening*, which involves fully concentrating on, understanding and responding to what is being said. The listener is active in trying to grasp the feelings of the person they are listening to and helping them to work out their problems, rather than passively listening [34]. This is key to building rapport, understanding and trust. Tips for active listening include subtle encouragement to show they are listening to the other person while keeping 'encouragers' (subtle actions or expressions which encourage the speaker to continue) at a minimum. Asking open-ended and non-leading questions, reflecting on what the other person has just said and maintaining good posture and eye contact are useful techniques. These can be enhanced by using effective pauses without needing to 'fill the gaps', and summarising or paraphrasing what the other person says to establish that they have understood. Drawing on their own, relevant experiences and talking about how they coped with those may be helpful, but they should be careful to avoid implying that they or other people have had it worse. The active listener should be mindful not to force the person to talk about things they may not be ready to discuss, not to try and alter their perceptions of the event, and not to re-traumatise the person. It is also important not to make any mention of feelings of shame or guilt unless the individual brings those up first. They should avoid exclamations of surprise, and avoid suggesting that it is weak or shameful to need help. They should also avoid 'why' questions, as these can make people defensive, as well as leading questions, digging for unnecessary information, preaching, interrupting, and patronising. Key advice would be to reassure the person that their feelings are normal and valid. However, if red flags come up, such as thoughts of self-harm, the individual should be helped to speak with an appropriately qualified professional.

Ongoing Psychological Issues

While the psychological symptoms of distress immediately following a traumatic experience tend to go away on their own with time (usually within 4 weeks) [35], in some cases, symptoms may worsen, and turn from 'distress' into 'disorder'. A minority of people will go on to develop mental health problems such as post-traumatic stress disorder, depression, anxiety, phobias or alcohol issues, which can significantly impair their functioning.

Post-Traumatic Stress Disorder

Key Points

While there are several mental health problems which can arise after experiencing a potentially traumatic event, by far the most commonly researched and believed to be the most central to post-event psychopathology is post-traumatic stress disorder, or PTSD [36, 37].

A diagnosis of PTSD is dependent on (i) being exposed to a traumatic event and (ii) suffering from distressing symptoms post-event [38]. Someone experiencing significant psychological distress after having experienced a *non*-traumatic stressor would instead likely be diagnosed with an adjustment disorder. This raises the question of what constitutes a 'traumatic event', and there remains some controversy in this area35. The Diagnostic and Statistical Manual of Mental Disorders-IV [39] stated that a traumatic incident had to include a response of helplessness, horror or fear. However, this failed to take into account individuals who certainly experienced potentially traumatic events but responded in an entirely rational way (for example, many people whose job roles include being regularly exposed to potentially traumatic events) [40]. This was inappropriate as it confused an individual's subjective response with the objective experience of exposure to a potentially traumatic event [41]. Therefore, the updated diagnostic criteria in 2013 removed the requirement for a response of helplessness, horror or fear.

The current diagnostic category for PTSD as described in the Diagnostic and Statistical Manual of Mental Disorders-5 [1] lists eight criteria which must be met for a diagnosis of PTSD to be made.

1. *Exposure to a traumatic event*—that is, an event which included exposure to death, the threat of death, serious injury, threat of serious injury, sexual violence, or threat of sexual violence. Exposure includes the direct experience of the event, direct witnessing of the event, learning that a close other has been exposed to actual or threatened trauma and repeated or extreme indirect exposure, usually in the course of professional duties.
2. *Persistent re-experiencing of the event*—this may be through involuntary thoughts, images, dreams, hallucinations or flashbacks.
3. *Avoidance of stimuli associated with the trauma*—this may involve avoidance of thoughts or feelings related to the event, avoidance of discussions of the event, avoidance of media coverage of the event, or avoidance of any places, people or other stimuli which trigger the person to recall the incident.
4. *At least two symptoms of negative alterations in cognition and mood*—any two of the following: inability to remember a particular (important) aspect of the event; persistent negative beliefs about the self, others or the world; persistent distorted cognitions about the cause or consequences of the event, leading to blame of the self or others; persistent negative emotions; loss of interest in usual activities; feelings of detachment from other people; and inability to experience positive emotions.
5. *At least two symptoms of negative alterations in arousal and reactivity*—any two of the following: irritable and angry outbursts; reckless or self-destructive behaviour; hyper-vigilance; exaggerated startle response; difficulties concentrating; disturbed sleep.
6. The above symptoms *persist for at least 1 month.*
7. The above symptoms *cause significant distress or impairment in function.*
8. The above symptoms *cannot be attributed to either another medical condition or the physiological effects of a substance.*

Understanding Factors Contributing to Psychological Distress and Disorder

Understanding the risk factors for post-traumatic mental health problems is essential, as this allows us to identify who is most vulnerable. We might, over-simplistically, simply expect that the higher the level of exposure to the potentially traumatic event, the more likely an individual is to experience long-term psychological problems. Unsurprisingly, people with a high level of exposure to the event (those who are closest to the incident and for more extended periods, or who are involved in the immediate rescue and care of victims and survivors, or witness severe injury or death) tend to suffer more psychological consequences than those who are further away from the incident or caught up in it for less time, or who do not witness such atrocities [42]. However, there are many other factors at play; we cannot automatically assume that those with high exposure will suffer psychological consequences, or that those with low exposure will not suffer. For example, while there has been a wealth of research on occupational groups at high risk of experiencing traumatic events, there are often strikingly low levels of mental health problems in such people. One study of police who dealt with the aftermath of the Madrid bombings found that only 1.2% of their participants were affected by post-traumatic stress after 5 weeks [40]. Other studies have reported much higher rates of mental health problems in similarly-affected employees [37]. So, it is clear that there are factors other than traumatic exposure itself which affect how people react to potentially traumatic events and whether or not they will develop psychological problems as a result.

Several comprehensive meta-analyses and systematic literature reviews have explored the risk factors for developing mental health disorders after experiencing a traumatic event. They have all noted that social and psychological factors are more significant predictors of mental health outcomes than demographic factors such as gender, age, race or education level [42–47].

Pre-Traumatic Event Predictors of Mental Health Outcomes

Key Points
There are several pre-event predictors of post-event mental health. A meta-analysis [47] identified prior trauma, prior psychological adjustment, and family history of psychopathology as risk factors for developing PTSD.

Previous experience of a traumatic event, even if it happened a long time ago, is associated with a higher risk of developing mental health problems. The more recent and relevant the experience, however, the more likely it is to matter, particularly if they have begun thinking about it again following the current trauma.

Stressful pre-disaster life events (such as divorce, bereavement, illness, work overload and any significant problems at home, work or with health) and prior mental health problems, in addition to family psychiatric history, are also predictive of mental health problems [46, 48]. It has been reported that the risk of experiencing mental health problems post-trauma increases with an increasing number of significantly stressful prior life events [49]. Childhood abuse is a particularly significant risk factor for mental health problems following exposure to a potentially traumatic event [46].

Peri-Traumatic Predictors of Mental Health

Key Points
An individual's experience and emotional responses during the potentially traumatic event can have a significant impact on the mental health symptoms they experience in the aftermath [47]. Feelings of risk or threat—in particular, thinking that one was going to die during the event—appear to be particularly important [42–44, 47].

Evidence suggests this is even more predictive of mental health problems post-incident than actual injuries experienced [50]. The longer the duration of time that the individual feels at risk, the worse their mental health outcomes are likely to be [51]. The critical factor here is about a significant threat to personal safety—whether the person felt unsafe, that their life was in danger, or that they *believed* they faced serious injury or death (even if they were not in fact at risk of either of these). Unsurprisingly, actual injury to the self or injury or death of close others is also predictive of poor mental health [42]. A study of fire-fighters [52] found an increase in PTSD risk with each additional death of a colleague experienced after the World Trade Center disaster in New York.

Also important are emotional reactions during the event. For example, studies of disaster workers have suggested that high levels of identification with the victims or imagining one's self or loved ones being victims are associated with poor post-disaster wellbeing [53, 54]. Peri-traumatic dissociation is also well-documented as predicting post-event mental health [42, 47, 55].

Social Support

Key Points
One of the key predictors of post-incident mental health is the quality of social support available during the recovery period [32, 42–45, 47].

A plethora of studies of military personnel have shown that unit cohesion, support from immediate managers and positive relationships with colleagues are associated with resilience. In contrast, poor support and poor cohesion are associated with mental health problems. Research on trauma-exposed organisations has shown that social support from colleagues and particularly managers is important for fostering resilience [42]. For this reason, the United Kingdom Psychological Trauma Society's guidelines for trauma-exposed organisations (2014) emphasises the importance of peer support and preparing those in managerial positions for supporting their staff.

Post-Event Coping Strategies

Coping strategies can generally be categorised as either positive or negative [56]. Negative coping strategies are ineffective, perpetuating stress rather than reducing it, and include deliberate avoidance of traumatic thoughts, denial of the experience, and self-destructive behaviours such as misuse of alcohol or drugs. These strategies appear to be associated with poorer mental health [42]. Positive coping strategies are effective in reducing feelings of stress, and include proactive coping, confrontive coping (such as planning, strategising or developing strategies to "beat" the problem), and planned problem-solving. Typically, positive coping strategies involve awareness of the situation; working towards a resolution of the problem; modifying behaviours to resolve the problem; and ultimately moving on with life [56]. These strategies tend to be associated with more positive mental health outcomes [42].

Often, people find themselves wanting to cope with their feelings by using alcohol, cigarettes, and/or prescription or recreational drugs. These can seem like an easy, quick way of escaping bad feelings and experiencing relief from stress. However, they are unhelpful long-term and can increase the chance of longer-term problems later by adversely affecting physical health, disrupting sleep patterns, negatively impacting relationships with others and potentially leading to addiction.

Post-Event Impact on Life

Key Points
If an individual experiences personal or professional loss as a result of the potentially traumatic event they appear to be at higher risk of mental health problems [42–44]. The more far-reaching the impact of the event on someone's life, the more likely they appear to suffer mental health problems. The impact may include property loss, job loss, financial problems, or insurance problems.

Multiple Exposures

It is also worth noting that exposure to multiple potentially traumatic events is another risk factor for mental health problems. Experiencing a singular traumatic event is known as Type I Trauma, while chronic exposure to multiple traumatic events over time is known as Type II Trauma [57]. Type II Trauma is often experienced by individuals working in occupations particularly at risk for trauma, such as emergency services and military personnel, humanitarian relief workers, healthcare professionals and journalists reporting from conflict zones or disaster scenes, as well as those frequently exposed to trauma vicariously such as therapists, child protection officers and social workers [58]. The chronic exposure experienced by those suffering from Type II Trauma can also lead to complex PTSD (C-PTSD) [38].

Early Detection of Trauma-Related Mental Health Disorders

Educating people about the symptoms of mental health problems (such as PTSD) is of utmost importance—if individuals cannot recognise symptoms in themselves or those close to them, then they will not recognise if they (or close others) need professional help.

Unfortunately, many people who might benefit from professional help after a traumatic event avoid seeking help even if they do acknowledge their symptoms, for a variety of reasons. Perhaps they are unaware of where to go for help, feel ashamed about admitting they are struggling, or hope the problem will go away on its own. Indeed, there is still a substantial amount of stigma surrounding mental health problems [59].

For this reason, in the cases of major incidents or disasters, a 'screen and treat' approach could be helpful, ensuring that everyone affected by the event is screened for potential mental health problems. The 2018 National Institute for Health and Care Excellence guidelines [20] recommend that the people responsible for coordinating disaster plans should screen all affected individuals.

After acts of terrorism in Tunisia, Paris and Brussels in 2015–2016, the English Department of Health funded an outreach programme to identify and support all residents of England who had been affected by any of these three incidents. Mental health questionnaires were mailed to all people known to be affected [60]. An overwhelming majority of those who responded (91.8%, $n = 195$) screened positive, according to the questionnaire scores, for at least one of PTSD, anxiety, depression, increased smoking or problematic drinking of alcohol. The screen and treat programme allowed for these people to be offered clinical assessment and, where necessary, subsequent referral for appropriate professional treatment. So it seems from this study that screen and treat programmes are beneficial in community settings. Still, it should be noted that only a small percentage of those affected by the incidents responded to the questionnaires, and issues relating to data protection limited the ability to identify and communicate with other people who may have benefitted from the screening. Similar problems arose from the UK's first use of the screen and treat approach, following the July 7th 2005 bombings in London. Agencies were reluctant to share the contact details of those affected with the screening team, and as a result, only a small percentage of those affected were screened [61]. However, community-based screen and treat programmes appear to be broadly successful for those who do take part, and more explicit policies around data sharing after major traumatic incidents may help.

It is important to note, however, that while there is reasonable evidence of community-based screen and treat programmes being effective, the same is not valid for post-incident, or post-deployment, screening programmes within organisational settings. Studies carried out in US troops suggest that military personnel identified as having a mental health problem through being screened after deployment did not experience any benefit. Indeed, a 2007 paper showed that US personnel who were screened, advised to obtain professional care and did so had poorer longer-term mental health than those who were encouraged to seek professional care, but who ignored the advice [62]. A randomised controlled study of post-deployment screening carried out in around 9000 UK military personnel, published in 2017, found screening had no impact on mental health status or help-seeking behaviour over a year after the screening was carried out [63]. It is likely that stigma as well as concerns about confidentiality, reputation and career impact, as well as fluctuating post-deployment mental health symptoms, all act to make psychological health screening within organisations ineffective.

Of course, some potentially traumatic events affect only a small number of people, or even only one person, and in such cases community screen and treat programmes would clearly not be used. In these cases, it is the people closest to the trauma-affected individual who are best placed to notice if the individual is in distress. It can be useful to compare their behaviour to their usual behaviour; are they acting differently, no longer taking part in their usual hobbies or activities, or withdrawing themselves from their usual social activities? Those especially close to the person may well notice changes in sleep and appetite, too. If they do feel that their loved one needs professional help, they should be supportive of this, and reassure the person that needing help does not imply instability or weakness.

In cases where individuals have experienced chronic exposure to trauma as a result of their occupational roles, or who by chance have experienced a 'one-off' traumatic event in the workplace, it may be their colleagues and/or manager who is best-placed to notice any problems and provide support [59]. It would, therefore, be helpful for any manager who finds themselves in the position of needing to support trauma-exposed staff to familiarise themselves with appropriate guidelines for treating traumatic stress [20, 64] and ensure that they can appropriately support staff who need it.

Treatment of Trauma-Related Mental Health Disorders

Key Points
If, after the 'active monitoring' period of 4 weeks, symptoms are persisting, formal mental health assessment and intervention may be needed. It may also be that specific therapy is indicated if someone presents with very severe and impairing symptoms before 4 weeks, although the evidence as to what works is less robust for treatments delivered during this period.

If, after active monitoring, someone is still struggling to cope with intense thoughts, feelings or physical reactions surrounding the incident; is feeling numb and detached; if their personal or professional life is suffering; if they are smoking or drinking to excess, or using drugs; if they have self-injurious thoughts or behaviours; if they have found themselves engaging in violent, aggressive or destructive behaviour; if they feel unable to enjoy life; or if they have vague signs of physical illness that cannot be explained and were not present before the trauma they should be assessed by a suitably trained professional. In these cases, it is recommended that people contact their GP or local mental health service. If they are suffering from a mental health disorder such as PTSD, it is essential they are treated by a professional mental health provider.

According to the NICE guidelines (2018), GPs should take responsibility for the initial assessment (including risk assessment and assessment of physical, psychological and social needs) and coordination of care. The guidelines recommend providing advice to patients (and their families and carers where appropriate) about common reactions to traumatic events, including the symptoms of PTSD and its course; assessment, treatment and support options; and where their care will take place. Treatment from specialists is likely to be required, and the guidelines suggest that GPs should support the transition to different services by providing the patient information about the service they are moving to and ensuring information is shared between all services involved. They should also include the patient and their carers or family if appropriate in meetings to plan the transition and address any specific worries the patient has about the transition.

Whilst there is mixed evidence for what kind of treatment is best for any one person, NICE guidelines helpfully clarify that evidence-based, trauma-focused therapies are the mainstay of any treatment approach, though different types of trauma may require different interventions. For example, one potential intervention (eye movement desensitisation and reprocessing) has been shown to be successful in some cases [65]. This intervention involves patients recalling an image representing the traumatic incident, along with the negative cognitive and bodily symptoms that come with that image, and following alternating eye movements while they do this, as a way of dampening the power of those emotionally charged memories and images. Although this has been shown to be successful for many types of trauma, NICE guidelines (2018) do not recommend it for use in people with war trauma. For people with non-combat-related trauma, when eye movement desensitisation and reprocessing is recommended, it must be based on a validated manual (i.e. be delivered in accordance with a previously agreed, evidence based and accepted structure) and be provided over 8–12 sessions (or more if required). It must also be delivered by trained practitioners with ongoing supervision, be delivered in a phased way and include psychoeducation about trauma responses, managing distressing symptoms, treating stressful memories and promoting alternative positive beliefs about the self. Each treatment session must repeat the eye movement stimulation until memories are no longer distressing and include the teaching of self-calming techniques for use between sessions.

Peer support groups can also be useful. The NICE guidelines (2018) recommend helping patients to access peer support groups if they want to, noting that these groups should always be led by people with mental health training. These sessions should be delivered in such a way that reduces the likelihood of exacerbating symptoms and provide useful information and help with accessing services.

Key Points

The most robust consistent evidence for the treatment of PTSD is for trauma-focused cognitive behavioural therapy [66, 67]. This may include exposure to the trauma in a safe way, such as by imagining or writing about the event to cope with feelings. It can also involve cognitive restructuring, which consists of the therapist helping the patient to look at the event in a more realistic way and reduce their feelings of guilt or shame.

Generally, 'talking therapies' which enable people to address their feelings about the event and improve their coping strategies, are recommended. NICE guidelines (2018) recommend four types of trauma-focused cognitive behavioural intervention: cognitive processing therapy, cognitive therapy for PTSD, narrative exposure therapy and prolonged exposure therapy. They note that all interventions should be based on a validated manual, be provided over 8–12 sessions (or more if required), be delivered by trained cognitive behavioural therapy practitioners with ongoing supervision from peers and include psychoeducation about trauma reactions, strategies for managing re-experiencing, and safety planning. They should also involve elaboration and processing of memories of the traumatic event, involve processing emotions related to the traumatic event (including shame and anger), involve re-structuring trauma-related meanings and help overcome avoidance of feelings. They should aim to re-establish normal functioning, prepare the patient for the end of treatment and include planning booster sessions if appropriate. Cognitive behavioural therapy can also be delivered online if the patient is deemed as not at risk of harm to themselves or others. Again, this type of intervention needs to be based on a validated programme and include guidance from a trained practitioner.

Medications are not usually the first line of treatment but can at times help lessen symptoms, particularly if coupled with therapy. The NICE guidelines (2018) suggest that medication should be a second-line strategy for people who do not want, or are not currently suitable for, talking therapies. There is some evidence that antidepressants such as paroxetine, sertraline and venlafaxine can help manage PTSD symptoms. The guidelines also recommend that specialists can consider the use of antipsychotics such as risperidone if the patient has disabling symptoms and behaviours, such as psychotic symptoms. Any pharmacological treatment should be reviewed regularly. Initial research on the effectiveness of pharmacological treatments for PTSD focused on benzodiazepines which were found to be ineffective and, at worst, could potentially lead to higher rates of PTSD [68]. Therefore, benzodiazepines are not recommended for use in the NICE guidelines (2018).

Often a combination of talking therapy and medication such as anti-depressants can be successful in treating mental health problems. It must be noted that talking therapies such as cognitive behavioural therapy are often delivered months after the trauma and are therefore significantly different from critical incident stress debriefing. Ideally, the treatment provided should help the patient understand and cope with their experience and their feelings; allow them to be able to relax; enable them to control their anger; return their sleep and diet habits to normal and teach the patient how to respond to reminders of the trauma without becoming distressed.

Summary

In the immediate aftermath of a potentially traumatic event, professional psychological help is not usually necessary or indeed recommended. While the majority of people affected by trauma will recover fully without psychological intervention, a minority will experience long-term mental health problems such as post-traumatic stress disorder and will need additional support. There are several pre-event, peri-event and post-event factors which are predictive of whether someone will go on to develop mental health problems. Perhaps most notably, a lack of social support and poor coping strategies are associated with poor mental health. Stigma around mental health, or simply not believing that professional help is needed, can stop people from seeking help even when they need it. Those who are still struggling to cope 4 weeks after the potentially traumatic event may benefit from talking therapies such as cognitive behavioural therapy and should be assisted to access professional help as often they fail to do so themselves.

Questions

1. What symptoms might people experience after a potentially traumatic event?
   (a) Fear, feeling depressed, feeling anxious
   (b) Confusion, poor attention, memory problems
   (c) Nausea, difficulty breathing, dizziness
   (d) All of the above

2. According to NICE PTSD management guidelines, what should someone do if they are experiencing non-severe symptoms of distress after a potentially traumatic event?
   (a) Seek professional help immediately
   (b) Monitor their symptoms and seek professional help if symptoms persist after a week
   (c) Monitor their symptoms and seek professional help if symptoms persist after four weeks
   (d) Monitor their symptoms and seek professional help if symptoms persist after six months

3. According to NICE guidelines, which of the following is NOT recommended for someone diagnosed with PTSD?
   (a) Prescription of benzodiazepines
   (b) Support groups
   (c) Cognitive behavioural therapy
   (d) Eye movement desensitisation and reprocessing

4. What should someone do if a loved one has recently experienced a potentially traumatic event?
   (a) Urge them to seek professional help immediately
   (b) Compare their behaviour to their usual behaviour and offer to listen to them/talk to them if they need it
   (c) Leave them alone
   (d) Ask them to describe the traumatic event in detail, in order to judge how much it might have traumatised them

5. What most commonly happens after a potentially traumatic event?
   (a) The majority of people are not affected at all
   (b) The majority of people experience some symptoms of distress, which improve on their own over time
   (c) The majority of people experience symptoms of distress which only improve with professional intervention
   (d) The majority of people are diagnosed with post-traumatic stress disorder

Answers

1. d
2. c
3. a
4. b
5. b

References

1. American Psychiatric Association, editor. Diagnostic and statistical manual of mental disorders: DSM-5. 5th ed. Washington, D.C: American Psychiatric Association; 2013. 947 p.

2. McManus S, Bebbington P, Jenkins R, Brugha T, NHS Digital, UK Statistics Authority. Mental health and wellbeing in England: Adult Psychiatric Morbidity Survey 2014: a survey carried out for NHS Digital by NatCen Social Research and the Department of Health Sciences, University of Leicester. 2016.
3. Walker S. Assessing the mental health consequences of military combat in Iraq and Afghanistan: a literature review: Soldiers mental health. Journal of Psychiatric and Mental Health Nursing [Internet]. 2010 Nov [cited 2020 Jan 20];17(9):790–6. Available from: https://doi.org/10.1111/j.1365-2850.2010.01603.x
4. Skogstad M, Skorstad M, Lie A, Conradi HS, Heir T, Weisaeth L. Work-related post-traumatic stress disorder. Occupational Medicine [Internet]. 2013 Apr 1 [cited 2020 Jan 20];63(3):175–82. Available from: https://academic.oup.com/occmed/article-lookup/doi/10.1093/occmed/kqt003
5. Bennett P. Levels of mental health problems among UK emergency ambulance workers. Emergency Medicine Journal [Internet]. 2004 Mar 1 [cited 2020 Jan 20];21(2):235–6. Available from: http://emj.bmj.com/cgi/doi/10.1136/emj.2003.005645
6. McCabe OL, Semon NL, Lating JM, Everly GS, Perry CJ, Moore SS, et al. An academic-government-faith partnership to build disaster mental health preparedness and community resilience. Public Health Rep [Internet]. 2014 Nov [cited 2020 Jan 20];129(6_suppl4):96–106. Available from: http://journals.sagepub.com/doi/10.1177/00333549141296S413
7. Bonanno GA. Loss, Trauma, and Human Resilience: Have We Underestimated the Human Capacity to Thrive After Extremely Aversive Events? American Psychologist [Internet]. 2004 [cited 2020 Jan 20];59(1):20–8. Available from: http://doi.apa.org/getdoi.cfm?doi=10.1037/0003-066X.59.1.20
8. Tedeschi RG, Calhoun LG. Posttraumatic Growth: Conceptual Foundations and Empirical Evidence. Psychological Inquiry [Internet]. 2004 Jan [cited 2020 Jan 20];15(1):1–18. Available from: http://www.tandfonline.com/doi/abs/10.1207/s15327965pli1501_01
9. Cannon WB. Bodily changes in pain, hunger, fear and rage: An account of recent researches into the function of emotional excitement. [Internet]. New York: D Appleton & Company; 1915 [cited 2020 Jan 20]. Available from: http://content.apa.org/books/10013-000
10. Steimer T. The biology of fear- and anxiety-related behaviors. Dialogues Clin Neurosci. 2002 Sep;4(3):231–49.
11. Dunn R, Brooks SK, Greenberg N. Psychological impact of traumatic events: guidance for trauma-exposed organisations. Occupational Health at Work [Internet]. 2015;12(1):17–21. Available from: https://www.kcl.ac.uk/kcmhr/publications/assetfiles/2015/Dunn2015.pdf
12. Horwitz AV. Distinguishing distress from disorder as psychological outcomes of stressful social arrangements. Health (London) [Internet]. 2007 July [cited 2020 Jan 20];11(3):273–89. Available from: http://journals.sagepub.com/doi/10.1177/1363459307077541
13. Mitchell JT. When disaster strikes...the critical incident stress debriefing process. JEMS. 1983 Jan;8(1):36–9.
14. Rose SC, Bisson J, Churchill R, Wessely S. Psychological debriefing for preventing post traumatic stress disorder (PTSD). Cochrane Common Mental Disorders Group, editor. Cochrane Database of Systematic Reviews [Internet]. 2002 Apr 22 [cited 2020 Jan 20]; Available from: http://doi.wiley.com/10.1002/14651858.CD000560
15. van Emmerik AA, Kamphuis JH, Hulsbosch AM, Emmelkamp PM. Single session debriefing after psychological trauma: a meta-analysis. The Lancet [Internet]. 2002 Sep [cited 2020 Jan 20];360(9335):766–71. Available from: https://linkinghub.elsevier.com/retrieve/pii/S0140673602098975
16. Wessely S, Rose S, Bisson J. Brief psychological interventions ('debriefing') for trauma-related symptoms and the prevention of post traumatic stress disorder. Cochrane Database Syst Rev. 2000;2:CD000560.
17. Kearns MC, Ressler KJ, Zatzick D, Rothbaum BO. Early Interventions For PTSD: A Review. Depress Anxiety [Internet]. 2012 Oct [cited 2020 Jan 20];29(10):833–42. Available from: http://doi.wiley.com/10.1002/da.21997
18. Bisson JI, Jenkins PL, Alexander J, Bannister C. Randomised controlled trial of psychological debriefing for victims of acute burn trauma. Br J Psychiatry [Internet]. 1997 July [cited 2020 Jan 20];171(1):78–81. Available from: https://www.cambridge.org/core/product/identifier/S0007125000147245/type/journal_article
19. Mayou RA, Ehlers A, Hobbs M. Psychological debriefing for road traffic accident victims: Three-year follow-up of a randomised controlled trial. Br J Psychiatry [Internet]. 2000 June [cited 2020 Jan 20];176(6):589–93. Available from: https://www.cambridge.org/core/product/identifier/S0007125000154698/type/journal_article
20. National Institute for Health and Care Excellence. Post-traumatic stress disorder. [Internet]. Manchester: National Institute for Health and Care Excellence; 2018 [cited 2020 Jan 20] p. 1–56. Available from: https://www.nice.org.uk/guidance/ng116
21. Gidron Y, Gal R, Givati G, Lauden A, Snir Y, Benjamin J. Interactive effects of memory structuring and gender in preventing posttraumatic stress symptoms. Randomized Controlled Trial [Internet]. 2007 Feb [cited 2020 Jan 20];195(2):179–82. Available from: https://insights.ovid.com/crossref?an=00005053-200702000-00014
22. Scholes C, Turpin G, Mason S. A randomised controlled trial to assess the effectiveness of providing self-help information to people with symptoms of acute stress disorder following a traumatic injury. Behaviour Research and Therapy [Internet]. 2007 Nov [cited 2020 Jan 20];45(11):2527–36. Available

from: https://linkinghub.elsevier.com/retrieve/pii/S0005796707001210
23. Greenberg N, Megnin-Viggars O, Leach J. Occupational health professionals and 2018 NICE post-traumatic stress disorder guidelines. Occupational Medicine [Internet]. 2019 Oct 1 [cited 2020 Jan 20];69(6):397–9. Available from: https://academic.oup.com/occmed/article/69/6/397/5579808
24. Whybrow D, Jones N, Greenberg N. Promoting organizational well-being: a comprehensive review of Trauma Risk Management: Table 1. OCCMED [Internet]. 2015 June [cited 2020 Jan 20];65(4):331–6. Available from: https://academic.oup.com/occmed/article-lookup/doi/10.1093/occmed/kqv024
25. Jones N, Burdett H, Green K, Greenberg N. Trauma risk management (TRiM): promoting help seeking for mental health problems among combat-exposed U.K. military personnel. Psychiatry. 2017;80(3):236–51.
26. Hunt E, Jones N, Hastings V, Greenberg N. TRiM: an organizational response to traumatic events in Cumbria Constabulary. Occupational Medicine [Internet]. 2013 Dec 1 [cited 2020 Jan 20];63(8):549–55. Available from: https://academic.oup.com/occmed/article-lookup/doi/10.1093/occmed/kqt113
27. Royal College of Psychiatrists. Coping after a traumatic event [Internet]. 2016 [cited 2020 Jan 20]. Available from: https://www.rcpsych.ac.uk/mental-health/problems-disorders/coping-after-a-traumatic-event
28. Norris FH, Watson PJ, Hamblen JL, Pfefferbaum BJ. Provider Perspectives on Disaster Mental Health Services in Oklahoma City. Journal of Aggression, Maltreatment & Trauma [Internet]. 2005 Apr 28 [cited 2020 Jan 20];10(1–2):649–61. Available from: http://www.tandfonline.com/doi/abs/10.1300/J146v10n01_22
29. Penedo FJ, Dahn JR. Exercise and well-being: a review of mental and physical health benefits associated with physical activity: Current Opinion in Psychiatry [Internet]. 2005 Mar [cited 2020 Jan 20];18(2):189–93. Available from: https://insights.ovid.com/crossref?an=00001504-200503000-00013
30. Hegberg NJ, Hayes JP, Hayes SM. Exercise Intervention in PTSD: A Narrative Review and Rationale for Implementation. Front Psychiatry [Internet]. 2019 Mar 21 [cited 2020 Jan 20];10:133. Available from: https://www.frontiersin.org/article/10.3389/fpsyt.2019.00133/full
31. Miles MS, Demi AS, Mostynaker P. Rescue workers' reactions following the hyatt hotel disaster. Death Education [Internet]. 1984 Oct [cited 2020 Jan 20];8(5–6):315–31. Available from: http://www.tandfonline.com/doi/abs/10.1080/07481188408252470
32. Brooks S, Amlôt R, Rubin GJ, Greenberg N. Psychological resilience and post-traumatic growth in disaster-exposed organisations: overview of the literature. J R Army Med Corps [Internet]. 2018 Feb 2 [cited 2020 Jan 20];jramc-2017-000876. Available from: http://jramc.bmj.com/lookup/doi/10.1136/jramc-2017-000876
33. Greenberg N, Thomas S, Iversen A, Unwin C, Hull L, Wessely S. Do military peacekeepers want to talk about their experiences? Perceived psychological support of UK military peacekeepers on return from deployment. Journal of Mental Health [Internet]. 2003 Dec [cited 2020 Jan 20];12(6):565–73. Available from: http://www.tandfonline.com/doi/full/10.1080/0963823031000l627928
34. Rogers CR, Farson RE. Active listening. 2015.
35. Greenberg N, Brooks S, Dunn R. Latest developments in post-traumatic stress disorder: diagnosis and treatment: Table 1. Br Med Bull [Internet]. 2015 June [cited 2020 Jan 20];114(1):147–55. Available from: https://academic.oup.com/bmb/article-lookup/doi/10.1093/bmb/ldv014
36. Breslau N, Chase GA, Anthony JC. The uniqueness of the DSM definition of post-traumatic stress disorder: implications for research. Psychol Med [Internet]. 2002 May [cited 2020 Jan 20];32(4):573–6. Available from: https://www.cambridge.org/core/product/identifier/S0033291701004998/type/journal_article
37. Neria Y, Nandi A, Galea S. Post-traumatic stress disorder following disasters: a systematic review. Psychol Med [Internet]. 2008 Apr [cited 2020 Jan 20];38(4):467–80. Available from: https://www.cambridge.org/core/product/identifier/S0033291707001353/type/journal_article
38. World Health Organization. International classification of diseases for mortality and morbidity statistics (11th Revision) [Internet]. World Health Organization; 2018 [cited 2020 Jan 20]. Available from: https://icd.who.int/browse11/l-m/en
39. American Psychiatric Association, editor. Diagnostic and statistical manual of mental disorders: DSM-IV. 4. ed., 7. print. Washington, DC; 1998. 886 p.
40. Miguel-Tobal JJ, Vindel AC, Iruarrízaga I, Ordi HG, Galea S. Psychopathological repercussions of the March 11 terrorist attacks in Madrid. Psychol Spain. 2005;9(1):75–80.
41. North CS, Suris AM, Davis M, Smith RP. Toward validation of the diagnosis of posttraumatic stress disorder. AJP [Internet]. 2009 Jan [cited 2020 Jan 20];166(1):34–41. Available from: http://psychiatryonline.org/doi/abs/10.1176/appi.ajp.2008.08050644
42. Brooks SK, Dunn R, Sage CAM, Amlôt R, Greenberg N, Rubin GJ. Risk and resilience factors affecting the psychological wellbeing of individuals deployed in humanitarian relief roles after a disaster. Journal of Mental Health [Internet]. 2015 Nov 2 [cited 2020 Jan 20];24(6):385–413. Available from: http://www.tandfonline.com/doi/full/10.3109/09638237.2015.1057334
43. Brooks SK, Dunn R, Amlôt R, Greenberg N, Rubin GJ. Social and occupational factors associated with psychological distress and disorder among disaster responders: a systematic review. BMC Psychol [Internet]. 2016 Dec [cited 2020 Jan 20];4(1):18. Available from: http://bmcpsychology.biomedcentral.com/articles/10.1186/s40359-016-0120-9

44. Brooks SK, Dunn R, Amlôt R, Rubin GJ, Greenberg N. Social and occupational factors associated with psychological wellbeing among occupational groups affected by disaster: a systematic review. J Mental Health [Internet]. 2017 July 4 [cited 2020 Jan 20];26(4):373–84. Available from: https://www.tandfonline.com/doi/full/10.1080/09638237.2017.1294732
45. Brooks SK, Dunn R, Amlôt R, Rubin GJ, Greenberg N. A systematic, thematic review of social and occupational factors associated with psychological outcomes in healthcare employees during an infectious disease outbreak. J Occup Environ Med [Internet]. 2018 Mar [cited 2020 Jan 20];60(3):248–57. Available from: http://Insights.ovid.com/crossref?an=00043764-201803000-00007
46. Brewin CR, Andrews B, Valentine JD. Meta-analysis of risk factors for posttraumatic stress disorder in trauma-exposed adults. J Consult Clin Psychol [Internet]. 2000 [cited 2020 Jan 20];68(5):748–66. Available from: http://doi.apa.org/getdoi.cfm?doi=10.1037/0022-006X.68.5.748
47. Ozer EJ, Best SR, Lipsey TL, Weiss DS. Predictors of posttraumatic stress disorder and symptoms in adults: A meta-analysis. Psychological Bulletin [Internet]. 2003 [cited 2020 Jan 20];129(1):52–73. Available from: http://doi.apa.org/getdoi.cfm?doi=10.1037/0033-2909.129.1.52
48. Cukor J, Wyka K, Jayasinghe N, Weathers F, Giosan C, Leck P, et al. Prevalence and predictors of posttraumatic stress symptoms in utility workers deployed to the World Trade Center following the attacks of September 11, 2001. Depress Anxiety [Internet]. 2011 Mar [cited 2020 Jan 20];28(3):210–7. Available from: http://doi.wiley.com/10.1002/da.20776
49. Biggs QM, Fullerton CS, Reeves JJ, Grieger TA, Reissman D, Ursano RJ. Acute stress disorder, depression, and tobacco use in disaster workers following 9/11. American Journal of Orthopsychiatry [Internet]. 2010 [cited 2020 Jan 20];80(4):586–92. Available from: http://doi.apa.org/getdoi.cfm?doi=10.1111/j.1939-0025.2010.01063.x
50. Ehlers A, Mayou RA, Bryant B. Psychological predictors of chronic posttraumatic stress disorder after motor vehicle accidents. J Abnormal Psychol [Internet]. 1998 Aug [cited 2020 Jan 20];107(3):508–19. Available from: http://doi.apa.org/getdoi.cfm?doi=10.1037/0021-843X.107.3.508
51. Maunder R, Lancee W, Balderson K, Bennett J, Borgundvaag B, Evans S, et al. Long-term psychological and occupational effects of providing hospital healthcare during SARS outbreak. Emerg Infect Dis [Internet]. 2006 [cited 2020 Jan 20];12(12):1924–32. Available from: http://wwwnc.cdc.gov/eid/article/12/12/06-0584_article.htm
52. Berninger A, Webber MP, Cohen HW, Gustave J, Lee R, Niles JK, et al. Trends of elevated PTSD risk in firefighters exposed to the world trade center disaster: 2001–2005. Public Health Rep [Internet]. 2010 July [cited 2020 Jan 20];125(4):556–66. Available from: http://journals.sagepub.com/doi/10.1177/003335491012500411
53. Hodgkinson PE, Shepherd MA. The impact of disaster support work. J Traum Stress [Internet]. 1994 Oct [cited 2020 Jan 20];7(4):587–600. Available from: http://doi.wiley.com/10.1002/jts.2490070407
54. Cetin M, Kose S, Ebrinc S, Yigit S, Elhai JD, Basoglu C. Identification and posttraumatic stress disorder symptoms in rescue workers in the Marmara, Turkey, earthquake. J Traum Stress [Internet]. 2005 Oct [cited 2020 Jan 20];18(5):485–9. Available from: http://doi.wiley.com/10.1002/jts.20056
55. Fullerton CS, Ursano RJ, Wang L. Acute stress disorder, posttraumatic stress disorder, and depression in disaster or rescue workers. AJP [Internet]. 2004 Aug [cited 2020 Jan 20];161(8):1370–6. Available from: http://psychiatryonline.org/doi/abs/10.1176/appi.ajp.161.8.1370
56. Seaward BL. Managing stress: principles and strategies for health and well being. 9th ed. Jones & Bartlett Learning: Burlington, MA; 2018.
57. Terr LC. Childhood traumas: an outline and overview. AJP [Internet]. 1991 Jan [cited 2020 Jan 20];148(1):10–20. Available from: http://psychiatryonline.org/doi/abs/10.1176/ajp.148.1.10
58. Sage CAM, Brooks SK, Greenberg N. Factors associated with Type II trauma in occupational groups working with traumatised children: a systematic review. Journal of Mental Health [Internet]. 2018 Sep 3 [cited 2020 Jan 20];27(5):457–67. Available from: https://www.tandfonline.com/doi/full/10.1080/09638237.2017.1370630
59. Brooks SK, Dunn R, Amlôt R, Rubin GJ, Greenberg N. Protecting the psychological wellbeing of staff exposed to disaster or emergency at work: a qualitative study. BMC Psychol [Internet]. 2019 Dec [cited 2020 Jan 20];7(1):78. Available from: https://bmcpsychology.biomedcentral.com/articles/10.1186/s40359-019-0360-6
60. Gobin M, Rubin GJ, Albert I, Beck A, Danese A, Greenberg N, et al. Outcomes of mental health screening for United Kingdom nationals affected by the 2015–2016 terrorist attacks in Tunisia, Paris, and Brussels: mental health screening after terrorist attacks. J Traum Stress [Internet]. 2018 Aug [cited 2020 Jan 20];31(4):471–9. Available from: http://doi.wiley.com/10.1002/jts.22317
61. Cabinet Office. Data protection and sharing guidance for emergency planners and responders. [Internet]. London: Cabinet Office; 2007 [cited 2020 Jan 20] p. 33. Available from: https://www.gov.uk/government/publications/data-protection-and-sharing-guidance-for-emergency-planners-and-responders
62. Milliken CS, Auchterlonie JL, Hoge CW. Longitudinal assessment of mental health problems among active and reserve component soldiers returning from the Iraq War. JAMA [Internet]. 2007 Nov 14 [cited 2020 Jan 20];298(18):2141. Available from: http://jama.jamanetwork.com/article.aspx?doi=10.1001/jama.298.18.2141

63. Rona RJ, Burdett H, Khondoker M, Chesnokov M, Green K, Pernet D, et al. Post-deployment screening for mental disorders and tailored advice about help-seeking in the UK military: a cluster randomised controlled trial. Lancet [Internet]. 2017 Apr [cited 2020 Jan 20];389(10077):1410–23. Available from: https://linkinghub.elsevier.com/retrieve/pii/S0140673616323984
64. United Kingdom Psychological Trauma Society. Traumatic stress management guidance: For organisations whose staff work in high risk environments. [Internet]. United Kingdom Psychological Trauma Society; 2014 [cited 2020 Jan 20]. Available from: http://www.ukpts.co.uk/site/assets/UKPTS-Guidance-Document-120614.pdf
65. Shapiro F. Eye movement desensitization: A new treatment for post-traumatic stress disorder. Journal of Behavior Therapy and Experimental Psychiatry [Internet]. 1989 Sep [cited 2020 Jan 20];20(3):211–7. Available from: https://linkinghub.elsevier.com/retrieve/pii/0005791689900256
66. Ehlers A, Clark DM. Post-traumatic stress disorder: The development of effective psychological treatments. Nordic Journal of Psychiatry [Internet]. 2008 Jan [cited 2020 Jan 20];62(sup47):11–8. Available from: http://www.tandfonline.com/doi/full/10.1080/08039480802315608
67. Kornør H, Winje D, Ekeberg Ø, Weisæth L, Kirkehei I, Johansen K, et al. Early trauma-focused cognitive-behavioural therapy to prevent chronic post-traumatic stress disorder and related symptoms: A systematic review and meta-analysis. BMC Psychiatry [Internet]. 2008 Dec [cited 2020 Jan 20];8(1):81. Available from: https://bmcpsychiatry.biomedcentral.com/articles/10.1186/1471-244X-8-81
68. Gelpin E, Bonne O, Peri T, Brandes D, Shalev AY. Treatment of recent trauma survivors with benzodiazepines: a prospective study. J Clin Psychiatry. 1996 Sep;57(9):390–4.

Correction to: Textbook of Acute Trauma Care

Peter Lax

Correction to: P. Lax (ed.), *Textbook of Acute Trauma Care*, https://doi.org/10.1007/978-3-030-83628-3

The original version of the book was inadvertently published with the following errors, and these have now been corrected and updated with this erratum:

Chapter 11 - The answer to question 1 on page 219 was previously given as A - The severity of brain injury. The correct answer is C - The intracranial relationship between pressure and volume. The answer on page 219 now appears correctly in the book as answer C.

Alex Psirides—missing third affiliation added to Contributors Page.

Alia Yaqub—affiliation error corrected in Contributors Page.

Shaun C. Moeller—affiliation error corrected in Contributors Page and Chapter Opening Page.

Ryan Fransman—affiliation error corrected in Contributors Page and Chapter Opening Page.

Robert Greig—post nominals removed from Contributors Page to keep in line with other authors.

Jake Turner—affiliation error corrected in Contributors Page and Chapter Opening Page.

Peter Lax—moved in Contributors Page between Timothy Knight and Caroline Leech.

Nicholas Freeman—removed from Contributors Page.

Amy Pearson—removed from Contributors Page.

Neil Roy—moved in the Contributors Page after Edward Rothera.

Clare Thompson—moved in the Contributors Page after Tim Stansfield.

The updated version of the chapters can be found at
https://doi.org/10.1007/978-3-030-83628-3_11
https://doi.org/10.1007/978-3-030-83628-3_15
https://doi.org/10.1007/978-3-030-83628-3_26

P. Lax (ed.), *Textbook of Acute Trauma Care*, https://doi.org/10.1007/978-3-030-83628-3_45